Infectious Diseases

Concise Textbook Series

- *Essential Neurology*, Second Edition, William Pryse-Phillips, M.D. and T.J. Murray, M.D.

- *Gynecology*, Ralph W. Hale, M.D. and John A. Krieger, M.D.

- *Nephrology*, Marvin Forland, M.D., Editor

- *Sexual Development and Disorders in Childhood and Adolescence*, Raymond M. Russo, M.D., Editor

- *Infectious Diseases*, Robert H. Waldman, M.D. and Ronica M. Kluge, M.D., Editors

Textbook of

Infectious Diseases

Editors

Robert H. Waldman, M.D.
Professor and Chairman, Department of Medicine
West Virginia University School of Medicine
Morgantown, West Virginia

Ronica M. Kluge, M.D.
Professor of Medicine
Director, Division of General Medicine and
Ambulatory Care
University of Texas Medical Branch
Galveston, Texas

MEDICAL EXAMINATION PUBLISHING CO., INC.
an Excerpta Medica company

Main entry under title:

Textbook of infectious diseases.

    Bibliography: p.
    Includes index.
    1. Communicable diseases. I. Waldman, Robert H.
(Date). II. Kluge, Ronica M. [DNLM: 1. Communicable
diseases. WC 100 C744]
RC111. T48 1983   616.9   83-7886
ISBN 0-87488-668-6

Printed in the United States of America

To Beth, Tom, Jenny, and especially Mike,
not only because they are my pride and joy, but also
because of their invaluable work on the index of this book.

Contents

vii

x   Contents

Contents   **xv**

Contributors

Edwin L. Anderson, M.D., West Virginia University Medical Center, Charleston Division, Charleston

Charles E. Andrews, M.D., Professor of Medicine, University of Nebraska Medical Center, School of Medicine, Omaha

John J. Barry, M.D., Assistant Professor of Medicine, West Virginia University Medical Center, Morgantown

Robert M. D'Alessandri, M.D., Associate Professor of Medicine; Section Chief, Comprehensive Medicine, Department of Medicine, West Virginia University School of Medicine, Morgantown

Stuart M. Deglin, M.D., Associate Professor of Medicine (Cardiology), West Virginia University School of Medicine, Morgantown

Roger G. Finch, M.B., Ch.B., M.R.C.P. (UK), M.R.C. Path., Consultant Physician in Microbial Diseases, The City Hospital, Nottingham, England; Senior Lecturer in Microbial Diseases, University of Nottingham, England; Honorary Consultant, Public Health Laboratory Service; Formerly Assistant Professor of Medicine, Department of Medicine, West Virginia University Medical Center, Morgantown

Melanie A. Fisher, M.D., Fellow in Infectious Diseases, Hospital of the University of Pennsylvania, Philadelphia

Rama Ganguly, Ph.D., Associate Professor, Department of Internal Medicine and Veterans Administration Medical Center, University of South Florida, Tampa

H. Preston Holley, Jr., M.D., Assistant Professor of Medicine, Division of Infectious Diseases, Medical University of South Carolina, Charleston

David L. Hoover, M.D., Department of Immunology, Walter Reed Army Institute of Research, Washington, District of Columbia

Rashida A. Khakoo, M.D., Associate Professor of Medicine; Acting Chief, Section of Infectious Diseases, West Virginia University Medical Center, Morgantown

Ronica M. Kluge, M.D., Professor of Medicine; Director, Division of General Medicine and Ambulatory Care, University of Texas Medical Branch at Galveston

Andrew P. Matragrano, M.D., Associate, Thoracic Medicine, Geisinger Medical Center, Danville, Pennsylvania

Enayatollah Osanloo, M.D., Assistant Professor of Medicine and Nephrology, Department of Medicine, West Virginia University School of Medicine and Medical Center, Morgantown

David A. Pitrolo, M.D., Internal Medicine Resident, West Virginia University Hospital, Morgantown

Gary R. Plotkin, M.D., F.A.C.P., Danville Internal Medicine, 115 South Main Street, Danville, Virginia

Larry G. Reimer, M.D., Assistant Professor of Medicine and Pathology; Director of Clinical Microbiology, West Virginia University Medical Center, Morgantown

James C. Reynolds, M.D., Assistant Professor, Department of Medicine, Hospital of the University of Pennsylvania, Philadelphia

Patrick A. Robinson, M.D., Chief, Infectious Disease Division, Department of Medicine, West Virginia University Medical Center, Charleston Division, Charleston

William F. Tarry, M.D., Fellow in Pediatric Urology, The Children's Hospital of Philadelphia; Instructor in Urology, The University of Pennsylvania School of Medicine, Philadelphia

Robert H. Waldman., M.D., Professor and Chairman, Department of Medicine, West Virginia University School of Medicine, Morgantown

Bruce A. Wallin, M.D., Associate Medical Director, Rheumatology/Immunology Group, Smithkline Beckman Corporation, Philadelphia, Pennsylvania

Preface

The *Textbook of Infectious Diseases* was conceived and written in order to provide a comprehensive, but not encyclopedic, text on infectious diseases for the student, resident, and practitioner. The aim of the editors and authors is to produce a volume, at reasonable cost, containing practical information to help the physician evaluate and treat patients with a possible infection, as well as material pertaining to prevention. Important and helpful information regarding microbiology and pathophysiology is also briefly included. Every attempt has been made to eliminate material which is not relevant to patient care.

Regarding the organization of the book, it is divided into four sections: a brief introduction, a section on basic principles of infection, another section on major categories of infectious diseases, and the final, and longest section, covering the specific organisms. This last section is subdivided according to the taxonomic classification of organisms causing infections. Some texts on infectious diseases are not organized in this fashion, but use either the "disease" type of approach or the "organism" type, or sometimes use parts of each. The problem with using only one of these approaches is that to adequately understand and be able to refer to aspects of infectious diseases, one must be able to refer to both the disease categories and the organism. For example, if one wants to learn about pneumococcal disease, it is preferable to be able to read chapters on pneumonia and meningitis, as well as a chapter on the organism *Streptococcus pneumoniae*. This does tend to make texts on infectious diseases rather long, with some redundancy. Hopefully, these disadvantages are kept to a minimum. The advantages of such a system are educationally beneficial and enable the practicing physician to deliver better medical care.

Part 1

INTRODUCTION

In 1900, four of the ten leading causes of death were infectious diseases. Even more impressive is that the top three leading causes of death were pneumonia, tuberculosis, and the infectious diarrheas; diphtheria was number 10 on the list. As an indication of the progress that has been made over the past 80 years, only one infectious disease is currently in that list, and that is pneumonia at number 5. The decrease in prevalence of infectious diseases has obviously had a great deal to do with the increased life expectancy that has occurred in "developed" countries during this century. While infectious diseases are less likely to cause death, except as a final event in the terminally ill, they still cause a great deal of morbidity (Tables I.1–I.3).

Two approaches have been and still are being used to battle infectious problems: (1) prevention, i.e., assisting the host defenses of the individual, and (2) treatment. Historically, the first has been much more effective, as one would expect. It should not go unnoticed, however, that the second has received a great deal more attention and funds in recent years.

A very brief historic review is in order to better appreciate the specific progress that has been made with respect to infectious diseases. The one person who can be clearly identified as having made the greatest contribution to the health of mankind is Edward Jenner. During the eighteenth century in Western Europe, approximately one-fourth of the population died of smallpox. This is approximately the same percentage of the population who currently die of cancer. However, whereas most cancer deaths are among the elderly, most smallpox deaths were among children or young adults; therefore, obviously, having even a greater impact on health. To imagine the impact of Jenner's development of vaccination, one would have to think, in modern terms, of a single individual who would develop a method of preventing all cancers. There have been other great advances in medical care, but none with as great an impact as Jenner's, and very few that can be associated so closely with the work of a single individual. The work that he started is of even greater interest since it has so recently come to fruition, with the final eradication of smallpox. This again is a unique event in our history.

The person who can be identified as probably having the second most important impact on our health is Louis Pasteur. Pasteur showed that microorganisms do not arise spontaneously but grow in a particular place only after contamination from elsewhere. This remarkable man also devised a procedure to attenuate bacteria so that they would not produce illness but would still stimulate the body's host defenses. It is interesting that Pasteur showed that these attenuated organisms were ineffective in treating a patient who was already ill with the disease. This, then, was the beginning of the split in the two arms of health care, prevention and therapy.

3

TABLE I.1   Death Rates in the United States, 1900 and 1970

| | 1900 | | 1970 | |
Causes	Deaths per 100,000	% of All Deaths	Deaths per 100,000	% of All Deaths
All	1659.0	100.0	940.2	100.0
Infectious diseases	541.0	32.6	37.9	4.0
Epidemic diseases	146.8	8.8	5.4	0.6
Tuberculosis	195.5	11.8	1.8	0.2
Meningitis	33.1	2.0	0.9	0.1
Pneumonia and influenza	165.6	10.0	29.8	3.2

TABLE I.2   Age-Specific Mortality, 1900 and 1970 Shown as Deaths per 1000

| | Age Group in Years | | | |
Years	1–4	15–24	45–54	65–74
1900	19.8	5.9	15.0	56.4
1970	0.8	1.3	7.3	35.8
Decline (%)	96.0	78.0	51.0	37.0

TABLE I.3   Observed Deaths Due to Infectious Disease and All Causes in Children in 1973 Compared with Deaths That Would be Expected at 1900 Rates

| Expected Versus Observed | Age Group in Years | | |
	1	1–4	5–14
1973 population risk	3,079,000	13,635,000	38,983,000
Deaths due to infectious disease			
Expected at 1900 rate	104,994	159,530	93,559
Observed in 1973	5,446	1,265	973
Deaths due to all causes			
Expected at 1900 rate	500,030	269,973	152,034
Observed in 1973	55,581	10,843	15,982

In the early part of this century, antisera developed against pneumococcal pneumonia and meningitis were found to be somewhat effective and raised the hope for therapeutic modalities to supplement the rapidly developing area of prevention. It was quickly discovered that each strain needed a specific antiserum to be effective.

With the development of the sulfonamides in the 1930s, the therapeutic era had arrived. In pneumococcal pneumonia the fatality rate dropped from 33 to 12%. Unfortunately, resistant strains began to appear.

In 1928, Fleming observed that a mold that contaminated a culture plate growing a *Staphylococcus* sp was surrounded by a growth-free zone. In 1941, the first patient was treated with penicillin and a beneficial response was noted. However, the patient died when the supply of penicillin was exhausted. With the development of more efficient ways of making large amounts of penicillin the pneumococcal pneumonia fatality rate dropped to 6%.

In this day of great interest in cost containment it is interesting to look at one aspect of medical economics with respect to penicillin. Thirty-five years ago penicillin cost $20.00/100,000 U. Today, $20.00 can buy approximately 1 billion U. Stated another way, 100,000 U today cost less than 1¢. This is an impressive decrease in the cost of medical care, even without taking into account a comparison of the value of $20.00 in 1945 to the lack of value that amount of money has today.

The next important advance in the treatment of infectious diseases resulted from the studies of Waksman with soil microbes. His studies resulted in streptomycin, the first effective antituberculous drug and, indirectly, in the class of aminoglycosides.

Despite these great advances, there have been accompanying problems. There has been a change in the kinds of microorganisms causing infections, i.e., resistant bacteria, and what previously had been rarely pathogenic bacteria have become an ever-increasing problem. This problem is almost entirely a result of the overuse of antibiotics. In addition, there is the important economic factor. Although, as mentioned earlier, the cost of penicillin has dropped precipitously, antibiotics have become the second most commonly used drugs in the United States, accounting for approximately one-sixth of all prescription drugs in total dollars. This amounts to over $1 billion/year, not including the expense of administration of the antibiotics or the profit to the pharmacies.

With control of most of the more severe bacterial infections, there has been more emphasis on diseases caused by viruses. The development of antiviral drugs has been difficult because in contrast to bacteria, viruses become incorporated into the metabolism of the invaded cell, thus it is almost impossible to affect the virus without harming the host cell. Definite progress is being made, however, and effective, safe antiviral drugs seem to be on the horizon. It should be emphasized that immunization continues to be the most important method for control of virus infections.

The final point in this introduction is to emphasize the areas of our greatest ignorance with respect to infectious diseases, i.e., information regarding their natural histories. Without this it is impossible to ascertain the benefit, or lack of it, of our various diagnostic and therapeutic maneuvers. Information in this area is very limited. For example, syphilis is an infectious disease that has been of tremendous interest for hundreds of years, yet it was not known until recently that 85% of untreated syphilis patients have a normal life expectancy, and 70% have absolutely no evidence of disease at the time of their death. An additional problem in this area is that there is an apparent alteration of the natural history of some of the more common infectious diseases. For example, salmonellosis, rheumatic fever, and scarlet fever seem to be decreasing in their severity and/or incidence, and this appears to be unrelated to the advent of antibiotic use. Finally, very little is known about the impact of infectious diseases other than their immediate mortality or morbidity. A few studies have been done in this area with respect to otitis media and its impact on learning, but this certainly is the most meager of beginnings for a very important area with respect to this and other important infectious diseases.

Part 2

GENERAL PRINCIPLES

1

FEVER
Robert M. D'Alessandri, M.D.

Introduction

The term *fever* has been used synonymously with disease itself. Although not a disease or diagnosis, an elevated temperature is one of the most primitive of the body's responses to disease and is the most constant of all clinical manifestations of infectious diseases. Unfortunately, it is often absent in the very young or the very old in situations in which one would expect a fever. Fever is also important because the termination of febrile response is usually associated with improvement in the patient's clinical condition and recovery.

Pathophysiology

Heat is normally produced in the skeletal muscles and liver and dissipated through the skin and lungs by convection, conduction, and radiation. Heat production and loss are controlled within narrow limits by the autonomic nervous system. The thermoregulatory center in the anterior hypothalamus senses small changes of temperature and initiates heat loss by vasodilation and sweating or heat conservation by vasoconstriction. During febrile episodes the *set point* at which body temperature is normally maintained is elevated. Body temperature rises to the new set point and once again body temperature is maintained at this level. In microbial diseases, endogenous pyrogen has been shown to act centrally at the anterior hypothalamus inducing vasoconstriction and fever. Granulocytes, and circulating and fixed tissue macrophages, produce endogenous pyrogen in response to various activators such as endotoxin, viruses, bacteria, inflammation, and antigen–antibody complexes. Lymphocytes produce lymphokines which induce other cells to release endogenous pyrogen. Endogenous pyrogen acts to reset the thermoregulator with resulting vasoconstriction and chills. Associated with the central action of endogenous pyrogen is an increase in prostaglandin E (PGE) levels in cerebrospinal fluid. When PGE is infused directly into the lateral ventricle, shivering, vasoconstriction, and elevation of body temperature occur. If prostaglandin inhibitors are administered, vasodilation and a fall in body temperature ensue. This suggests that prostaglandins may act as the molecular mediators of the febrile response and may account for the antipyretic action of salicylates, acetominophen, and indomethacin. Not all febrile states are mediated by endogenous pyrogen. In thyroid storm and pheochromocytoma there are reduced heat loss and fever as a result of direct peripheral activation of thermoregulatory mechanisms. In heat stroke and central nervous system (CNS) lesions, the hypothalamic thermoregulatory center malfunctions with resetting of the set point upward with resultant fever.

As the temperature rises, chills and rigors reflexly occur as a result of vasoconstriction and rapid cooling of the skin. With each degree Farenheit rise in body temperature above normal there is an approximately 8% rise in basal metabolic rate, an increase in heart rate of about 10 beats per minute, an increase in respiratory rate, and augmented renal and hepatic blood flow. In prolonged febrile states respiratory alkalosis may soon be followed by metabolic acidosis owing to the increased catabolic activity of the host. Despite these physiologic alterations there are no pathologic changes in the CNS with sustained temperatures less than 106°F. In fact, temperatures of 106-108° sustained for as long as 8-10 hr are rarely associated with any permanent CNS effects. Following downward resetting of the thermoregulatory center, rapid heat dissipation occurs. Sweating occurs and may be quite profuse. Antipyretics can reproduce the cycle of chills to sweats repeatedly if administered inappropriately (dosage schedule too infrequent) to patients with sustained temperature elevations.

Manifestations of Fever

Clinical

As previously mentioned, tachycardia, chills, and sweating are physiologic responses to fever. In certain disease states such as typhoid fever, yellow fever, and in certain patients with cardiac failure, the respiratory and cardiac rates often are not elevated proportionately to the height of the temperature. In pneumococcal pneumonia the respiratory rate may be increased disproportionately to the degree of fever. In addition to these manifestations associated with fever, patients frequently notice a vague sense of warmth, may feel flushed, or may have headaches.

Delirium and altered mental status may accompany high fever or may be the only manifestation of infection in the elderly. Febrile convulsions occur only in children. Adults with fever and a convulsive disorder must be assumed to have an underlying CNS pathology.

Fever blisters, caused by herpesvirus type I, are commonly associated with febrile episodes related to certain infectious diseases such as pneumococcal pneumonia, meningococcal meningitis, and typhoid fever. Although termed fever blisters, the reactivation of this herpesvirus infection is probably more related to the stress associated with the illness rather than to the presence of fever itself.

Increased fluid losses via the skin and the respiratory tract as a result of fever, and decreased intake as a result of anorexia and altered mental status, may lead to severe dehydration. This should be suspected in all elderly pyrexic patients.

Body Temperature Variations

Body temperature exhibits a diurnal variation with the highest daily temperatures in the late afternoon and early evening and the lowest temperatures in the early morning hours. This pattern is not established until the second year of life. Physiologic temperature elevations occur in response to exercise (as high as 102-104°F), menses, eating, and emotional disturbances. In the very young and the elderly, cold environmental temperatures may cause a marked reduction in body temperature.

In clinical practice oral and rectal temperatures are recorded as reflective of body temperature. Oral temperatures may be falsely lowered by mouth breathing, drinking or eating cold substances, and shock. Drinking or eating hot substances, chewing, and smoking may falsely elevate oral temperatures.

Rectal temperatures are usually 0.5-1°F higher than oral temperatures. Rectal temperatures are most frequently used in children, in adults with altered mental status, or when oral temperatures are invalid for the previously mentioned reasons. Also possibly apocryphal, it has been stated that an occasional patient may falsely elevate a rectal temperature by voluntary constriction of the muscles in the rectal area.

In special cases axillary, skin, urine, or tympanic membrane temperatures are used. Of these, urine and tympanic membrane thermometry are the most accurate reflections of body temperature. When determining urine temperature, a prewarmed vessel is used to collect the urine and the temperature recorded immediately. This represents an excellent method for checking on spurious or factitious fever.

Fever Patterns

Fever is defined as an increase in body temperature over the normal range owing to a disease process and not from environmental or physiologic factors. *Intermittent fever* is a daily fever spike followed by a return to normal body temperature. This is also called hectic fever and is often associated with pyogenic abscesses, gram-negative bacteremia, and disseminated tuberculosis. *Remittent fever* is elevated body temperature that does not return to normal. The changes in temperature are not as marked as in the intermittent fever pattern. *Sustained fever* is a continuous temperature elevation with less variation in temperature than that seen in the remittent fever pattern. Pneumococcal pneumonia, typhoid fever, and meningococcal meningitis often cause this fever pattern. Antipyretics may convert a sustained pattern to a hectic or remittent pattern. *Relapsing or recurrent fever* is characterized by periods of fever (either intermittent, remittent, or sustained) followed by periods of normal temperature. This pattern is frequently seen in patients with lymphoma (Pel-Ebstein fever) and in patients with brucellosis.

Factitious fevers are spurious temperature elevations produced by the patient and not associated with any underlying organic disease process. Hyperpyrexia means body temperature higher than 41°C (106°F) and is rarely caused by infectious agents.

Fever of unknown origin (FUO) or prolonged fever requires the presence and documentation of fever for at least 3 weeks, with nondiagnostic inhospital studies. A rigid definition is necessary because the designation of FUO requires a lengthy and expensive hospital workup. Only one-third of patients with FUO will have an infectious etiology. Neoplasia, connective tissue disorders, drugs, factitious fever, and miscellaneous causes account for most of the remaining etiologies.

Factitious fever may be difficult to determine. Such findings as a normal sedimentation rate, failure of the pulse to rise with fever, and careful monitoring of rectal and/or urine temperatures should be among the initial steps in the diagnostic plan. In addition, a detailed drug history including prescribed, social, and over-the-counter drugs must be reviewed.

Laboratory tests of initial import include a white blood cell count, urinalysis, sedimentation rate, and chest roentgenogram. Serologic tests may be useful when ordered specifically (as opposed to a panel of "febrile agglutinins"). Cultures and stains (where applicable) of blood, urine, and sputum for bacteria, fungus, and acid-fast organisms should be performed. Other body fluids such as cerebrospinal fluid (CSF), bone marrow, ascites, and pleural fluid should be similarly cultured and stained. Tuberculin skin testing should be performed. Other skin tests such as histoplasmin or coccidioidin should not be performed, since skin testing with these agents may elevate serologic titers.

More invasive procedures and exploratory surgical operations are indicated when less invasive studies have proved nondiagnostic and when the probability of diagnosis is high. Patients who are deteriorating rapidly often require direct invasive procedures to make a speedy diagnosis. In certain special cases it may be necessary to begin treatment before a definitive diagnosis is established. In general, however, therapeutic trials should not be done.

Management

As body temperature rises a number of physiologic effects are noted, such as chills, tachycardia, and hyperventilation. Therefore, the natural tendency is to treat fever and return body temperature to normal levels. There are a number of reasons why this may not be the best approach.

Fever may have some survival value. In lizards, which as poikilotherms maintain body temperature at environmental temperature, survival following challenge with pathogenic bacteria is inversely proportional to body temperature. Lizards maintained in higher than normal environmental temperatures had increased survival when compared with lizards similarly challenged but maintained at physiologic or below physiologic temperatures. In addition, many bacteria and viruses tolerate high body temperatures poorly. For example, influenza viruses do not replicate at temperatures above 38°C. Fever therapy was once very popular for treatment of syphilis.

Fever is also an important sign of infection, or at least indicates that disease is present. As already noted, fever curves are of little use as diagnostic aids but are useful in following the response to treatment. There is potential toxicity associated with all antipyretic drugs. Also, the rapid lowering of body temperature may be related to the development of seizures in children. Antipyretics may increase the patient's symptomatic awareness of fever if not properly prescribed.

Antipyretics are indicated in febrile patients with preexisting heart disease in whom the increased metabolic rate may have deleterious effects. In patients with a history of seizures or with CNS lesions, antipyretics may be important in preventing febrile convulsions. In addition, antipyretics may improve cerebral function in febrile patients. When using antipyretics, small doses should be prescribed every 3 or 4 hr around the clock. This minimizes wide temperature variations and provides maximum symptom relief for the patient. Since fever is but a manifestation of underlying disease, therapy is best directed to the disease process causing the fever rather than to the fever itself.

Selected Bibliography

Aduan, R. P., Fauci, A. S., Dale, H. C., Herzberg, J. H., and Wolff, S. M.: Factitious fever and self-induced infection. *Ann Intern Med* 90:230-242, 1979.

Atkins, F. and Bodel, P.: Fever. *N Engl J Med* 286:27-34, 1972.

Bernheim, H. A. and Kluger, M. J.: Fever: Effect of drug-induced antipyresis on survival. *Science* 193:237-238, 1976.

Dinarello, C. A. and Wolff, S. M.: Pathogenesis of fever in man. *N Engl J Med* 298:607-612, 1978.

Keusch, G. T.: Fever. To be or not to be. *N Y State J Med* 76:1998-2001, 1976.

Klastersky, J. and Kass, E. H.: Is suppression of fever or hypothermia useful in experimental and clinical infectious diseases? *J Infect Dis* 121:81-86, 1970.

Ledger, W. J. and Kriewall, T. J.: The fever index. A quantitative indirect measure of hospital-acquired infections in obstetrics and gynecology. *Am J Obstet Gynecol* 115: 514-520, 1973.

Milton, A. S.: Modern views on the pathogenesis of fever and the mode of action of antipyretic drugs. *J Pharm Pharmacol* 28:393-399, 1976.

Petersdorf, R. G., and Beeson, P. B.: Fever of unexplained origin: Report of 100 cases. *Medicine* 40:1-30, 1961.

2

APPROACH TO THE PATIENT WITH FEVER
Ronica M. Kluge, M.D.

Introduction

Fever is one of the most common symptoms of disease and, historically, one of the earliest recognized. Fever most frequently heralds the presence of an infectious process, but also may accompany a number of diseases not known to be caused by microorganisms. Parenthetically, it should be noted that some infectious diseases are not generally associated with fever, e.g., leprosy, cholera, and venereal diseases. This chapter will suggest a common sense approach to the patient with fever including special reference to fever of undetermined origin.

The Febrile Patient

In any febrile patient, regardless of age or underlying medical condition, a basic question must be considered: Is the fever related to an infection? Most infections are accompanied by fever, and in some cases, fever may be the only sign/symptom of an infection. However, there are a variety of noninfectious conditions that can be associated with fever. Another important consideration in the initial evaluation of the febrile patient is an assessment of the acuteness and severity of the process causing the fever. Lastly is the consideration regarding intervention: Is specific therapy available and must it be initiated swiftly to be beneficial?

Most patients presenting with fever have other symptoms and signs which give the evaluator a sense of direction, e.g., rigor, pleuritic chest pain, and purulent sputum in acute bacterial pneumonia. The evaluation process, therefore, must begin with a pertinent history and physical examination. Frequently, the diagnosis is made from information obtained in the history and physical examination and is merely confirmed by appropriate laboratory studies. The clinical setting (age, other diseases, exposures, travel history, etc.) can be extremely important. Baseline laboratory data will include complete blood count, white cell differential, and urinalysis. Radiologic examination may be appropriate, e.g., chest x-ray in pneumonia or tuberculosis. Appropriate specimens should be obtained for Gram stain and routine culture; special stains and cultures are requested if fungal, mycobacterial, or certain viral infections are suspected.

Usually by this point, self-limited infectious illnesses and simple, treatable infectious diseases have been diagnosed and appropriate therapy can be initiated. More serious infections may require further diagnostic procedures, e.g., lumbar puncture, blood cultures, paracentesis, before the best treatment can be decided. Meningitis, septicemia, and peritonitis should be considered medical emergencies requiring the most rapid assessment and institution of therapy. Detailed recommendations for the diagnosis of various infections can be found in the appropriate chapters.

Fever of Undetermined Origin (FUO)

Many clinicians consider the patient with FUO to pose the greatest challenge to their diagnostic abilities. The most important point to be made here is that a systematic approach to the problem is necessary. First and foremost, satisfy the criteria for the syndrome of FUO: illness of 3 weeks or more; temperature of 38.4°C or higher on several occasions; diagnosis uncertain after 1 week of investigation. For children, a duration of 2 weeks is generally accepted, the other criteria being the same.

There can be no substitute for the most complete history and the most thorough physical examination. Furthermore, both should be repeated at frequent intervals during the course of the evaluation. Patients frequently remember some pertinent bit of history days after the first questioning, and new symptoms or signs can appear at anytime. All aspects of the history must be considered carefully, with special attention directed to travel (domestic or foreign), animal exposure, use of alcohol or other drugs, life-style (camping, backpacking, hunting), family history (thyroid disease, Mediterranean fever), allergy history, prior medical problems, and dental or surgical procedures. Even the most minor and/or transient complaint might be of importance, e.g., transient skin rash in systemic lupus, or mild abdominal discomfort in lymphoma or intraabdominal abscess. In addition to the meticulous physical examination which is done at the time of presentation, certain areas should be reexamined daily: skin, eyes, nail beds, lymph nodes, abdomen, lungs, and heart.

The presence of fever and its pattern must be documented. It is not uncommon to have a patient referred for an FUO workup fail to manifest fever in the hospital. This may be related to disappearance of a self-limited infectious or other process, or to unwarranted concern about normal variation in temperature. The fever pattern may be of value in selected cases: factitious fever, malaria, cyclic neutropenia, Hodgkin's disease, or CNS damage. Factitious fever is usually a diagnosis by exclusion, but certain features may give early clues to this possibility: absence of appropriate tachycardia; marked hyperpyrexia (> 41°C); lack of diurnal variation; or discrepancy between simultaneous body and urine temperatures. When the release of malarial parasites from erythrocytes is synchronized, a recognizable fever pattern may emerge, but this is not seen in newly infected patients, or in those from nonendemic areas. History of possible exposure (travel, transfusion, or IV narcotics) and positive blood smears will help make this diagnosis. Patients with cyclic neutropenia frequently have fever during the nadir of their neutrophil counts, which occurs about every 3 weeks. Pel-Ebstein fever, described in occasional patients with Hodgkin's disease, is the pattern in which fever occurs every evening for several days, alternating with days or weeks without fever. Profound CNS damage is frequently associated with sustained fever; this may be related to the impairment of hypothalamic temperature regulation.

Basic laboratory investigations (Table 2.1) for patients with FUO begin with a complete blood count, white cell differential, erythrocyte sedimentation rate (ESR),

TABLE 2.1   Nonspecific Clues from the Laboratory in Patients with FUO

Monocytosis

> Bacterial endocarditis
> Tuberculosis
> Brucellosis
> Solid tumor
> Hodgkin's disease
> Inflammatory bowel disease

Lymphocytosis

> Tuberculosis
> Infectious mononucleosis
> Cytomegalovirus infection

Leukopenia

> Miliary tuberculosis
> Brucellosis
> Lymphoma
> Systemic lupus erythematosus

Elevated ESR

> Giant cell arteritis
> Rheumatic fever
> Still's disease
> Lymphoma
> Subacute bacterial endocarditis

Elevated alkaline phosphatase

> Obstructive/infiltrative disease of the liver
> Hypernephroma
> Still's disease
> Subacute thyroiditis
> Hodgkin's disease
> Giant cell arteritis

Rheumatoid- factor positive

> Subacute bacterial endocarditis

liver function tests, antistreptolysin O, rheumatoid factor, antinuclear antibody, serum uric acid, calcium and phosphorus, urinalysis, stool guaiac, and chest roentgenogram. Obtain three to six specimens of blood for aerobic and anaerobic culture over 24-48 hr. Place skin tests for tuberculosis and appropriate controls (may use SK/SD, mumps, candida, or trichophyton antigens). Obtain a serum sample to freeze as "acute" specimen ("convalescent" serum in 10-14 days), and urine and other body fluid specimens (pleural, peritoneal, CSF), for routine bacterial, as well as fungal and acid-fast stains and cultures. If, at this point, the tests have yielded neither a diagnosis nor a direction, proceed with other noninvasive studies (Table 2.2): radiologic studies of gastrointestinal and genitourinary tracts; ultrasound scans of the abdomen with special reference to biliary tract, pancreas, kidneys, and lymph nodes, and a liver-spleen scan. Additional noninvasive studies may be of benefit: abdominal CT, ventilation/perfusion lung scan, bone scan, panorex of the mandible, or a gallium scan.

More aggressive diagnostic studies (Table 2.3) are indicated in the patient with persistent fever, especially if accompanied by weight loss or other clinical deterioration. A biopsy of the bone marrow, liver, and lymph node should be done, and the specimens examined histologically and sent for culture. Temporal artery or other biopsies are indicated in the proper clinical setting, as is pulmonary or celiac axis angiography. Usually by this time at least 2 weeks have elapsed and it is appropriate to send the paired acute and convalescent sera for study: brucella, cytomegalovirus, mycoplasma, Q fever, toxoplasmosis, EB virus, trichinosis, psittacosis, typhoid fever, histoplasmosis.

Exploratory laparotomy, once considered the final step in the FUO evaluation, has fallen out of favor in recent years. There is ample evidence to suggest that this procedure is of value only in those patients who have a sign, symptom, or laboratory abnormality related to the abdomen. It should not be carried out otherwise because the return does not warrant the attendant risks.

The usual causes of FUO in adults and children are listed in Table 2.4. Several points deserve emphasis: The speed of your diagnostic evaluation should be related directly to the patient's degree of illness; patients with FUO who remain undiagnosed at the time of discharge from the hospital seem to do well with many defervescing spontaneously and few being found subsequently to have serious disease; patients with FUO frequently have uncommon presentations of common disease. If the patient shows progressive clinical deterioration, a therapeutic trial may be considered. As the therapies differ greatly and may adversely affect the outcome of some diseases, the clinician must have at least a strong suspicion as to which disease process is being treated (Table 2.5). Patients with giant cell arteritis who receive steroids, and patients with Still's disease or rheumatic fever who receive salicylates have a dramatic response, frequently becoming afebrile within 24-48 hr. Constitutional symptoms and the ESR are slower to respond, taking days to weeks. A therapeutic trial for suspected tuberculosis should include two or three drugs and should be continued for at least 3 weeks before being considered a failure. Patients being treated for presumptive endocarditis should receive antibiotics for at least 2 weeks before therapy is discarded as being of no benefit.

TABLE 2.2   Noninvasive Diagnostic Tests for the Patient with FUO

Chest roentgenogram

>   Apical fibrosis, pleural or parenchymal calcifications
>   Miliary pattern

Blood cultures

>   Obtain three to six aerobic/anaerobic specimens
>   Endovascular infection
>   Osteomyelitis

Skin tests

>   PPD plus control (SK/SD, mumps, candida, or trichophyton)
>   Tuberculosis
>   Anergic states

GI x-rays

>   Whipple's disease
>   Tuberculous enteritis
>   Neoplasm
>   Diverticulitis
>   Crohn's disease
>   Ulcerative colitis

IVP and renal ultrasound

>   Hypernephroma
>   Tuberculosis
>   Intrarenal/perinephric abscess
>   Retroperitoneal nodes

Liver/spleen scan and ultrasound

>   Splenomegaly
>   Neoplasm
>   Abscess
>   Gallbladder disease

Echocardiography

>   Endocarditis
>   Atrial myxoma

Abdominal CT, ultrasound, gallium scan

>   Abdominal/retroperitoneal masses, abscesses, or
>   lymphadenopathy

Ventilation/perfusion lung scan

>   Recurrent pulmonary emboli

TABLE 2.2 (Cont'd)

Acute/convalescent sera

Q fever
Cytomegalovirus
Toxoplasmosis
Brucellosis
Trichinosis
Psittacosis
Infectious mononucleosis

Lumbar puncture

Cryptococcosis
Tuberculosis

Bone survey/scan

Osteomyelitis
Carcinoma

Panorex

Dental abscess

TABLE 2.3   Invasive Diagnostic Tests for the Patient with FUO

Pulmonary angiography

Recurrent pulmonary emboli

Celiac axis angiography

Polyarteritis nodosa

Liver biopsy

Hepatoma	Sarcoidosis
Metastatic carcinoma	Brucellosis
Lymphoma	Hepatitis
Miliary tuberculosis	

Bone marrow biopsy

Lymphoma	Histoplasmosis
Miliary tuberculosis	Brucellosis

Lymph node biopsy

Lymphoma
Tuberculosis
Sarcoidosis

TABLE 2.3 (Cont'd)

Temporal artery biopsy

Giant cell arteritis

Exploratory laparotomy

N.B. (Likely to be helpful *only* if there is
objective clinical evidence of abdominal disease)

Abscesses	Tuberculosis
Lymphoma	Crohn's disease
Arteritis	

TABLE 2.4   Causes of FUO*

Disease	Adults	Children
Infection	35	60
Neoplasm	20	2
Connective tissue diseases	15	7
Miscellaneous	25	15
No diagnosis	5	16

* Approximate percentage of total cases

TABLE 2.5   Therapeutic Trials in the Patient with FUO

Steroids	Giant cell arteritis
Salicylates	Still's disease
	Rheumatic fever
Antimicrobials	Tuberculosis
	Infective endocarditis

Selected Bibliography

Aduan, R. P., Fauci, A. S., Dale, D. C., Herzberg, J. H., and Wolff, S. M.: Factitious fever and self-induced infection. *Ann Intern Med* 90:230-242, 1979.

Bernheim, H. A., Block, L. H., and Atkins, E.: Fever: Pathogenesis, pathophysiology and purpose. *Ann Intern Med* 91:261-270, 1979.

Brewis, E. G.: Child care in general practice; undiagnosed fever. *Br Med J* 5427: 107-109, 1965.

Dechovitz, A. B. and Moffet, H. L.: Classification of acute febrile illnesses in childhood. *Clin Pediatr* 7:649-653, 1968.

Effersoe, P.: Fever of unknown origin: A follow-up study of 34 patients discharged without diagnosis. *Dan Med Bull* 15:240-244, 1968.

Ellman, L.: Bone marrow biopsy in the evaluation of lymphoma, carcinoma and granulomatous disorders. *Am J Med* 60:1-7, 1976.

Esposito, A. L. and Gleckman, R. A.: A diagnostic approach to the adult with fever of unknown origin. *Arch Intern Med* 139:575-579, 1979.

Feigin, R. D. and Shearer, W. T.: Fever of unknown origin in children. *Curr Prob Pediatr* 6:1-65, 1976.

Ferrucci, J. T., Jr.: Body ultrasonography. *N Engl J Med* 300:538-542, 590-602, 1979.

Habibian, M. R., Staab, E. V., and Matthews, H. A.: Gallium citrate Ga[67] scans in febrile patients. *JAMA* 233:1073-1076, 1975.

Jacoby, G. A. and Swartz, M. N.: Fever of undetermined origin. *N Engl J Med* 289:1407-1410, 1973.

Lentle, B. C., Russel, A. S., Percy, J. S., Scott, J. R., and Jackson, F. I.: Bone scintiscanning updated. *Ann Intern Med* 84:297-303, 1976.

Levitt, R. G., Biello, D. R., Sagel, S. S., Stanley, R. J., Aronberg, D. J., Robinson, M. L., and Siegel, B.: Computed tomography and ^{67}Ga citrate radionuclide imaging for evaluating suspected abdominal abscess. *Am J Roentgenol* 132: 529-534, 1979.

McClung, H. J.: Prolonged fever of unknown origin in children. *Am J Dis Child* 124:544-550, 1972.

Murray, H. W., Tuazon, C. U., Guerrero, I. C., Claudio, M. S., Alling, D. W., and Sheagren, J. N.: Urinary temperature. A clue to early diagnosis of factitious fever. *N Engl J Med* 296:23-24, 1977.

Musher, D. M., Fainstein, V., Young, E. J., and Pruett, T. L.: Fever patterns. Their lack of clinical significance. *Arch Intern Med* 139:1225-1228, 1979.

Petersdorf, R. G.: Fever of unknown origin. *Ann Intern Med* 70:864–866, 1969.

Petersdorf, R. G. and Beeson, P. B.: Fever of unexplained origin: Report on 100 cases. *Medicine* 40:1–30, 1961.

Pettersson, T.: Fever of obscure origin: A follow-up investigation of 88 cases. *Acta Med Scand* 171:575–583, 1962.

Schimmelpfenning, R. W., Jr. and Chusid, M. J.: Illnesses associated with extreme elevation of the erythrocyte sedimentation rate in children. *Clin Pediatr* 19:175–178, 1980.

Simon, H. B.: Extreme pyrexia. *JAMA* 236:2419–2421, 1976.

Vickery, D. M. and Quinnell, R. K.: Fever of unknown origin. An algorithmic approach. *JAMA* 238:2183–2188, 1977.

Wyler, D. J.: Diagnostic implications of markedly elevated erythrocyte sedimentation rate: A reevaluation. *South Med J* 70:1428–1430, 1977.

3

PHAGOCYTES AND HOST DEFENSE
Rama Ganguly, Ph.D.

Origin and Nature of Phagocytic Cells

When the physical and chemical barriers of primary host defense mechanisms are overcome by an invading microorganism, two important phagocytic cells are called into play: polymorphonuclear leukocytes (PMNs) and mononuclear phagocytes. In the early nineteenth century, Metchnikoff recognized these two major groups of phagocytes as microphages and macrophages, respectively. These cells, also called the professional phagocytes, possess specialized receptors for the Fc portion of IgG molecules as well as for activated complement C3. Microorganisms with IgG or activated C3 on their surface are more easily phagocytosed by attachment to these receptors. There are other phagocytic cells (so called nonprofessional phagocytes) that also participate in the ingestion of microbial organisms under certain conditions, e.g., endothelial cells, epithelial cells, and fibroblasts, but these are devoid of any specialized receptors for mediation of phagocytic functions.

The PMNs are produced in huge numbers (10^9-10^{11} cells daily), and they circulate in the blood for 6-7 hr after their release from the bone marrow. They possess numerous enzymes and antimicrobial substances contained in lysosomes, which are granules in the cytoplasm. The PMNs leave the circulation by squeezing through endothelial cell junctions and they survive in tissue for only a few days.

Mononuclear phagocytes also originate in the bone marrow. After 1-2 days in circulation, they further differentiate into macrophages upon entering the surrounding tissues by migration through the vessel walls. These cells are dispersed throughout the body and may be of two kinds: fixed or wandering. The fixed cells are found primarily along the blood vessels in the liver, spleen, bone marrow, and lymph nodes. They are collectively referred to as the reticuloendothelial system. The wandering macrophages, also called tissue macrophages, are found in the alveoli and the peritoneal cavity. Like PMNs, the macrophages also possess lysosomal enzymes and often the myeloperoxidase enzyme system. Mature macrophages possess many times more lysosomal enzymes than do the monocytes. The life span of macrophages is measured in weeks to months. Macrophages are not end-stage cells and are capable under certain conditions of synthesizing new DNA and multiplying.

Antimicrobial Mechanisms of Phagocytic Cells

In response to an inflammatory stimulus, the PMNs characteristically are the first to arrive at the site of inflammation. The mononuclear phagocytes arrive later, explained at least in part by their slower migration. On the other hand, PMNs are short-lived and therefore, in chronic infection, they are replaced by the long-lived macrophages. Certain bacteria, like the tubercle bacillus and brucellae, specifically attract macrophages to the site of infection. They are phagocytosed by macrophages but are able to prevent, in the nonsensitized hosts, degranulation of the macrophages upon phagocytosis. These organisms are classic examples of pathogens capable of intracellular proliferation inside the phagosome (the vacuole containing the phagocytosed particle) and result in chronic persistent infection. The macrophages with the intracellular pathogens form walled-off nodules surrounded by connective tissues - probably as a measure to prevent spread of infection. These are called granulomas. Another very important role of the macrophage is its participation as a helper cell in the immune response of lymphocytes. Macrophages probably process and present the antigen in proper form to the immunocompetent cells, the B and T lymphocytes. Not only do they activate lymphocytes through the production of soluble factors (e.g., lymphocyte-activating factor) in response to the antigenic stimuli, but they are also capable of being activated in response to the soluble factors produced by lymphocytes - the lymphokines. Lymphokine-stimulated macrophages become sticky and metabolically more active and spread out in appearance. They possess enhanced bactericidal capacity and are called *angry macrophages.* Thus a *feed-back* mechanism exists between the macrophage and the lymphocyte in the afferent limb of the immune response.

Intracellular killing of pathogens proceeds through four interrelated stages: chemotaxis, opsonization, ingestion, and killing. Chemotaxis is the process of directed movement of the phagocytic cells to the site of inflammation. Factors responsible for this directed movement are mostly of host origin. The complement system plays an important role as the source of such leukotactic factors (C3a and C5a, C567) which work in concert with another complement derivative C3b as an oposonin (vide infra). Leukotactic factors also may be derived from leukocytes, including sensitized lymphocytes. Other nonspecific leukotactic factors are known, e.g., trypsin, plasmin, and bacterial proteases.

Phagocytosis of bacteria requires interaction between the microbes and certain humoral factors before the interaction with the phagocytic membrane. These humoral factors, collectively termed *opsonins,* are specific or natural antibodies against the microbe, the complement-derived component C3b, and other cofactors such as tuftsin. The latter is a gamma globulin moiety produced by the spleen which coats PMNs and stimulates phagocytosis.

The process of ingestion rapidly follows attachment of the microbial cell to the phagocyte. The leukocytic membrane completely surrounds the bacterium within a phagocytic vacuole (called *phagosome)* and the cytoplasmic granules discharge their contents into the newly formed vacuole resulting in the formation of a *phagolysosome.* The phagocytic event is accompanied by a burst of metabolic activity within the PMN and in this process stored glycogen is metabolized. Glucose (derived from the glycogen of PMNs) is metabolized by both the glycolytic and the hexose monophosphate shunt (HMS) pathways. This generates reduced co-enzymes, i.e., NADH (by glycolysis) and NADPH (by HMS metabolism). Upon re-oxidation of these reduced coenzymes large amounts of H_2O_2 are formed. This H_2O_2 diffuses from the cytoplasm of the phagocyte into the phagolysosome where in conjunction with the myeloperoxidase enzyme and halide ions (from the phago-cyte), it aids in bacterial killing. Experimental evidence indicates that PMNs also produce superoxide anion (O_2^-) during the phagocytic event. This O_2^- is ex-tremely toxic for the internalized microbial cell. Superoxide dismutase forms H_2O_2 from O_2^- by oxidation. Phagocytosis can also proceed in absence of oxy-gen. Lactoferrin and cationic proteins of PMNs probably aid in bacterial killing under anaerobic conditions. Over 60 different enzymes have been recognized in the lysosomes, e.g., proteases, lipase, carbohydrases, RNase, DNase, acid phospha-tase, and myeloperoxidase, to name just a few. Lysozyme hydrolyzes the cell-wall mucopeptides of certain bacteria.

Patients with bacterial infections have increased metabolic activities of their PMNs as well as higher turnover of their hydrogen ions. This property of the leu-kocytes has been utilized in developing laboratory tests useful for clinical diagno-sis. Nitroblue tetrazolium (NBT) is a colorless, soluble dye in the oxidized state but upon reduction converts into formazan which is a blue insoluble compound. Therefore, PMNs from patients with bacterial infection reduce NBT in an accel-erated manner and the blue cytoplasmic precipitate thus formed in large number of cells becomes visible under the light microscope.

Defects in Phagocytes

Phagocytic disorders may be due to extrinsic and/or intrinsic defects. The ex-trinsic defects may arise from

1. Deficiencies of opsonin secondary to deficiencies of antibody and comple-ment factors
2. Suppression of the total number of phagocytic cells by immunosuppressive agents
3. Interference of phagocytic activities by steroids or other drugs
4. Suppression of the total number of PMNs in circulation due to the pres-ence of autoantibodies against their surface antigens

The intrinsic defects of phagocytic functions are related to the enzymatic/ metabolic activities of the phagocytic cells that are required in their bactericidal activities. These defects may result in a wide range of clinical presentations from mild recurrent skin infections to severe, overwhelming, and fatal systemic infec-tions. Characteristically, these patients suffer usually from bacterial infections; viral and protozoal infections are not common problems in them. Table 3.1 lists various types of phagocytic dysfunctions according to the proposed classification by a committee of the World Health Organization.

Evaluation of the phagocytic functions can be done in a patient using numer-ous tests in vivo or in vitro or both. These include: quantitative nitroblue tetra-zolium (NBT) test, quantitative intracellular-killing curve determination, and chemotaxis, random migration, and glass-wool adherence of the phagocytes.

Narcotic drugs such as morphine are known to interfere with the HMS pathway and thus intracellular killing by PMNs. It is, therefore, not surprising that patients requiring long-term narcotic therapy or drug addicts have lower general host re-sistance to infections. Defective macrophage functions also occur in various nu-tritional deficiencies, especially in acute protein-caloric malnutrition. Thymic

TABLE 3.1   Phagocytic Dysfunction Classification

---

1. Chronic granulomatous disease

2. Glucose-6-phosphate dehydrogenase deficiency

3. Myeloperoxidase deficiency

4. Chediak-Higashi syndrome

5. Job's syndrome

6. Tuftskin deficiency

7. "Lazy leukocyte syndrome"

8. Elevated IgE, defective chemotaxis, eczema, and
    recurrent infections

---

involution, as well as marked leukopenia, may occur in such conditions thus resulting in enhanced susceptibility to infections.

Chronic granulomatous disease (CGD) of children is associated with susceptibility to infection with unusual organisms normally of low virulence, e.g., *Staphylococcus epidermidis, Serratia marcescens, Aspergillus.* The CGD patients show
an X-linked inheritance pattern (a female variant occurs) and onset of symptoms
is usually by 2 years of age. Draining lymphadenitis, hepatosplenomegaly, pneumonia, osteomyelitis, and abscesses are common clinical findings. The enzymatic
deficiency in CGD is either NADH or NADPH oxidase or NADH reductase, resulting in abnormal intracellular metabolism of neutrophils, decrease in oxygen consumption, H_2O_2 production, and phagocytic killing. Aggressive diagnostic measures and therapy are required for long-term survival and functional ability of such
patients.

Glucose-6-phosphate dehydrogenase deficiency is associated with decrease in
HMS pathway activities and H_2O_2 production in white cells. Thus these patients
also are unable to kill certain organisms in a normal manner similar to that of
CGD patients. Myeloperoxidase deficiency in patients is also associated with delayed killing of organisms by the phagocytes. These patients show enhanced infections from certain microbes such as *Candida* and staphylococci.

Chediak-Higashi syndrome, associated with repeated infections, results from
the presence of giant lysosomes in the PMNs and their precursors, promyelocytes.
The characteristic abnormality of giant cytoplasmic granular inclusions in white
blood cells and platelets may be observed on routine peripheral blood smears under
a light microscope. Neutrophil chemotaxis, phagocytic killing, and microtubule
functions also have been described as abnormal in these patients. This syndrome
is a multisystem, autosomal-recessive disorder with recurrent bacterial infections
with a variety of organisms. The prognosis is poor. Hepatosplenomegaly, partial
albinism, central nervous system abnormalities, and a high incidence of lymphoreticular malignancies are usual findings. There is no treatment other than specific
antibiotic therapy for the infecting organisms. Finally, neutropenia associated
with defective chemotactic response of neutrophils is observed in patients with

"lazy leukocyte syndrome." The Rebuck window test shows abnormal in vivo inflammatory response in these patients. These patients do not show an increase in the number of WBC following epinephrine or endotoxin stimulation. Phagocytic cells from these individuals also show defective random migration. They suffer from severe bacterial infections. Treatment with specific antibiotics is required.

Selected Bibliography

Allen, R. C.: Evaluation of serum opsonic capacity by quantitating the initial chemiluminescent response from phagocytosing polymorphonuclear leukocytes. *Infect Immun* 15:828-833, 1977.

Barbior, B. M., Kipnes, R. S., and Curnutte, J. T.: Biological defense mechanisms. The production by leukocytes of superoxide: A potential bactericidal agent. *J Clin Invest* 52:741-744, 1973.

Berlin, R. D., Fera, J. P., and Pfeiffer, R.: Reversible phagocytosis in rabbit polymorphonuclear leukocytes. *J Clin Invest* 63:1137-1144, 1979.

Bridges, R. A., Berendes, H., and Good, R. A.: A fatal granulomatous disease of childhood. *Am J Dis Child* 97:387-408, 1959.

Dechatelet, L. R.: Oxidative bactericidal mechanisms of polymorphonuclear leukocytes. *J Infect Dis* 131:295-303, 1975.

Ganguly, R., Durieux, M. F., and Waldman, R. H.: Macrophage function in vitamin C-deficient guinea pigs. *Am J Nutr* 29:762-765, 1976.

Keusch, G. T., Douglas, S. D., Braden, K., and Geller, S. A.: Antibacterial functions of macrophages in experimental protein calorie malnutrition (2 parts). *J Infect Dis* 138:125-133, 134-142, 1978.

Klebanoff, S. J.: Intraleukocytic microbicidal defects. *Ann Rev Med* 22:39-62, 1971.

Moulder, J. W.: Intracellular parasitism: Life in an extreme environment. *J Infect Dis* 130:300-306, 1974.

Scully, C. M. and Lehner, T.: Bacterial and strain specificities in opsonization, phagocytosis and killing of *Streptococcus mutans*. *Clin Exp Immunol* 35:128-132, 1979.

Shear, H. L., Nussenzweig, R. S., and Bianco, C.: Immune phagocytosis in murine malaria. *J Exp Med* 149:1288-1298, 1979.

Sixbey, J. W., Fields, B. T., Sun, C. N., Clark, R. A., and Nolan, C. M.: Interactions between human granulocytes and *Blastomyces dermatitis*. *Infect Immun* 23:41-44, 1979.

Stossel, T. O.: Phagocytosis (3 parts). *N Engl J Med* 290:717-723, 774-781, 833-839, 1974.

Weaver, E. A., Tsuda, H., Goldblum, R. M., Goldman, A. S., and Davis, C. P.: Relationship between phagocytosis and immunoglobulin A release from human colostral macrophages. *Infect Immun* 38:1073-1077, 1982.

4

IMMUNITY TO INFECTIOUS DISEASES

Rama Ganguly, Ph.D. and Robert H. Waldman, M.D.

Immunity to infectious diseases refers to the capacity enjoyed by an organism to remain unaffected by harmful microbial agents present in the environment and within. The variety of microbial agents that can cause infection is extremely large, possessing many pathogenic mechanisms. Host defense mechanisms are also multiple, being specific and nonspecific, local and systemic, as well as humoral and cellular (Table 4.1). In this chapter, the resistance mechanisms will be considered under two categories: (1) nonspecific, or natural, and (2) specific, or acquired.

Natural Immunity

There are many components which act as nonspecific or innate factors of immunity. The mucociliary escalator of the respiratory tract, for example, plays a significant role in the discharge of microorganisms from the body, either being coughed out or swallowed and excreted in the bowel contents. Similarly, salivary secretions dispose of many potential pathogenic agents in the mouth. Various enzymes, chemicals, and antimicrobial agents that exert significant protective roles are produced in body fluids. These include lysozyme, salivary glycolipids, acidity of the stomach, secretions of the skin and vagina, and spermine as well as zinc in seminal plasma. The endogenous microbial flora interact with natural host factors and among themselves to prevent pathogenic colonization and to sustain the balance of this ecosystem which exists on normal healthy mucosae. For many pathogens, attachment of the agent to specific membrane receptor sites is of crucial importance. Their affinity for host cells may be inhibited by many nonspecific humoral factors. Phagocytic cells, especially those of the respiratory tract, stay in a constant state of activation because of frequent antigenic bombardment.

TABLE 4.1   Postulated Immune Mechanisms Responsible for Protection

| Infection | CMI | Humoral | | Unknown |
		Systemic	Secretory	
Viruses				
Picornaviruses	–	+	+	
Myxoviruses	+/–	+/–	+/–	
Poxviruses	+	–	–	
Hepatitis viruses	+/–	+	–	
Bacteria				
Bedsonias and rickettsiae				+
Eubacteria	–	+	+/–	
Mycobacteria	+	–	–	
Fungi	+	–	–	
Protozoa				+

Once the local defenses are breached (Table 4.2) by the infective agent, the polymorphonuclear leukocyte and monocyte/macrophage systems are called into play. They initiate the inflammatory process at the site of deposition of the agents or may carry them to regional lymph nodes. Their functions are enhanced by chemotaxis and opsonization. Complement-mediated bacteriolysis without phagocytosis is another mode of host defense. Agglutination of microbial agents by circulating nonspecific factors enhances clearance of the pathogen from the blood stream through phagocytosis. Finally, fever has been recognized as a possible mode of natural defense. Thus, application of analgesics for suppression of fever needs careful reevaluation. Examples of various factors of natural host defenses are shown in Table 4.3.

Acquired Immunity

Acquired immunity results from natural disease processes (active natural immunity), from artificial exposure to attenuated or inactivated pathogens or their toxoids (active artificial immunity), or from receiving antibody, sensitized lymphocytes, or their soluble products from an immune donor (passive immunity). An

TABLE 4.2   Some Conditions Compromising Mechanical Defense
             Barrriers Against Infection

Urinary bladder instrumentation

Indwelling venous catheterization

Surgical procedures

Burns

Tracheostomy

TABLE 4.3   Nonspecific Immunity

Physical	Epithelial surfaces, ciliary movement, peristalsis
Biochemical	Lysozyme, basic polypeptides, properdin, β-lysins, plakins, leukins
Cellular	Phagocytes, reticuloendothelial system, inflammation
Others	Body temperature, oxygen tension in tissues, antagonism of indigenous flora

---

example of the latter is the transfer of IgG in utero from mother to fetus (passive natural immunity). When such a transfer takes place under artificial conditions, such as the injection of gamma globulin, it results in passive artificial immunity.

Acquired immunity, whether active or passive, natural or artificial, may be T-cell and/or B-cell mediated. Each of these may, in turn, be either systemic and/or secretory in nature. Systemic and secretory immune functions operate, at least partially, independently of each other.

Humoral Immunity (Tables 4.4 and 4.5)

Understanding of the role of humoral immunity has emerged largely from studies of patients having agammaglobulinemia, who demonstrate exceptional susceptibility to encapsulated pyogenic pathogens, e.g., *Streptococcus pneumoniae, Haemophilus influenzae, S. pyogenes, Neisseria meningitides,* and *Pseudomonas aeruginosa.*   Children with this type of immunodeficiency rarely become infected during the first 6 months of life because they are protected by antibodies derived in

TABLE 4.4   Some Properties of Immunoglobulin Classes

Property	IgM	IgG	IgA	IgD	IgE
Molecular weight (x 10^{-3})	900	150	160/400	150	190
Sedimentation coefficient	19	7	7/11	7	8
Half-life in serum (days)	5	23	6	3	2.5
Earliest Ab* in primary immune response	+				
Most abundant Ab in most late responses		+			
Prominent in external secretions			+		+
Transported across placenta		+			
Active in complement fixation by					
Classical pathway	++	+			
Alternate pathway	+	+	+	+	+

*Ab = antibody

TABLE 4.5   Serum Immunoglobulin Levels at Various Ages

Age	% of Adult Level*		
	IgM	IgG	IgA
2-4 mo	45	32	10
5-8 mo	61	39	19
9-14 mo	82	57	23
2-3 yr	84	72	40
5-6 yr	88	87	68
11-12 yr	94	98	85
15-16 yr	120	104	96

*Mean adult levels: IgM 100 mg%, IgG 1100 mg%, IgA 180 mg%

utero. Treatment of these children with injections of gamma globulin has been
only partially successful, since serum IgG may be easily replaced; however, there
has been no successful methodology developed for the replacement of secretory
IgA. Thus these patients eventually develop the sequelae of severe and repeated
respiratory tract infections.

The first immunoglobulin class of antibody that develops following interaction
with an antigen is IgM (Figure 4.1). Immunoglobulin M may be the only class
formed in response to certain large immunogens with repeating antigenic determinants on their surface, e.g., pneumococcal capsular polysaccharide, cell walls
of gram-negative bacilli, bacterial flagellae, and surfaces of viruses. When IgM
reacts with an antigen, complement is activated so effectively that a single antibody molecule can cause cell lysis. The IgM antibodies are 20-1000 times more
potent in agglutination, bacterial killing, and opsonization when compared with
IgG antibody. Although fetuses are capable of synthesizing IgM, levels are very
low at birth, but rise quickly thereafter as a result of antigenic stimulation. Therefore one way of detecting intrauterine infection is to measure the IgM levels in
cord blood.

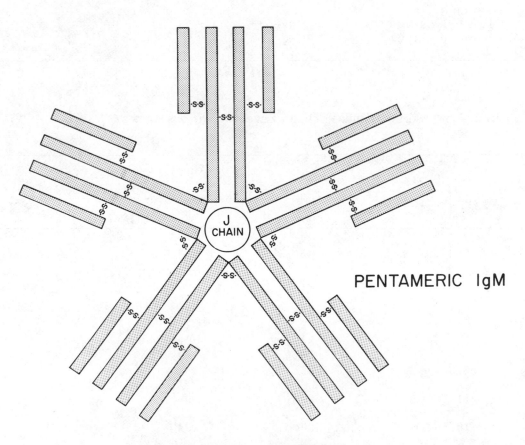

FIGURE 4.1   Model of IgM.

Immunoglobulin G (IgG) (Figure 4.2) constitutes 85% of the total serum immunoglobulin. Most of the antibody to gram-positive pyogenic bacteria, certain
viruses, and toxins in adult serum belong to this class. It crosses the placenta and
accounts for much of the acquired resistance of the newborn during the first 6
months of life.

Immunoglobulin A (IgA) comprises only 10% of serum immunoglobulins, but
abounds in mucosal secretions, where it is the principal mediator of protection
against infection. Secretory IgA has been demonstrated to be locally produced
and is detected in greater quantities, relative to serum, in saliva, colostrum, tears,
and respiratory, gastrointestinal, and genitourinary secretions. Its structure in
serum is that of a monomer, i.e., analogous to IgG, containing two heavy and two
light chains. However, in secretions it is mainly found in the form of a dimer, and
possesses two additional polypeptide chains – secretory component, which is unique
to secretory IgA, and a J chain, which is found on both IgM and secretory IgA (Figures 4.3 and 4.4). The structure of IgA appears to be adapted to the purpose of
mucosal immunity, as it has somewhat increased resistance to digestion by proteolytic enzymes and reducing agents. Secretory IgA antibody protects against
mucosal viral infections by inhibiting attachment and penetration of the viruses
into mucosal epithelial cells. In addition to protecting against viruses that only
infect mucosal surfaces, it acts as an initial barrier to the portal of entry of invasive viral infections such as polio, measles, and rubella. Secretory IgA antibody
also appears to protect against bacterial infections. This seems to be accomplished by the inhibition of bacterial adherence to mucosal cells. Unable to attach

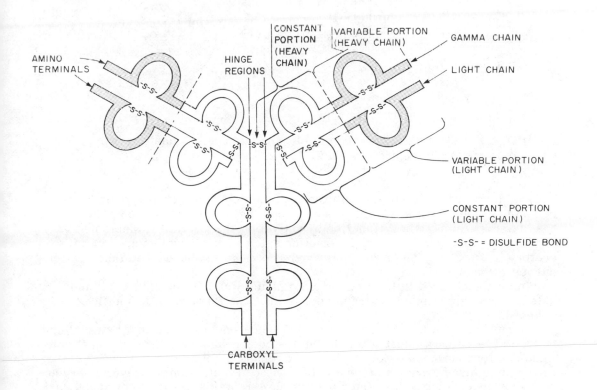

FIGURE 4.2   Model of IgG.

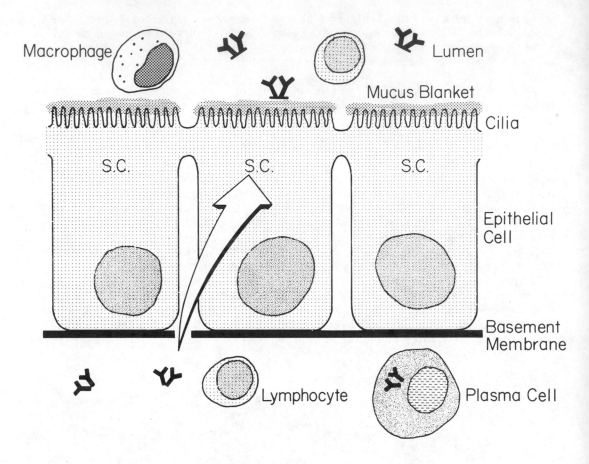

FIGURE 4.3   Schematic drawing of cells and immune mechanisms of mucosal surfaces, such as the respiratory tract.

and maintain intimate contact with the epithelial cells, most pathogenic bacteria become harmless. Although secretory IgA does not appear to fix complement by the classic pathway, it may function by activating the alternate complement pathway, or there may be some interaction between the complement system, secretory IgA antibody, and lysozyme, which is present in abundance in most external secretions.

Immunoglobulin D (IgD) is an immunoglobulin which is found in small and variable amounts in serum and extracellular fluids. The function of IgD antibodies is unknown.

Immunoglobulin E (IgE) is found in very small amounts in serum, extracellular fluid, and secretions. Most of the IgE in the body is attached to tissue mast cells. Although found in small amounts, IgE is extremely potent since it causes release of the contents of granules in mast cells. These granules contain several very active substances, such as histamine and the slow-reacting substance of anaphylaxis. Immunoglobulin E is the reaginic antibody, responsible for immediate hypersensitivity reactions. It is also thought that IgE has some relationship to protection

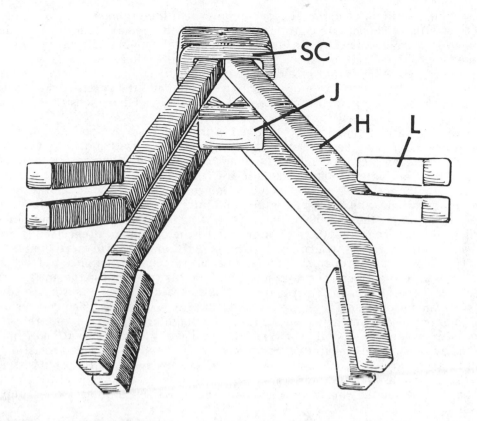

FIGURE 4.4   Model of secretory IgA. SC = secretory component; J = J chain; H = heavy chain; L = light chain.

against some parasitic infestations, but the mechanism is unclear. Although serum IgE levels are elevated in many patients with allergic diseases, e.g., eczema, the highest levels are found in people with intestinal parasitism.

Cellular Immunity

Acquired immunity to some infectious agents does not result from the classic mechanism in which specific antibody interferes with infectivity or pathogenicity by combining with the invading organism or its toxic products. There is no evidence, for example, that microorganisms are influenced by antibody while they are protectively accommodated within the cytoplasm of host cells, unless the microorganism has left specific antigens on the surface of the host cell. Antibody can only neutralize intracellular microbes, particularly viruses, while they are in transit from one host cell to the next. This is effective mainly against those viruses that, following replication within the host cell, cause cell lysis. In addition, some bacteria and protozoa are quite unaffected by antibody, even when they exist extracellularly. Protection in these situations depends upon cell-mediated immunity (CMI), i.e., that immune system which leads to an alteration of the intracellular milieu, changing it from one in which the organism may prosper, to one that will not support its continued survival. Cell-mediated immunity includes those processes in which thymus-derived sensitized lymphoid cells (T cells) effect antigen recognition and response. In addition to protection against many microorganisms, CMI is important as a defense mechanism against neoplastic growth, and also plays the central role in allograft rejection and the graft-versus-host reaction. The classic clinical test for CMI is the delayed hypersensitivity skin reaction.

Cell-mediated immunity is comprised of two principal components, macrophages and T lymphocytes. When a pathogen enters the system of a previously sensitized individual, a small number of T lymphocytes accumulate and become activated. These activated cells release into the surrounding extracellular fluid several physiologically active effectors, including migration-inhibitory, chemotactic, blastogenic, cytotoxic, and transfer factors, and interferon(Table 4.6). The result of these mediators is the attraction and retention of macrophages and other nonsensitized lymphocytes at the site of growth of the organism. Recruited lymphocytes become activated, transform into blast cells, and liberate more *lymphokines* into the area. Thus through mediators, an amplification of the initial effect occurs. The initial antigen recognition by the T cell is specific for the antigen to which the T cell has been sensitized, but this specific reaction results in a sequence of nonspecific effects, e.g., activation of macrophages. The end result is development of delayed hypersensitivity and a heightened resistance to the specific microorganism, as well as unrelated organisms. Hence, activation of macrophages by BCG, an attenuated *Mycobacterium,* can lead to enhanced resistance both to *M. tuberculosis,* and *Listeria monocytogenes* or *Bordetella pertussis.* Such activation can also lead to increased resistance to viruses. On the other hand, it has been observed that many viral and bacterial diseases cause temporary suppression of CMI.

Activated macrophages have several characteristics, including increased "stickiness," enhanced phagocytic capacity, increased number and size of cytoplasmic organelles, increased oxygen consumption, increased activity of the hexose monophosphate shunt, and increased H_2O_2 production. Sensitized T cells also have "killer" function. Cytotoxic T cells specifically recognize foreign surface antigens on cells and kill the cell following direct contact by an as yet unknown mechanism.

TABLE 4.6   Some Products of Activated Lymphocytes

Migration-inhibitory factor

Macrophage-aggregating factor

Chemotactic factor

Blastogenic factor

Interferon

Transfer factor

In addition to the cells of the monocyte/macrophage line, which are essential for the protective role of CMI against many different pathogens, the other major phagocytic cell of the body is the neutrophilic granulocyte or polymorphonuclear leukocyte. The neutrophil is important in the functioning of humoral immunity, along with antibody (usually IgG) and complement. When IgG antibody reacts with its antigen, the complement system is activated, leading to the release of several factors that attract neutrophils (chemotaxis) and make the antigen more readily phagocytized (opsonization). Increased susceptibility to infection is clearly related to quantitative or qualitative defects in neutrophils, whether this defect is a result of disease or of therapy (Table 4.7). Both neutrophils and macrophages serve a protective mechanism nonspecifically, i.e., without antibody or T cells reacting with antigens. However, the activity of these phagocytic cells is tremendously increased by the specific immune reactions.

Interferon, which may be considered a lymphokine, is an inhibitor of viral replication, as well as a modulator of immune reactions. Interferon is produced by both lymphoid and nonlymphoid cells, and is stimulated by a wide variety of viruses and nonviral substances. There are at least three interferons with different chemical, physical, immunologic, and biologic properties, all with antiviral activity but perhaps with different immunomodulating properties.

Passive Immunization (Tables 4.8 and 4.9)

Situations in which passive administration of antibody is useful are: (1) insufficient time for active immunization, e.g., administration of antisera to the bacterial toxins that are responsible for tetanus or botulism; (2) no vaccine is available, as is the case for hepatitis A virus infection; (3) immune deficiency states wherein passive administration of human gamma globulin has been shown to be beneficial in alleviating recurrent infections; and (4) inhibition of antibody production, e.g., administering gamma globulin to inhibit the host's own defense mechanisms. The latter is generally considered undesirable; however, in certain situations, excellent use of this basic immunologic principle has been made. Rh disease is caused by maternal anti-Rh antibody crossing the placenta and hemolyzing fetal Rh-positive red cells. As prophylaxis against this disorder, anti-Rh antibody is administered to the mother, thus inhibiting production of her own Rh antibody.

TABLE 4.7   Conditions Causing Impaired Phagocytic Function

Decreased numbers of polymorphonuclear leukocytes

Drug-induced granulocytopenia, including antitumor therapy

Myelophthisic processes

Defective function

Chronic granulomatous disease

Acidosis

Corticosteroid therapy

TABLE 4.8   Indications for Passive Administration of Gamma Globulin

---

Insufficient time for active immunization to be effective

    Tetanus

    Botulism

No vaccine available

    Pooled serum must contain sufficient antibody, as a result of random selection or screening of donors

    Hepatitis A

Immunization with live virus vaccine contraindicated

Humoral immune deficiency diseases involving IgG

Suppression of patient's antibody production (Rh disease)

TABLE 4.9   Disadvantages of Gamma Globulin Therapy

Protection is of short duration

Large doses cannot be given

Unpredictable uptake from injection site

Immunoglobulins are potentially immunogenic

Exogenous gamma globulin may inhibit endogenous synthesis

Side effects: sterile abscess, fibrosis, rare anaphylactic-type reaction

Painful and expensive

The mother is not sensitized and will not react with the rapid production of large amounts of anti-Rh antibody during a subsequent pregnancy.

There are basically two different types of passively administered gamma globulin: a randomly collected, relatively low-titer preparation and a specifically stimulated, very high-titer one. High-titer, specific gamma globulin preparations directed against tetanus, rabies, and type B hepatitis are available. The other gamma globulin is used primarily for patients with low or absent production.

There are a number of disadvantages of passive immunization. Protection is of short duration, the half-life of passively administered IgG being about 3 weeks.

However, under field conditions, protection against hepatitis A virus persists for considerably longer than this. The recommended dosage interval for gamma globulin for prophylaxis against hepatitis A is 4-6 months in endemic areas. Immunoglobulins are themselves immunogens, especially serum from other species. Horse serum, the major source of antitetanus antiserum for many years, was the classic cause of serum sickness. Human immunoglobulins are also immunogenic, although this is rarely of clinical importance. Gamma globulin injections are painful and expensive.

The use of transfer factor may be considered as passive cell-mediated immunity. Transfer factor results in the recruitment of noncommitted T lymphocytes. When lymphocytes are obtained from a donor and are lysed, the debris removed, and the supernatant dialyzed, transfer factors to all antigens to which that person is sensitized are obtained in the dialysate. When these transfer factors are injected into another person, the recipient's noncommitted T lymphocytes are recruited, and the recipient shows evidence of CMI to those antigens for several months. Thus transfer factor use is actually a combination of passive sensitization and active participation by the recipient's own T cells. Transfer factor has been used experimentally with some success in treating such diseases as mucocutaneous candidiasis, coccidioidomycosis, and chronic hepatitis B infection.

Active Immunization (Table 4.10)

The purpose of active immunization is to stimulate the individual's own protective mechanisms. To do this rationally, the protective mechanisms should be known. Unfortunately, there are few incidences in infectious diseases where the protective mechanisms have been elucidated completely. One of the few examples is tetanus, in which serum antibody to the toxin is known to be protective. Despite the fact that little is known about the mechanism of protection in most infectious diseases, from a practical point of view, the central question is whether or not a vaccine works. Determining this is often fairly difficult. Some vaccines were introduced into general use before they were critically assessed, and at about the same time the great advances were being made in other general public health measures. When the diseases for which some vaccines were given decreased, the vaccines were widely accepted as being efficacious. The improvement in hygienic conditions in this country may have been partially, or completely, responsible for the decrease. Measuring the immune response to administration of a vaccine may, or may not, correlate with protection. The measurement of serum antibody has too often been assumed to correlate with vaccine efficacy. Serum antibody is the easiest variable to measure, but it has been proved to play a protective role in very few infectious diseases.

A recent area of interest in immunization is the route of vaccine administration. The most common method of vaccine administration has been the parenteral route, although alternate routes have been used for many years. In the Middle Ages, the Turks and Chinese used intranasal immunization with crusts from smallpox lesions. This is believed to be the first example of immunization in history. Because the most convenient method for assessing a vaccine's effectiveness has been the measurement of serum antibody, the parenteral route for immunization has usually been used; however, one recent highly successful immunization has been given by an alternate route, i.e., the oral attenuated polio vaccines. The route of immunization should depend upon the immune host defense mechanism that is responsible or is thought to be responsible for protection. If the stimulation of serum antibody is the aim of immunization, the subcutaneous, intramuscular, or intradermal immunization would be most efficient. However, if secretory

TABLE 4.10   Factors in Vaccine Development

Factor	Comment
Evaluating effectiveness	
Widespread use coinciding with decreased incidence of disease	May have nothing or little to do with vaccine, but may be due to other factors, such as generally improved public health
Measuring an immune response, such as serum antibody	The measured immune response may have nothing or little to do with protection, since protective mechanism is known with certainty for very few infections
Field trials	Controlled studies of vaccine efficacy against naturally occurring disease; difficult and expensive to carry out
Challenge studies	Controlled studies of vaccine efficacy, usually induced disease rather than naturally occurring disease; easier to carry out since fewer people can be used, but may not represent the natural situation very well
Route of immunization	Should be chosen relative to type of immune response desired, i.e., systemic vs secretory
Live (attenuated) vs killed (inactivated) vaccines	
Live	*Advantages*: more intense and durable immune responses, fewer doses of vaccine needed
	Disadvantages: more care in handling necessary (especially important in underdeveloped parts of world where refrigeration not always available); more dangerous with respect to reversion to virulence or administration of an adventitious agent

antibody or cell-mediated immunity on secretory surfaces is the source of immunity, then local application of the antigen such as by nosedrops, aerosol, oral ingestion, intravaginally or eyedrops would be most effective. Another question concerns the stimulation of humoral immunity vs CMI. Currently, it remains largely unanswerable, since with most infectious diseases, the exact importance of humoral vs cellular mechanisms is unknown. Even if it were known, there is little information regarding the methodology of immunization to ensure that one or the other form of immunity results.

Another important consideration in evaluating vaccines is the duration of protection. In most instances, it is desirable to give a vaccine once and obtain lifelong immunity. This is not an unrealistic goal, since many infectious diseases, e.g., measles, render the individual immune for life. It is generally felt that live, attenuated vaccines give longer immunity than do killed vaccines. However, there is little firm evidence to support this. There are no controlled studies in which a live, attenuated vaccine has been compared with the killed vaccine. The comparison of the live, attenuated, oral polio vaccine with the killed, injected vaccine is not appropriate to answer this question because in addition to the difference in live vs killed organisms, the route of administration of vaccine is different. Although there are no direct studies comparing the two, the general results with the live, attenuated measles vaccine have been superior to those of the killed measles vaccine. However, this probably is not due to a difference in the duration of protection, but rather to the poorly understood hypersensitivity reaction which is induced by the killed measles vaccine.

TABLE 4.11   Recommendations Regarding Immunization for Foreign Travel

---

Current with respect to tetanus toxoid, diphtheria toxoid, and poliomyelitis

Yellow fever: attenuated vaccine, 0.5 ml subcutaneously, booster within prior 10 yrs, available only at approved centers - for travel to Africa and South America

Cholera: killed vaccine, 0.5 ml followed by 1.0 ml booster 4-6 weeks later, intramuscularly; booster every 6 mo - Asia, Middle East

Hepatitis: passive immunization with human gamma globulin, 0.01 ml/lb q 2-3 mo, or 0.05 ml/lb q 4-6 mo - travel to endemic area

Optional, depending on rural or urban epidemicity in location

   Typhoid: killed vaccine 0.5 ml subcutaneously x 2, 4-6 wk apart

   Plague: killed vaccine, 0.5 ml intramuscularly x 2, 4-6 wk apart

   Rabies: preexposure, human diploid cell vaccine, three doses on days 0, 7, and 21

TABLE 4.12   Precautions in Use of Vaccines

Hypersensitivity reactions:	to egg proteins - vaccines grown in eggs (typhus, rabies, yellow fever, and influenza rarely)
	to antibiotics or preservatives - check package insert
Immunocompromised host:	should not receive live attenuated viral vaccines; household contacts should be immunized only with caution, since some vaccine viral strains may be transmissible
Febrile patients:	should usually be deferred, to avoid vaccine side-effects from being confused with underlying illness, or vice versa
Pregnancy:	live attenuated viral vaccines should be avoided, because of theoretical or proven risk to fetus

Selected Bibliography

Allansmith, M., McClellan, B. H., Butterworth, M., and Maloney, J. R.: The development of immunoglobulin levels in man. *J Pediatr* 72:276-290, 1968.

Artenstein, M. S.: The current status of bacterial vaccines. *Hosp Pract* 8:49-56, 1973.

Bernheim, H. A. and Kluger, M. J.: Effect of drug-induced antipyresis on survival. *Science* 193:237-239, 1976.

Dunnick, J. K. and Galasso, G. J.: From the National Institutes of Health. Clinical trials with endogenous interferon. *J Infect Dis* 139:109-123, 1979.

Edsall, G.: Present status of pertussis vaccination. *Practitioner* 215:310-314, 1975.

Ganguly, R., Cusumano, C. L., and Waldman, R. H.: Suppression of cell-mediated immunity after infection with attenuated rubella virus. *Infect Immun* 13:464-469, 1976.

Ganguly, R., Ogra, P. L., Regas, S., and Waldman, R. H.: Rubella immunization of volunteers via the respiratory tract. *Infect Immun* 8:497-502, 1973.

Ganguly, R. and Waldman, R. H.: Local immunity and local immune responses. *Prog Allergy* 27:1-68, 1980.

Gold, R., Lepow, M. L., Goldschneider, I., Draper, T. F., and Gotschlich, E. C.: Kinetics of antibody production to group A and group C meningococcal polysaccharide vaccines administered during the first six years of life: Prospects for routine immunization of infants and children. *J Infect Dis* 140:690-697, 1979.

Hanson, L. A.: Transfer factor – A new form of immunotherapy. *Acta Med Scand* 198:1-3, 1975.

Kasper, D. L., Onderdonk, A. B., Crabb, J., and Bartlett, J. G.: Protective efficacy of immunization with capsular antigen against experimental infection with *Bacteroides fragilis*. *J Infect Dis* 140:724-731, 1979.

Kilbourne, E. D.: Influenza as a problem in immunology. *J Immunol* 120:1447-1452, 1978.

Kirkpatrick, C. H.: Properties and activities of transfer factor. *J Allergy Clin Immunol* 55:411-421, 1975.

Krugman, S. and Katz, S. L.: Childhood immunization procedures. *JAMA* 237:2228-2230, 1977.

Lauteria, S. F., Kantzler, G. N., High, P. C., Lee, J. D., and Waldman, R. H.: An attenuated influenza virus vaccine: Reactogenicity, transmissibility, immunogenicity and protective efficacy. *J Infect Dis* 130:380-383, 1974.

Madoff, M. A. and Gleckman, R. A.: Immunizations: Where the money should be. *J Infect Dis* 133:230-232, 1976.

Meiklejohn, G.: Smallpox: Is the end in sight? *J Infect Dis* 133:347-352, 1976.

Melnick, J. L.: Vaccines and vaccine policy: The poliomyelitis example. *Hosp Pract* 13:41-47, 1978.

Moulden, J. W.: Intracellular parasitism: Life in an extreme environment. *J Infect Dis* 130:300-306, 1974.

Notkins, A. L.: Viral infections: Mechanisms of immunologic defense and injury. *Hosp Pract* 9:62-75, 1974.

Purcell, R. H.: The viral hepatitides. *Hosp Pract* 13:51-63, 1978.

Ramsey, E. W., Brandes, L. J., Jacob, K. H. A., and Goldenberg, G. J.: An evaluation of the peripheral leukocyte migration inhibition test as a correlate of delayed cutaneous hypersensitivity. *Cell Immunol* 23:334-341, 1976.

Sabin, A. B.: Immunization. Evaluation of some currently available and prospective vaccines. *JAMA* 246:236, 1981.

Salk, J. and Salk, D.: Control of influenza and poliomyelitis with killed virus vaccine. *Science* 195:834-847, 1977.

Stossel, T. P.: Phagocytosis. *N Engl J Med* 290:717-723, 1974.

Stossel, T. P., Root, R. K., and Vaughan, M.: Phagocytosis in chronic granulomatous disease and the Chediak-Higashi syndrome. *N Engl J Med* 286:120-123, 1972.

Stuart-Harris, C. H.: The influenza virus and the human respiratory tract. *Rev Infect Dis* 1:592-599, 1979.

Stuart-Harris, C. H.: The principles and practices of immunization. *Practitioner* 215:285-293, 1975.

Wakelin, D.: Immunity to intestinal parasites. *Nature* 273:617-620, 1978.

Waldman, R. H. and Ganguly, R.: Immunity to infections on secretory surfaces. *J Infect Dis* 130:419-440, 1974.

Zuckerman, A. J. and Howard, C. R.: Toward hepatitis B vaccines. *Bull N Y Acad Med* 51:491-500, 1975.

5

BASIC PRINCIPLES OF ANTIBIOTIC USAGE
Roger G. Finch, M.B.

Although the widespread application of antibacterial substances to treat infections is less than 40 years old, the successful application of molds to superficial skin infections dates back to antiquity. The term *antibiotics* was coined by Vuillemin, in 1889, who observed antagonism between bacteria, and this was the basis for the observation by Fleming in 1929, who noted inhibition of growth of staphylococci by the mold *Penicillium*.

Waksman defined an antibiotic as a " . . . chemical substance produced by microorganisms and possessing the ability to kill or inhibit the growth of bacteria and other microorganisms when present in high dilution." More than half of the available antibiotics are derived from fungi belonging to the *actinomycetes* with smaller contributions from other fungi, bacteria, plants, lichens, and animals. Only a very small percentage of the several thousands of antibiotics described have been used therapeutically.

In addition to the antibiotics, several chemotherapeutic agents such as nalidixic acid, trimethoprim, and the sulfonamides, which do not originate from microorganisms, are also able to inhibit the growth of microorganisms. Several of these agents have been synthesized while several antibiotics remain only partly synthesized. The term antimicrobial agents embraces both the terms antibiotic and chemotherapeutic agents. However, common usage frequently employs the term *antibiotic* for all antimicrobial agents.

The fundamental principle of antimicrobial chemotherapy is the selective toxicity of an agent on the metabolism of a microbe. The ideal agent should possess high activity, be nontoxic to the host, have a narrow antimicrobial spectrum, preferably be able to be synthesized, and finally, should be inexpensive. At present no drug meets these criteria, although penicillin, in the nonhypersensitive patient, comes the closest to fulfilling them. Some antibiotics are toxic to mammalian cells and have been found useful in the treatment of malignant disease, e.g., actinomycin D, daunorubicin, and mithramycin.

Mode of Action

Antimicrobial drugs act by interfering with bacterial (1) cell-wall synthesis, (2) cell membrane integrity, (3) protein synthesis, (4) nucleic acid structure and function, or (5) metabolic function, to produce either a lethal (bactericidal) or inhibitory (bacteriostatic) effect. Table 5.1 summarizes some examples of antibacterials according to their site and type of action.

Bactericidal and Bacteriostatic Effect of Antibiotics

Antibiotics that are bactericidal produce microbial death and lysis, and include the penicillins, cephalosporins, and aminoglycosides. In contrast, bacteriostatic drugs inhibit microbial multiplication without killing that organism, hence once the drug is removed from the environment the microorganism can start to replicate once more. Bacteriostatic agents include chloramphenicol and the tetracyclines. Such agents rely on host defenses, particularly phagocytic cells, to eliminate microorganisms from the body. Some drugs such as erythromycin are bacteriostatic at low concentrations and bactericidal at higher concentrations.

The selection of a bactericidal drug is important when treating infections associated with either a functional or absolute impairment of phagocytosis. In bacterial endocarditis phagocytic cells are unable to penetrate the infected vegetations; and granulocytopenia, particularly below $500/mm^3$, is associated with a high prevalence of potentially fatal bacteremia.

Selective Toxicity

To be used therapeutically it is essential that the drug should be inhibitory or lethal to the microorganism and not to the host. Sulfonamides inhibit microbial synthesis of folic acid, essential for purine and nucleic acid synthesis, by competitive inhibition of para-aminobenzoic acid. Humans, unlike bacteria, require exogenous preformed folic acid, and hence sulfonamides are selectively toxic to bacteria.

In contrast the aminoglycoside antibiotics, such as gentamicin, are both nephrotoxic and ototoxic to humans at concentrations that are not much higher than the levels necessary to inhibit bacteria. For example, the minimum inhibitory concentration (MIC) for many pathogenic gram-negative bacteria lies between 1 and 4 µg/ml, while toxic effects are associated with levels in excess of 12 µg/ml, thus the margin between efficacy and toxicity is small. The ratio of the toxic dose to the effective dose is known as the *therapeutic index*. The higher this index is the safer the drug. Penicillin has a high therapeutic index and gentamicin a low therapeutic index.

Narrow-Spectrum and Broad-Spectrum Antibacterials

Antibacterials are traditionally separated into either narrow-spectrum or broad-spectrum drugs, although this division is artificial and of doubtful usefulness. Penicillin is the classic example of a narrow-spectrum drug being lethal to gram-positive cocci (staphylococci and streptococci), gram-negative cocci (*Neisseria* spp) and gram-positive bacilli (*Clostridium*). However it is also active against many anaerobic bacteria, with the notable exception of *Bacteroides fragilis*.

TABLE 5.1   Action of Selected Antibacterial Drugs on Cell Function

Site/Function Inhibited	Drug(s)	Specific Metabolic Effect
Cell-wall synthesis	Penicillins; cephalosporins	Inhibit transpeptidase thus preventing cross-linking of cell-wall peptidoglycan
	Bacitracin	Inhibits dephosphorylation of lipid pyrophosphate thus impairing regeneration of lipid carrier
	Vancomycin	Inhibits peptidoglycan synthetase and polymerization of linear peptide
Cell membrane functions	Colistin; polymixin B	Bind and disrupt membrane phospholipids by detergent action
DNA and RNA synthesis	Nalidixic acid	Interferes with DNA template-DNA polymerase complex
	Rifampin	Inhibits DNA-dependent RNA polymerase
Inhibition of folic acid synthesis	Sulfonamide	Inhibits dihydropteroate synthetase thereby producing competitive inhibition of para-aminobenzoic acid
	Trimethoprim	Inhibition of enzyme dihydrofolate reductase
Inhibition of protein synthesis	Aminoglycosides	Act on 30S ribosome producing nonsense proteins from misreading of mRNA
	Chloramphenicol; erythromycin; clindamycin	Acts on 50S ribosome to inhibit peptide bonding
	Tetracycline	Acts on 30S ribosome to inhibit binding of amino-acyl-tRNA

In contrast, ampicillin and the cephalosporins are considered broad-spectrum agents since they have clinical efficacy against several gram-negative bacteria in addition to their action on gram-positive and gram-negative cocci. The aminoglycosides are also considered broad-spectrum because of their efficacy in the treatment of a wide range of infections caused by gram-negative bacteria, including *Pseudomonas aeruginosa*. Chloramphenicol is truly a broad-spectrum antibacterial with therapeutic activity against most gram-positive and gram-negative facultative and anaerobic pathogenic bacteria.

Principles of Antimicrobial Therapy

The selection of an appropriate antimicrobial drug is dependent upon both an accurate clinical and microbiologic diagnosis, the known efficacy of the agent in such a situation, favorable pharmacokinetics, and predictable adverse effects.

The initial clinical diagnosis is of necessity presumptive and is confirmed subsequently when laboratory information becomes available. The anatomic site of the infection often provides clues to the possible etiology. For example, lobar pneumonia is of sudden onset and is frequently caused by *Streptococcus pneumoniae* which is sensitive to penicillin. The diagnosis should, however, be confirmed by the examination of sputum for the presence of gram-positive diplococci on smear and culture of *S. pneumoniae*. It is always desirable to culture infected material *before* chemotherapy so that treatment can be made more certain by the isolation, identification, and antibacterial susceptibility testing of the pathogen(s).

Initial guidance for therapy is based on presumptive diagnosis and awareness of the likely pathogens, although much information can be gained by examination of a stained smear of the infected material. Knowledge of the likely pathogen and its usual sensitivity pattern permits initial selection of therapy, which may require modification once laboratory information becomes available. The importance of making a clinical and microbiologic diagnosis is to avoid unnecessary use of chemotherapy. For example, many upper respiratory tract infections are of viral origin and therefore unresponsive to antibacterial chemotherapy. Apart from being inappropriate, such use is expensive and carries a risk of adverse reactions.

Adjunctive Treatment

Adequate drainage of infected material is also necessary if treatment is to be successful. Undrained pus, obstruction within the urinary or respiratory tracts, and the presence of foreign bodies including bladder catheters, intravenous devices, and prosthetic implants all are potential causes for the failure of chemotherapy. These obstructions should be drained or removed although the management problems associated with removing an infected hip prosthesis may justify a course of intensive antibiotics in the hope of saving the prosthesis.

Single and Combined Therapy

In general, it is preferable to use a single agent, which should be the least toxic and most effective agent for a given situation. Ideally the spectrum should be narrow to avoid major alterations of the normal flora with resulting superinfection. Despite this general rule there are situations where combined therapy is indicated. Such situations include: (1) the need for a synergistic antimicrobial effect, (2) the prevention of drug resistance, (3) the treatment of truly mixed infection, or (4) the initial blind treatment of suspected yet unconfirmed infection.

Synergy

Drugs in combination may either be synergistic, antagonistic, or additive. A synergistic effect is one in which the minimal inhibitory concentration (MIC) to the drugs in combination is less than the MIC to each agent alone. The usual criteria for synergy requires a reduction of the MIC to one-fourth of the original MIC. In general, combinations of bactericidal drugs show a synergistic effect, e.g., penicillin plus gentamicin.

The value of synergistic inhibition of bacterial growth is well known in the treatment of enterococcal endocarditis in which drugs such as penicillin or ampicillin in combination with gentamicin are of proven value. The combination of trimethoprim-sulfamethoxazole is also synergistically inhibitory to a wide range of bacteria.

In contrast, some drugs may show antagonism in vitro. For example, the combination of a bactericidal drug such as penicillin and a bacteriostatic agent such as tetracycline has been reported in one study to be antagonistic in vivo in the treatment of pneumococcal meningitis, although many authorities doubt the validity of this.

Many drugs in combination simply show an additive effect, thus little advantage is gained over use of the single agent. However, it is occasionally advantageous to use such a combination to reduce the amount of two drugs that both have toxic side effects.

Prevention of Drug Resistance

It is uncommon for chemotherapy to fail owing to the emergence of drug-resistant strains. Nonetheless, in the treatment of tuberculosis it is well recognized that primary resistance to many commonly used antituberculous drugs can exist among a minority population of the strains. If a single agent were to be used then these strains can survive and subsequently be responsible for the failure of chemotherapy. Primary resistance to two or more drugs is rare and hence, the proven value of combined therapy in the treatment of tuberculosis.

Truly Mixed Infections

These are uncommon except for infections associated with intestinal or female genital tract sepsis where a mixture of both anaerobic and facultative bacteria is common, and each has a differing sensitivity pattern.

Initial Chemotherapy

Life-threatening or rapidly progressive infections cannot await the results of culture and sensitivity testing of microbiologic samples before treatment is commenced. The choice of agent is of necessity "blind" although the selection should be made from an assessment of the likely pathogenic organism in a given clinical situation, i.e., an educated guess. The choice of agent should also take into consideration host factors such as malignancy, granulocytopenia, indwelling vascular devices, and whether or not the infection is related to mucosal surfaces which suggests the possibility that anaerobic bacteria may be important. Some commonly used combinations of drugs for such initial therapy include a penicillinase-resistant penicillin, (e.g., methicillin, cloxacillin, dicloxacillin, oxacillin, or nafcillin) or a cephalosporin (e.g., cefazolin or cefamandole) in combination with an aminoglycoside (e.g., gentamicin or tobramycin). If anaerobic bacteria are thought to be contributing to the infection then clindamycin or chloramphenicol may be added, although some cephalosporins such as cefoxitin have useful activity against anaerobic bacteria. In the granulocytopenic patient combinations that have been widely used are carbenicillin or ticarcillin in conjunction with an aminoglycoside such as gentamicin or tobramycin, since gram-negative bacteria including *P. aeruginosa* are important in this group of patients.

Whenever antibiotics are started in this blind fashion it is imperative to assess the patient clinically for response and also to recognize that the initial choice of chemotherapy may need modification once laboratory information becomes available.

Pharmacologic Factors

Successful chemotherapy is dependent upon the drug reaching the infecting micro-organism in concentrations sufficient to inhibit or kill. Several factors operate to produce this result and include absorption, distribution, metabolism, and excretion.

Absorption

Most drugs, including antibiotics, are absorbed from the proximal small intestine and as such are dependent upon the physicochemical properties of the drug molecule. In general, most drugs are either weak bases or weak acids which either ionize and are therefore water soluble or remain un-ionized and essentially lipid soluble. The pKa of the drug and the pH of the intestinal tract are important determinants of these responses. For example, gentamicin is highly water soluble and not absorbed from the bowel. In contrast, the sulfonamides are weak acids with a low molecular weight and are readily absorbed.

Many antibiotics are acid labile, e.g., methicillin, several cephalosporins, and erythromycin, and are inactivated in the presence of normal gastric acid. This can be overcome by modifying the drug to produce its salt or ester, or by coating the agent which is released subsequent to its passage through the stomach. Erythromycin base, for example, is more acid tolerant in the form of the stearate or the ethylsuccinate, while clindamycin palmitate survives the gastric acidity to be hydrolyzed later by esterases present in the gut mucosa. Hydroxylation can also enhance absorption and is demonstrated by the improved blood levels of amoxicillin when compared with its parent compound, ampicillin.

The presence of food in the stomach can also affect the rate of absorption of many antibiotics. In general, most antibacterials should be administered 0.5-1 hr before food or 2 hr after a meal. Some drugs, most notably the aminoglycosides, are not absorbed to any significant degree from the bowel.

The presence of other drugs can interfere with the absorption of certain antibiotics. For example, tetracycline absorption is impaired by chelation with calcium ions present in milk or antacid mixtures.

Drug absorption following intramuscular injection is usually rapid and is due to penetration of capillary walls by diffusion. This depends upon the lipid solubility of the agent. Lipid-insoluble molecules, in contrast, pass through pores in the capillary endothelium. Absorption of a drug such as penicillin can be slowed by injecting it in a poorly soluble state as with procaine or benzathine penicillin, which produces sustained although low serum levels.

Distribution

Distribution of antibacterials in the various body fluids is similarly dependent upon the ionizability and lipid solubility of the drug. Aminoglycosides are highly water soluble and therefore have a small volume of distribution which corresponds to the extracellular fluid space. This contrasts with griseofulvin which is highly lipid soluble and as such is distributed throughout most body tissues.

The blood supply in health and its supply in disease are also important determinates of drug penetration. Avascular areas, such as the aqueous humor, are penetrated poorly, whereas inflammation frequently enhances the degree of penetration of a drug, as is seen with inflammation of the meninges and the penetration of penicillin.

Another factor affecting the distribution of antimicrobial agents is the degree to which they are absorbed or *bound* to plasma proteins. There is marked variation in the extent of protein-binding among these drugs and even within the members of a group of antibiotics. For example, methicillin is approximately 30% protein-bound whereas cloxacillin is about 95% protein-bound. Protein-binding is a reversible process, thus the constant release of bound drug to the free form maintains the equilibrium. A protein-bound drug does not cross the placenta, blood-brain barrier, or glomerular membrane and hence can have an important effect on the distribution of a drug between plasma and tissues. Nonetheless, there is little in vivo evidence to suggest that the variation in protein-binding between drugs belonging to the same group has an effect on their therapeutic efficacy.

Metabolism

Antibiotics, in keeping with other drugs, undergo oxidation, reduction, or hydrolysis before conjugation, which results in acetylation, methylation, glucuronidation, or sulfate formation. The rate of metabolism will determine the percentage of unchanged drug excreted in either the urine or bile.

Some drugs, such as the aminoglycosides, are not metabolized but are excreted in the urine in the unchanged state. Drug metabolism can be influenced by the presence of other enzyme-inducing drugs as well as by the maturity of hepatic enzymes. For example, barbiturates can result in lower levels of doxycycline through enzyme induction, while the failure to conjugate chloramphenicol can cause cardiovascular collapse in the premature infant.

Excretion

Antibacterial agents are excreted primarily in the urine or in the bile, although other body fluids, including breast milk, are minor routes of excretion.

Renal excretion is dependent upon the processes of glomerular filtration, tubular secretion, and tubular absorption. Impaired glomerular filtration will prolong the elimination of drugs, such as the aminoglycosides, for which this is the main route of excretion. Lipid solubility is crucial for tubular reabsorption and as such is affected by urinary pH. For example, the sulfonamides are weak acids and are more readily excreted in an alkaline urine. Tubular excretion can be decreased by probenecid, thereby producing higher blood levels of certain antibiotics such as the penicillins and cephalosporins.

Alteration of drug dosage in renal failure is very much dependent upon both the metabolism and excretion of the drug. Those excreted almost totally by glomerular filtration, such as the aminoglycosides, require very careful control, whereas other drugs that do not accumulate require no adjustment and include erythromycin, clindamycin, and doxycycline. Other agents, such as the penicillins and cephalosporins, require some dose modification in severe renal impairment, although adverse effects with these agents are uncommon.

Drug Resistance

Drug resistance may be *primary (intrinsic)* or *secondary (acquired).*   Primary resistance implies the lack of the appropriate target or inability of the drug to reach
such a target within the bacterial cell. For example, gentamicin is without effect
on anaerobic bacteria since its penetration and effect on bacteria are an oxygen-
requiring process, while amphotericin B binds to sterols present in the fungal cell
membrane but absent in bacteria.

Acquired drug resistance developing during therapy is uncommon, but does occur in patients infected with *Staphylococcus aureus* treated with erythromycin.
Drug-sensitive strains are eliminated, allowing drug-resistant strains to multiply
and predominate. Such drug resistance may arise spontaneously by mutation or
may be transferred from another bacterium, usually by a process of conjugation.

Conjugation between bacteria allows the transfer of extrachromosomal pieces
of DNA, known as *plasmids,* from one bacterium to another. Plasmids code for
enzymes, such as *penicillinase,* which determine drug resistance. Such resistance
coding may be for either single or multiple antibiotics. For this reason plasmids
are also referred to as *R-* or *resistance factors* and are responsible for drug resistance among gram-negative bacteria. Epidemics of shigellosis and salmonellosis within the community and hospital infections with Enterobacteriaceae and *P.
aeruginosa* have increasingly been recognized to be associated with such drug-
resistant strains.

Adverse Reactions

It is unfortunate that no drug therapy is without risk of adverse reactions. The incidence and severity vary from drug to drug and from patient to patient and a
knowledge of such effects should be considered before selecting chemotherapy.
Such adverse reactions may be (1) allergic, (2) idiosyncratic, (3) due to alterations
in the host's normal flora, or (4) toxic in origin.

Allergic reactions range from the trivial to the fatal and are most commonly
seen with the penicillins and cephalosporins. Most manifestations take the form
of a variety of skin eruptions, although acute anaphylaxis, serum sickness-like syndrome and drug fever may occur.

Idiosyncratic reactions may or may not be genetically determined. Chloram-
phenicol-induced marrow aplasia is rare and unpredictable whereas hemolysis, in
association with sulfonamide use, may be the result of glucose-6-phosphate dehydrogenase deficiency. Similarly, slow acetylators of isoniazid have an increased
incidence of peripheral neuropathy compared with rapid acetylators.

Gastrointestinal intolerance is the most common side effect and produces
symptoms of nausea, epigastric discomfort, and diarrhea. The diarrhea may be
either a response to direct irritation of the bowel following alteration of the normal flora or due to enterocolitis associated with *S. aureus* or *Candida albicans*
overgrowth. Such effects are seen in association with broad-spectrum agents such
as tetracycline and ampicillin. Pseudomembranous colitis is a specific adverse reaction associated with a characteristic macroscopic and microscopic picture resulting from the effects of *Clostridium difficile* toxin on the bowel. It has been
associated with a variety of antibiotics, although clindamycin has the greatest
potential for allowing such bacterial overgrowth and toxin production.

Organ toxicity occurs with certain drugs. For example, the aminoglycosides
are well known for toxic effects on the kidney and on the ear in which they can
produce both deafness and vestibular disturbances. Jaundice of the cholestatic
variety occasionally accompanies prolonged use of erythromycin estolate, while

chloramphenicol is notorious for its potentially fatal suppression of bone marrow. Table 5.2 summarizes some of the many toxic reactions associated with use of a variety of antimicrobial agents. Fortunately, few of these toxic reactions are life-threatening and they usually are self-limiting. Fatalities are associated with bone marrow aplasia, fulminating hepatoxicity, pseudomembranous colitis, and the Stevens-Johnson syndrome. Immediate hypersensitivity reactions, such as anaphylaxis to penicillin and its derivatives, also produce fatalities, and thus stress the need to inquire about a previous history of allergy, particularly in individuals with an atopic tendency.

Toxicity can be minimized by an awareness of such adverse reactions, careful clinical and laboratory monitoring, and the use of antibiotic assays of blood levels of toxic drugs followed by appropriate dosage adjustment. Failing the availability of drug assay, then dosage adjustment should be in accordance with renal function and is aided by nomograms which take into account body weight, age, sex, and serum creatinine.

Prophylactic Use of Antibacterial Agents

Antibiotic prophylaxis is widely used and of unquestioned efficacy in the prevention of such diseases as malaria and tuberculosis in recent tuberculin converts. However, in the wider field of bacterial prophylaxis, the use of antibacterials still provokes widespread controversy because much prescribing in the name of prophylaxis is of unproven efficacy.

For successful chemoprophylaxis the infection to be prevented should be caused by a known organism or organisms, whose sensitivity is predictable, and the practice should be of proven efficacy and carry a minimum risk of toxicity. The use of penicillin prophylaxis for recurrent S. pyogenes sore throats in patients with a previous history of rheumatic fever fulfills these criteria.

Certain surgical operations, such as colorectal surgery, carry a high risk of infectious complications from the fecal flora. It is therefore common practice for mechanical cleansing of the bowel to be used in conjunction with oral antibiotics such as neomycin and erythromycin. This is known to reduce the incidence of postoperative wound infections. Topical antibiotics may be supplemented with systemic prophylaxis with agents effective against both the aerobic and anaerobic flora. Hysterectomy also has a high risk of wound infection and similarly justifies the use of systemic chemoprophylaxis.

In these surgical situations systemic chemoprophylaxis aims at producing bactericidal concentrations of drug at the site of the operation during the immediate perioperative period and for about 24 hr postoperatively. The initial dose is therefore given 1-2 hr before surgery. Adverse reactions are uncommon, and the reduction in wound infection is gratifying.

Infections complicating prosthetic implant surgery, notably cardiac valve replacement, can have devastating and fatal effects. Although it is difficult to confirm the efficacy of chemoprophylaxis, it is commonly employed.

Dosage and Duration of Chemotherapy

The dosage of antibiotic necessary to cure an infection is not reliably known. As a rule the aim is to produce levels at least fourfold higher than the MIC of the causative bacterium. With drugs, such as the penicillins, the levels achieved are often manyfold higher than this. However, with the aminoglycosides it is not uncommon to fall short of such a margin when treating gram-negative bacteria, which have a relatively high MIC.

TABLE 5.2   Selected Side Effects to Some Common Antibiotics

Adverse Reaction	Antimicrobial Agent
Hypersensitivity reactions	Penicillins, cephalosporins, clindamycin, amphotericin B, trimethoprim-sulfamethoxazole, sulfonamides
Skin	
Rashes	Penicillins, cephalosporins, clindamycin, sulfonamides, neomycin
Stevens-Johnson	Sulfonamides, penicillin
Photosensitivity	Tetracycline, nalidixic acid
Lungs	
Pulmonary eosinophilia	Sulfonamide
Pulmonary fibrosis	Nitrofurantoin
Gut	
Nausea, vomiting, diarrhea	Erythromycin, ampicillin, cephalexin, nitrofurantoin, nalidixic acid, tetracyclines
Enterocolitis	Tetracycline, ampicillin, chloramphenicol
Pseudomembranous colitis	Clindamycin, ampicillin, cephalosporins
Hematologic	
Bone marrow suppression	Sulfonamides, chloramphenicol, trimethoprim-sulfamethoxazole, penicillin, cephalosporins, nalidixic acid
Hemolysis	Sulfonamides, penicillins, cephalosporins, nalidixic acid, nitrofurantoin
Megaloblastic marrow	Trimethoprim-sulfamethoxazole, nitrofurantoin, penicillin, cephalosporins
Platelet dysfunction	Carbenicillin
Hepatotoxicity	Erythromycin, tetracycline, oxacillin, nitrofurantoin, isoniazid, rifampin
Nephrotoxicity	Aminoglycosides, tetracycline, vancomycin, methicillin, cephaloridine, sulfonamides
Neurotoxicity	
Peripheral neuropathy	Nitrofurantoin, isoniazid, metronidazole
Benign intracranial hypertension	Nalidixic acid, tetracycline
Neuromuscular blockade	Aminoglycosides
Ototoxicity	Aminoglycosides, vancomycin, erythromycin
Tooth-staining	Tetracyclines
Superinfection	Tetracycline, ampicillin, cephalosporins, chloramphenicol
Metabolic	Na-carbenicillin, K-penicillin

In addition, there are few infections for which the duration of treatment is known with any reliability. It is generally believed that for acute infectious processes treatment should continue for 48 hr beyond the time of clinical resolution. However, there are many exceptions to this rule. For example, *S. pyogenes* pharyngitis requires 10 days treatment, osteomyelitis requires at least 4 weeks of therapy, and infective endocarditis also requires at least 4 weeks of treatment to reduce the chance of relapse. Uncomplicated bacteriuria responds very rapidly to chemotherapy; 4-day treatment appears to be as effective as 10 days, and recent evidence suggests that even single-dose treatment may be satisfactory. Pulmonary tuberculosis is effectively controlled by 12-month continuous chemotherapy while even shorter courses probably will prove efficacious.

Failure of Chemotherapy

Failure of chemotherapy can occur for a variety of drug, host, and microbial reasons. The drug may be ineffective through primary or, less commonly acquired resistance. It may also fail to penetrate to the site of infection because of its pharmacokinetic properties. Inadequate dosing may operate, so that increasing the dosage or using a parenteral preparation may prove effective. Host factors associated with a poor response to treatment include failure of cell-mediated, phagocytic, or humoral immunity. Granulocytopenia of less than $500/mm^3$ is associated with a high risk of fatal bacteremia. Under these circumstances it is important that bactericidal and not bacteriostatic drugs be used.

Chemotherapy also may fail as a result of the normal host's response to infection. Abscess formation, eschar, and granulation tissue all impair diffusion of antimicrobial agents. Under these circumstances surgical drainage or debridement are essential adjuncts to chemotherapy.

Finally the diagnosis may be incorrect, or secondary infection with opportunistic organisms, such as fungi, may have developed. Several malignant, collagen-vascular, and noninfectious conditions may present with fever, and clinical and laboratory reevaluation should bear these noninfectious conditions in mind.

Selected Bibliography

Abramowics, M. (ed.): *Handbook of Antimicrobial Therapy.* Medical Letter, Inc., New Rochelle, NY, 1981.

Barrett, S. P. and Watt, P. J.: Antibiotics and the liver. *J Antimicrob Chemother* 5:337, 1979.

Bennett, W. M., Muther, R. S., Parker, R. A., Feig, P., Morrison, G., Golper, T. A., and Singer, I.: Drug therapy in renal failure: Dosaging guidelines for adults. Part 1: Antimicrobial agents, analgesics. *Ann Intern Med* 93:62, 1980.

Buckwold, F. J. and Ronald, A. R.: Antimicrobial misuse - Effects and suggestions for control. *J Antimicrob Chemother* 5:129, 1979.

Hoeprich, P. D.: Current principles of antimicrobic therapy. *Obstet Gynecol* 55: 1215, 1980.

Parker, C. W.: Drug therapy: Drug allergy. *N Engl J Med* 292:511, 1975.

6

ANTIMICROBIAL THERAPY
Roger G. Finch, M.B.

β-Lactam Antibiotics

The β-lactam antibiotics include the penicillins and cephalosporins and make up the largest group of antibiotics in clinical use. By modifying the basic molecular structure a wide range of drugs has been produced resulting either in improvements in microbiologic activity, in pharmacokinetics, or in a reduction in toxic side effects.

   The penicillins and cephalosporins have a different basic structure (Figure 6.1), yet share the β-lactam ring which characterizes this group of agents. The most recent discovery is the monobactams, a class of agents which have the basic β-lactam ring alone.

The Penicillins

The penicillins originated from the parent compound penicillin, a natural antibiotic first recognized by Fleming and later isolated and purified by Chain and Florey in Oxford, England, in 1940. Penicillin was isolated from the mold *Penicillium notatum*. It is now purified from *P. chrysogenum* which provides a higher yield. The structure of penicillin G, benzylpenicillin, consists of the basic 6-amino-penicillanic acid nucleus in which a β-lactam ring is linked to a thiazolidine ring. Figure 6.2 shows the penicillins in common use and shows how they are related to this basic structure.

Mode of Action

The penicillins interfere with cell-wall synthesis by inhibition of transpeptidation in the final cross-linking of adjacent peptidoglycan strands. This results in a

56

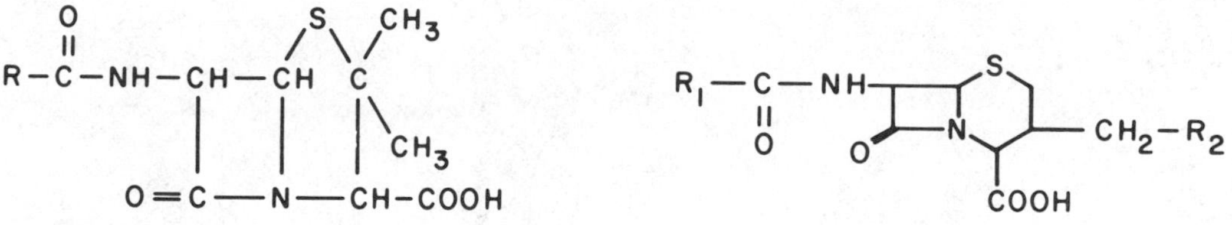

$$O = C - N - CH - COOH$$

A.   B.

FIGURE 6.1   The basic chemical structure of the penicillins and cephalosporins.
(A) Penicillin nucleus. (B) Cephalosporin nucleus.

weakened cell wall which lyses as the internal osmotic pressure within the bacterium increases.

Penicillin G (Benzylpenicillin)

  Spectrum of Activity

Penicillin G was the first penicillin to be used widely. It is extremely active
against streptococci including *Streptococcus pneumoniae,* group A, B, C, and G
hemolytic streptococci and many of the oral viridans streptococci. However,
group D streptococci other than *S. bovis* are relatively resistant. Against staphylococci the situation is different. Very few hospital strains are now susceptible
and only 20-30% of community strains remain sensitive. This is due to the widespread ability of staphylococci to produce the β-lactamase enzyme *penicillinase.*
This enzyme inactivates the drug by hydrolysing the β-lactam ring.
  Penicillin is also active against *Neisseria meningitidis* and most strains of
N. gonorrhoeae, although here again penicillinase-producing strains have steadily
increased in number following the importation of such strains from Southeast
Asia and West Africa.
  Other aerobic and facultative bacteria susceptible to penicillin include *Bacillus anthracis, Erysipelothrix rhusiopathiae, Listeria monocytogenes* and *Pasteurella* spp.
  Many anaerobic bacteria are extremely sensitive to penicillin: the clostridia;
anaerobic cocci such as peptococci and peptostreptococci; and many strains of
bacteroides, with the exception of *Bacteroides fragilis,* which also produces β-
lactamase.

  Pharmacology

Benzylpenicillin usually is administered parenterally. However, oral administration of large doses can produce therapeutic tissue concentrations despite the substantial degree of hydrolysis by gastric acid. The drug is promptly absorbed from
the intramuscular site to produce high blood concentrations and rapid diffusion
into many body tissues and serosal surfaces. It crosses the placenta but penetrates
poorly into the CSF in the absence of inflammation. However, in meningitis therapeutic concentrations are readily achieved and vary according to the degree of
inflammation. Penicillin also may be given by the intrathecal route, although caution is necessary since excessive dosaging may produce convulsions.

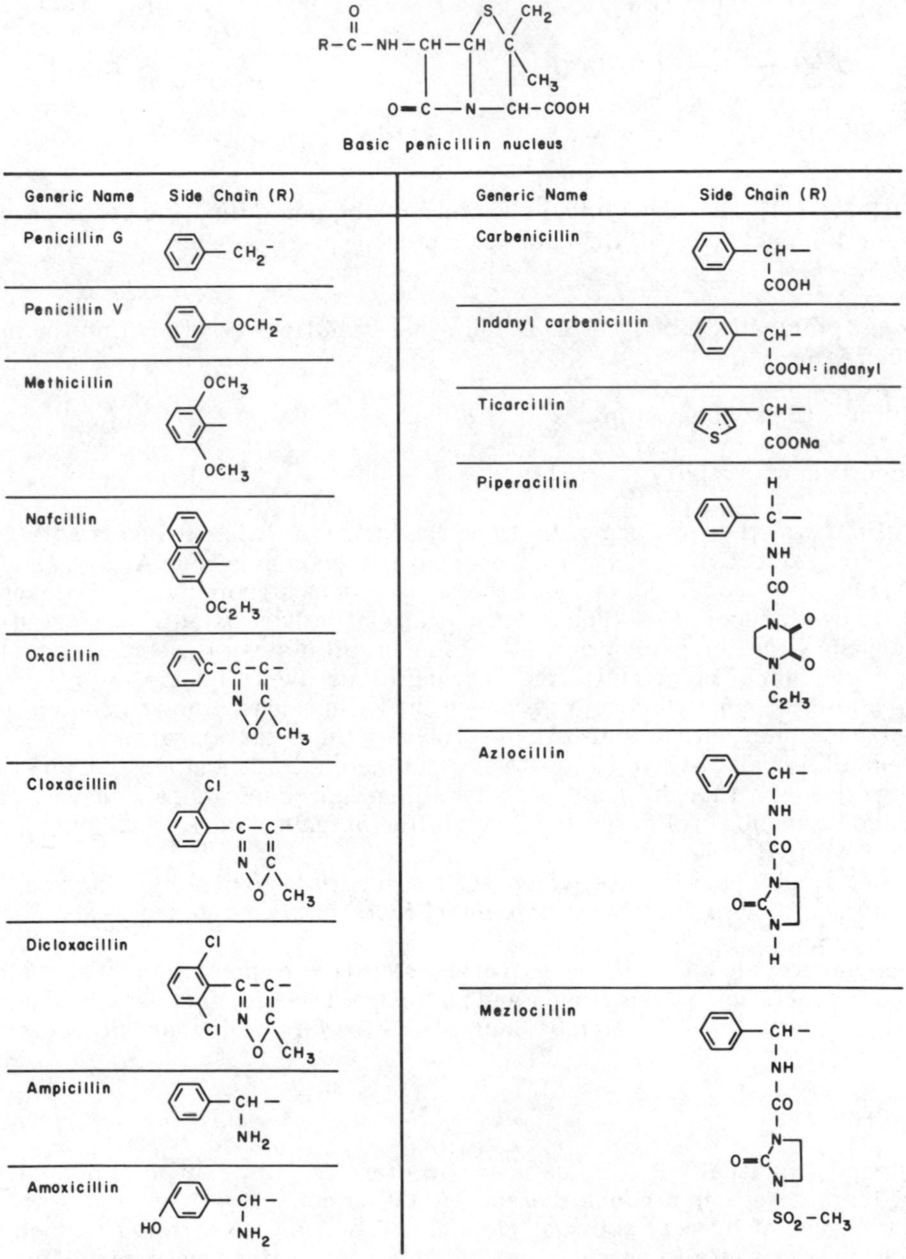

FIGURE 6.2   Chemical structure of the penicillins in clinical use.

The plasma half-life is short, being approximately 40 min. Penicillin is excreted by the kidneys where approximately 60% is eliminated by the tubules. This mechanism may be blocked by probenecid thus producing more sustained blood and tissue levels.

The short half-life of penicillin led to the introduction of procaine penicillin G and benzathine penicillin G for intramuscular use. The former produces peak concentrations at 2 hr and therapeutic levels for 24 hr, while the latter produces sustained but low concentrations for a period in excess of 2 weeks, making this a suitable agent for the prophylaxis of rheumatic fever.

Owing to the instability of penicillin G to gastric acid, phenoxymethyl penicillin (penicillin V) and subsequently phenethicillin were introduced. These are derivatives of penicillin G and are slightly less active microbiologically. There is considerable variation in the rate and degree of absorption of these agents, with food, in particular, lowering peak concentrations. Phenethicillin produces higher serum concentrations than penicillin V.

Clinical Use

Penicillin is highly active and generally well tolerated. It is the drug of choice in the treatment of pneumococcal infections such as pneumonia, meningitis, and septicemia. In addition, meningococcal meningitis and septicemia respond well, although elimination of nasopharyngeal carriage is unreliable, and alternative agents are necessary.

Penicillin is the treatment of choice for syphilis and gonorrhea, although the increasing resistance of gonococci to penicillin has required the use of alternative agents for these infections in some situations.

Penicillin is active against most oral bacteria, including the viridans streptococci, and is used to treat endocarditis caused by such organisms.

Other forms of endocarditis caused by oral streptococci and by enterococci are more resistant to penicillin and require the synergistic action of a combination of penicillin with an aminoglycoside such as gentamicin.

For other streptococcal infections, notably those caused by group A, B, C, and G β-hemolytic streptococci, penicillin is also the agent of choice. Serious infection requires parenteral therapy although *S. pyogenes* pharyngitis often responds to oral penicillin V.

Penicillin is active against many anaerobic bacteria although *B. fragilis* is resistant. Where mixed infections arise from the oropharyngeal flora, as in the case of aspiration pneumonia or lung abscess, penicillin is often effective. Other anaerobic infections such as gas gangrene require prompt surgical attention; however, penicillin is recommended to eradicate the residual vegetative forms of *Clostridium perfringens* or other clostridia. The drug is also used prophylactically in patients undergoing lower-limb amputation who have underlying peripheral vascular disease to prevent postoperative gas gangrene. Actinomycosis is another anaerobic infection for which penicillin is recommended, although treatment is often protracted.

Other less common infections that respond to penicillin are leptospirosis, anthrax, and yaws.

Penicillin is used in the chemoprophylaxis of *S. pyogenes* infections in those who have sustained a previous attack of rheumatic fever. It is also used in patients with established valvular heart disease or other cardiovascular abnormalities that render them vulnerable to infective endocarditis caused by oral streptococci which may produce a bacteremia following orodental surgery.

Adverse Reactions

Penicillin is a well-tolerated drug. The most frequent adverse reaction is hyper-sensitivity, although direct toxic reactions occur occasionally. Hypersensitivity reactions are due to prior sensitization either following therapeutic exposure or from contact with penicillin in the environment or in foods. Hypersensitivity reactions vary in frequency among the penicillins, being most common with procaine penicillin. Fatal anaphylaxis is reported to occur in 1:50,000-67,000 patients treated.

Hypersensitivity reactions are divided into *immediate, accelerated,* and *delayed* reactions. The immediate reactions occur within a few minutes, and in their most severe form produce anaphylaxis which in extreme instances is accompanied by laryngeal edema and cardiovascular collapse. Other less severe manifestations include pruritus, rhinitis, wheezing, urticaria, angioedema, and hypotension. The accelerated reaction occurs within 3 days of administration and produces an urticarial eruption that only occasionally produces laryngeal edema. Such reactions are rarely fatal. The late reactions occur beyond the 3-day period, may not be manifested for weeks, and can occur after treatment has stopped. Various skin eruptions including maculopapular, vesicular, bullous, urticarial, and exfoliative dermatoses occur. Pruritus is common. Furthermore, a serum sickness-like syndrome may result in fever, arthralgia, generalized lymphadenopathy, and splenomegaly.

Penicillin hypersensitivity is related to the formation of antigenic breakdown products known as *major* and *minor* determinants. The former includes penicilloyl derivatives, while the latter includes sodium benzylpenicilloate and benzylpenicillin itself. These agents act as haptens and stimulate antibody formation which is widely detectable in the population. The immediate hypersensitivity reactions are mediated by antibodies to the minor determinants while the intermediate and delayed reactions correlate better with the presence of antibodies to the major determinants. Skin-testing with penicilloylpolylysine (PPL) indicates hypersensitivity to the major determinants but is not an accurate predictor of acute anaphylaxis.

In general, hypersensitivity to one penicillin indicates hypersensitivity to all penicillins. Furthermore, owing to structural similarities there is the risk of cross-hypersensitivity to the cephalosporins. This risk, in the order of 10%, is greatest in patients exhibiting immediate hypersensitivity to the penicillins. Therefore, prescribing cephalosporins for patients with a past history of penicillin hypersensitivity demands careful evaluation.

Penicillin also may produce neurotoxicity. This occurs with very large dosages, particularly when underlying renal insufficiency coexists. Furthermore, direct intrathecal injection of more than 20,000 U has induced convulsions.

Finally, excessive sodium- or potassium-loading may be a problem in patients with renal insufficiency who receive large doses of parenteral penicillin.

The Broad-Spectrum Penicillins

Ampicillin and its hydroxy derivative, amoxicillin, are broad-spectrum penicillins. More recently several esters of ampicillin have been produced which are prodrugs and include hetacillin and metampicillin. Hetacillin is a product of ampicillin and acetone, while metampicillin is a formaldehyde derivative of ampicillin. Both agents are rapidly hydrolyzed to ampicillin in the gut.

Spectrum of Action

Ampicillin is slightly less active than penicillin against facultative gram-positive cocci, such as staphylococci, β-hemolytic streptococci, and *S. pneumoniae*. Like penicillin it is inactivated by penicillinase, hence most hospital and many community strains of *Staphylococcus aureus* are resistant. Its advantage over penicillin is its activity against enterococci, *Haemophilus influenzae, Escherichia coli,* indole-negative *Proteus* spp, *Salmonella,* and *Shigella* spp. Indole-positive *Proteus* spp and *P. aeruginosa* are resistant as are most strains of *Klebsiella pneumoniae*. In recent years resistance to ampicillin has been increasingly recognized among strains of *H. influenzae, E. coli, Salmonella,* and *Shigella* spp. Ampicillin, like penicillin, is highly active against both gonococci and meningococci, although the penicillin-resistant strains of *N. gonorrhoeae* also will be resistant to ampicillin.

Other susceptible organisms include *L. monocytogenes, Clostridium* spp and many other anaerobic bacteria, although *B. fragilis* is resistant.

Pharmacology

Ampicillin is absorbed from the upper gastrointestinal tract producing peak serum concentrations at 2 hr of 5 μg/ml following a 500-mg dose. Food delays the absorption of ampicillin but not amoxicillin, which produces peak serum concentrations approximately twice those of ampicillin. Both drugs are available for parenteral administration.

Ampicillin is distributed widely in the body including joint, pleural, peritoneal, and amniotic fluids and bronchial secretions. The concentration in kidney tissue varies according to renal function. In chronic pyelonephritis, for example, tissue concentrations are significantly lower than in the normal kidney. In the absence of meningitis very little ampicillin is detectable in the CSF, in contrast to the situation in meningitis when therapeutic concentrations are produced. Both ampicillin and amoxicillin are partly excreted in the bile, provided there is no obstruction to flow. Renal excretion predominates and results in high concentrations in the urine.

Clinical Use

Ampicillin has been used in the treatment of a wide range of infections. Amoxicillin may have certain advantages in the treatment of bacterial upper respiratory tract infection and typhoid fever. However, the ampicillin prodrugs have no great therapeutic advantage, despite their better absorption, but they do have the benefit of causing less diarrhea.

Ampicillin is effective in the treatment of both upper and lower urinary tract infection; the majority of pathogens are susceptible. Resistance among enterobacteria, however, is increasing.

Respiratory tract infections such as otitis media, sinusitis, pneumonia, and exacerbations of chronic bronchitis are often caused by *S. pneumoniae* and *H. influenzae* against which ampicillin is active. Amoxicillin achieves better concentrations in the middle ear and may be preferred. Penicillin remains preferable for the treatment of pneumococcal infections because of fewer side effects and lower cost.

Ampicillin is widely used to treat meningitis caused by *S. pneumoniae, N. meningitidis, H. influenzae,* group B *streptococcus, L. monocytogenes,* and susceptible strains of *E. coli,* employing dosages of 50-200 mg/kg/day. However, the recognition of β-lactamase-producing strains of *H. influenzae* has led to the more frequent substitution of chloramphenicol.

Ampicillin is used to treat serious shigellosis provided the organism is sensitive. Ampicillin and in particular amoxicillin have proved effective in the treatment of typhoid and paratyphoid fever. Amoxicillin in dosages of 6 g/day has produced cure rates comparable to chloramphenicol. Oral ampicillin in high dosage is sometimes effective in eliminating persistent biliary excretion of *S. typhi*.

Ampicillin is also effective as single-dose oral therapy of gonorrhea using 3.5 g combined with probenecid. Pharyngeal infections are less responsive to this regimen. Biliary tract infections often respond to ampicillin, although *Klebsiella* spp and increasing numbers of *E. coli* are resistant.

Adverse Reactions

Hypersensitivity reactions are common to all the penicillins. However, rashes occur in approximately 5-7% of persons receiving ampicillin. Such rashes are often maculopapular and may resemble measles. Urticaria also occurs. Rashes are less frequent with amoxicillin. It has been suggested that protein impurities or polymers may be responsible for the higher prevalence of rashes with ampicillin in comparison with penicillin. The prevalence of rash is extremely high in patients suffering from infectious mononucleosis. Up to 95% of these patients will develop an eruption which is presumed to be secondary to the altered immune state associated with infectious mononucleosis. Such sensitivity is also seen with amoxicillin and cephalexin and also may occur in other viral infections such as cytomegalovirus. This usually does not reflect lifelong hypersensitivity to the penicillins. Ampicillin rashes also occur more frequently in patients with lymphoproliferative diseases.

Gastrointestinal intolerance producing nausea, vomiting, and in particular diarrhea occurs with both the oral and intravenous ampicillins. With oral treatment the prevalence varies from 5 to 20%. A lower prevalence of diarrhea (about 2%) is seen with amoxicillin.

Superinfection by resistant organisms such as ampicillin-resistant gram-negative bacteria, *S. aureus,* and more frequently *C. albicans* resulting in oral, gastrointestinal, or vaginal candidiasis, may occur. Other adverse reactions are those common to the penicillins.

Penicillinase-Resistant Penicillins

Penicillin resistance among *S. aureus* became widespread soon after the antibiotic was introduced and was due to inactivation of the antibiotic by penicillinase produced by the organism. By modifying the side chain, the β-lactam ring was protected from inactivation. The drugs so formed include methicillin, the isoxazolyl penicillins, oxacillin, cloxacillin and dicloxacillin, and also nafcillin.

Antibacterial Spectrum

These agents are all active against *S. aureus* and *S. epidermidis* including the penicillinase-producing strains. Methicillin is the least active and dicloxacillin the most active. Resistance to penicillinase activity is greatest for methicillin and nafcillin, which gives the latter a possible advantage over the other agents. Staphylococci resistant to methicillin are also resistant to the other agents in this group.

More recently a new form of resistance to the penicillins, known as *tolerance,* has been recognized in *S. aureus.* There is a deficiency in killing which has occasionally had clinical significance and is due to inhibition of the autolytic enzyme system within the cells.

Methicillin-resistant strains have increased in prevalence recently. They are resistant to all the penicillinase-resistant penicillins but are usually susceptible to vancomycin. *Streptococcus pyogenes, S. pneumoniae,* β-hemolytic streptococci, and many viridans streptococci also are susceptible, although enterococci are resistant. Such activity is lower than for penicillin, which remains the preferred drug for such infections.

Methicillin was the first penicillinase-stable penicillin. It is inactivated by gastric acid and must therefore be infused intravenously over 10 min, although the intramuscular route also may be used. Eighty percent of the drug is excreted unchanged into the urine by glomerular filtration and tubular secretion. Plasma methicillin is about 30% bound to protein, the lowest percentage for any of the penicillins.

The isoxazolyl penicillins are acid-resistant and orally absorbed. Oxacillin is 5-methyl-3-phenyl-4-isoxazolyl penicillin. Absorption of cloxacillin and particularly dicloxacillin is greater than that of oxacillin and is related to the additional chlorine atoms present in these agents. Absorption is best in the fasting state. The isoxazolyl penicillins are also used parenterally. Approximately 20-30% of the drugs are excreted unchanged in the urine while 10% are excreted in the bile. Blood levels of cloxacillin are approximately twice those for oxacillin. There are small variations in the rate of metabolism and excretion. The isoxazolyl penicillins are all highly protein-bound. However, it is difficult to substantiate any therapeutic advantage between them.

Nafcillin is also acid-resistant but its absorption is relatively poor. It is mostly used parenterally. The drug is slightly less protein-bound than the isoxazolyl penicillins. However, claims for superior efficacy of this agent remain theoretical and unsubstantiated clinically.

Clinical Use

The agents are primarily used to treat staphylococcal infections caused by penicillin-resistant organisms. Their activity against *S. pyogenes* renders them useful in situations where it is difficult to differentiate clinically between staphylococcal or streptococcal infection, e.g., cellulitis. In general, oxacillin and nafcillin are used parenterally while cloxacillin and dicloxacillin are mainly oral agents, despite the existence of oral and injectable formulations of these drugs. Methicillin is now less commonly used.

Adverse Reactions

Hypersensitivity reactions common to the penicillins also apply to this group of agents. In addition, a reversible hypersensitivity interstitial nephritis is more common with methicillin and recognized by the occurrence of proteinuria, hematuria, uremia, and eosinophilia. Neutropenia also has been observed with methicillin and oxacillin. Reversible hepatotoxicity, which on biopsy has the appearances of a nonspecific hepatitis, has been seen with oxacillin.

Carbenicillin and Ticarcillin

Carbenicillin and ticarcillin are broad-spectrum penicillins active against many gram-negative bacteria including *P. aeruginosa.* In addition, many anaerobic bacteria including *B. fragilis* are susceptible. Ticarcillin is similar to carbenicillin but is more active against *P. aeruginosa.* Not all gram-negative bacteria are susceptible. *Enterobacter, Serratia-Providencia* spp and some strains of *Klebsiella* spp are resistant, as are strains of staphylococci.

In general, resistance to carbenicillin is usually intrinsic so that the drug has remained useful in treating serious pseudomonal infections. In this situation they are frequently combined with gentamicin or tobramycin to produce synergistic inhibition. This appears to be effective in vivo when treating pseudomonal infections in patients with granulocytopenia.

Both carbenicillin and ticarcillin are relatively inactive and must be given in large doses, about 30 g/day for carbenicillin, about 18 g/day for ticarcillin. These drugs are excreted unchanged by the kidney, thus dosage modification is necessary in renal failure.

An orally absorbed indanyl ester of carbenicillin also is available which is rapidly hydrolyzed and excreted in the urine. Serum concentrations are low and it is inappropriate for the treatment of systemic infections, but it is effective in urinary tract infections.

Adverse Reactions

In addition to hypersensitivity reactions, a variety of other adverse reactions are recognized and include neurotoxicity, hypersensitivity hepatitis, and disturbances of fluid balance as a consequence of sodium-loading. Both carbenicillin and ticarcillin contain approximately 4.7 mEq of sodium per gram. This may precipitate cardiac failure and pulmonary edema in patients with compromised cardiac or renal function, and is more of a problem with carbenicillin since it must be given in larger doses than ticarcillin.

Occasionally, bleeding disorders occur with carbenicillin owing to altered platelet function and aggregation. Carbenicillin in high concentrations can inactivate gentamicin in vitro and occasionally in vivo. Therefore, the drugs should not be mixed and should be administered at separate sites at separate times.

Mezlocillin, Azlocillin, and Piperacillin

Three new agents have been recently tested which are mainly indicated for the treatment of gram-negative infections. Mezlocillin and azlocillin are ureidopenicillins and are chemically related. Piperacillin is an aminobenzylpenicillin derivative and has a similar antimicrobial spectrum to carbenicillin.

Spectrum of Activity

Mezlocillin is active against the Enterobacteriaceae and has modest activity against *P. aeruginosa.* It is more active than carbenicillin against *Proteus, Enterobacter,* and *Klebsiella* spp; *H. influenzae* and *Neisseria* spp; and anaerobic bacteria such as *B. fragilis* are also susceptible.

Azlocillin has a similar spectrum of activity to mezlocillin but is more active against *P. aeruginosa.* Both mezlocillin and azlocillin are synergistically inhibitory to *P. aeruginosa* and other gram-negative bacilli when combined with an aminoglycoside.

Piperacillin is a broad-spectrum agent effective against gram-positive cocci including pneumococci, group A streptococci, *S. faecalis* and staphylococci, although penicillinase-producing strains of staphylococci are resistant. In addition the Enterobacteriaceae are inhibited although some strains of *E. coli* are resistant. It is more active than the other β-lactams against *P. aeruginosa.*

Clinical Use

These agents have been evaluated in a wide variety of infections. Piperacillin is effective in the treatment of gram-negative infections and may be useful when an aminoglycoside is contraindicated. However, the lack of universal susceptibility of *E. coli* means that single-agent therapy in life-threatening infections may not be appropriate.

Mezlocillin also is highly active against gram-negative bacteria although less active against *P. aeruginosa*. Here again its area of use is as an alternative to carbenicillin or ticarcillin, when aminoglycosides are contraindicated. Azlocillin has a similar spectrum of activity but is primarily limited to the treatment of infections caused by *P. aeruginosa*.

The Cephalosporins

Cephalosporins and penicillins both share the β-lactam ring. However, cephalosporins differ from the penicillins since the basic structure is 7-aminocephalosporanic acid. This consists of a β-lactam and dihydrothiazine ring. Cephalosporins were isolated from the mold *Cephalosporium acremonium* from which have been derived a large number of agents with varying pharmacokinetic and antibacterial properties. Like penicillins the cephalosporins are bactericidal and inhibit cell-wall synthesis.

The cephamycins are structurally similar to the cephalosporins although derived from *Streptomyces* spp and will be discussed in this section. Cefoxitin is the best known agent in this group.

Spectrum of Activity

Injectable Cephalosporins

The cephalosporins in general are active against gram-positive cocci including staphylococci and streptococci but excluding enterococci, although as in the case of penicillin, enterococci may be synergistically inhibited by a cephalosporin and an aminoglycoside. The cephalosporins also are active against facultative gram-negative bacteria, although such activity varies according to their stability to β-lactamase inactivation. These enzymes are widely distributed among gram-negative bacteria. The earlier cephalosporins such as cephalothin, cephaloridine, and cefazolin are generally active against *E. coli* and indole-negative *Proteus* spp, but not *Klebsiella* spp and many other Enterobacteriaceae. The subsequent introduction of cefamandole and cefuroxime both with enhanced β-lactamase stabililty has extended the spectrum of activity to include most *Klebsiella* spp. These cephalosporins are also very active against *Haemophilus*. All of these agents are active against both penicillin-sensitive and penicillin-resistant strains of staphylococci; however, methicillin-resistant staphylococci are usually also resistant to these agents. Both cefuroxime and cefamandole inhibit anaerobic bacteria, although *B. fragilis* is often resistant.

Cefoxitin is less active against gram-positive cocci than cephalothin. However, its activity against anaerobic gram-positive cocci and most strains of *B. fragilis* makes this a useful agent in the treatment of anaerobic infections. In addition, it is active against facultative gram-negative bacteria including *E. coli,* indole-positive *Proteus,* and *Klebsiella* spp, and some strains of *Serratia marcescens.*

The most recent cephalosporins include cefotaxime and moxalactam, which are extremely resistant to β-lactamase inactivation and possess remarkable activity against many gram-negative bacteria. This is achieved with some reduction

·in activity against staphylococci. The Enterobacteriaceae, *Neisseria* spp, and *H. influenzae* are extremely susceptible. Cefotaxime also is highly active against *S. pneumoniae* and β-hemolytic streptococci, but not enterococci. Of interest is the activity of these cephalosporins against *P. aeruginosa* which is modest, but preludes further developments in the cephalosporins.

Oral Cephalosporins

The oral cephalosporins include cephalexin, cephradine, cefaclor, cephaloglycin, and cefadroxil. None of the oral cephalosporins is comparable in activity to injectable preparations. Their activity against gram-positive bacteria is modest and is also limited against gram-negative bacteria. There are minor differences among the various drugs. Cefaclor is more active against *H. influenzae* and *S. aureus*.

Pharmacokinetics

The injectable cephalosporins are rapidly distributed throughout the body tissues although CSF penetration by the earlier cephalosporins, such as cephalothin, is poor even when the meninges are inflamed. Cephalothin and cephapirin have short half-lives of about 40 min and are therefore given in large doses every 4-6 hr. Cefazolin on the other hand is more stable with a half-life of 1.5-2 hr and produces high serum and tissue concentrations.

Cefotaxime and moxalactam are also widely distributed throughout the body and appear to result in therapeutic concentrations within the CSF.

The oral cephalosporins are acid-stable and absorbed from the upper bowel. Serum concentrations range from 10 to 20 μg/ml after a 500-mg dose, and the half-lives are in the order of 45 min.

The cephalosporins are excreted primarily through the kidneys by both glomerular filtration and tubular secretion which may be blocked by probenecid. Some of the cephalosporins, such as cephalothin, cephacetrile, and cefotaxime undergo partial desacetylation in the liver. The desacetyl metabolite has some microbiologic activity. In the case of cefotaxime this may accumulate in advanced renal insufficiency if the dose is not reduced. Biliary concentration of the cephalosporins vary but are lower for cephradine and higher for cefazolin and cefuroxime.

Clinical Use

The cephalosporins have been extensively used in the treatment of a wide variety of common infections. They remain an effective alternative to penicillin in selected hypersensitive patients, although there is a risk of cross-hypersensitivity occurring. This is recognized in approximately 10% of patients treated with cephalosporins who have a past history of penicillin hypersensitivity.

Cephalosporins have been useful in the treatment of gram-negative infections either alone or in combination for their synergistically inhibitory activity against *K. pneumoniae*. The injectable cephalosporins also have been used extensively in conjunction with an aminoglycoside, ticarcillin or carbenicillin, for the management of febrile and presumedly infective episodes in patients who are granulocytopenic.

Anaerobic infections have been successfully treated with cefamandole and particularly cefoxitin, although they are less active than clindamycin, chloramphenicol, or metronidazole.

The newer injectable cephalosporins, moxalactam and cefotaxime, are extremely active against many gram-negative bacilli, except *P. aeruginosa,* and may provide an alternative to the aminoglycosides. They may be effective in the treatment of gram-negative bacillary meningitis, but further studies are necessary.

The oral cephalosporins tend to have relatively low activity but have achieved popularity in the treatment of urinary tract and soft tissue infections in patients who are unable to tolerate other agents.

Adverse Reactions

In general, the cephalosporins are a well-tolerated group of antibiotics. Hypersensitivity reactions occur in approximately 5% of patients and are manifest by rashes, which are frequently morbilliform; fever; eosinophilia; urticaria; and occasionally anaphylaxis. The oral cephalosporins produce minor degrees of gastrointestinal intolerance including diarrhea.

Local tolerance to the injectable agents varies. Both cephalothin and cefoxitin are painful by the intramuscular route; the former should be avoided by this route while the latter is given with a local anesthetic.

Nephrotoxicity occurs with dosages in excess of 6 g/day of cephaloridine. Such nephrotoxicity takes the form of acute tubular necrosis and is potentiated by the simultaneous use of a loop diuretic or other nephrotoxic antibiotic. Nephrotoxicity has also been reported when cephalothin is used in conjunction with an aminoglycoside. This remains unproved. The newer cephalosporins appear to be free from nephrotoxicity.

A disulfiram reaction has been described between alcohol and some cephalosporins, including moxalactam. However, this is unlikely to be of much clinical significance.

Tetracyclines

The tetracyclines are a large family of broad-spectrum antibiotics active against many common bacteria, rickettsiae, mycoplasmas, and chlamydiae. There are minor differences in activity between the various agents, and pharmacokinetic differences separate some of these agents.

The various tetracyclines include chlortetracycline, oxytetracycline, demeclocycline, methacycline, minocycline, and doxycycline. These agents are structurally similar and derived from *Streptomyces* spp. They are bacteriostatic at therapeutic concentrations and act by interfering with protein synthesis at the 30S ribosomal subunit, with consequent interference with the binding of transfer RNA to messenger RNA.

Spectrum of Activity

Tetracyclines are active against gram-positive bacteria, but resistance among staphylococci, pneumococci and *S. pyogenes* has increased, particularly in the former. The tetracyclines also are active against many gram-negative bacteria including *E. coli, Enterobacter* and *Klebsiella* and *Proteus* spp. *Serratia marcescens* and *P. aeruginosa* are usually resistant. Most strains of *H. influenzae* and *Neisseria* spp are susceptible. Resistance is increasing among *Shigella* spp.

The tetracyclines also have clinically useful activity against anaerobic bacteria, although more effective agents are generally preferred. Other bacteria susceptible to the tetracyclines include *Mycoplasma pneumoniae, Ureaplasma ureolyticum, Rickettsia, Coxiella burnetii,* and chlamydiae.

Pharmacology

The tetracyclines are absorbed from the upper gut although food impairs absorption. In addition, the divalent cations magnesium, calcium, and aluminum, present in antacid, and ferrous compounds interfere with absorption, since tetracycline forms stable chelates with these ions.

Once absorbed, the tetracyclines are widely distributed throughout the body, although the meninges are poorly penetrated, even when inflamed. The tetracyclines are metabolized by the liver, excreted in the bile, and then enter the gut where they may be reabsorbed into the enterohepatic circulation to be subsequently cleared again by the liver or kidneys. Renal excretion is unimportant for doxycycline and minocycline, thus making them of value in the treatment of patients with underlying renal insufficiency.

Tetracyclines are incorporated into maturing teeth and bones. In the former case, oxidation may produce yellow or brown discoloration. This is preventable if tetracyclines are avoided in children under the age of 8 years.

Clinical Use

The tetracyclines formerly were widely used in the treatment of many common infections. However, increased resistance and the availability of more active alternative agents have limited their use. Their current indications include the treatment of atypical pneumonia such as psittacosis and mycoplasmal infections, although erythromycin is often preferred for the latter. Rickettsial infections respond well to the tetracyclines.

The tetracyclines are used to treat a variety of venereal infections, i.e., granuloma inguinale, nongonococcal urethritis caused by either chlamydiae or *U. ureolyticum,* and as alternative therapy for the treatment of gonorrhea and syphilis.

Other infections caused by *Chlamydia trachomatis,* namely inclusion conjunctivitis and lymphogranuloma venereum, also respond to tetracyclines. Relapsing fever, brucellosis, melioidosis, plague, tularemia, and chancroid are other less common indications.

Tetracyclines also are used as protracted low-dose therapy for acne. They are also alternative agents for managing infective exacerbations of chronic bronchitis and in treating urinary tract infections.

Individual tetracyclines have specific actions. Minocycline is effective in the chemoprophylaxis of *N. meningitidis* by its ability to eliminate nasopharyngeal carriage. Unfortunately, the high incidence of vestibular side effects limits its use. Demeclocycline is used in the management of the syndrome of inappropriate ADH secretion since high-dose therapy reverses the effects of this condition by its ability to induce a state of nephrogenic diabetes insipidus.

Side Effects

The tetracyclines have been used extensively and generally are well tolerated. Among the adverse reactions, gastrointestinal intolerance is prominent. Nausea, vomiting, diarrhea, and superinfection with *C. albicans* resulting in oral and gastrointestinal candidiasis are all recognized. Vaginal candidiasis may also result, while *S. aureus* enterocolitis is fortunately uncommon.

The effect of tetracyclines on teeth has been mentioned. There is a differential risk of dental staining among the tetracyclines: it is least for oxytetracycline. This can be avoided if tetracyclines are not prescribed for children under the age of 8 years. Tetracyclines also may be nephrotoxic. First, preexisting renal insufficiency may be aggravated, possibly due to the antianabolic effect of tetracycline. It is more common in the elderly and may be irreversible. In addition, degraded tetracyclines are tubulotoxic and can induce a Fanconi-like syndrome while demeclocycline, as mentioned earlier, can induce nephrogenic diabetes insipidus. Doxycycline appears to be devoid of nephrotoxicity and is preferred in patients with preexisting renal insufficiency.

Hepatotoxicity is uncommon but produces effects ranging from reversible elevation of liver enzymatic activity to acute fatty necrosis of the liver which, although rare, is reported with the use of intravenous tetracyclines during pregnancy. Caution should be exercised in patients with liver dysfunction and alternative agents considered.

Uncommon side effects include photosensitivity and other skin eruptions, marrow toxicity, benign intracranial hypertension, and vestibular toxicity with minocycline.

Chloramphenicol

Chloramphenicol is a broad-spectrum antibiotic originally derived from *Streptomyces venezuelae* but now synthesized. It is mainly bacteriostatic although against some bacteria it is bactericidal. It acts by binding to the 50S ribosomal subunit thus interfering with peptide bonding and protein synthesis.

Thiamphenicol is a substituted derivative of chloramphenicol which has improved pharmacokinetics but appears to be devoid of marrow toxicity. Thiamphenicol is not available in the United States.

Spectrum of Activity

Chloramphenicol is active against gram-positive cocci, although some *S. aureus* are resistant. Most Enterobacteriaceae including *Salmonella* spp, *H. influenzae*, *Neisseria* spp, and nearly all anaerobic bacteria are susceptible. It is also active against mycoplasmas, chlamydiae, and rickettsiae, but not mycobacteria or *P. aeruginosa*. It is bactericidal against *H. influenzae*, gram-positive cocci, and the *Neisseria* spp.

Resistance to chloramphenicol is either intrinsic or due to enzymatic inactivation by chloramphenicol acetyltransferase. This latter method appears to be the mechanism of resistance among occasional strains of *H. influenzae*. Transferable resistance occurs and has been responsible for an epidemic of chloramphenicol-resistant typhoid fever.

Pharmacokinetics

Chloramphenicol is rapidly absorbed from the upper gastrointestinal tract and achieves serum concentration comparable with those achieved by intramuscular injection with peak serum concentrations of 8-13 μg/ml 2 hr after a 1-g dose.

Chloramphenicol is widely distributed throughout the body, including the CSF and brain, where therapeutic concentrations appear even in the absence of meningitis. Chloramphenicol is glucuronidated in the liver before excretion in the urine, although some free drug is also present. Where liver function is either immature or impaired, concentrations of the free drug accumulate and these are responsible for some of the toxic effects.

Clinical Use

Chloramphenicol is effective in the treatment of a wide range of infections. However, the risk of marrow toxicity now restricts its use to life-threatening infections where alternative treatment is either not available or is less effective. Such diseases include typhoid fever and other septicemic salmonelloses and the treatment of ampicillin-resistant *H. influenzae* infections. It is also indicated for the treatment of serious anaerobic infections, most notably those caused by *B. fragilis*, although alternative agents exist. It is of value in the treatment of meningococcal, pneumococcal, and *L. monocytogenes* meningitis in patients hypersensitive to the penicillins.

Chloramphenicol is an alternative agent for the treatment of plague, tularemia, melioidosis, and rickettsial infections. Topical chloramphenicol is used to treat superficial eye and ear infections.

Adverse Reactions

The most serious side effect of chloramphenicol treatment is marrow toxicity which presents in two forms. First, there is dose-related bone marrow suppression which causes progressive anemia and subsequently, leukopenia and thrombocytopenia. This occurs when the daily dosage exceeds 4 g or the serum concentrations exceed 25 µg/ml. This form of suppression is reversible and is thought to be due to inhibition of protein synthesis in stem cells.

The more serious form of marrow toxicity is aplastic anemia which is idiosyncratic and is about 80% fatal. The prevalence varies from 1:25,000 to 1:40,000 courses of treatment. It may occur during treatment or weeks to months after treatment has ceased. It rarely follows intravenous use.

Another potentially serious adverse reaction is the "grey syndrome" which occurs in premature infants for whom large doses of chloramphenicol have been prescribed. Immaturity of hepatic conjugating enzymes results in high concentrations of free drug with subsequent cardiovascular collapse in extreme cases.

Less serious side effects include gastrointestinal intolerance and occasionally hypersensitivity reactions. Optic neuritis and ototoxicity also have been described.

Clindamycin

Clindamycin and lincomycin are bactericidal antibiotics derived from *Streptomyces lincolnensis*. Clindamycin is the chlorinated derivative of lincomycin and is both more active and better absorbed from the gut than lincomycin, which it has now largely replaced. Both drugs were widely used before the relationship between antibiotic-associated colitis and the use of clindamycin was recognized. Clindamycin is now restricted to the treatment of serious or life-threatening infections where alternative agents are inappropriate.

Clindamycin and lincomycin inhibit bacterial protein synthesis in a fashion similar to erythromycin and chloramphenicol by binding to the 50S ribosomal subunit.

Spectrum of Activity

Clindamycin and lincomycin are active against staphylococci, β-hemolytic streptococci, and pneumococci among the gram-positive bacteria. They have little activity against enterococci although *S. bovis* is susceptible.

One of the most important features of its activity is the broad-spectrum action of clindamycin against most obligate anaerobic bacteria. Its activity against clostridia is less predictable and some strains of *C. perfringens* are resistant.

Clindamycin is also active against *Corynebacterium diphtheriae*, *Nocardia* spp, and *B. anthracis*. It is also active against *Plasmodium falciparum* and has been used in the treatment of chloroquine-resistant cases of *P. falciparum* malaria.

Pharmacology

Clindamycin is available orally as the hydrochloride and the palmitate. The latter is inactive but is rapidly hydrolyzed to active clindamycin within the gut. Absorption produces peak concentrations of approximately 5 µg/ml after a 300-mg dose. The half-life is approximately 2.5 hr. The drug is widely distributed throughout the body tissues and crosses the placenta although penetration of the brain and CSF is poor. Clindamycin penetrates bone and has achieved popularity in the treatment of staphylococcal osteomyelitis. Lincomycin, on the other hand, is less well absorbed from the gut although food does not interfere with the absorption of either drug.

Both agents are metabolized by the liver, following which approximately 90% of the drugs is excreted by the kidneys. Dose modification is necessary in severe liver disease or when renal function is markedly impaired.

Clinical Indications

The recognition that antibiotic-associated colitis is an adverse reaction of clindamycin has limited its use. It remains a highly effective agent for the treatment of both staphylococcal and β-hemolytic streptococcal infections and may be used to treat such infections in patients who are hypersensitive to the penicillins and cephalosporins. The use of clindamycin for treating bone and joint infections still has its advocates, although alternative agents are available.

The most important clinical use remains the treatment of obligate anaerobic infections, in particular those related to the gastrointestinal and female genital tracts where *B. fragilis* is a common pathogen. Under these circumstances, the drug is usually combined with an aminoglycoside effective against the facultative bacteria.

Lincomycin has no therapeutic advantages over clindamycin which has largely replaced it.

Adverse Reactions

The gut is the most important target for the adverse reactions of both lincomycin and clindamycin. Diarrhea occurs in up to 25% of the patients taking clindamycin. Antibiotic-associated colitis may progress to pseudomembrane formation. This may occur during treatment with clindamycin or after treatment has ceased. It is recognized clinically by the development of diarrhea, often with blood and mucus. On endoscopic examination the mucosa is edematous with scattered plaques of necrotic tissue. The latter, along with PMNs and fibrin, make up the pseudomembrane. The colitis is the result of toxin production by *C. difficile*, which is allowed to multiply with the suppression of the usual normal flora. Although clindamycin is the drug most commonly associated with this side effect, being reported in as many as 10% of patients receiving the antibiotic, many other agents also have been associated with the condition. Antibiotic-associated colitis usually responds to oral vancomycin which is active against *C. difficile*. Relapses have been described.

Other adverse reactions to clindamycin include hypersensitivity rashes, neutropenia, and reversible hepatotoxicity.

Erythromycin

Erythromycin is a macrolide antibiotic derived from *Streptomyces erythraeus*. It consists of a large lactam ring to which is attached an amino sugar desosamine and cladinose, a neutral sugar. Erythromycin base is partly inactivated by gastric acid, and therefore various salts and esters have been developed to overcome this. Erythromycin is also available for intravenous use as the lactobionate or gluceptate.

Erythromycin inhibits polypeptide synthesis by binding to the 50S ribosomal subunit and interfering with translocation. The ribosomal receptor site overlaps with those for chloramphenicol and clindamycin, hence erythromycin prevents the binding of these antibiotics.

Erythromycin is either bactericidal or bacteriostatic. It is usually bactericidal against staphylococci, pneumococci, and *H. influenzae*.

Spectrum of Activity

Erythromycin is active against staphylococci, β-hemolytic streptococci, *S. pneumoniae* and most oral viridans streptococci. Its activity against enterococci is unpredictable. Erythromycin is also active against some gram-positive aerobic bacilli such as *L. monocytogenes, C. diphtheriae,* and *B. anthracis.* It is also active against *Neisseria* spp. Its activity against *H. influenzae* is variable.

Strict anaerobic bacteria such as peptococci, peptostreptococci, and several gram-positive bacilli are susceptible. However, *Bacteroides* spp are less predictably susceptible, although *B. melaninogenicus* is usually sensitive. *Clostridium tetani* and *C. perfringens* are usually sensitive.

In addition, erythromycin is active against *Legionella pneumophila* and other *Legionella* spp and also *M. pneumoniae,* which makes this agent popular in the treatment of these atypical pneumonias. Erythromycin is also active against *Chlamydia trachomatis* and *Treponema pallidum.*

Resistance to erythromycin became common among *S. aureus* soon after it was introduced. Currently, erythromycin is active against most staphylococci. *Streptococcus pyogenes* resistance is uncommon in the United States.

Pharmacology

Erythromycin base is unstable in acid and to avoid such inactivation it is frequently prescribed as an enteric-coated preparation. Alternatively, various salts and esters such as erythromycin stearate, erythromycin ethylsuccinate, and erythromycin estolate, which are stable to gastric acid, are prescribed. Erythromycin stearate liberates active erythromycin to produce a blood concentration comparable with that of the base. The estolate, on the other hand, is more lipid-soluble and more completely absorbed, producing higher serum concentrations. Intravenous erythromycin lactobionate and gluceptate have half-lives of approximately 70-100 min.

Erythromycin is widely distributed throughout the body tissues and can be demonstrated in pleural and ascitic fluid, bronchial secretions, and the middle ear. Penetration into the CSF is poor, even in the presence of meningitis.

Erythromycin is metabolized in the liver and is excreted mainly in the bile from whence some enterohepatic recirculation occurs. Only approximately 5% is excreted in the urine.

Clinical Use

Erythromycin has been available for many years and has remained a popular antibiotic for the treatment of pediatric infections because toxicity is low. More recently the identification of *L. pneumophila* as a cause of atypical pneumonia has resulted in an increase in erythromycin use.

Erythromycin is active against staphylococci and streptococci and is a useful alternative to the penicillins for the treatment of skin and soft-tissue infections. It is also effective in the treatment of pneumococcal pneumonia.

Erythromycin is also alternative therapy for the treatment of gonorrhea, syphilis, and nongonococcal urethritis. Neonatal ophthalmia caused by *C. trachomatis* has been treated with systemic erythromycin combined with topical tetracycline ointment.

One important primary indication is the treatment of *M. pneumoniae* and *L. pneumophila* respiratory infections. Erythromycin is somewhat more effective than tetracycline in the treatment of mycoplasmal pneumonia although excretion of viable bacteria often persists despite clinical resolution.

Other indications for erythromycin include the treatment of nasopharyngeal carriers of *C. diphtheriae* and for the chemoprophylaxis of siblings of patients with established pertussis. It has no effect on the established disease.

Finally, erythromycin in combination with neomycin is an effective preoperative bowel preparation in patients undergoing colon surgery, reducing the incidence of postoperative infection.

Side Effects

Erythromycin is remarkably well tolerated and side effects are few. The most frequent side effect is gastrointestinal intolerance, producing nausea, vomiting, and sometimes diarrhea. Local phlebitis from the intravenous preparation is not uncommon, while the intramuscular injection is painful.

Hepatotoxicity occurs with erythromycin estolate but rarely with other preparations. Cholestatic jaundice due to a hypersensitivity reaction usually follows prolonged or repeated use of erythromycin estolate. There are occasional reports of reversible ototoxicity.

Aminoglycosides

The aminoglycoside antibiotics include streptomycin, neomycin, kanamycin, gentamicin, tobramycin, amikacin, sisomicin, and netilmicin. This group of antibiotics has a common aminocyclitol structure to which are attached amino sugars. More correctly they are called aminoglycosidic aminocyclitols, which differentiates them from spectinomycin which is also an aminocyclitol but not an aminoglycoside. All are derivatives of *Streptomyces* spp, with the exception of gentamicin and sisomicin which are derived from *Micromonospora* spp, which is the explanation for their different spelling. Amikacin is a derivative of kanamycin and netilmicin is semisynthetically derived from sisomicin.

The aminoglycosides are bactericidal and interfere with protein synthesis by binding to the 30S ribosomal subunit thus producing misreading of the genetic coding. It remains debatable whether or not this is their sole mode of action.

Nonetheless, the penetration of the cytoplasmic membrane is an aerobic energy-dependent process which explains the failure of the aminoglycoside antibiotics to inhibit obligate anaerobic bacteria.

Spectrum of Activity

Aminoglycosides are most active against facultative gram-negative bacilli belonging to the Enterobacteriaceae. The more recently introduced aminoglycosides gentamicin, tobramycin, amikacin, and netilmicin are also active against *P. aeruginosa* and other *Pseudomonas* spp. There are minor differences in activity between these agents: gentamicin is the most active against the Enterobacteriaceae, whereas tobramycin is most active against *P. aeruginosa*. Modest activity is exhibited against *S. aureus* although they are not primarily antistaphylococcal agents. All aminoglycosides lack activity against obligate anaerobic bacteria and streptococci. However, synergistic inhibition of enterococci and also other strains of β-hemolytic streptococci may be demonstrated by the penicillins, cephalosporins, and vancomycin in combination with gentamicin, tobramycin, or amikacin. These same aminoglycosides are also synergistically inhibitory against *P. aeruginosa* when combined with carbenicillin or ticarcillin.

The aminoglycosides also show varying activity against *Mycobacterium* spp. Streptomycin was used as a first-line agent for the treatment of *M. tuberculosis* infections. Both kanamycin and amikacin are occasionally used for the treatment of various mycobacterial infections.

Resistance among the aminoglycosides is an increasing problem and may be caused by problems with permeability of the drug or from enzymatic inactivation. The mechanisms of resistance vary. For example, with streptomycin a single-step mutation produces high-level resistance, while low-level resistance reflects impaired uptake of the drug. Low-level resistance among enterococci can be overcome by combining penicillin with an aminoglycoside. Strains with high-level resistance are not thus inhibited.

Enzymatic inactivation of the aminoglycosides appears to be increasing. These enzymes are primarily present among the Enterobacteriaceae and *Pseudomonas* spp and are plasmid transmitted. There are three classes of enzyme: aminoglycoside acetyltransferases, phosphotransferases, and nucleotidyltransferases (formerly adenyltransferase). They act by attacking the basic ring structure at various points thus destroying the activity of the aminoglycoside. Aminoglycosides vary in their susceptibility to enzymatic inactivation; it is greatest for kanamycin and least for amikacin. Amikacin is at present susceptible to only a single acetyltransferase enzyme. Amikacin is therefore often active against strains resistant to other aminoglycosides, although the problem of permeability resistance still remains.

Pharmacology

The aminoglycosides are lipid-soluble and not absorbed from the gastrointestinal tract to any degree, unless there is mucosal ulceration. They are therefore parentally administered with the exception of neomycin which is restricted to topical use owing to its unacceptable toxicity when used systemically. Peak concentrations occur approximately 1 hr after an intramuscular injection. The half-life in patients with normal renal function is 2 hr with the exception of streptomycin (3 hr). The drugs are widely distributed throughout the extracellular fluid compartment and are poorly protein-bound. Their low lipid solubility is responsible for the poor concentrations within CSF and brain tissue. The CSF concentrations of gentamicin may be increased by intrathecal or intraventricular injection. The drugs are excreted unchanged by the kidney by glomerular filtration and hence, dosage modification is essential in renal insufficiency if toxic levels are to be avoided.

Nephrotoxicity is the most readily recognized adverse effect of the aminoglycosides. It is identified biochemically by a rise in the BUN and serum creatinine levels while the urine excretion of brush-border enzymes such as alanine aminopeptidase indicates tubular damage. Fortunately most episodes of nephrotoxicity are reversible. The potential for nephrotoxicity varies somewhat among the aminoglycosides, being low for streptomycin, kanamycin, tobramycin, and probably netilmicin. The occurrence of nephrotoxicity is reduced by avoiding excessive dosage, repeated courses of aminoglycoside, and the concurrent use of nephrotoxic combinations such as furosemide and possibly cephalothin.

Other adverse reactions are relatively uncommon and include rashes, eosinophilia, marrow and liver toxicity, and neuromuscular blockade from a curare-like effect. The potential for neuromuscular blockade varies being greatest for neomycin and uncommon with the more recently introduced aminoglycosides. This side effect is potentiated by the simultaneous use of muscle relaxants or the presence of myasthenia gravis.

Individual Aminoglycosides

Streptomycin

Streptomycin was the first aminoglycoside used and proved valuable in the treatment of both gram-negative bacillary infections and tuberculosis. Nevertheless, its use has decreased since more active and less toxic agents are available. It is still indicated, however, for the treatment of tularemia, plague, brucellosis, usually in combination with a tetracycline, and as an alternative to penicillin G in the treatment of rat-bite fever. It is also an alternative agent for the treatment of chancroid, granuloma inguinale, and shigellosis. Severe hypersensitivity rashes and hepatitis with fever can occur in addition to renal toxicity and ototoxicity.

Neomycin

Neomycin is now limited to topical use because of unacceptable systemic toxicity. As a topical agent it has been used to control staphylococcal skin infections, usually in combination with polymyxin and bacitracin, with or without corticosteroids. However, topical use is not without risks since skin sensitization and the emergence of drug-resistant organisms can occur. Oral neomycin is used in liver failure to reduce the nitrogen load from gut bacteria and as part of the preoperative bowel preparation in combination with erythromycin.

Kanamycin

With the availability of gentamicin the use of kanamycin has diminished substantially. It remains effective in the treatment of gram-negative bacillary infections and as a reserve drug for the treatment of tuberculosis. *Pseudomonas aeruginosa* is resistant.

Gentamicin

Gentamicin is the most widely used aminoglycoside. Its advantage over earlier aminoglycosides includes high activity and efficacy in treating serious gram-negative bacillary infections including those caused by *P. aeruginosa* in most body tissues, although penetration into the CSF remains poor.

Gentamicin also has been used topically for the treatment of burns and superficial infections of the ear and eye. However, topical use has been associated with an increase in resistance of gram-negative bacilli, and such use is not encouraged.

Oral gentamicin in combination with vancomycin and nystatin has been used to decontaminate the gut of patients with malignant disease rendered neutropenic by cytotoxic chemotherapy. Such use has had equivocal results and many patients find the regimen unpalatable.

Dosage must take into account age, body weight, and renal function if therapeutic concentrations are to be achieved and toxic concentration avoided. Various methods for determining and maintaining the appropriate therapeutic concentration have been described. They include nomograms and formulae, but in general, a patient with normal renal function can be prescribed 3-5 mg/kg/day in three divided doses. *Trough* (or valley) serum concentrations immediately before the next dose should be less than 2 µg/ml and peak concentrations should not exceed 12 µg/ml. In the newborn, the dosage must take account of the maturity of the kidneys as well as the weight of the infant. Other factors may affect gentamicin concentrations, including fever, which may reduce serum concentrations, and anemia, which elevates them. Whenever possible, the drug serum concentration should be determined by enzymatic, microbiologic, or radioimmunoassay.

Tobramycin

Tobramycin has a pharmacokinetic and activity spectrum similar to gentamicin and therefore, its indications for use and its dosage are similar. Its activity against *P. aeruginosa* is two- to fourfold greater than gentamicin. It appears to be slightly less ototoxic and nephrotoxic. It has the advantage of being active against some gentamicin-resistant strains of *P. aeruginosa*.

Amikacin

Amikacin is derived from kanamycin and thus has similar pharmacokinetics. However, it is microbiologically more active with a spectrum that includes *P. aeruginosa*. It also is extremely resistant to inactivation by most aminoglycoside-inactivating enzymes and is therefore useful in the treatment of gram-negative bacillary infections resistant to other aminoglycosides. Synergistic inhibition of *P. aeruginosa* can also be demonstrated when amikacin is combined with carbenicillin or ticarcillin.

Netilmicin and Sisomicin

Netilmicin and sisomicin are two new aminoglycosides. Netilmicin is claimed to be less toxic than gentamicin and to be active against gentamicin-resistant bacteria. Sisomicin resembles gentamicin very closely in its microbiologic activity and pharmacokinetics. It is unlikely that either drug will replace the existing aminoglycosides.

Vancomycin

Vancomycin is a glycopeptide antibiotic derived from *Streptomyces orientalis*. It is bactericidal and acts by binding to and inhibiting cell-wall synthesis. It has a narrow spectrum of activity confined to *Staphylococcus aureus, S. epidermidis, Streptococcus pyogenes, S. pneumoniae,* viridans streptococci, and corynebacteria.

Streptococcus faecalis is synergistically inhibited by vancomycin and gentamicin. Vancomycin is also active against clostridia, including *C. difficile*.

Pharmacokinetics

Vancomycin is poorly absorbed from the gut and must be administered intravenously. Intramuscular administration is too painful. The normal half-life is about 6 hr although in anephric patients a single 1-g dose provides therapeutic concentrations for approximately 10 days. Normally about 80% of the drug is excreted unchanged by the kidney. The drug is widely distributed throughout the tissues and crosses the meninges when they are inflamed. The drug is not removed by peritoneal or hemodialysis.

Clinical Use

Vancomycin has had increased use for the treatment of serious staphylococcal infections in patients hypersensitive to the β-lactam antibiotics or in the treatment of methicillin-resistant staphylococcal infections. It is also useful in the treatment of staphylococcal infections of intravascular shunts in patients undergoing hemodialysis.

Vancomycin has been used to treat antibiotic-associated colitis caused by toxin-producing strains of *C. difficile*. Vancomycin may be used in the chemoprophylaxis of infective endocarditis in patients, who are hypersensitive to penicillin, undergoing operative procedures which predispose to streptococcal bacteremia.

Adverse Reactions

Vancomycin is nephrotoxic and ototoxic and is irritating to the veins thus thrombophlebitis occurs. Rapid intravenous infusion may cause hypotension, tachypnea, nausea, vomiting, and flushing.

Spectinomycin

Spectinomycin is an aminocyclitol antibiotic isolated from *Streptomyces spectabilis*. Although related to other aminocyclitols it is not an aminoglycoside. It acts on the 30S ribosomal subunit thus inhibiting protein synthesis.

Spectrum of Activity

Spectinomycin, although restricted to the treatment of gonococcal infections, is also active against many *E. coli*, *K. pneumoniae*, *Enterobacter* spp, and *H. influenzae*. However, this activity is modest, and other agents are preferred.

Pharmacology

Spectinomycin must be given by intramuscular injection. A single 2-g dose produces serum concentrations of 100 µg/ml. The drug is excreted primarily through the kidneys in the unchanged state. Protein-binding is minimal.

Clinical Use

Spectinomycin is used in a single 2-g dose for the treatment of anogenital gonorrhea caused by penicillinase-producing strains of N. *gonorrhoeae* or in those patients who have failed to respond to other agents and in whom alternative drugs are contraindicated. Unfortunately, spectinomycin is not effective in the treatment of gonococcal pharyngitis, but may be used to treat disseminated gonococcal infection, when caused by penicillinase-producing strains. Its safety in pregnancy or childhood has not been established.

Side Effects

These are uncommon although local intolerance may occur following intramuscular injection. Other minor complaints include nausea and unsteadiness. Nephrotoxicity or ototoxicity do not appear to be problems.

The Sulfonamides

The sulfonamides are among the earliest of the antimicrobial agents. They have been used in the treatment of a wide variety of infections, and drugs are available for oral, parenteral, and topical use. Sulfamethoxazole has been combined with trimethoprim to produce a sequentially and often synergistically inhibitory mixture, effective in the treatment of a wide variety of bacterial and *Pneumocystis carinii* infections.

The sulfonamides are bacteriostatic and interfere with bacterial folic acid synthesis by competitive inhibition of para-aminobenzoic acid by blocking the enzyme dihydrofolic acid synthetase. This interferes with purine synthesis and hence nucleic acid formation. The sulfonamides are selective since humans can use preformed folic acid in the diet, whereas bacteria must manufacture it from para-aminobenzoic acid.

Spectrum of Activity

The sulfonamides are broad-spectrum agents active against many gram-positive and gram-negative bacteria. However, resistance has seriously limited their effectiveness against many bacteria. In addition to antibacterial activity the sulfonamides have some effect on protozoa.

Streptococci are susceptible although enterococci are resistant. Staphylococci are moderately susceptible. *Neisseria meningitidis* and N. *gonorrhoeae* were extremely sensitive but unfortunately resistance, particularly among meningococci, is now widespread. Many of the Enterobacteriaceae are susceptible although resistance has increased.

Salmonella and *Shigella* spp are also less sensitive than formerly. Strains of *Pseudomonas* are occasionally susceptible. Other bacteria that are sensitive include C. *trachomatis* and *Nocardia* spp. As mentioned, the sulfonamides are also active against some protozoa including *Toxoplasma gondii* and P. *falciparum*. Difficulties can arise with the laboratory testing of sulfonamide susceptibility if the medium is not free from antagonists such as thymine and thymidine. In addition, the inoculum size is critical.

Pharmacology

The many preparations of sulfonamide can be conveniently separated into those that are orally administered and those that are topically applied. The oral agents are further subdivided into short-, intermediate-, and long-acting preparations according to their absorption and duration of action. The short-acting sulfonamides include sulfadiazine, sulfamethizole, and sulfasoxazole. An intermediate-acting sulfonamide is sulfamethoxazole, which is well absorbed from the gut but slowly excreted, thus twice daily dosage is sufficient. This agent is used in combination with trimethoprim. The long-acting sulfonamide sulfamethoxydiazine has a half-life of 35 hr.

Oral sulfonamides are well absorbed from the gut and distributed widely throughout most body fluids and cavities. Furthermore, the short-acting sulfonamide, sulfadiazine, achieves high CSF concentrations even in the absence of inflammation. The placenta is crossed and the drug is detectable in breast milk. Protein-binding varies widely, from 20 to 90%.

The sulfonamides are conjugated in the liver and are excreted by the kidneys by glomerular filtration and tubular secretion in both the free and conjugated forms. The short-acting sulfonamides are rapidly excreted and achieve high urine concentrations. However, the long-acting preparations are more slowly excreted. Tubular reabsorption takes place, particularly if the urine is acid. Under these circumstances the sulfonamides are less soluble and may form crystal precipitates, a problem which was more common with the earlier sulfonamides. This can result in an obstructive uropathy.

Clinical Use

The sulfonamides are now used far less than formerly owing to the availability of more active and less toxic agents. Drug resistance, particularly among meningococci and enterobacteria also has contributed to this reduced use. Urinary tract infections caused by susceptible bacteria respond well to sulfisoxazole and sulfamethizole because they produce high urinary concentrations. Meningococcal meningitis was previously treated very effectively with sulfadiazine. Group A streptococcal infections were formerly treated with sulfonamides, which have also been used for long-term prophylaxis of streptococcal pharyngitis in patients who have had rheumatic fever. Nonetheless, penicillin is usually preferred.

Gastrointestinal shigellosis responds to oral sulfonamides, although here again increased drug resistance has limited the value of these agents. Other indications for the sulfonamides include lymphogranuloma venereum, nocardiasis, and chancroid, although alternative agents are available. Other antimicrobial uses of sulfonamides include the treatment of chloroquine-resistant *P. falciparum* infections in combination with pyrimethamine and quinine. The combination of sulfadoxine and pyrimethamine has proved helpful for the chemoprophylaxis of *P. falciparum* malaria in South East Asia and other parts of the world where chloroquine-resistant malaria exists.

Another use for the sulfonamides is in the treatment of inflammatory bowel disease. The well-absorbed sulfonamide sulfapyridine is combined with salicylic acid to form salicylazosulfapyridine(sulfasalazine) which is effective maintenance treatment for patients with ulcerative colitis in remission. Sulfasalazine is absorbed from the upper bowel and excreted in the bile and back into the gut where bacteria act on the compound to separate it into sulfapyridine and 5-aminosalicylic acid. Sulfapyridine is subsequently reabsorbed and excreted in the urine whereas the 5-aminosalicylic acid is excreted in the feces and is probably the active constituent of the compound, the sulfonamide simply acting as a carrier.

Topical sulfonamides have been used in the management of burns to prevent pseudomonal infection. Various preparations have been used including mafenide and silver sulfadiazine.

Adverse Reactions

Unfortunately, the sulfonamides not uncommonly produce adverse reactions which range from the trivial to the life-threatening. Various hypersensitivity reactions occur, particularly rashes, which may be maculopapular, urticarial, exfoliative dermatitis, erythema multiforme, or occasionally the Stevens-Johnson syndrome, which may be fatal. Erythema nodosum also occurs and appears to be more common with the long-acting sulfonamides.

Other serious adverse reactions are hematologic dyscrasias. Agranulocytosis is fortunately less common with the more recent agents. Other reactions include aplastic anemia, hemolytic anemia, and thrombocytopenia. Methemoglobinemia complicated the use of some earlier compounds.

Nephrotoxicity, most notably crystalluria, occurred with the earlier relatively insoluble sulfonamides, but it is now uncommon. Adequate hydration and alkalinization of the urine minimizes this risk.

Less frequent adverse reactions include a drug-induced lupus syndrome, polyarteritis nodosum, and hypersensitivity hepatotoxicity. Jaundice may also occur in the newborn due to the displacement of bilirubin from protein-binding sites by the sulfonamides. The drug is therefore contraindicated in late pregnancy and in the neonate.

Trimethoprim-Sulfamethoxazole

Trimethoprim is a synthetic chemotherapeutic agent with bacteriostatic antimicrobial properties in its own right. It interferes with purine synthesis in the same metabolic pathway as the sulfonamides by inhibiting the enzyme dihydrofolate reductase. Since it shares similar pharmacokinetic properties with sulfamethoxazole the drugs have been combined in a fixed-ratio preparation.

Spectrum of Activity

Trimethoprim is active against staphylococci, *S. pneumoniae, S. faecalis,* and β-hemolytic streptococci, as well as viridans streptococci. It has modest activity against *N. gonorrhoeae* and *N. meningitidis* but good activity against *H. influenzae, E. coli, K. pneumoniae, Enterobacter, Proteus, Nocardia, Salmonella,* and *Shigella* spp. It is relatively inactive against *P. aeruginosa* and anaerobic bacteria.

In combination with sulfamethoxazole synergistic inhibition is demonstrable against most trimethoprime-susceptible bacteria. Gonococci differ by being more susceptible to sulfamethoxazole than they are to trimethoprim. Trimethoprim-sulfamethoxazole is also active against *Coxiella burnetii, Pneumocystis carinii,* and *Toxoplasma gondii.*

Sulfonamide-resistant bacteria may be only inhibited by trimethoprim in some instances. There is concern that trimethoprim resistance will increase and this has been confirmed in Finland and the United Kingdom where trimethoprim-sulfamethoxazole has been used for some years.

Pharmacology

Trimethoprim is combined with sulfamethoxazole in a fixed ratio of 1:5 (each tablet contains 80 mg of trimethoprim and 400 mg of sulfamethoxazole). This produces a plasma ratio of 1:20 which is usually optimal for synergistic activity. Trimethoprim, like the sulfonamide, is readily absorbed from the gut and widely distributed throughout the body fluids and also enters the CSF in the presence of meningitis. The half-life of trimethoprim is between 10 and 14 hr and therefore matches the pharmacokinetics of sulfamethoxazole. Trimethoprim is excreted in the urine mostly in the unchanged state, although a small amount is conjugated. The urinary concentration varies according to the pH since trimethoprim is a weak base and urine excretion is inversely proportioned to pH. Biliary levels are approximately 50% of the plasma levels.

Clinical Use

The combining of trimethoprim with sulfamethoxazole has substantially increased the spectrum of activity of the sulfonamides. Urinary tract infections acquired in the community or hospital usually respond well. However, it is unlikely that the combination is synergistic within the urine since high concentrations of both trimethoprim and the sulfonamide are present and are active in their own right. Nonetheless, the drug is a useful alternative to ampicillin and has been used in the chemoprophylaxis of recurrent urinary tract infections. It also has been used prophylactically to prevent urinary tract infections after prostatectomy.

Trimethoprim-sulfamethoxazole has been widely used in the treatment of typhoid fever and other salmonella infections. It appears to be as effective as chloramphenicol and provides alternative treatment of chloramphenicol-resistant strains of *S. typhi*.

Many acute bacterial respiratory infections including bacterial exacerbations of chronic bronchitis have been effectively treated with trimethoprim-sulfamethoxazole, with cure rates similar to those of tetracycline and ampicillin. Other indications for trimethoprim-sulfamethoxazole include gonorrhea, lymphogranuloma venereum, and acute brucellosis. It has been helpful in the treatment of chronic brucellosis, although cure is not universal. Another indication is infection with *Mycobacterium marinum*.

Among protozoal infections, *P. carinii* pneumonia responds to high-dose treatment with trimethoprim-sulfamethoxazole where 20 mg/kg of trimethoprim and 100 mg/kg of sulfamethoxazole per day are more effective than pentamidine isethionate. The drug also has been used successfully as prophylaxis against *P. carinii* infections in children with acute lymphoblastic leukemia, when infection rates are high. The drug has been used in malaria and toxoplasmosis with some success in uncontrolled trials.

Trimethoprim-sulfamethoxazole has been used for chemoprophylaxis of bacterial infections in patients with myeloproliferative or lymphoproliferative malignancies who are undergoing cytoxic chemotherapy that renders them granulocytopenic. In this situation it has reduced the number of febrile infective episodes.

Adverse Reactions

The side effects of trimethoprim-sulfamethoxazole are frequently those associated with the use of the sulfonamide. Nevertheless, some adverse reactions appear to be related to the combined preparation. Gastrointestinal intolerance is associated with high dosages. Hematologic effects associated with the dual interruption of folic acid metabolism have produced megaloblastic bone marrow changes and macrocytic anemias. Bone marrow suppression which may affect any cell line has been recognized. Such adverse reactions are more frequent with prolonged treatment or in patients receiving immunosuppressive therapy.

Hypersensitivity rashes occur in 1.6-8% of patients. Most of these are due to the sulfonamide component and similarly vary in their severity. Although uncommon, true trimethoprim hypersensitivity can occur. The safety of the drug has not been established in pregnancy. Other adverse effects include hepatic necrosis, polyneuropathy, and pseudomembranous colitis. The drug interacts with phenytoin by prolonging the half-life, and potentiates the effects of warfarin by inhibiting its metabolism.

Metronidazole

Metronidazole belongs to the nitromidazole drugs. It is an interesting agent because it was originally introduced as an antiprotozoal agent for the treatment of *Trichomonas vaginalis* infections and was subsequently found to have activity against other protozoa, most notably *Entamoeba histolytica, Giardia lamblia,* and *Balantidium coli.* A chance observation that acute gingivitis improved in a patient receiving metronidazole for a coincidental trichomonal vaginitis led to the evaluation of the drug's antibacterial effect against obligate anaerobic bacteria. The drug also has radiosensitizing properties.

The exact mode of action of metronidazole remains uncertain. Evidence exists that the nitro group is reduced in both protozoa and anaerobic bacteria and that the drug acts as an electron acceptor. The electron transport proteins of the ferridoxin and flavodoxin variety are probably important in this process and are absent in aerobic bacteria. Metronidazole is selectively taken up by anaerobic bacteria and oxygen markedly inhibits this process. It is postulated that the products of metronidazole reduction are inhibitory to protein and nucleic acid synthesis.

Spectrum of Activity

As mentioned, metronidazole is only active against obligate anaerobic bacteria. Aerobic, facultative, and microaerophilic bacteria are uniformly resistant. The drug is particularly active against *Bacteroides* spp and fusobacteria, most *Clostridium* spp, peptococci, and peptostreptococci. Resistance among anaerobic bacteria is rare.

Pharmacology

Metronidazole is administered orally and is well absorbed, producing serum concentrations of approximately 11 μg/ml following a 500-mg dose. The drug is also available for intravenous administration. The drug is widely distributed throughout the body and is detectable in therapeutic concentrations in the brain and CSF.

Metronidazole is oxidized and glucuronidated in the liver and excreted in the urine, mostly in the metabolized state. Fifteen percent of the orally administered dose is detectable in the feces. The method of assay of metronidazole can produce marked differences in concentrations, being greater for the polarographic method than for the microbiologic assay, reflecting the detection of total as opposed to active drug.

Clinical Use

Metronidazole was originally introduced for the oral treatment of genitourinary
T. vaginalis infections for which it is highly effective. Recurrences may occur,
and hence it is important to treat both sexual partners. Drug resistance has only
recently been described and is extremely uncommon.

Metronidazole is also effective for the treatment of most forms of amebiasis. It is highly effective for both amebic abscesses and acute amebic dysentery.
However, the treatment of asymptomatic cyst excretion is less predictable and
alternative agents are available (see Chapter 119). Metronidazole is also effective in the treatment of dracontiasis.

Metronidazole is now being used increasingly for both the treatment and
prophylaxis of anaerobic bacterial infections, particularly those infections where
B. fragilis is commonly present. Such infections include those associated with
the gastrointestinal and female genital tracts. It also is effective for the treatment of anaerobic central nervous system, chest, skin, and soft-tissue infections.

Many such infections are caused by a mixture of anaerobic and facultative
aerobic bacteria and therefore, metronidazole is combined with another antibiotic, such as an aminoglycoside or a cephalosporin, active against the aerobic organisms. Metronidazole is available for oral and intravenous use and has only recently been approved for the treatment of anaerobic infections in the United
States, but worldwide experience has been substantial. It is preferred by many to
both clindamycin and chloramphenicol in the treatment of anaerobic infection because these two agents are associated with significant side effects.

Metronidazole has also been demonstrated to be effective in the prophylaxis
of postoperative anaerobic infections in patients undergoing elective large bowel
surgery and hysterectomy.

Adverse Reactions

Metronidazole has been used extensively for the treatment of trichomoniasis for
nearly 20 years and has been well tolerated. The most common side effects are
gastrointestinal and include a metallic taste, nausea, and occasionally abdominal
pain, which may interrupt treatment. More serious side effects include a peripheral neuropathy which is usually reversible, skin rashes, pruritus, headache, depression, and a reversible neutropenia. An "Antabuse-reaction" also may occur if
alcohol is taken simultaneously.

The drug has been plagued by anxiety over observations of bacterial muto-
genicity and carcinogenic effects in rats administered high doses of metronidazole
for prolonged periods. The relevance of these findings to humans remains uncertain and clinical evidence for carcinogenic or teratogenic effects is absent.

The cost of this and other antibiotics is stated in Table 6.1.

Polymyxins

The polymyxins are a group of bactericidal polypeptide antibiotics obtained from
Bacillus polymyxa. Among the polymyxins, polymyxin B and polymyxin E, otherwise known as colistin, have been used clinically.

The polymyxins are active against many gram-negative bacteria including
E. coli, Enterobacter, Klebsiella, Salmonella, Shigella, and also *P. aeruginosa.*
All *Proteus* spp are resistant to polymyxins as are many anaerobic bacteria and
most gram-positive and gram-negative cocci. Classic strains of *Vibrio cholerae*
are sensitive to polymyxins but the El Tor biotype is resistant. Synergistic inhibition of Enterobacteriaceae has been demonstrated for polymyxins and trimethoprim-sulfamethoxazole.

TABLE 6.1   Antibiotic Costs

Drug	Dose/Day	Cost* ($)
Gentamicin	240 mg	28
Tobramycin	240 mg	33
Chloramphenicol	4 g	42
Amikacin	1.5 g	63
Clindamycin	1.8 g	65
Carbenicillin	30 g	75
Cefoxitin	8 g	88
Cefamandole	8 g	90
Ticarcillin	18 g	90
Piperacillin	18 g	124
Metronidazole	4 g	168
Cefotaxime	8 g	183
Moxalactam	8 g	196

*Wholesale, September, 1982, per day

The methanesulfonates of polymyxin B and colistin are less active in vitro but are less toxic and therefore, preferred for parenteral use.

Polymyxin B sulfate may be given parenterally either by intramuscular injection or continuous infusion. Bolus injection is to be avoided. Colistin methanesulfonate (colistimethate) may also be given by intramuscular or intravenous administration. The polymyxins accumulate in renal failure; hence dose reduction is necessary. Polymyxin B sulfate is also available for topical application in various solutions and creams, often in combination with bacitracin and neomycin. It also has been used as a urinary tract irrigant.

Both polymyxin B and colistin are now used infrequently for the treatment of systemic infections owing to the availability of more effective and less toxic drugs such as the aminoglycosides. Nonetheless, they are occasionally used for the treatment of serious *P. aeruginosa* infections, in combination with other antipseudomonal agents.

The topical use continues with various creams, ointments, sprays, and drops for superficial infections and also as a wound or bladder irrigant. However, the evidence for their efficacy remains equivocal, although toxicity does not appear to be a problem.

The important adverse reactions of systemically administered polymyxins are neurotoxicity and nephrotoxicity which are dose related. Neurotoxicity may be acute and follow intravenous bolus injection. More important is neuromuscular blockade which may impair respiration and is not reversed by neostigmine, but may improve with calcium. Nephrotoxicity occurs in up to 20% of patients and is recognized by elevation of the BUN and serum creatinine levels and the presence of proteinuria and hematuria. Acute tubular necrosis may develop, is more frequent when other nephrotoxic agents are used, and fortunately is usually reversible.

Bacitracin

Bacitracin is a peptide antibiotic derived from *Bacillus licheniformis* and was formerly used systemically for the treatment of staphylococcal infections. However, it is now considered too toxic for other than topical application. Bacitracin is active against staphylococci, *S. pyogenes,* and some gram-negative bacteria. It interferes with cell-wall synthesis and is bactericidal. Currently it is used in various topical antibiotic preparations such as creams, ointments, and aerosol sprays in combination with neomycin and polymyxin B.

Nalidixic Acid

Nalidixic acid is a synthetic derivative of 1,8-naphthyridine. The drug is bactericidal and interferes with DNA, RNA, and protein synthesis, although the exact mode of action is unknown.

Nalidixic acid is inhibitory to most Enterobacteriaceae. However, it is inactive against *P. aeruginosa* and gram-positive cocci. Resistance may develop in vitro and has emerged in vivo, related to low urinary concentrations. Overall resistance to nalidixic acid remains uncommon.

The drug is orally administered and well absorbed producing peak serum concentrations of 21-50 µg/ml, 2 hr after a single 1-g dose. It is rapidly glucuronidated by the liver, and about 90% is excreted by the kidney in the inactive conjugated form. The remaining fraction is unchanged drug and active hydroxy metabolite. Very little drug is detectable in other sites. Urinary concentrations are 50-500 µg/ml on a regimen of 1 g every 6 hr. The drug is highly protein-bound.

Nalidixic acid is confined to the treatment of urinary tract infections caused by susceptible bacteria. Serum concentrations are inadequate to treat systemic infection. The drug is not concentrated in the prostate and is not helpful in the management of bacterial prostatitis. It has been used for the chemoprophylaxis of urinary tract infections, although trimethoprim-sulfamethoxazole is generally preferred.

The drug is usually well tolerated although occasional gastrointestinal symptoms occur. In renal failure the active drug does not accumulate, but the conjugate does and may be responsible for toxicity. The drug is contraindicated in patients with advanced liver disease. Neurotoxicity may result in intracranial hypertension, confusion, depression, excitement, as well as headache, drowsiness, giddiness, and occasionally grand mal seizures.

Nitrofurans

The nitrofurans include nitrofurantoin, nitrofurazone, and furazolidone. They are nitroheterocyclic drugs which are related to the nitroimidazoles, of which metronidazole is one, and the nitrothiazoles which include niridazole used in the treatment of schistosomiasis. The mode of action of the nitrofurans remains uncertain, although DNA may be damaged or bacterial enzymes inhibited.

The nitrofurans are active against gram-negative bacilli, although *P. aeruginosa* is resistant. Staphylococci and *S. faecalis* are also susceptible and there is some activity against anaerobic bacteria. Although resistant strains occur, there has not been a notable increase in resistance over the years, and plasmid mediated resistance has not been reported.

Nitrofurantoin is the most widely used member of the nitrofurans. Oral administration of the crystalline or macrocrystalline form is readily absorbed from the upper gastrointestinal tract. However, serum concentrations are low since the drug is rapidly degraded and excreted in the urine where therapeutic concentrations are achieved. In the presence of renal failure urinary concentrations fall to subtherapeutic levels, hence the drug is contraindicated in renal failure. There is little difference in the excretion of the crystalline or macrocrystalline forms.

Among the other nitrofurans, furazolidone has been used orally in the treatment of gastrointestinal salmonella and shigella infections while nitrofurazone is available for topical use, particularly in patients suffering from burns or requiring skin grafting.

Nitrofurantoin is the only commonly used member of this group and its primary indication is for the treatment of susceptible urinary tract infections. There is no indication for the parenteral use of this drug. Nitrofurantoin also has been used in the chemoprophylaxis of recurrent urinary tract infection. Resistance does not appear to develop and the gastrointestinal flora is little affected.

Gastrointestinal intolerance, producing nausea, vomiting, and upper abdominal discomfort, is relatively frequent, although diarrhea is uncommon. The macrocrystalline preparation is claimed to be better tolerated. Hypersensitivity reactions are uncommon but present with rashes, drug fever, and eosinophilia. Nitrofurantoin may also produce an acute pneumonitis, characterized by cough, dyspnea, fever, and infiltrates on radiographic examination. This reaction tends to occur soon after administration and is probably allergic. Less frequently, a progressive diffuse interstitial pneumonitis with pulmonary fibrosis has followed long-term therapy. This may be only partly reversible.

Other side effects include peripheral neuropathy, which is more common in patients on long-term treatment and with renal insufficiency, hepatotoxicity, hemolytic and megaloblastic anemia, bone marrow depression, and an Antabuse-reaction.

Methenamine

Methenamine is a chemotherapeutic agent which is inactive until hydrolyzed in an acid environment (pH 5.5) to formaldehyde and ammonia. The former is the active agent and has well-known bactericidal properties by denaturing DNA and protein. The drug is used for the treatment of urinary tract infections provided the urinary pH can be maintained low enough for hydrolysis to occur.

Formaldehyde is active against all bacteria. However, in the treatment of urinary tract infections caused by *Proteus* spp the urine is generally too alkaline for sufficient breakdown and production of formaldehyde.

Methenamine is readily absorbed from the upper gastrointestinal tract and distributed widely throughout the body but remains inactive since formaldehyde is not produced at normal body pH. The drug is readily excreted in the urine. To produce an acid urine, methenamine is available as a mandelic acid or hippuric acid salt which renders the urine more acid.

Methenamine as the mandelate or hippurate is restricted to the treatment of urinary tract infections. Owing to the availability of more active agents these salts are not commonly used. They may be of benefit in long, suppressive treatment of urinary tract infections once the urine has been rendered sterile by another agent.

Gastrointestinal intolerance may occur but in general the compounds are well tolerated. Nonetheless, the generation of formaldehyde within an inflamed bladder may of itself produce symptoms of dysuria, frequency, and hematuria.

Selected Bibliography

Barza, M.: Antimicrobial spectrum, pharmacology, and therapeutic use of antibiotics. II. Penicillins. *Am J Hosp Pharm* 34:57, 1977.

Barza, M. and Miao, P. V. W.: Antimicrobial spectrum, pharmacology, and therapeutic use of antibiotics. III. Cephalosporins. *Am J Hosp Pharm* 34:621, 1977.

Barza, M. and Schiefe, R. T.: Antimicrobial spectrum, pharmacology, and therapeutic use of antibiotics. I. Tetracyclines. *Am J Hosp Pharm* 34:49, 1977.

Barza, M. and Schiefe, R. T.: Antimicrobial spectrum, pharmacology and therapeutic use of antibiotics. IV. Aminoglycosides. *Am J Hosp Pharm* 34:723, 1977.

Cook, F. V. and Farrar, W. E.: Vancomycin revisited. *Ann Intern Med* 88:813, 1978.

Gleckman, R., Alvarez, S., and Joubert, D. W.: Drug therapy reviews: Nalidixic acid. *Am J Hosp Pharm* 36:342, 1979.

Gleckman, R., Alvarez, S., and Joubert, D. W.: Drug therapy reviews: Nitrofurantoin. *Am J Hosp Pharm* 36:342, 1979.

Gleckman, R., Alvarez, S., Joubert, D. W., and Matthew, S. J.: Drug therapy reviews: Methenamine mandelate and methenamine hippurate. *Am J Hosp Pharm* 36:1509, 1979.

Gleckman, R., Alvarez, S., and Joubert, D. W.: Drug therapy reviews: Trimethoprim-sulfamethoxazole. *Am J Hosp Pharm* 36:893, 1979.

Neu, H. C. (ed.): Tetracyclines: A major appraisal. *Bull N Y Acad Med* 54:141, 1978.

Neu, H. C.: The new beta-lactamase-stable cephalosporins. *Ann Intern Med* 97:408, 1982.

Nicholap, P.: Erythromycin: Clinical review. I. Clinical pharmacology. *N Y State J Med* 77:2088, 1977.

7

TREATMENT OF VIRAL INFECTIONS
Robert H. Waldman, M.D.

The need for antiviral drugs is obvious. Since viral infections are so common, causing a tremendous amount of morbidity and some mortality, one could ask why a country that can put a man on the moon cannot do a better job of developing safe and effective antiviral agents. The reason is severalfold:

1. Most important is the intimate biochemical relationship between the viral replication process and the normal metabolic processes of the host cell. Stated another way, the virus actually becomes a part of the host cell, or more accurately, takes over the metabolism of the cell.
2. There are very few enzymes unique to viral replication. This means that there are very few steps in the viral life cycle having enzymes that could be potentially blocked without harming the host cell.
3. There is a disappointing lack of correlation between in vitro studies, animal models, and results in humans. It is unclear why this is true, but to some extent this may be because certain drugs do not penetrate well into tissues, and/or there are metabolic differences between cells of different species or even between different organs in the same species.
4. There have been no outstanding successes that would help in selecting model test systems. This is in contradistinction to the antibacterial area, where the early success with penicillin led to the development of the test systems that have been used for the identification, isolation, and evaluation of virtually all successive antibacterial agents.
5. Viruses mutate readily, leading to ease in appearance of resistant strains.

The steps in viral infection are outlined in Table 7.1. As should be obvious, the earlier in the process that an antiviral agent works, the better the expected results with respect to effectiveness and lack of toxicity for the host cell.

TABLE 7.1   Steps in Viral Infections

---

1. Attachment

2. Penetration

3. Uncoating

4. DNA viruses code for mRNA (transcription)

5. Synthesis of viral proteins (translation)

6. Replication of viral nucleic acid

7. Assembly

8. Release

For convenience, this chapter will be divided into two main sections: specific, meaning the use of agents that are more or less specific for viral infections; and nonspecific approaches, i.e., general approaches to the care of patients with viral infections. Agents or therapeutic approaches that are specific for a certain viral infection will be mentioned only briefly, with reference to the chapter dealing with that infectious agent.

Specific Therapy

This section will be subdivided into a discussion of those agents mainly used for disseminated viral infections, and a subsection dealing with localized infections.

Disseminated Infections

Adenine Arabinoside (Vidarabine or Vira-A)

Vidarabine is approved for the treatment of herpes simplex encephalitis and also may be beneficial against others of the herpes group of viruses. In people with compromised host defenses who are infected with herpes zoster, vidarabine leads to accelerated clearing of virus from vesicles, cessation of new vesicle formation, and a shorter time to total pustulation. It is most effective when given in the first 6 days. Significant benefit can only be shown in patients with reticuloendothelial neoplasia because these patients are at a greater risk for dissemination. Patients with normal host defenses have such a low risk of an adverse outcome that there is little benefit to be derived from treatment. In a double-blind study comparing vidarabine and placebo, by day 5, 46% of the placebo group showed improvement, whereas 83% of the drug group were improved (Table 7.2).

In herpes simplex encephalitis, vidarabine reduced the mortality from 70 to 28%. No benefit could be demonstrated in patients who were already comatose at the start of therapy. Therefore, it is of great importance to make the diagnosis early and begin prompt therapy.

TABLE 7.2   Pain in Immunocompromised Patients with Herpes Zoster Treated with Adenine Arabinoside (Ara-A)

	Treatment Group		
Response	Ara-A	Placebo	P
Improved	83%	46%	0.001
No change or worse	17%	54%	

The recommended dose is 15 mg/kg/day for 10 days, given as continuous or every 12-hr infusions. There is minimal clinical toxicity, mainly related to the gastrointestinal tract and bone marrow suppression. Toxicity is due to the mode of action of the drug, which is to decrease normal synthesis of DNA, leading to decreased production of the DNA virus in the host cells. The drug also affects DNA synthesis by other cells in the host, particularly those which are rapidly dividing as are those of the gastrointestinal tract and bone marrow.

There have been case reports suggesting that the drug is effective in encephalitis caused by cytomegalovirus and varicella virus, but lacking suitable controls these are hard to interpret.

Acyclovir

Acylovir is a newly available antiviral agent that is of great interest, not only because of its effectiveness but also because of its unique mechanism of action. Acyclovir is phosphorylated by viral thymidine kinase to acyclovir monophosphate, which is further phosphorylated to acyclovir triphosphate. This compound inhibits viral DNA polymerase and is also incorporated into viral DNA. Uninfected cells convert very little acyclovir to acyclovir triphosphate. The ointment form of acyclovir has been tested in double-blind trials of genital and oral herpes simplex, and there has been some benefit shown. The drug is also absorbed orally, thus it may be useful as an oral agent against the herpes group of viruses. Acyclovir is relatively nontoxic, but has been reported to cause renal damage. There is also the concern that herpes simplex virus may develop resistance during the course of treatment.

Cytosine Arabinoside

An analogue of adenine arabinoside, cytosine arabinoside has been ineffective in controlled clinical trials.

Rifampicin

Rifampicin, which is effective against a wide spectrum of infectious agents, also inhibits RNA-dependent DNA polymerase of certain viruses, particularly the oncornaviruses, and blocks synthesis of viral protein. It has some tissue culture activity against pox- and herpesviruses. There have been no clinical trials published.

Methisazone

Methisazone, which inhibits synthesis of structural proteins necessary for completion of viral assembly, is specific for smallpox and will be discussed in Chapter 69.

Localized Viral Infections

2^1-Deoxy-5-Iodouridine (Idoxuridine or IDU)

Idoxuridine is somewhat effective in herpetic keratitis and will be discussed in more detail in Chapter 66.

Amantadine

Amantadine is specific for influenza A virus infection and will be discussed in more detail in Chapter 48. An experimental agent, *ribavirin* may have some degree of effectiveness against influenza viruses, and possibly other viruses, such as hepatitis B. Most of its testing has been done with respect to influenza; therefore it also will be discussed in Chapter 48.

Other agents have been tested for use in localized herpes simplex infections such as *Ara-A, trifluorothymidine, trichlorthymidine, photodynamic inactivation, and phosphonoacetic acid,* and these will be discussed in Chapter 66.

Nonspecific Therapy

One of the most interesting developments in the treatment of viral infections has been the use of immune enhancers. This approach is very appealing, since it would work to improve the host defenses, thereby avoiding the toxicity of the antiviral agents which, almost by necessity, have an effect on the metabolism of the host's cells. There are several problems with this approach, however, and among these are that while a great deal is known about immunology as related to viral infections, we are still far from knowing exactly what mechanisms protect us against infection and, possibly different, the mechanisms that cause viral infections to end. In addition, the immune response is extremely complicated, and it is difficult to know if one will obtain a beneficial result by enhancing it. For example, should one be stimulating helper T cells or suppressor T cells and is it possible to differentially stimulate one and not the other?

Levamisole

The most widely studied immune enhancer has been levamisole. This agent appears to restore immune function particularly cell-mediated immunity in animals and people with impaired function. It seems to have little or no enhancing activity in people with normal immune responses. In a study that has very many interesting aspects, but at the same time is open to many potential criticisms, a group of children with recurrent upper respiratory infections were placed on either placebo or levamisole. During the course of the winter, the severity of their symptoms was subjectively compared with the previous winter. In the placebo group, about 7% felt much better than the previous year, whereas in the levamisole group, 54% were much better.

Inosiplex (Isoprinosine)

Inosiplex is another drug that has been shown to have immunoenhancing activity. Clinical trials have led to mixed results, but in one interesting study with induced rhinovirus infection in volunteers, there was a 70% reduction in symptoms in the Isoprinosine group and of potentially greater importance, it was shown that the drug worked therapeutically, i.e., after challenge, as well as when used prophylactically. In artificially induced influenza virus infection, in several trials, Isoprinosine has been shown to be effective, either when started before challenge or after. Isoprinosine has also been shown to give dramatic results in children with subacute sclerosing panencephalitis (SSPE). The mechanism of action of Isoprinosine is complex but may be related to the fact that it seems to enhance the T-cell responses, both in normal and in immunosuppressed subjects.

Transfer Factor

Transfer factor is a small-molecular-weight substance produced by T lymphocytes in response to a mitogen or to a specific antigen. The transfer factor's function is to recruit uncommitted T cells so that they function as "sensitized" lymphocytes, reacting to the specific antigen. Transfer factor can be prepared from donors who have potent cell-mediated immunity (CMI) to a virus. When this transfer factor is administered to a recipient who is infected with that virus theoretically, since CMI is probably the most important host defense mechanism in all but a few viral infections, the infected person should be better able to handle the infection. However, the results have not lived up to expectations, although case reports suggesting benefit in hepatitis B, cytomegalovirus, and other viral infections, have been published.

Gamma Globulin

The effectiveness of gamma globulin (i.e., IgG preparations) in preventing or modulating certain viral infections would seem to argue against the earlier statement about the importance of CMI. However, it is probable that various types of host defenses have a major or minor role in all infections, i.e., that while "certain instruments may have lead parts, all of them are important in the complex symphony" which is our immune system. Gamma globulin preparations may be *nonspecific,* i.e., pooled from randomly selected donors, or *specific,* prepared from donors known to have high titers of antibody against the pathogen. The latter is preferable in most situations, with the former effective if antibody is possessed at reasonable titers by most people. Table 7.3 shows the situations in which gamma globulin has been shown to be effective. One limitation on the use of gamma globulin has been the inability to use it intravenously because in the preparation process aggregation of the IgG occurs. This aggregated IgG may fix complement when given intravenously, leading to vascular collapse on occasion. Newer preparations are available which avoid this aggregation, and therefore higher titers of antibody might be attained in a seriously ill recipient.

Interferon

Interferon is a class of proteins capable of inhibiting virus replication in vertebrate cells. Interferon is produced in host cells in response to a wide range of stimuli, including viruses, other intracellular parasites, and synthetic polynucleotides. It is effective by inducing an intracellular polypeptide which interferes with translation of viral-coded messages. This agent appears to be effective

TABLE 7.3   Use of Immune Serum Globulin (Gamma Globulin)
In Viral Infections

Shown to be effective in prevention or modification
of measles, hepatitis A, and hepatitis B

Possibly effective

Prevention of rubella in pregnancy
Modification of varicella

"Specific" (high-titer antibody) human immune globulin
preparations

Licensed

Mumps immune globulin
Rabies immune globulin
Vaccinia immune globulin
Hepatitis B immune globulin

Under development

Rubella immune globulin
Zoster immune globulin
Western equine encephalitis immune globulin

---

during the first 3-4 days of viral infection, at which time the host cells become
refractory to the action of interferon for a short time. It is nonimmunogenic but
is not without side effects, although some or most of these side effects may actually be a result of contaminating substances which are invariably found in
batches of interferon.

Three interferons can be distinguished chemically and antigenically. Human
leukocyte interferon is induced in leukocytes obtained from blood donors who have
been virally stimulated. This interferon is a glycoprotein made up of two components with a total molecular weight of approximately 35,000. Human fibroblast
interferon, also a glycoprotein, has a molecular weight of about 20,000. It has
been prepared from cultured fibroblasts stimulated with a synthetic polynucleo-
tide. Immune interferon is produced primarily by T lymphocytes in response to
antigens or mitogens.

Interferon administration, in the large doses necessary to treat viral infections, nearly always causes fever, liver-function test abnormalities, as well as
malaise, fatigue, anorexia, mild hair loss, reversible leukopenia, and thrombocytopenia. In most of the well-controlled, published studies on interferon
therapy, the benefit has been modest at best (Table 7.4). The side effects that
are seen with interferon make it questionable whether or not the slight clinical
benefit, on balance, is worthwhile. This question would be pertinent even if interferon production were easy and inexpensive; however currently, this is not the
case. Adequate amounts of interferon are difficult and expensive to produce.

TABLE 7.4   Interferon in Treatment of Herpes Zoster in Patients with Cancer

	Placebo	Interferon
Spread in primary dermatome	↑2.5 x 3.9 days	↑1.5 x 1.6 days
Distal cutaneous spread	5/15	0/15
Postherpetic neuralgia	5/14	5/14

The material that is currently undergoing clinical testing is extremely heterogeneous, and it is even questionable if the observed effects are due to interferon or to some other factor that may be contaminating the material.

A way around some of the problems mentioned above is the use of "genetic engineering." There is work on using a plasmid containing the DNA code for production of interferon that might be introduced into an easily grown bacterium. This could make it possible to produce very large amounts of interferon much more economically. Another alternative approach is the use of interferon inducers, i.e., inducing the person to produce his/her own endogenous interferon. Polyriboinosinic-polyribocytidylic acid is an effective interferon inducer, but it is too toxic for general use. Propanediamine derivatives have been somewhat successful, when given intranasally, in inducing a local interferon which can protect against rhinovirus infection. A problem with interferon inducers is that there is a hyporesponsive state that develops for several days after the administration of the inducer, but this problem may be solved by the finding that, at least in mice, prostaglandins reverse the hyporesponsive state.

Another question that might be raised about interferon is that if it works, why does the viral infection not cure itself. This might be the main mechanism whereby viral infections cease, but some viruses, hepatitis B being a good example, are sensitive to the action of interferon but are poor inducers. Thus these viruses do not induce enough interferon in the host to have a significant effect on the course of the infection, but exogenous interferon, or more potent interferon inducers, might be of great benefit.

Ascorbic Acid

Ascorbic acid (vitamin C) has received a great deal of public notice in the past few years especially with respect to prevention or treatment of respiratory viral infections. Therefore, this subject will be discussed in more detail in Chapter 11.

Antipyretics

Although on the surface it would seem to be a mundane question, the role of antipyretics in the general supportive care of a patient with a viral infection is of potentially great importance with respect to morbidity. Adding to the relevance of the question is that it is widely accepted that aspirin or acetaminophen should be used, almost in a reflex manner, in any patient with a cold or other mild to moderate viral or bacterial illness. Add to this, the tremendous advertising campaign that innundates the homes of Americans telling them: "Most doctors recommend Tylenol or Bayer aspirin for the treatment of colds or flu." Certainly these agents lower the temperature and relieve aches and pains, and if there is no evidence that they are harmful, then this would certainly be a justification for their use. Unfortunately, despite the widespread use for many years, the data are extremely meager.

From the theoretical point of view, one could make a fairly good argument against the use of antipyretics. Fever might be a normal host defense mechanism since this complex pathophysiologic mechanism probably developed evolutionally to serve some useful purpose. Most infectious agents grow best at 37°C, and grow much less well, or not at all, at 38-40°C. Viruses are especially sensitive to temperatures above 37°C. In fact, influenza virus grows best at 36°C, and rhinovirus at 33°C. So one could argue that fever is important in limiting the growth of viral agents in the body. Therefore bringing down the temperature might be adverse to the host. In addition, there is experimental evidence that aspirin is somewhat of an immunosuppressant agent.

There is also some experimental evidence in both animals and humans that lowering the body temperature has an adverse effect on the outcome of certain infections. In one study in human volunteers infected with rhinovirus, the group that was given aspirin had a longer duration of infection than did the group that was given placebo.

In summary, with respect to antipyretics, there are certainly insufficient data to come to any conclusion, and therefore it would be inappropriate to recommend antipyretics not be used because they certainly are effective in lowering the body temperature when fever might be at a dangerous level, as in young infants, and they ease many of the symptoms of mild viral infections. On the other hand, it would seem prudent to recommend their judicious use, especially with respect to situations where they would not be expected to be useful such as rhinorrhea or cough. Also controversial is the role of aspirin in the pathogenesis of Reye's syndrome.

Another classic recommendation in the management of mild to moderate viral infections is the use of bed rest. There is neither theoretical nor experimental evidence that rest is of any therapeutic value, other than the psychologic benefit that might accrue to the patient, and the public health value of removing an infected person from society. Attempts to show a deleterious effect of exercise on the course of hepatitis have been unsuccessful.

Selected Bibliography

Balfour, H. H., Jr., Groth, K. E., McCullough, J., Kalis, J. M., Marker, S. C., Nesbit, M. E., Simmons, R. L., and Najarian, J. S.: Prevention or modification of varicella using zoster immune plasma. *Am J Dis Child* 131:693-696, 1977.

Borden, E. C.: Interferons: Rationale for clinical trials in neoplastic disease. *Ann Intern Med* 91:472-479, 1979.

Cheeseman, S. H., Rubin, R. H., Stewart, M. D., et al.: Controlled clinical trial of human leukocyte interferon in renal transplantation. 1. Effects on cytomegalovirus and herpes simplex virus infections. *N Engl J Med* 300:1345-1349, 1979.

Ch'ien, L. T., Benton, J. W., Buchanan, R. A., and Alford, C. A.: Adenine arabinoside treatment of severe pox and herpetic infections of man. *Pediatr Res* 6:384, 1972.

Corey, L., Reeves, W. C., Chaing, W. T., et al.: Ineffectiveness of topical ether for the treatment of genital herpes simplex virus infection. *N Engl J Med* 299:237, 1978.

Felber, T. D., Smith, E. B., Knox, J. M., Wallis, C., and Melnick, J. L.: Photodynamic inactivation of herpes simplex. *JAMA* 223:289-292, 1973.

Field, A. K., Young, C. W., Kraoff, I. H., Tytell, A. A., Lampson, G. P., Nemes, M. M., and Hilleman, M. R.: Induction of interferon in human subjects by poly I:C. *Proc Soc Exp Biol Med* 136:1180-1186, 1971.

Galbraith, M. B., Oxford, J. S., Schild, G. G., and Watson, G. I.: Protective effect of aminoadamantane on influenza A_2 infections in the family environment. *Ann N Y Acad Sci* 173:29-43, 1970.

Greenbag, H. B., Pollard, R. B., Luturk, L. I., et al.: Effect of human leucocyte interferon on hepatitis B virus infection in patients with chronic active hepatitis. *N Engl J Med* 295:517-522, 1976.

Hill, D. A., Baron, S., Perkins, J. C., Worthington, M., VanKirk, J. E., Mills, J., Kapikian, A. Z., and Chanock, R. M.: Evaluation of an interferon inducer in viral respiratory disease. *JAMA* 219:1179-1184, 1972.

Hilleman, M. R.: Double-stranded RNAs (poly I:C) in the prevention of viral infections. *Arch Intern Med* 126:109-124, 1970.

Pazin, G. J., Armstrong, J. A., Lam, M. T., Tan, G. C., Jannetta, P. J., and Ho, M.: Prevention of reactivated herpes simplex infection by human leukocyte interferon after operation on the trigeminal root. *N Engl J Med* 301:225-230, 1979.

Pitt, H. A. and Costrini, A. M.: Vitamin C prophylaxis in marine recruits. *JAMA* 241:980, 1979.

Stevens, D. A., Jordan, G. W., Waddell, T. F., and Merigan, T. C.: Adverse effect of arabinoside on disseminated zoster in a controlled trial. *N Engl J Med* 289:873-878, 1973.

Waldman, R. H. and Ganguly, R.: Effect of CP-20,961, an interferon inducer, on upper respiratory tract infections due to rhinovirus type 21 in volunteers. *J Infect Dis* 138:531-535, 1978.

Weinstein, L. and Chang, T.: The chemotherapy of viral infections. *N Engl J Med* 289:725-730, 1973.

Whitley, R. J., Ch'ien, L. T., Dolin, R., Galasso, G. J., and Alford, C. A., Jr.: Adenine arabinoside therapy of herpes zoster in the immunosuppressed. *N Engl J Med* 294:1193-1199, 1976.

Whitley, R. J., Soong, S. G., Dolin, R., Galasso, G. J., Ch'ien, L. T., and Alford, C. A.: Adenine arabinoside therapy of biopsy-proved herpes simplex virus encephalitis. *N Engl J Med* 297:289-294, 1977.

8

ANTIMICROBIAL USE IN RENAL OR LIVER DISEASE
Ronica M. Kluge, M.D.

Introduction

The basic pharmacologic principles related to absorption, distribution, metabolism, and excretion of antimicrobial agents are outlined in Chapter 5. This chapter will discuss the factors to be considered in modifying antimicrobial therapy for patients with renal or liver dysfunction. Because the kidney and liver serve as the major, if not the only, routes for excretion and/or inactivation of antimicrobial agents, one must know the patient's renal and kidney function both before and during administration of the drugs.

Renal Disease

Most antimicrobial agents are eliminated primarily by the kidneys; these drugs require modification of dosage and/or dose interval in the face of renal failure (Table 8.1). Some antimicrobials are contraindicated in renal failure (Table 8.2). Other antimicrobials are excreted or detoxified primarily by the liver and do not require dosage modification in the patient with renal dysfunction (Table 8.3)

Make an initial assessment of the patient's renal function based on the serum creatinine level and the creatinine clearance if at all possible. Patients with mild to moderate renal dysfunction are those with a serum creatinine level of 1.5–5.0 mg/dl and a creatinine clearance of 20–80 ml/min. Patients with severe renal impairment have a serum creatinine level above 5 mg/dl and a clearance of less than 20 ml/min. Antimicrobial dosages can be modified by decreasing the unit dose or by increasing the interval between doses. Table 8.4 outlines recommended dosage modifications for the most commonly used antimicrobials in the face of varying degrees of renal impairment. Table 8.5 lists those antimicrobials

TABLE 8.1   Antimicrobials that Require Dosage Modification in
Patients with Renal Dysfunction

Mild to moderate dysfunction

Aminoglycosides	Cephalexin
Carbenicillin	Polymyxins
Ticarcillin	Vancomycin
Cefazolin	5-Flucytosine

Severe dysfunction

Penicillin	Cefoxitin
Ampicillin	Lincomycin
Methicillin	Isoniazid
Cephalothin	Ethambutol
Cefamandole	Trimethoprim-sulfamethoxazole

TABLE 8.2   Antimicrobials that Are to be Avoided in Patients
with Renal Dysfunction

Cephaloridine	Nalidixic acid
Tetracycline	Neomycin
Methenamine mandelate	Para-aminosalicylic acid
Nitrofurantoin	Spectinomycin

Long-acting sulfonamides

TABLE 8.3   Antimicrobials that Do Not Require Dosage Modification in
Patients with Renal Dysfunction

Chloramphenicol	Oxacillin
Clindamycin	Cloxacillin
Erythromycin	Dicloxacillin
Doxycycline	Nafcillin
Rifampin	Amphotericin B

Miconazole

TABLE 8.4   Dose Modifications for Selected Antimicrobials in Patients with Renal Dysfunction

Drug	Dose Modification Mild to Moderate	Dose Modification Severe
Penicillin G	None	1.0-1.5 million U q6h
Ampicillin	None	0.5-1.0 g q8h
Methicillin	None	1.0-2.0 g q8h
Carbenicillin	3.0g q4h	2.0 g q12h
Ticarcillin	None	2.0 g q12h
Cephalothin	None	1.0 g q8h
Cefazolin	0.5g q12h	0.5g q24h
Cefamandole	None	1.0 g q12h
Cefoxitin	None	1.0 g q12h
Cephalexin	None	250-500 mg q12h
Streptomycin	0.5 g qd	0.5 g q3d
Kanamycin	7.5 mg/kg q (serum creatinine X 9) h*	
Gentamicin	1.5 mg/kg q (serum creatinine X 8) h*	
Tobramycin	1.5 mg/kg q (serum creatinine X 6) h*	
Amikacin	7.5 mg/kg q (serum creatinine X 9) h*	
Polymyxin	2.5 mg/kg x 1 dose, then 1 mg/kg q3-7d	
Colistin	150 mg qd	150 mg q2-4d
Vancomycin	1 g qd	1 g q7d
Trimethoprim-sulfamethoxazole	1 tab q12h	1 tab q24h
Isoniazid	None	200 mg qd
Ethambutol	None	5-10 mg/kg qd
5-Flucytosine	37.5 mg/kg q12h	37.5 mg/kg qd

*May wish to give half the dose at half the calculated interval

TABLE 8.5   Antimicrobials That Require a Further Dose After Hemodialysis

Aminoglycosides	Sulfonamides
Cephalosporins	Chloramphenicol
Penicillin	Trimethoprim
Ampicillin	Cycloserine
Carbenicillin	Ethambutol
Ticarcillin	5-Flucytosine

TABLE 8.6   Antimicrobials That Require Dosage Modifications in Patients with Liver Dysfunction

Drug	Modification
Tetracycline	Reduce to one-third to one-half normal, or avoid
Erythromycin	Estolate and proprionate forms to be avoided
Clindamycin	Reduce to one-third to one-half normal
Isoniazid	Reduce to one-half to two-thirds normal
Rifampin	Reduce to one-half to two-thirds normal, or avoid
Chloramphenicol	Reduce to one-third to one-half normal

that are hemodialyzed in significant amounts, thereby requiring an additional dose after hemodialysis. It is extremely important to continue close monitoring of the patient's renal function during therapy and to make further dosage modifications as needed. Whenever possible, determination of peak and trough serum concentrations of the antibiotic should be made to assist in maintenance of appropriate levels without courting additional renal toxicity. Most hospital laboratories can now measure aminoglycoside levels with a high degree of accuracy; serum concentrations of other antimicrobials may be available from reference laboratories.

Liver Disease

Those antimicrobial agents that are primarily excreted or detoxified by the liver probably should be administered in reduced dosage to patients with preexisting liver disease (Table 8.6). There are few data on which to base the calculated reductions; these recommendations represent a "best guess." Functional liver cell mass, obstruction to bile flow, and inducible oxidative enzyme systems are important factors governing drug metabolism in patients with liver disease. The presence of ascites increases the extracellular fluid volume and therefore the distribution volume of some antibiotics (e.g., penicillins, aminoglycosides). If the patient's albumin is decreased, there may be more free antibiotic available in the serum. In the patient with acute hepatitis, metabolism of the drug may be impaired. It must be remembered that drugs metabolized primarily in the liver may also be hepatotoxic.

The ideal way to follow patients with liver disease who require treatment with antimicrobials detoxified by the liver would be to obtain periodic serum samples for drug concentrations. Unfortunately, these measurements are not available in the usual hospital laboratory.

Selected Bibliography

Appel, G. B. and Neu, H. C.: The nephrotoxicity of antimicrobial agents. *N Engl J Med* 296:663-670, 722-728, 784-787, 1977.

Barrett, S. P. and Watt, P. J.: Antibiotics and the liver. *J Antimicrob Chemother* 5:337-348, 1979.

Bennett, W. M., Muther, R. S., Parker, R. A., Feig, P., Morrison, G., Golper, T. A., and Singer, I.: Drug therapy in renal failure: Dosing guidelines for adults. *Ann Intern Med* 93:62-89, 1980.

Dulger, R. J., Lindholm, D. D., Murray, J. S., and Kirby, W. M. M.: Effect of uremia on methicillin and oxacillin blood levels. *JAMA* 187:319-322, 1964.

Cheigh, J. S.: Drug administration in renal failure. *Am J Med* 62:555-563, 1977.

Czerwinski, A. W., Pedersen, J. A., and Barry, J. P.: Cefazolin plasma concentrations and urinary excretion in patients with renal impairment. *J Clin Pharmacol* 14:560-566, 1974.

Davies, M., Morgan, J. R., and Anand, C.: Administration of ticarcillin to patients with severe renal failure. *Chemotherapy* 20:339-341, 1974.

Fass, R. J. and Saslaw, S.: Clindamycin: Clinical and laboratory evaluation of parenteral therapy. *Am J Med Sci* 263:369-382, 1972.

Garcia, M. J., Dominguez-Gil, A., Tabernero, J. M., and Tomero, J. A. S.: Pharmacokinetics of cefoxitin in patients with normal or impaired renal function. *Eur J Clin Pharmacol* 16:119-124, 1979.

Hoffman, T. A., Cestero, R., and Bullock, W. E.: Pharmacodynamics of carbenicillin in hepatic and renal failure. *Ann Intern Med* 73:173-178, 1970.

Humbert, G., Spyker, D. A., Fillastre, J. P., and Leroy, A.: Pharmacokinetics of amoxicillin: Dosage nomogram for patients with impaired renal function. *Antimicrob Agents Chemother* 15:28-33, 1979.

Jusko, W. J., Lewis, G. P., and Schmitt, G. W.: Ampicillin and hetacillin pharmacokinetics in normal and anephric subjects. *Clin Pharmacol Ther* 14:90-99, 1972.

Kirby, W. M. M., DeMaine, J. B., and Serril, W. S.: Pharmacokinetics of the cephalosporins in healthy volunteers and uremic patients. *Postgrad Med J* 47(supp.):41-46, 1971.

Leroy, A., Humbert, G., Oksenhandler, G., Fillastre, J. P.: Pharmacokinetics of aminoglycosides in subjects with normal and impaired renal function. *Antibiotics Chemother* 25:163-180, 1978.

Maher, J. F.: Principles of dialysis and dialysis of drugs. *Am J Med* 62:475-481, 1977.

Mellin, H. E., Welling, P. G., and Madsen, P. O.: Pharmacokinetics of cefamandole in patients with normal and impaired renal function. *Antimicrob Agents Chemother* 11:262-266, 1977.

Moellering, R. C., Jr., Krogstad, D. J., and Greenbelt, D. J.: Vancomycin therapy in patients with impaired renal function: A nomogram for dosage. *Ann Intern Med* 94:343-346, 1981.

Nauta, E. H. and Mattie, H.: Dicloxacillin and cloxacillin: Pharmacokinetics in healthy and hemodialysis subjects. *Clin Pharmacol Ther* 20:98-108, 1976.

Reidenberg, M. M. and Drayer, D. E.: Drug therapy in renal failure. *Ann Rev Pharmacol Toxicol* 20:45-54, 1980.

Rudnick, M., Morrison, G., Walker, B., and Singer, I.: Renal failure, hemodialysis and nafcillin kinetics. *Clin Pharmacol Ther* 20:413-423, 1976.

Shils, M. E.: Renal disease and the metabolic effects of tetracycline. *Ann Intern Med* 58:389-408, 1963.

Spyker, D. A., Thomas, B.L., Sande, M. A., and Bolton, W. K.: Pharmacokinetics of cefaclor and cephalexin: Dosage nomograms for impaired renal function. *Antimicrob Agents Chemother* 14:172-177, 1978.

Suhrland, L. G. and Weisberger, A. S.: Chloramphenicol toxicity in liver and renal disease. *Arch Intern Med* 112:747-754, 1963.

Van Scoy, R. E. and Wilson, W. R.: Antimicrobial agents in patients with renal insufficiency. *Mayo Clin Proc* 52:704-706, 1977.

Weinstein, L. and Dalton, A. C.: Host determinants of response to antimicrobial agents. *N Engl J Med* 279:467-473, 1968.

9

BASIC BACTERIOLOGY
Roger G. Finch, M. B.

Introduction

The ability to isolate and identify pathogenic microorganisms from clinical specimens is an essential part of the diagnosis and management of infectious diseases. In addition, environmental sampling, including samples from persons who are suspected carriers of pathogenic microorganisms, provides epidemiologic information for the recognition and control of both hospital-acquired disease and public health hazards of an infectious nature.

Reliable information is dependent upon the quality of sampling, the speed of delivery to the laboratory, as well as the quality of the many laboratory techniques aimed at isolation and identification of pathogenic organisms.

Correct interpretation of culture results is vital for patient care and requires an understanding of the range of pathogens associated with specific disease processes, such as pneumonia and urinary tract infections, as well as an awareness of the normal microbiologic flora at a particular site. The interrelationship between the normal flora and hospital microbial flora is such that many infections are caused by such organisms that have become part of the patient's own normal flora. This occurs most frequently when the ecological balance is disturbed by disease or treatment such as the use of broad-spectrum antibiotics, corticosteroid drugs, or immunosuppressive therapy.

Other diagnostic techniques include a variety of serologic tests aimed at detecting microbial antigens in body fluids or measuring the host's responses. Such antibody responses are by their nature usually of retrospective value only.

Another important area for the laboratory is determining the susceptibility of pathogenic microorganisms to antimicrobial agents appropriate to the disease. Some bacteria, such as streptococci, have predictable sensitivity patterns but many, particularly gram-negative facultative* bacteria, show a wide range of resistance to antibiotics.

Sample Collection

The collection of material for microbiologic staining and culture should ensure that it is processed in the optimum manner to yield information that is either diagnostic or confirmatory of a disease process and compatible with the clinical assessment of the patient. General points to consider are:

1. Whenever possible collect samples for cultures before antimicrobial drugs are used
2. Collection into sterile containers or by sterile swabs avoiding contamination by patient's own normal flora
3. Collection of material such as blood, spinal fluid, joint fluid, ascites, or pleural effusion requires strict attention to aseptic technique
4. Prompt delivery of samples to the laboratory is essential to prevent loss of fastidious, or overgrowth of the hardier, organisms and thereby prevent misleading culture results (refrigeration of urine specimens is particularly important if semiquantitative culture techniques are to be of value)
5. Transport media are valuable for the preservation of fastidious organisms such as *Neisseria gonorrhoeae* and anaerobic bacteria (Stuarts, Carey Blair, and Transgrow transport media)
6. Pus is best aspirated in a glass needle and syringe and the needle occluded using a sterile rubber bung (this method along with prompt delivery to the laboratory, increases the chances of isolating strict anaerobic bacteria from clinical samples)
7. Correct identification of the samples and the provision of relevant clinical information, including any antibiotics in use, permits the laboratory to process the sample appropriately
8. Serologic testing frequently relies on a fourfold rise in antibody titer so that acute serum as well as convalescent samples are necessary.

Direct Examination and Staining

The value of immediate examination of a specimen submitted for culture cannot be stressed too strongly. The information is available rapidly and can both provide diagnostic evidence and suggest a therapeutic approach at least 1 day sooner than can cultural techniques.

Macroscopic Examination

A sample may be purulent, nonpurulent, serosanguinous, or hemorrhagic. Sputum is a good example for which direct inspection frequently can differentiate a salivary from a truly mucoid or purulent sample. Similarly, direct examination of spinal fluid may show turbidity, which is usually related to the cell count, and

---

*Under anaerobic or low oxygen conditions these bacteria attack carbohydrates fermentatively, but given adequate oxygen they utilize the tricarboxylic acid cycle for production of energy.

suggests a pyogenic meningitis. Pigment-producing organisms can stain purulent material: pyocyanin from some strains of *Pseudomas aeruginosa* produces a greenish tinge to purulent material. A foul odor is an important feature of pus containing anaerobic bacteria. Furthermore, if a swab of the pus fluoresces brick-red under ultraviolet light, this suggests the presence of *Bacteroides melaninogenicus.*

Microscopy

Microscopy of clinical specimens is exceedingly useful in determining the presence and morphology of bacteria and in providing an estimate of their concentration. Such staining also provides a means of classification. In addition to visualizing bacteria the cellular response can be seen and is useful in many clinical situations; e.g., the differential cell count on spinal fluid can indicate a "viral" vs "pyogenic" type of meningitis.

A variety of microscopic techniques can assist in the recognition of certain bacteria. For example, the presence of spirochetes in a syphilitic chancre can be visualized by dark-field microscopy. Fluorescent microscopy using a variety of antibody conjugates can provide rapid identification of certain bacteria such as *Streptococcus pyogenes* and *N. gonorrhoeae.*

However, the most common method of visualizing bacteria is to use the stain first described by Gram.

Gram Stain

Gram-positive organisms retain crystal violet after washing in acetone-alcohol and appear blue, whereas gram-negative bacteria, having more permeable cell walls, lose the dye and then take up the counter stain safranin and appear red. This immediately permits a morphologic distinction between cocci and bacilli and their stained appearance.

Acid-Fast Stains

These include the original Ziehl-Neelson stain and the Kinyoun modification. Mycobacteria possess a high lipid content and do not stain by Gram's method. However, by using a strong dye and heat they can retain the dye in spite of attempts to decolorize with acid-alcohol. They are therefore acid-fast. The usual stain employed is carbolfuchsin. The Kinyoun modification includes a detergent and therefore eliminates the need for heat. In addition to mycobacteria certain other organisms will also take up the stain, e.g., *Nocardia* spp. These appear morphologically distinct from mycobacteria; however, neither can be identified with certainty except by cultural methods.

Romanowsky Stains

These include both the Wright's and Giemsa stains. These are particularly useful for demonstrating parasites, such as those of malaria in peripheral erythrocytes and histoplasma in tissues. Furthermore, cellular morphology is shown well and permits differentiation of polymorphonuclear from mononuclear cells. Multinucleate giant cells also may be demonstrated in vesicular fluid from patients suffering from varicella-zoster or herpes simplex infections. This is known as the Tzanck preparation.

Others

India Ink

The India ink preparation is another useful technique for the demonstration of capsulated organisms such as *Cryptococcus neoformans* in cerebrospinal fluid. The capsule is seen as a clear halo around the yeast.

Capsule-Swelling or Quellung Test

A simple slide test, the quellung test, enables a bacterium to be serotyped using commercially available type-specific antiserum. Capsules of homologous strains become refractile and readily visible by light microscopy. Organisms that can thus be typed include capsulated strains of *Haemophilus influenzae*, *Streptococcus pneumoniae*, *Neisseria meningitidis*, and *Klebsiella* spp.

Specific Samples

Blood

Collection

Blood is collected from a peripheral vein, preferably in the antecubital fossa or distal to it following adequate skin disinfection with 70% alcohol, 2% iodine, or an iodophor, and inoculated immediately into liquid media suitable for the growth of aerobic, facultative anaerobic, or obligate anaerobic bacteria. Commonly employed media include brucella, thioglycolate, and trypticase soy broth. Commercially available broths frequently contain an atmosphere of carbon dioxide and 0.025% sodium polyanethol sulfonate (SPS) which is an anticoagulant with anti-complementary and antiphagocytic properties. The ratio of SPS to blood is critical and should be between 1:10 and 1:20. This ratio will determine the volume of blood to be collected. Studies determining the number of blood cultures necessary to diagnose bacteremia have shown that one set (aerobic and anaerobic bottle) produces a diagnostic yield of 75%, two sets 89%, and three sets 98%. Therefore, one or two sets is adequate for most clinical situations. Repeat cultures may be necessary if bacteremia has been suppressed by prior antibiotic use.

Isolation

Blood cultures are usually incubated in an atmosphere of 10% CO_2 at 35°-37°C, examined daily for growth, and subcultured at regular intervals such as 24 hr, 48 hr, and 7 days. Subculture is carried out on blood or chocolate agar, incubated in 10% CO_2 for aerobes and on blood agar for anaerobes. Prolonged incubation up to 4 weeks may be necessary for the isolation of fastidious organisms such as brucellae. Commercially available systems utilize ^{14}C-labeled glucose which when metabolized by multiplying bacteria permits the detection of $^{14}CO_2$. The system is fully automatic and allows early detection of bacteremia.

The most common blood culture isolates are staphylococci, streptococci, *Neisseria* spp, *P. aeruginosa*, *H. influenzae*, *E. coli*, *Proteus* spp, and anaerobic gram-negative rods such as *Bacteroides* spp. However, most bacteria pathogenic to man have been isolated from blood, and hence it is important to assess any positive culture result in the light of the clinical picture. "Contaminants" are bacteria introduced into the blood culture system either at the time of sample collection from inadequate skin preparation or through faulty handling in the laboratory during sample processing, notably with subculturing techniques. Diphtheroids, *S. epidermidis* and *Bacillus* spp are the most frequently isolated contaminants; however, such bacteria can assume a pathogenic role and this should be considered whenever they are isolated repeatedly from a patient with suspected infection.

Urine

Collection

The urine is sterile in health but readily supports the growth of a wide range of fecal organisms. Urinary tract infections are a common problem and rely for their diagnosis on the identification and quantitation of the pathogen. Counts of greater than 100,000 organisms/ml of urine indicate "significant" bacteriuria in a promptly processed sample or in one that has been refrigerated at 4°C within 1 hr of voiding. Counts of 10^3-10^5 of a single pathogen indicate possible, or probable infection and justify repeat sample processing.

Proper sample collection of urine is critical for diagnosis. It should be free from contamination by the normal flora of the urethra or introitus. A variety of urine collection methods are available and include a midstream specimen in the male after adequate cleansing of the glans, a clean catch sample in the female after thorough cleansing of the vulva, and a catheter sample of urine obtained by needle aspiration of the predisinfected catheter tubing in those patients with chronic indwelling catheters. It is rarely justified to catheterize a patient for the sole purpose of obtaining urine for microscopy and culture. Occasionally in the young or the bedridden elderly, a suprapubic needle aspiration of bladder urine may be the only means to obtain an uncontaminated sample.

Isolation

Microscopy of the Gram-stained or unstained sediment is helpful in determining the presence of red and white blood cells, casts, crystals, and bacteria.

Culturing on an inhibitory medium such as MacConkey or EMB agar assists in the identification of pathogens and inhibits swarming of *Proteus* spp. A semiquantitative method using a standard 0.01 ml loop provides a means of determining the bacterial count. Identification and antibiotic sensitivity testing are essential and are discussed later.

Common urinary tract pathogens reflect the normal facultative flora of the individual. *Escherichia coli, Proteus* spp, enterococci, *Klebsiella* spp, *P. aeruginosa* and *S. epidermidis* are the most common isolates although other gram-negative bacteria and yeasts can also be responsible.

Sterile pyuria is a feature of tuberculosis infection of the urinary tract. For diagnosis it is important to culture the sediment of three consecutive early morning urine samples.

The reliability of a single, clean urine sample is almost 100% in the male. In the female this figure is about 80%, and by repeat urine sampling 90 and 100% reliability can be attained when two and three cultures, respectively, are cultured.

Sputum

The human defense mechanisms maintain the bronchial airways sterile in health below the level of the carina. However, unless the mouth and oropharynx are bypassed, expectorated sputum is always contaminated to lesser or greater degrees by the normal flora of these sites.

Collection

A sputum sample for bacteriologic examination should be freshly expectorated. Salivary samples are inadequate and the culture results can be misleading. In the uncooperative, unconscious, or postoperative patient, physical methods of posturing and percussing the patient can assist with sputum collection. Early morning sputum samples are the most rewarding for the diagnosis of tuberculosis, although swallowed sputum can be sampled by early morning gastric lavage with saline or by taking laryngeal swabs under direct vision.

In the individual patient from whom it is considered important to obtain sputum free from contamination with oropharyngeal flora, transtracheal aspiration of sputum through the cricothyroid membrane can prove useful.

Processing

Sputum samples should be Gram stained promptly to determine the adequacy of the specimen as reflected by the preponderance of polymorphonuclear compared with oral squamous cells. Information concerning the presence or absence of bacteria, their morphology, and relative abundance is invaluable in making an initial assessment of the possible etiologic agents. Special stains such as the Ziehl-Neelson or its Kinyoun modification are necessary for demonstrating the presence of acid-fast bacilli.

Sputum is cultured on blood agar and chocolate blood agar which will support the growth of the majority of pathogenic bacteria. In addition, MacConkey agar is helpful for the isolation of gram-negative bacteria. It is unnecessary and misleading to culture sputum for anaerobic bacteria unless the sample was obtained by transtracheal aspiration or by surgical means.

If fungal infection is suspected clinically then culturing on Sabouraud dextrose agar is indicated. Lowenstein-Jensen egg medium remains the most useful for the culture of mycobacteria. It is not normal practice to culture for fastidious pathogens, such as *Mycoplasma pneumoniae,* which require special media to support growth.

Common bacterial respiratory pathogens include *S. pneumoniae, H. influenza,* and to a lesser extent *S. aureus, P. aeruginosa, Serratia marcescens* and *Klebsiella* spp. The isolation of *E. coli, Proteus* spp, *Acinetobacter* spp, and *Enterobacter* spp frequently reflects colonization in debilitated patients or in those who have received antimicrobial chemotherapy. Nonetheless, they can on occasion, be truly pathogenic.

Mycobacterium tuberculosis and other mycobacteria are also important pathogens. Fungi such as *Candida albicans, Aspergillus* spp, and *Cryptococcus neoformans* are diagnosed occasionally, usually in immunosuppressed patients. Thus, these fungi are considered opportunistic.

Pus

Collection

Purulent material should be collected in a sterile container and sent to the laboratory promptly for staining and culture. Pus in communication with or adjacent to mucous membranes can be anticipated to contain bacteria making up the normal flora, particularly anaerobic bacteria. In these situations, samples should be aspirated by syringe and needle and the contents dispatched immediately to the laboratory. Alternatively, an anaerobic transport system can be employed utilizing an oxygen-free environment. If pus cannot be obtained, then a swab of infected material should be placed in a transport medium, of which several are available commercially.

Processing

Microscopic examination of the stained material is useful for an initial assessment of the sample; it will indicate the presence or absence of bacteria, determine their morphology and tinctorial characteristics, and suggest the possibility of anaerobic bacteria if it appears polymicrobial in nature.

Other physical characteristics which may be useful diagnostically are the feculent smell of anaerobic pus, brick-red fluorescence under ultraviolet light which is characteristic of *B. melaninogenicus,* and the presence of sulfur granules in actinomycosis that can then be crushed between two glass slides and stained to show the characteristic morphology.

Media for the processing of purulent material usually include blood agar, EMB or MacConkey agar, and thioglycollate broth. If mycobacteria or fungi are suspected then appropriate media are inoculated.

Cerebrospinal Fluid

Collection

The necessity for adequate skin disinfection before collecting cerebrospinal fluid (CSF) cannot be stressed too strongly. The fluid should be examined macroscopically for turbidity, blood-staining, or xanthochromia. If the tap is traumatic the least blood-stained aliquot should be used to determine the cell count. If fungal or tuberculous meningitis is suspected a large volume, up to 10 ml, is desirable to improve the chance of isolating the organism. A simultaneous blood glucose determination is helpful in interpreting the CSF glucose findings.

Processing

Microscopic examination should include a cell count and differential white cell analysis before centrifugation. The sample is then centrifuged for 15 min at 2500 rpm and the sediment used for smear and culture and the supernatant for glucose and protein analysis and serologic tests. For mycobacterial or *H. influenzae* meningitis and in situations where there is a low concentration of pathogens in the CSF, centrifugation may have to be increased to $10,000 \times g$ for 60 min, although 30 min is usually adequate.

The use of 0.45 μm membrane filters is helpful for concentrating CSF samples when fungal meningitis is suspected. A nigrosin or India ink preparation of the sediment is a valuable means for determining the presence of capsulated yeasts such as *C. neoformans.*

Culture media appropriate for CSF include blood agar, chocolate blood agar, Sabouraud dextrose agar, and Lowenstein-Jensen medium.

Serologic tests on CSF can be useful for the diagnosis and monitoring of certain infections, e.g., cryptococcal antigen and antibody detection. Counterimmunoelectrophoresis (CIEP) has been popularized in recent years as a means of detecting bacterial antigens in the CSF and providing a rapid means (less than 1 hr) of diagnosis. This can be particularly useful in patients who have a negative smear and culture (e.g., patients who have been treated with antibiotics before collecting CSF).

Haemophilus influenzae, N. meningitidis, and *S. pneumoniae* are numerically the most important causes of pyogenic meningitis. However, in the neonate *E. coli* and group B streptococci are the most important pathogens. Other pathogens include *Listeria monocytogenes* and *S. aureus. Staphylococcus epidermidis* and facultative gram-negative bacilli cause infection following neurosurgical procedures.

Feces

Collection

For the recognition of enteric pathogens a fresh stool sample, promptly delivered to the laboratory, will provide the highest chance of isolation. Swabs are less reliable and care must be taken to ensure that the anal sphincter is penetrated in obtaining the specimen.

If the clinical situation suggests the possibility of food poisoning, then a sample of the ingested food also should be examined. Enteric pathogens may be excreted intermittently; therefore it is important to obtain repeat stool specimens. This applies particularly to identification of the "carrier" stage for bacteria such as salmonellae.

Processing

The majority of fecal pathogens are facultative aerobic bacteria, although *C. perfringens* can cause food poisoning. The anaerobic flora outnumbers the aerobic and facultative flora by approximately 100:1. It is therefore generally unrewarding to culture stools for anaerobic microorganisms.

Gross and microscopic examination of the sample is useful for determining the presence of blood and mucus and for identifying leukocytes. These are commonly present in the dysenteries and salmonella infections as opposed to their absence in intoxications and viral infections.

The Gram stain is a rapid means whereby the clinical suspicion of enterocolitis secondary to either *S. aureus* or *C. albicans* can be supported before cultural confirmation.

A variety of selective and enrichment media are employed for the recognition of pathogenic enteric bacteria (Table 9.1). Biochemical and serologic tests are carried out on the pure isolate for further speciation and identification. The large number of antigenically distinct *Salmonella* serotypes precludes routine serotyping in laboratories other than reference centers; however, the use of pooled antisera permits an initial identification.

Escherichia coli is responsible for many instances of travelers' diarrhea as a result of heat-stable and heat-labile enterotoxin production. The identification of these toxins is still an activity of reference or research laboratories.

Serum Fluids (Joint, Bursal, Pleural, Pericardial Fluid, and Ascites)

Collection

Serous body fluids are sterile normally and require adequate skin disinfection before their aspiration. Prompt delivery to the laboratory will ensure the survival of fastidious organisms such as *Neisseria* spp and anaerobic bacteria.

TABLE 9.1   Media for Recognition of Pathogenic Enteric Bacteria

Media	Organism Isolated
Desoxycholate citrate MacConkey EMB SS	*Salmonella* *Shigella* colorless colonies *Proteus* (lactose-negative) Other gram-negative bacilli: red or dark purple (lactose-positive)
Thiosulfate citrate bile sucrose (TCBS)	*V. cholerae*
Phenylethyl alcohol blood agar	*S. aureus*

Processing

Microscopic examination is carried out in a similar manner to the handling of CSF. Measurement of the protein and glucose content, as well as determining the amount of lactic acid dehydrogenase (LDH) present, is helpful in differentiating exudate from transudate and in supporting the presence or absence of a pyogenic process. The fluid is cultured anaerobically, in 10% CO_2; and for fungi and mycobacteria when clinically appropriate.

Bone marrow samples can be processed in a similar manner. The invasive nature of the procedure makes it imperative that aerobic, anaerobic, fungal, and mycobacterial cultures be set up if there is the possibility of an infectious process.

Nasopharyngeal Cultures

These cultures include both throat cultures for pathogens such as *S. pyogenes, Corynebacterium diphtheriae, N. meningitidis,* and *N. gonorrhoeae,* and nasal cultures for the isolation of *Bordetella pertussis.*

Collection

Throat swabs should be collected under direct vision with a good light; the tonsils and fauces are swabbed vigorously while rotating the swab. Nasal swabs for determining *S. aureus* carriage are collected by sampling both nasal vestibules.

Pernasal swabs using flexible wire with cotton or Dacron tips are the best method for the bacteriologic confirmation of pertussis although the "cough plate" whereby secretions are collected by directly coughing onto fresh blood agar plates can also be rewarding.

Processing

Inoculation onto sheep blood agar is a satisfactory means of identifying *S. aureus,* hemolytic streptococci, and *N. meningitidis.* If gonorrhea is suspected, then Thayer-Martin medium is indicated. Tellurite agar is required for the recognition of *C. diphtheriae* and Bordet-Gengou media for *B. pertussis* and *B. parapertussis.* If epiglottitis is suspected and appropriate swabs taken, these should be cultured on chocolate blood agar for the isolation of *H. influenzae.*

There is little value in Gram-staining nasopharyngeal swabs owing to the presence of the normal microbiologic flora. However, for the diagnosis of Vincent's angina or stomatitis it is necessary to demonstrate the presence of *Fusobacterium* and spirochetes in a Gram-stained smear.

Direct fluorescent microscopy of throat swabs has been used as a rapid means of demonstrating the presence of *S. pyogenes,* by employing an appropriate fluorescein-labeled conjugate.

Identification of Microorganisms

A brief review of common laboratory methods will be described. Further information is available by consulting the references cited.

A prerequisite for identification is the ability to culture the pathogen. The media appropriate for a variety of clinical samples have been discussed. These require incubation in air with or without 5-10% carbon dioxide or in an atmosphere free from oxygen for obligate anaerobes. The optimum temperature is usually 35-37°C, reflecting the normal body temperature. Some microorganisms grow best at 20°C, including most fungi. The majority of aerobic and facultative bacteria grow well if incubated for 24 hr. Some require more prolonged incubation, notably the obligate anaerobes for which 5 days or more may be necessary.

The colonial appearance, pigment production, hemolysis, and pH alteration as demonstrated by change in indicator color, are all essential clues to the assessment of individual microorganisms. The Gram-stained appearance of emulsified colonies or broth suspensions is an important initial means for determining morphology and tintorial appearance. This will be the basis for a summary of the main characteristics of the microorganisms most frequently encountered in clinical specimens.

Gram-Positive Cocci

Staphylococcus Aureus and *S. Epidermidis*

These occur in clusters or singly and produce smooth, opaque, round colonies on blood agar. The colonies are white, creamy, or yellow and may produce a small zone of clear (β-) hemolysis. They are differentiated by the presence or absence of the enzyme coagulase. Coagulase-positive *S. aureus* will form a coagulum if incubated for 4 hr or longer in plasma. Coagulase-negative *S. epidermidis* produces no coagulum. Phage-typing of *S. aureus,* and occasionally *S. epidermidis,* is carried out for epidemiologic purposes, particularly for the identification of nosocomial epidemics.

Micrococcus species are sometimes confused with *S. epidermidis.* They occasionally produce urinary tract infection, endocarditis, and infections of cerebrospinal fluid shunts. They tend to produce tetrads on the Gram stain.

Streptococcus

The genus *Streptococcus* includes a variety of species recognized by their ability or inability to hemolyze red blood cells. On Gram stain they appear in pairs or chains. This genus also includes *S. pneumoniae* and the enterococci. Hemolysis on sheep blood agar can be complete (β-hemolysis) giving a clear translucent zone around individual colonies, partial (α-hemolysis) producing a zone of green hemolysis, or there may be no apparent hemolysis (δ-hemolysis). α-Hemolytic streptococci are a heterogeneous group of bacteria, most frequently found in the oropharynx as part of the normal flora. They are frequent causes of bacterial endocarditis. β-Hemolytic streptococci include *S. pyogenes* which can be differentiated from other β-hemolytic strains by means of a bacitracin-containing disc which inhibits growth of *S. pyogenes* on a blood agar plate. This test is approximately 95% reliable since it is rare for other β- hemolytic streptococci to be inhibited by bacitracin. Nonhemolytic (δ) streptococci include many enterococci that are more resistant to heat, acid pH, and grow well on MacConkey agar. They are found in the gastrointestinal and female genital tracts and are responsible for both urinary tract infections and bacterial endocarditis.

Streptococcus pneumoniae grows well on blood agar in 10% CO_2 producing a small zone of α-hemolysis around the colonies. It is readily soluble in bile and this fact is utilized in a simple disc test. Optochin-impregnated discs will inhibit growth of pneumococci, thus differentiating them from most other viridans streptococci.

Streptococci are also classified by the Lancefield system in which the group-specific cell-wall antigen is extracted, using heat and acidification, and reacted with rabbit group-specific antisera. Many of the groupable streptococci are further subdivisible by identifying other protein antigens. This approach is extremely important for epidemiologic studies.

The anaerobic streptococcus, *Peptostreptococcus,* is commonly found in pus associated with gastrointestinal and female genital tract infections. It is important to differentiate the strictly anaerobic streptococcus from those which require carbon dioxide for their growth (capnophilic). Certain antimicrobials used for treating strictly anaerobic strains are inactive against these microaerophilic and capnophilic strains.

Gram-Negative Cocci

Neisseria

Both *N. gonorrhoeae* and *N. meningitidis* are gram-negative diplococci. Both organisms poorly tolerate drying and cooling and should be cultured promptly on blood or chocolate blood agar and incubated in 5-10% carbon dioxide. *Neisseria gonorrhoeae* is usually isolated on Thayer-Martin medium which is a selective preparation that includes vancomycin, colistin, and nystatin which inhibit the normal flora of the genital area allowing recognition of *N. gonorrhoeae*. A variety of transport media such as the Transgrow system permits survival of the gonococcus if immediate processing is not possible. *Neisseria gonorrhoeae* ferments glucose alone which differentiates it from *N. meningitidis* which ferments both glucose and maltose. Both species are oxidase-positive. A fluorescent antibody test with conjugated rabbit antiserum is a useful confirmatory test for *N. gonorrhoeae.*

A number of other *Neisseria* spp are found in the oropharynx and are rarely pathogenic. Anaerobic gram-negative cocci belong to the genus *Veillonella* and are rare causes of human infections.

Gram-Positive Bacilli

Both spore-forming and nonsporulating bacilli are included in this category. The former includes *Bacillus* and *Clostridium* spp.

Bacteria of the genus *Bacillus* are widely distributed and frequent causes of laboratory contamination, *B. subtilis* being the most common. *Bacillus anthracis* is the cause of anthrax.

The genus *Clostridium* contains a large number of species characterized by their requirement for anaerobiasis and the production of a wide variety of toxins. In addition, under adverse conditions they produce spores which are extremely durable and resistant to heat and drying. *Clostridium tetani* and *C. botulinum* produce potent neurotoxins that can be demonstrated using mouse inoculation studies, while those responsible for gas gangrene, notably *C. perfringens, C. septicum, C. novyi,* and *C. bifermentans,* produce several tissue toxins that can be used for identification. Their fermentative and proteolytic characteristics are responsible for the gas production and tissue destruction so characteristic of gas gangrene. *Clostridium difficile* is associated with pseudomembranous colitis following the use of antibiotic therapy. The toxin is demonstrable in the stool using a tissue cytotoxicity test neutralizable with antiserum.

The genus *Corynebacterium* includes a large number of species present in the normal flora of the mouth, female genital tract, and skin. These are grouped under the term *diphtheroids.* They appear palisaded on Gram stain and frequently simulate Chinese lettering. They are rarely pathogenic and are frequent causes of contaminated specimens such as blood cultures. On the other hand, *C. diphtheriae* is responsible for diphtheria. Its pathogenicity lies in its ability to elaborate a potent exotoxin that is formed by certain strains. Three subspecies are recognized based on colonial appearance and other factors and are termed *mitis, intermedius,* and *gravis.* However, the critical factor clinically is the production of the exotoxin which can be demonstrated using an immunoprecipitin test.

Listeria monocytogenes is recognized by its ability to produce hemolysis on blood agar, and its motility at room temperature and absence of motility at 35°C. The organism may be dismissed mistakenly as a contaminant owing to its morphologic similarities to diphtheroids on Gram-staining.

Actinomyces are slow-growing, strict anaerobes, while *Nocardia* also grow slowly but aerobically. They have a branching appearance on Gram stain and also take up an acid-fast stain. Actinomycotic pus frequently contains 1-2 mm golden *sulfur* granules which when crushed and Gram-stained show typical morphology. Speciation requires biochemical analysis.

Other anaerobic gram-positive bacilli which rarely cause clinical infection include *Lactobacillus* spp, *Eubacterium,* and *Bifidobacterium.*

Gram-Negative Bacilli

Haemophilus influenzae is pleomorphic with coccobacillary forms which are pale staining. It is the most common member of this genus and grows well on chocolate blood agar or agar supplemented with both X (NAD) and V (hemin) factors. Capsulated strains can be serotyped. Serotype b is the most frequent variety and is responsible for meningitis, arthritis, cellulitis, osteomyelitis, and epiglottitis. Noncapsulated strains are found in association with otitis media and exacerbations of chronic bronchitis with purulent sputum production. *Haemophilus parainfluenzae* differs in its nutritional requirements and is rarely pathogenic for humans.

The Enterobacteriaceae family includes many facultative genera responsible for clinical infections. It includes *Escherichia, Shigella, Salmonella, Klebsiella, Enterobacter, Serratia, Proteus,* and some less well-known genera such as

Acinetobacter, Citrobacter, and *Providencia. Escherichia, Klebsiella,* and *Proteus* are part of the normal flora of the gut and are responsible for urinary tract infections, abdominal infections, and gram-negative bacteremia. This family also includes the enteric pathogens belonging to the genera *Salmonella* and *Shigella.* All of the genera ferment glucose and grow well on laboratory media, including MacConkey and EMB agar which inhibit many gram-positive bacteria and also permit a differentiation into lactose and nonlactose fermenting bacteria, the latter including most strains of *Salmonella* and *Shigella.* Further identification includes biochemical and serologic testing. Agglutination tests are important in the speciation of both salmonellae and shigellae following an initial series of biochemical tests. *Proteus* spp are separated by their ability to ferment indole and other sugars.

Pseudomonas spp of which *P. aeruginosa* is the most important in clinical medicine, has a characteristic fruity odor and ability to produce two pigments, pyocyanin and fluorescin. Pseudomonads are strict aerobes and are also oxidase-positive, which is useful in differentiating them from the Enterobacteriaceae which are facultative anaerobes.

Vibrio are gram-negative motile bacilli and appear comma shaped on Gram stain. They grow well on selective media such as TCBS. *Vibrio cholerae* and its biotypic variant *V. cholerae* var. *El Tor* ferment lactose slowly. In addition, *V. cholerae* is identified by slide agglutination with Ogawa and Inaba antisera to confirm the serotype.

The anaerobic gram-negative bacilli include many genera but those of frequent clinical significance are *Bacteroides* and *Fusobacterium* which are nonsporing, obligate anaerobes found in the gastrointestinal and female genital tracts. Identification and speciation depends upon the Gram stained appearance, biochemical analysis, and susceptibility to selected antibiotics. Gas-liquid chromatography can identify volatile fatty acids produced by bacterial metabolism and is another useful method for the speciation of anaerobic bacteria. The main species are *B. fragilis* and *B. melaninogenicus. Fusobacterium* is remarkably pleomorphic and has four species which are found in clinical specimens.

Mycobacteria

Tuberculosis may be caused by the classic mycobacteria, *M. tuberculosis* and *M. bovis,* and less commonly by the atypical (anonymous) mycobacteria which include the photochromogens *M. kansasii* and *M. marinum,* the scotochromogen *M. scrofulaceum,* the nonphotochromogens *M. intracellulare* and *M. xenopi,* and the rapid grower *M. fortuitum.* The classic mycobacteria grow slowly, taking up to 30-40 days to produce colonies. Most of the atypical mycobacteria tend to grow more rapidly, within 1-3 weeks, while the rapid growers produce colonies within 3-7 days.

Specimens for mycobacterial culture frequently contain low concentrations of bacteria. Thus three serial samples of sputum or urine are necessary. Early morning specimens are best because they contain the highest concentration of bacteria. Decontamination of the specimen with sodium hydroxide is often carried out, following concentration by centrifugation. Uncontaminated samples such as CSF and pleural fluid simply require concentration.

Careful microscopy of all specimens suspected to contain mycobacteria is essential because the results of culture are not available for several weeks in most instances. Microscopy is either carried out on Ziehl-Neelsen- (Z-N) or Kinyoun-stained samples or by fluorescent microscopy using an auramine stain which permits rapid examination of specimens. Specimens are cultured on media containing egg; Lowenstein-Jensen medium is the best known. Cultures are incubated in the dark at 37°C for up to 10 weeks. Identification relies on the rate of growth, pigment production, colonial morphology, and various biochemical reactions.

Antimicrobial Susceptibility Testing

Once a pathogenic microorganism is isolated in pure culture, it is important to know which antibiotics are likely to be useful for treatment. Some bacteria are consistently susceptible to certain antibiotics and make susceptibility testing unnecessary except under unusual circumstance; *S. pneumoniae* and *S. pyogenes* are good examples. They are sensitive to penicillin and therefore rarely tested in the laboratory, although in recent years relatively resistant pneumococci have caused sporadic infection.

Many bacteria have unpredictable sensitivity patterns, particularly the gram-negative facultative bacilli. Therefore, the standardized method of Kirby and Bauer was developed. In this method the test strain, using a standardized inoculum, is surface seeded onto Mueller-Hinton agar. On the surface of the agar are placed discs impregnated with known concentrations of the antibiotics to be tested and the plate is then incubated overnight. The antibiotic diffuses out of the disc into the medium to produce a zone of growth inhibition. The diameter of the zone site is recorded and compared with that obtained from a wide range of organisms whose zone size and minimum inhibitory concentration have been determined.

A control plate using a reference organism such as *S. aureus* (ATCC 25723) or *E. coli* (ATCC 25922) is set up daily and the zone diameter noted and compared with reference standards as part of the quality control of such tests. The test strain can then be stated to be *sensitive, intermediate,* or *resistant* to that antibiotic.

The importance of careful technique and standardization needs strong emphasis. Problems encountered with the methods can be related to the inoculum, failure to use Mueller-Hinton agar or to check its pH, and the use of improperly stored or outdated discs. Furthermore, slow-growing, anaerobic, and nutritionally fastidious organisms are not suitable for testing by this method.

Under certain clinical situations it is helpful to know more accurately the susceptibility of a given organism. The common method employed is to test for the minimum inhibitory concentration (MIC) defined as the least amount of antibiotic necessary to inhibit the growth of a bacterium under carefully controlled circumstances in vitro. The usual method uses Mueller-Hinton broth or other appropriate medium in a series of tubes containing twofold differences in the concentration of the antibiotic being used, and to which is added a standardized inoculum of the bacterium to be tested. Following overnight incubation the tubes are examined for growth and the first tube without growth indicates the concentration of antibiotic which is the MIC. By further subculturing, on agar, the broth from the tubes showing no visible growth and again incubating overnight, the concentration of antibiotic that is actually bactericidal can be determined. This is called the minimum bactericidal concentration.

Other Tests

Other laboratory tests useful for the treatment of certain infections include the assay of antibiotic in serum or other body fluids. This is important to ensure that adequate levels of an antibiotic are being achieved and further, in the case of toxic agents, that harmful levels are not being exceeded.

Another laboratory test appropriate for the management of infections, such as bacterial endocarditis, is to determine the killing ability of the patient's serum while receiving antibiotic treatment using the bacterium responsible for his infection. Serum is tested just before and approximately 1 hr after administration of the drug to correspond with expected *trough* and *peak* levels of the antibiotic. A *peak* dilution inhibitory to the bacterium of 1:8 or 1:16 is believed to be adequate for the management of most infections.

Selected Bibliography

Davis, B. D., Dulbecco, R., Eisen, H. N., Ginsberg, H. S., Wood, W. B., and McCarty, M.: *Microbiology,* 3rd edition. Harper & Row, Hagerstown, 1980.

Finegold, S. M. and Martin, W. J.: *Bailey & Scott's Diagnostic Microbiology,* 6th edition. C. V. Mosby Co., St. Louis, 1982.

Lennette, E. H., Spaulding, E. H., and Truant, J. P.: *Manual of Clinical Microbiology,* 3rd edition. American Society of Microbiology, Washington, DC, 1980.

MacFaddin, J. F.: *Biochemical Tests for Identification of Medical Bacteria,* 2nd edition. William & Wilkins Co., Baltimore, 1980.

Washington, J. A., II: Blood cultures: Principles and techniques. *Mayo Clin Proc* 50:91, 1975.

10

LABORATORY DIAGNOSIS OF VIRAL INFECTIONS
Robert H. Waldman, M.D.

The specific diagnosis of viral infections presents a special challenge to the clinician and to the diagnostic laboratory. This is especially striking when compared
with the great strides that have been made in the laboratory diagnosis of bacterial
and fungal infections. Among the problems facing the physician trying to make a
specific diagnosis of a viral infection are the paucity of distinctive clinical syndromes that allow the physician to make an accurate bedside diagnosis, the expense and time consumed by available diagnostic procedures, and the benign and
self-limited nature of most viral infections usually resulting in a well patient by
the time the diagnosis is finally made. Contributing to the frequent irrelevancy
of knowing the exact diagnosis, is that there are very few specific modalities of
therapy for viral infections.

The purpose of this chapter, therefore, is not to discuss in detail the various
ways a research virology laboratory may go about diagnosing a viral infection, but
simply to present a few basic principles for diagnosing viral infections, with the
hope and expectation that within several years better procedures will be found to
make more rapid diagnoses, at a time when more chemotherapeutic agents will be
available (Table 10.1)

The exact diagnosis of viral infections occasionally can be made on the basis
of clinical findings. There are a few viral infections in which the clinical features
are distinctive enough to allow one to make a diagnosis in the proper clinical setting. As with most other types of infectious disease, these "proper clinical set-
ings" include the age of the patient, the season of the year, the geographic area,
etc. Examples of such viral infections are those caused by the herpesviruses, and
measles, mumps, and smallpox viruses.

Aside from the clinical picture presented by the patient, the diagnosis sometimes can be made on epidemiologic grounds. This is based on the observation that

TABLE 10.1   Precautions in Interpretation of Results from
Viral Diagnostic Laboratory

Virus Isolation

False-positive

Viral contaminant present in isolation system, most commonly in tissue culture

Bacterial contamination being mistaken for a positive effect in isolation system, e.g., causing cytopathic effect on tissue culture or death of inoculated test egg or animal

Virus present but not cause of disease, either because persistent or reactivated virus from prior infection (e.g., herpes simplex) or patient is infected with two viruses simultaneously

False-negative

Sample handled incorrectly - wrong timing (too late or too early), wrong specimen (incorrect site), improper transport, incorrect isolation procedures

Serology

False-positive

Nonspecific inhibitors (e.g., influenza virus inhibitors are present in nearly all sera)

Double infection

Cross-reacting antigens lead to antibody rise

Recent immunization

False-negative

Improper testing: incorrect timing (specimens obtained too late, convalescent sera obtained too soon), testing done incorrectly (wrong test used, incorrect antigen)

Persistent antigen leading to immune complexes and "soaking-up" of antibody

Nonspecific inhibitors mask antibody response

---

in an epidemic of a viral disease, almost all similar illnesses are caused by the same agent. Examples of this are influenza virus epidemics, epidemic exanthems caused by enteroviruses, and epidemic pleurodynia. Another epidemiologic situation in which the diagnosis can be made with some certainty is a situation in which there is a special set of epidemiologic events, such as jaundice in a drug abuser, or croup in an infant.

One should not forget that the routine clinical laboratories may be of great help in evaluating a patient with a possible viral infection. The best example of this is the white blood cell count and blood smear because it has been recognized for many years that patients who clinically have an infection and have a low or normal white count, are more likely to be infected with a virus. Lymphocytosis and atypical lymphocytes are usually seen in patients with viral infections, particularly patients infected with Epstein-Barr (EB) virus, cytomegalovirus, or early in the course of hepatitis A or B virus infection. On the other hand, it must be remembered that every patient with atypical lymphocytes does not have a viral infection. Patients with drug reactions, particularly patients receiving phenytoin (Dilantin), will not infrequently have atypical lymphocytes.

Obtaining and Handling of Specimens

The first question that must be asked with respect to obtaining specimens for the special virology laboratory is which material from the patient's body will be sent for evaluation. This depends on the type of clinical syndrome exhibited by the patient. In patients with primarily a respiratory illness, the best virus yield is obtained from throat gargles or nasal washings. The latter is not usually practical since it requires some degree of skill to do and causes a bit of discomfort for the patient. The throat swab is definitely of less value as far as sensitivity is concerned. Undoubtedly of more clinical relevance is obtaining specimens in patients with possible central nervous system viral infection. For these patients spinal fluid and a stool specimen or rectal swab are the most likely to give useful information. In patients with a viral exanthem, again a stool specimen or rectal swab should be obtained. If an arbovirus infection is suspected, then whole blood must be sent for culture. In patients with a vesicular exanthem, an aspirate or scraping of the lesion should be used.

The handling of the specimen or specimens is even more important than with the most fastidious bacterial species, since most viruses very quickly become non-infectious without susceptible tissue in which to grow. Therefore, specimens should be transported immediately to the virology laboratory, preferably on ice. If more than a few minutes will transpire before the specimen can be taken to, or processed by, the laboratory, the specimen should be frozen at -70°C. If the specimen must be shipped to a distant site, it should be packed in dry ice or liquid nitrogen. A recent advance, which has great potential for improving the yield from these specimens, is the use of transport tubes which contain a small amount of tissue culture. These transport tubes should be taken to the bedside and can be inoculated immediately and then sent to the diagnostic laboratory with the virus already beginning to replicate. Of course, these transport tubes containing tissue cultures should not be sent on ice or frozen. Virus isolation and identification are made by: (1) identifying the cytopathic effect of viruses on tissue culture; (2) making use of the fact that tissue culture cells infected with certain viruses will absorb fairly strongly some species of red blood cells to their surface; (3) neutralization, by specific antisera, of the ability of the virus to infect living tissue, whether it is in an experimental animal, an embryonated egg, or tissue culture; or (4) the use of fluorescein-tagged specific antisera to "stain" infected tissue culture (Table 10.2). As mentioned earlier, this process is expensive and fairly time consuming, requiring 4-5 days under the best circumstances.

There are two very recent advances in viral identification which eventually may be very helpful and practical in rapid diagnosis of viral infections. The first of these is immune electron microscopy. Although this is still a rather expensive technique and is used only in research laboratories, it might enable a clinical virology laboratory to make an etiologic diagnosis within hours. The principle of the technique is to mix a material in which viruses are sought, such as a stool filtrate, with specific antisera. The antibody causes the specific virus particles to agglutinate, thereby making them easier to find upon electron microscopic examination, following centrifugation.

The other new technique is the enzyme-linked immunosorbent assay (ELISA). This technique can be used either to detect viral antigen in a specimen or to measure viral antibodies. It is relatively inexpensive and quite sensitive, and in addition, requires only small amounts of material. It is also rapid, giving a result within several hours. The ELISA technique uses an enzyme to measure the binding of antigen to antibodies. Examples of the use of the ELISA technique are in the more sensitive and rapid detection of hepatitis A and B antigens, and in particular, the e antigen of hepatitis B (HBeAg). In addition, the ELISA technique has been used to measure antibody to measles, rubella, and herpes, replacing the older methods for measuring antibody to these viruses.

Serologic Testing

Another method for diagnosis of viral infections is the use of serologic testing, i.e., the measurement of antibody to the viral agent. In most situations it is necessary to show a significant increase (usually fourfold or greater) in antibody between the time the patient is first seen (acute specimen) and another blood specimen is obtained 2-3 weeks later (convalescent serum). Other specimens, such as various external secretions, have been used in the research laboratory to detect a rise in antibody in response to a viral infection, but the only clinically relevant specimen currently used is serum. One exception to the general rule of obtaining acute and convalescent sera is infectious mononucleosis in which one specimen only is necessary for the detection of heterophil antibody.

People often have antibody present in the acute serum sample. This may be a result of prior infection, or of infection with viruses with cross-reacting antigens. Therefore, antibody in the acute sample, in most situations, is difficult to interpret.

TABLE 10.2   Use of Immunofluorescence in Rapid Diagnsis of Viral Infection

Specimen	Example
Brain (biopsy)	Rabies, herpes simplex
Corneal scraping	Herpes simplex
Vesicle scraping	Varicella, herpes simplex
Blood leukocytes	Measles, cytomegalovirus
Liver (biopsy)	Hepatitis B

In some situations, but again largely in research laboratories, antibody that is the result of remote infections has been differentiated from the acute development of antibody, by making use of the fact that IgG antibody is more consistent with the former, while IgM antibody indicates a much more recent rise in titer.

One practical point is that serum must be kept sterilely at 4°C or frozen between the time it is collected and the measurements are performed, otherwise incorrect results may be found.

The obvious limitation of the serologic diagnosis of viral infections with respect to any help in management of an individual patient is this time delay. With most viral infections, the patient has recovered by the time the convalescent serum sample is to be obtained and the tests performed. Therefore, serology is mainly used for epidemiologic and investigative purposes. An important exception to this is the use of serologic testing to make a diagnosis for which some particular therapeutic measure might be indicated, for example rubella in a pregnant woman.

Criteria for Laboratory Diagnosis of Viral Infections

As mentioned before, the two primary criteria for diagnosis of viral infections are virus isolation and/or fourfold or greater rise in serum antibody titer. With respect to the latter, one is sometimes faced with the problem of a high titer of antibody in both the acute and the convalescent specimen, or one only has a convalescent specimen. In this situation, the lack of a fourfold or greater rise in titer may still be significant if the viral disease is a rare one, if the antibody is not long-lasting, if it can be determined that the antibody is of the IgM class, or by testing contacts of the patient and showing that they have virologic or serologic evidence of the disease.

To avoid having to wait for the convalescent serum specimen, an epidemiologic technique, which is sometimes of value, is to compare the titers of people with the acute illness with those of other patients who have recovered from the illness. This technique is used to identify influenza virus epidemics in a shorter period than would be possible if one had to wait until acute and convalescent specimens from the same individuals were obtained and tested.

Summary

There is unquestionably a need for more rapid methods for diagnosing viral infections (Table 10.3). These no doubt will result as more antiviral agents become available, especially if these drugs are specific for certain viral infections (i.e., "necessity is the mother of invention"). One can give a pertinent example of such a need at the present time: it would be tremendously helpful to have a better method for rapidly diagnosing herpes simplex encephalitis, rather than having to resort to a brain biopsy, now that there is a drug which has been shown to be effective in this viral infection.

TABLE 10.3   Laboratory Diagnosis of Some Viral Infections

Disease	Etiologic Agent	Specimen(s)	Test(s)
Adenovirus	(30 serotypes)	Throat and/or conjunctival swabs, pharyngeal washing	Virus isolation in tissue culture
		Blood	Serology - CF, neutralization, hemagglutination
Croup	Parainfluenza	Throat and/or nasal swab or washing	Virus isolation in tissue culture
Cytomegalovirus	CMV	Urine, saliva, throat swab	Virus isolation - human embryo fibroblasts
		Blood	Serology - CF
Dengue		Blood	Serology - neutralization, HI and CF
Encephalitis	Japanese B; St. Louis, Western and Eastern equine; Venezuelan; herpes simplex (see below)	Brain biopsy	Virus isolation
		Blood	Serology
Hepatitis	A	Blood	Serology - immune adherence hemagglutination
		Stool	Virus identification - immunoelectronmicroscopy
	B	Blood	Detection of viral antigens - HB_SAg, e antigen; measurement of antibodies to these antigens by several different techniques
	non-A, non-B	None	

Table 10.3 (Cont'd)

Disease	Etiologic Agent	Specimen(s)	Test(s)
Herpes labialis Genital herpes Gingivostomatitis	Herpes simplex	Vesicle fluid, saliva, throat washing or swab, spinal fluid	Virus isolation - embryonated eggs, lab animals, tissue culture
Encephalitis		Brain biopsy	Immunofluorescence
		Blood	Serology - CF, neutralization (nearly all adults have serum antibody)
Herpangina Pleurodynia Respiratory tract or gastrointestinal infection	Coxsackie virus A and B	Throat, nasal, stool	Virus isolation- tissue culture, suckling mice
		Blood	Serology - neutralization
Aseptic meningitis		Blood	Serology - CF, neutralization
Infectious mononucleosis	Epstein-Barr	Blood smear Blood	Atypical lymphocytes Serology
Influenza	A, B, C	Throat, nasal	Virus isolation - embryonated eggs, tissue culture
		Blood	Serology - hemagglutination inhibition, CF
Mumps		Saliva, spinal fluid	Virus isolation - embryonated eggs, tissue culture
		Blood	Serology - CF, hemagglutination inhibition
Poliomyelitis		Stool, throat	Virus isolation - tissue culture
		Blood	Serology - CF, neutralization

Table 10.3 (Cont'd)

Disease	Etiologic Agent	Specimen(s)	Test(s)
Rabies		Brain tissue	Smears for Negri bodies Immunofluorescence Virus isolation – mice
Yellow fever		Blood	Serology – neutralization Virus isolation mice
		Liver tissue	Histology – midzonal necrosis and "Councilman" bodies

Selected Bibliography

Evans, A. S.: New discoveries in infectious mononucleosis. *Mod Med* 42:18–24, 1974.

Kapikian, A. Z., Feinstone, S. M., Purcell, R. H., Wyatt, R. G., Thornhill, P. S., Kalica, A. R., and Chanock, R. M.: Detection and identification by immune electron microscopy of fastidious agents associated with respiratory illness, acute nonbacterial gastroenteritis and hepatitis A. *Perspect Virol* 9:9, 1975.

McCracken, A. W. and Newman, J. T.: The current status of the laboratory diagnosis of viral diseases of man. *Crit Rev Lab Clin Med* 5:331, 1975.

11

VIRAL UPPER RESPIRATORY INFECTIONS
Robert H. Waldman, M.D.

Respiratory infections are the most common acute illnesses in the United States (Table 11.1) Fortunately, they are nearly always brief and mild, but the total morbidity is immense. The average adult has two to five upper respiratory infections each year with an average duration of 5-7 days each. Children, and adults in frequent contact with children, have respiratory infections with even greater frequency.

Etiology (Table 11.2)

The rhinovirus group accounts for about one-third of upper respiratory infections. There are about 90 serotypes of this small, acid-labile, ether-resistant, RNA virus which grows best at 33°C. There are 30-40 strains of coxsackievirus. Patients who have respiratory infections caused by this group of viruses more often have systemic illness. Viruses from this group also may cause aseptic meningitis, myocarditis, herpangina, and epidemic pleurodynia. Coxsackieviruses are a more frequent cause of viral respiratory infections in the summer and autumn. The strains most commonly associated with respiratory infection are A21 and B2, 3, 4, and 5. There are about 40 strains of echovirus. Similar to coxsackieviruses, infection with echovirus often is associated with systemic manifestations, especially a rash, enteritis, or aseptic meningitis. Other RNA viruses that fairly commonly cause respiratory infection are the myxoviruses, the paramyxoviruses, and the coronaviruses. These are discussed in more detail in Chapters 48, 51, 52 and 57.

Among the DNA viruses, only the adenoviruses are frequently associated with respiratory infections. Types 4 and 7 cause acute respiratory disease of military recruits, a syndrome similar to the common cold, but more severe and more

TABLE 11.1   Incidence and Type of Acute Illnesses in the United States*

Category of Acute Illness	Percentage
Infectious diseases	
Upper respiratory tract infections	31.3
Influenza	19.7
Digestive	5.7
Virus (unspecified)	4.6
Pneumonia	3.0
Common childhood	1.9
Others	5.4
Subtotal:	71.6
Injuries	14.6
All other acute diseases	13.8
Total:	100.0

*From current estimates, Health Interview Survey 1970

commonly associated with a modest fever. Adenovirus type 3 causes pharyngo-conjunctival fever and epidemic pharyngitis, types 3 and 7 cause conjunctivitis, and type 8 causes epidemic keratoconjunctivitis. Overall, adenoviruses cause fewer than 5% of viral respiratory infections.

Even in the best of studies, in approximately 40% of respiratory infections presumed to be of viral etiology, a virus cannot be isolated nor does a rise in serum antibody indicate the cause of the infection.

Epidemiology

According to the National Health Suvey, viral respiratory infections constitute 83% of all acute infectious problems. The incidence of the common cold is 1.2–6.2 per person each year, depending on the age group. Upper respiratory infections are responsible for 80% of all lost school days and 40% of all lost work days.

Viral respiratory infections are highly contagious, with spread usually occurring by fairly close person-to-person contact, either by aerosol droplets or by touching contaminated inanimate objects. Rhinovirus has been studied fairly extensively with respect to touching contaminated environmental surfaces and then self-inoculation of the nasal mucosa. Alternatively, transmission can occur by direct hand-to-hand contact. This has important public health implications, because it is very possible that the most effective way of decreasing the incidence of viral respiratory infections, at least those caused by rhinovirus, would be to carefully avoid contaminating one's hands with nasal or pharyngeal secretions, to

TABLE 11.2   Etiologic Agents and Clinical Manifestations of
Human Respiratory Infections

Agents	Serotypes	Most Important Clinical Manifestation(s)
Myxoviruses		
Influenza	A and B	Influenza
Parainfluenza	1, 2, 3, and 4	Croup in infants and young children
Respiratory syncytial	–	Bronchiolitis and/or pneumonia in infants
Coronavirus	≥ 3	Common cold
Picornaviruses		
Coxsackievirus	≥ 10	Febrile pharyngitis in children, upper respiratory infection in military recruits
Rhinovirus	≥ 90	Common cold
Adenovirus	1, 2, 3, 4, 5, 7, 14, and 21	Upper or lower respiratory infection, mainly in children and military recruits
Mycoplasma pneumoniae		Pneumonia in children and young adults

practice thorough hand-washing, and to avoid inoculating oneself by touching the upper respiratory tract. With other viruses, for example coxsackievirus, spread by the airborne route has been documented by carrying out studies of volunteers separated by a wire mesh screen, and then infecting one of the groups and showing that the group on the other side of the screen became infected after the appropriate incubation period.

There is a striking seasonal variation, and during the December to February period, 50% of people will have a respiratory viral infection. During the comparable June to August period, only 20% of people will have such an infection. This is accounted for by the predominance of rhinoviruses and coronaviruses as the causative agents. The cause of this seasonal pattern is unknown; however, some of the factors that have been suggested are the more crowded conditions that occur in cold weather; the dryness of the air due to heating of our homes and places of work leading to drying of the mucous membranes, possibly leading to decreased resistance; and finally, poorer ventilation, leading to persistence of aerosol droplets in the air. There is no evidence that exposure to cold per se leads to increased susceptibility.

Patients with chronic bronchitis have increased severity of illness when in-fected by most of the viruses associated with respiratory infections. The explana-tion for this might be that the viruses gain access to the lower respiratory tract because of alterations in the normal structural host defenses. In addition, there is a question about the role of these viruses in the progression of the disease proc-ess in these patients.

The incubation period of the various viral respiratory infections is generally short, i.e., in the order of 2-4 days. As mentioned earlier, the range of host sus-ceptibility is very narrow, with most of the viruses able to replicate and cause ill-ness only in humans. Children are the important reservoirs and vectors.

Viral respiratory infections are frequent illnesses because of the large number of viral serotypes; also because reinfection may occur with the same virus sero-type. The latter is particularly true of coronaviruses and respiratory syncytial virus.

Diagnosis

The signs and symptoms of viral respiratory infections vary from patient to pa-tient, and from infection to infection in the same patient. This has led to the fairly artificial division of viral respiratory infections into various syndromes as shown in Table 11.3. There is a large overlap, and thus it is not always easy, or of any clinical importance, to differentiate between the various syndromes. The ex-planation of the variability in clinical presentation is multifactorial, including the propensity of different viruses to preferentially infect different areas of the re-spiratory tract; differing virulence of the viral strains; and differences in the size of viral inocula, the particle size of the aerosolized droplets that are inhaled, un-derlying disease of the respiratory tract causing differing susceptibilities, and the immune status of the individual.

TABLE 11.3   Spectrum of Illness Caused by Some Respiratory Viruses

Agents	Cold	Febrile URI	Influenza-like	Croup	Pneumonia	Bronchiolitis
Rhinovirus	++++	++				
Coxsackie virus A21	++++	+++	++			
Influenza A	+	++	++++	+++	++	
Respiratory syncytial	++	++	+	+	+++	+++
Parainflu-enza 3	++	++	+	+	++++	
Parainflu-enza 1	++	++	+++	++++	++++	

Rhinovirus tends to cause a benign illness characterized by little or no fever, little in the way of systemic manifestations, and cough is an uncommon or relatively unimportant symptom (the "common cold"). With influenza virus infection, rhinorrhea is usually a minor manifestation, but cough, fever, and myalgias are more prominent. In a single individual, however, simply on the basis of the clinical manifestations, one cannot differentiate the virologic causes of most acute upper respiratory infections. Thus an individual patient with a low-grade fever, mild sore throat, sneezing, and stuffy and runny nose, might be infected with any of the viruses causing respiratory infections (Table 11.4).

TABLE 11.4   Respiratory Illnesses and Predominant Causative Viruses

Respiratory Tract Illness	Important Etiologic Agents
Common cold	
Without fever	Rhinovirus, parainfluenza, adenovirus, respiratory syncytial, Coxsackie A21
With fever	Rhinovirus, parainfluenza, adenovirus, coronavirus, respiratory syncytial, influenza A and B, Coxsackie A21
Sore throat	
Without white spots	Adenovirus types 1,2,3,4,5, and 7; Coxsackie A2,4,5,6,8,10, and B2,3,5; herpes hominis type 1
With white spots	Adenovirus types 1,2,3,4,5, and 7
With blisters	Coxsackie A2,4,5,6,8
Ear infection	Adenovirus types 1,2,3,5, and 6; parainfluenza; respiratory syncytial
Conjunctivitis	Adenovirus types 3,7,8, and 19; enterovirus 70
Laryngitis/croup	Parainfluenza types 1,2, and 3; influenza A and B;
Tracheobronchitis	Parainfluenza types 1,2, and 3; influenza A and B; adenovirus types 1,2,3, 4,5, and 7
Bronchiolitis	Respiratory syncytial; parainfluenza types 1 and 3
Pneumonia	Respiratory syncytial; parainfluenza types 1,2, and 3; adenovirus types 1, 2,3,5, and 7; influenza A and B

The most important differential diagnosis is to rule out streptococcal pharyngitis since, at the present time, that is the only common infectious agent causing upper respiratory infection for which there is specific beneficial therapy (diphtheria is uncommon, and amantadine as therapy for influenza A is of marginal benefit). Therefore, a throat culture should be obtained on any patient who has a sore throat as a significant symptom and who is ill enough to have sought medical care. It is also important to ensure that lower respiratory infection is not present, and this should be easily accomplished with a careful history, physical examination, and a chest roentgenogram if appropriate.

Attempts at viral isolation and serologic tests are of interest to the clinical investigator, but currently of no benefit to the patient because the results will not be available until the patient has recovered, and there is nothing that would change the management of the patient even if the results were available instantaneously. When chemotherapeutic agents that are specific for certain viruses become available, then rapid and specific diagnosis of the cause of viral respiratory infections will be necessary.

Also important in the differential diagnosis is allergic or vasomotor rhinitis, which can give similar nasal symptoms. It should be possible to rule these out on the basis of the patient's history. Other diseases to be considered are bacterial sinusitis, otitis media, Vincent's angina, infectious mononucleosis, and diphtheria.

Prognosis and Complications

The major complication of viral respiratory infections is bacterial superinfection. This complication may manifest itself as bacterial sinusitis, otitis media, bronchitis, or pneumonia. Pneumonia is particularly common following influenza. Lower respiratory bacterial complications are more common in smokers and in patients with chronic respiratory diseases. Otitis media and sinusitis are more common in children.

Differentiating viral from bacterial pneumonia is a difficult task. Patients with viral pneumonia tend to have more of an interstitial infiltrate, the distribution is not lobar, the cough is more likely to be dry, and the physical findings tend to be scanty in relationship to the chest x-ray findings. Fever is likely to be lower and the white count should be normal or slightly elevated with more of a lymphocytosis, less of a granulocytosis, or a shift to the left. Chilliness may be present in viral infections, including viral pneumonias, but shaking chills are exceedingly uncommon, and a history of rigor almost always means bacterial pneumonia with bacteremia unless aspirin, which may precipitate a chill, has been given.

The organisms that most often cause superinfection are the opportunistic bacteria commonly found in the respiratory tract, i.e., the pneumococcus, *Haemophilus influenzae,* and, less commonly, *Staphylococcus aureus.* There are several pathogenic factors that may contribute to the development of bacterial superinfection. Probably the most important is the impairment of normal host defense mechanisms that results from epithelial damage, thereby impairing the normal mucociliary apparatus. In addition to this impairment of bacterial removal, the inflammation that results from a viral respiratory infection leads to increased transudation of protein and fluid, providing a better culture medium for the bacteria. If the increased secretions become dried, obstruction of the many tubes and orifices in the respiratory tract may develop, resulting in bacterial growth behind the obstruction. Viral infections also have been shown to be immunosuppressive, but this is of unknown practical significance. The role of various medications should not be overlooked. For example, aspirin is an immunosuppressant. It also lowers the body temperature which may be an important host defense mechanism, and patients receiving aspirin shed virus longer than do controls, suggesting that the viral infection may be more severe when aspirin is used. Codeine, found in many cough medicines, suppresses the cough reflex which is important in protecting the lower respiratory tract. Thus the use of codeine may increase the chance of bacterial superinfection of the lower respiratory tract.

With respect to the development of bacterial infection of the sinuses and middle ear, it is unknown whether direct viral invasion of these areas is necessary for subsequent bacterial infection, or whether the important pathogenetic mechanism is simply the edema and inflammation of the orifices, leading to inadequate drainage. The latter is probably more important.

A recent study, which is of considerable theoretical interest, showed that *S. aureus* and the pneumococcus have increased adherence to mucosal cells during viral respiratory infections.

The most important group of patients with respect to these complications are those with chronic cardiopulmonary disease, in whom even the mildest viral respiratory infection can cause very significant morbidity and mortality.

Immunology and Prevention

There has been great interest in host susceptibility to infection, particularly with respect to viral respiratory infections. As mentioned before, there has been no experimental evidence to show that exposure to cold is a factor in susceptibility to these infections, nor have other forms of stress, such as inadequate sleep, been shown to be of importance.

The role of various immune functions has been studied extensively, and it would appear that both antibody and cell-mediated immunity play some role in protection. Serum antibody may be important in protecting against some of the viruses; however, secretory antibody has been shown to be more relevant in rhinovirus and parainfluenza virus infections.

As for immunization, the only vaccine that is available is that for prevention of influenza. Vaccines may be developed against some of the agents in the future, but with the exception of potential ones against parainfluenza and respiratory syncytial viruses in young children, the cost of developing the vaccines and their likelihood for success, and the lack of severity of the viral respiratory infections in terms of morbidity and mortality, would seem to indicate that the cost/benefit ratio is against their development. Chemotherapy for prophylaxis of respiratory viral infections is a distinct possibility and will be discussed briefly in the next section. As was mentioned earlier, common hygienic measures such as avoiding hand contact with the upper respiratory tract and compulsive hand-washing might be quite effective in decreasing the spread.

Therapy

Antiviral chemotherapy has been covered in Chapter 6. It must be emphasized that any agent used as prophylaxis or therapy for viral respiratory infections must be so safe that it could be made available without a prescription, not only because of the mild nature of the disease but also because of time constraints. If one had to see a doctor, get a prescription, and have it filled, then the illness would probably either be over or have progressed to the point that the chemical would be ineffective.

With respect to nonspecific forms of therapy, there is no evidence that bed rest is of benefit, other than decreasing the spread of viral infection by removing the virus shedder from society. Fluid replacement is of great importance, because dried secretions are uncomfortable and may lead to obstruction of various tubes and ostia in the upper and lower respiratory tract. Optimal fluid replacement can be obtained with water, juices, soft drinks which do not contain caffeine, or warm liquids, the classic one being chicken soup. Caffeine-containing fluids such as colas, coffee, tea, or chocolate, probably are not good at maintaining hydration because caffeine is a mild diuretic. Alcohol-containing fluids, while making the patient feel better, are also not beneficial for hydration because alcohol inhibits secretion of antidiuretic hormone.

Decongestants should be used judiciously since they may shrink swollen mucous membranes leading to better drainage, but they also tend to dry the mucous membranes, leading to inspissation of the secretions.

The use of antibiotics in the prevention of bacterial complications of viral respiratory infections is controversial. The early use of antibiotics could theoretically increase the chance of bacterial superinfection by suppressing the normal flora of the respiratory tract, leading to colonization with more dangerous organisms. Obviously, when patients have bacterial pneumonia, sinusitis, or otitis media, antibiotics should be used. However, whether or not antibiotics should be used when patients have no fever, only an increased purulent sputum production, or increased purulent nasal discharge, is questionable. A fairly good compromise, pending more definitive study, might be to undertake a short course of antibiotics if a patient has not significantly improved on about day 5, or has improved and then has become worse with increased sputum production, a change in sputum from fairly clear to purulent, or a purulent discharge from the anterior nares or the nasopharynx. Tetracycline, ampicillin, amoxicillin, or the fixed combination of trimethoprim-sulfamethoxazole should be used because the most common organisms are the pneumococcus and *H. influenzae*.

A final controversial issue is the use of ascorbic acid (vitamin C). Rather than discuss in detail the various and conflicting studies that have been carried out in an attempt to quantitate the protective and/or therapeutic benefit, if any, resulting from the use of large doses of vitamin C, suffice it to say that we simply do not know. My interpretation of the data is that there is a small but real beneficial effect of vitamin C. On the other hand, gastrointestinal upset may result from the large doses of vitamin C usually recommended, and there are some potential harmful effects of long-term use, including renal calculi, osteoporosis, and interactions with other drugs. I would neither encourage nor discourage the use of vitamin C.

Selected Bibliography

Chalmers, T. C.: Effects of ascorbic acid on the common cold. An evaluation of the evidence. *Am J Med* 58:532, 1975.

D'Alessio, D. J., Peterson, J. A., Dick, C. R., and Dick, E. C.: Transmission of experimental rhinovirus colds in volunteer married couples. *J Infect Dis* 133: 28-36, 1976.

Douglas, R. G., Jr., Lindgren, K. M., and Couch, R. B.: Exposure to cold environment and rhinovirus common cold: Failure to demonstrate effect. *N Engl J Med* 279:743, 1968.

Gwaltney, J. M., Jr. and Hendley, J. O.: Rhinovirus transmission, one if by air, two if by hand. *Am J Epidemiol* 107:357, 1978.

Hendley, J. O., Wenzel, R. P., and Gwaltney, J. M.: Transmission of rhinovirus colds by self-inoculation. *N Engl J Med* 288:1361-1364, 1973.

Holmes, M. J., Reed, S. E., Stott, E. J., and Tyrrell, D. A. J.: Studies of experimental rhinovirus type 2 infections in polar isolation and in England. *J Hyg* 76:379, 1976.

Jackson, G. G. and Muldoon, R. L.: Viruses causing common respiratory infections in man. *J Infect Dis* 127:328-355, 1973.

Monto, A. S. and Bryan, E. R.: Susceptibility to rhinovirus infection in chronic bronchitis. *Am Rev Resp Dis* 118:1101-1103, 1978.

Panusarn, C., Stanley, E. D., Dirda, V., Rubenis, N., and Jackson, G. G.: Prevention of illness from rhinovirus infection by a topical interferon inducer. *N Engl J Med* 291:57-61, 1974.

Perkins, J. C., Tucker, D. N., Knopf, H. L. S., Wenzel, R. P., Kapikian, A. Z., and Chanock, R. M.: Comparison of protective effect of neutralizing antibody in serum and nasal secretions in experimental rhinovirus type 13 illness. *Am J Epidemiol* 90:519-526, 1969.

Smith, C. B., Purcell, R. H., Bellanti, J. A., and Chanock, R. M.: Protective effect of antibody to parainfluenza type 1 virus. *N Engl J Med* 275:1145, 1966.

Waldman, R. H. and Ganguly, R.: Effect of CP-20,961 an interferon inducer, on upper respiratory infections due to rhinovirus type 20 in volunteers. *J Infect Dis* 138:531, 1978.

Waldman, R. H. and Ganguly, R.: Therapeutic efficacy of inosiplex (Isoprinosine) in rhinovirus infection. *Ann N Y Acad Sci* 284:153, 1977.

West, S., Brandon, B., Stolley, P., and Rumrill, R.: A review of antihistamines and the common cold *Pediatrics* 56:100-107, 1975.

12

SINUSITIS
Robert H. Waldman, M.D.

Sinusitis is an inflammation of the paranasal sinuses. It is a troublesome, often recurrent, and common condition, estimated to occur in at least 25% of people. It may be either acute or chronic, but the common feature of both is that the disease results from inadequate drainage of the sinus. This inadequate drainage may be secondary to allergy, to swollen mucosae from a viral infection, or from some other type of obstructing lesion, with the result that bacteria gain entrance into the space and multiply. Acute sinusitis is characterized by pressure, pain, local tenderness (particularly in the cheek and upper teeth), and relatively minimal fever. Radiographic examination reveals an air-fluid level in the affected sinus.

Chronic sinusitis is characterized by a purulent discharge, either nasally or down the posterior pharynx, and local pain. Radiographic examination reveals a thickened mucosa. Chronic sinusitis is often a result of local irritation, as from cigarette smoke.

Etiology

Most bacterial infections of the sinuses, other than those of dental origin, are secondary to virus infection causing swollen mucous membranes and obstruction to drainage. The sinus then becomes colonized by organisms found in the normal flora. The most common organisms isolated are pneumococci, streptococci, *Haemophilus influenzae,* and staphylococci (Table 12.1). Among several studies, the results of sinus cultures vary widely at least in part due to differing techniques, particularly with respect to attempts to isolate anaerobes. Normal healthy sinuses are invariably negative for bacteria. Some workers have concluded that there is no significant difference between the microbial flora in acute and chronic sinusitis;

TABLE 12.1   Etiologic Agents in Sinusitis (%)

Organism(s)	Acute	Chronic
Pneumococci	20-35*	5-15
H. influenzae	15-30	3-10
Streptococci (aerobes and anaerobes)	5-35	10-25
Other anaerobes	5-10	25-30
S. aureus	3-6	5-15
No growth	20-25	25-60

*Range from various studies, percentage of patients from whom organism was isolated

however, others have shown that in acute sinusitis pure cultures are usually found, while in chronic sinusitis there is a tendency to isolate a mixed growth of organisms. It would also appear that pneumococci and H. influenzae are isolated less commonly in chronic sinusitis, that anaerobes are more common, and that anaerobes may account for the much higher incidence of "no bacterial isolate" from cases of chronic sinusitis. Other workers have found L forms, which are bacterial variants that replicate with defective or absent cell walls, usually in areas with high osmotic concentrations. They can be isolated only by using special techniques not usually employed in the ordinary hospital bacteriology laboratory.

On rare occasions viruses or fungi have been isolated from patients with acute or chronic sinusitis.

Epidemiology and Pathogenesis

As indicated previously, sinusitis is a common condition, accounting for about a million work days lost each year in the United States. Contributory factors are lower socioeconomic conditions, infections of the upper respiratory tract and of the teeth, and associated pulmonary diseases.

Although acute rhinitis is by far the most common factor in the development of acute sinusitis, pharyngitis, tonsillitis, and adenoiditis, all can serve as a focus of infection. Because of the close proximity of the maxillary sinus to the teeth, it is not surprising that odontogenic infection accounts for about 10% of cases of maxillary sinusitis. This leads to the clinical point that in patients with maxillary sinusitis the condition of the teeth should not be overlooked.

The known relationship between sinus infections and diseases of the chest, including chronic bronchitis, asthma, bronchiectasis, and cystic fibrosis, raises the difficult question of cause and effect, i.e., is the sinusitis important in the etiology of bronchiectasis, or vice versa? This question is impossible to answer at the present time.

Another contributing factor is trauma, including fractures of the sinuses, foreign bodies, and barotrauma. Anatomic abnormalities, such as a deviated nasal septum resulting from trauma, also predispose to the development of sinusitis because of interference with normal drainage.

It has been postulated that acute sinusitis can result from swimming in contaminated water. It is thought that during diving or jumping into the water, bacteria may be forced into the sinuses. Furthermore, even if the water is not contaminated, it is felt that chemical rhinitis as a result of disinfectants in swimming pool water may cause enough mucosal irritation and edema to lead to secondary bacterial sinusitis.

Sinusitis is most common in the maxillary sinus, followed by ethmoid, frontal, and sphenoidal, in that order. Often, however, there is simultaneous involvement of more than one sinus.

Diagnosis

The diagnosis is usually based on clinical findings. Symptoms include both general (fever, malaise, and headache) and local ones. The local symptoms, in the early stages, may consist only of a feeling of discomfort in the postnasal space, with clear nasal passages, but this quickly gives way to nasal obstruction on the side of the sinusitis, with loss of vocal resonance. A nearly constant symptom is nasal or postnasal discharge, with the former early in the course of illness, becoming postnasal later on. Patients may complain of olfactory disturbances, unpleasant taste, and/or epistaxis. Pain is localized or is referred along branches of the nerves involved in the inflammation. Maxillary pain is characteristically described by drawing the finger from the inner canthus of the eye downward across the cheek under the eye. It also radiates along the upper alveolus and is referred to the teeth or gums on the infected side. Ethmoidal pain is localized over the bridge of the nose and inner canthus of the eye. Patients also have a feeling of tenderness of the eyeball and pain behind the eye aggravated by eye movements. Sphenoidal sinusitis causes occipital or vertical headaches, and usually there is pain behind the eye, but the eye itself is not tender. The pain of frontal sinusitis is localized mainly to the forehead and is nearly always associated with generalized headaches.

Patients with chronic sinusitis may have any of these symptoms and signs, and in addition, often have pharyngitis and/or laryngitis, due to the continuous drainage of infected purulent material; chronic bronchitis; mild nausea, thought to be due to the swallowing of large amounts of infected secretions; and/or conjunctivitis, which can be a result of obstruction of the lacrimal tract.

In frontal sinusitis, pressure over the floor of the sinus just above the inner canthus usually elicits pain. In maxillary sinusitis, there may be slight flushing and swelling of the cheek, which may spread to the lower eyelid.

On examination of the anterior or posterior nasal passages, localized areas of red, shiny, and swollen mucosa in the neighborhood of the ostia of the infected sinus may be seen. If one sees pus flowing from the ostium of a sinus, this is very good evidence of sinusitis. However, if pus is seen trickling down the middle turbinate or bulla ethmoidalis, it would not be clear which particular sinus was infected.

Transillumination can be used to examine the maxillary and frontal sinuses. An abnormality is noted if the light transmission is decreased, this usually being detectable only by comparing the right and left sides. To examine the maxillary sinuses, a bright light is placed tightly against the skin over each of the maxillary sinuses with the patient's mouth widely open. The strength of the light transmission is observed to the side of the roof of the mouth. To examine the frontal sinuses, the bright light is placed on the inner aspect of the roof of the orbit, and the light transmission is observed over the frontal sinuses, i.e., on each side of the lower part of the forehead. In my experience, transillumination has not been a helpful way to make the diagnosis of sinusitis.

The laboratory is of minimal help in diagnosing sinusitis. It is impractical to obtain sinus cultures on every patient with acute sinusitis. Gram stain and cultures of nasal secretions have been used, but careful evaluation reveals that they have almost no relationship to the organism that is causing the sinusitis. In chronic sinusitis, aspiration of the sinus fluid for culture and sensitivities should be carried out by a physician skilled in the procedure. The material should be cultured for both aerobes and anaerobes.

Roentgenography has been shown to have an accuracy of approximately 80-85% in diagnosing sinusitis. The radiologic findings of fluid levels within the sinuses, opaque sinuses (suggesting that the sinus is filled with pus), and a thickened mucosal lining, all are suggestive of sinusitis but are not pathognomonic.

The differential diagnosis includes:

1. Dental neuralgia: can be differentiated with a careful dental examination.
2. Temporomandibular neuralgia: this is caused by strain on the temporomandibular joint by abnormalities in the bite mechanism or clenching the teeth, and probably can be differentiated on the basis of the location of the pain and a careful history and observation of the patient.
3. Trigeminal neuralgia: pain is over the fifth cranial nerve distribution only.
4. Migraine: a history of similar pain on previous occasions will usually differentiate.
5. Temporal arteritis: the location of the pain and tenderness will usually differentiate.
6. Other infectious diseases: erysipelas may cause confusion because of the swelling and redness over a cheek, along with headache and fever. This should be differentiable on the basis of the swelling and stippling of the skin surface. Other infectious diseases that might be confused are extremely rare, e.g., nasal diphtheria and typhoid fever.

Treatment

As with other infectious diseases that have been covered in this section, the basic principles are adequate drainage, appropriate antibiotic therapy, and a general conservative approach to therapy since the prognosis without treatment is extremely good. Surgical procedures should be avoided unless absolutely necessary.

Antibiotic therapy is empirical, based on a knowledge of the likely pathogens. Seven to ten days of ampicillin or tetracycline is usually successful. Studies have shown that ampicillin reaches higher concentrations in the sinus secretions than do other antibiotics tested. Of special note is that cephalosporin levels in the sinus secretions are particularly low. Medical drainage, using decongestants, should certainly be given an adequate trial before more aggressive therapy is undertaken. Topical decongestant nosedrops also may be helpful. Antihistamines should be used if there is a history suggestive of an allergic component underlying the illness.

In patients who are failures on medical therapy (i.e., the patient is deteriorating), surgical drainage, with cultures of the aspirated fluid, should be carried out by a physician skilled in the procedure.

The management of chronic sinusitis depends principally on whether or not the lining mucosa has been chronically and irreversibly damaged by repeated infection. If recovery of the mucosal lining is possible, treatment should be conservative and consist of adequate drainage by medical or minor surgical procedures such as antral washouts. If recovery of the mucosal lining is not possible, surgery is inevitable. The surgical procedure can be one of two types: (1) all of the diseased mucous membrane is excised and a good drainage system is created; (2) obliteration of the sinus cavity.

Finally, it is important to emphasize that the underlying causes of sinusitis, such as infected teeth, allergies, or mechanical obstruction, must be corrected.

Complications

Sinusitis is complicated by involvement or dissolution of the bony walls of the sinus, leading to spread of the infection into adjacent orbital or intracranial tissues. Due to widespread use of antibiotics, complications are uncommon, but when they do occur they usually follow an acute exacerbation of chronic sinusitis. The most common complication is orbital inflammatory disease. Eyelid edema is the earliest sign of orbital involvement. At this stage, there is usually minimal sinus pain or eye discomfort. Treatment involves decongestants and parenteral antibiotics.

Orbital cellulitis is characterized by diffuse inflammation, pain, limitation of eye movement, chemosis (conjunctival edema), proptosis, and impairment of visual acuity. Treatment of this complication is high-dose intravenous antibiotics, decongestants, and warm compresses, or alternatively, surgical drainage plus antibiotics. Antibiotic therapy should be continued for 4-6 weeks, although after stabilization of the patient, the route of antibiotic administration can be switched to oral.

With orbital abscess, the patient has internal and external ophthalmoplegia, impaired vision, chemosis, and proptosis. Patients have central scotomata, rapidly progressing to complete loss of vision. Orbital apex syndrome results from posterior orbital inflammation and is characterized by the classic triad of ophthalmic nerve anesthesia, internal and external ophthalmoplegia, and amaurosis secondary to optic neuritis or atrophy. Both of these latter complications are extremely serious and require the care of an experienced ophthalmologist as well as a generalist with considerable experience in infectious diseases.

Cavernous sinus thrombosis presents as high fever, chills, signs of meningeal irritation, and the patient appears extremely toxic. The use of heparin is controversial, both because of lack of evidence of benefit, and also because of the problem with hemorrhagic infarctions resulting from venous thrombosis. Other intracranial complications are epidural abscess, or brain abscess.

Osteomyelitis was common in the preantibiotic era, but fortunately is rare today. The frontal bone is the most commonly involved, and treatment, as with other types of osteomyelitis, requires prolonged antibiotic therapy.

With all of these complications, early diagnosis is important, and can only be obtained if the primary care physician has a high index of suspicion, and carries out careful ophthalmologic and neurologic examinations.

Prevention and Immunology

Sinus secretions contain mainly IgA which is produced locally in response to infection. There seems to be a relationship between the concentration of IgA antibody and recovery from infection.

It makes sense that decongestants and antihistamines might be beneficial in preventing sinusitis in patients who have upper respiratory infections. However, this has never been proved to be the case. Nonetheless, use of these drugs is recommended, especially in patients with recurrent sinusitis, or patients in whom an allergic component is felt to be significant in the pathogenesis of the sinusitis.

Selected Bibliography

Axelsson, A.: Treatment of acute maxillary sinusitis. A comparison of four different methods. *Acta Otolaryngol* 70:71-76, 1970.

Axelsson, A.: Treatment of acute maxillary sinusitis. II. A comparison of five further methods. *Acta Otolaryngol* 72:148-154, 1971.

Axelsson, A.: Concentration of antibiotics in sinus secretions. Doxycycline and spiramycin. *Ann Otol Rhinol Laryngol* 82:44-48, 1973.

Axelsson, A.: The concentration of antibiotics in sinus secretions. Ampicillin, cephradine and erythromycin estolate. *Ann Otol Rhinol Laryngol* 83:323-331, 1974.

Axelsson, A. and Jensen, C.: The roentgenologic demonstration of sinusitis. *Am J Roentgenol Radium Ther Nucl Med* 122:621-627, 1974.

Baily, B.: Management of sinus infections. *Am Fam Physician* 8:100-107, 1973.

Bhattacharyya, T.: Incidence of bacteria, L-form and mycoplasma in chronic sinusitis. *Acta Otolaryngol* 74:293-296, 1972.

Bjorkwall, T.: Bacteriological examinations in maxillary sinusitis. *Acta Otolaryngol* 83(suppl):1, 1950.

Carenfelt, C.: Pneumococcal antibodies in maxillary sinus secretion. *Scand J Infect Dis* 9:277, 1977.

Frederick, J.: Anaerobic infection of the paranasal sinuses. *N Engl J Med* 290: 135-137, 1974.

Gnarpe, H. and Lundberg, C.: Preliminary report: L-phase organisms in maxillary sinus secretions. *Scand J Infect Dis* 3:257-259, 1971.

McNeil, R.: Comparison of the findings on transillumination, x-ray and lavage of the maxillary sinus. *J Laryngol* 77:1009, 1963.

Rantanen, T.: Double-blind trial of doxycycline in acute maxillary sinusitis. A clinical and bacteriological study. *Acta Otolaryngol* 76:58-62, 1973.

Rulon, J.: Sinusitis in children. *Postgrad Med* 48:107-112, 1970.

Sanders, S.: Allergic rhinitis and sinusitis. *Otolaryngol Clin N Am* 4:565-578, 1971.

Urdal, K. and Berdal, P.: The microbial flora in 81 cases of maxillary sinusitis. *Acta Otolaryngol* 37:20, 1949.

13

OTITIS MEDIA AND EXTERNA
Robert H. Waldman, M.D.

Otitis Media

Otitis media is an inflammation of the mucosal lining of the middle ear and can be divided into various types, including acute otitis media, thought to be nearly always of infectious origin; secretory or serous otitis media, from which microorganisms usually cannot be cultured; and various forms of chronic otitis media. This section will concern itself primarily with acute otitis media, a common condition, mainly in children, which can lead to serious, and even life-threatening consequences. The most troublesome aspect of acute otitis media is that of recurrences which result in progressive loss of hearing.

Etiology

There is a strong relationship between acute otitis media and common respiratory viral infections. There is a particularly strong correlation between adenoviral and respiratory syncytial viral epidemics, especially in infants under 1 year of age. Another frequent association is with measles: 10% of children with measles develop acute otitis media. However, actual isolation of viral agents from middle ear fluids in patients with acute otitis media can rarely be accomplished. It is thought that acute otitis media occurs as a secondary complication of the common respiratory viral infections, not as a result of primary infection by the viruses of the mucosa of the middle ear.

Bacterial agents are commonly found, with one or more bacterial strains isolated from aspirated middle ear fluid 70-80% of the time. Stated another way, despite the very best in culture techniques, including searching for anaerobic organisms, 20-30% of the fluids are sterile. These patients with sterile middle ear

144

fluids appear clinically no different from patients from whom positive isolates are obtained, and it is believed that most of these represent patients in whom the organisms are extremely fastidious, or in whom the organisms have died in the usual course of events of the disease. Table 13.1 shows the composite results of several studies determining the most common organisms isolated from patients with acute otitis media. The pneumococcus is the most common organism found, although there are data which suggest that the pneumococcus generally does not play a primary pathogenic role in the disease. As mentioned earlier, it appears that a viral infection sets the stage, with secondary bacterial infections causing the disease. Pneumococcal otitis media tends to be accompanied by more pain and fever. The *Haemophilus influenzae* strains are usually rough, unencapsulated, and untypable. Anaerobes are commonly found, sometimes in pure culture, but often mixed with other anaerobes or with aerobes.

With respect to the bacterial distribution among age groups, earlier studies suggested that *H. influenzae*, *Staphylococcus aureus*, and various gram-negative organisms were more common in neonates and young children; however, more recent studies have not supported this, showing the same bacterial distribution in younger children as in older ones. *Staphylococcus aureus*, while being relatively rare in initial attacks, is more common with recurrent episodes of the disease.

In patients with chronic otitis media, it is not uncommon to find enteric gram-negative organisms such as *Proteus, Klebsiella, Enterobacter,* and *Pseudomonas* spp.

TABLE 13.1   Bacteria Found Most Commonly in Middle Ear Fluid in Patients with Acute Otitis Media

Organism	% of Patients
Pneumococci	25-75
*H. influenzae**	15-30
Anaerobes (peptococci and propionibacteria)	20-30
Group A streptococci	2-10
S. aureus	1-5
Less common: gram-negative enteric bacteria, myco-bacteria, corynebacteria, and *N. catarrhalis*	

*15-40% of *H. influenzae* are ampicillin-resistant

Pathogenesis

As previously mentioned, acute otitis media is preceded most commonly by a viral upper respiratory infection, leading to secondary bacterial growth on the mucosa of the middle ear. As is common with respect to infections of other semiclosed spaces of the body, infection of the middle ear occurs when the normal drainage pathway is blocked. This normal drainage occurs via the eustachian tubes. In infants and young children, the eustachian tube is relatively short and straight, and therefore, bacteria have easier access than in older individuals. In addition, in younger individuals, there is more abundant lymphatic tissue surrounding the nasopharyngeal opening of the eustachian tube, with consequent obstruction common with lymphatic hypertrophy. Another anatomic predisposition is seen with the frequent association of acute otitis media with the occurrence of cleft palate.

Thus it is easy to see that with viral upper respiratory infection edema and transient lymphatic enlargement occur, leading to partial obstruction of the eustachian tube. If there are potentially pathogenic bacteria in the upper respiratory tract, the coughing and sneezing which occur with the viral respiratory infection, or with even the normal swallowing activity, may force secretions containing bacteria into the eustachian tube, but these secretions are unable to drain back normally into the nasopharynx. The bacteria then are able to multiply and cause infection. The usual time course from the onset of symptoms of a viral upper respiratory infection to the onset of acute otitis media is 5-10 days.

Epidemiology

More than 75% of children will have one or more attacks of acute otitis media, with the first attack almost always occurring before 10 years of age. The commonness of this disease is attested to by the results of one survey in which acute otitis media accounted for about 25% of visits to a pediatrician in children under 6 years of age. About half of neonates in the first year of life will have acute otitis media. Many of these neonates will have multiple attacks in the succeeding year or two after the first attack. The incidence of attacks decreases with age, and the disease is uncommon in adults.

From the association with acute upper respiratory viral infections, it is not surprising that otitis media is most common during the winter months.

Clinical Diagnosis

The most important aspect of the diagnosis is visualization of the eardrum. This makes the diagnosis difficult at times. Overdiagnosis results when the observer sees what appears as a reddened and/or bulging drum in a child who has been crying or who has a respiratory infection but not otitis media.

Because of the importance of seeing the drum clearly, cerumen should be removed if necessary. Bulging will occur first in the area of the pars flaccida (Shrapnell's membrane), because it is the least rigid part of the drum. Most experts feel that redness is a less important criterion than is bulging. As the disease progresses and pressure increases, the entire drum may be distorted, leading to disappearance of the light reflex. While pain and fever may not be present earlier, at this point, with bulging of the entire drum, nearly all patients have those findings.

Visualization is unnecessary in patients who have recently had spontaneous perforation of their drum, leading to a profuse mucopurulent discharge. In these patients cleaning the ear canal sufficiently to visualize the drum causes unnecessary trauma to the child. In this setting the differential diagnosis of otitis media and otitis externa may be slightly difficult, except that in the latter there is extreme pain of the ear canal.

In addition to pain which occurs in as few as one-fourth of the patients, especially if diagnosed and treated early, and fever which occurs in 40-70%, other symptoms are pulling at the ear by the patient, nausea, and vomiting.

Some writers in this area recommend pneumatic otoscopy as a more sensitive method for diagnosing early acute otitis media. This may be especially helpful in differentiating acute otitis media from viral myringitis, a fairly common finding in acute viral respiratory infection, but in which there is no fluid behind the drum and the pneumatic otoscopy is normal.

Laboratory Diagnosis

Culture of all cases is impractical since in the usual clinical situation the diagnosis is made on clinical grounds, and antibiotic therapy is begun empirically based on knowledge of the usual pathogens. After spontaneous perforation, culture is useful only if obtained very soon, i.e., within the first 8 hours. Pharyngeal and nasopharyngeal cultures are worthless in determining the bacterial etiology. If myringotomy is performed, a culture from the tip of the myringotomy knife is accurate and should be performed.

Treatment

As with most common infectious problems, there are a few basic principles underlying the proper therapeutic approach to acute otitis media: (1) most importantly, adequate drainage must occur; (2) appropriate antibiotic therapy used in appropriate dosages and for an adequate length of time to eradicate the offending organism/organisms; (3) since the natural history of the untreated disease is that approximately 97% of patients will recover completely, therapy must be safe, and it must be remembered that (a) a lot of patients are being treated with no benefit to them in order to prevent complications in that very small 3%; and (b) evaluation of therapy is difficult because nearly any therapeutic approach, assuming it is not strikingly harmful, will lead to overwhelming success.

With respect to drainage, there is considerable controversy over the question of the necessity of surgical drainage and moreover, which procedure should be done, i.e., myringotomy or tympanocentesis. These relatively invasive procedures may be of benefit, not only because they drain the infected site, but because they enable obtaining material for culture. Although there are differences between authorities in this area, it would seem prudent to recommend drainage in the following situations: (1) All newborns (to obtain material for culture since the infecting organism may be one of the less common; (2) children who are seriously ill or toxic, (3) patients who are not responding to more conservative management; (4) patients who develop acute otitis media while on antibiotics; (5) those who develop suppurative complications (see later discussion); and (6) patients who are immunocompromised. Another value of myringotomy is that it is beneficial for the immediate relief of severe pain.

Drainage may be enhanced by medical means, i.e., use of decongestants. Although they have not been proved effective, they are probably beneficial, are quite safe, and are recommended. The addition of antihistamines to the decongestant regimen, either separately or in combination preparations, has theoretical merit for several reasons: the possible relationship of allergic reactions to the lymphatic hypertrophy and mucosal edema, and the decongestive and sedative actions of antihistamines. However, recent studies indicate no benefit, either prophylactically or therapeutically.

Antibiotic therapy usually is empiric and is aimed at the most common bacterial pathogens found in this disease, i.e., the pneumococcus, *H. influenzae,* streptococci, both aerobes and anaerobes, and the various other anaerobic agents. The antibiotic which best fits the bill is ampicillin, 50-100 mg/kg/day in four divided doses for 10-14 days, or alternatively, equivalent doses of amoxicillin. In patients who are allergic to penicillin, erythromycin, 30-50 mg/kg/day plus a sulfonamide, 100 mg/kg/day, or the fixed combination of sulfamethoxazole and trimethoprim is quite effective.   The general expense of the various regimens is summarized in Table 13.2.

A variable problem is ampicillin-resistant *H. influenzae.* The incidence of these resistant organisms seems to vary with geographic location and the season of the year, but the most recent data indicate that 15-40% of the isolates are resistant. Where the incidence is low, it would not seem to be a large enough problem to stop using ampicillin or amoxicillin. Where the problem is of greater magnitude, two alternatives are reasonable, either the use of penicillin-sulfonamide combination, or sulfamethoxazole-trimethoprim combination routinely, or the use of one of those alternatives, or chloramphenicol, only if the patient does not seem to be showing a response after 48 hr of ampicillin or amoxicillin.

The old approach of using penicillin in patients over 4 or 5 years of age, based on the belief that *H. influenzae* infection was rare in older children, cannot be supported by more recent data.

The effects of antibiotics on the clinical illness are not striking. Clinicians should remember that the main purpose of antibiotic therapy in otitis media is to prevent sequelae, although even with respect to this, antibiotics may have no effect on the incidence of recurrences.

Complications

The most dreaded complication of otitis media before the antibiotic era was spread of the infection causing mastoiditis, meningitis, and/or brain abscess. However, these complications are rare today and represent the most important contribution

TABLE 13.2   Cost to Pharmacist of Antibiotics to Treat Average 10 Kg Child with Otitis Media

Antibiotic	Dosage	Cost ($)
Amoxicillin	62.5 mg (1/2 tsp) t.i.d.	2.00
Trimethoprim; sulfamethoxazole	40 mg; 200 mg (5 ml) b.i.d.	2.35
Ampicillin	125 mg (5 ml) q.i.d.	2.80
Erythromycin plus sulfisoxazole	100 mg (1/2 tsp) q.i.d. 375 mg (3/4 tsp) q.i.d.	4.80
Cefaclor	125 mg (5 ml) t.i.d.	8.25

that antibiotic therapy has made in relation to this disease. More common complications, and ones that antibiotics have had little or no impact upon, are persistence of the inflammation and relapse. In reference to the latter, the relapse rate is about 20% within 2 months, is higher if the causative organism is *H. influenzae,* and is unrelated to whether or not a myringotomy was performed. An important contributory factor may be the presence of underlying allergic disease, causing recurrent obstruction of the eustachian tube. Therefore with recurrences strict attention should be paid to this possibility.

Persistent effusion is common, occurring in 10-60% of patients. This complication is more common in younger patients and in whites. If the persistent effusion lasts for more than 2-4 months, myringotomy is usually recommended. Medical treatment consists of decongestants and antihistamines.

Another complication is a perforated eardrum. This complication probably requires no specific therapy, although some experts recommend a combination steroid-antibiotic eardrop. There is no evidence that this has been efficacious, and 3-5% of recipients of these drops develop hypersensitivity to the antibiotic component.

A poorly studied, yet potentially very important complication of acute otitis media is the problem of acquisition of learning and language skills, personality development, etc. Certainly acute otitis media is the most frequent cause of conductive hearing loss in children, and studies have shown that it may be associated with impaired cognitive development.

Rarer, but more life threatening complications of acute otitis media are mastoiditis, meningitis, facial nerve palsy, suppurative labyrinthitis, and lateral sinus thrombophlebitis. A mild mastoiditis probably occurs in all cases of acute otitis media. However, significant mastoiditis is manifest by recurrence of pain, low-grade fever, mastoid tenderness, and continued drainage of purulent material from the ear. On physical examination there is an outward and downward displacement of the pinna. The treatment is high doses of antibiotics intravenously; adequate drainage of the middle ear; topical antibiotic-steroid drops, the purpose of which is to shrink the mucosa to aid in drainage; and surgery. Meningitis is a serious complication which must be kept in mind, especially in infants with acute otitis media.

If a patient develops a facial nerve palsy the treatment is immediate myringotomy plus high-dose intravenous antibiotics and steroids (80 mg prednisone for 7 days with gradual tapering). Surgical decompression should be carried out if the patient does not respond or if nerve conduction studies show degeneration of the nerve.

Suppurative labyrinthitis is manifested by sudden loss of cochlear and vestibular function. The treatment is high-dosage intravenous antibiotics, myringotomy, close observation for intracranial spread, and surgical drainage of the labyrinth at the first indication of meningitis. Lateral sinus thrombophlebitis is manifest by the classic finding of a "picket-fence" type of fever, i.e., fever spikes once or twice each day. This complication often leads to brain abscess. Treatment is high-dose intravenous antibiotics, surgical drainage, and removal of all infected material. Since infarction of cerebral tissue from venous thromboses tends to be hemorrhagic, anticoagulants should not be used.

Prevention - Immunology

The immunology of the middle ear may be of some importance in understanding the normal host defenses against acute otitis media. In normal individuals, there are no antibody manufacturing cells detectable in the mucosa. In otitis media, the fluid contains antibodies of all immunoglobulin classes, but has high concentrations of secretory IgA. In patients with serous otitis media, the middle ear mucosa contains many IgA-producing cells. However, there currently is no proof as to what protective immune mechanism(s) if any, develop(s) following the infection.

Of great recent interest has been the use of prophylactic antibiotics in very high-risk groups, e.g., Eskimos. Studies have shown a decrease in the number of recurrent bouts of otitis media in children given prophylactic ampicillin or sulfisoxazole. However, more studies are needed before a definite recommendation can be given. Since about 6% of colds in young children lead to acute otitis media, it would seem reasonable to use decongestants, or a decongestant-antihistamine mixture during colds to prevent the development of acute otitis media. This approach, however rational, has not been useful in well-controlled studies.

Tonsilloadenoidectomy has been proposed as a way of preventing recurrent otitis media, and this may be necessary. However, it would seem appropriate to try prophylactic antibiotics first. Tympanostomy tubes are fairly commonly used to provide constant drainage; however, they have never been shown to be beneficial, and they certainly are traumatic to the child as well as being expensive.

With the recent introduction on the market of pneumococcal vaccine, the question arises as to its usefulness in preventing pneumococcal otitis media. Certainly the vaccine is well tolerated, but there are no published studies showing its efficacy in preventing acute otitis media. In addition, children under 2 years of age do not have a consistent immune response to the vaccine and therefore, it might be expected to provide poor protection in this group, the one that most needs the protection.

Tuberculous Otitis Media

This is a rare disease today which is characterized by chronic painless discharge, chronic mastoiditis, and progressive deafness. The diagnosis is made by staining and culture of the discharge.

Seromucinous Otitis Media

The hallmark of seromucinous otitis media is a sterile effusion. This disorder is questionably related to prior acute otitis media with incomplete antibiotic treatment. The prevalence seems to be increasing and is seen in 1-4% of children. Occasional viral isolates have been detected, in particular parainfluenza and respiratory syncytial viruses.

One hypothesis as to the etiology of seromucinous otitis media is that it is an allergic reaction. Eosinophils are commonly, but not invariably found. IgE is usually absent in the fluid.

The clinical picture is one of conduction deafness, usually bilateral, insidious onset, usually only detected at the time of entrance to school, and the physical finding of an opaque drum with increased vasculature and loss of mobility. Seeing a fluid level is diagnostic, but it is not commonly found.

The fluid is of variable consistency, from thin to "glue-like," the color is clear to green, and there are many cells, mainly polymorphonuclear leukocytes and macrophages.

The treatment is surgical drainage. Most of the patients have a mild hearing loss with about 20% having permanent clinical deafness. Ten to twenty percent have to be reoperated on.

Otitis Externa

Otitis externa is a skin infection of the external auditory canal and auricle of the ear. It is usually a localized infection, but may be associated with a generalized condition such as psoriasis or herpes zoster.

Otitis externa is most commonly a bacterial infection, with *Pseudomonas aeruginosa* and *Streptococcus pyogenes* isolated more than any other agents. In some series, 10% of the infections are caused by fungi, particularly *Aspergillus niger* and *Candida albicans;* however, it is not clear if they are actually causing the infection, or if they simply colonize the already infected skin. Otitis externa may be a result of herpes zoster, varicella, or herpes simplex virus. Infection with one of the viruses is distinctive in that vesiculations or hemorrhagic blebs may be seen. Otitis externa also may be associated with allergic skin reactions, trauma, other dermatitides such as seborrheic dermatitis or eczema, or some combination of these etiologic factors.

The disease usually begins with trauma to the skin, such as placing an object in the external canal in an attempt to clean it. The disease is more common in hot and humid weather and following swimming or showering. This is explained on the basis of wetness and higher temperatures providing a good culture medium for the bacteria or fungi which are omnipresent in the external canal.

The clinical manifestations are swelling of the auricle and the external auditory canal, pain and tenderness, particularly with pulling on the pinna, but usually absence of systemic manifestations such as fever and leukocytosis.

The diagnosis is strictly clinical based on the signs and symptoms. A purulent discharge usually indicates a bacterial cause. Culture may be obtained for bacteria and fungi, but this usually is not necessary because the results are hard to interpret, the question is always arising as to whether or not organisms that are isolated are really pathogenic; and in almost all cases the culture results would not influence the therapeutic approach.

The treatment is first to cleanse the affected area with a mild saline solution, decrease the inflammation with steroid drops, and administer topical antibiotics. The latter two can be accomplished using a combination of antibiotics and corticosteroids in a solution which is administered several times a day using a cotton wick to ensure that the solution penetrates deeply into the auditory canal and maintains contact with the affected area. In selecting the antibiotic, the important criteria are that the antibiotic or antibiotics are effective against both pseudomonads and streptococci, and that the chance of sensitization, leading to an allergic reaction, is small.

In more severe cases, if pre- or postauricular cellulitis is present, systemic antibiotics should be used. If the infection does not resolve promptly, i.e., within 3-5 days, one should suspect an underlying problem such as seborrheic dermatitis or habitual mechanical irritation.

Prevention is accomplished with good hygiene, guarding against trauma to the external auditory canal, and keeping the ear canal dry during warm, humid weather, or following swimming or showering. This can be accomplished by the use of 70% alcohol on a cotton wick.

Malignant Otitis Externa

This is a fulminate form of otitis externa, characterized by pain, edema, purulent discharge, and loss of hearing. The pain is deep and boring, and worse at night. Patients who are predisposed to this severe illness are the elderly, diabetics, and patients who are malnourished, anemic, with severe atherosclerosis, or who have had frostbite. This affliction leads to extension beyond the canal with resultant chondritis and osteomyelitis. Radiologic examination reveals soft-tissue swelling and, with advanced cases, bony erosions. Neurologic changes eventually result, with facial nerve palsy. The differential diagnosis includes benign or malignant tumors of the area.

The pathogen is almost always *P. aeruginosa,* although *Aspergillus* has been reported on occasion. Treatment involves control of the diabetes if present, full doses of intravenous gentamicin (or tobramycin) and ticarcillin (or carbenicillin) for 10-14 days, and careful cleaning of the external canal. Aspergillus infection would require amphotericin B therapy. Surgical debridement may be indicated.

Selected Bibliography

Chandler, J. R.: Malignant external otitis. *Laryngoscope* 78:1259-1294, 1968.

Cowan, D. L. and Brown, M. J. K. M.: Seromucinous otitis media and its sequelae. *J Laryngol Otol* 88:1237, 1974.

Dermot, J., Durcan, R. T. S., Goodchild, R.T.S., and Weingraf, C.: Otitis externa - A report on a multicentre clinical trial. *J Laryngol Otol* 82:379, 1968.

Holm, V. A. and Kunze, L. H.: Effect of chronic otitis media on language and speech development. *Pediatrics* 43:833, 1969.

Howie, V. M., Ploussard, J. H., and Lester, R. L., Jr.: Otitis media: A clinical and bacteriological correlation. *Pediatrics* 45:29, 1970.

Howie, V. M., Ploussard, J. H., and Sleyer, J.: Comparison of ampicillin and amoxicillin in the treatment of otitis media in children. *J Infect Dis* 129: 5181, 1974.

Kaplan, G. J., Fleshman, J. K., Bender, T. R., et al.: Long-term effects of otitis media: A ten-year cohort study of Alaskan Eskimo children. *Pediatrics* 52: 577-585, 1973.

Maynard, J. E., Fleshman, J. K., and Schopp, C. F.: Otitis media in Alaskan Eskimo children. Prospective evaluation of chemoprophylaxis. *JAMA* 219:597, 1972.

Nilson, B. W., Poland, R. L., Thompson, R. S., Morehead, D., Baghdossarian, A., and Carver, D. H.: Acute otitis media: Treatment results in relation to bacterial etiology. *Pediatrics* 43:351, 1969.

Olson, A. L., Klein, S. W., Charney, E., et al.: Prevention and therapy of serous otitis media by oral decongestant: A doubleblind study in pediatric practice. *Pediatrics* 61:679, 1978.

Paparella, M. M.: Pathology of sensorineural hearing loss in otitis media. *Ann Otol* 81:632-647, 1972.

Perrin, J. M., Charney, E., MacWhinney, J. B., et al.: Sulfisoxazole as chemoprophylaxis for recurrent otitis media. A doubleblind crossover study in pediatric practice. *N Engl J Med* 291:667, 1974.

Reed, W. P.: The immunologic substrate: Role of local and systemic immunity in the head and neck. *Otolaryngol Clin N Am* 9:581, 1976.

Roddey, D. F., Jr., Earle, R., Jr., and Haggerty, R.: Myringotomy in acute otitis media: A controlled study. *JAMA* 197:849-853, 1966.

Schwartz, R., Rodriguez, W. J., Khan, W. N., and Ross, S.: Acute purulent otitis media in children older than 5 years. *JAMA* 238:1032-1033, 1977.

Shurin, P. A., Pelton, S. I., Donner, A., and Klein, J. O.: Persistence of middle-ear effusion after acute otitis media in children. *N Engl J Med* 300:1121-1123, 1979.

Zinkus, P. W., Gottlieb, M. I., and Schapiro, M.: Development and psychoeducational sequelae of chronic otitis media. *Am J Dis Child* 132:1100-1104, 1978.

14

PHARYNGITIS, EPIGLOTTITIS, DEEP NECK INFECTIONS, AND PERITONSILLAR ABSCESSES
David L. Hoover, M.D.

Pharyngitis

Pharyngitis, soreness of the throat usually accompanied by objective findings of erythema, exudate, or enlarged cervical lymph nodes, may be caused by the agents noted in Table 14.1.

Streptococcus Pyogenes

Group A streptococcal pharyngitis is important both numerically, accounting for approximately one-third of the cases and because of its suppurative and nonsuppurative complications. The disease itself is generally self-limited, lasting less than 5 days with or without therapy. Suppurative complications, uncommonly seen since the widespread use of antibiotics, include peritonsillar and retropharyngeal abscesses, sinusitis, and otitis media. The nonsuppurative complications, rheumatic fever and acute poststreptococcal glomerulonephritis, are both probably immunologically mediated. Rheumatic fever may be the result of a host response stimulated by a streptococcal antigen immunologically cross-reactive with the myocardium or heart valve, and may occur after infection with one of many M protein serotypes (Chapter 83). The incidence of this complication is highly variable, at the most on the order of 3% in certain epidemics. In recent years, rheumatic fever has become a much less common disease. Poststreptococcal glomerulonephritis is probably the result of streptococcal antigen-antibody complex deposition in the glomerular basement membrane and follows infection of the skin or pharynx with nephritogenic strains of several M types, especially types 12, 1, 4, 25, and 41.

Clinical differentiation of streptococcal from nonstreptococcal pharyngitis is inaccurate, although the presence of fever, tender cervical lymphadenopathy, and

154

TABLE 14.1   Causes of Pharyngitis

Bacterial

   Group A *S. pyogenes*
   N. gonorrhoeae
   C. diphtheriae
   M. pneumoniae

Viral

   Adenovirus
   Epstein-Barr virus
   Others

---

pharyngeal exudate, and the absence of cough favor a streptococcal causality. Causation of pharyngitis by streptococci is most firmly established by demonstrating an antibody rise to streptococcal enzymic secretory products or cell-wall components. Interpretation of throat cultures is difficult, since 10-20% of asymptomatic individuals are pharyngeal carriers of group A streptococci. For practical purposes, however, patients with pharyngitis and a positive throat culture for group A streptococci should be treated as having a streptococcal infection. For effective treatment to prevent rheumatic fever and suppurative complications, antibiotics (penicillin or erythromycin) must be given for 10 days. A single intramuscular injection of benzathine penicillin achieves this goal with elimination of organisms in 90% of the patients (Table 14.2). Treatment has not been shown to prevent glomerulonephritis.

When a patient has repeated, severe attacks of streptococcal pharyngitis, the question of tonsillectomy may be raised. The usefulness of this approach in decreasing streptococcal sore throats is controversial at best, and is further clouded by the possible immunologic consequences of tonsillectomy. Polio vaccine-induced secretory IgA and IgG levels in nasopharyngeal secretions have been reported to decrease following tonsillectomy; poliovirus immunization in tonsillectomized children produces lower specific secretory IgA levels than in children with intact tonsils. There also may be an association between tonsillectomy and Hodgkin's disease, but there is no clear causal relationship.

TABLE 14.2   **Eradication of Streptococci in Patients with Pharyngitis**

Penicillin	Treatment Failure (Approximate %)
7-day course	31
10-day course	18

Neisseria Gonorrhoeae

Infection of the pharynx with N. gonorrhoeae is most often asymptomatic, occurring primarily in persons who practice fellatio. Clinical pharyngitis with nonspecific findings may occasionally be seen, however. Disseminated gonococcal infection may develop with the pharynx as the only apparent source of infection. Penicillin is the treatment of choice. Spectinomycin may be ineffective in eradicating the organism from this site.

Corynebacterium Diphtheriae

Pharyngitis due to C. diphtheriae occurs primarily in children, especially in those lacking adequate immunization. Sore throat and gradually rising fever are the most common presenting complaints. On examination, a dirty gray-green membrane which resists removal may be seen on the pharynx, tonsils, or tonsillar pillars in approximately three-fourths of the patients. Cervical edema, sometimes severe enough to cause a "bull-neck" appearance, is a frequent finding. Severe complications include airway obstruction and toxin-mediated myocarditis and cranial and peripheral neuropathies. In the unimmunized, the case-fatality rate from diphtheria is about 13%, seven times the rate of those with an adequate immunization history. Prompt antitoxin administration upon clinical suspicion of disease remains the primary mode of therapy. Erythromycin or penicillin should be given to eliminate the organism from patients and their culture-positive contacts.

Mycoplasma Pneumoniae

This organism causes approximately 5% of cases of pharyngitis in adolescents and young adults. Signs and symptoms are nonspecific unless associated with other characteristics of mycoplasmal infection such as myringitis or pneumonia. Generally, antimicrobial therapy for pharyngitis alone is not indicated because of the uncertainty of diagnosis and the benign nature of the disease.

Adenoviruses

The adenoviruses are a common cause of febrile exudative pharyngitis in children and young adults. Conjunctivitis, often unilateral, is frequently present. Cervical adenopathy is usual. In military recruits, epidemics may occur, and have been associated particularly with types 4 and 7.

Epstein-Barr Virus

The Epstein-Barr (EB) virus causes pharyngitis, usually with prominent cervical adenopathy, in nearly all patients with infectious mononucleosis. Approximately one-third of the cases have tonsillar or pharyngeal exudates. Sore throat, especially of more than 3-day duration, accompanied by fever, fatigue, adenopathy, and hepatic or splenic enlargement in an adolescent or young adult should strongly suggest the diagnosis, which may be confirmed by appropriate serologic tests. Treatment is symptomatic. In the unusual case in which marked tonsillar enlargement threatens the airway, particularly in children, a short course of systemic corticosteroids may result in dramatic improvement. The long-term effects of such therapy, however, in terms of latent virus infection, oncogenicity, etc., are unknown and worrisome because of the association of EB virus with lymphoma.

Other Viruses

Parainfluenzae, echo- and coxsackieviruses also may be responsible for pharyngitis. Pharyngitis may accompany the mononucleosis syndrome caused by cytomegalovirus. Herpes simplex virus may cause vesicular and ulcerative lesions in the pharynx either as a manifestation of primary infections or in the immunocompromised host.

Epiglottitis

Epiglottitis, inflammation of the epiglottis and supraglottic tissues, occurs most often in children 2-6 years of age. A growing number of cases, however, has been reported in otherwise healthy adults. Blood cultures are positive for *Haemophilus influenzae,* type b in over 90% of the cases. Similarly, cultures of the epiglottis or pharynx usually reveal *Haemophilus* as well as normal pharyngeal flora. In adults *S. pneumoniae* and *H. parainfluenzae* also have been implicated as causative agents. The typical patient is febrile and complains of soreness of the throat out of proportion to signs of pharyngeal inflammation. With advancing disease, painful dysphagia and a muffled voice occur. The patient sits up, leans forward, protrudes the head, and drools saliva. Acute upper airway obstruction may occur with extreme rapidity. The disease tempo is swift in children, with symptoms developing over hours. In adults, complaints may be present for 2 or more days. Upon serious consideration of the diagnosis attempts to examine the epiglottis should be made only in the immediate presence of personnel and facilities for tracheal intubation. On examination, the bright red epiglottis is edematous, with edema extending to the aryepiglottic folds. In adults an epiglottic abscess may be present. Lateral x-ray films of the neck, not usually necessary for diagnosis, show enlargement of the epiglottic abscess and "hourglass deformity" of the laryngeal vestibule. Peripheral blood leukocytosis and neutrophilia are usual. In children, management consists of immediate securing of the airway either by tracheal intubation or by tracheostomy, and parenteral administration of chloramphenicol. With this approach, the high case-fatality rate noted with observation and emergency intervention in children should be reduced to 1% or less. In adults, due to a larger airway and slower disease progression, close observation, airway humidification, and antibiotic administration may suffice. Epiglottic abscesses should be drained. Despite bacteremia, distant foci of infection are uncommon, although epiglottitis associated with pneumonia, meningitis, sinusitis, and otitis media has been rarely reported.

Deep Neck Infections

Deep neck infections occur primarily in one of three fascial compartments. Infections of the lateral pharyngeal and retropharyngeal spaces are usually secondary to suppuration of lymph nodes that drain the sinuses, middle ear, teeth, and pharynx. The most common causative organisms are group A *S. pyogenes, S. pneumoniae,* and *Staphylococcus aureus.* Anaerobes including *Bacteroides fragilis* may be present alone or with aerobes. Prevertebral abscesses are most often secondary to cervical osteomyelitis. *Staphylococcus aureus* is the most common offender in this region, although *Mycobacterium tuberculosis* has been important in the past. Retropharyngeal and prevertebral abscesses present with fever and symptoms of airway or esophageal obstruction, neck pain, and often a bulging posterior pharynx. In retropharyngeal infections, the bulge frequently is unilateral.

Soft-tissue films of the neck show soft-tissue swelling anterior to the cervical vertebrae. Lateral pharyngeal abscess presents with similar complaints but trismus is common, as are anterior cervical swelling and bulging of the lateral pharyngeal wall.

If pyogenic deep neck infections are diagnosed early before fluctuance appears, administration of a penicillinase-resistant semisynthetic penicillin in high doses may result in cure. Most patients, however, will require drainage. Complications of deep neck abscesses include mediastinitis, carotid artery erosion with hemorrhage, internal jugular vein septic thrombophlebitis, and asphyxia. Retropharyngeal abscesses may rupture anteriorly, causing aspiration of pus and subsequent pneumonitis.

Peritonsillar Abscess

Peritonsillar abscesses occur as a complication of pharyngitis or tonsillitis, primarily in young adults. Symptoms, which often begin after the inciting superficial infection has subsided, include soreness of the throat, with pain often referred to the ear, dysphagia, dysarthria, and trismus. Examination discloses erythema of the tonsil and its pillars. The uvula, soft palate, and tonsil are displaced medially. Culture of pus may yield group A streptococci, but often only the usual pharyngeal flora including anaerobes may be grown.

Treatment consists of incision and drainage, often followed by tonsillectomy. The latter may be performed at the time of initial drainage or deferred for several weeks. Penicillin should also be administered. Complications of peritonsillar abscesses are those of the deep neck abscesses which may result from extension of infection.

Selected Bibliography

Streptococcal Pharyngitis

Glezen, W. P., et al.: Group A streptococci, mycoplasmas, and viruses associated with acute pharyngitis. *JAMA* 202:455-460, 1967.

Kaplan, E. L., et al.: Diagnosis of streptococcal pharyngitis: Differentiation of active infection from the carrier state in the symptomatic child. *J Infect Dis* 123:490-501, 1971.

Rammelkamp, C. H., Jr.: Epidemiology of streptococcal infections. *Harvey Lect* 51:113-142, 1957.

Siegel, A. C., Johnson, E. E., and Stollerman, G. H.: Controlled studies of streptococcal pharyngitis in a pediatric population. I. Factors related to the attack rate of rheumatic fever. *N Engl J Med* 265:559-566, 1961.

Wannamaker, L. W.: Perplexity and precision in the diagnosis of streptococcal pharyngitis. *Am J Dis Child* 124:352-358, 1972.

Gonococcal Pharyngitis

Becker, G. D. and Wernicke, A. M.: Gonococcal pharyngitis. *Ann Otol* 83:550-554, 1974.

Fuimara, N. J., Wise, H. M., and Many, M.: Gonorrhoeal pharyngitis. *N Engl J Med* 276:1248-1250, 1967.

Wiesner, P. J., Tronca, E., Bonin, P., et al.: Clinical spectrum of pharyngeal gonococcal infection. *N Engl J Med* 288:181-185, 1973.

Diphtheria

Brooks, G. F., Bennett, J. V., and Feldman, R. A.: Diphtheria in the United States, 1959-1970. *J Infect Dis* 129:172-178, 1974.

Fisher, A. M. and Cobb, S.: The clinical manifestations of the severe form of diphtheria. *Bull Johns Hopkins Hosp* 84:297-325, 1948.

McCloskey, R. V., et al.: The 1970 epidemic of diphtheria in San Antonio. *Ann Intern Med* 75:495-503, 1971.

Naiditch, M. J. and Bowers, A. G.: Diphtheria. *Am J Med* 17:229-245, 1954.

Mycoplasma Pharyngitis

Denny, F. W., Clyde, C. W., and Glezen, W. P.: *Mycoplasma pneumoniae* disease: Clinical spectrum, pathophysiology, epidemiology and control. *J Infect Dis* 123:74-92, 1971.

Evans, A. S., Allen, V., and Sueltmann, S.: *Mycoplasma pneumoniae* infections in University of Wisconsin students. *Am Rev Respir Dis* 96:237-244, 1967.

Mogabgab, W. J.: *Mycoplasma pneumoniae* and adenovirus respiratory illnesses in military and university personnel, 1959-1966. *Am Rev Respir Dis* 97:345-358, 1968.

Adenoviral Pharyngitis

Bell, J. A., et al.: Pharyngoconjunctival fever. Epidemiological studies of a recently described disease entity. *JAMA* 157:1083, 1955.

Brandt, C. D., et al.: Infections in 18,000 infants and children in a controlled study of respiratory tract disease. I. Adenovirus pathogenicity in relation to serologic type and illness syndrome. *Am J Epidemiol* 90:484, 1969.

Fox, J., Hall, C., and Cooney, M.: The Seattle virus watch. VIII. Observations of adenovirus infections. *Am J Epidemiol* 105:362, 1977.

Pereira, M. S.: Adenovirus infections. *Postgrad Med J* 49:798-801, 1973.

Epiglottitis

Baxter, J. D. and Pashley, N. R. T.: Acute epiglottitis – 25 years' experience in management. The Montreal Children's Hospital. *J Otolaryngol* 6:473–476, 1977.

Chow, A. W., et al.: *Hemophilus parainfluenzae* epiglottitis with meningitis and bacteremia in an adult. *Am J Med Sci* 267:365–368, 1974.

Gorfinkel, H. J., Brown, R., and Kabins, S. A.: Acute infectious epiglottitis in adults. *Ann Intern Med* 70:289–294, 1969.

Hawkins, D. B., et al.: Acute epiglottitis in adults. *Laryngoscope* 83:1211–1220, 1973.

Margolis, C. Z., Colletti, R. B., and Brundy, G.: *Hemophilus influenzae* type b: The etiologic agent in epiglottitis. *J Pediatr* 87:322–323, 1975.

Ossoff, R. H. and Wolff, A. P.: Acute epiglottitis in adults. *JAMA* 244:2639, 1980.

Robineau, M., et al.: *Haemophilus parainfluenzae* epiglottitis with positive blood cultures in an adult. *Scand J Infect Dis* 5:229–231, 1975.

Whisnant, J. K., et al.: Host factors and antibody response in *Haemophilus influenzae* type b meningitis and epiglottitis. *J Infect Dis* 133:448–455, 1976.

Neck Infections

Beck, A. L.: Deep neck infections. *Ann Otol Rhinol Laryngol* 56:439–481, 722–765, 1947.

Bryan, C. S., et al.: Retropharyngeal infection in adults. *Arch Intern Med* 134:127–130, 1974.

Johnson, J. T. and Tucker, H. M.: Recognizing and treating deep neck infection. *Postgrad Med* 59:95–100, 1976.

McCurdy, J. A., Jr.: Peritonsillar abscess. A comparison of treatment by immediate tonsillectomy and interval tonsillectomy. *Arch Otolaryngol* 103:414–415, 1977.

Richards, L.: Retropharyngeal abscess. *N Engl J Med* 215:1120–1130, 1936.

15

TRACHEOBRONCHITIS, LARYNGOTRACHEOBRONCHITIS (CROUP), BRONCHIOLITIS, AND BRONCHIECTASIS
David L. Hoover, M.D.

Bronchiolitis

Bronchiolitis is a common lower respiratory tract infection in infants and children, occurring mostly in those under 2 years of age. Respiratory syncytial virus accounts for approximately 70% of the cases, followed by parainfluenza type 3 virus. Children over 2 years of age are more likely to have infection with parainfluenza type 1 or adenovirus. Still later in childhood *Mycoplasma pneumoniae* may be the causative agent.

The role of various host factors in the pathogenesis of bronchiolitis is uncertain. Younger infants have more severe disease than older infants. Older children or adults rarely develop bronchiolitis, despite frequent infection with respiratory syncytial virus. Clinical expression of the disease may be due to the relatively narrower small airways in infants. Immunologic factors, however, may also be important.

Primarily a mucosal infection of small bronchi and bronchioles, bronchiolitis presents with little evidence of systemic toxicity, although low-grade fever is present in about one-half of the cases. Plugging of small airways with desquamated epithelial cells and mucus leads to the characteristic findings of tachypnea, wheezing, subcostal or intercostal retractions, and evidence of air-trapping in the lungs. Localized pulmonary infiltrates and rales may occur, although these most often are due to atelectasis. A patchy interstitial pneumonia also may accompany the disease. Hypoxemia, due mostly to ventilation-perfusion imbalance, is generally present. An etiologic diagnosis may be made by cultural or serologic methods appropriate for the suspected agents. Therapy, however, is entirely supportive, consisting primarily of adequate oxygenation and hydration. Adrenal corticosteroids, antibiotics, and β-adrenergic agents have no demonstrated efficacy in treatment.

Respiratory isolation of cases may be an important adjunct to prevent noso-comial spread of infection. Adverse sequelae of bronchiolitis include bronchiolitis obliterans and bronchiectasis. The case-fatality rate is approximately 1%, with the highest rate occurring in infants under 6 months of age. A possible role for this disease in predisposing to chronic adult respiratory ailments has been sug-gested but not yet clearly demonstrated.

Tracheobronchitis

Acute tracheobronchitis may accompany upper respiratory infection with most of the numerous agents of respiratory disease. The overwhelming majority of tra-cheobronchitis infection is virus induced, except in young adults, in whom *M. pneu-moniae* is more common. *Salmonella typhi* and *Bordetella pertussis* may cause bronchitis as their primary manifestation of disease. Other potential pathogens including *Streptococcus pneumoniae, Haemophilus influenzae, Staphylococcus aureus* and enteric gram-negative rods may be found in the sputum during acute bronchitis. Their pathogenic role, however, is uncertain.

Typical signs and symptoms include cough, with scant sputum production de-veloping late, retrosternal burning or soreness, and variable constitutional symp-toms of fever, myalgia, and lassitude. Rhonchi or localized wheezing may be present, but rales denote pneumonitis. Chest x-rays are normal or show nonspe-cific prominence of lung markings. These clinical manifestations reflect the ef-fect of infection on ciliated respiratory epithelium, as observed in experimental models. First, the normal cephalad beating of cilia is slowed, impairing the nor-mal clearance of mucus. Persistent infection leads to sloughing of epithelium and migration of inflammatory cells into the submucosal areas. Within a short time, denudation of the airway wall occurs. With control of the invader, regeneration of epithelium begins, reestablishing normal clearance mechanisms. Microbial invasion of epithelial cells is not always required for the development of mucosal abnor-malities. *Mycoplasma pneumoniae* and *B. pertussis,* for example, cause similar clinical and pathologic abnormalities in the absence of cell penetration.

Acute tracheobronchitis is generally a self-limited disease. Inhalation of hu-midified air and administration of salicylates may reduce chest discomfort, cough, and systemic manifestations. Internal hydration is more important than inhalation as a method for maintaining low sputum viscosity. Expectorants, such as glyceryl guaiacolate, also may be of value for the same reason, but the dose necessary to effect a more liquid sputum is two to four times that recommended on the bottle of the commonly used over-the-counter preparation. Codeine is an effective cough suppressant but should be used only if sputum production is absent. Bron-chitis due to specific bacterial pathogens should be treated with appropriate anti-microbial agents. Cough and abnormalities of gas exchange, perhaps reflecting undetected bronchiolitis, may persist for several weeks to months following an episode of acute viral bronchitis. Recovery is, however, generally complete.

Laryngotracheobronchitis (Croup)

Croup is a manifestation of laryngeal, tracheal, and bronchial infection of chil-dren approximately 3 months to 3 years of age. Parainfluenza viruses, especially type 1, and influenza A and B viruses account for most of the cases. Many other respiratory tract viruses as well as *M. pneumoniae* also have been implicated.

Infection generally begins in the nasal mucosa, with progressive caudal spread. The most significant major airway alterations occur in the subglottic area. There, where the submucosa is loosely bound to supporting structures, inflammatory cellular infiltrate, mucosal edema, and sloughing and deposition of fibrinous debris combine to cause airway narrowing. Little expansion of the larynx can occur because of the completely encircling cartilaginous rings of the cricoid cartilage. Infection of the bronchi causes interference with mucociliary clearance and accumulation of debris and secretions which may further narrow the subglottic passage. Such a narrowed airway results in increased work of breathing, a high-pitched cough, and inspiratory stridor. Finally, terminal airway narrowing due to bronchiolar infection results in ventilation-perfusion inequalities. The increased work of breathing is therefore aggravated by the increased respiratory drive resulting from hypoxemia.

Clinically, the expression of disease correlates with the location of infection. After 2 or 3 days of coryza or pharyngitis, a sharp, harsh, brassy cough develops, frequently accompanied by roughened voice or less commonly, aphonia. The onset is frequently at night; severity may decrease during the day. Inspiratory stridor and supraclavicular retractions follow. The rate of respiration increases but depth decreases. If the condition is severe, respiratory fatigue eventually develops, which may culminate in acute respiratory failure. Fever is common, but the child does not appear systemically ill. Examination of the chest discloses wheezes and stridor. Rales and signs of consolidation may be present if the causative agent has also caused pneumonia. The white blood cell count and differential usually are normal. Bronchoscopy shows a normal epiglottis. The subglottic area is narrowed with epithelium ranging from pale to dark red. Fibrinopurulent debris is variably present. Anteroposterior and lateral x-rays of the soft tissues of the neck show narrowing in the subglottic region, with a normal epiglottis. Among hospitalized patients, 80% have arterial hypoxemia.

The most important differential diagnosis is that between croup and epiglottitis. More gradual onset, characteristic cough, association with preceding upper respiratory infection, and absence of drooling salivation favor the former diagnosis. Neck x-rays and direct visualization of the epiglottis (only with personnel and facilities for endotracheal intubation immediately present) may be used to confirm a doubtful diagnosis. The presence of a laryngeal or pharyngeal membrane should suggest the possibility of diphtheria, particularly in the unimmunized patient. Foreign-body aspiration may present as stridor and dyspnea and should be considered in the differential diagnosis.

Treatment remains controversial. The use of room temperature humidification is a time-honored, if unproven, remedy. Racemic epinephrine administration via the airway has had a variable effect in controlled trials, but may be of benefit. The value of short-term, high-dose corticosteroids is unclear. Antibiotics play no role except in the rare event of bacterial superinfection. Oxygen should be administered to maintain the $pAO_2 \geq 60$ mmHg. The onset of respiratory failure requires endotracheal intubation.

The duration of stridor and dyspnea is usually 3-4 days. Cough, however, may persist for a week or more. In general, about 5% of patients will require ventilatory support. Mortality, due almost entirely to respiratory failure, should be less than 3%. No definitive data are available regarding long-term effects of croup on respiratory function.

Bronchiectasis

Bronchiectasis is a chronic, suppurative condition of dilated bronchi, manifested by purulent sputum which is often blood streaked but rarely fetid. The diagnosis may be suspected from the history of pronounced chronic sputum production with occasional febrile exacerbations. Physical examination may disclose coarse rales or rhonchi over the involved area. Signs of consolidation are variable. Plain chest radiographs may show linear streaking, especially at the bases, and occasionally collapse or consolidation. Confirmation of the diagnosis may be obtained by bronchography.

Sinusitis frequently accompanies bronchiectasis, but its pathogenetic significance remains obscure in most cases. Predisposing factors have in common impairment of mucociliary clearance in the bronchi. Patients with some forms of the disease, including Kartagener's syndrome (bronchiectasis, sinusitis, and situs inversus), possess respiratory epithelial cilia which are immotile owing to ultrastructural defects. Other familial cases are due to defective airway supporting structures. Bronchopulmonary aspergillosis may first become evident because of associated bronchiectasis. Prior pulmonary infections such as tuberculosis, pertussis, measles, and other viral and bacterial pneumonias may likewise destroy the ciliated epithelium or damage connective tissue leading to bronchial dilatation. As a result of these insults, colonization and infection occur with a variety of organisms, particularly *H. influenzae, S. pneumoniae,* aerobic gram-negative bacilli, and anaerobes. These bacteria in turn further impair local defenses, completing an unfortunate cycle. Interruption of this cycle by early and adequate treatment of pulmonary infections, use of broad-spectrum antibiotics in established disease, postural drainage, and resection of localized involvement has contributed to a marked decline in the incidence and severity of the condition. If untreated or uncontrolled, however, complications include respiratory insufficiency, amyloidosis, and metastatic infection, particularly brain abscess.

Selected Bibliography

Bronchiolitis

Aherne, W., Bird, T., Court, S. D. M., Gardner, P. S., and McQuillin, J.: Pathological changes in virus infections of the lower respiratory tract in children. *J Clin Pathol* 23:7-18, 1970.

Foy, H. M., Cooney, M. K., Maletzky, A. J., and Grayston, J. T.: Incidence and etiology of pneumonia, croup and bronchiolitis in pre-school children belonging to a prepaid medical care group over a four-year period. *Am J Epidemiol* 97:80-92, 1973.

Fulginiti, V. A. (Chairman): Workshop on bronchiolitis. *Pediatr Res* 11:209-270, 1977.

Glezen, W. P., Loda, F. A., Clyde, W. A., Seria, R. J., Schaffer, C. I., Conley, W. G., and Denney, F. W.: Epidemiologic patterns of acute lower respiratory tract disease of children in a pediatric group practice. *J Pediatr* 78:397-406, 1971.

Hall, C. B., Douglas, R. G., Geiman, J. M., and Messner, M. K.: Nosocomial respiratory syncytial virus infections. *N Engl J Med* 293:1343-1346, 1975.

Kattan, M., Keene, T. G., Lapierre, J. G., et al.: Pulmonary function abnormalities in symptom-free children after bronchiolitis. *Pediatrics* 59:683-688, 1977.

Leer, J. A., Green, J. L., Heimlich, E. M., Hyde, J. S., Moffett, H. L., Young, G. A., and Barron, B. A.: Corticosteroid treatment in bronchiolitis: A controlled, collaborative study in 297 infants and children. *Am J Dis Child* 117: 495-503, 1969.

Reilly, C. M., Stokes, J., McClelland, L., Cornfield, D., Hamparian, V. V., Ketler, A., and Hilleman, M. R.: Studies of acute respiratory illnesses caused by respiratory syncytial virus. 3. Clinical and laboratory findings. *N Engl J Med* 264:1176-1182, 1961.

Sims, D. G., Downham, M. A. P. S., Gardner, P. S., et al.: Study of 8-year-old children with a history of respiratory syncytial virus in infancy. *Br Med J* 1: 11-14, 1978.

Whol, M. E. B. and Chenick, V.: Bronchiolitis. *Am Rev Respir Dis* 118:759-781, 1978.

Bronchiectasis and Tracheobronchitis

Bjerkestrand, G., Digrances, A., and Schreiner, A.: Bacteriological findings in transtracheal aspirates from patients with chronic bronchitis and bronchiectasis. *Scand J Respir Dis* 56:201-207, 1975.

Bradshaw, II. H., Putney, F. J., and Clerf, L. H.: The fate of patients with untreated bronchiectasis. *JAMA* 116:2561-2563, 1941.

Cate, T. R., Roberts, J. S., Russ, M. A., and Pierce, J. A.: Effects of common colds on pulmonary function. *Am Rev Respir Dis* 108:858-865, 1973.

Dascomb, H. E., and Hilleman, M. R.: Clinical laboratory studies in patients with respiratory disease caused by adenovirus (RI-APC-ARD agents). *Am J Epidemiol* 94:280-289, 1971.

Field, C. E.: Bronchiectasis. *Arch Dis Child* 44:551-561, 1969.

Gwaltney, J. M., Hendly, J. O., Simon, G., and Jordan, W. S.: Rhinovirus infections in an industrial population. II. Characteristics of illness and antibody response. *JAMA* 202:494-500, 1967.

Hall, W. J., Hall, C. B., and Speers, D. M.: Respiratory syncytial virus in adults. Clinical, virologic and pulmonary function studies. *Ann Intern Med* 88:203-205, 1978.

Monto, A. S. and Cavallaro, J. J.: The Tecumseh study of respiratory illness. II. Patterns of occurrence with respiratory pathogens, 1965-1969. *Am J Epidemiol* 94:280-289, 1971.

Powell, D. A., Hu, P. C., Wilson, M., Collier, A. M., and Baseman, J. B.: Attachment of *Mycoplasma pneumoniae* to respiratory epithelium. *Infect Immun* 13: 959-966, 1976.

Sasaki, Y., Togo, Y., Wagner, N. H., Hornick, R. B., Schwartz, A. W., and Proctor, D. F.: Mucociliary function during experimentally induced rhinovirus infection in man. *Ann Otol* 82:203-211, 1973.

Stott, N. H. and West, R. R.: Randomized controlled trial of antibiotics in patients with cough and purulent sputum. *Br Med J* 2:556-559, 1979.

Laryngotracheobronchitis (Croup)

Adair, J. C., Ring, W. H., Jordan, W. S., and Elwyn, R. A.: Ten-year experience with IPPB in the treatment of acute laryngotracheobronchitis. *Anesth Analg* 50:649-655, 1971.

Brenneman, J., Clifton, W. M., Frank, A., and Holinger, P.: Acute laryngotracheobronchitis. *Am J Dis Child* 55:667-695, 1938.

Davison, F. W.: Acute laryngeal obstruction in children. *JAMA* 171:1301-1305, 1959.

Foy, H. J., Cooney, M. K., Maletzky, A. J., and Graystone, T. J.: Incidence and etiology of pneumonia, croup and bronchiolitis in preschool children belonging to a prepaid medical care group over a four-year period. *Am J Epidemiol* 97:80-92, 1973.

Glezen, W. P. and Denney, F. W.: Epidemiology of lower respiratory disease in children. *N Engl J Med* 288:498-505, 1973.

Hall, C. B., Geiman, J. M., and Breese, B. B.: Parainfluenza viral infections in children: Correlation of shedding with clinical manifestations. *J Pediatr* 91: 194-198, 1977.

Leipzig, B., Oski, F. A., Cummings, C. W., Stockman, J. A., and Swender, P.: Efficacy of steroids in treatment of croup. *J Pediatr* 94:194-196, 1979.

Newth, C. J. L., Levison, H., and Bryan, A. C.: The respiratory status of children with croup. *J Pediatr* 81:1068-1073, 1972.

Rabe, E. F.: Infectious croup. I. Etiology. *Pediatrics* 2:255-265, 1948.

Rabe, E. F.: Infectious croup. II. "Virus croup." *Pediatrics* 2:415-427, 1948.

Westley, C. R., Cotton, E. K., and Brooks, J. G.: Nebulized racemic epinephrine by IPPB for the treatment of croup. *Am J Dis Child* 132:484-487, 1978.

16

PNEUMONIA
Ronica M. Kluge, M.D.

Pneumonia, infection of the lung parenchyma, was once the leading cause of death in this country. It still is responsible for 10% of all hospital admissions. A cause of considerable morbidity and some mortality, the disease requires the physician to act quickly to identify the most likely etiologic agent and initiate appropriate therapy.

Etiology

Almost any microbial agent can cause pneumonia (Tables 16.1-16.4). Community-acquired pneumonia in the adult is due to *Streptococcus pneumoniae* (the pneumococcus) in most cases. Although this agent is responsible for about half of bacterial pneumonia in children, *Haemophilus influenzae* and *Staphylococcus aureus* are frequently causative. In contrast, hospital-acquired bacterial pneumonias are more likely to be due to various gram-negative bacilli. Viral agents can cause primary pneumonias or lead to bacterial superinfections. *Mycoplasma pneumoniae* is the most common agent causing pneumonia in children and young adults. *Chlamydia* and a recently discovered bacterium, *Legionella,* have assumed importance as etiologic agents in pneumonia in infants and adults, respectively. Rarer causes of pneumonia include Q fever, actinomycetes, fungi, *Mycobacterium tuberculosis,* and various parasites.

TABLE 16.1   Bacterial Causes of Community-Acquired Pneumonias

	Percentage*	
Agent	Adults	Children
Pneumococcus (*S. pneumoniae*)	90	50
S. aureus	5	16
S. pyogenes	2	2
K. pneumoniae	3	1
H. influenzae	1	32

*% of bacterial pneumonias

TABLE 16.2   Viral Causes of Pneumonia

Agent	Adults	Children
Influenza	Common	Infrequent
Adenovirus	Common	Infrequent
Respiratory syncytial	Not seen	Common
Parainfluenza	Infrequent	Common
Other	Rare	Rare

TABLE 16.3   Fungal Causes of Pneumonia

Aspergillus	*C. neoformans*
Candida	*H. capsulatum*
C. immitis	*Mucor*

TABLE 16.4   Miscellaneous Causes of Pneumonia

M. pneumoniae	C. burnetii
Actinomycetes	M. tuberculosis
Chlamydia	P. carinii
L. pneumophila	Parasites
Anthrax	Melioidosis
Brucella	Plague
Tularemia	

Epidemiology

The pneumococcus, *H. influenzae*, various streptococcal species, and *S. aureus* are common inhabitants of the upper respiratory tract. Transmission of these organisms occurs via droplets (sneeze, cough). Gram-negative bacilli, usually acquired in the hospital, colonize the respiratory tract when patients have been receiving antibiotics, steroids, or antimetabolites, and when patients require ventilatory support. Viral agents and mycoplasmas also spread by droplets; viruses are transferred commonly by hand-to-hand contact. Chlamydia are acquired by infants during passage through the birth canal. Psittacosis organisms are transmitted from birds to humans in aerosols. The less frequent causes of pneumonia are also acquired via aerosol in most instances (Table 16.5). Occasionally the agent may reach the lung through the hematogenous route, but most often respiratory pathogens are aspirated from air or the oropharynx into the lungs.

The incubation period for most bacterial and viral pneumonias is thought to be short, 1-3 days. Exceptions to this are chlamydial pneumonia in newborns (1-2 months) and mycoplasma (2-3 weeks).

Bacterial pneumonias can occur at all seasons, although they are most prevalent during winter and early spring. Viral and mycoplasmal pneumonias tend to cluster in fall and winter months, whereas, Legionnaire's disease is seen in late summer and fall. Other agents cause pneumonia in a sporadic fashion.

The attack rates of bacterial pneumonia are highest at the extremes of age. Mycoplasma tends to affect older children and young adults. Fungal pneumonias tend to occur in immunocompromised individuals and in patients on long-term, broad-spectrum antibiotics.

Pathogenesis

In the healthy individual the lung is protected from microbial invasion by a number of mechanisms. These include: filtration and humidification of air in the upper airways; intact cough and epiglottic reflexes; entrapment and removal of organisms by mucous secretion and ciliary movement; cellular immunity (alveolar macrophages, T lymphocytes, polymorphonuclear leukocytes); and humoral immunity

TABLE 16.5   Environmental Factors in Unusual Pneumonias

Agent	Factor
Anthrax	Cattle, swine, horses, wool, hides
Brucellosis	Abattoir worker, veterinarian
Melioidosis	Travel to S.E. Asia, S. America
Plague	Squirrels, chipmunks, rabbits, rats
Tularemia	Rabbits, squirrels, infected flies, or ticks
Psittacosis	Birds
Leptospirosis	Rats, dogs, cats, cattle, swine
Q fever	Goats, cattle, swine
Legionnaire's	Soil, water-cooling equipment

TABLE 16.6   Factors Predisposing to Pneumonia

Congenital anomalies: cleft palate, tracheoesophageal fistula, sequestration of lung

Congenital/acquired immune defects

Alteration in level of consciousness: seizures, stroke, anesthesia, intoxication, trauma

Depressed pulmonary clearance: cigarette smoke, hypoxemia, acidosis, ethanol, uremia

Steroids and immunosuppressive agents

Mechanical obstruction

(opsonins, antibodies, complement). When one of these mechanisms is breached, defective, or rendered incompetent, microorganisms can gain access to the lung and establish infection. Certain factors known to predispose to the development of pneumonia are listed on Table 16.6.

Bacterial pneumonias begin with an acute inflammatory response with hyperemia, exudation of edema fluid, deposition of fibrin, and egress of polymorphonuclear leukocytes into the alveoli. Later, there is an increase of macrophage activity. Some bacterial organisms provoke a more fulminant, necrotizing process, e.g., anaerobic bacteria and *Klebsiella pneumoniae*. Mycoplasmas, viruses and *Pneumocystis* cause an interstitial pneumonitis. Fungal organisms produce a number of different effects in the lung: *Cryptococcus* causes little reaction, whereas *Coccidioides* or *Aspergillus* may result in necrosis and cavity formation.

Diagnostic Features

Clinical

The symptoms of chills, fever, cough, sputum production, and pleuritic chest pain are common to pneumonias caused by a wide variety of microbial organisms. Table 16.7 offers some points useful in differentiating bacterial from viral or mycoplasmal pneumonias. Early administration of appropriate antibiotics to the patient with a bacterial pneumonia should promote quick resolution of the process and decrease the incidence of complications. Distinguishing features of the most common bacterial and viral pneumonias are presented in Table 16.8.

TABLE 16.7 Diagnostic Clues to Separate Bacterial from Viral/Mycoplasmal Pneumonias

Factor	Bacterial	Viral/Mycoplasmal
Onset of symptoms	Sudden	Gradual
Rigors	Common	Uncommon
Fever	High	Low-grade
Cough	Productive	Paroxysmal, non-productive
Sputum	Purulent	Mucoid, if present
Pleuritic chest pain	Common	Uncommon
Signs of consolidation on physical	Common	Rare
Sputum Gram stain	Neutrophils, abundant bacteria	Mononuclear cells, rare bacteria
WBC, differential	Elevated with immature neutrophils	Normal
Chest x-ray	Consolidation	Patchy infiltrates

TABLE 16.8   Distinguishing Features of Acute Pneumonias Due to Bacterial And Viral Organisms

Agent	Fever	Rigors	Cough	Sputum/Gram Stain	WBC/mm³	Other Clues
Pneumococcus	Variable, 100-106°F usually sustained	Severe, usually single, chill at onset	Productive; pleuritic chest pain	Rusty (bloody) and/or purulent; gram-positive diplococci	15-30,000 with left shift	Preceding URI common; herpes labialis frequent; multilobar involvement 10-30%
Staphylococcus	102-106°F; hectic or sustained	Multiple	Productive; pleuritic chest pain	Purulent, may be blood-streaked; gram-positive cocci in clusters	>15,000 with left shift	Affects infants, elderly, debilitated; may follow influenza; pneumatoceles; empyema, abscess common
Streptococcus	104°F or higher; hectic	Multiple	Productive; pleuritic chest pain	Purulent, may be blood-streaked; gram-positive cocci in chains	20-30,000 with left shift	Pleural effusion and empyema common; often follows influenza
H. influenzae, b	Variable	Infrequent	"Croup" in children, wheezing	Purulent; gram-negative coccobacilli	15-30,000 with left shift	Preceding URI; seen in patients with chronic lung or heart disease, alcoholism, splenectomy; multilobar involvement, empyema common

Organism	Temperature	Bacteremia	Cough	Sputum	WBC	Clinical features
Klebsiella	101–102°F	Multiple	Productive, pleuritic chest pain	Mucopurulent, may be bloody; gram-negative bacilli with thick capsules	20–40,000 with left shift	Affects upper lobes, dense infiltrate, abscesses; seen in diabetics, alcoholics and patients with chronic lung disease
Other gram-negative bacilli	Usually high; may be absent in elderly, debilitated	Multiple	Productive	Purulent; gram-negative bacilli	Variable	Affects infants, elderly, debilitated, alcoholics, diabetics, those on antibiotics, steroids or immunosuppressive agents, ventilators
Anaerobes (aspiration)	Variable, often low grade	Infrequent	Productive	Purulent and foul-smelling; mixed flora	Variable	Periodontal disease and altered state of consciousness; lung abscess, empyema common
Mycoplasma	101–104°F	Occasional	Paroxysmal, usually non-productive	Mucoid, if present; rare polys and no bacteria on stain	10,000 or less	Children and young adults; physical unimpressive although x-ray shows patchy infiltrates; may have bullous myringitis; cold agglutinin-positive 50%; hemolytic anemia occasionally
Legionella	103–106°F	Multiple	Nonproductive; pleuritic chest pain	Mucoid, if present; rare polys and no bacteria on stain	10–25,000; 50% with left shift	Myalgias, abdominal pain and headache; CNS, liver and renal abnormalities; patchy infiltrates and consolidation on x-ray
Chlamydia	None or low-grade	None	Staccato, with wheezing	No bacteria on stain	Absolute increase in eosinophils	Affects infants ages 1–4 mo; 50% with conjunctivitis; on x-ray diffuse infiltrates and hyperinflation

TABLE 16.8 (Cont'd)

Agent	Fever	Rigors	Cough	Sputum/Gram Stain	WBC/mm^3	Other Clues
Psittacosis	Variable	Infrequent	Productive, pleuritic chest pain	Mucoid, bloody, no bacteria on stain	Depressed in 25%	Headache, myalgias prominent; macular rash, splenomegaly may be present; contact with birds
Tuberculosis	100–102°F, remittent or intermittent	Rare	Variable, usually productive	Purulent; gram stain not helpful; acid-fast stain positive	Less than 10,000	Seen in children and the elderly; may be rapidly progressive; exposure to known TB source
Influenza	103–105°F	Uncommon	Nonproductive, hacking nature	Scant, may be bloody; rare polys and no bacteria on stain	10–15,000	Seen in patients with chronic lung and heart disease, pregnancy; profound dyspnea, cyanosis; seen in fall and winter
Adenovirus	Low-grade	Rare	Variable	Scant; no organisms or polys on stain	Less than 10,000	Associated with severe conjunctivitis; epidemic in closed populations
Echovirus	Low-grade	Rare	Variable	Scant; no organisms or polys on stain	Less than 10,000	Rash; seen in summer
Respiratory syncytial	101–104°F	Rare	Variable; frequent wheezing	Scant; no organisms or polys on stain	10–20,000	Seen primarily in children
Parainfluenza	101–104°F	Rare	Variable; may have "croup"	Scant; no organisms or polys on, stain	Less than 10,000	Seen primarily in children
Varicella	Up to 105°F	Rare	Harsh, nonproductive	Scant, though may be bloody; no organisms	Less than 10,000	Rare in children; affects 15–30% of adults with varicella; nodular densities on x-ray, later calcify

The clinical setting cannot be overemphasized. For example, the otherwise healthy individual who acquires pneumonia in the community is likely to have pneumococcus, mycoplasma, or perhaps a virus as the causative agent. The hospitalized patient may have pneumonia due to staphylococci or to gram-negative bacilli. The immunocompromised host is subject to more exotic organisms (fungi, *Pneumocystis,* parasites) in addition to the usual hospital organisms. This patient population may develop pneumonias from "nonpathogens" such as *Neisseria (Branhamella) catarrhalis* or have multiple, simultaneous infective agents present.

Laboratory

Basic laboratory examination for the patient with pneumonia includes white blood cell count and differential, sputum for appropriate stains and cultures, and a chest roentgenogram. The patient suspected of having a bacterial or fungal pneumonia should also have blood sent for culture. Counterimmunoelectrophoresis of respiratory secretions may be helpful in distinguishing patients with pneumococcal pneumonia from those who are carriers of the pneumococcus. A wet mount of the sputum will reveal *Strongyloides stercoralis* larvae in that disease. Silver stain is needed to demonstrate *Pneumocystis carinii.* *Legionella pneumophila* can be demonstrated in the sputum using an immunofluorescent-staining technique. Transtracheal aspirate is useful in some cases (Table 16.9). Bronchoscopy with

TABLE 16.9   Transtracheal Aspiration

Indications
  No sputum being produced

  No clear diagnosis from expectorated sputum

  Poor response to antibiotics chosen on basis of expectorated sample

Contraindications
  Hypoxia/hypercapnia

  Uncooperative patient

  Violent coughing

  Bleeding diathesis

Complications
  Hemoptysis

  Subcutaneous/mediastinal emphysema

  Aspiration

  Soft-tissue infection at site

washings, brushings, and/or transbronchial biopsy may be useful in obtaining material for diagnosis. Occasionally, percutaneous or open lung biopsy will be necessary. Serology can be diagnostic for many viral pneumonias as well as for mycoplasmal and Legionnaire's. These tests are useful only in retrospect as acute and convalescent samples are needed to detect a significant rise in antibodies.

Differential

The differential diagnosis for pneumonias includes pulmonary embolus, congestive heart failure, carcinoma (primary, metastatic, or lymphangitic), pneumoconiosis, sarcoidosis, radiation, transfusion reaction (white cells), drug toxicity [nitrofurantoin (Furadantin), bleomycin, methotrexate, etc.], hypersensitivity pneumonitis, pulmonary sequestration, and aspiration of foreign body. In most cases the history and physical examination will rule out these noninfectious etiologies.

Complications

The complications of pneumonia vary somewhat depending on the causative agent, but include effusion and empyema, pneumothorax, metastatic infection, lung abscess/cavity formation, bronchiectasis, parenchymal or pleural fibrosis, and superinfection.

Therapy

General supportive measures should include adequate hydration and nutrition, oxygen therapy, and good pulmonary toilet. In some instances, ventilatory support is required. Table 16.10 outlines specific antimicrobial therapy for the most common infective pneumonias. These choices are meant as a guide only; you may have a particular problem with resistance in your hospital or community which would alter these recommendations. Once culture results and antibiotic sensitivities are available from the laboratory, you may need to change to a more appropriate agent.

Prevention

Specific preventive measures against pneumonias have centered around the use of vaccines. The best studied and most widely used are influenza and pneumococcal vaccines. Vaccines against several other agents are being investigated. Details of prevention can be found in chapters dealing with each specific microbe.

Prognosis

The prognosis of pneumonia varies greatly depending on the age and underlying condition of the patient and the specific etiologic organism. Mortality figures are listed in Table 16.11.

TABLE 16.10   Antimicrobial Therapy for Pneumonia

Cause	Drug of Choice	Alternative Drug(s)
Pneumococcus	Penicillin	Erythromycin
Staphylococcus	Penicillinase-resistant penicillin	Clindamycin, cephalosporin
Streptococcus	Penicillin	Erythromycin
H. influenzae, b	Ampicillin*	Chloramphenicol
Klebsiella	Aminoglycoside + cephalosporin	Either drug alone
Other gram-negative bacilli	Aminoglycoside	Chloramphenicol, newer cephalosporins
Anaerobes (aspiration)	Penicillin	Erythromycin
Mycoplasma	Erythromycin	Tetracycline
Legionella	Erythromycin	Ampicillin
Chlamydia	Sulfonamides	Erythromycin
Psittacosis	Tetracycline	Erythromycin
Tuberculosis	Isoniazid + 1-2 others	Rifampin
Influenza A	Amantadine	None
Actinomycosis	Penicillin	Erythromycin
Nocardia	Sulfonamides	Erythromycin
Q fever	Tetracycline	Erythromycin
Pneumocystis	Trimethoprim-sulfamethoxazole	Pentamidine
Fungi	Amphotericin B	Flucytosine, miconazole, ketoconazole

*If ampicillin-resistant H. influenzae is a significant problem in your area, begin treatment with chloramphenicol

TABLE 16.11   Mortality in Adults with Pneumonia

Agent	Rate (%)
Pneumococcus	2-10
Staphylococcus	10-20
Klebsiella	25-50
Pseudomonas	35-80
Legionella	15-20
Influenza	80-90

Selected Bibliography

Bartlett, J. G.: Anaerobic bacterial pneumonitis. *Am Rev Respir Dis* 119:19-23, 1979.

Bays, B. B., Thomas, G. D., Leonard, J. S., Jr., Southern, P. M., Jr., Pierce, A. K., and Sanford, J. P.: Gram-negative bacillary necrotizing pneumonia: A bacteriologic and histopathologic correlation. *J Infect Dis* 120:687-697, 1969.

Beem, M. O. and Saxon, E. M.: Respiratory-tract colonization and a distinctive pneumonia syndrome in infants infected with *Chlamydia trachomatis.* *N Engl J Med* 296:306-310, 1977.

Briggs, D. D., Jr.: Pulmonary infections. *Med Clin N Am* 61:1163-1183, 1977.

Broome, C. V., Cherry, W. B., Winn, W. C., Jr., and MacPherson, B. R.: Rapid diagnosis of Legionnaire's disease by direct immunofluorescent staining. *Ann Intern Med* 90:1-4, 1979.

Bynum, L. J. and Pierce, A. K.: Pulmonary aspiration of gastric contents. *Am Rev Respir Dis* 114:1129-1136, 1976.

Chandler, F. W., Hicklin, M. D., and Blackmon, J. A.: Demonstration of the agent of Legionnaire's disease in tissue. *N Engl J Med* 297:1218-1220, 1977.

Congeni, B. L. and Nankervis, G. A.: Diagnosis of pneumonia by counterimmunoelectrophoresis of respiratory secretions. *Am J Dis Child* 132:684-687, 1978.

Cunha, B. A. and Quintiliani, R.: The atypical pneumonias. *Postgrad Med* 66:95-102, 1979.

Denny, F. W., Clyde, W. A., Jr., and Glezen, W. P.: *Mycoplasma pneumoniae* disease: Clinical spectrum, pathophysiology, epidemiology, and control. *J Infect Dis* 123:74-92, 1971.

Eichenwald, H. F.: Pneumonia syndromes in children. *Hosp Prac* 11:89-96, 1976.

Finland, M.: Pneumonia and pneumococcal infections, with special reference to pneumococcal pneumonia. *Am Rev Respir Dis* 120:481-502, 1979.

Fisher, A. M., Trever, R. W., Curtin, J. A., Schultze, G., and Miller, D. F.: Staphylococcal pneumonia: A review of 21 cases in adults. *N Engl J Med* 258:919–928, 1958.

Geckler, R. W., Gremillion, D. H., McAllister, C. K., and Ellenbogen, C.: Microscopic and bacteriological comparison of paired sputa and transtracheal aspirates. *J Clin Microbiol* 6:396–399, 1977.

Ginsburg, C. M., Howard, J. B., and Nelson, J. D.: Report of 65 cases of *Haemophilus influenzae b* pneumonia. *Pediatrics* 64:283–286, 1979.

Graham, W. G. B and Bradley, D. A.: Efficacy of chest physiotherapy and intermittent positive-pressure breathing in the resolution of pneumonia. *N Engl J Med* 299:624–627, 1978.

Greenfield, S., Teres, D., Bushnell, L. S., Hedley-Whyte, J., and Feingold, D. S.: Prevention of gram-negative bacillary pneumonia using aerosol polymyxin as prophylaxis. *J Clin Invest* 52:2935–2940, 1973.

Guckian, J. C. and Christensen, W. D.: Quantitative culture and Gram stain of sputum in pneumonia. *Am Rev Respir Dis* 118:997–1005, 1978.

Harrison, H. R., English, M. G., Lee, C. K., and Alexander, E. R.: *Chlamydia trachomatis* infant pneumonitis. *N Engl J Med* 298:702–708, 1978.

Kirby, B. D., Snyder, K. M., Meyer, R. D., and Finegold, S. M.: Legionnaire's disease: Clinical features of 24 cases. *Ann Intern Med* 89:297–309, 1978.

Levine, D. P. and Lerner, A. M.: The clinical spectrum of *Mycoplasma pneumoniae* infections. *Med Clin N Am* 62:961–978, 1978.

Lewallen, K. R., McKinney, R. M., Brenner, D. J., Moss, C. W., Dail, D. H., Thomason, B. M., and Bright, R. A.: A newly identified bacterium phenotypically resembling, but genetically distinct from *Legionella pneumophila:* An isolate in a case of pneumonia. *Ann Intern Med* 91:831–834, 1979.

Martone, W. J., Marshall, L. W., Kaufmann, A. F., Hobbs, J. H., and Levy, M. E.: Tularemia pneumonia in Washington, DC. *JAMA* 242:2315–2317, 1979.

McDade, J. E., Shepard, C. C., Fraser, D. W., Tsai, T. R., Redus, M. A., Dowdle, W. R., and Laboratory Investigative Team: Legionnaire's disease: Isolation of a bacterium and demonstration of its role in other respiratory disease. *N Engl J Med* 297:1197–1203, 1977.

McNeely, D. J., Kitchens, C. S., Kluge, R. M.: Fatal *Neisseria (Branhamella) catarrhalis* pneumonia in an immunodeficient host. *Am Rev Respir Dis* 114:399–402, 1976.

Pasculle, A. W., Myerowitz, R. L., and Rinaldo, C. R., Jr.: New bacterial agent of pneumonia isolated from renal-transplant recipients. *Lancet* 2:58–61, 1979.

Pennington, J. E. and Miler, J. J.: Evaluation of a new polyvalent *Pseudomonas* vaccine in respiratory infections. *Infect Immun* 25:1029–1034, 1979.

Pennington, J. E., Reynolds, H. Y., and Carbone, P. P.: Pseudomonas pneumonia. *Am J Med* 55:155-160, 1973.

Scanlon, G. T. and Unger, J. D.: The radiology of bacterial and viral pneumonias. *Radiol Clin N Am* 11:317-338, 1973.

Schoenbaum, S. C. and Weinstein, L.: Respiratory infections in pregnancy. *Clin Obstet Gynecol* 22:293-300, 1979.

Shulman, J. A., Phillips, L. A., and Petersdorf, R. G.: Errors and hazards in the diagnosis and treatment of bacterial pneumonias. *Ann Intern Med* 62:41-58, 1965.

Singer, C., Armstrong, D., Rosen, P. P., Walzer, P. D., and Yu, B.: Diffuse pulmonary infiltrates in immunosuppressed patients. *Am J Med* 66:110-120, 1979.

Stevens, R. M., Teres, D., Skillman, J. J., and Feingold, D. S.: Pneumonia in an intensive care unit. *Arch Intern Med* 134:106-111, 1974.

Stratton, C. W., Hawley, H. B., Horsman, T. A., Tu, K. K., Ackley, A., Fernando, N. K., and Weinstein, M. P.: *Hemophilus influenzae* pneumonia in adults. *Am Rev Respir Dis* 121:595-598, 1980.

Thorsteinsson, S. B., Musher, D. M., and Fagan, T.: The diagnostic value of sputum culture in acute pneumonia. *JAMA* 233:894-895, 1975.

Tillotson, J. R. and Finland, M.: Bacterial colonization and clinical superinfection of the respiratory tract complicating antibiotic treatment of pneumonia. *J Infect Dis* 119:597-624, 1969.

Tillotson, J. R. and Lerner, A. M.: Pneumonias caused by gram-negative bacilli. *Medicine* 45:65-76, 1966.

Wallace, R. J., Jr., Musher, D. M., and Martin, R. R.: *Hemophilus influenzae* pneumonia in adults. *Am J Med* 64:87-93, 1978.

17

LUNG ABSCESS
Charles E. Andrews, M. D.

Introduction

Primary lung abscess is defined as a parenchymal, suppurative process seen as a cavitary lesion, often with a fluid level on roentgenograms of the chest. The signs and symptoms of pulmonary infections are similar regardless of the location or the causative organism. A variety of diseases may present as a cavitary lesion on the chest roentgenogram as listed in Table 17.1. This section is concerned with primary lung abscess and other listed conditions will be considered only as they relate to this entity.

Lung abscesses may be classified conveniently into three groups on the basis of their pathogenesis. Table 17.2, adapted from Schackter, lists three groups: (1) primary, (2) opportunistic, and (3) hematogenous. The prevalence of lung abscess in the general population is unknown, but undoubtedly has decreased since the advent of antibiotics. The primary type of lung abscess associated with oral sepsis and aspiration occurs most frequently and accounts for up to 90% of the patients.

Etiology and Pathogenesis

Oropharyngeal secretions contain approximately 10^7 aerobic and 10^8 anaerobic bacteria per milliliter. These organisms represent a complex microbial population which is restricted in composition and location.

The distal airways and pulmonary parenchyma usually are sterile due to effective lung defense mechanisms. Bacteria can enter the lung via inhaled air, aspirated oropharyneal or other secretions, or the blood. Inhaled air normally contains relatively few organisms, while 0.01 ml of aspirated oropharyngeal secretions contains 10^5 aerobic and 10^6 anaerobic bacteria. Fifty percent of normal

TABLE 17.1   Diseases That May Present as a Cavitary Lesion on the
Chest Roentgenogram

Primary lung abscess

Tuberculosis

Fungi including:
    histoplasmosis
    blastomycosis
    coccidioidomycosis
    aspergillosis

Carcinoma, primary or metastatic

Infected cyst

Infected bullae

Nontuberculosis granulomatous disease

Extension of a subphrenic process

Pulmonary infarction

---

subjects and 70% of subjects with impaired consciousness will aspirate small volumes of oropharyngeal secretions while asleep. Thus most bacterial infections of the lung are probably secondary to aspirated oropharyngeal contents.

Classic studies have demonstrated the tendency for aspirated secretions to produce disease in the gravity-dependent segments of the lung, especially the posterior segments of the upper lobes and the superior segments of the lower lobes. After aspiration of these organisms, a pneumonitis occurs with fluid and inflammatory cells in the alveoli. Later a fibrosing inflammation occurs. Necrotizing pneumonia and lung abscess represent progression of simple pneumonitis; empyema may be a complication of either.

In a primary lung abscess, infections occur because an excessive number of organisms overwhelm the defense mechanisms of the lung. Patients with a lung abscess classified as opportunistic or secondary to an endobronchial lesion, have a different situation in which the defense mechanisms are defective and cannot handle the usual small numbers of organisms to which the lung is exposed.

Embolism to the lung may lead to infarction. The infarcted area becomes an ideal culture medium for the growth of anaerobic bacteria and the subsequent development of lung abscess. It has been estimated that 3% of initially sterile infarcts become infected. Occasionally, the embolus itself is infected and leads directly to abscess formation. This is most likely to occur following bowel surgery, septic abortion, pelvic septic thrombophlebitis, or narcotism.

TABLE 17.2   Classification of Lung Abscess by Pathogenesis

Primary

    Oral sepsis and decreased cough reflex

        Alcohol
        Anesthesia
        Drugs
        Seizures
        Neurologic disorders
        Coma

    Esophageal disorders often with oral sepsis

        Diverticula
        Achalasia
        Strictures
        Motility disorders
        Cancer

    Endobronchial obstruction

        Cancer
        Foreign body

    Postnecrotizing pneumonia

Opportunistic

    Newborn

        Prematurity
        Congenital abnormalities of the heart or lung

    Elderly

        Blood dyscrasias
        Cancer of the lung and oropharynx
        Treatment with steroids
        Postoperatively

    Nosocomial

Hematogenous

    Septicemia

    Pulmonary infarct

        Bland
        Septic

Diagnosis (Table 17.3)

Patients with the primary type lung abscess have an insidious onset and protracted course. Their illness usually starts with malaise, fatigue, fever, and cough. In 25% of the cases there is a history of loss of consciousness which could have been associated with aspiration. Within 1 or 2 weeks, the cough becomes productive of purulent, foul-smelling sputum and may be associated with hemoptysis. Anorexia and weight loss occur and the patient appears chronically ill. Symptoms may be present for 1 day to months before medical attention is sought. Males predominate 3:1 and a history of alcoholism or epilepsy is frequently obtained. Evidence of poor oral hygiene including periodontitis and gingivitis is usually present. Lung abscess can occur in the edentulous patient but it is unusual and often associated with carcinoma. Leukocytosis and anemia are common.

A roentgenogram of the chest is usually diagnostic. The abscess appears as a thick-walled, radiolucent area 1-8 cm in diameter, frequently with an air-fluid level. It may be surrounded by a soft-appearing infiltrate. The location of the lesion depends upon the position of the patient when aspiration occurred. The right lung is involved twice as frequently as the left. Usually either the posterior segment of an upper lobe or the superior segment of a lower lobe is involved. Multiple small abscesses in the lower lobes are suggestive of septic emboli.

It is sometimes difficult to differentiate between a peripheral lung abscess and empyema. The correct diagnosis must be made as soon as possible to institute drainage of the empyema. Several roentgenographic features suggest empyema as the proper diagnosis (Table 17.4). Ultrasound studies are useful in clarifying the diagnosis in these patients. Computed axial tomography (CAT) scanning of the thorax will probably be helpful with accumulation of more experience with this type of disease process.

Sputum Gram stain and routine culture should be done and are worthwhile, even though results in the primary type of community-acquired lung abscess do not correlate well with results of cultures when specimens are obtained by transtracheal aspiration. Results of routine studies may be more useful in planning treatment for patients with opportunistic lung abscess, especially those caused by

TABLE 17.3   Characteristics of Patients with Lung Abscess*

Characteristic	Approximate %
Aspiration	75
Weight loss (average 9 lb)	55
Fever (average minimum 101.9°F rectally)	95
Leukocytosis (average $\sim$ 15,000/mm^3)	90
Anemia (average hematocrit 35%)	90

*Adapted from *Am Rev Respir Dis* 109:510, 1974

**TABLE 17.4   Roentgenographic Features Which Suggest Empyema
Rather Than Lung Abscess**

Presence of pleural effusions on an earlier film

Extension of the air-fluid level to the chest wall

Extension of the lesion across fissure line

A tapering border of the air-fluid pocket

Location of the air pocket in the posterior costophrenic sulcus

A cavity of unequal dimension

---

nosocomial agents, secondary to bronchial obstruction, and those few primary abscesses which do not respond to initial treatment. Careful and appropriate culture of secretions obtained by transtracheal aspiration, before the patient receives antibiotic therapy, usually will yield the responsible aerobic and anaerobic organisms (Table 17.5). In the patient with a typical history and physical and roentgenographic findings of a community-acquired lung abscess, the risk of a complication from transtracheal aspiration is probably greater than the chance of not responding to routine initial treatment with penicillin. Invasive aspiration and percutaneous needle lung aspiration should be considered in those patients with opportunistic lung abscess or in those with unusual clinical features.

Even though the clinical picture and roentgenographic findings in lung abscess and tuberculosis have many similarities, it is not difficult to make the correct diagnosis. An acid-fast stain of the sputum from patients with cavitary tuberculosis is nearly always positive for the organism and is sufficient evidence to warrant antituberculous treatment while awaiting culture results.

Bronchoscopy should be limited to carefully selected patients: to obtain secretions for culture, to rule out bronchogenic carcinoma or other causes of bronchial obstruction, or to aid the drainage of pus from the abscess. Materials obtained during the usual bronchoscopic procedure are contaminated by secretions from the oropharynx. The use of a wire brush retracted within telescoping cannulas with a distal occlusion may eliminate contamination and make bronchoscopy a more useful technique to determine the organisms involved in lower respiratory tract infections.

The incidence of bronchogenic carcinoma presenting as a lung abscess varies from 10 to 40%. One analysis of 56 patients with lung abscess associated with malignancy found that 62% were due to necrosis and central cavitation of the tumor, and 30% were secondary to bronchial obstruction.

Aspiration may occur in patients with esophageal disease. Appropriate evaluation of the gastrointestinal tract should be done in those patients with lung abscess and a history suggestive of disease in this area.

TABLE 17.5   Bacteriology of Lung Abscess

Organisms	Approximate % of Cases
Anaerobic	90
Cocci	
Peptostreptococcus	40
Peptococcus	25
Others	15
Gram-negative bacilli	
F. nucleatum	50
B. melaninogenicus	45
B. fragilis	15
Others	10
Gram-positive bacilli	
Eubacterium spp	20
Propionibacterium spp	10
≥ 1 anaerobe, no aerobic organisms	60
Aerobic and facultative	
Gram-positive cocci	25
Gram-negative bacilli	
P. aeruginosa	10
Klebsiella spp	8
H. influenzae	4
Pure culture of one of above	25

Treatment and Prognosis

The primary, community-acquired type of lung abscess responds to single-drug antibiotic therapy in spite of the variety of organisms present. The treatment of choice is intravenous penicillin G, 4-8 million U/day. When the patient becomes afebrile and clinically improved, the drug may be given by the oral route. Treatment must be continued until the chest radiograph is clear or shows only a small residual lesion. This may require 6 weeks, by 12 weeks 90-95% of patients have complete resolution. Clindamycin is an acceptable alternative agent in this disease, if the patient is allergic to penicillin.

As with any abscess, pus should be drained. Because most lung abscesses are connected to a bronchus, appropriate physical therapy and postural drainage are usually adequate. Bronchoscopy has been used as an adjunctive therapy for drainage. If the abscess continues to enlarge, does not drain, and/or the patient remains toxic, bronchoscopy should be done. The passage of a radiopaque angiographic catheter through the bronchoscope into the abscess with subsequent irrigation and drainage may be helpful.

In patients with lung abscess of the opportunistic type or secondary to bronchial obstruction, one-drug therapy may not be adequate. Infection with *Pseudomonas aeruginosa* and *Staphylococcus aureus,* in addition to the anaerobic organisms, are likely to be important in these patients. An aminoglycoside or penicillinase-resistant penicillin should be given, as sensitivity tests indicate.

Since the advent of antibiotic therapy, the indications for surgery in lung abscess have virtually disappeared (Table 17.6).

Dental treatment may be indicated as a preventive measure.

In the opportunistic group, therapy must be directed toward the patient's underlying disease. The nature of the disease and its response to therapy largely determine the outcome of the lung abscess. Mortality in the primary type of lung abscess is approximately 2-10%, but approaches 75% in all others.

TABLE 17.6   Indications for Surgery in Patients with Lung Abscess

Drainage of empyema secondary to lung abscess
if tube drainage is inadequate

To differentiate lung abscess from carcinoma
if other approaches are unsuccessful

Life-threatening hemoptysis

Selected Bibliography

Abernathy, R. S.: Antibiotic therapy of lung abscess: Effectiveness of penicillin. *Chest* 53:592-598, 1968.

Adams, F. V. and Kolodny, E.: M-mode ultrasonic localization and identification of fluid-containing pulmonary cysts. *Chest* 75:330-333, 1979.

Bartlett, J. G. and Fingold, S. M.: Anaerobic infections of the lung and pleural space. *Am Rev Respir Dis* 110:56-77, 1974.

Bartlett, J. G., Gorback, S. L., Tally, F. P., and Fingold, S. M.: Bacteriology and treatment of primary lung abscess. *Am Rev Resp Dis* 109:510-518, 1974.

Block, A. J., Wagley, P. F., and Fisher, A. M.: Delayed closure of lung abscess: A re-evaluation of the indication for surgery. *Johns Hopkins Med J* 125:19-24, 1969.

Brock, R. C.: Studies in lung abscess, Part VI: Lung abscess and bronchial carcinoma. *Guy's Hosp Rep* 97:75-86, 1948.

Connors, J. P., Roper, C. L., and Ferguson, T. B.: Transbronchial catheterization of pulmonary abscess. *Ann Thorac Surg* 19:254-260, 1975.

Estrera, A. S., Platt, M. R., Mills, L. J., and Shaw, R. R.: Primary lung abscess. *J Thorac Cardiovasc Surg* 79:275-282, 1980.

Friedman, P. J. and Hellekaut, A. G.: Radiologic recognition of bronchopleural fistula. *Radiology* 124:289-295, 1977.

Gibbons, R. J., Spinell, D. M., and Skobe, Z.: Selective adherence as a determinant of the host tropisms of certain indigenous and pathogenic bacteria. *Infect Immun* 13:238-246, 1976.

Gorback, S. L. and Bartlett, J. B.: Anaerobic infections. *N Engl J Med* 290:1177-1184, 1237-1246, 1289-1294, 1974.

Harber, P. and Terry, P. B.: Fatal lung abscess: Review of 11 years experience. *South Med J* 74:281-283, 1981.

Huxley, E. J., Vcroslov, J., Gray, W. R., et al.: Pharyngeal aspiration in normal adults and patients with depressed consciousness. *Am J Med* 64:564-568, 1978.

Irwin, R. S., Garrity, F. L., Erickson, A. D., Corrao, W. M., and Kaemmerlen, J. R.: Sampling lower respiratory tract secretions in primary lung abscess. *Chest* 79:559-565, 1981.

Johanson, W. G., Jr. and Harris, G. D.: Aspiration pneumonias, anaerobic infections and lung abscess. *Med Clin N Am* 64:385-394, 1980.

Perlman, L. V., Kerner, E. and D'Esopo, N.: Clinical classification and analysis of 97 cases of lung abscess. *Am Rev Respir Dis* 99:390-398, 1969.

Rowe, L. D., Keane, W. M., Jafek, B. W., and Atkins, J. P.: Transbronchial drainage of pulmonary abscess with flexible fiberoptic bronchoscope. *Laryngoscope* 89:122-128, 1979.

Schackter, E. N.: Suppurative lung disease: Old problems revisited. *Clin Chest Med* 2:41-49, 1981.

Schackter, E. N., Knesman, H., and Putman, C.: Diagnostic problems in suppurative lung disease. *Arch Intern Med* 136:167-171, 1976.

Shafron, R. D., and Tate, C. F.: Lung abscess: A five-year evaluation. *Chest* 52:12-18, 1968.

Teague, R. B., Wallace, R. J., Jr., and Awe, R. J.: The use of quantitative sterile brush culture and Gram stain analysis in the diagnosis of lower respiratory tract infection. *Chest* 79:157-161, 1981.

Weiss, W.: Cavity behavior in acute, primary non-specific lung abscess. *Am Rev Respir Dis* 108:1273-1275, 1973.

Weiss, W. and Cherniak, M. S.: Acute non-specific lung abscess: A controlled study comparing oral and parenterally administered penicillin G. *Chest* 66:348-351, 1974.

Wimberly, N., Faling, L. J., and Bartlett, J. G.: A fiberoptic bronchoscopy technique to obtain uncontaminated lower airway secretions for bacterial culture. *Am Rev Respir Dis* 119:337-343, 1979.

18

EMPYEMA
Ronica M. Kluge, M.D.

Empyema is simply defined as pus in the pleural space. The condition can be acute or chronic and may be related to an infection in the lung or to another focus of infection, contiguous or distant.

Etiology (Table 18.1)

The bacteriology of empyema is different today than it was in the preantibiotic era. The microbes will vary somewhat depending on the patient's age and the clinical setting. The shift over time has been from predominantly pneumococci to staphylococci and gram-negative bacilli. The difference is at least partly due to the change in processes predisposing to empyema. Before the introduction of antibiotics, empyema most frequently occured as a consequence of community-acquired pneumonia; today, empyema occurs following trauma, surgery, or as a complication of infection elsewhere, especially in the abdomen.

Other organisms can cause empyema: *Mycobacterium tuberculosis,* actinomycetes, fungi, and rarely parasites such as ameba. Details can be found in the specific chapters about these microbes.

Epidemiology

When the empyema follows a community-acquired pneumonia, it is likely to be due to pneumococci. Empyemas following hospital-acquired pneumonia usually are caused by staphylococci, gram-negative bacilli, and anaerobes. In infants and young children, empyema usually is due to the staphylococcus, and anaerobes are seen rarely.

TABLE 18.1   Current Etiology of Empyema

Organisms	Adult	Child
S. pneumoniae	12-15*	2-5
Other streptococci	3-5	2
S. aureus	25-35	75-90
H. influenzae	0-5	1
Gram-negative bacilli	15-30	2
Anaerobes	15-35	1

*Numbers are percentages

Before antibiotics were available 70% of empyema was seen in patients under the age of 30 years; today, only 35% of empyema occurs in patients under 30. Antecedent infections are documented in 50-60% of the cases. Seventy percent of empyemas follow pneumonia, and 15-20% occur after surgery. Other predisposing causes are listed in Table 18.2. There is a slight seasonal variation, following that of pneumonia, with the highest incidence in winter months.

Pathogenesis

Bacteria or other microbes enter the pleural cavity by a number of routes: contiguous spread (pulmonary infection, leakage from a bronchial stump, or esophageal anastamosis), bronchopleural fistula, hematogenous, lymphatic, direct from trauma or thoracentesis, across the diaphragm, or from lymph node drainage. In the presence of infection and inflammation, there is increased permeability of capillaries which allows exudation of fluid into the pleural space. This process evolves with the polymerization of fibrin, the attraction of large numbers of leukocytes, and the beginning of fibroblast proliferation. At this point the empyema

TABLE 18.2   Factors Predisposing to Empyema

Pneumonia	Bronchiectasis
Thoracic surgery	Asthma
Tumor	Foreign body
Spontaneous pneumothorax	Dental extraction
Lung or subdiaphragmatic abscess	Tonsillectomy

may be loculated and difficult to drain. When not removed, the exudate eventually may become organized into a thick, constricting peel, or may rupture spontaneously into the lung parenchyma or through the chest wall (empyema necessitans).

Diagnostic Features

Clinical

The first signs and symptoms of empyema are essentially those of the underlying disease process. The most common symptoms are listed in Table 18.3. In many cases of anaerobic empyema the onset is insidious and the patient cannot pinpoint the date his symptoms began. Infants and young children may manifest empyema as an exacerbation of respiratory distress symptoms. The older child appears more ill and in greater respiratory difficulty.

The physical examination findings are those of a pleural effusion: decreased/absent breath sounds, dullness to percussion, and decreased/absent tactile fremitus. The degree of respiratory distress is frequently a reflection of the size of the empyema.

Laboratory

The peripheral white blood cell count is normal (20%) or elevated (80%) and shows a loft shift toward immature forms. Blood cultures yield the causative organism in 5-25% of cases.

Confirmation of the diagnosis depends upon demonstration of pleural fluid and examination of same. Chest roentgenograms should include PA, lateral, and decubitus views for the highest return. A lateral decubitus film is especially good

TABLE 18.3   Clinical Features of Empyema

Feature	% of Cases
Fever	80
Dyspnea	60
Chest pain	50
Weight loss	25
Chills	25
Hemoptysis	15
Night sweats	12

for detecting smaller effusions and for differentiating pleural thickening from fluid. Ultrasound is useful for exact localization of loculated pockets of fluid; this technique can also distinguish between fluid and fibrosis.

Aspiration of nonloculated empyema can be accomplished by needle or catheter; if there is concern about loculated fluid, the aspiration should be done under ultrasound guidance. The pleural fluid should be analyzed for white blood cells (total and differential), red blood cells, protein, glucose, LDH, amylase, specific gravity, and pH. Gram, fungal, and acid-fast stains should be done and the fluid cultured for aerobes, anaerobes, fungi, and tubercle bacilli. Anaerobic empyema is usually extremely malodorous.

It is not wise to use a single laboratory test to define empyema. A helpful constellation is listed in Table 18.4.

Additional diagnostic tests may be necessary in selected patients, e.g., pleural biopsy for histologic and microbiologic examination in patients with tuberculosis, and counterimmunoelectrophoresis of pleural fluid when the clinical situation has been modified by previous antibiotics. Computerized tomography, sinograms, or bronchograms may be indicated.

Differential Diagnosis

Empyema must be distinguished from the other causes of exudative pleural effusions: malignancy, embolism with infarction, pancreatitis, rheumatoid lung.

TABLE 18.4   Characteristics of Infected Pleural Fluid

White blood cells $\geq$ 2500/mm^3

White cell differential
      Polys predominate = bacterial
      Lymphs predominate = fungal, TB

Protein $\geq$ 3.0 g/dl, ratio P/S* 0.5

Glucose   50% that of serum

LDH $\geq$ 200 IU, ratio P/S* 0.6

Specific gravity $\geq$ 1.018

pH $\leq$ 7.2

Positive culture

*Ratio of pleural fluid to serum content

Grossly bloody effusions occur primarily in pleural malignancies, pulmonary infarction, or trauma. Cytologic examination of pleural fluid will detect malignant
cells. Patients with rheumatoid effusions have extremely low glucose (<20 mg/
dl) and depressed complement in the pleural fluid. Pleural effusions related to
pancreatitis contain elevated amylase levels.

Complications

Empyema is accompanied by a variety of complications. Those related directly
to the lung include pleural peel requiring decortication, lung abscesses, and bronchopleural fistula. The other complications result from contiguous or distant
spread of the infection, such as purulent pericarditis, peritonitis from diaphragmatic rupture, rib osteomyelitis, bacteremia, meningitis, septic arthritis.

Therapy

The two most important aspects of therapy are adequate drainage of the infected
material and appropriate antimicrobial agents. Drainage may be effected by
closed or open methods; generally the closed methods are attempted first. Repeated needle aspiration may be sufficient, but often an intercostal tube must be
inserted and controlled by water seal or by continuous suction. Occasionally, rib
resection and open drainage may be necessary. A chest tube is usually required
for 7-10 days.

The choice of antibiotics is dependent upon the susceptibilities of the organism causing the empyema. Initial choice can be guided by the results of the Gram
stain (or other stains). Whenever possible a single agent should be administered;
the duration of therapy is at least 3-4 weeks. There is no advantage to instillation of antibiotics into the pleural space, and this should not be attempted.

The introduction of proteolytic enzymes or fibrinolytic agents into the pleural space has not been proved effective in promoting drainage and may be associated with marked systemic reactions.

Prevention and Immunology

Early and appropriate treatment of pneumonia and good surgical technique are
ways to prevent the occurrence of empyema. The use of pneumococcal vaccine
in high-risk individuals may help to decrease the incidence of empyema.

Considerable controversy surrounds the notion that development of empyema
following thoracotomy for cancer might improve survival from the tumor. The
theory proposed is that the infection activates the host's cellular immune system
which then acts in a nonspecific fashion to destroy the remaining cancer cells.
Data on this from several sources are conflicting and it is doubtful if a conclusive
clinical trial could be carried out.

Prognosis

Several poor prognostic features are listed in Table 18.5. The mortality figures
compare with a range of 3-10% in patients who are less than 50 years of age, have
a single gram-positive organism, no underlying disease process, and who acquired
their empyema outside the hospital.

TABLE 18.5   Poor Prognostic Indicators in Empyema

Indicator	% Mortality
Age > 50 years	30
Multiple organisms	41
Gram-negative bacilli	42
Underlying illness	44
Hospital-acquired empyema	50

Selected Bibliography

Agostoni, E.: Mechanics of the pleural space. *Physiol Rev* 52:57-128, 1972.

Bartlett, J. G., Gorbach, S. L., Thadepalli, H., and Finegold, S. M.: Bacteriology of empyema. *Lancet* 1:338-340, 1974.

Bechamps, G. L., Lynn, H. B., and Wenzl, J. E.: Empyema in children: Review of Mayo Clinic experience. *Mayo Clin Proc* 45:43-50, 1970.

Brohee, D., Vanderhoeft, P., and Smets, P.: Lung cancer and postoperative empyema. *Eur J Cancer* 13:1429-1436, 1977.

Davis, W. C. and Johnson, L. F.: Adult thoracic empyema revisited. *Am Surg* 44: 362-368, 1978.

Finland, M. and Barnes, M. W.: Changing ecology of acute bacterial empyema: Occurrence and mortality at Boston City Hospital during 12 selected years from 1935 to 1972. *J Infect Dis* 137:274-291, 1978.

Finland, M. and Barnes, M. W.: Duration of hospitalization for acute bacterial empyema at Boston City Hospital during 12 selected years from 1935 to 1972. *J Infect Dis* 138:520-530, 1978.

Fishman, N. H. and Ellertson, D. G.: Early pleural decortication for thoracic empyema in immunosuppressed patients. *J Thorac Cardiovasc Surg* 74:537-541, 1977.

Landay, M. J. and Conrad, M.R.: Lung abscess mimicking empyema on ultrasonography. *Am J Roentgenol* 133:731-734, 1979.

Light, R. W., Girard, W. M., Jenkinson, S. G., and George, R. B.: Parapneumonic effusions. *Am J Med* 69:507-512, 1980.

Light, R. W., MacGregor, M. I., Luchsinger, P. C., and Ball, W. C., Jr.: Pleural effusions: The diagnostic separation of transudates and exudates. *Ann Intern Med* 77:507-513, 1972.

Nilsson, B. S., Broberg, S., Larsen, F., and Mellner, C.: Diagnosis and treatment of empyema. *Scand J Respir Dis* 102(suppl):202-204, 1978.

Ramilo, J., Harris, V. J., and White, H.: Empyema as a complication of retro-pharyngeal and neck abscesses in children. *Radiology* 126:743-746, 1978.

Ruckdeschel, J. C., Codish, S. D., Stranahan, A., and McKneally, M. F.: Postoperative empyema improves survival in lung cancer. *N Engl J Med* 287:1013-1017, 1972.

Sahn, S. A.: Pleural manifestations of pulmonary disease. *Hosp Prac* 16:73-89, 1981.

Sahn, S. A., Taryle, D. A., and Good, J. T., Jr.: Experimental empyema. *Am Rev Respir Dis* 120:355-361, 1979.

Siegel, J. D., Gartner, J. C., and Michaels, R. H.: Pneumococcal empyema in childhood. *Am J Dis Child* 132:1094-1096, 1978.

Sullivan, K. M., O'Toole, R. D., Fisher, R. H., and Sullivan, K. N.: Anaerobic empyema thoracis. *Arch Intern Med* 131:521-527, 1973.

Weese, W. C., Shindler, E. R., Smith, I. M., and Rabinovich, S.: Empyema of the thorax then and now: A study of 122 cases over four decades. *Arch Intern Med* 131:516-520, 1973.

19

ENDOCARDITIS AND ENDARTERITIS
Stuart M. Deglin, M.D.

Definition

Infective endocarditis and endarteritis are infections of the heart valves or of the internal surface of the heart or a blood vessel.

The disorder should ideally be described by the infectious agent involved, the activity of the process (i.e., healed or active), and the site of infection. The terms acute and subacute are sometimes used to differentiate between rapidly progressive and the less virulent forms of bacterial endocarditis. It should be realized that the clinical course cannot be uniformly predicted by the infecting organism and that any case of infective endocarditis may result in serious cardiac damage or peripheral complications. Nevertheless, it is worthwhile to recognize that the most inherently pathogenic organisms such as *Staphylococcus aureus,* *Streptococcus pneumoniae,* and *Neisseria gonorrhoeae* not only often cause a rapidly progressive form of the disease but are virulent enough to cause endocarditis in the absence of a preexisting structural cardiac abnormality.

Etiology

The organisms responsible for infective endocarditis include bacteria, fungi, and rickettsiae. Parasitic endocarditis has been reported and viral endocarditis also has been postulated to occur. Bacterial endocarditis is by far the most common. In the preantibiotic era almost two-thirds of the cases were due to nonpneumococcal streptococci followed by pneumococci, staphylococci, and gonococci. However, with the advent of antibiotics, cardiac surgery, and widespread intravenous narcotic abuse the spectrum of organisms responsible for endocarditis has changed.

In a series collected between 1962 and 1973, *S. aureus* was the single most common causative organism (30%), and nonpneumococcal and nonenterococcal *Streptococcus* spp accounted for another 30%. Ten percent were due to enterococci, 10% were culture-negative and the remainder were caused by *S. epidermidis,* pneumococcus, gram-negative bacilli, anaerobic organisms, fungi, and other unusual grampositive pathogens (Table 19.1).

Epidemiology

Epidemiologic studies show a lower incidence of hospitalizations for infective endocarditis in the antibiotic era as opposed to earlier years. It is not certain whether this reflects an actual decrease in occurrence of the disease or more successful therapy in community settings from whence cases are less likely to be reported.

While recent reports show an increase in the mean age at which endocarditis occurs, it continues to be a problem in the pediatric age group. In patients under the age of 25 there is usually an associated congenital cardiac malformation. About one-fifth of patients with infective endocarditis have previously undergone cardiac surgery and half of these have had prosthetic heart valves. In 60-75% of cases there is a recognized underlying abnormality of the cardiovascular system and rheumatic valvular disease remains the most common underlying disease. Eight to fifteen percent of cases occur in drug addicts.

TABLE 19.1   Infective Endocarditis – Etiologic Agents

Agent	Approximate % of Cases			
	All Patients	Addicts	Prosthetic Valves	
			Early	Late
Viridans streptococci	40	10	6	25
S. aureus	20	50	20	15
S. fecalis	10	8	4	9
S. epidermidis	7	2	25	25
Gram-negative bacilli	7	15	20	10
Fungi (mainly *Candida*)	2	10	10	6
Diphtheroids	2	2	8	4
Others	4	2	2	2
No organism	10	5	5	5

Pathogenesis and Pathology

There are two major factors which are usually necessary for the development of infective endocarditis: the responsible organism must enter the blood and in 60–75% of cases there is an underlying structural abnormality of the cardiovascular system.

Established infections of other systems such as pneumonia, urinary tract or wound infections, arteriovenous shunt infections in dialysis patients, and septic phlebitis may be associated with bacteremia and then endocarditis. On the other hand, transient bacteremia due to various procedures and manipulations is common and may result in infective endocarditis. Causes of transient bacteremia which have been associated with endocarditis include dental extraction or cleaning; urologic procedures, particularly if the urine is infected; and manipulation of infected intrauterine contraceptive devices. There are numerous other causes of transient bacteremia including some everyday activities such as tooth brushing or use of oral irrigation devices, and other less routine experiences such as vaginal delivery of an infant and most endoscopic examinations.

Other than those associated with urologic manipulations, most bacteremias go unrecognized and are inconsequential. Their likelihood of producing endocarditis depends upon the organism involved, the type of underlying cardiac disease present, and probably the intensity and duration of bacteremia. Gram-positive cocci demonstrate greater adherence to endothelial surfaces than do gram-negative organisms and therefore present a greater risk of endocarditis to patients with valvular disease. The enterococcus is generally considered to be the most common cause of endocarditis following urologic procedures even though it is responsible for only about one-third of the bacteremias following these manipulations. *Staphylococcus aureus* is a particularly virulent organism and is the most likely one to cause infective endocarditis in the absence of underlying heart disease.

Prosthetic heart valves appear to be susceptible to a wider variety of organisms including gram-negative rods and *S. epidermidis.* Indwelling intravenous cannulas and pressure-monitoring catheters are other potential sources of bacteremia and endocarditis, particularly in the early postoperative period in patients requiring a prosthetic heart valve.

Intravenous drug abuse is another cause of infective endocarditis. Drug addicts rarely have underlying cardiac disease and have a disproportionately high incidence of *S. aureus, Candida,* and gram-negative rods as the responsible organism. The skin is the most likely source of the organism in these patients rather than the drugs themselves or the injection paraphernalia, but contaminants in the drugs may cause endothelial injury which serves as a nidus for infection.

There are certain sites at which infective endocarditis is particularly likely to develop and certain underlying cardiac disorders with which it is likely to be associated. These are listed in Table 19.2. The circulatory characteristics of these sites have been described as high-velocity flow through a narrow orifice with a large pressure gradient. It is postulated that these conditions disrupt laminar flow just distal to the orifice, resulting in endothelial damage and an increased local bacterial count. Atrial septal defect is an example of a congenital lesion very rarely associated with infective endocarditis because it lacks the high pressure gradient.

The initial lesion of infective endocarditis appears to be a platelet-fibrin aggregate. In an active vegetation there is a middle layer composed primarily of bacteria surrounded by an outer layer of fibrin.

TABLE 19.2   Common Forms of Underlying Heart Disease in Infective
Endocarditis and Endarteritis

Aortic regurgitation

Mitral regurgitation

Congenital aortic stenosis (bicuspid valve)

Prosthetic heart valves

Tricuspid regurgitation

Ventricular septal defects

Patent ductus arteriosus

Coarctation of the aorta

Arteriovenous fistula

Diagnostic Features

Clinical

Infective endocarditis is commonly classified as acute or subacute. The differentiation is sometimes, but not always, useful since there is a great deal of overlapping of organisms, clinical features, and prognosis.

Acute infective endocarditis often appears suddenly with high fever, chills,
and diaphoresis, but emboli or hemodynamic complications may cause the initial
signs. It is usually caused by a virulent organism, most commonly *S. aureus*. Other
virulent organisms that usually cause acute endocarditis include pneumococcus,
gonococcus, and fungi, but less virulent organisms such as viridans streptococci
also may cause an abrupt clinical presentation. The more aggressive organisms
may infect previously normal hearts, and 40–50% of the cases occur in the absence
of previously recognized heart disease. Precipitating events such as dental ex-
tractions are often absent. Because endocarditis in drug addicts is most often due
to *S. aureus,* these patients commonly have an acute clinical course.

Subacute infective endocarditis is characterized by an insidious onset with a
history of fatigue, malaise, weight loss, and low-grade fever for weeks to months.
The classic history of dental or genitourinary tract manipulations is more likely
to be present. The fever may be continuous or intermittent. Fever may be absent
in the presence of intracerebral or subarachnoid bleeding, severe congestive heart
failure, uremia, or most commonly administration of antibiotics, salicylates, or
corticosteroids.

Heart murmurs are present in 85% of the cases. Variation in the intensity of a
previously existing murmur often reflects changes in temperature or progression of
anemia and may occur under many clinical circumstances in the absence of infective endocarditis. A new murmur of aortic, mitral, or tricuspid regurgitation, however, suggests active infection. In two-thirds of cases of right-sided endocarditis
there is no heart murmur.

Petechiae are much less common now than in the preantibiotic era and are found in less than 40% of the cases. Subungual hemorrhages are now more often due to trauma than to infective endocarditis and should only be considered significant if observed to develop in the absence of trauma.

Osler's nodes are small, raised, tender, discolored areas usually occurring in the pads of the fingers or toes. They may last for only hours. They are seen in only 10-25% of the patients. The Janeway lesion is a small, painless, erythematous lesion occurring on the palms and soles and is seen in less than 5% of the patients.

Splenomegaly is present in 25-55% of the cases. Retinal lesions are present in less than 10% of the cases and include exudates and oval shaped hemorrhages with a pale center (Roth's spots).

The clinical and laboratory features of infective endocarditis are outlined in Table 19.3.

TABLE 19.3   Clinical and Laboratory Features of Infective Endocarditis

Feature	Frequency (%)
Constitutional symptoms	90-100
Fever	85-100
Heart murmur	60-95
Petechiae	30-70
Heart failure	25-65
Splenomegaly	23-57
Neurologic abnormalities	30
Arthralgias	25
Osler's nodes	10-23
Janeway lesions	0-5
Roth's spots	2-4
Elevated erythrocyte sedimentation rate	95-100
Positive blood cultures	80
Rheumatoid factor	50-80
Anemia	40-80
Leukocytosis	50-65
Microscopic hematuria	50
Echocardiographic abnormalities	34

Laboratory

Laboratory findings in infective endocarditis include nonspecific hematologic and serologic abnormalities, abnormal echocardiography, as well as positive blood cultures and other microbiologic determinations. The frequency of laboratory abnormalities is included in Table 19.3.

Leukocytosis usually is present in acute endocarditis but may be absent in one-third to one-half of patients with subacute bacterial endocarditis. The mistake must not be made of excluding infective endocarditis as a diagnostic possibility because of a normal white blood count. Normochromic, normocytic anemia is a common finding. Rheumatoid factor is present in over half of the patients with subacute bacterial endocarditis and correlates with disease activity of over 6-week duration. The role played by this IgM antibody in the host response is unclear. Microscopic hematuria is found in approximately 50% of the cases.

Large vegetations due to infective endocarditis sometimes can be visualized by means of M-mode echocardiography. Visualization of vegetations implies a poor prognosis and suggests the need for surgical intervention. Echocardiography can also provide hemodynamic information, e.g., early closure of the mitral valve reflects severe aortic regurgitation.

The causative organism of infective endocarditis is isolated in over 80% of the cases. In most cases the first blood culture will reveal the organism. For the patient with a subacute presentation, most authorities suggest obtaining three to six separate cultures over a 24-hr period, both to maximize the chances of determining the etiologic agent and to avoid attaching undue significance to a contaminant if only one of five cultures is positive. Because bacteremia is continuous in endocarditis the timing of cultures is not critical. There is no advantage in obtaining arterial over venous blood for culture. Every attempt must be made to avoid contamination of blood culture specimens by skin flora. The venapuncture site should be first prepared with alcohol and then with iodine solution. Cultures should be handled in such a way that anaerobic organisms, fungi, other unusual organisms, and cell-wall-deficient varients can be isolated.

One important cause of negative blood cultures in infective endocarditis is prior use of antibiotics. If blood cultures are negative in patients suspected of having endocarditis who have received antibiotics before hospital admission, it is desirable to repeat cultures on several consecutive days following cessation of the antibiotics.

Other techniques that may detect blood stream invasion with bacteria include examination of buffy coat smears, histologic examination of vegetations which embolize to peripheral arteries, and demonstration of teichoic acid antibodies (in patients with staphylococcal endocarditis).

Differential Diagnosis

Since any of the complications associated with endocarditis (congestive failure, embolization, glomerulonephritis, etc.) may be responsible for the presenting features of infective endocarditis, the differential diagnostic possibilities are numerous (Table 19.4). In addition, the nonspecific clinical features of subacute bacterial endocarditis may cause it to be confused with any number of systemic illnesses. In the absence of such typical features as development of a new heart murmur or a source of bacteremia, diagnosis of endocarditis depends upon suspicion of the disease and use of appropriate laboratory studies.

TABLE 19.4   Differential Diagnosis of Infective Endocarditis

---

Acute rheumatic fever

Marasmic endocarditis

Systemic lupus erythematosus

Vasculitis

Atrial myxoma

Atrial thrombus

Hypernephroma

Carcinoid

Cytomegalovirus infection in patients
recently having valve replacement

Treatment

High concentrations of antibiotic are needed to cure infective endocarditis. In-travenous therapy usually is required to achieve adequate serum concentrations of the drug. Quantitative sensitivities (serum "cidal" level or Schlicter test) should be performed using serial tube dilutions of the patient's serum. Optimal therapy requires the serum to be bactericidal at a 1:8 dilution at the peak of serum anti-biotic concentration. Since therapy must usually be continued for 4-6 weeks, cost, efficacy, and toxicity must all be considered in choosing antibiotics.

Some experts suggest the addition of gentamicin 5 mg/kg/day to penicillin therapy for viridans streptococcal endocarditis; when combination therapy is used, a 3-week course of treatment is considered adequate. There is in vitro and in vivo evidence to suggest that the combination of gentamicin plus an antistaphylococcal penicillin is synergistic against *S. aureus* and this combination is an alternative therapy for *S. aureus* endocarditis. Some patients with endocarditis caused by highly penicillin-sensitive viridans streptococci have been treated successfully with penicillin alone for just 2 weeks. In some instances, it may be possible to switch the patient to oral antibiotics to complete therapy. In such cases, it is nec-essary to assure serum cidal levels of antibiotic in a dilution of 1:8.

When the clinical picture suggests endocarditis but blood cultures are nega-tive, or if therapy must be begun before the results of blood cultures are available and there is no evidence to point to a particular organism, treatment may be in-itiated with penicillin, 12 million U daily, and an aminoglycoside. Alterations in therapy can be made when culture results are available. Table 19.5 outlines sug-gested treatment regimens for the most common organisms causing infective endocarditis.

Surgery now plays an important role in the treatment of many patients with infective endocarditis. Heart failure that is difficult to manage with the basic modalities of digitalis and diuretics is the most common indication for surgery,

TABLE 19.5   Regimens for Treatment of Bacterial Endocarditis

Organism	Antibiotic and Daily Dose	Alternative for Penicillin Allergy and Daily Dose	Duration of Therapy
Viridans streptococcus and nonenterococcal group D streptococcus	Penicillin G IV 10-12 million U	Vancomycin, 2 g	2-4 wk
Enterococcus	Penicillin G 10-18 million U or ampicillin IV 8 g, plus streptomycin IM 1 g or gentamicin 5 mg/kg	Vancomycin IV, 2 g and streptomycin IM, 1 g or gentamicin IV, 5 mg/kg	4-6 wk
S. aureus	Nafcillin IV 12 g; or oxacillin IV 12 g	Vancomycin IV, 2 g	6 wk
Aerobic gram-negative rods	Gentamicin IV, 5 mg/kg; or tobramycin, 5 mg/kg		6 wk
Fungi	Amphotericin B, increase to 1 mg/kg		Total dose of 2 g or more

generally aortic or mitral valve replacement. Recent reports indicate that early surgical intervention is warranted in patients who develop heart failure associated with infective endocarditis, and in infections with organisms that are particularly resistant to therapy, such as *Candida, Pseudomonas,* and *Serratia marcescens,* and in the presence of repeated embolic episodes.

Prevention

In animal models, high-dose antibiotic administration before inoculation with organisms has been useful in preventing infective endocarditis. Extrapolation of these data to humans provides the regimens suggested in Table 19.6.

In patients with susceptible cardiac lesions, antibiotic prophylaxis is recommended for all dental procedures including cleaning. When practical, the intravenous route is suggested. For dental and upper respiratory tract procedures, viridans streptococci are the organisms against which therapy is primarily directed. Alternative regimens are suggested for patients who have prosthetic heart valves or those who have been taking daily penicillin for rheumatic fever prophylaxis.

Antibiotic prophylaxis before instrumentation of the gastrointestinal and genitourinary tract is aimed primarily against enterococci. Percutaneous liver biopsy, proctoscopy, sigmoidoscopy, barium enema, upper gastrointestinal tract endoscopy, pelvic examination, dilatation and curettage of the uterus, and uncomplicated insertion of intrauterine devices rarely have been associated with development of infective endocarditis and probably do not require prophylaxis.

Complications and Prognosis

Most fatalities in infective endocarditis are the result of complications which may occur despite eradication of the organism from the blood. Congestive heart failure is the most common cause of death (61% of fatalities). The outcome is most commonly the result of aortic or mitral insufficiency including aortic-to-right ventricular communication. Apparent valvular stenosis with obstruction to blood flow also may result from large vegetations, particularly common with fungal infections. Myocardial abscesses, particularly common in *S. aureus* endocarditis, may cause conduction disturbances, arrhythmias, or signs of continuing infection despite vigorous therapy. Embolization of fragments of vegetations may result in myocardial, cerebral, splenic, renal, or retinal infarction. Fungal endocarditis is noted for particularly large, friable vegetations which may embolize to the large arteries. Glomerulonephritis complicating infective endocarditis appears to be the result of immune-complex deposition. Sterile and, less commonly, purulent meningitis may occur in association with infective endocarditis.

In the preantibiotic era the mortality from infective endocarditis was 98%. Currently this entity still causes a 30% mortality despite appropriate therapy. Features associated with poor prognosis include congestive heart failure, infection with resistant organisms (fungi, gram-negative enteric organisms), or with staphylococci on the left side of the heart, and infection of prosthetic heart valves.

TABLE 19.6   Infective Endocarditis Prophylaxis

Dental procedures and surgical procedures of the upper respiratory tract

No Penicillin Allergy

Congenital heart disease or native valvular disease	Prosthetic heart valves *or* already on daily penicillin prophylaxis for rheumatic fever
Aqueous penicillin G 1 million U IM *plus* procaine penicillin 600,000 U IM 30-60 min before procedure. Then penicillin V 500 mg p.o. q6h x 8 doses *or* Penicillin V 2.0 g p.o. 30-60 min before procedure and then 500 mg p.o. q6h x 8 doses	Aqueous penicillin G 1 million U IM *plus* procaine penicillin 600,000 U IM *plus* streptomycin 1 g IM 30-60 min before procedure. Then penicillin V 500 mg p.o. q6h x 8 doses

Penicillin Allergy

Vancomycin 1 g IV over 30-60 min before procedure. Then erythromycin 500 mg p.o. q6h x 8 doses

or

Erythromycin 1 g p.o. 1.5-2 hr before procedure. Then 500 mg p.o. q6h x 8 doses

Genitourinary or gastrointestinal tract surgery or instrumentation

No Penicillin Allergy

Aqueous penicillin G 2 million U IM or IV *or* ampicillin 1.0 g IM or IV 30-60 min before procedure and then q8-12h x 2 doses	*plus*	Gentamicin 1.5 mg/kg IM or IV 30-60 min before procedure and then q8h x 2 doses *or* streptomycin 1.0 g IM 30-60 min before procedure and then q12h x 2 doses

Penicillin Allergy

Vancomycin 1.0 g IV over 30-60 min before procedure *plus* streptomycin 1.0 g IM 30-60 min before procedure (may repeat both drugs in 12 hr)

Selected Bibliography

AHA Committee Report: Prevention of bacterial endocarditis. *Circulation* 56: 139A, 1977.

Bayer, A. S., Theofilopoulos, A. N., Tillman, D. B., Dixon, F. J., and Guze, L. B.: Use of circulating immune complex levels in the serodifferentiation of endo-carditic and nonendocarditic septicemias. *Am J Med* 66:58, 1979.

Berger, S. A., Weitzman, S., Edberg, S. C., and Casey, J. I.: Bacteremia after the use of an oral irrigation device. *Ann Intern Med* 80:510-511, 1974.

Black, S., O'Rourke, R. A., and Karliner, J. S.: Role of surgery in the treatment of primary infective endocarditis. *Am J Med* 56:357-369, 1974.

Casey, J. and Miller, M. H.: Infective endocarditis. Part II. Current therapy. *Am Heart J* 96:263-269, 1978.

Everett, E. D. and Hirschmann, J. V.: Transient bacteremia and endocarditis prophylaxis. A review. *Medicine* 56:61-77, 1977.

Gould, K., Ramirez-Ronda, C. H., Holmes, R. K., and Sanford, J. P.: Adherence of bacteria to heart valves in vitro. *J Clin Invest* 56:1364-1370, 1975.

Gutman, R. A., Striker, G. E., Gilliland, B. C., and Cutler, R. E.: The immune complex glomerulonephritis of bacterial endocarditis. *Medicine* 51:1-25, 1972.

Kaplan, E. L., Rich, H., Gersony, W. I., and Manning, J.: A collaborative study of infective endocarditis in the 1970's. *Circulation* 59:327-335, 1979.

Lerner, P. I.: Infective endocarditis - A review of selected topics. *Med Clin N Am* 58:604-622, 1974.

Lerner, P. I. and Weinstein, L.: Infective endocarditis in the antibiotic era. *N Engl J Med* 274:199-206, 259-266, 323-331, 388-393, 1966.

Levy, R. L. and Hong, R.: The immune nature of subacute bacterial endocarditis (SBE) nephritis. *Am J Med* 54:645-652, 1973.

MacGregor, R. R. and Beaty, H. N.: Evaluation of positive blood cultures: Guide-lines for early differentiation of contaminated from valid positive cultures. *Arch Intern Med* 130:84-87, 1972.

Parrillo, J. E., Borst, T. C., Mazur, M. H., Iannini, P., Klempner, M. S., Moeller-ing, R. C., Jr., and Anderson, S. E.: Endocarditis due to resistant viridans streptococci during oral penicillin chemoprophylaxis. *N Engl J Med* 300:296, 1979.

Pazin, G. J., Peterson, K. I., Griff, E. W., Shaver, J. A., and Ho, M.: Determina-tion of site of infection in endocarditis. *Ann Intern Med* 82:746-750, 1975.

Pelletier, L. L. and Petersdorf, R. G.: Infective endocarditis: A review of 125 cases from the University of Washington Hospitals, 1963-1972. *Medicine* 56: 287-313, 1977.

Pesanti, E. L. and Smith, I. M.: Infective endocarditis with negative blood cultures. *Am J Med* 66:43-50, 1979.

Pruitt, A. A., Rubin, R. H., Karchmer, A. W., and Duncan, G. W.: Neurological complications of bacterial endocarditis. *Medicine* 57:329, 1978.

Ramirez-Ronda, C. H.: Adherence of glucan-positive and glucan-negative streptococcal strains to normal and damaged heart valves. *J Clin Invest* 62:808, 1978.

Rapaport, E.: The changing role of surgery in the management of infective endocarditis. *Circulation* 58:598-599, 1978.

Richardson, J. V., Karp, R. B., Kirklin, J. W., and Dismukes, W. E.: Treatment of infective endocarditis: A ten-year comparative analysis. *Circulation* 58: 589-597, 1978.

Rise, E., Smith, J. F., and Bell, J.: Reduction of bacteremia after oral manipulations. *Arch Otolaryngol* 90:106-109, 1969.

Rodbard, S.: Blood velocity and endocarditis. *Circulation* 27:18-28, 1963.

Stewart, J. A., Silimperi, D., Harris, P., Wise, N. K., Fraker, T. D., Jr., and Kissio, J. A.: Echocardiographic documentation of vegetative lesion in infective endocarditis: Clinical implications. *Circulation* 61:374-380, 1980.

Tuazon, C. U. and Sheagren, J. N.: Teichoic acid antibodies in the diagnosis of serious infections with *Staphylococcus aureus*. *Ann Intern Med* 84:543-546, 1976.

Wann, L. S., Dillon, J. C., Weyman, A. E., and Feigenbaum, H.: Echocardiography in bacterial endocarditis. *N Engl J Med* 295:135-139, 1976.

Weinstein, L. and Rubin, R. H.: Infective endocarditis - 1973. *Prog Cardiovasc Dis* 16:239-274, 1973.

Williams, R. C., Jr. and Kunkel, H. G.: Rheumatoid factor, complement, and conglutinin aberrations in patients with subacute bacterial endocarditis. *J Clin Invest* 41:666-675, 1962.

Wilson, L. M.: Etiology of bacterial endocarditis before and since the introduction of antibiotics. *Ann Intern Med* 58:946-952, 1963.

Wilson, W. R., Thompson, R. L., Wilkowske, C. J., Washington, J. A., II, Guiliani, E. R., and Geraci, J. E.: Short-term therapy for streptococcal infective endocarditis. *JAMA* 245:360-363, 1981.

20

PERICARDITIS
Stuart M. Deglin, M.D.

Definition

Pericarditis is an inflammatory reaction of the pericardium often occurring in association with a similar myocardial process.

Etiology

Infective pericarditis may be viral, bacterial, tuberculous, fungal, mycoplasmal, or parasitic in etiology, but over half of the cases are probably viral. Many viruses have been implicated as etiologic agents of pericarditis, but coxsackievirus B is the most common. The most common etiologic agents of purulent pericarditis are *Staphylococcus aureus, Streptococcus pneumoniae, Haemophilus influenzae,* and *Candida* and *Aspergillus* spp although many other organisms occasionally cause this disorder.

Epidemiology

The incidence of viral pericarditis is uncertain because of the difficulty in confirming the diagnosis. Most authorities agree that the majority of cases of *acute benign* or *idiopathic* pericarditis are probably viral in origin. Despite the advent of cardiothoracic surgery and immunosuppressive drugs, the occurrence of purulent pericarditis has decreased in the antibiotic era. Tuberculous pericarditis has decreased along with the underlying disease itself and occurs in approximately 8% of cases of pulmonary tuberculosis.

Pathogenesis and Pathology

Viruses are assumed to reach the pericardium via the bloodstream, but may enter the pericardium from the myocardium, which can be the site of primary infection.

Purulent pericarditis is invariably a complicating factor of another process. The most common pathogenesis is contiguous spread of infection from preexisting disease in the lung, pleura, or mediastinum. In these cases local acute inflammation occurs in the parietal pericardium adjacent to the site of infection. This is followed by accumulation of exudate in the pericardial space. It has been proposed that alternate routes of spread may be by septic microemboli from a pulmonary focus or by systemic bacteremia. In recent years, the initial infection has most often been associated with cardiothoracic surgical operations, immunosuppressive therapy, esophageal rupture due to neoplastic disease, and infective endocarditis. Thirteen percent of the cases of fatal infective endocarditis have pericarditis. The mechanisms for development of pericarditis in these cases include extension of inflammation from (1) ring abscess, (2) mycotic aneurysm, (3) septic coronary arterial embolus, or (4) myocardial abscess. Of the rarely reported cases of amebic pericarditis, all have spread from a hepatic abscess.

Tuberculous pericarditis probably develops by hematogenous dissemination or by lymphatic spread from involved mediastinal lymph nodes. It progresses from a stage of granulomatous reaction with diffuse fibrin deposition to a stage of pericardial effusion. Fibrous thickening may progress over a period of many years to cause chronic constrictive pericarditis.

Diagnostic Features

Clinical

The findings of acute pericarditis usually occur in association with symptoms and signs of the underlying disease. For example, the chest discomfort of acute idiopathic (probably viral) pericarditis may follow an upper respiratory tract infection.

Chest pain is one of the few complaints that can be attributed to the pericarditis itself. The pain is classically retrosternal in location and often radiates into the neck or the left upper extremity. It is sharp and is exacerbated by breathing, trunk motion, and the supine position. Often it is relieved, at least partially, by sitting up and leaning forward.

One of the first auscultatory findings of pericarditis is a pericardial friction rub. This is a high-pitched, scratchy sound best heard along the left sternal border. There may be one, two, or three components corresponding to atrial systole, ventricular systole, and ventricular diastole. It is difficult to be certain that the sound is a pericardial rub if only one component is present.

Other findings in acute pericarditis are those due to pericardial effusion, if it occurs. The effects of pericardial effusion depend in part upon its rate of accumulation. Rapid accumulation of only a few hundred milliliters can result in cardiac tamponade, while over 1 L may develop gradually in the absence of dramatic physical findings. One finding, when pericardial fluid does not cause tamponade, is a disparity between the apical impulse and the beginning of dullness to percussion of the left cardiac border. Ewarts' sign is an area of bronchial breathing below the left scapular angle seen with a large pericardial effusion or with cardiac enlargement of any cause.

When a pericardial effusion exerts enough pressure to impede cardiac filling, cardiac tamponade develops. Dyspnea is a common symptom but typical orthopnea usually is not present. Physical findings of cardiac tamponade include distended neck veins which sometimes become even more distended during inspiration, hepatosplenomegaly, lower extremity edema, pulsus paradoxus, and systemic hypotension.

When the situation progresses to chronic constrictive pericarditis, chest pain is usually absent but evidence of elevated venous pressure including ascites and edema is usually present.

Laboratory

The diagnosis of viral pericarditis depends upon a fourfold rise in titer of neutralizing antibodies against the specific virus in the first week or two after onset of illness or perhaps a twofold rise if the initial titer is high. Since the viremic stage may be over by the time cardiac manifestations develop, it may be difficult to isolate the virus, although this should be attempted from throat washings, stool specimens, or pericardial fluid samples.

The most direct diagnostic technique in purulent pericarditis is isolation of the organism from pericardial fluid. Culture techniques must be used that will allow isolation of anaerobic, fungal, and acid-fast organisms. In about 50% of the cases of tuberculous pericarditis, mycobacteria can be isolated from the fluid. Gram stain and acid-fast stain should be performed immediately after obtaining the fluid.

Serologic studies may help in the recognition of acute histoplasmosis, the stage of the disease in which most cases of pericarditis occur. Other fungal etiologies can be confirmed serologically, but this is of necessity a delayed diagnosis.

The white blood cell count of pericardial fluid will reveal a polymorphonuclear leukocytosis in fully developed cases and glucose values are often low compared with those of the blood.

In the presence of pericarditis, isolation of organisms from the blood or another source, or histologic evidence, as in the case of tuberculosis, is of value.

In acute pericarditis typical electrocardiographic changes are diffuse ST segment elevation during the first several days of illness, followed by T wave inversion. Large effusions may cause a decrease in QRS amplitude. Electrical alternans is suggestive of tamponade. Atrial arrhythmias may be seen during acute pericarditis but are usually transient.

As pericardial fluid accumulates the chest roentgenograms will demonstrate an enlarging cardiac silhouette in the absence of pulmonary congestion. Pericardial calcification is seen in 50% of cases of constrictive pericarditis. Angiocardiography, cardiac blood pool imaging with radioisotope labeled albumin, and intravenous injection of carbon dioxide, all have been largely replaced by echocardiology for the demonstration of pericardial effusion. Echocardiography is a sensitive, reliable, and rapid technique for detecting and estimating the size of pericardial effusion. It is noninvasive and can be performed serially to follow changes in fluid volume.

There are distinctive findings of constrictive pericarditis at cardiac catheterization including the classic diastolic dip-and-plateau pressure configuration in the ventricles and equalization of right atrial, right ventricular, pulmonary artery end-diastolic, and pulmonary wedge pressures.

Differential Diagnosis

The chest pain of acute pericarditis must be differentiated from acute myocardial infarction, spontaneous pneumothorax, pleuritis, and mediastinal emphysema. In myocardial infarction the pain is usually dull or pressure-like and is not related to respiration as is the case with pericarditis. Development of significant Q waves on the electrocardiogram makes the diagnosis of myocardial infarction in most cases, and myocardial scanning with technetium pyrophosphate is a sensitive technique for confirming transmural acute myocardial infarction. Only if there is transmural damage would a pericardial rub be present in myocardial infarction, and in these cases the laboratory studies indicated earlier can provide the differentiation from acute pericarditis.

Pleuritis is associated with only a pleural friction rub, and there are no characteristic ECG findings. Dissection of air into the mediastinum can be seen on roentgenograms in mediastinal emphysema; this point makes the differentiation from pericarditis easy, even though mediastinal emphysema is associated with a sound simulating a friction rub.

Infective pericardial effusion must be differentiated from those due to neoplasm, trauma, uremia, postmyocardial infarction syndrome, and adverse reactions to drugs. The setting of a preexisting thoracic infection or thoracic surgery immediately suggests purulent pericarditis and examination of the fluid is necessary.

Treatment

There is no specific treatment for viral pericarditis. Aspirin is usually successful in relieving chest pain, but occasionally indomethacin or corticosteroids are required.

Purulent pericarditis requires intravenous antibiotic therapy based on the offending organism. Dosages should be similar to those used for other life-threatening systemic infections, but intrapericardial installation of antibiotics is not necessary. Surgical drainage of the pericardial space is almost always necessary both for the control of infection and prevention of cardiac tamponade.

Antimicrobial treatment of tuberculous pericarditis is addressed in Chapter 104. The role of corticosteroids in preventing chronic constrictive pericarditis remains controversial.

If cardiac tamponade occurs, prompt needle aspiration of fluid is lifesaving.

Pericardial resection is required if constrictive pericarditis causes disabling symptoms.

Complications and Prognosis

Viral pericarditis is usually benign and self-limited. Most cases are associated with some element of myocardial involvement, and this may occasionally result in severe cardiomyopathy. Rarely, the disease may end in constrictive pericarditis.

The results of therapy for purulent pericarditis vary, depending in part upon the type of underlying disease. A review of 26 patients with purulent pericarditis between 1960 and 1974 from the Massachusetts General Hospital revealed a 77% overall mortality. There were no survivors in patients with contiguous spread from postoperative infections or infective endocarditis. On the other hand, patients with pneumococcal pericarditis who are treated promptly with both systemic antibiotics and surgical drainage have excellent survival. The mortality of untreated pneumococcal pericarditis, however, approaches 100%.

The most devastating potential complication of purulent and tuberculous pericarditis is chronic constrictive pericarditis with its associated impairment of cardiac output and often striking manifestations of venous congestion. Surgical therapy is required in these cases.

Selected Bibliography

Guimares, A. C., Vinhaes, L. A., Filho, A. S., Esteves, J. P., and Abreu, W. N.: Acute suppurative amebic pericarditis. *Am J Cardiol* 34:103-106, 1974.

Hahn, R. S., Holman, E., and Frerichs, J. B.: The role of the bronchial artery circulation in the etiology of pulmonary and pericardial suppuration. *J Thorac Surg* 27:121-129, 1954.

Horowitz, M. S., Schultz, C. S., Stinson, E. B., Harrison, D. C., and Popp, R. L.: Sensitivity and specificity of echocardiographic diagnosis of pericardial effusion. *Circulation* 50:239-247, 1974.

Kauffman, C. A., Watanakunakorn, C., and Phair, J. P.: Purulent pneumococcal pericarditis: A continuing problem in the antibiotic era. *Am J Med* 54:743-750, 1973.

Oill, P. A., Bayer, A. S., Criley, J. M., Blaufuss, A. H., and Fisher, L.: Infectious disease emergencies. *West J Med* 125:119-136, 1976.

Rooney, J. J., Crocco, J. A., and Lyons, H. A.: Tuberculous pericarditis. *Am J Med* 72:73-81, 1970.

Rubin, R. H. and Moellering, R. C.: Clinical, microbiologic, and therapeutic aspects of purulent pericarditis. *Am J Med* 59:68-78, 1975.

Sainnani, G. S., Krompotic, E., and Slodki, S. J.: Adult heart disease due to the Coxsackie virus B infection. *Medicine* 47:133-147, 1968.

Tan, J. S., Holmes, J. C., Fowler, N. O., Manitsas, G. T., and Phair, J. P.: Antibiotic levels in pericardial fluid. *J Clin Invest* 53:7-12, 1974.

21

MYOCARDITIS
Stuart M. Deglin, M.D.

Definition

Infective myocarditis is the direct infiltration of myocardial cells or their interstitium by infectious agents or by inflammatory cells in response to these agents.

Etiology

Myocarditis may be caused by almost any infectious agent including bacteria, viruses, fungi, mycoplasmas, and parasites. Worldwide, the most common myocardial infection is Chagas' disease, caused by *Trypanosoma cruzi*. In the United States viruses, particularly coxsackie-, echo-, and polioviruses, are the most common cause of myocarditis.

Epidemiology

The prevalence of some types of myocarditis is difficult to determine because many cases are asymptomatic or go unnoticed in the wake of noncardiac disease caused by the same organism. Thus, while electrocardiographic abnormalities consistent with myocarditis occur in 10-33% of cases of common infectious diseases, clinical manifestations of heart disease are much less common.

Similarly, in the acute stages of Chagas' disease, electrocardiograms are rarely recorded because the clinical syndrome is mild. If carefully sought, however, electrocardiographic abnormalities indicating myocarditis are common. Approximately 30% of patients with Chagas' disease develop clinically important chronic myocardial disease after 10-20 years. In some endemic areas in South America, the prevalence of Chagas' disease is an astounding 100% of people over 60 years of age. Myocarditis is present in 10-25% of cases of diphtheria, and in 4-10% of routine autopsies.

Pathology and Pathogenesis

The pathologic findings in infective myocarditis depend upon the responsible organism. In most forms of viral myocarditis histologic examination reveals myofiber necrosis, mononuclear cell infiltrates, and cardiac dilatation. Rubella myocarditis differs in that intracellular vacuolation is prominent in the absence of interstitial inflammation. Eosinophilic intranuclear inclusion bodies are typical of varicella myocarditis. There is usually a latent period between systemic viral infection and the appearance of clinical myocarditis. This suggests the operation of an autoimmune mechanism. Viral particles may be identified in myocardial tissue but usually only early in the course of myocarditis.

Bacterial myocarditis has an even wider spectrum of pathologic findings and pathogenetic mechanisms. Diphtheritic myocarditis is caused by an endotoxin which alters cellular respiration. There is resultant myocytolysis, intracellular fat accumulation, and glycogen depletion. Conduction system necrosis is particularly prominent. Myocardial tuberculosis usually is seen as a direct extension of disease from hilar lymph nodes to the right atrium and consists of caseating granulomas. There is also a rare diffuse interstitial infiltrative form of tuberculous myocarditis. The myocarditis of acute rheumatic fever is part of the immunologic response to pharyngeal infection by the group A β-hemolytic streptococci. The typical pathologic finding is the Aschoff body. The pathologic features of meningococcal myocarditis are similar to those in other areas of the body and include petechiae, hemorrhages, and capillary thromboses, probably due to endotoxin. Release of toxic substances is also implicated in the pathogenesis of myocarditis due to typhoid fever and tetanus. Myocardial abscess formation may complicate infections due to staphylococci and occasionally those due to pneumococci and gonococci. This usually represents a complication of bacterial endocarditis. Either diffuse or localized myocardial gummas may be present in syphilis. Spirochetes are present in the myocardium in congenital, but not late-acquired syphilis.

Vasculitis is a common pathologic finding in all of the rickettsial diseases but there is little impairment of cardiovascular function because the myofibers are preserved.

Infestation of the myocardium is the pathologic mechanism in most forms of parasitic myocarditis. *Trypanosoma cruzi* results in particularly striking inflammation and degeneration of autonomic ganglia and the cardiac conduction system. The myocardial damage due to malaria is primarily the result of vascular occlusion by organisms and parasitized red blood cells.

Diagnostic Features

Clinical

It is likely that relatively mild cases of myocarditis due to an underlying infection are often missed clinically, in part because nonspecific findings such as fatigue, fever, and tachycardia are attributed to the systemic disease.

The most common manifestations of myocarditis are those of congestive heart failure but even in these cases dyspnea, fatigue, and pulmonary rales may be attributed to an associated pneumonitis.

Persistent tachycardia disproportionate to the degree of fever and persisting even with resolution of fever should arouse suspicion of myocardial disease. Atrial and ventricular tachyarrhythmias as well as conduction disturbances often cause palpitations and syncope. Unexpected sinus bradycardia may occur in association with typhoid fever.

Chest pain, if present, is usually pleuritic and reflects the simultaneous involvement of epicardium and pericardium. Pericardial friction rubs may be present in myocarditis for the same reason. Occasionally pressure-like chest pain reminiscent of angina pectoris is present. The angina pectoris may occur in malaria because of vascular occlusion by parasites and parasitized red blood cells.

Particularly in viral myocarditis, the cardiac manifestations often begin a week or more after the clinical peak of the systemic infection. Viral myocarditis is almost invariably associated with symptoms of myalgia.

Laboratory

The typical electrocardiographic abnormalities of myocarditis are identical to those described for pericarditis in Chapter 20. Less specific ST segment and T wave abnormalities are even more common. Occasionally there are abnormal Q waves on the ECG, causing a pseudomyocardial infarction pattern. Arrhythmias of any kind may be seen on electrocardiogram and are nonspecific, but atrioventricular and intraventricular conduction disturbances developing in association with a systemic illness point toward myocardial involvement. Chest roentgenography and echocardiography show cardiac enlargement if heart failure has supervened and the echocardiogram will demonstrate any pericardial fluid if there is associated pericarditis. Two-dimensional echocardiography is useful in directing intracardiac thrombi.

Cardiac enzymes may be elevated in myocarditis and isoenzyme determinations confirm the myocardial origin.

Specific etiologic diagnosis requires skillful use of the microbiologic and serologic laboratories.

Differential Diagnosis

Chest pain, arrhythmias, and heart failure with new onset following a systemic infection make the diagnosis of infective myopericarditis fairly clear. The differential diagnosis becomes more extensive when myocarditis results in chronic congestive heart failure.

Myocardial disease due to an infectious agent must first be differentiated from one of the more common forms of heart disease (coronary heart disease, hypertensive heart disease, rheumatic heart disease, and pericardial disease) and then from noninfective cardiomyopathies.

Coronary Heart Disease

Patients with congestive heart failure due to coronary disease have invariably sustained extensive transmural myocardial infarction at some time and have a history and electrocardiographic findings consistent with those events. The absence of coronary risk factors such as diabetes mellitus, hyperlipidemia, family history of coronary disease, hypertension, and cigarette smoking provides some evidence in favor of primary myocardial disease.

Hypertensive Heart Disease

A history of sustained systolic and diastolic hypertension, hypertensive abnormalities of the ocular fundus, and left ventricular hypertrophy shown by electrocardiography and echocardiography all weigh against primary myocardial disease.

Rheumatic Heart Disease

Heart failure in these patients is usually associated with evidence of valvular abnormalities such as mitral stenosis and aortic regurgitation. On the other hand, mitral and tricuspid regurgitation may be due to ventricular dilatation of any cause.

Pericardial Disease

In most cases of pericarditis there is an associated element of epicardial disease. Nevertheless, when pericardial constriction is predominant the clinical findings are mainly those of elevated venous pressure, and cardiac catheterization shows typical hemodynamic alterations.

When historic, diagnostic, and laboratory criteria suggest a cardiomyopathy the etiologic differential diagnosis is extensive. Neuromuscular diseases such as pseudohypertrophic and myotonic muscular dystrophy are associated with congestive heart failure. The associated clinical features are usually clear. Systemic lupus erythematosus and progressive systemic sclerosis are commonly associated with myocardial involvement. The systemic features of these diseases and serologic studies usually allow the diagnosis to be made. The heart may be involved in either primary amyloidosis or in the form secondary to multiple myeloma or chronic inflammatory diseases. In the latter form the underlying disease provides a clear diagnostic clue. When congestive heart failure of uncertain cause occurs in a relatively young person, the demonstration of amyloid deposits in rectal or gingival biopsies suggests cardiac amyloidosis.

Hemochromatosis may be associated with heart failure. Physical findings of hepatomegaly, skin pigmentation, and laboratory evidence of diabetes mellitus suggest this diagnosis. The serum iron and iron-binding capacity can be used to calculate transferrin saturation. This is invariably greater than 80% in hemochromatosis and these studies should be included in the evaluation of patients with heart failure of uncertain cause.

Heavy alcohol consumption is a cause of chronic cardiomyopathy. The diagnosis is made by history. This is to be distinguished from acute beriberi heart disease due to thiamine deficiency.

There are many drugs that cause cardiomyopathy such as daunorubicin and doxorubicin. History of administration of drugs with cardiomyopathic potential is the most useful way of clarifying the etiology of heart failure in these patients.

Treatment

Specific treatment of the underlying infection is available in bacterial or fungal infections and in some parasitic diseases. No effective specific therapy is available for Chagas' disease in the chronic stage or for systemic viral illness.

Bed rest has long been suggested as an adjunctive measure in acute myocarditis. In the patient with chronic heart failure due to a previous or inactive infection moderate physical activity should be encouraged, within the limits of patient tolerance.

Most therapy for myocarditis is aimed at the major complications: heart failure, arrhythmias, and thromboembolism. The commonly employed treatment for heart failure of any cause is used including digitalis glycosides, diuretics, and dietary salt restriction. In more difficult cases vasodilators may be of value.

Tachyarrhythmias are often difficult to suppress in the presence of active inflammation. In view of the possibility of sudden death, monitoring in an intensive care unit is useful as long as serious arrhythmias persist. Arrhythmias may respond to antiarrhythmic drugs more readily if congestive heart failure can be controlled. Bradyarrhythmias, usually due to atrioventricular conduction disturbances, may require temporary or permanent pacemaker support if the heart rate is slow enough to cause hemodynamic compromise.

If thromboembolic events complicate myocarditis, anticoagulants are indicated, and prophylactic anticoagulation is commonly employed in patients with severe chronic cardiomyopathies because of the high incidence of embolic complications.

Prevention

The myocarditis of diphtheria and poliomyelitis are now rarely seen because of immunization of children. Chagas' disease can only be approached by means of improving sanitation and living conditions in endemic areas.

Patients with cardiac and pulmonary disease should be immunized against influenza since this disease poses a serious threat to them even if myocarditis does not occur.

Prognosis and Complications

Viral myocarditis is most often benign in adults and recovery is usually complete. In one study, by Gerzen et al., of 45 patients who developed electrocardiographic abnormalities in conjunction with a variety of acute infectious processes, all had normal exercise tolerance after a 6- to 68-month follow-up. However, chronic congestive heart failure and permanent conduction disturbances may occur. Sudden death has occurred in cases of viral myocarditis. The heart failure syndrome due to coxsackievirus B myocarditis is more frequently fatal in neonates and usually occurs in nursery epidemics.

Myocarditis is the most common cause of death in diphtheria. The development of bundle-branch block carries a 50% mortality and complete atrioventricular block is associated with an 80-100% mortality .

The acute myocarditis of Chagas' disease is mild and usually followed by complete clinical recovery. However, following a latent period (10-20 years) chronic Chagas' disease appears as progressive heart failure; tachyarrhythmias, which not infrequently result in sudden death; and conduction disturbances including complete atrioventricular block, which also carries a grave prognosis.

Since *Trichinella spiralis* does not encyst in the heart, the myocarditis of trichinosis is transient, and persistent cardiac disease is unlikely.

Mural thrombi developing in dilated cardiac chambers make systemic and pulmonary embolic events a risk when myocarditis of any etiology results in congestive heart failure.

In summary, the three major causes of morbidity and mortality in myocarditis are intractable congestive heart failure, intractable arrhythmias, and embolic events.

Selected Bibliography

Burch, G. E. and Giles, T. D.: The role of viruses in the production of heart disease. *Am J Cardiol* 29:231–240, 1972.

Deglin, S. M., Deglin, J. M., and Chung, E. K.: Drug induced cardiovascular disease. *Drugs* 14:29–40, 1977.

DeMaria, A. N., Neumann, A., Bommer, W., Weinert, L., Grehl, T., DeNardo, S., Amsterdam, E. A., and Mason, D. T.: Left ventricular thrombi identified by cross-sectional echocardiography. *Ann Intern Med* 90:14–18, 1979.

Fowler, N. O.: Classification and differential diagnosis of the myocardiopathies. *Prog Cardiovasc Dis* 7:1–16, 1964.

Gerzen, P., Holmgren, G. B., and Zetterquist, S.: Acute myocarditis: A follow-up study. *Br Heart J* 34:575–583, 1972.

Harris, L. C. and Nghiem, Q. X.: Cardiomyopathies in infants and children. *Prog Cardiovasc Dis* 15:255–287, 1972.

Harvey, W. P., Segal, J. P., and Furel, T.: The clinical spectrum of primary myocardial disease. *Prog Cardiovasc Dis* 7:17–42, 1964.

Lewes, D., Rainford, D. J., and Lane, W. F.: Symptomless myocarditis and myalgia in viral and mycoplasma infections. *Br Heart J* 36:924–932, 1974.

Morales, A. R., Vichidbandha, P., Chandruang, P., Evans, H., and Beurgeois, C. H.: Pathologic features of cardiac conduction disturbances in diphtheritic myocarditis. *Arch Pathol* 91:1–7, 1971.

Rosenbaum, M. D.: Chagasic myocardiopathy. *Prog Cardiovasc Dis* 7:199–225, 1964.

Sainini, G. S., Krompotic, E., and Slodki, S. J.: Adult heart disease due to the Coxsackie virus B infection. *Medicine* 47:133–147, 1968.

22

SUPPURATIVE THROMBOPHLEBITIS
Robert H. Waldman, M.D.

Suppurative or septic thrombophlebitis is a bacterial or fungal infection of veins, associated with thrombus formation and sepsis. The thrombosis and occlusion of the vein, along with the bacterial growth, lead to the vein becoming a purulent cavity. The prognosis in this disease is extremely grave. Most cases today are a result of infected intravenous plastic catheters. Other types of suppurative thrombophlebitis, i.e., pelvic, cavernous sinus, and pylephlebitis (suppurative thrombophlebitis of the portal vein) are extremely rare.

Etiology

The agents most often isolated from patients with suppurative thrombophlebitis are shown in Table 22.1. The organisms do not seem to be related to the patient's preexisting skin flora, and contamination at the time of insertion of the plastic catheter may be a major source of the infection.

Epidemiology and Pathogenesis

We are in the midst of a major epidemic of serious infections secondary to the use of intravenous administration of fluids, blood, and nutritional substances, as well as intravenous tubes for monitoring purposes. Insertion of an intravenous catheter breaks one of the most important host defense mechanisms, i.e., the intact skin. Bacterial colonization of intravenous devices occurs at a rate of 30–80% (Table 22.2). Bacteremia occurs in 2-4%. The source and significance of the bacteria on the intravenous catheter have not definitely been established; however, there is a correlation between having an infected catheter and the subsequent

TABLE 22.1   Organisms Isolated from Patients with Suppurative Thrombophlebitis

Organisms	Percentage
Klebsiella-Enterobacter group	40
Providencia spp	20
Proteus spp	20
S. marcescens	12
S. aureus	12
P. aeruginosa	8
E. coli	8
Candida spp	8

TABLE 22.2   Intravenous Catheters

Day	% Positive Culture*	% with Sepsis
1	12	0.0
2	24	0.3
3	29	0.7
4	33	2.9

*From catheter tip upon removal

development of phlebitis. Nonetheless, for reasons that are not clear, about half of infected intravenous catheters are not associated with clinical phlebitis. The most important figures, however, are that about 40 million Americans are hospitalized each year, about one-fourth receive some sort of intravenous therapy, and sepsis is related to this intravenous therapy in about 25,000 patients each year. A much smaller number have suppurative thrombophlebitis, which is at the most severe end of the spectrum of disease associated with intravenous catheter use.

Factors that have been shown to favor the development of infected intravenous catheters are shown in Table 22.3. During a transient bacteremia, organisms may be trapped within the loosely organized clot that almost always forms around plastic catheters within the first 24 hours. Four to ten percent of intravenous fluid mixtures contain culturable microorganisms. Five percent dextrose solution supports growth of only a few organisms, but those include members of the tribe

TABLE 22.3   Factors Related to Development of Infected
                        Intravenous Catheters

Patient already septic
Transient bacteremia from another source
Irrigating or otherwise manipulating an occluded,
      leaking, or infiltrated catheter
Contaminated fluid being administered
Total parenteral nutrition
Burned patient
Length of time catheter remains in place
Cancer patient
Corticosteroids and/or other immunosuppressive therapy
Plastic cannulas (as opposed to steel)
Intravenous therapy in lower extremity

Klebsielleae, which are the organisms most commonly found in suppurative thrombophlebitis. With respect to total parenteral nutrition, a minor point, but one of
some interest, is the possible relationship to granulocytic abnormalities that may
result from folic acid and phosphate depletion which commonly occurs in these
patients. In burned patients, suppurative thrombophlebitis is the most common
cause of death due to infection, developing in as many as 8% of these patients.

The source of the organisms has not been definitely established. More than
half of all health workers have coliform organisms on their hands, again those of
the tribe Klebsiellcae being the most common. In addition, these organisms on
the hands of health workers are usually resistant to most antibiotics.

Why there is the relationship between development of suppurative thrombophlebitis and plastic, as opposed to steel, cannulas is unknown. This may be related to the length of time the plastic cannulas remain in place, the general degree of debility of the patients, and the larger bore of the cannulas that are usually used.

Suppurative thrombophlebitis less commonly results from local extension of
infection, such as skin infections, particularly furuncles. These are particularly
dangerous when they occur in the face, because they may lead to cavernous sinus
thrombophlebitis. The latter also may result from other infections in the area,
such as sinusitis or otitis media. Pelvic vein suppurative thrombophlebitis is associated with pelvic infections, which may be secondary to gynecologic surgery,
abortion, or parturition.

Diagnosis

The diagnosis is a clinical one, and should be suspected in any patient who is septic and who has, or has recently had, an intravenous catheter in place. There are
usually signs and symptoms of inflammation over the involved vein, although this
aspect may be made more difficult if the patient is on immunosuppressive therapy,
and/or has an impaired level of consciousness.

If an intravenous catheter is in place, when it is removed and the vein is
"milked-down" peripherally, one can often extrude a small drop of pus. This is
diagnostic of suppurative thrombophlebitis. There may not be a firm cord present since the vein is purulent and not completely filled with clot.

Septic emboli, usually to the lung, are found in nearly half of all patients, and their occurrence should make one very suspicious of the diagnosis of suppurative thrombophlebitis.

Pelvic suppurative thrombophlebitis follows surgery or parturition by 7-14 days in most cases, and patients have fairly nonspecific signs and symptoms, with high fever, rigors, abdominal pain, and nausea and vomiting. Abdominal and pelvic examinations also are fairly nonspecific in most cases, although occasionally the involved tender vein can be palpated.

The diagnosis of suppurative thrombophlebitis in any area is often made on the basis of a patient with positive blood cultures, in an appropriate setting, who fails to respond to appropriate antibiotics.

Treatment

In a patient with signs or symptoms of local inflammation, or with unexplained fever and an intravenous catheter in place within the preceding week or so, remove and culture the catheter and, in addition, obtain blood cultures. It has been proposed that quantitative cultures of the catheter tip are helpful in differentiating significant from trivial contamination, and therefore it may be helpful to roll the catheter tip across a blood agar plate rather than placing it in a broth solution, with heavy growth probably indicating serious infection.

In the clinical situation just described, the patient should be started on therapy with a penicillinase-resistant penicillin and aminoglycoside. If the patient does not respond, i.e., becomes more septic within 24-28 hr, strong consideration should be given to the diagnosis of suppurative thrombophlebitis. A careful examination of the intravenous catheter sites should be carried out, and if there is any indication that suppurative thrombophlebitis might be present, exploratory surgery should be done. At the time of surgery, ligation and complete removal of infected veins and tributaries must be accomplished.

In contradistinction to superficial suppurative thrombophlebitis, i.e., that secondary to intravenous catheters, pelvic suppurative thrombophlebitis can be cured with medical therapy. Because of the usual causative organisms, i.e., anaerobic streptococci and *Bacteroides,* chloramphenicol or clindamycin plus an aminoglycoside, or ampicillin plus chloramphenicol should be administered intravenously. The use of heparin is controversial, with a review of the reported cases in the literature suggesting that its use may be beneficial; however, there are no controlled studies supporting this. If the patient does not respond to antibiotic therapy, a trial of heparin should be administered before surgical intervention is considered.

Prognosis and Complications

As already mentioned, medical treatment alone for superficial suppurative thrombophlebitis is not effective since nearly all patients will die of persistent bacteremia or septic emboli. Even with medical and surgical treatment the mortality is still high, probably in the range of 30-50%.

The major complication is septic embolization, most characteristically to the lung, manifested on chest roentgenogram by small, scattered, rapidly extending areas of infiltrate which can be confused with bronchopneumonia.

TABLE 22.4   General Principles

Intravenous catheters should be used only when less dangerous methods are not possible

Catheter must be inspected daily

Catheter must be removed after 48 hr, except under special circumstances

Three-way stopcocks should be avoided if possible; at least, should be changed every 24 hr, because they provide a portal of entry for bacteria or fungi

Forced irrigation should be avoided because of possibility of thromboembolism

TABLE 22.5   Recommended Technique for Intravenous Catheter Placement

Prepare area with antiseptic solution

Use sterile drapes and gloves

Apply antibiotic ointment to the site after insertion

Anchor catheter securely

Apply sterile dressing

"Date" catheter

Prevention

Prevention (Tables 22.4 and 22.5) is essentially related to minimizing the factors which are listed in Table 22.3. Intravenous catheters should be used as infrequently as possible, and under no circumstance simply for the convenience of medical or nursing staff. They should be inserted under aseptic conditions with secure anchoring of the cannula. The use of local application of antibiotic ointments certainly has not been definitely proved but probably should be undertaken. If cannulas are placed under emergency situations where sterile technique is not possible, then the cannula should be replaced at the first opportunity. Insertion sites should not be wrapped so extensively that they cannot be easily inspected, and they should be inspected daily with reapplication of the antibiotic ointment. The patient should be questioned regarding pain at the site, and palpation for tenderness or a cord should be done.

Selected Bibliography

Collin, J., Collin, C., Constable, F. L., et al.: Infusion thrombophlebitis and infection with various cannulas. *Lancet* 2:150–153, 1975.

Collins, R. N.: Suppurative pelvic thrombophlebitis. *Am J Obstet Gynecol* 108: 681–687, 1970.

Collins, R. N., Braum, P. A., Zinner, S. H., and Kass, E. H.: Risk of local and systemic infection with polyethylene intravenous catheters: A prospective study of 213 catheterizations. *N Engl J Med* 279:340, 1968.

Ferguson, R. L., Rosett, W., Hodges, G. R., et al.: Complications with heparin lock needles. A prospective evaluation. *Ann Intern Med* 85:583, 1976.

Goldmann, D. A., Maki, D. G., Rhame, F. S., Kaiser, A. B., Tenney, J. H., and Bennett, J. V.: Guidelines for infection control in intravenous therapy. *Ann Intern Med* 79:848, 1973.

Irwin, G. R., Jr., Hart, R. J., and Martin, C. M.: Pathogenesis and prevention of intravenous catheter infections. *Yale J Biol Med* 46:85, 1973.

Maki, D. G.: Preventing infection in intravenous therapy. *Anesth Analg* 56:141, 1977.

Maki, D. G., Goldmann, D. A., and Rhame, F. S.: Infection control in intravenous therapy. *Ann Intern Med* 79:867–887, 1973.

Maki, D. G., Weise, C. E., and Sarafin, H. W.: A semiquantitative culture method for identifying intravenous-catheter-related infection. *N Engl J Med* 296: 1305–1309, 1977.

Pruitt, B. A., Stein, J. M., Foley, F. D., et al.: Intravenous therapy in burn patients. Suppurative thrombophlebitis and other life-threatening complications. *Arch Surg* 100:399, 1970.

Stein, J. M. and Pruitt, B. A., Jr.: Suppurative thrombophlebitis. A lethal iatrogenic disease. *N Engl J Med* 282:1452, 1970.

23

VIRAL GASTROENTERITIS
Ronica M. Kluge, M.D.

Viruses are thought to be responsible for a majority of acute gastroenteritis episodes in infants and children and have been proved the causative agent in a number of outbreaks among adults. Other infectious causes of diarrhea are discussed
in Chapter 24.

Microbiology

Rotaviruses and 27-nm Norwalk-like agents are the most common viruses associated with gastroenteritis syndromes. Occasionally enteroviruses or adenoviruses
have been incriminated (Table 23.1)

Rotaviruses have a double-stranded RNA genome, a spherical shape, and a
double-shelled capsid. The complete virion is about 70 nm in diameter. These
viruses are known to cause acute diarrheal disease in many newborn and young
animal species, including humans. The human rotavirus strains share a number of
antigens with those of animals, but can be distinguished by use of specific immunofluorescence and enzyme-linked immunosorbent assay tests. Efforts to cultivate human rotaviruses have been disappointing. At least three serotypes have
been described.

The Norwalk, Hawaii, and Montgomery County Maryland (MC) agents are 27-
nm particles which are isometric and both acid and ether stable. The nucleic acid
content of the genome has not yet been determined (whether DNA or RNA). While
the Norwalk and MC agents seem related, the Hawaii agent is antigenically distinct. Other 27-nm particles have been recovered from patients in England; these
agents are related to, but distinct from, the Norwalk and Hawaii agents.

TABLE 23.1   Etiologic Agents

Proven	Probable
Rotavirus	Coronaviruses
Norwalk agent	Adenoviruses
Hawaii agent	Echoviruses
	Coxsackievirus A
	Reoviruses

Epidemiology

Rotaviruses are ubiquitous, found throughout the world, and in most every mammalian species. In humans these viruses appear to cause symptomatic gastroenteritis primarily in the child aged 6 months to 2 years. Rotaviruses are responsible for 40-55% of diarrheal episodes in this age group. The disease is seasonal with the highest incidence occurring during the winter months. Spread is thought to occur by the fecal-oral route; hospital-acquired rotavirus infections account for 20-30% of cases. The incubation period is 2-4 days. Up to 50% of adults in contact with children who have rotavirus-induced diarrhea will show serologic evidence of infection; only 10-30% of these adults will be symptomatic.

The Norwalk-like agents have been associated with acute epidemic diarrheal disease of short duration (12-24 hr). The primary attack rate is $\sim$ 50%, while that among contacts is $\sim$ 30%.

The incubation period is 1-2 days. Adults and school-aged children are affected.

Pathogenesis and Pathophysiology

The histologic changes that occur in the intestinal tract as a result of rotavirus infection have been determined on rather limited human material and in extensive animal studies. Mucosal changes range from mild to severe and include shortening and blunting of villus projections, mononuclear cell infiltration of the lamina propria, swelling of mitochondria, and irregularity of microvillae. The viruses penetrate and multiply in the enterocytes of the small intestine. The damaged cells release large numbers of virus particles into the lumen; these cells are also sloughed. Animal data suggest that malabsorption and enzyme deficiencies related to the cell damage result in diarrhea. In the experimental model, histologic changes return to normal within 48-72 hr of the onset of symptoms.

There are no good animal models for the disease caused by Norwalk-like agents. Consequently, the histopathology has been documented in normal volunteers with experimentally induced infection. Microscopic changes include shortening and blunting of the villus projections, distorted microvillae, swollen mitochondria, crypt hypertrophy, and intracellular edema. Malabsorption occurs during the acute illness. The histologic changes persist for at least 4 days after illness subsides but return to normal by 2 weeks. More severe histologic changes seem to be associated with more severe illness.

Diagnostic Features

Clinical

Rotavirus infections range from a very mild to occasionally fatal illness. The disease occurs primarily in children between the ages of 6 months and 2 years. The predominant symptoms include diarrhea (100%), vomiting (96%), fever (77%), and dehydration (83%); the older child may complain of abdominal pain. The course of the disease is 3-5 days. Adults generally have asymptomatic infections when exposed to rotaviruses (Table 23.2).

The Norwalk-like agents are associated with the abrupt onset of nausea and vomiting, followed promptly by abdominal pain and diarrhea; low-grade fever is present in $\sim$ 50%. The disease occurs primarily in adults and school-aged children. The duration is no longer than 12-36 hr.

Laboratory

Routine laboratory tests in patients with viral gastroenteritis are likely to be normal. Dehydration may cause changes in serum sodium, blood urea nitrogen, or hematocrit. Fecal leukocytes may be present in 10-15% of infants and children with viral gastroenteritis but rarely are seen in adults. Immune electron microscopy can be used to demonstrate virus particles in the stool, but it is not generally available. A serologic diagnosis of rotavirus or Norwalk-like agent illness can be confirmed by indirect hemagglutination-inhibition assay or radioimmunoassay; rotavirus infection also can be diagnosed by enzyme-linked immunosorbent assay. Neither group of viruses can be recovered by current culture techniques.

TABLE 23.2 Distinguishing Clinical Features of Viral Gastroenteritis

	Rotavirus	Norwalk-like Agents
Age	6 mo-2 yr	Adults, school-aged children
Incubation period	2-4 days	1-2 days
Diarrhea	++++	++
Vomiting	++	++++
Abdominal pain	++	++
Fever	+++	+
Duration of symptoms	3-5 days	12-36 hr

Differential Diagnosis

Viral gastroenteritis must be distinguished from other infectious causes of diarrhea (see Chapter 24). The presence of fever suggests the possibilities of invasive diseases such as those caused by *Salmonella* or *Shigella* spp; when fever is absent, a toxin-mediated disease is possible, such as that related to staphylococci or to *Clostridium perfringens.* Fecal leukocytes strongly suggest inflammation of the colon, likely to be seen in shigellosis, invasive *Escherichia coli,* or amebiasis and in noninfectious inflammatory bowel disease such as ulcerative colitis or pseudomembranous colitis. Stool culture can rule out the presence of bacterial pathogens; ova and parasites also should be looked for in selected individuals.

Complications

The complications of viral gastroenteritis are primarily related to the development of dehydration and electrolyte abnormalities and therefore, are more likely to occur in the very young or very old. The deaths reported (fortunately rare in this country) are due to profound dehydration leading to cardiovascular collapse. Rare complications include gastrointestinal bleeding, Henoch-Schönlein purpura, encephalitis, and hemolytic-uremic syndrome.

Therapy

Therapy is limited to supportive measures including aggressive replacement of fluid and electrolyte losses. Oral replacement with sucrose- or glucose-electrolyte solutions may be adequate. Some clinicians advocate removal of milk and other lactose-containing foods from the diet during the acute episode. Enteric precautions/isolation should be employed for patients who require admission to the hospital to prevent nosocomial spread of the infection.

Immunology and Prevention

The ubiquitous nature of rotavirus is confirmed by the fact that 90% of children aged 2 years or older have serologic evidence of previous infection with the agent. This may explain why rotavirus infection in the adult is usually asymptomatic.

In contrast, experimental infection with the Norwalk agent fails to induce long-lasting protection for subsequent challenge. Serum antibody to Norwalk agent peaks 2–3 weeks after infection and persists for 6–14 weeks, waning thereafter. The presence or amount of serum antibody does not correlate with protection, indicating that other factors must be important to immunity in this disease.

In the future, prevention may be possible by vaccines. Currently, good hygiene and enteric isolation are the only useful methods for preventing spread of viral gastroenteritis.

Prognosis

Viral gastroenteritis is a self-limited illness, provided fluid and electrolyte losses are replaced.

Selected Bibliography

Adler, J. L. and Zickl, R.: Winter vomiting disease. *J Infect Dis* 119:668–673, 1969.

Agus, S. G., Dolin, R., Wyatt, R. G., Tousimis, A. J., and Northrup, R. S.: Acute infectious nonbacterial gastroenteritis: Intestinal histopathology. *Ann Intern Med* 79:18–25, 1973.

Bishop, R. F., Davidson, G. P., Holmes, I. H., and Ruck, B. J.: Virus particles in epithelial cells of duodenal mucosa from children with acute nonbacterial gastroenteritis. *Lancet* 2:1281–1283, 1973.

Blacklow, N. R. and Cukor, G.: Viral gastroenteritis. *N Engl J Med* 304:397–406, 1981.

Blacklow, N. R., Dolin, R., Fedson, D. S., Dupont, H. L., Northrup, R. S., Hornick, R. B., and Chanock, R. M.: Acute infectious nonbacterial gastroenteritis: Etiology and pathogenesis. *Ann Intern Med* 76:993–1008, 1972.

Carlson, J. A. K., Middleton, P. J., Szymanski, M. T., Huber, J., and Petric, M.: Fatal rotavirus gastroenteritis: Analysis of 21 cases. *Am J Dis Child* 132: 477–479, 1978.

Davidson, G. P., Bishop, R. F., Townley, R. R. W., et al.: Importance of a new virus in acute sporadic enteritis in children. *Lancet* 1:242, 1975.

Dolin, R., Larry, A. G., Wyatt, R. G., Thornhill, T. S., and Gardner, J. D.: Viral gastroenteritis induced by the Hawaii agent. *Am J Med* 59:761–768, 1975.

Donta, S. T.: Changing concepts of infectious diarrheas. *Geriatrics* 30:123–126, 1975.

Drachman, R. H.: Acute infectious gastroenteritis. *Pediatr Clin N Am* 21:711–737, 1974.

Eichenwald, H. F. and McCracken, G. H., Jr.: Acute diarrheal disease. *Med Clin N Am* 54:443–453, 1970.

Estes, M. K. and Graham, D. Y.: Epidemic viral gastroenteritis. *Am J Med* 66: 1001–1007, 1979.

Harris, J. C., Dupont, H. L., and Hornick, R. B.: Fecal leukocytes in diarrheal illness. *Ann Intern Med* 76:697–703, 1972.

Holdaway, M. D.: Management of gastroenteritis in early childhood. *Drugs* 14: 383–389, 1977.

Holmes, I. H.: Viral gastroenteritis. *Prog Med Virol* 25:1–36, 1979.

Hughes, J. M., Merson, M. H., and Pollard, R. A., Jr.: Food-borne disease outbreaks in the United States, 1973. *J Infect Dis* 132:224–228, 1975.

Kim, H. W., Brandt, C. D., Kapikian, A. Z., Wyatt, R. G., Arrobio, J. O., Rodriguez, W. J., Chanock, R. M., and Parrott, R. H.: Human reovirus-like agent infection. Occurrence in adult contacts of pediatric patients with gastroenteritis. *JAMA* 238:404-407, 1977.

Moffet, H. L., Shulenberger, H. K., and Burkholder, E. R.: Epidemiology and etiology of severe infantile diarrhea. *J Pediatr* 72:1-14, 1968.

Nalin, D. R., Mata, L., Varga, W., et al.: Comparison of sucrose with glucose in oral therapy of infant diarrhoea. *Lancet* 1:277, 1978.

Palmer, D. L., Koster, F. T., Rafiqul Islam, A. F. M., Mizanur Rahman, A. S. M., and Sack, R. B.: Comparison of sucrose and glucose in the oral electrolyte therapy of cholera and other severe diarrheas. *N Engl J Med* 297:1107-1110, 1977.

Parrino, T. A., Schreiber, D. S., Trier, J. S., Kapikian, A. Z., and Blacklow, N. R.: Clinical immunity in acute gastroenteritis caused by Norwalk agent. *N Engl J Med* 297:86-89, 1977.

Pickering, L. K., DuPont, H. L., Olarte, J., et al.: Fecal leukocytes in enteric infections. *Am J Clin Pathol* 68:562-565, 1977.

Plotkin, G. R., Kluge, R. M., and Waldman, R. H.: Gastroenteritis: Etiology, pathophysiology and clinical manifestations. *Medicine* 58:96-114, 1979.

Portnoy, B. L., DuPont, H. L., Pruitt, D., Abdo, J. A., and Rodriguez, J. T.: Antidiarrheal agents in the treatment of acute diarrhea in children. *JAMA* 236:844-846, 1976.

Rodriguez, W. J., Kim, H. W., Brandt, C. D., Yolken, R. H., Richard, M., Arrobio, J. O., Schwartz, R. H., Kapikian, A. Z., Chanock, R. M., and Parrott, R. H.: Common exposure outbreak of gastroenteritis due to type 2 rotavirus with high secondary attack rate within families. *J Infect Dis* 140:353-357, 1979.

Schreiber, D. S., Blacklow, N. R., and Trier, J. S.: The small intestinal lesion induced by Hawaii agent acute infectious nonbacterial gastroenteritis. *J Infect Dis* 129:705-708, 1974.

Thornhill, T. S., Kalica, A. R., Wyatt, R. G., Kapikian, A., and Chanock, R.: Pattern of shedding of the Norwalk particle in stools during experimentally induced gastroenteritis in volunteers as determined by immune electron microscopy. *J Infect Dis* 132:28-34, 1975.

Widerlite, L., Trier, J. S., Blacklow, N. R., and Schreiber, D. S.: Structure of the gastric mucosa in acute infectious nonbacterial gastroenteritis. *Gastroenterology* 68:425-430, 1975.

Wyatt, R. G., Kapikian, A. Z., Thornhill, T. S., Sereno, M. M., Kim, H. W., and Chanock, R. M.: In vitro cultivation in human fetal intestinal organ culture of a reovirus-like agent associated with nonbacterial gastroenteritis in infants and children. *J Infect Dis* 130:523-528, 1974.

24

ENTEROCOLITIS
Gary R. Plotkin, M.D.

Enterocolitis is inflammation of the mucous membrane of variable portions of both the small and large intestines. Diarrhea is an increase in the frequency, fluidity, or volume of bowel movements relative to the usual habits of an individual, while dysentery consists of frequent bowel movements accompanied by blood and mucus with tenesmus or abdominal pain on defecation. Neonatal necrotizing enterocolitis is an acute fulminant disease characterized by focal or diffuse ulceration and necrosis of the distal small bowel and colon with formation of intramural gas (pneumatosis intestinalis). The acute inflammatory enteritides consist of specific infectious and noninfectious processes involving the distal small bowel and colon (Table 24.1). The syndromes of necrotizing enterocolitis of the newborn and pseudomembranous enterocolitis also may have microbiologic etiologies. In view of the large number of etiologic agents responsible for enterocolitis, the following discussion will review those organisms which are of historic interest or which are more commonly encountered in the United States.

Microbiology and Epidemiology

The shigellae infect humans and certain other primates, and in most instances shigellosis will be traceable to a symptomatic or asymptomatic human host. Since few *Shigella* organisms are required to cause clinical illness, the organism may spread by human-to-human contact without interposition of a vehicle such as food, water, or milk. Besides direct fecal-oral transmission, the dissemination of the organism may be enhanced by poor sanitation with contamination of water or food including milk, cheese, watercress, and fruit pies. Epidemics have been described in custodial institutions and aboard cruise ships. In the more developed

TABLE 24.1   Infectious Agents Causing Enterocolitis

Bacteria

Shigella spp	*C. fetus*
Salmonella spp	*V. parahemolyticus*
E. coli	*S. aureus*
Yersinia spp	*C. perfringens*
N. gonorrhoeae	spirochetes

Chlamydia

lymphogranuloma venereum

Fungi

Candida spp	*S. schenckii*
C. neoformans	*Aspergillus* spp
P. brasiliensis	*C. immitis*
H. capsulatum	Mucoraceae
B. dermatitidis	

Parasites

E. histolytica	*T. trichiura*
B. coli	schistosomes
G. lamblia	*E. vermicularis*
Cryptosporidium	*T. spiralis*

---

countries, shigellosis is usually an endemic contact-spread infection affecting children below the age of 10 years. *Shigella dysenteriae* 1 has caused epidemic disease in Central America and the Indian subcontinent while *S. sonnei* is the most common species of *Shigella* isolated in Western Europe, Japan, and North America including the United States.

Salmonellae are gram-negative, flagellated, nonencapsulated, nonsporulating, facultatively anaerobic bacilli of the family Enterobacteriaceae. The three species consist of *S. typhi, S. choleraesuis,* and *S. enteritidis;* the latter contains more than 1700 serotypes. The frequency of both *S. typhi* and non-typhi salmonella infections peaks during the summer months, although a substantial number of cases of salmonellosis occur throughout the year. The highest incidence of salmonella infections correlates with outbreaks of food poisoning; age-specific attack rates are highest in those under 20 and over 70 years of age.

In the United States typhoid fever is relatively uncommon compared with cases of non-typhi salmonellosis. Since humans are probably the only reservoir of *S. typhi,* typhoid fever usually follows ingestion of water or food contaminated by feces from a chronic carrier or symptomatic individual. Direct human-to-human transmission may occur via the fecal-oral route, and flies and dust physically transporting the bacteria may be sources of infection in endemic areas. Epidemics of typhoid fever in industrial societies have been traced to human fecal contamination of spaghetti, corned beef, and milk products.

Non-typhi *Salmonella* spp are primarily pathogens of lower animals. These organisms can be transmitted less commonly from human to human via the fecal-oral route. Nontyphoidal salmonellae have been isolated from almost all animal species including chicken, duck, turkey, dove, pigeon, starling, flea, cockroach, tick, louse, tortoise, whale, seal, parrot, sparrow, house fly and hamster. The most important factor involved in the transmission of nontyphoidal salmonellae in the United States perhaps has been the increasing trend toward mass processing and distribution of food products. Poultry, eggs, dairy products, beef, and pork constitute the main foods responsible for dissemination of *Salmonella* organisms. The conditions required for initiation of a foodborne outbreak of salmonellosis include a reservoir of the infective agent, contamination of a food item capable of supporting bacterial growth, suitable temperature and time for bacterial multiplication, and ingestion of a large enough number of organisms by susceptible persons. Acquisition of nontyphoidal *Salmonella* organisms from water contaminated with animal or human excreta occurs but is less common compared with *S. typhi.*

The reservoir of infection among domestic animals is important in the epidemiology of nontyphoidal salmonellosis. Animal-to-animal transmission may occur or animal feeds containing salmonella-contaminated fishmeal or by-products of the meat packing industry may be sources of infection among animals. Additionally, processing equipment, abattoirs, and packing plants become contaminated from infected carcasses and thus serve to contaminate the uninfected meats being processed.

Outbreaks commonly occur in institutions such as acute-care hospitals, pediatric wards, newborn nurseries, nursing homes, psychiatric hospitals, and institutions for the retarded. Common vehicles of nosocomial outbreaks are a variety of foods such as poultry, eggs, meat, dry coconut, protein food supplements, and yeast. Outbreaks also have been traced to pharmacologic or diagnostic preparations including thyroid, pituitary, adrenal, cortical, pancreatic, and liver extracts, carmine dye, pepsin, gelatin, bile salts, vitamins, and platelets. Cross-infection with spread by person-to-person contact or by fomites is responsible for many of the outbreaks in newborn nurseries, pediatric wards, and hospitalized adults. Diagnostic devices, e.g., fiberoptic endoscopes, and hospital personnel who are carriers of *Salmonella* also have been implicated.

The enteroinvasive *Escherichia coli* strains belong to certain somatic O serogroups and are often associated with diarrhea which clinically resembles bacillary dysentery. The O serogroups which mainly contain "dysentery-producing" strains are 28 ac, 112 ac, 124, 136, 143, 144, 152, and 164. These strains of *E. coli* are frequently atypical in their biochemical reactions and may be nonlactose to late-lactose fermenters, anaerogenic, or nonmotile. Clinical laboratories may report these strains as *Shigella.* Such tests as lysine decarboxylase or the utilization of sodium citrate and sodium acetate will enable one to correctly differentiate *E. coli* from *Shigella* spp. Accurate identification is important epidemiologically.

During investigations of diarrhea affecting American troops in the Mediterranean area during 1944 and 1945, *E. coli* O 124 was isolated from foodhandlers and individuals with diarrhea. An outbreak of dysentery-like disease which occurred among schoolchildren in London in 1949 also was due to *E. coli* O 124, and the epidemiology suggested a foodborne infection. Probably the largest outbreak due to enteroinvasive *E. coli* O 124 occurred in the United States in 1971 when approximately 400 persons experienced diarrhea following the ingestion of imported

French (Camembert) cheese. *Escherichia coli* O 124 also has been associated with sporadic cases and small outbreaks of diarrhea in Eastern Europe, India, Brazil, and Japan. These outbreaks mainly involve adults and children, but not neonates. This contrasts with the epidemiologic patterns of nonenteroinvasive strains of *E. coli* since these affect neonates, especially those in nurseries. *Escherichia coli* O 164 was initially isolated from the stools of a British prisoner in 1946, and since that time strains have been recovered from sporadic cases of diarrhea in numerous countries. The remaining O serogroups 28 ac, 112 ac, 136, 143, 144, and 152 have been reported from sporadic cases and small outbreaks of dysentery-like disease from various countries; however, the epidemiology has not been as thoroughly studied as *E. coli* O 124 and O 164.

    Yersinia are aerobic and facultatively anaerobic, noncapsulated coccobacillary or rod-shaped, gram-negative bacteria that are nonmotile at 37°C; however, *Y. pseudotuberculosis* and *Y. enterocolitica* are motile at 22-25°C and have peritrichous flagella. *Yersinia enterocolitica* was initially isolated during a period from 1933 to 1947 in New York State from 11 patients with cervical adenitis, enteritis, and terminal ileitis. Further isolation in the United States was not reported until 1968; however, the organism subsequently has been recognized more frequently. In contrast, over 1000 cases of yersiniosis were diagnosed in the Scandinavian countries between 1964 and 1971. Human infections due to *Y. enterocolitica* are ubiquitous and also have been reported from other parts of Europe, Africa, Canada, and Asia. *Yersinia enterocolitica* is a zoonotic bacterium which has been isolated from guinea pigs, rabbits, swine, chinchillas, cows, horses, sheep, deer, rats, monkeys, dogs, cats, beavers, mink, raccoons, various birds, fleas, mussels, and oysters. The organism has also been recovered from milk, water specimens such as well water, streams, and various foods including salad vegetables, ground beef, pork, sausage, lamb, and giblets. The mode of transmission of *Y. enterocolitica* is not completely understood; however, it can be isolated from the feces of various animals incriminated in the contamination of food and water. Fecal-oral transmission may occur in humans; healthy human carriers have been described although uncommonly.

    Campylobacter organisms were previously placed in the genus *Vibrio* because of their morphologic similarity to *V. cholerae*; that is, both are thin, motile, curved, gram-negative rods. However, there are major differences in biochemical and growth characteristics and in DNA base nucleotide content between *V. cholerae* and the organisms now classified as campylobacters. *Campylobacter* is derived from the Greek words meaning curved (campylo) and rod (bacter). There are three species within the genus *Campylobacter (C. fetus, C. sputorum,* and *C. fecalis)* and three subspecies of *C. fetus* (ss. *fetus,* ss. *intestinalis,* and ss. *jejuni).* The latter two subspecies are human pathogens.

    The two subspecies *C. fetus intestinalis* and *jejuni* appear to infect different age groups; that is, 96% of the former occur in adults, and 60% of the latter are isolated from stools of infants under 1 year of age. The epidemiology of campylobacter enteritis is complex and is not entirely known. Strains of *C. fetus* are found in a variety of animal hosts including poultry, calves, swine, birds, sheep, dogs, and cats; however, not all of these strains may cause human enteritis. Venereal transmission, contamination of food and water, and contact with infected animals, especially chickens and dogs, all have been cited as possible sources of human infection. Transmission of infection with foods may involve cross-contamination of salad and uncooked poultry and meats. Ingestion of raw beef liver or raw milk also has been implicated in human cases of diarrhea due to *C. fetus.* Placental transfer or exposure at delivery may account for infection in the fetus or newborn. Additionally, person-to-person spread by the fecal-oral route has been suggested by an outbreak of diarrhea which occurred in a nursery. Campylobacters have been associated with diarrhea in the United States, England, Scotland, Rwanda, Belgium, Canada, South Africa, Sweden, and Australia.

Other vibrio-like organisms may be divided into: (1) *Vibrio cholerae* (both classic and El-Tor biotypes), (2) nonagglutinating vibrios (vibrios which do not agglutinate in *V. cholerae* O group 1 antiserum), (3) halophilic vibrios (*V. parahemolyticus* and *V. alginolyticus)*, and (4) halophilic, lactose-positive *Vibrio*. Strains of nonagglutinable or non-O1 *V. cholerae* have been isolated from seafood and saltwater and produce gastrointestinal symptoms mimicking those of true cholera, that is, a profuse, watery-type diarrhea. Uncommonly, patients develop dysentery-like symptoms including abdominal cramps and bloody diarrhea. Epidemiologically, raw oysters harvested from or near Oyster Bay, Wakulla County, Florida, have been incriminated as the vehicle of transmission in two patients who presented with bloody diarrhea and whose stool specimens contained non-O1 *V. cholerae* organisms.

Vibrio parahemolyticus is a marine halophilic organism first isolated in 1950 from postmortem specimens from patients who died during a foodborne outbreak traced to semidried sardines in Japan. This organism has been repeatedly isolated from seafood products during summer food-poisoning outbreaks in Japan but has also been reported as a cause of gastrointestinal illness in India, Thailand, Malaysia, Panama, Great Britain, and the United States.

Enteritis necroticans, a hemorrhagic necrotizing jejunitis, was first described in Germany after World War II as a new epidemic disease called "Darmbrand" which meant "fire in the bowels." In 1961 a similar condition called "Pig-Bel" was recognized in New Guinean highlanders after pig feasting. Enteritis necroticans has been shown to be due to *Clostridium perfringens* type C.

Lymphogranuloma venereum (LGV) is a venereal disease caused by *Chlamydia trachomatis* (serotypes L-1, L-2, L-3) and usually involves the genitalia and regional lymph nodes but may also produce significant rectal disease. Lymphogranuloma venereum is endemic in Asia, Africa, and South America, but as many as 500 cases each year are reported in the United States. It occurs more frequently in men than in women and especially in persons of low socioeconomic status living in the Southeast United States, in male homosexuals, and in persons returning from endemic regions outside the United States. Besides being sexually transmitted, LGV can be spread by fomites, laboratory accidents, and nonsexual contact. The reservoirs are probably individuals with asymptomatic or symptomatic urethral, cervical, or anorectal infection.

Amebiasis is acquired by the ingestion of *Entamoeba histolytica* cysts. Common modes of transmission include contaminated water or fresh vegetables. Most outbreaks have been traced to a water supply contaminated by sewage; however, direct fecal-oral transmission is more frequent in mental institutions. Infected food handlers do not appear to be significant sources of transmission. Amebiasis occurs throughout the world, and infection rates can exceed 50% in countries or localities where sanitary facilities and hygienic practices are unsatisfactory. Amebiasis is endemic in most countries, and a history of foreign travel is not necessary for consideration of this diagnosis.

Balantidium coli is a ciliated protozoan belonging to the subphylum Ciliophora. Many mammals harbor this organism but the pig and less commonly, the rat are probably the common sources of infection in man. Human infection is more common in New Guinea, Micronesia, Southern Russia, and parts of South and Central America.

Giardia lamblia is a flagellated protozoan which causes a cosmopolitan infection that under unsanitary and tropical conditions can reach prevalence rates of up to 20%. A familial clustering of infection is common, suggesting direct fecal-oral transmission. Several epidemics of symptomatic giardiasis have been recorded. One occurred in 1965-1966 among skiers at Aspen, Colorado, and was traced to contamination of well water by sewage. American visitors to the Soviet Union, especially Leningrad, have often become infected with *G. lamblia,* and epidemiologically the attack rates were higher among those who had drunk tap water.

The formation of pseudomembranes on the surface of the small or large intestine represents a nonspecific response to injury and various agents have been incriminated including heavy-metal poisoning, intestinal obstruction, abdominal surgery, shock, bowel ischemia, ischemic cardiovascular disease, bronchopneumonia, uremia, *Staphylococcus aureus,* and antibiotics. The use of broad-spectrum antibiotics, especially chloramphenicol and tetracycline, was first associated in 1950s with an enterocolitis in which *S. aureus* was cultured from the stool or pseudomembrane. The occurrence of staphylococcal enterocolitis was sporadic between the years 1950 and 1965; however, the relationship between *S. aureus* in the stool and intestinal pseudomembrane formation is now being questioned because an overgrowth of this organism is common in stools of patients who are receiving broad-spectrum antimicrobial agents. Because of the renewed interest during the past several years, antibiotic-associated pseudomembranous colitis has been intensely investigated and has been associated with clindamycin, lincomycin, ampicillin, penicillin G, cephalosporins, tetracycline, streptomycin, chloramphenicol, erythromycin, metronidazole, and trimethoprim-sulfamethoxazole. Clindamycin-associated pseudomembranous colitis has been the most extensively studied form of the disease and prevalence data have shown considerable differences ranging from 0.01 to 10%. No readily identifiable patient-risk factor has been found and both oral and parenteral clindamycin have been implicated. However, clustering of cases of antibiotic-associated colitis has been reported and epidemiologically may represent cross-infection. Toxigenic *Clostridium difficile,* a gram-positive, obligately anaerobic bacillus, has been implicated as the major cause of antibiotic-associated pseudomembranous colitis; however, this organism also can be part of the normal intestinal flora of healthy persons. Presumably antibiotics permit the emergence of *C. difficile* while suppressing the competing flora.

Neonatal necrotizing enterocolitis is a disease seen preponderantly in hospitalized premature infants. Its epidemiology is similar to an infectious disease, i.e., cases have often been clustered in time and location, and some outbreaks have appeared to be limited by instituting various control measures such as patient isolation.

Pathogenesis and Pathology (Tables 24.2 and 24.3)

The effect of an intestinal pathogen is modified by a complex interplay between host and environment, and internal physiologic and defense factors moderate the microorganism's ability to survive and cause disease. Gastric acidity, peristalsis, mucous barrier, and Paneth's cell lysozymes are important defense mechanisms. Within the lumen of the large intestine, there is a stable resident flora which is naturally resistant to alteration. Specific receptor sites on the intestinal tissue or in the mucus permit the attachment of organisms or toxins, thus enabling various pathophysiologic events to be initiated.

Traditionally, bacterial pathogens that cause diarrhea in humans (see Table 24.2) have been divided into three groups depending upon their characteristic interaction with the intestinal mucosa. The first group of pathogens, typified by *V. cholerae* and enterotoxigenic *E. coli* strains, produces their disease through

TABLE 24.2   Pathogenesis of Bacterial Diarrheas

Pathogen	Bacterial-Mucosal Interaction	Pathogenic Mechanism	Localization
V. cholerae, *E. coli*	No invasion	Enterotoxin production	Small bowel
Shigella spp, *E. coli*	Penetration, intraepithelial multiplication	Mucosal inflammation with destruction	Initially small bowel, later colon
Salmonella spp	Penetration into submucosa	Inflammation of the lamina propria	Small bowel and colon

multiplication in the small intestine followed by release of an exotoxin which causes loss of fluid and electrolytes. In this type of illness there is no mucosal invasion. The second group of pathogens, exemplified by shigellae and nonenterotoxin-producing strains of *E. coli,* invades and destroys the colonic epithelium. Salmonellae constitute the third group of intestinal pathogens. Even though intestinal epithelial invasion involving the small bowel and colon occurs with the salmonellae, extensive destruction of the intestinal mucosa does not result. It has become evident that this classification is greatly oversimplified and perhaps no longer valid.

Evidence from recent experimental studies indicated that clinical shigellosis involves both the small bowel and colon. While no invasion of jejunum occurs, many organisms are present in the lumen with resultant water and electrolyte secretion. Several strains of *S. dysenteriae* 1, *S. flexneri,* and *S. sonnei* have been shown to produce a cell-free toxin which causes secretion of isotonic fluid by the small intestine, perhaps by activating the adenylate cyclase-cyclic AMP system. These events may explain the initial phase of watery diarrhea that is seen clinically in shigellosis. The human colon, however, appears to be refractory to the biologic effects of shigella toxin. Intact bacteria penetrate human colonic epithelial cells and must multiply therein to produce disease, possiby a result of toxin production intracytoplasmically.

The pathologic process of shigellosis is essentially an inflammatory response to the mucosal invasion by the organism. This primarily involves the colon, although the terminal ileum may occasionally be affected. On proctosigmoidoscopy the mucosa is inflamed, granular, edematous, and friable, with variable degrees of bleeding. There may also be ulcerations which can penetrate to the muscularis mucosae.

Strains of *S. typhimurium* have been studied in the ligated rabbit ileal loop model to determine the mechanisms whereby bacteria which invade the gastrointestinal mucosa evoke fluid secretion. The organisms employed differed in various biologic attributes including the ability to invade the epithelium, multiply within the mucosa, elicit an acute inflammatory reaction, and disseminate across the intestinal wall. Some strains provoked small-intestinal fluid secretion, although these did not elaborate enterotoxin. Only those strains that invaded the mucosa were accompanied by either inflammation or fluid secretion, while noninvasive strains produced neither histologic abnormalities nor fluid secretion. Additionally, there was no correlation between the ability of invasive organisms to

TABLE 24.3   Food Poisoning

Pathogen	Pathogenesis	Incubation Period	Symptoms	Usual Source
S. aureus	Heat-stable toxin	2–6 hr	Nausea, vomiting, cramps, little or no fever, diarrhea in ∿ one-third cases	Pastries, meat left unrefrigerated
C. perfringens	Heat-stable toxin	6–12 hr	Diarrhea, cramps, little or no fever	Meat or gravy kept warm for several hours
C. botulinum	Heat-labile toxin	Hours to days	Gastrointestinal followed by neurologic	Home-canned foods
Salmonella spp	Infection	12–36 hr	Diarrhea, abdominal pain, fever	Inadequately cooked animal products; fecal contamination
Shigella spp	Infection	1–3 days	Water, mucoid and/or bloody diarrhea, fever	Fecal-oral

evoke fluid secretion and the intensity of mucosal inflammation, the number of intramucosal salmonellae, or in the ability to disseminate from the rabbit ileum. These observations suggested that mucosal invasion may be a necessary factor for the intestinal fluid loss in salmonellosis. A bacterial property or factor in addition to invasion of the gastrointestinal mucosa seemed to contribute to this fluid loss. This factor may induce fluid secretion by stimulating the prostaglandin and/or adenylcyclase-cyclic AMP system(s). In an experimental model involving rabbit ileal loops, indomethacin completely inhibited intestinal fluid secretion mediated by *S. typhimurium;* however, indomethacin failed to alter the local invasiveness of the microorganism. The postulated mechanisms of this action of indomethacin to prevent ileal loop secretion included: (1) inhibition of prostaglandin synthesis or prostaglandin-mediated adenylcyclase activation, (2) membrane-stabilizing actions, and/or (3) effects upon cyclic AMP protein kinase. An enterotoxic factor isolated from cultures of *S. enteritidis* appeared to possess various properties similar to the heat-stable and heat-labile enterotoxins of *E. coli.* Both invasion and enterotoxin may be prerequisites for production of diarrhea in salmonellosis.

Rectal biopsies from patients with salmonellosis have revealed abnormalities ranging from mucosal edema and hyperemia, with and without petechial hemorrhages, to mucosal friability with slough formation. There is dilatation and congestion of capillaries in the mucosa and submucosa, and focal collections of polymorphonuclear or mononuclear leukocytes are present in the lamina propria and in the lumen of mucosal capillaries. The crypts may contain abscesses. Histologic changes in the distal small bowel especially involving Peyer's patches range from mild hyperplasia to necrosis and ulceration with infiltration of polymorphonuclear and/or mononuclear leukocytes.

Enteroinvasive *E. coli* invades the colonic mucosa of adults thus leading to inflammation and superficial ulceration resembling shigellosis. These strains of *E. coli* produce a dysentery-like disease, and on sigmoidoscopy one observes ulcerations. Several strains of *E. coli* isolated during outbreaks of infantile enteritis neither produce classic heat-labile or heat-stable enterotoxin nor penetrate epithelial cells. These strains may cause diarrhea by as yet unrecognized toxin(s).

Various experimental systems involving clinical isolates of *Y. enterocolitica* have been employed to further delineate the organism's modes of pathogenicity. Enterotoxin produced by many isolates of *Y. enterocolitica,* especially at temperatures of 30°C or lower, resembles the heat-stable enterotoxin of *E. coli,* i.e., it is stable at 100°C for 15 minutes, is active in the infant mouse and rabbit ileal loop systems but not in the Y1 adrenal cell assay, and its molecular weight varies from 1000 to 10,000. The invasiveness of *Y. enterocolitica* also resembles *E. coli.* Pathologically *Y. enterocolitica* produces a terminal ileitis, and in adults the ileum has a coarse, irregular, or nodular mucosa with occasional ulcerations. Endoscopically the rectosigmoid area may reveal erythema, edema, and aphthoid ulcerations. Microscopic examination of colonic biopsy specimens demonstrates ulcerations or chronic nonspecific inflammation with infiltration by mostly mononuclear cells and lymphocytes.

The pathogenesis of campylobacter enteritis is unknown. The frequent early occurrence of profuse, watery diarrhea suggests a small-bowel secretory component; however, the finding of stools containing blood and mucus suggests mucosal damage due to an invasive organism. The principal sites of infection are the jejunum and ileum, and these areas may appear hemorrhagic and necrotic. Uncommonly, the colon may be involved and mimic acute ulcerative colitis.

Clostridium perfringens type C strains isolated from patients with enteritis necroticans produce an enterotoxin; however, pathologically the disease largely involves the jejunum and is characterized by a patchy, gangrenous enteritis with intramural gas. There may also be submucosal, subserosal, mesenteric, and lymph node gas.

Primary amebic lesions begin in the colon as minute erosions or microulcers located at the top of a mucosal nodule. This nodule is caused by central necrosis with surrounding edema and a narrow margin of inflammatory reaction consisting of plasma cells, lymphocytes, and eosinophils. Since the muscular layers of the colon are relatively resistant to amebic invasion, the necrotic process extends laterally and produces the characteristic flask-shaped ulcer. Trophozoites are found in large numbers at the junction of viable tissue cells and necrotic debris. Absence of a generalized mucosal inflammatory reaction is characteristic of uncomplicated invasive amebic disease. Occasionally trophozoites invading the colon induce a proliferative host response with formation of a granulomatous mass known as an ameboma.

Giardiasis is mainly an infection of the small bowel, and histologic studies of the jejunal and duodenal mucosa in symptomatic patients may be normal or reveal mild to severe partial villous atrophy and extensive cellular infiltration of the lamina propria with lymphocytes, plasma cells, and polymorphonuclear leukocytes. Microscopically, G. lamblia is seen adhering by its flattened ventral surface to the epithelium of the villi and crypts; however, mucosal invasion does occur occasionally. The pathogenesis of diarrhea in giardiasis is not known.

In antibiotic-associated pseudomembranous colitis, one usually observes gross or microscopic evidence of characteristic pseudomembranes lining the colonic mucosa. The gross lesions reveal exudate, punctate, raised, yellowish-white plaques, and between these plaques the mucosa is edematous and hyperemic. With time the plaques enlarge and may coalesce over extensive segments. The lesions are located mainly in the colon, and small-bowel involvement is unusual. Mild cases show focal necrosis with polymorphonuclear cells and an eosinophilic exudate in the lamina propria. Disrupted glands containing mucin and acute inflammatory cells surmounted with pseudomembranes composed of fibrin, mucin, and polymorphonuclear cells may be seen. There are areas of normal mucosa, and the inflammatory changes are limited to the superficial half of the lamina propria. In severe cases there is complete structural necrosis with extensive involvement of the lamina propria and a thick pseudomembrane. There is no evidence of bacterial invasion involving the bowel mucosa or pseudomembrane.

Bacteriologic studies in tissue culture assays support the etiologic role of C. difficile in antibiotic-associated pseudomembranous colitis. Supernates of stool specimens from affected patients usually contain a cytotoxin that is neutralized with C. sordellii antitoxin. This cytotoxin has been rarely recovered from individuals without gastrointestinal complications related to antibiotic usage. Additionally, stool cultures from patients with antibiotic-associated pseudomembranous colitis usually grow C. difficile, which is found infrequently in the fecal flora of healthy individuals. This toxin is a high-molecular-weight protein of 600,000 and appears to cause changes in the permeability of cells in tissue cultures.

Neonatal necrotizing enterocolitis is characterized by focal or diffuse ulceration and necrosis of the distal small intestine and colon and accumulation of air in the bowel wall (pneumatosis intestinalis) or within the peritoneum (pneumoperitoneum). The entire intestine, however, can be involved, with the most common site being the ileum. Pathologically, small perforations may be present and covered with deposits of fibrin or exudate. Surgical inspection reveals ulcers, hemorrhages, infarcted segments, and irregular mucosal patterns. Stenotic lesions may remain after resolution of neonatal necrotizing enterocolitis. Organizing thrombi are found in the mesenteric arteries and venules. Even though transmural disease leading to perforation is common, when necrosis is limited to the mucosa or submucosa, healing may occur by epithelialization, fibroblastic proliferation, and granulation tissue.

A variety of factors have been implicated in the etiology of neonatal necrotizing enterocolitis, including prematurity, ingestion of infected amniotic fluid,
segmental volvulus, mucosal injury, endotoxin, localized Shwartzman reaction,
infection, gastrointestinal ischemia, and oral feedings.

Diagnostic Features and Complications (Tables 24.4 and 24.5)

Clinically, shigellosis initially presents as an acute, febrile, watery diarrhea generally accompanied by abdominal cramps. After 1-3 days the illness usually progresses to the colonic or dysenteric phase in which the stool becames scant,
bloody, and mucoid, and intestinal cramps are severe. Tenesmus occurs with each
bowel movement. However, about 50% of patients never develop bloody diarrhea.
Shigellosis is usually a self-limited disease in the normal host; however, intestinal
perforation with peritonitis may occur. The epidemic of Shiga (S. dysenteriae 1)
dysentery in Central America during 1969-1971 was characterized by a severe
constellation of symptoms including rapid progression to bloody diarrhea within
24 hr in 70% of patients and to dysentery in 50%. This degree of severity of
symptomatology was much greater than expected with either S. flexneri or S.
sonnei. In some patients with Shiga dysentery the mucoid intestinal discharge was
in such copious amounts that the stool appeared like "red currant jelly." In such
patients large segments of colonic mucosa were denuded, friable, congested, and
hemorrhagic.

TABLE 24.4   **Incubation Period and Duration of Illness for
Enteric Pathogens**

Agent	Incubation Period	Duration of Illness
S. aureus	1-6 hr	8-24 hr
C. perfringens	4-24 hr	< 24 hr
V. parahemolyticus	2-48 hr	24-72 hr
E. coli	4-24 hr	24-72 hr
B. cereus	8-16 hr	12 hr
Salmonella spp	8-72 hr	5-7 days
Viruses	16-36 hr	1-2 days
C. botulinum	8 hr-8 days	days to weeks
Shigella spp	1-3 days	2-20 days
E. histolytica	1 day-2 wk	3 days to several weeks

TABLE 24.5   Clinical Features of Acute Diarrheal Disease Useful in Differential Diagnosis

Clinical Features	Shigella	Entero-pathogenic E. coli	Salmonella (excluding typhoid fever)	S. typhi	V. cholerae	Viral
Age	6 mo-6 yr (rare in neonate)	0-5 yr	Any age	Any age	Any age	Any age
Diarrhea in household	Common (>50%)	No	Variable	Variable	Variable	Variable
Onset	Abrupt	Gradual	Variable	Gradual	Abrupt	Abrupt
Vomiting as a prominent symptom	Absent	Uncommon	Common	Uncommon	Occasional	Common
Fever (>102°F)	Common	Absent	Variable	Common	Absent	Uncommon
Respiratory symptoms	Common (bronchitis)	Absent	Uncommon	Common, nonproductive cough	Absent	Common (upper respiratory)
Convulsion	Common	Rare	Rare	Occasional	Occasional	Rare
Anal sphincter	Lax tone (rarely rectal prolapse)	Normal	Normal	Normal	Normal	Normal
Stools						
Consistency	Watery	Loose, slimy	Loose, slimy	Loose	Watery	Loose
Odor	Relatively odorless	Foul	Foul (rotten eggs)	Foul	Innocuous	± Mal-odorous
Blood	Common	Rare	Rare	Occasional	None	Rare
Color	Yellow green (almost colorless in severe cases)	Green	Green	Brown	Clear, rice water	Variable
Mucus	Present	Variable	Variable	Variable	Absent	Absent

There is nothing pathognomonic about the triad of fever, abdominal pain, and watery diarrhea to implicate *Shigella* as the causative agent. The specific diagnosis can be suspected when the illness progresses to dysentery. Shigellosis usually spreads within households; however, identification of a sporadic case can be a difficult diagnostic problem.

Occasionally adults will develop fever, headache, and stiff neck as the presenting signs of shigellosis. Cerebrospinal fluid is usually normal; however, there may be a mononuclear cellular response with normal sugar and protein levels and negative culture. Central nervous system manifestations, especially seizures, are more common in children and may actually antedate the gastrointestinal manifestations. Symptoms such as cough, coryza, or pleuritic pain may occur in shigellosis, as well as petechial or morbilliform cutaneous lesions and erythematous areas resembling rose spots. A hemolytic-uremic syndrome may be caused by the Shiga bacillus and has been reported in Bangladeshi children. Additionally, Reiter's syndrome, dehydration, keratoconjunctivitis, iritis, nonsuppurative or suppurative arthritis, osteomyelitis, bacteriuria, and vaginitis have occurred in shigellosis.

The peripheral white count may be elevated and there may be azotemia in shigellosis. Bacteremia, which is not common, does not necessarily lead to progressive disease or to metastatic foci of infection. Clotting values may reveal disseminated intravascular coagulopathy in patients infected with *S. dysenteriae* 1. In shigellosis, sigmoidoscopic examination reveals varying degrees of mucosal hyperemia, friability, and ulceration, but these findings are not diagnostic. During the colonic phase, stool generally contains polymorphonuclear leukocytes and red blood cells. The specific diagnosis of intestinal shigellosis can only be established by stool cultures. Salmonella-shigella (S.S.) agar may suppress the growth of many shigellae, and therefore one should also use MacConkey and either xylose-lysine-deoxycholate (XLD) or Hektoen enteric (HE) agars.

After an incubation period of 6-48 hr, headache, malaise, nausea, vomiting, and diarrhea appear abruptly in salmonellosis. Abdominal pain is frequent and can be mild to severe, and fever and shivering may be present. The clinical features of large-volume, watery stools with colicky periumbilical abdominal pains are indicative of small-bowel involvement, but dysenteric features such as frequent small-volume bloody movements, tenesmus, and tenderness over the sigmoid are often present. In uncomplicated cases, the acute stage usually terminates within 48 hr, although it may be prolonged and the patient may not feel well for several more days. Dehydration in severe cases may lead to hypotension, oliguria, and uremia.

Potentially all salmonellae are capable of invading the intestinal mucosa and causing septicemia or a typhoid-like syndrome (enteric fever). Possible sequelae of this bacteremia include splenomegaly, endocarditis, meningitis, osteomyelitis, pyelonephritis, and focal abscesses in the gastrointestinal tract and other organs. In enteric fever the diarrhea may be mild and transient, and thus the patient may present with headache, malaise, enlarged spleen, and unexplained pyrexia.

Diagnosis of gastrointestinal salmonellosis is dependent upon a positive stool culture since none of the signs or symptoms are pathognomonic. Fecal leukocytes (Table 24.6) and red blood cells may be present. In *S. typhi* infection the stool may contain mononuclear leukocytes, whereas in nontyphoid salmonellosis the cells may be neutrophils. Epidemic diarrhea traced to a common foodborne source should suggest the diagnosis of salmonellosis.

By virtue of their ability to penetrate the intestinal mucosa, strains of enteroinvasive *E. coli* produce dysentery which is clinically identical to shigellosis and is usually self-limiting. Since normal stool contains *E. coli,* cultures of fecal material as routinely performed in most clinical microbiology laboratories usually

TABLE 24.6   Fecal Leukocytes in Diarrheal Diseases

Predominant Cell	Approximate % of Total WBCs	Disease
Polymorphonuclear	90 (∿ 10% eosinophils)	Ulcerative colitis
	85	Invasive *E. coli*;
	85	shigellosis;
	75	nontyphoid salmonellosis
Mononuclear	95 Variable	Typhoid fever; amebic dysentery
None		Viral enterocolitis; cholera; normals

are not helpful in enabling one to diagnose enterocolitis caused by *E. coli*. As previously discussed, enteroinvasive *E. coli* are frequently atypical in their biochemical reactions and may be misidentified as *Shigella*. Epithelial invasion by *E. coli* may be demonstrated in the laboratory using the Sereny test in which living suspensions of bacteria are instilled into the eye of a guinea pig. Positive strains produce an ulcerative keratoconjunctivitis. Alternative tests for enteroinvasive *E. coli* include the ability of the organism to invade and multiply in HeLa cells or in monolayers of Hep-2 cells.

The clinical manifestations of yersiniosis are protean and range from the asymptomatic carrier state to overwhelming sepsis and death. Most commonly *Y. enterocolitica* produces various gastrointestinal symptoms. In children under 5 years, diarrhea is mild, self-limiting, and may mimic salmonellosis or shigellosis. Fever, vomiting, and/or abdominal pain may occur in 60-80% of these children. The stool may be profuse and watery or, uncommonly, bloody. Polymorphonuclear leukocytes may or may not be present. Diarrhea usually ceases after 2 weeks, but it may last several months. Intestinal ulcerations with perforation and peritonitis have been described. Over the age of 5 years, abdominal pain in the right iliac fossa is more common and may mimic acute appendicitis. Exudative pharyngitis and tonsillitis may present concomitantly with the gastrointestinal manifestations.

Arthritis caused by *Y. enterocolitica* is more common in adults, is generally antedated by abdominal symptoms, and may be mono- or polyarticular in nature. The synovial fluid is usually sterile; however, occasionally *Y. enterocolitica* may be isolated from the aspirate. Individuals with histocompatibility locus HLA-B27 have a greater incidence of arthritis after infection with *Y. enterocolitica*.

Yersiniosis presenting as a bacteremic syndrome usually occurs in patients compromised by malnutrition, carcinoma, leukemia, aplastic anemia, hemoglobinopathy, diabetes mellitus, renal or hepatic insufficiency, hemochromatosis, or immunosuppressive therapy. However, bacteremia in apparently otherwise healthy individuals has also been described. Miscellaneous manifestations of yersiniosis

include osteomyelitis, cholecystitis, pneumonia, lung abscesses, iritis, panophthal-
mitis, Parinaud's oculoglandular syndrome, meningitis, urethritis, thyroiditis, glomerulonephritis, myocarditis, thrombophlebitis at indwelling catheter site, Reiter's-like syndrome, hemolytic anemia, cellulitis, maculopapular and erysipelas-
like skin eruptions, erythema nodosum, hepatitis, and localized abscesses involving skin, neck, liver, spleen, and lymph nodes. *Y. enterocolitica* also has been isolated from urine, wounds, peritoneal fluid, and pharynx.

Recovery of *Y. enterocolitica* from such specimens as blood or cerebrospinal
fluid is uncomplicated, but isolation from feces can be problematic because of
overgrowth by normal flora. The ability of *Yersinia* to grow in water at temperatures of 4 and 25°C enables one to isolate this organism from samples containing
other gram-negative bacteria. Media should be incubated at 22, 25, and 37°C,
and optimal recovery from fecal material may be further enhanced by suspension
of the sample in 0.067 M phosphate buffered saline at pH 7.6 and incubating at
4°C for 4 weeks. Weekly subculture of the fecal-saline mixture on MacConkey or
brain heart infusion agars increases the chances of recovering *Y. enterocolitica*.

The incubation period for campylobacter enteritis ranges from 1.5 to 10 days.
Diarrhea may be preceded by a febrile prodromal period, malaise, headache, dizziness, backache, myalgias, abdominal pain, and occasionally rigors. The abdominal pain is periumbilical and cramping and simulates appendicitis, mesenteric
adenitis, intussusception, and visceral perforation. After 1.5 days, the stools rapidly become liquid, foul-smelling, and watery. Blood sometimes appears in the
stools after 1-2 days, and many patients experience a feeling of urgency or incontinence. Thus campylobacter enterocolitis may mimic salmonellosis or shigellosis.
The diarrhea lasts for about 2-3 days; however, relapses may occur. Patients with
campylobacter enterocolitis who have undergone abdominal surgery because of
signs and symptoms suggestive of an acute abdomen, have had acute inflammation
of the ileum, jejunum, and associated mesenteric lymph nodes. Complications of
systemic campylobacteriosis have included sepsis, endocarditis, meningitis, thrombophlebitis, pericarditis, peritonitis, salpingitis, septic arthritis, and pulmonary and
chest wall abscesses.

The stool in campylobacter enteritis may contain acute inflammatory and red
blood cells, and the organism microscopically appears spirally curved and gram-
negative. This bacteria may be isolated from fecal material by employing blood
or Columbia agars with added antimicrobials to prevent overgrowth by the normal
fecal flora. Since *C. fetus* is microaerophilic, cultures are ideally incubated in an
atmosphere of 5% oxygen, 10% carbon dioxide, and 85% nitrogen.

The few patients reported with enterocolitis secondary to non-O1 *V. cholerae*
(nonagglutinable) or halophilic lactose-positive *Vibrio* organisms did not have
signs or symptoms that were pathognomonic. Epidemiologically, however, there
was a history of recent shellfish ingestion or exposure to salt water. The halophilic lactose-fermenting *Vibrio* spp will grow readily on thiosulfate-citrate bile
salts sucrose (TCBS) agar and on heart infusion or MacConkey agars. Non-O1 *V.
cholerae* is biochemically indistinguishable from *V. cholerae* O group 1 and can be
grown on MacConkey and TCBS agars. Clinically the gastrointestinal illness associated with *V. parahemolyticus* ranges from a nonspecific watery diarrheal syndrome to dysentery with bloody and/or mucoid stools. Diagnosis is therefore microbiologic, and isolation of the pathogen from stool specimens can be achieved
by employing TCBS agar.

Enteritis necroticans is characterized clinically by anorexia, severe abdominal
pain, bloody diarrhea, vomiting, prostration, and hypotension; however, it also may
present in a mild form. Since the symptoms are not pathognomonic, the diagnosis is suggested epidemiologically. Acute complications may include ileus, strangu-
lation, and bowel perforation with peritonitis, while late sequelae consist of

obstruction, fistulas, malabsorption, and fibrosis with stenosis. The course of the disease is often too fulminant for detection of air in the bowel wall radiologically.

Many patients with *E. histolytica* infections are asymptomatic. Mild disease or nondysenteric colitis can cause anorexia, malaise, weight loss, abdominal pain, flatulence, tenesmus, and alternating episodes of mild diarrhea and constipation. In amebic dysenteric colitis, bowel movements may number 12–18 daily, contain blood-streaked mucus or large amounts of blood, and be associated with chills, night sweats, weakness, nausea, vomiting, anorexia, fever, and weight loss. Occasionally, a localized amebic ulceration may occur in the cecum or appendix and produce pain in the right lower abdomen with minimal diarrhea. Rarely invading amebic trophozoites can produce an exuberant reaction of the connective tissue with edema and development of a mass of granulation tissue called an ameboma. This usually occurs in the rectosigmoid or cecal portions of the colon and often is not associated with diarrhea. Pain is the most common symptom, and the lesion may bleed easily and produce obstruction, intussusception, or volvulus. A rare fulminating form of amebic colitis is manifested by profuse diarrhea, anorexia, nausea, vomiting, abdominal tenderness, and rectal tenesmus. The patient may be dehydrated, toxic, and febrile. The fulminant process is more likely to occur in elderly, debilitated, or immunosuppressed individuals. Additionally, toxic megacolon, perforation, and massive necrosis with sloughing of mucosal casts can occur.

Sigmoidoscopy is valuable for diagnosing intestinal amebiasis. Ulcerations may be seen but are not pathognomonic; however, sigmoidoscopy enables one to obtain specimens for parasitic examination. The best material for demonstration of trophozoites, in decreasing order of preference, is exudate from ulcers, blood-streaked exudate in the lumen and liquid feces. Amebic trophozoites should be identified only by experienced personnel. A variety of serologic tests are available for detecting antibodies resulting from invasive amebic disease; however, these tests remain positive for varying periods of time even after successful treatment. The degree of positivity does not differentiate extraintestinal from intestinal disease or even dysenteric from asymptomatic intestinal infections. False-negative tests also occur.

Clinically, balantidiasis is very similar to amebiasis; however, there is a greater tendency to bowel perforation, especially in severe cases. Mild illness may present as intermittent diarrhea consisting of blood-stained feces. Diagnosis is dependent upon finding trophozoites in the stool.

The most common symptoms in giardiasis are poorly localized abdominal discomfort and distention, colic, borborygmi, flatulence, nausea, and frequent loose stools. The illness may last for only a few days or may continue intermittently for 2–3 months. More severely affected patients may develop steatorrhea. In giardiasis there may be secondary lactase insufficiency and/or malabsorption of carotene, vitamin B_{12}, fat, and D-xylose. Giardiasis may be diagnosed by stool examination. If stool specimens are negative, trophozoites may be obtained by duodenal aspiration or by the use of a recoverable nylon yarn swallowed in a weighted capsule.

Most patients with antibiotic-associated pseudomembranous colitis have diarrhea, usually lacking visible blood and mucus. Microscopic examination of the stool reveals neutrophils. Patients may also present with abdominal cramps and tenderness, fever, and peripheral leukocytosis. Common complications include hypoalbuminemia and electrolyte imbalance. Symptoms often begin 4–10 days after initiation of antimicrobial treatment; however, they can occur either after one dose of the antibiotic or after the drug has been discontinued. The natural course of the disease is also variable. Most patients will improve as soon as the antibiotic is discontinued, whereas in those whose symptoms began after cessation of the antibacterial agent, diarrhea is prolonged and systemic complaints are persistent. Antibiotic-associated pseudomembranous colitis is a pathologic diagnosis which requires gross or microscopic evidence of pseudomembranes within the colon. Proctosigmoidoscopy usually enables one to observe the pseudomembranes; however, there are a few patients in whom the rectosigmoid area is uninvolved. In these patients colonoscopy demonstrates characteristic lesions in other areas of the colon. The tissue culture assay of stools for a cytotoxin which can be neutralized by *C. sordellii* antitoxin has become a helpful diagnostic test.

Neonatal necrotizing enterocolitis may present as a benign illness with minimal signs and symptoms; however, the most frequent early manifestations are abdominal distention and gastric retention of formula from previous feedings. Bile-stained emesis, melena, hematochezia, and abdominal tenderness appear later. Necrotizing enterocolitis may develop over 1 or 2 days in those with a history of poorly tolerated feedings, or it may progress over the course of a few hours with rapid progression and fatal outcome. Associated manifestations include temperature instability, apnea, bradycardia, mottling, cyanosis, shock, and disseminated intravascular coagulation. Early abdominal roentgenograms may demonstrate an ileus with dilated loops of bowel, but serial films will show pneumatosis intestinalis, portal venous gas, or free intraabdominal air.

Differential Diagnosis

Since many of the infectious causes of enterocolitis produce similar signs and symptoms, the differential diagnosis of profuse, watery diarrhea or dysentery would include such agents as bacteria, chlamydiae, spirochetes, mycobacteria, and parasites. Shigellosis can mimic ulcerative colitis, amebic enterocolitis, acute diverticulitis, cholecystitis, pyelonephritis, pneumonia, dengue fever, aseptic meningitis, delirium tremens, or a herniated intervertebral disk. Gastrointestinal salmonellosis must be differentiated from shigellosis, invasive and enterotoxigenic *E. coli* infection, and staphylococcal food poisoning. *Yersinia, Campylobacter,* and nonagglutinable *Vibrio* spp produce similar clinical manifestations and can simulate the inflammatory bowel diseases. Clinically, enteritis necroticans is similar to acute shigellosis, food-poisoning syndromes, antibiotic-associated pseudomembranous colitis, and ulcerative colitis. The differential diagnosis of tuberculous enterocolitis includes carcinoma, amebiasis, appendiceal abscess, and occlusive vascular disease.

Amebiasis should usually be considered in the evaluation of chronic diarrhea especially when the feces contain blood-streaked mucus or exudate. More common differential diagnostic possibilities include bacterial and viral enteritis, inflammatory bowel disease, carcinoma of the colon, and irritable colon syndrome. In contrast to shigellosis, onset of amebiasis is usually more gradual, chills are rare, fever is absent to mild, diarrhea is less severe, and the feces contain moderate numbers of epithelial and mononuclear cells and eosinophils. Inflammatory bowel disease produces diffuse or segmental inflammation, irregular ulcerations, or pseudopolypoid changes. Amebic ulcers are found and often appear on an otherwise normal mucosa. However, *E. histolytica* can cause intestinal thumbprinting and pseudopolypoid changes in the colonic mucosa and can occur in association with carcinoma of the colon.

Clinically, giardiasis has to be distinguished from irritable bowel syndrome, cholecystitis, and various malabsorption syndromes including tropical sprue and celiac disease. In giardiasis, serum folate levels may be depressed but anemia is unusual. Glossitis, tetany, and osteomalacia as manifestations of malabsorption in giardiasis are very rare.

Before its recognition as a definite entity, neonatal necrotizing enterocolitis may have been misdiagnosed as intestinal infarction, peritonitis, appendicitis, idiopathic gastrointestinal perforation, or ischemic enteritis. Clinical presentation of necrotizing enterocolitis may mimic neonatal sepsis; signs and symptoms common to both include apnea, bradycardia, temperature instability, cyanosis, lethargy, gastric retention, bloody stools, and erythema and tenderness of the abdominal wall.

Treatment

Treatment of diarrhea and enterocolitis involves supportive measures especially replacement of fluids and electrolytes. In the normal adult many of the previously reviewed bacterial agents generally cause a mild and self-limited illness, and therefore antimicrobials are not necessary except when the illness involves extraintestinal sites. Antibiotics are indicated (Table 24.7) when severe shigella enterocolitis occurs in infants, elderly, and the debilitated. Additionally, antibacterial agents may be administered if shigellosis is occurring in epidemic form within an institution.

Therapy of enteritis necroticans consists of bowel decompression, fluid and electrolyte replacement, and resection of the involved bowel if there is persistence of paralytic ileus, sepsis, or diffuse peritonitis. *Clostridium perfringens* type C antiserum may be helpful. Elective surgery for intestinal obstruction may be required up to 6 months after the acute illness.

Management of antibiotic-associated colitis includes rehydration, electrolyte replacement, and supportive care. The antibiotic should be discontinued and antiperistaltic drugs avoided. Most patients will recover with these modalities; however, some will continue to remain symptomatic. In the latter group of patients, cholestyramine or vancomycin orally has been generally efficacious. Cholestyramine may act by binding the cytotoxin produced by *C. difficile*. The mode of action of vancomycin is not known; however, virtually all strains of *C. difficile* are susceptible to this antibiotic. Vancomycin is the drug of choice in the treatment of antibiotic-associated pseudomembranous colitis.

Supportive care and judicious use of surgery are crucial in the management of neonatal necrotizing enterocolitis. Systemic antibiotics which are active against enteric pathogens should be administered when there is evidence of peritonitis or sepsis. A reasonable antibiotic choice is ampicillin or penicillin plus gentamicin or tobramycin.

Immunology

The gastrointestinal tract contains an immunologic system that functions somewhat independently from the systemic immune mechanism and consists of: (1) plasma cells and lymphocytes dispersed throughout the mucosal lamina propria, (2) Peyer's patches which are collections of T and B lymphocytes with germinal centers, and (3) mesenteric lymph nodes. The lamina propria plasma cells produce predominantly IgA antibody which is selectively transferred to the mucosal surface where it is the major secreted immunoglobulin. IgA coproantibody occurs mainly in the 11S form and IgG and IgM also may be produced locally. The intestinal plasma cells, which are derived from precursors in Peyer's patches, migrate as immunoblasts in the thoracic duct lymph and after entering the systemic circulation, home to the lamina propria of the gut. The local intestinal immune system may protect against various antigens encountered at the mucosal surface, and

TABLE 24.7 Antibiotic Treatment of Enterocolitis

Agent	Usual Case of Mild-Moderate Severity	Severe or Protracted	Systemic Infection	Comments
Shigella spp	None	Ampicillin, tetracycline, or trimethoprim-sulfamethoxazole	–	May possess plasmids coding for multiple antibiotic resistance
Salmonella spp	None	None	Ampicillin, chloramphenicol, or trimethoprim-sulfamethoxazole	Antibiotics may prolong duration of excretion of organism
E. coli	None	None	Ampicillin or aminoglycosides	
Yersinia spp	None	None	Chloramphenicol or aminoglycosides	
Campylobacter spp	None	Erythromycin or tetracycline	–	
V. parahemolyticus	None	Penicillin or tetracycline	–	
Amebiasis	Diiodohydroxyquin	Diiodohydroxyquin plus metronidazole or emetine		
B. coli	Tetracycline			
G. lamblia	Quinacrine			

serum antibodies including IgG, IgM, and IgA may also be transferred to the mucosal surface. The exact role of immune mechanisms in the control of the gut flora is unknown. In patients with selective IgA deficiency in the serum, the bacterial flora of the small intestine and feces is normal. Additionally, local cell-mediated immunity may be important in the pathogenesis of various gastrointestinal infections.

Circulating humoral and cellular immune mechanisms probably do not have significant protective action against the enterocolitis produced by *Salmonella* and presumably their actions in host defense begin after the microorganism has penetrated the mucosa. The systemic immune system may have an indirect benefit by controlling bacteremia and recirculation of the organism from the bile or pancreatic ducts to the intestine.

Intestinal antibody responses to *Shigella* spp and *E. coli* have been demonstrated but the function of the secretory IgA has not been established. An experimental shigella vaccine administered orally has been quite effective in field trials in Yugoslavia. Infants immunized orally with strains of *E. coli* may contain IgA and IgM antibodies in their duodenal aspirates; however, the role of these immunoglobulins in immunity is unknown.

Clinical observations of reinfections with *E. histolytica* have suggested that minimal protective immunity occurs. Humans who are reinfected respond with elevated indirect hemagglutination titers, and the titers may remain persistently high after successful treatment. Cell-mediated immunity may be more important in limiting the extent of tissue invasion.

Symptomatic giardiasis may be associated with immunodeficiency syndromes, especially common variable hypogammaglobulinemia. Serum immunoglobulin levels are usually normal in randomly selected patients with either symptomatic or asymptomatic giardiasis; however, significantly lower levels of jejunal secretory IgA exist in many symptomatic patients.

Prevention

Humans are born immunologically immature, and the major systemic immune deficiencies in neonates include decreased opsonization and chemotaxis. In premature infants there also is decreased transplacental transfer of immunoglobulins. During the neonatal period, infants have both minimal detectable antibody present within the small intestine and IgA-producing plasma cells in the lamina propria. Since the structural integrity of the small bowel is immature in the preterm infant, the absorption of various antigens may be enhanced in this age group. With prematurity the local immunologic responsiveness may be delayed thus enabling the development of necrotizing enterocolitis.

There is evidence suggesting that breast milk may be protective against infectious and necrotizing enterocolitis in infants when administered fresh. The protective factors in human breast milk may include *Lactobacillus bifidus* growth factor, antistaphylococcal factor, lysozyme, lactoperoxidase, lactoferrin, interferon, complement, antitrypsin, secretory IgA, IgG, IgM, lymphocytes, macrophages, and neutrophils. *Lactobacillus bifidus* inhibits intestinal colonization by coliforms, whereas secretory IgA may prevent the mucosal binding of certain bacteria and/or enterotoxins and may initiate bacterial agglutination. Lysozyme induces bacterial cell-wall lysis, and lactoperoxidase with hydrogen peroxide have bactericidal activity. Lactoferrin binds bacterial growth factors. Additionally, lymphocytes, monocytes, and neutrophils may enhance cell-mediated immunity and phagocytosis locally within the gastrointestinal tract.

Prevention of shigellosis and salmonellosis is partly dependent upon restricting the activities of individuals excreting the microorganism, e.g., carriers should not be employed as food handlers. Within an institution patients should be isolated and enteric precautions should be enforced. Good personal hygiene is probably the most important aspect in the prevention of enterocolitis caused not by just *Shigella* and *Salmonella* spp but by most enteric pathogens including *E. histolytica* and *G. lamblia.* Control of salmonellosis among animals represents an enormous task, and hygienic conditions in food-processing establishments must be stringently controlled. Since experimentally immunization with parenteral typhoid vaccine appears protective for individuals living in endemic areas, vaccination should be considered for travelers to these areas and laboratory personnel handling *S. typhi.*

Prognosis

Most cases of enterocolitis due to infectious agents are either benign and self-limited or respond to specific therapeutic modalities, thus the overall prognosis remains excellent. Mortality occurs mainly in the very young and old and in other groups who are compromised immunologically. Profound dehydration and major electrolyte imbalances which are refractory to treatment are the principal causes of morbidity and mortality.

Selected Bibliography

Ammann, A. J. and Hong, R.: Selective IgA deficiency: Presentation of 30 cases and a review of the literature. *Medicine* 50:223-236, 1971.

Barker, W. H. Jr. and Gangarosa, E. J.: Food poisoning due to *Vibrio parahaemolyticus. Ann Rev Med* 25:75-81, 1974.

Bartlett, J. G.: Antibiotic-associated colitis. *Clin Gastroenterol* 8:783-801, 1979.

Bennett, A.: Cholera and prostaglandins. *Nature* 231:536, 1971.

Black, R. E., Jackson, R. J., Tsai, T., Medvesky, M., Shayegani, M., Feeley, J. C., MacLeod, K. I. E., and Wakelee, A. M.: Epidemic *Yersinia enterocolitica* infection due to contaminated chocolate milk. *N Engl J Med* 298:76-79, 1978.

Blake, P. A., Merson, M. H., Weaver, R. E., Hollis, D. G., and Heublein, P. C.: Disease caused by a marine *Vibrio.* Clinical characteristics and epidemiology. *N Engl J Med* 300:1-5, 1979.

Blaser, M. J., Berkowitz, I. D., LaForce, F. M., Cravens, J., Reller, L. B., and Wang, W-L. L.: Campylobacter enteritis: Clinical and epidemiologic features. *Ann Intern Med* 91:179-185, 1979.

Bolen, J. L., Zamiska, S. A., and Greenough, W. B., III: Clinical features in enteritis due to *Vibrio parahemolyticus. Am J Med* 57:638-641, 1974.

Brodsky, R. E., Spencer, H. C., Jr., and Schultz, M. G.: Giardiasis in American travelers to the Soviet Union. *J Infect Dis* 130:319-323, 1974.

Butzler, J. P. and Skirrow, M. B.: Campylobacter enteritis. *Clin Gastroenterol* 8:737–765, 1979.

Carpenter, C. C. J.: Cholera and other enterotoxin-related diarrheal diseases. *J Infect Dis* 126:551–564, 1972.

Dupont, H. L. and Hornick, R. B.: Clinical approach to infectious diarrheas. *Medicine* 52:265–270, 1973.

DuPont, H. L., Sullivan, P., Evans, D. G., Pickering, L. K., Evans, D. J., Vollet, J. J., Ericsson, C. D., Ackerman, P. B., and Tjoa, W. S.: Prevention of traveler's diarrhea (emporiatic enteritis): Prophylactic administration of subsalicylate bismuth. *JAMA* 243:237–241, 1980.

Evans, N.: Pathogenic mechanisms in bacterial diarrhoea. *Clin Gastroenterol* 8: 599–623, 1979.

Formal, S. B., DuPont, H. L., and Hornick, R. B.: Enterotoxin diarrheal syndrome. *Ann Rev Med* 24:103–110, 1973.

Gemski, P., Jr., Takeuchi, A., Washington, O., and Formal, S. B.: Shigellosis due to *Shigella dysenteriae* 1. Relative importance of mucoid invasion vs. toxin production in pathogenesis. *J Infect Dis* 126:523–530, 1972.

Giannella, R. A., Gots, R. E., Charney, A. N., Greenough, W. B., III, and Formal, S. B.: Pathogenesis of salmonella-mediated intestinal fluid secretion. Activation of adenylate cyclase and inhibition by indomethacin. *Gastroenterology* 69:1238–1245, 1975.

Grady, G. F. and Keusch, G. T.: Pathogenesis of bacterial diarrheas. *N Engl J Med* 285:831–841, 891–900, 1971.

Guerrant, R. L., Lahita, R. G., Winn, W. C., Jr., and Roberts, R. B.: Campylobacteriosis in man: Pathogenic mechanisms and review of 91 bloodstream infections. *Am J Med* 65:584–592, 1978.

Harris, J. C., Dupont, H., and Hornick, R. B.: Fecal leukocytes in diarrheal illness. *Ann Intern Med* 76:697–703, 1972.

Hughes, J. M., Hollis, D. G., Gangarosa, E. J., and Weaver, R. E.: Non-cholera vibrio infections in the United States. Clinical, epidemiologic, and laboratory features. *Ann Intern Med* 88:602–606, 1978.

Juniper, K.: Amoebiasis. *Clin Gastroenterol* 7:3–29, 1978.

Keusch, G. T.: Shigella infections. *Clin Gastroenterol* 8:645–662, 1979.

Kliegman, R. M.: Neonatal necrotizing enterocolitis: Implications for an infectious disease. *Pediatr Clin N Am* 26:327–344, 1979.

Knight, R.: Giardiasis, isosporiasis and balantidiasis. *Clin Gastroenterol* 7:31–47, 1978.

Kohl, S.: *Yersinia enterocolitica* infections in children. *Pediatr Clin N Am* 26: 433–443, 1979.

Konowalchuk, J., Speirs, J. I. and Stavric, S.: Vero response to a cytotoxin of *Escherichia coli*. *Infect Immun* 18:775–779, 1977.

Kosloske, A. M.: Necrotizing enterocolitis in the neonate. *Surg Gynecol Obstet* 148:259–269, 1979.

Kosloske, A. M., Ulrich, J. A., and Hoffman, H.: Fulminant necrotizing enterocolitis associated with clostridia. *Lancet* 2:1014–1016, 1978.

Lake, A. M. and Walker, W. A.: Neonatal necrotizing enterocolitis: A disease of altered host defense. *Clin Gastroenterol* 6:463–480, 1977.

Lambert, M. E., Schofield, P. F., Ironside, A. G., and Mandal, B. K.: Campylobacter colitis. *Br Med J* 1:857–859, 1979.

Levine, M. M., Bergquist, E. J., Nalin, D. R., Waterman, D. H., Hornick, R. B., Young, C. R., and Sotman, S.: *Escherichia coli* strains that cause diarrhoea but do not produce heat-labile or heat-stable enterotoxins and are noninvasive. *Lancet* 1:1119–1122, 1978.

Maki, M., Gronroos, P., and Vesikari, T.: In vitro invasiveness of *Yersinia entero-colitica* isolated from children with diarrhea. *J Infect Dis* 138:677–680, 1978.

Pai, C. H. and Mors, V.: Production of enterotoxin by *Yersinia enterocolitica*. *Infect Immun* 19:908–911, 1978.

Pai, C. H., Mors, V., and Toma, S.: Prevalence of enterotoxigenicity in human and nonhuman isolates of *Yersinia enterocolitica*. *Infect Immun* 22:334–338, 1978.

Palmer, D. L., Koster, F. T., Rafiquel Islam, A. F. M., et al.: Comparison of sucrose and glucose in the oral electrolyte therapy of cholera and other severe diarrheas. *N Engl J Med* 297:1107–1110, 1977.

Plotkin, G. R., Kluge, R. M., and Waldman, R. H.: Gastroenteritis: Etiology, pathophysiology and clinical manifestations. *Medicine* 58:95–114, 1979.

Rettig, P. J.: Campylobacter infections in human beings. *J Pediatr* 94:855–864, 1979.

Rowe, B.: The role of *Escherichia coli* in gastroenteritis. *Clin Gastroenterol* 8: 625–644, 1979.

Santulli, T. V., Schullinger, J. N., Heird, W. C., Gongaware, R. D., Wigger, J., Barlow, B., Blanc, W. A., and Berdon, W. E.: Acute necrotizing enterocolitis in infancy: A review of 64 cases. *Pediatrics* 55:376–387, 1975.

Sack, D. A., Kamisky, D. C., Sack, R. B., et al.: Prophylactic doxycycline for traveler's diarrhea. *N Engl J Med* 298:758–763, 1978.

Taylor, P. R., Weinstein, W. M., and Bryner, J. H.: *Campylobacter fetus* infection in human subjects. Association with raw milk. *Am J Med* 66:779-783, 1979.

Tedesco, F. J.: Antibiotic associated pseudomembranous colitis with negative proctosigmoidoscopy examination. *Gastroenterology* 77:295-297, 1979.

Torphy, D. E. and Bond, W. W.: *Campylobacter fetus* infections in children. *Pediatrics* 64:898-903, 1979.

Turnbull, P. C. B.: Food poisoning with special reference to Salmonella - its epidemiology, pathogenesis and control. *Clin Gastroenterol* 8:663-714, 1979.

Ulshen, M. H. and Rollo, J. L.: Pathogenesis of *Escherichia coli* gastroenteritis in man - another mechanism. *N Engl J Med* 302:99-101, 1980.

Walder, M.: Susceptibility of *Campylobacter fetus* subsp. *jejuni* to twenty antimicrobial agents. *Antimicrob Agents Chemother* 16:37-39, 1979.

Walker, W. A.: Antigen absorption from the small intestine and gastrointestinal disease. *Pediatr Clin N Am* 22:731-746, 1975.

Walker, W. A.: Host defense mechanisms of the gastrointestinal tract. *Pediatrics* 57:901-916, 1976.

Welsh, J. K. and May, J. T.: Anti-infective properties of breast milk. *J Pediatr* 94:1-9, 1979.

25

DIVERTICULITIS
Gary R. Plotkin, M.D.

Definition

Diverticula are herniations or saccular protrusions of one or more layers of the walls of the intestine. They may be found at all levels of the gastrointestinal tract but are most common in the sigmoid colon. Diverticulitis is an inflammatory complication of diverticulosis and results from either micro- or macroperforation.

Epidemiology and Pathogenesis

The incidence of diverticular disease increases with advancing years; the disorder affects mainly those over the age of 40. The incidence increases from 5% in the fifth decade to approximately 50% in the ninth decade. Colonic diverticula can be demonstrated in 8% of the adult population. A dramatic rise in the prevalence of diverticular disease has occurred in the more economically developed nations of the West, whereas, diverticulosis is rare in rural Africa or Asia. The prevalence of the disease in each developing country seemingly varies directly with its state of economic development. A racial predilection does not appear to play a role since the incidence of diverticular disease increases with time in those native Africans or Japanese who settle in the Western countries. Epidemiologic data suggest that a diet low in fiber parallels the prevalence of diverticulosis.

Pathologically, diverticulitis represents chronic inflammation and lymphoid hyperplasia in the mucosa at the diverticulum apex and may result from inspissated fecal material within the lumen. The inflammatory process may spread beyond the serosa of the diverticula (peridiverticulitis) thus producing a focus of granulation tissue, inflammatory cells, or fibrotic tissue within the peritoneum.

Diagnosis

Clinical symptoms and physical findings in diverticulitis are dependent upon the extent of extradiverticular inflammation. Predominant symptoms include lower abdominal pain which can be either intermittent or steady. Fever and chills often are present. Occasionally, the patient will present with a brief episode of diarrhea. Pericolitis, however, may cause colonic obstruction with constipation, abdominal distention, anorexia, and nausea. If the inflammatory bowel process is contiguous with the bladder or ureter, then the patient's symptoms may stimulate a urinary tract infection. Less commonly, the patient may present with sepsis from a ruptured diverticulum.

On physical examination, the patient with diverticulitis has lower-quadrant abdominal tenderness, usually on the left, with or without a palpable mass. Since the inflammatory process may involve the peritoneum, direct and rebound tenderness may be elicited. Rectal examination may reveal a tender mass, which results from an inflamed sigmoid or pelvic abscess. None of the symptoms or physical findings is pathognomonic.

The peripheral white blood cell count is usually elevated with a left shift. Plain abdominal roentgenograms can be normal, or reveal free air beneath the diaphragm or paralytic ileus secondary to peritonitis. Proctosigmoidoscopy is either normal or demonstrates an extraluminal mass which completely or partially obstructs the lumen. Whether or not a barium enema should be done during the acute phase of diverticulitis remains controversial. However, roentgenographic evidence of diverticulitis includes barium outside a diverticulum, delineation of a paracolic or intramural mass, or presence of a fistulous tract originating in the colon. Proctosigmoidoscopy, colonoscopy, and barium enema are not entirely benign in diverticular disease; however, they are employed to eliminate other clinically similar conditions, including inflammatory bowel disease and carcinoma. The urine in diverticulitis may contain red or white cells if there is contiguous involvement of the urinary tract, and occasionally an intravenous pyelogram may demonstrate a fistula between the colon and bladder or ureter. Abdominal sonography, computed axial tomography, or gallium scan may prove useful for detecting intraabdominal abscesses secondary to diverticulitis.

Episodes of pain produced by diverticulosis may mimic those of diverticulitis. A palpable sigmoid loop in diverticulosis also can simulate an inflammatory mass secondary to diverticulitis; however, fever, leukocytosis, and signs of peritoneal irritation suggest diverticulitis. A barium enema enables one to differentiate diverticulitis from diverticulosis since, in the former, one usually observes barium outside of a diverticulum or evidence of a fistula or mass. Other diseases that should be considered are inflammatory bowel disease, ischemic colitis, and carcinoma of the colon. The latter, like diverticulitis, may cause luminal narrowing, rectal bleeding, obstruction, fistula formation, abdominal mass, or perforation. Localized abdominal tenderness, leukocytosis, and fever favor diverticulitis, while chronic rectal bleeding and weight loss are more common in colonic carcinoma. However, diverticular disease may coexist with carcinoma. Once the acute episode of diverticulitis subsides, proctosigmoidoscopy, colonoscopy, and barium enema often help in eliminating the possibility of a concomitant carcinoma. Many times diverticulitis cannot be differentiated from colonic carcinoma and exploratory laparotomy becomes necessary.

Complications and Prognosis

Diverticulitis may be associated with partial or complete intestinal obstruction affecting either the small or large bowel. Obstruction of the small bowel is due to edema and kinking secondary to a pericolic mass or abscess. Diverticulitis may cause complete large-bowel obstruction either by intramural abscess, pericolic fibrosis, or by marked angulation of the pelvic colon secondary to adhesions between a pericolic mass and the lateral pelvic wall. Pericolic fibrosis results usually from chronic diverticulitis.

In acute phlegmonous diverticulitis, the inflammatory process is confined to the immediate pericolic tissues; however, a variant form known as gangrenous sigmoiditis represents anaerobic cellulitis of the sigmoid mesocolon with massive edema and black discoloration of the tissues. Diverticulitis may also result in a pericolic abscess, i.e., the inflammatory process is usually situated within the confines of the mesocolic fat but occasionally it may be found outside the mesocolon with small bowel, omentum, and adjacent parietal peritoneum forming the abscess walls. The abscess will either resolve with conservative management or will rupture into the bowel lumen, peritoneal cavity, bladder, or vagina. Peritonitis resulting from diverticulitis may either be localized or diffuse. Other abdominal complications of diverticulitis include portal septicemia, suppurative pyelophlebitis, and hepatic, subphrenic, and intraabdominal abscesses.

Formation of fistulas is a common complication of diverticular disease and may occur in as many as one-fifth of the patients with diverticulitis. Colovesical fistulas account for approximately 50% of them and are more common in men. Women are less prone because of the protection afforded the bladder by the uterus and broad ligaments. Symptoms and signs of a colovesical fistula include pneumaturia, fecaluria, dysuria, pyuria, hematuria, and bacteriuria. Cystoscopy, proctosigmoidoscopy, and barium enema are important in the diagnosis.

Colocutaneous fistula usually complicates an abdominal operation for diverticulitis and occurs in 6% of such patients. Coloenteric fistulas, which comprise about 10% of all fistulas associated with diverticulitis, commonly involve the ileum and occur in patients who have other fistulas or history of sepsis. A colovaginal fistula may occur in patients who have previously undergone hysterectomy and present clinically as a medically refractory vaginal discharge. The uterus is usually resistant to fistula formation. Diverticulitis has uncommonly caused necrotizing fasciitis of the lower extremity or abdominal wall.

The natural history, prevention, and prognosis of diverticular disease are not completely known. Many patients remain asymptomatic, and there is obviously an unidentified number of patients who probably have minor symptoms but do not seek medical advice. At the other extreme is a subset of patients who require hospitalization for medical and/or surgical treatment. When diverticular disease occurs in those under 35 years, it often presents in an aggressive form with a high complication rate. Individuals over the age of 60 also have a high morbidity and mortality. Persistent symptoms usually are more common in patients with total colonic involvement than in those with disease localized to the sigmoid; however, symptoms cannot be correlated either with the size or with the total number of diverticula.

Between 10 and 25% of patients with colonic diverticula will eventually develop peridiverticular inflammation. There is a poor correlation between the clinical features and the pathologic findings of diverticular disease. Twenty-five percent of patients who are treated conservatively for the initial inflammatory attack will require additional hospitalization and more than 70% will continue to have intermittent symptoms between the acute attacks. Fifty percent of patients who require readmission will be hospitalized within 1 year of the first attack and

90% within 5 years. Medical treatment of recurrent disease is less effective than for the initial attack, and complications are more common in those with recurrent episodes of diverticulitis. Finally, since diverticular disease is so highly variable, the long-term benefits of medical management including a high-fiber diet remain unknown.

Treatment

As previously mentioned, epidemiologic data suggest that a low-fiber diet may be responsible for diverticular disease. However, before the development of this concept, the treatment was a low-roughage diet, the purpose being to avoid obstructing or irritating a diverticula with harsh residue. It is now generally accepted that increased intraluminal pressure in the colon, prolonged intestinal transit time and reduced stool weight are factors in diverticular disease. Thus an increased intake of unrefined fiber is recommended both for prophylaxis and therapy of diverticular disease. Bulk agents derived from semisynthetic polysaccharides, mucilaginous seeds, seed coats, and mucilaginous gums have been recommended. Nonetheless, whether or not any dietary manipulations can prevent or reverse diverticula or prevent the development of diverticulitis remains unknown.

Anticolinergic agents, local application of heat, and nonopiate analgesics have been employed in alleviating colonic spasm and pain in diverticular disease. Purgatives such as mineral oil and bile salts should be avoided. Without well-controlled studies, it is difficult to determine the efficacy of therapeutic modalities.

Approximately two-thirds to three-fourths of patients treated successfully medically for the first attack of acute diverticulitis do not have recurrent symptoms or hospital admissions. Therapeutic maneuvers for acute diverticulitis are directed toward resting the colon to alleviate inflammation, spasm, and obstruction. Such measures include nasogastric suction and intravenous fluids. The patient with diverticulitis must be closely observed for localized or diffuse peritonitis and sepsis.

The role of antimicrobial therapy in diverticular disease is variable. Parenteral antibiotics have been employed and are indicated in treating such complications of diverticulitis as bacteremia, diffuse peritonitis, and intraabdominal, hepatic, and pericolic abscesses. The normal colonic bacterial flora is responsible for these infections and consequently is polymicrobial and includes facultative and obligate anaerobes (*E. coli, Proteus, Klebsiella, Citrobacter, Pseudomonas aeruginosa, enterococcus, Bacteroides* spp including *fragilis, Fusobacterium, Peptostreptococcus, Clostridium perfringens, Eubacterium, Bifidobacterium,* and *Actinomyces*). Parenteral penicillin or ampicillin plus gentamicin or tobramycin are active against the previously mentioned bacteria, excluding most strains of *B. fragilis*. The latter organism is inhibited by clindamycin or chloramphenicol. Whether or not oral absorbable, nonabsorbable, or parenteral antibiotics are beneficial in diverticulosis or uncomplicated diverticulitis remains unknown.

The traditional indications for operative intervention in patients with diverticular disease are recurrent diverticulitis, perforation, enlarging mass or abscess, persistent obstruction, fistula, refractory hemorrhage, generalized peritonitis, and the inability to differentiate carcinoma. When a fistula is present, a diverting colostomy alone is usually insufficient, and the fistula and adjacent bowel should be resected.

Selected Bibliography

Berman, P. M. and Kirsner, J. B.: Current knowledge of diverticular disease of the colon. *Am J Dig Dis* 17:741–759, 1972.

Brodribb, A. J. M.: Treatment of symptomatic diverticular disease with a high-fiber diet. *Lancet* 1:664–666, 1977.

Byrne, J. J. and Hennessy, V. L., Jr.: Diverticulitis of the colon. *Surg Clin N Am* 52:991–999, 1972.

Connell, A. M.: Dietary fiber and diverticular disease. *Hosp Pract* 11:119–124, 1976.

Connell, A. M.: Pathogenesis of diverticular disease of the colon. *Adv Intern Med* 22:377–395, 1977.

Eastwood, M. A., Smith, A. N., Brydon, W. G., and Pritchard, J.: Comparison of bran, ispaghula, and lactulose on colon function in diverticular disease. *Gut* 19:1144–1147, 1978.

Galbut, D. L., Gerber, D. L., and Belgraier, A. H.: Spontaneous necrotizing fasciitis. Occurrence secondary to occult diverticulitis. *JAMA* 238:2302, 1977.

Hinchey, E. J., Schaal, P. G. H., and Richards, G. K.: Treatment of perforated diverticular disease of the colon. *Adv Surg* 12:05–109, 1978.

Hodgson, W. J. B.: The placebo effect. Is it important in diverticular disease? *Am J Gastroenterol* 67:157–162, 1977.

Kirwan, W. O., Smith, A. N., McConnell, A. A., Mitchell, W. D., and Eastwood, M. A.: Action of different bran preparations on colonic function. *Br Med J* 4:187–189, 1974.

Larson, D. M., Masters, S. S., and Spiro, H. M.: Medical and surgical therapy in diverticular disease. A comparative study. *Gastroenterology* 71:734–737, 1976.

Mendeloff, A. I.: Dietary fiber and human health. *N Engl J Med* 297:811–814, 1977.

Meyers, M. A., Alonso, D. R., Morson, B. C., and Bartram, C.: Pathogenesis of diverticulitis complicating granulomatous colitis. *Gastroenterology* 74:24–31, 1978.

Morson, B. C.: Pathology of diverticular disease of the colon. *Clin Gastroenterol* 4:37–52, 1975.

Painter, N. S., Almeida, A. Z., and Colebourne, K. W.: Unprocessed bran in treatment of diverticular disease of the colon. *Br Med J* 2:137–140, 1972.

Painter, N. S. and Burkitt, D. P.: Diverticular disease of the colon, a 20th century problem. *Clin Gastroenterol* 4:3–21, 1975.

Sethbhakdi, S.: Pathogenesis of colonic diverticulitis and diverticulosis. *Postgrad Med* 60:76–81, 1976.

26

HEPATITIS
H. Preston Holley, Jr., M.D.

Definition

Hepatitis is an acute inflammation of the liver which results in some degree of hepatocyte necrosis. This chapter will be concerned with hepatitis caused by the hepatitis viruses. The spectrum of disease caused by these viruses is extremely variable and may be totally asymptomatic, acute, subacute, chronic, or fulminant resulting in death.

Etiology

The most common causes of viral hepatitis are hepatitis A virus (HAV, formerly "infectious hepatitis"), hepatitis B virus (HBV, formerly "serum hepatitis") (Table 26.1), and a relatively newly recognized entity, non-A, non-B hepatitis (NANBH), which resembles hepatitis A and B clinically and is probably caused by two or more viruses which have not yet been characterized. Other viruses have been associated with hepatitis, but these are less common.

Epidemiology

Hepatitis A

Hepatitis A virus is found worldwide, but the exact prevalence of the disease in different countries is hard to estimate because of inadequate reporting systems in much of the world. Even in the United States surveys suggest that viral hepatitis is underreported. Approximately 30,000 cases of hepatitis A are reported

TABLE 26.1   Nomenclature of the Hepatitis Viruses

Viral Antigens	Associated Antibodies
Hepatitis A virus (HAV)	
Hepatitis A antigen (HA Ag)	Antibody to HA Ag (anti-HA)
Hepatitis B virus (HBV)	
Hepatitis B surface antigen (HBsAg)	Antibody to HBsAg (anti-HBs)
Hepatitis B core antigen (HBcAg)	Antibody to HBcAg (anti-HBc)
Hepatitis B "e" antigen (HBeAg)	Antibody to HBeAg (anti-HBe)
Hepatitis B delta antigen (HBdAg)	Antibody to HBdAg (anti-HBd)

annually, but it has been estimated that at least twice as many cases of icteric hepatitis A occur annually, and several times this number have subclinical infection.

Hepatitis A virus is spread by the fecal-oral route, usually by person-to-person contact. Infection is readily transmitted in areas of overcrowding and poor sanitation. Common-source outbreaks most commonly result from fecal contamination of water and food by infected persons during the incubation period when large quantities of HAV are shed in the feces. Several outbreaks have been associated with shellfish which frequently are served raw or poorly cooked. Nursery school, day-care center and other institutional outbreaks are probably due to the poor hygiene of young children and the close contact among such persons. Transmission by blood transfusion or by parenteral inoculation is rare. No viremic carrier state of HAV infection has been described as there has been for HBV infection.

Hepatitis B

Hepatitis B virus is found worldwide. Approximately 16,000 cases are reported annually in the United States, but many cases are not reported. The reported prevalence of HBV infection in the United States has been stable over the past few years.

Spread of HBV infection occurs via parenteral and nonparenteral means. Parenteral injection of blood or blood products from an infected person by blood transfusion, contaminated needle-stick, or other means is an important method of transmission. There is a large reservoir of HBV carriers (over 175 million in the world) which make up 20% of the population in some tropical areas and are a major public health problem. In the United States less than 0.5% of the population has persistent HBV infection. Medical, dental, and laboratory personnel are at much greater risk of parenteral transmission than the general population. Today, transmission by blood transfusion is not common.

Since the introduction of screening of blood for transfusion for the presence of hepatitis B surface antigen (HBsAg, a marker of the virus), there has been a decrease in transfusion-associated HBV infection but not in the overall prevalence of hepatitis B. Transmission of HBV by inoculation may occur during medical and dental procedures; acupuncture; ear-piercing; tattooing; sharing of needles, razors, or other objects; or during laboratory accidents involving spillage of contaminated blood.

Studies have identified HBsAg in blood, certain plasma fractions, saliva, menstrual and vaginal discharges, semen, amniotic fluid, colostrum, breast milk, and occasionally in urine, feces, bile, sweat, tears, spinal fluid, pleural fluid, and ascitic fluid. It is not surprising that contact-associated transmission is believed to be a major mode of HBV infection. Epidemiologic studies in areas of the world with a high prevalence of HBV infection support this notion. Familial clustering of HBV infection has been well documented. Recent studies have also provided circumstantial evidence for sexual transmission. In one study 18% of spouses of patients with acute hepatitis B contracted the infection with no infection in other family members. Also, a significant excess of cases of hepatitis B has been found in two promiscuous groups: male homosexuals and patients with venereal diseases and their sexual contacts.

Vertical transmission has been suggested by careful studies of pregnant women who had active hepatitis during pregnancy. The risk of transmission to the child was much greater if the mother's infection occurred during the last trimester of pregnancy. It remains unclear whether the child is actually infected in utero or during or after delivery. Although in utero infection can occur, this appears to occur only rarely.

Non-A, Non-B Hepatitis

Since specific markers for the non-A, non-B hepatitis viruses are not available, the epidemiology of this form of hepatitis has not been well studied. Transmission by the parenteral route has clearly been demonstrated in several outbreaks related to blood transfusions, transfusions of serum concentrates, needle-sticks, and in experimental animals. Indeed these viruses are probably responsible for about 80% of posttransfusion hepatitis. Several reports of multiple episodes of hepatitis in parenteral drug abusers suggest that parenteral transmission is likely responsible, but nonparenteral means cannot be ruled out in many of these cases. A viremic carrier state has been described in a patient whose sera was shown to be infective for 6 years.

Person-to-person transmission has been suggested in studies of the seroepidemiology of viral hepatitis in Costa Rica. Reports from the United States also suggest that up to 25% of patients hospitalized with sporadic hepatitis have NANBH infection. Many of these patients have no known parenteral exposure.

Pathogenesis and Pathology

The pathologic changes in acute hepatitis A and B are indistinguishable. All components of the liver are involved. Two constant pathologic features are seen in acute hepatitis: hepatocyte necrosis and histiocytic periportal inflammation. Necrosis occurs mainly in the central zone of the lobule around the central vein, and in fatal fulminant cases the entire lobule is involved.

Inflammation varies and usually is more intense in the portal areas, with mononuclear cells predominating. Polymorphonuclear cells and a few eosinophils also may be present. The architecture of the lobules is often distorted but the reticulum remains intact so that when regeneration occurs the lobule is reconstructed. In cases of chronic hepatitis, due to HBV or non-A, non-B viruses, the integrity of the lobule may be lost. Signs of bile stasis occur in all cases with jaundice but do not occur in anicteric cases. Subsequent changes, even postnecrotic cirrhosis, can occur without preceding jaundice.

Two types of chronic hepatitis may result from hepatitis B infection, chronic persistent hepatitis (CPH) and chronic active hepatitis (CAH). The CPH is usually a benign, nonprogressive disease characterized by chronic portal inflammation with little or no fibrosis. Rarely, CPH has been reported to progress to CAH. In CAH there is a chronic inflammatory infiltration of plasma cells and lymphocytes in the portal areas extending into the parenchyma. There also is moderate or severe piecemeal necrosis with loss of the limiting plate and bridging hepatic necrosis in some patients. Multilobular bridging necrosis has prognostic significance since it is often associated with development of cirrhosis or a more severe course of CAH. Unfortunately the changes seen are not pathognomonic of CAH and can be seen in drug-induced hepatitis, Wilson's disease, and occasionally primary biliary cirrhosis.

Diagnostic Features

Clinical Manifestations

In general, hepatitis due to HAV, HBV, and NANBH viruses are clinically similar and require serologic testing for specific diagnosis (see Chapter 72). Most patients have a period of nonspecific complaints called the prodrome. This prodrome is usually short (average 2-7 days) with hepatitis A but longer (average 14-28 days) with hepatitis B. Symptoms are nonspecific and may include weakness, anorexia, myalgias, headache, photophobia, and arthralgias. Pharyngitis, cough, and coryza are more common with hepatitis A. Fever is also common in hepatitis A but unusual with hepatitis B. Arthritis, angioedema, urticaria, or rash occur in a small percentage of cases due to hepatitis B. Nausea and vomiting usually appear a few days before the onset of jaundice. Aversion to the taste of cigarettes or specific foods is common. Many patients also complain of a fullness in the right upper quadrant. Darkening of the urine is commonly noticed before the onset of jaundice, even with a total serum bilirubin of less than 1 mg/dl.

The icteric phase begins with the appearance of jaundice. Anorexia, malaise, and weakness may worsen. Other symptoms generally improve although nausea and vomiting may persist and require hospitalization for hydration in more severe cases. Pruritus may appear with increasing jaundice but is usually temporary. The liver and spleen are often palpable.

The convalescent phase begins with a decrease in jaundice and improvement of symptoms, particularly the return of appetite and a general feeling of improvement. The liver and spleen return to normal size. Recovery is usually complete in 90-95% of patients in 6 months.

Fulminant hepatitis, on the other hand, is a life-threatening form of hepatitis which can be associated with any of the hepatitis viruses but is most common with HBV infection (accounting for about two-thirds of the cases). The onset may be that of typical hepatitis or may be that of acute hepatic failure. One of the clinical hallmarks is the small liver or decreasing liver size during the course of illness. There also is usually progressive jaundice but some patients have died before jaundice was clinically evident. Transaminase levels are usually markedly elevated but may fall with progressive liver destruction. Hypoglycemia occasionally occurs with massive hepatic necrosis. Another important finding is the alteration in mental status due to hepatic encephalopathy which can progress to obtundation and coma. Survival is related to the severity of the encephalopathy and also the age of the patient (lower survival in patients over 40). Overall mortality is 60-90%. Early recognition and specific supportive measures can decrease mortality, and survival often results in complete resolution of the hepatitis.

A small percentage of patients with hepatitis B develop immune-complex diseases which seem to have different pathogenic mechanisms. These include a serum sickness-like syndrome, polyarthritis and skin rashes, polyarteritis, polymyalgia rheumatica, glomerulonephritis, and immune-complex liver disease. The actual incidence of these complicating illnesses associated with HBV infection is unknown.

Chronic hepatitis has been associated with hepatitis B and NANB hepatitis but not with hepatitis A. The serology and relationship with hepatoma are discussed in Chapter 72.

Laboratory

The serology of the hepatitis viruses is discussed in Chapter 72.

Tests of liver function are helpful to follow the course of hepatitis, but the values do not correlate with severity of the disease. The serum transaminase levels begin to rise about 1 week before, or coincidentally with, the onset of clinical symptoms, with the SGPT level usually being higher than that of SGOT. The peak SGPT levels are usually from 500 to 5000 IU. Bilirubin levels rise subsequently and may continue to rise even after the transaminase peak has been reached. Peak bilirubin levels are characteristically reached in 2-3 weeks and maximum values are usually less than 10 mg/dl in uncomplicated acute hepatitis. The serum bilirubin most commonly falls to normal more rapidly than the transaminases. In 5-10% of patients the transaminase levels remain slightly elevated for several months.

The serum alkaline phosphatase may be normal or slightly elevated, and the prothrombin time may be slightly prolonged but usually not more than 5 sec. Serum bile acids are elevated in the acute phase of hepatitis. Serum albumin often remains normal or slightly decreased. Alpha-fetoprotein (AFP) has been found in some sera during the course of acute hepatitis. The highest values have been seen in patients with viral bridging necrosis. The significance of this "embryonic" protein in hepatitis is unknown.

There may be minimal hematologic changes during acute hepatitis. Occasionally anemia due to Coombs'-negative hemolysis occurs, usually in persons with glucose-6-phosphate dehydrogenase (G-6-PD) deficiency. The reticulocyte count may be slightly elevated. Aplastic anemia is rare but has been reported in about 200 patients following HAV infection. During acute hepatitis, mild leukopenia with a relative lymphocytosis is sometimes seen. Atypical lymphocytes (usually <10%) may be seen. Leukocytosis greater than 12,000 is uncommon unless there is fulminant hepatitis or severe bridging necrosis.

Differential Diagnosis

Acute hepatitis A or B usually can be diagnosed serologically, as discussed in Chapter 72. Unfortunately, there is no commercially available test for the specific diagnosis of NANBH. Therefore this diagnosis depends on the exclusion of HAV, HBV, and other causes of hepatitis. Epstein-Barr virus (EBV) and cytomegalovirus (CMV) both can present with hepatitis indistinguishable clinically from illness due to the hepatitis viruses. Serologic tests are available for EBV and CMV and a demonstration of a fourfold titer rise with time would confirm the diagnosis (as will be discussed later).

Drug-induced hepatitis, alcoholic hepatitis, primary biliary cirrhosis, and a variety of other disorders leading to hepatic necrosis can mimic viral hepatitis. A history of drug or alcohol ingestion may be helpful. In alcoholic hepatitis the SGOT often is twice as high as the SGPT, and the absolute SGPT level rarely exceeds 100 IU. A hepatitis picture may be caused by other infections that can produce hepatocellular injury such as bacterial infections (e.g., leptospirosis, gram-negative sepsis, etc.), parasitic infections (e.g., malaria, toxoplasmosis, *Entamoeba histolytica*), and rickettsial infections (e.g., Q fever and typhus). Ischemic changes due to hypotension, congestive heart failure, or anorexia can also mimic hepatitis when they result in centrolobular hepatic necrosis. The differential can be greatly narrowed in most cases by a thorough evaluation of the patient including a complete history and physical examination. A liver biopsy is generally not indicated unless there is severe progressive dysfunction and other diagnoses seem likely, or the patient has documented viral hepatitis but liver functions remain abnormal for greater than 3 months suggesting chronic hepatitis.

Other Viruses Causing Hepatitis

Cytomegalovirus

Cytomegalovirus (CMV) infection is commonly asymptomatic. Involvement of the liver may occur in such infections as well as being usually seen in clinically apparent illness. Syndromes of CMV infection with hepatitis include congenital CMV infection, CMV mononucleosis, postperfusion syndrome, posttransfusion hepatitis, granulomatous hepatitis, and disseminated infection in immunosuppressed patients.

Typically the hepatitis is mild and anicteric. Clinical symptoms usually include malaise, fever, myalgias, weakness, and headache. Hepatosplenomegaly occurs in a small percentage of patients. Cervical adenopathy is uncommon and may be helpful in clinically differentiating CMV from Epstein-Barr virus infection. Laboratory aspects include a relative lymphocytosis with atypical lymphocytes, elevated transaminase (usually < 300), and mildly elevated alkaline phosphatase. Cytomegalovirus can be cultured frequently from urine during the illness, and viruria may persist for many weeks.

Liver biopsy specimens usually show mononuclear cell infiltrates in the portal triads and lobular sinusoids. Focal hepatocellular necrosis and a patchy mononuclear inflammatory reaction may be seen. Noncaseating epithelioid granulomas are sometimes seen.

The diagnosis is confirmed by demonstrating a fourfold rise (or fall) in the CMV complement-fixation titer (with or without a positive CMV culture) and the absence of serologic changes suggesting another etiology.

Epstein-Barr Virus

Anicteric hepatitis is a common finding in the infectious mononucleosis syndrome caused by Epstein-Barr virus (EBV). Serum transaminase levels are elevated in over 90% of the cases and alkaline phosphatase in over 50%. Jaundice occurs in less than 10%. Pathology of the liver shows patchy focal necrosis with a mononuclear infiltrate in the portal areas and in the sinusoids. Hepatic failure has only rarely been reported.

The EBV may be transmitted by blood transfusion and has been one of the causes of posttransfusion hepatitis which must be ruled out to establish the diagnosis of NANB hepatitis. Serology usually will distinguish EBV hepatitis from anicteric viral hepatitis. A fourfold or greater rise in EBV titer or a positive differential heterophile absorption test will help establish the diagnosis. The course of the hepatitis generally is self-limited and mild although it can persist for several weeks.

Herpes Simplex

Herpes simplex virus (HSV) rarely causes hepatitis, and when it does, involvement is part of disseminated herpes simplex infection. Both HSV-1 and HSV-2 have been associated with disseminated infection and hepatitis. The patients are usually immunocompromised. Severe infections have been associated with fever, leukopenia, hypotension, progressive hepatic failure, and disseminated intravascular coagulation. Pathologic specimens have shown areas of coagulation necrosis in the liver with little acute inflammation. Cowdry's type A inclusion bodies (eosinophilic nuclear inclusions surrounded by a clear halo) have been described. These patients typically have obvious herpetic skin or mucosal lesions, and esophagitis is common. Diagnosis includes serologic evaluation and cultures for HSV. Mild liver function abnormalities are usually present.

Yellow Fever Virus

Yellow fever is an acute disease caused by the arthropod-borne yellow fever virus. The disease occurs in South and Central America and in sub-Saharan Africa. The incubation period is 3-6 days following the bite of an infected mosquito (Aedes aegypti). Abrupt onset of chills, fever, headache, malaise, myalgias, nausea, and vomiting occur and last for about 3 days. A brief remission usually lasting for several hours to days follows. Then patients develop fever, jaundice, petechiae, and often a bleeding diathesis with hematemesis from bleeding points in the stomach and duodenum. The liver function tests are abnormal with elevated transaminase, direct and indirect bilirubin, and prolonged prothrombin time. Liver biopsy shows hepatocellular necrosis of the midzonal portion of the liver with intracellular Councilman bodies. There is little if any inflammatory cell infiltrate even with severe panlobular damage. Mortality is variable but may be as high as 60%.

The diagnosis should be suspected in patients who present with a fulminant type of hepatitis and a history of recent travel to or through an endemic area and no history of yellow fever vaccination. Diagnosis can be made by culture, serology, or histopathologic changes.

Lassa Virus

This arenavirus is responsible for Lassa fever, an acute febrile illness characterized by fever, chilliness, malaise, myalgia, and diarrhea. Other symptoms such as severe sore throat, headache, epigastric pain, vomiting, and cough may be seen.

Physical examination may reveal petechiae, cervical lymphadenopathy, conjunctival suffusion, and occasionally a central macular rash. Laboratory findings include leukopenia, proteinuria, and elevated liver function tests (SGOT, SGPT, LDH). The CPK level also may be elevated, and the electrocardiogram may show evidence of myocarditis. The hepatitis has not been extensively studied because of the infectious risk. The mortality appears to be very high.

The disease is found in western Africa and can be spread from person to person. Suspected patients with a history of recent travel to an endemic area should be placed in strict isolation. Diagnosis may be made serologically or by culture. Virus has been found in the serum and urine for the first 2-3 weeks of illness, and attempts to isolate the virus should only be made by experienced laboratories equipped with class 4 maximum containment facilities. All body fluid and blood specimens should be handled with extreme caution.

Immunoprophylaxis of Viral Hepatitis

The official recommendations for immunoprophylaxis of viral hepatitis are made by the Public Health Service Advisory Committee on Immunization Practices (ACIP) and have been published by the Centers for Disease Control (1981). These recommendations are similar in many respects to earlier ones proposed by that committee (1977). Seeff and Hoofnagle (1979) have reviewed the earlier recommendations and suggested some alternatives based on their interpretation of the available literature. (This author agrees with some of their recommendations and therefore, these alternative recommendations are included in the tables.)

Human immune globulin (IG) (formerly ISG, or gamma globulin), given intramuscularly or subcutaneously, is the agent of choice for prevention of type A hepatitis (Table 26.2). Some studies have shown greater efficacy with doses higher than those recommended by the ACIP. Anti-HAV titers in lots of IG are not standardized; thus some authors recommend a higher dose. No hepatitis A vaccine is available.

Table 26.3 shows the recommendations published by the CDC and alternative recommendations for immunoprophylaxis against hepatitis B infection. Screening serology (HBsAg and anti-HBs) is advisable in all persons who are to receive hepatitis B prophylaxis because positive evidence of previous HBV infection would negate the necessity for prophylaxis (Table 26.4). If the results of such screening will not be available within 7 days of a *definite* exposure (e.g., contaminated needle-stick), it is advisable to give the first dose of high-titer hepatitis B immune globulin (HBIG) as soon as possible and to base the need for the second dose on the pending serology. Prevention of hepatitis B is still controversial, partially because of the high cost of HBIG and partially because some studies have shown that currently available IG (with measurable anti-HBs) may be as effective as HBIG in some situations. The Bureau of Biologics is currently considering a recommendation that all IG produced in the United States be required to contain a standardized minimal anti-HBs titer. Presently no measurable anti-HBs titer is required in IG, but most, if not all, lots have some antibody.

A new hepatitis B vaccine is available which is prepared from the plasma of hepatitis B carriers and consists of noninfectious purified HBsAg. Immunization results in the development of only anti-HBs. The vaccine has been shown to be safe and highly protective against HBV infection in randomized placebo-controlled trials. Because it is weakly immunogenic, several doses are required. It is likely that periodic booster doses will be necessary to maintain good antibody levels. High-risk persons such as medical and dental personnel, persons dealing with blood or blood products, hemodialysis patients, and others should be considered for the vaccine. Trials are currently in progress evaluating the efficacy of passive-active immunity with HBIG and the hepatitis B vaccine.

Without specific tests for diagnosing non-A, non-B hepatitis, the value of prophylactic immune globulins is unknown. Some authors recommend prophylaxis in cases of needle-stick or mucosal exposure to blood from a patient with NANBH and in patients receiving numerous units of transfused blood or human serum concentrates (e.g., factor VIII, factor IX). Human immune globulin in a single dose of 0.06 ml/kg has been suggested, but there is no good evidence that this is effective. Since most posttransfusion hepatitis is due to NANBHV, the elimination of high-risk blood and donors might reduce the incidence of disease. Recently the Transfusion-Transmitted Viruses Study Group has reported a significant association between transfusion of blood containing an elevated alanine aminotransferase (ALT) and the subsequent development of NANBH in recipients of such blood. Thirty-three percent of recipients of a single unit of blood with an ALT > 45 IU and 91% of those receiving two such units developed NANBH compared with 8% who received

TABLE 26.2   Immunoprophylaxis for Prevention of Type A Hepatitis Using Human Immune Globulin (IG)

Recommended for Use	Type of Exposure	Circumstances of Exposure	Dose[1] (ml/kg) [Alternate Dose][2]	Number of Doses
Yes	Postexposure	Close contact with persons having acute hepatitis A (households, sexual contacts, prisons, institutions for mentally retarded, day-care centers)	0.02 [0.06][2]	1
Yes	Preexposure	Travelers to tropical and developing countries who will depart from ordinary tourist routes.		
		Visit < 3 mo	0.02 [0.06]	1
		Visit > 3 mo	0.06 [0.06]	Every 5 mo [Every 4 mo]
		Handlers of nonhuman primates	0.05 [0.06]	Every 4–6 mo [Every 4 mo]
No	Postexposure	Casual school, office, factory or hospital contacts (unless an epidemic develops)	None	None
		Common-source exposure	None	None

[1]Advisory Committee on Immunization Practices: *MMWR* 30(34):423–435, 1981
[2]Seff, L. B. and Hoofnagle, J. H.: *Gastroenterology* 77:161–182, 1979

TABLE 26.3   Immunoprophylaxis for Prevention of Type B Hepatitis

Recommended for Use	Type of Exposure	Circumstance of Exposure	Agent and Dosage[1] [Alternate Regimen][2]	Number of Doses
Yes	Postexposure	Acute exposure to HBsAg (accidental needle-stick or mucosal exposure)	HBIG, 0.06 ml/kg [HBIG, 5 ml]	Two (one immediately - within 7 days and second, same dose 25–30 days later)
[Yes][2]	[Postexposure]	[Sexual contacts of persons with acute hepatitis B during previous 1 mo]	[HBIG, 5 ml]	[as above]
Yes	Postexposure	Infants born to HBsAg positive mother	HBIG, 0.5 ml	Three, at birth (within 24 hr) and same dose at 3 and 6 mo
No	Preexposure	Hemodialysis units, custodial institutions for the mentally retarded (if it is used IG is recommended)	IG, 0.05–0.07 ml/kg	Every 4 mo

[1]Advisory Committee on Immunization Practices: *MMWR* 30(34):423–435, 1980
[2]Seeff, L. B. and Hoofnagle, J. H.: *Gastroenterology* 77:161–182, 1979

TABLE 26.4   Interpretation of Hepatitis B Antigen and Antibody Profile

Antigen	Antibody	Meaning
HBsAg+	–	Early acute illness
HBsAg+ HBeAg+	–	Early acute illness
HBsAg+ HBeAg+	Anti-HBc + Anti-HBe – Anti-HBs –	Acute illness or chronic carrier state
HBsAg+ HBeAg–	Anti-HBc + Anti-HBs –	Acute illness probably resolving or chronic carrier state
–	Anti-HBc + Anti-HBe + Anti-HBs –	Convalescence (called "window phase," is seen for 1 to several weeks following resolution of clinical illness)
–	Anti-HBc + Anti-HBe + Anti-HBs +	Recovery state, no longer infectious
–	Anti-HBc + Anti-HBs + Anti-HBe –	Recovery

no units with an ALT > 45 IU. The risk of developing NANBH after transfusion was also greater with paid donor blood, especially that coming from commercial agencies, than with volunteer blood.

Therapy of Viral Hepatitis

Acute Hepatitis

Treatment of acute viral hepatitis is supportive. A high-calorie, vitamin-supplemented, balanced diet is recommended. Restricted activity has generally been recommended during acute illness but there is no evidence that this hastens recovery or prevents chronic liver disease. It is prudent to avoid vigorous exercise, however, for several weeks. Sedatives and other drugs metabolized in the liver should be avoided if possible.

Hospitalization is sometimes required for prolonged anorexia, nausea, and vomiting, or severe cases. Patients with type A hepatitis should be placed on enteric isolation and blood precautions. Patients with type B or suspected NANB hepatitis should be on blood precautions. A private room is usually not necessary unless the patient is incontinent of feces.

Studies using ACTH or corticosteroids in acute hepatitis have not shown them to be beneficial and they are not recommended.

Fulminant Hepatitis

Patients with massive hepatic necrosis need intensive support with a severely restricted protein diet, management of hypoglycemia with glucose administration, and control of gastrointestinal bleeding. Maintenance of the airway is essential and if respiratory failure is imminent, endotracheal intubation is necessary. Intravenous nutrition with vitamin supplementation, especially thiamine, is necessary. Depression of clotting factors made in the liver is a characteristic finding and bleeding is common. Infusion of cimetidine has been shown to decrease gastrointestinal bleeding but does not influence survival. Fresh-frozen plasma should be used only as necessary to control bleeding episodes. Cleansing of the bowel to reduce ammonia formation has been standard therapy in hepatic encephalopathy. Either neomycin (1 g every 4-6 hr orally or by nasogastric tube) or lactulose (30-50 ml every 2 hr until diarrhea occurs, then every 4-6 hr to keep the stool pH < 6) may be used. Corticosteroids are of no proven benefit and the risks weigh against their use. Infusion of immune serum globulin has *not* been shown to be of benefit.

Experimental centers have undertaken heroic measures in an attempt to reverse fulminant hepatic failure and these include: plasmapheresis, exchange transfusions, hemodialysis, or peritoneal dialysis, cross-circulation with human volunteers or nonhuman primates, hemoperfusion over charcoal, and polyacrylonitrite-membrane hemodialysis. The only controlled trial was using exchange transfusion and there was no therapeutic benefit.

Chronic Hepatitis

Chronic persistent hepatitis does not require therapy. Chronic active hepatitis (CAH) may cause symptomatic episodes with marked malaise, fever, and increases in transaminase and bilirubin. If the biopsy of the liver shows chronic active hepatitis, a course of steroid therapy for several months may be tried. Prednisolone 15 mg daily has been suggested by Sherlock. The disease is not usually reversible and CAH often progresses to cirrhosis or liver failure, although steroid therapy may slow the progression. A recent prospective controlled study in HBsAg-positive patients with CAH showed a deleterious effect of prednisolone on the course of their disease. Thus in patients who have CAH with HBsAg in the blood, steroids should probably be avoided.

Because of the severe outcome of chronic active hepatitis, investigators have turned their attention to more specific modes of therapy. Studies using some agents are promising but all are still investigational, including transfer factor, interferon, levamisole, adenine arabinoside (ara-A), ribavirin, and (+)-cyanidanol-3. No form of therapy has proved to be very effective thus far. Controlled trials with various drugs and combinations of antiviral and immunotherapy are underway at the present time.

Selected Bibliography

Aach, R. D., Szmuness, W., Mosley, J. W., Hollinger, F. B., Kahn, R. A., Stevens, C. E., Edwards, V. M., and Werch, J.: Serum alanine aminotransferase of donors in relation to the risk of non-A, non-B hepatitis in recipients. The Transfusion-Transmitted Viruses Study. *N Engl J Med* 304:989-994, 1981.

Acute Hepatic Failure Study Group: Failure of specific immunotherapy in fulminant type B hepatitis. *Ann Intern Med* 86:272-277, 1977.

Advisory Committee on Immunization Practices: Immune globulins for protection against viral hepatitis. *Morbid Mortal Wk Rep* 26:425-428, 441-442, 1977.

Advisory Committee on Immunization Practices: Immune globulins for protection against viral hepatitis. *Morbid Mortal Wk Rep* 30:423-435, 1981.

Bradley, D. W.: Hepatitis A virus infection. Pathogenesis and serodiagnosis of acute disease. *J Virol Meth* 2:31-45, 1980.

Clarke, J., Craig, R. M., Saffro, R., Murphy, P., and Yokoo, H.: Cytomegalovirus granulomatous hepatitis. *Am J Med* 66:264-269, 1979.

Dienstag, J. L., Alaama, A., Mosley, J. W., Redeker, A. G., and Purcell, R. H.: Etiology of sporadic hepatitis B surface antigen-negative hepatitis. *Ann Intern Med* 87:1-6, 1977.

Eron, L., Kosinski, K., and Hirsch, M. S.: Hepatitis in an adult caused by herpes simplex virus type 1. *Gastroenterology* 71:500-504, 1976.

Favero, M. S., Maynard, J. E., Leger, R. T., Graham, D. R., and Dixon, R. E.: Guidelines for the care of patients hospitalized with viral hepatitis. *Ann Intern Med* 91:872-876, 1979.

Fawaz, K. A., Grady, G. F., Kaplan, M. M., and Gellis, S. S.: Repetitive maternal-fetal transmission of fatal hepatitis B. *N Engl J Med* 293:1357-1359, 1975.

Francis, D. P. and Maynard, J. E.: The transmission and outcome of hepatitis A, B, and non-A, non-B: A review. *Epidemiol Rev* 1:17-31, 1979.

Grady, G. F., Lee, V. A., Prince, A. M., Gitnick, G. L., Fawaz, K. A., Vyas, G. N., et al.: Hepatitis B immune globulin for accidental exposures among medical personnel: Final report of a multicenter controlled trial. *J Infect Dis* 138:625-637, 1978.

Gregory, P. B., Knauer, C. M., Kempson, R. L., and Miller, R.: Steroid therapy in severe viral hepatitis. A double-blind, randomized trial of methylprednisolone versus placebo. *N Engl J Med* 294:681-687, 1976.

Hadler, S. C., Sorley, D. L., Acree, K. H., Webster, H. M., Schable, C. A., Francis, D. P., and Maynard, J. E.: An outbreak of hepatitis B in a dental practice. *Ann Intern Med* 95:133-138, 1981.

Hadler, S. C., Webster, H. M., Erben, J. J., Swanson, J. E., and Maynard, J. E.: Hepatitis A in day-care centers: A community-wide assessment. *N Engl J Med* 302:1222-1227, 1980.

Hoofnagle, J. H., Gerety, R. J., Tabor, E., Feinstone, S. M., Barker, L. F., and Purcell, R. H.: Transmission of non-A, non-B hepatitis. *Ann Intern Med* 87:14-20, 1977.

Iber, F.: Easier decisions in viral hepatitis for the practitioner. *JAMA* 245:849, 1981.

Koff, R. S.: *Viral Hepatitis.* John Wiley & Sons, New York, 1978, p. 242.

Krugman, S. and Gocke, D. J.: *Viral Hepatitis.* W. B. Saunders Co., Philadelphia, 1978, p. 147.

Krugman, S., Overby, L. R., Mushahwar, I. K., Ling, C-M., Frosner, G. G., and Deinhardt, F.: Viral hepatitis type B: Studies on natural history and prevention re-examined. *N Engl J Med* 300:101-106, 1979.

Lam, K. C., Lai, C. L., Trepo, C., and Wu, P.C.: Deleterious effect of prednisolone in HBsAg-positive chronic active hepatitis. *N Engl J Med* 304:380-386, 1981.

Lauer, J. L., Van Drunen, N. A., Washburn, J. W., and Balfour, H. H., Jr.: Transmission of hepatitis B virus in clinical laboratory areas. *J Infect Dis* 140: 513-516, 1979.

Leichtner, A. M., LeClair, J., Goldmann, D. A., Schumacher, R. T., Gewolb, I. H., and Katz, A. J.: Horizontal nonparenteral spread of hepatitis B among children. *Ann Intern Med* 94:346-349, 1981.

Maupas, P., Chiron, J. P., Barin, F., Coursaget, P., Goudeau, A., Perrin, J., Denis, F., and Diop Mar, I.: Efficacy of hepatitis B vaccine in prevention of early HBsAg carrier state in children. *Lancet* 1:289-292, 1981.

McAuliffe, V. J., Purcell, R. H., and Gerin, J. L.: Type B hepatitis. A review of current prospects for a safe and effective vaccine. *Rev Infect Dis* 2:470-492, 1980.

Meek, E. S. and O'Connor, M. L.: Hepatitis B: A review. *Crit Rev Clin Lab Sci* 7:49-98, 1976.

Mosley, J. W.: Epidemiology of viral hepatitis: An overview. *Am J Med Sci* 270: 253-270, 1975.

Mosley, J. W., Redeker, A. G., Feinstone, S. M., and Purcell, R. H.: Multiple hepatitis viruses in multiple attacks of acute viral hepatitis. *N Engl J Med* 296: 75-78, 1977.

Prince, A. M., Szmuness, W., Mann, M. K., Vyas, G. N., Grady, G. F., Shapiro, F. L., Suki, W. N., Freidman, E. A., Avram, M. M., and Stenzel, K. H.: Hepatitis B immune globulin. Final report of a controlled, multicenter trial of efficacy in prevention of dialysis-associated hepatitis. *J Infect Dis* 137:131-144, 1978.

Redeker, A. G.: Viral hepatitis: Clinical aspects. *Am J Med Sci* 270:9-16, 1975.

Rubin, E.: Acute and chronic viral hepatitis. *Fed Proc* 38:2665-2673, 1979.

Scullard, G. H., Pollard, R. B., Smith, J. L., Sacks, S. L., Gregory, P. B., Robinson, W. S., and Merigan, T. C.: Antiviral treatment of chronic hepatitis B virus infection. I. Changes in viral markers with interferon combined with adenine arabinoside. *J Infect Dis* 143:772-783, 1981.

Seeff, L. B. and Hoofnagle, J. H.: Immunoprophylaxis of viral hepatitis. *Gastroenterology* 77:161-182, 1979.

Seeff, L. B., Zimmerman, J. H., Wright, E. C., Finkelstein, J. D., Garcia-Pont, P., Greenlee, H. B., et al.: A randomized, double blind controlled trial of the efficacy of immune serum globulin for the prevention of post-transfusion hepatitis. *Gastroenterology* 72:111-121, 1977.

Stern, H.: Cytomegalovirus and EB virus infections of the liver. *Br Med Bull* 28: 180-185, 1972.

Szmuness, W., Much, M. I., Prince, A. M., Hoofnagle, J. H., Cherubin, C. E., Harley, E. J., and Block, G. H.: On the role of sexual behavior in the spread of hepatitis B infection. *Ann Intern Med* 83:489-495, 1975.

Tabor, E., Seeff, L. B., and Gerety, R. J.: Chronic non-A, non-B hepatitis carrier state. Transmissible agent documented in one patient over a six-year period. *N Engl J Med* 303:140-143, 1980.

Villarejos, V. M., Provost, P. J., Ittensohn, O. L., McLean, A. A., and Hilleman, M. R.: Seroepidemiological investigations of human hepatitis caused by A, B, and a possible third virus. *Proc Soc Exp Biol Med* 152:524-528, 1976.

Villarejos, V. M., Visona, K. A., Eduarte, C. A., Provost, P. J., Hilleman, M. R.: Evidence for viral hepatitis other than type A or type B among persons in Costa Rica. *N Engl J Med* 293:1350-1352, 1975.

Winn, W. C., Monath, T. P., Murphy, F. A., and Whitfield, S. G.: Lassa virus hepatitis. Observations on a fatal case from the 1972 Sierra Leone epidemic. *Arch Pathol* 99:599-604, 1975.

Zuckerman, A. J.: The three types of human viral hepatitis. *Bull WHO* 56:1-20, 1978.

Zuckerman, A. J. and Howard, C. R.: *Hepatitis Viruses of Man.* Academic Press, New York, 1979, p. 269.

27

HEPATIC ABSCESS
Roger G. Finch, M.B.

Definition

Pyogenic liver abscess is an acute or subacute suppurative infection of the liver parenchyma resulting in local or systemic symptoms. It is caused by a wide variety of bacteria either alone, or as part of a polymicrobial infection, which usually reflects an intraabdominal source for the infection.

Etiology

The bacteria associated with liver abscess are usually of enteric origin, i.e., *Escherichia coli,* anaerobic or microaerophilic streptococci, *Bacteroides* spp, and *Fusobacterium nucleatum.* Other bacteria less commonly found are *Klebsiella* spp, *Proteus* spp, *Staphylococcus aureus,* and *Pseudomonas aeruginosa.* Improved methods for the isolation and identification of anaerobic microorganisms have confirmed their presence in about 50% of the cases of liver abscess and they are probably responsible for the reports of "sterile abscess."

Epidemiology

Pyogenic liver abscess is an uncommon condition with prevalence based on hospital admissions and autopsy series that varies from 0.05 to 0.5%. It is frequently unsuspected in life and only recognized at autopsy. It is associated with advancing age and is found more often in males than females. There appears to be no racial predisposition.

Pathogenesis and Pathology

Pyogenic liver abscess results from infection of the liver parenchyma by a wide range of bacterial pathogens, which reach the liver by one of several routes. These include (1) the portal venous system (portal pyemia) secondary to abdominal sepsis, most notably appendicitis, diverticulitis, and umbilical sepsis; (2) the systemic route via the hepatic artery; (3) ascending cholangitis from biliary tract sepsis; (4) penetrating injuries of the liver; (5) direct spread from contiguous structures such as subphrenic abscess, empyema of the gallbladder, pancreatic abscess, perinephric abscess, or an abscess secondary to a perforated viscus. Appendicitis, diverticulitis, and ascending cholangitis are the most frequent predisposing conditions. There is also an association between metastatic malignant diseases to the liver, from gastrointestinal tumors, and hepatic abscess. The right lobe of the liver is most commonly involved reflecting its predominant blood flow. Abscesses are frequently multiple or multiloculated, although solitary abscesses are found.

Diagnostic Features

Clinical

Systemic manifestations of sepsis are often present with fever, sweats, chills, and rigors. Anorexia, nausea, weight loss, and malaise also may be present. Local manifestations include right upper quadrant pain with tenderness to palpation and percussion over the liver, which may or may not be enlarged. Subcapsular abscess may produce pleuritic chest pain and cough. Both clinical and radiographic findings may indicate elevation of the right hemidiaphragm, sometimes with an effusion and occasionally, consolidation of the right lower lobe. Jaundice may or may not be clinically apparent and there may be few features to suggest hepatic disease, which accounts for delays or failure to diagnose the disease.

Laboratory

Laboratory investigations reveal a polymorphonuclear leukocytosis in two-thirds of patients, with acceleration of the sedimentation rate and variable degrees of anemia. Tests of liver function are frequently remarkably normal with little or no elevation of the transaminases. On the other hand, serum alkaline phosphatase is usually mildly elevated unless there is more pronounced biliary tract obstruction. As the illness progresses hypoalbuminemia develops. Both a rising serum alkaline phosphatase and a falling serum albumin, particularly if the latter is less than 2 g/100 ml, indicate a poor prognosis. Serum vitamin B_{12} levels may be markedly elevated and reflect release secondary to the destruction of liver tissue.

Blood cultures, which are positive in up to 50% of the cases, should always be obtained and set up for anaerobic as well as aerobic pathogens. Bacteremia is more frequently associated with multiple hepatic abscesses than with solitary ones.

Plain radiographs of the abdomen may confirm the presence of hepatomegaly, but gas within an abscess cavity is rarely seen on the plain radiograph. The chest radiograph may show an elevated hemidiaphragm, obliteration of the costophrenic angle from an effusion of varying size, and occasional consolidation or atelectasis at the right base.

Ultrasound and radionuclide scans of the liver are the most valuable investigations. Both techniques can detect lesions down to 2 cm in diameter. In addition to strongly suggesting the diagnosis, they can both locate and indicate if there are single or multiple abscesses present. They also are extremely valuable in differentiating intrahepatic abscesses from subdiaphragmatic or subhepatic abscesses.

Other more invasive techniques include selective celiac angiography, which can aid in the differentiation of vascular neoplasms from avascular abscesses or cysts.

The diagnosis may occasionally be made by blind needle biopsy of the liver when the patient is under investigation for fever of unknown origin. A liver biopsy is not usually recommended unless preparations for immediate surgery are made beforehand.

Differential Diagnosis

Several other pyogenic conditions may mimic intrahepatic abscess. These include subdiaphragmatic and subhepatic abscess, perinephric abscess, ascending cholangitis, and empyema of the gallbladder. Among malignant conditions, primary hepatocellular carcinoma can closely simulate an hepatic abscess, as can metastatic malignant disease. Amebic liver abscess tends to have a more insidious onset and is considered in Chapter 123.

Treatment

The management of liver abscess is primarily surgical. Incision and drainage of the abscess or abscesses usually result in prompt resolution of symptoms. The surgical approach will be determined by the location of the abscess. Occasionally with multiple-abscess formation complete drainage of the abscess material may not be feasible. Needle aspiration has also proved successful.

Antimicrobial therapy is an important adjunct to surgery and needs to be given in full dosages for extended periods. Although occasional reports have suggested antimicrobial therapy alone may be effective, this experience is not universal and failures have been reported.

Antimicrobial-sensitivity testing of blood and pus isolates are a useful guide to the selection of appropriate agents. Ampicillin is frequently effective in the management of *Escherichia coli* infections and will also adequately cover the penicillin-sensitive anaerobic organisms, namely peptostreptococci and *Bacteroides* spp other than *B. fragilis.* It will also be effective against the microaerophilic streptococci that have been associated with liver abscess, such as *Streptococcus milleri.* Either chloramphenicol, clindamycin, or metronidazole would also be appropriate therapy for the treatment of anaerobic hepatic abscess.

The duration of therapy has not been established, but it is recommended that at least 4 weeks therapy should be given following surgical drainage. Treatment should be guided by clinical response, resolution of biochemical abnormalities, and may be aided by repeat hepatic scans to show shrinkage of the abscess cavity.

Complications and Prognosis

Systemic complications are primarily those of septicemia and shock, particularly if the abscess is associated with gram-negative bacillemia. Rupture of the abscess will produce peritonitis and carries the risk of metastatic abscess formation.

Occasionally rupture has occurred into the pleural cavity to produce an empyema. Portal vein thrombosis and portal hypertension are rare complications.

With early diagnosis and a combined therapeutic approach (surgical drainage plus appropriate antimicrobials) mortality still approaches 25-30%.

Selected Bibliography

Bateman, N. T., Eykyn, S. J., and Phillips, I.: Pyogenic liver abscess caused by *Streptococcus milleri*. *Lancet* 1:657-659, 1975.

Berger, L. A. and Osborne, B. R.: Treatment of pyogenic liver abscesses by percutaneous needle aspiration. *Lancet* 1:132-134, 1982.

Herbert, D. A., Rothman, J., Simmons, S., Fogel, D. A., Wilson, S., and Ruskin, J.: Pyogenic liver abscesses: Successful nonsurgical therapy. *Lancet* 1:134-136, 1982.

Pitt, H. A. and Zuidema, G. C.: Factors influencing mortality in the treatment of pyogenic hepatic abscess. *Surg Gynecol Obstet* 140:228-324, 1975.

Ramson, J. H. C., Madayag, M. A., Localio, S. A. and Spencer, S. C.: New diagnostic and therapeutic techniques in the management of pyogenic liver abscesses. *Ann Surg* 181:508-517, 1975.

Rubin, R. H., Swartz, M. N., and Malt, R.: Hepatic abscess: Changes in clinical, bacteriologic and therapeutic aspects. *Am J Med* 57:601-610, 1974.

Sabbaj, J., Sutter, V. L., and Finegold, S. M.: Anaerobic pyogenic liver abscess. *Ann Intern Med* 77:629-638, 1972.

28

CHOLECYSTITIS AND CHOLANGITIS
Gary R. Plotkin, M.D.

Cholecystitis, which may be acute or chronic, is a pathologic diagnosis; i.e., histologically, the wall of the gallbladder is characterized by various degrees of inflammation. Cholangitis may be defined as inflammation of the bile ducts and is most commonly associated with a common duct stone. Two clinical forms of acute cholangitis have been described: suppurative obstructive and nonsuppurative types.

Microbiology

The exact role of infection in the pathogenesis of various disorders involving the gallbladder and biliary tree has long been controversial. Although bacteria of many types, including Enterobacteriaceae and obligate anaerobes, may be found in both the contents and wall of gallbladders in the presence of cholecystitis, choledocholithiasis, or cholelithiasis, they also occur in the absence of inflammation and obstruction. Bacteria in concentrations of 10^5/ml or higher may exist in the biliary tract of asymptomatic individuals. However, the incidence of bactibilia is higher in acute cholecystitis than in chronic and is especially high when there is obstruction of the bile duct. The organisms found in the gallbladder are similar to those in the normal intestinal flora, and it has been postulated that the bacteria reach the biliary tree by an ascending route. Bacteria also may be excreted by the liver into bile or colonize the biliary system from the hematogenous or lymphatic routes. It has been postulated that asymptomatic bactibilia becomes manifested clinically either as cholangitis or empyema of the gallbladder following surgery, obstruction, and percutaneous or operative cholangiography. Of the anaerobic bacteria, *Clostridium perfringens* and *Bacteroides fragilis* are the most commonly isolated in patients with empyema of the gallbladder or sepsis from a biliary tract focus. Whether or not infection is an important cause of uncomplicated acute cholecystitis is unknown. Bacterial invasion of the gallbladder may be a secondary phenomenon occurring after acute cholecystitis has developed because of obstruction, chemical irritation, or vascular occlusion. Estimates of the incidence of positive cultures in acute cholecystitis vary from a few to 75%, with the higher percentage being associated with diabetes mellitus or advanced age. Bacteria less commonly isolated from acutely inflamed gallbladders include *Brucella, Acinetobacter, Salmonella, Arizona, Haemophilus, Yersinia,* and *Mycobacterium.* Fungi also have been cultured from surgically removed gallbladders.

Emphysematous cholecystitis is a rare form of acute, usually gangrenous, cholecystitis in which gas is demonstrated within the lumen and wall of the gallbladder and frequently with the concomitant pericholecystic infiltration of gas. This type of infection is caused by a mixture of facultative and obligate anaerobes with *Clostridium perfringens* being most frequently isolated.

Acute cholangitis results from the invasion of an obstructed biliary tree by enteric organisms, most commonly *Escherichia coli, Klebsiella, Streptococcus, Enterobacter, Pseudomonas, Citrobacter, Bacteroides, Staphylococcus, Proteus,* and *Clostridium.* The term cholangitis lenta signifies a rare hematogenous form of suppurative cholangitis associated with endocarditis in the absence of biliary obstruction. Gram-negative septicemia with or without endotoxic shock may be associated with the acute suppurative obstructive form of cholangitis.

Nonbacterial pathogens have been associated with various disorders of the gallbladder, and ascariasis and infestation by liver flukes are the most important and prevalent parasitic diseases of the biliary system. Other parasites including *Entamoeba histolytica, Trichomonas,* and *Taenia saginata* also have been identified in duodenal biliary drainage and in gallbladders removed at operation. *Giardia lamblia* has also been associated with cholecystitis.

Pathogenesis and Pathology

The pathogenesis of acute cholecystitis is only partially understood, i.e., acute inflammation of the gallbladder may be due to vascular insufficiency or induced by various chemical or mechanical factors. More than 90% of acute cholecystitis is associated with cholelithiasis; however, 50% of the patients with gallbladder stones may remain asymptomatic. Nevertheless, the initiating event in acute cholecystitis usually is obstruction of the cystic duct by a gallstone. Also, stagnant bile probably exerts an irritant inflammatory action on the gallbladder mucosa. Further injury of the gallbladder is induced by high intraluminal pressures generated by the cystic duct obstruction. This increased pressure results in collapse of the nutrient blood vessels within the gallbladder wall, and thus ischemia occurs. Whether the presence of bacteria represents a primary initiating event or a secondary phenomenon remains unknown. Bacterial invasion may intensify or propagate the inflammatory changes once they are initiated by the aforementioned factors.

The pathogenesis of acute acalculous cholecystitis which occurs in 2-10% of all patients with acute cholecystitis remains an enigma. Kinked cystic duct, periductal adhesions, enlarged cystic node, tortuous cystic artery, and pancreatic reflux have been implicated as etiologic agents. Acalculous cholecystitis occurs in association with congenital anomalies of the biliary or vascular systems, vasculitis, debilitation, diabetes mellitus, hypertension, congestive heart failure, cor pulmonale, arteriosclerosis, malignancies, and in the postpartum, postsurgical, and posttrauma patient.

Cholangitis is associated with common duct obstruction and bacteria in the bile. The word ascending often is used to describe the pathogenesis of infection, i.e., from the alimentary canal. However, the mechanisms whereby the extrahepatic biliary tract becomes infected are unknown. Lymphatic and hematogenous routes, as well as hepatic excretion of bacteria filtered from the portal vein, also may be involved in producing cholangitis. It has been postulated that the chills and fever of cholangitis are due to bacteria being regurgitated into the bloodstream from the bile ducts. Cholangitis occurs more frequently with bile duct stricture and common duct stones than with carcinomas of the papilla and pancreas. Choledocholithiasis, besides producing cholangitis, may cause pressure necrosis of the duct resulting in a fistula, bile peritonitis, or hemobilia.

Nonsuppurative cholangitis, which is the most common type of acute cholangitis, usually is caused by calculous biliary obstruction, parasites, biliary stricture, or periampullary malignancy. Movement of stones within the common bile duct may account for the intermittent nature of acute nonsuppurative cholangitis. The ductal obstruction results in jaundice, biliary colic, and perhaps infection of stagnated bile, as well as occasionally bacteremia. The latter may account for the chills and fever.

In acute suppurative obstructive cholangitis, purulent material accumulates under increasing pressure in the biliary tract. A common duct stone is the initiating event in most patients, but malignancies of the biliary tree or pancreas, stricture, pancreatitis, and parasites also may be precipitating factors. Acute suppurative cholangitis may or may not follow the nonsuppurative form. The bile ducts are dilated above the site of obstruction, have inflammatory thickening of their walls, and may contain purulent material. In suppurative obstructive cholangitis the liver tends to be diffusely enlarged and congested with degrees of necrosis varying from central lobular degeneration to multiple abscesses. Liver biopsies reveal pericholangitis with acute and chronic inflammatory cells within, and adjacent to, the portal tracts. Proliferation of bile ducts is present, and the inflammatory cellular infiltration extends from the portal tracts into the liver parenchyma.

Diagnosis

Clinical

The typical attack of acute cholecystitis usually commences with acute abdominal pain and tenderness and may mimic previous episodes of self-limited biliary colic. The pain initially is either poorly localized or maximally felt in the epigastrium or left upper quadrant. Later, the pain moves to the right-upper quadrant, increases in severity and is associated with anorexia and vomiting. This pattern of visceral pain reflects parietal involvement as the gallbladder becomes inflamed. Rarely, the pain may be more intense in the back or shoulder rather than in the abdomen. If local infection or systemic sepsis occurs, the patient may experience chills or even present in shock.

The clinical findings in acute cholecystitis are variable. The temperature usually ranges from 99 to 102°F, and a higher value should suggest suppurative complications. As the patient breathes in deeply while the physician palpates the right subcostal region, pain is elicited and inspiratory arrest occurs momentarily (Murphy's sign). In a few patients, especially the elderly, local findings are not very impressive, and symptoms consist of mild anorexia and abdominal discomfort. In other individuals, however, abdominal guarding and localized rebound tenderness are prominent and complications including empyema or perforation of the gallbladder and sepsis are likely to develop. In approximately one-third of the patients with acute cholecystitis the gallbladder is palpable as a tender mass and is usually enlarged in those experiencing their first attack. When a right upper quadrant mass or fullness is recognized, one must consider emphysematous cholecystitis, localized perforation of the gallbladder with pericholecystic abscess, and carcinoma of the gallbladder. The latter may coexist with acute or subacute cholecystitis. Many patients admitted for treatment of acute cholecystitis present with dehydration, peritonitis, reflex paralytic ileus with abdominal distention, and even sepsis and shock. Jaundice is present in about 20% of patients with acute cholecystitis.

An unexplained fever may be due to subacute or chronic cholecystitis or perforated gallbladder without specific symptoms or abnormal physical findings. These patients are often debilitated or elderly. Rarely, fever may be secondary to subhepatic abscess following an earlier attack of cholecystitis.

The clinical definition of cholangitis comprises Charcot's triad, which consists of right upper quadrant abdominal pain, jaundice, and fever with chills. The duration and severity of cholangitis may be variable, i.e., an attack can be either transient, self-limited, and mild, or sustained and associated with sepsis. Pain may be absent and jaundice usually appears within 24 hr. An enlarged and palpable gallbladder is unusual in patients with choledocholithiasis since the gallbladder is usually scarred and nondistensible from previous chronic cholecystitis. The presence of a palpable, nontender gallbladder in a jaundiced patient (Courvoisier's law) suggests that the biliary obstruction is secondary to a malignancy. Hepatic enlargement may be detected in calculous biliary obstruction, and mild to moderate tenderness often is present in the right upper quadrant during the acute attack.

In nonsuppurative cholangitis, which is the most common form, blood cultures are frequently positive but the patient is not toxic, and the severe symptoms subside either spontaneously or with medical treatment within 24-28 hr. Acute suppurative obstructive cholangitis consists of unremitting severe cholangitis with bacteremia, and mental confuson, lethargy, and septic shock are prominent features. It is about one-tenth as frequent as the nonsuppurative form.

Laboratory

With respect to laboratory diagnosis, elevations of serum conjugated bilirubin, alkaline phosphatase and transaminases in association with abdominal pain are highly suggestive of biliary tract disease. Approximately 75% of patients with acute cholecystitis and common duct obstruction have elevated levels of serum transaminase, and the values are higher than those with acute cholecystitis without choledocholithiasis.

In patients with acute cholecystitis, plain roentgenograms of the abdomen often demonstrate localized ileus or air-fluid levels in the right upper quadrant. Radiopaque gallstones may comprise 10-30% of all gallstones and thus may be detected by abdominal roentgenograms. Occasionally, radiolucent clefts on the plain radiograph may indicate gallstones and occur as a result of gas accumulating in the center of the stone. Obstruction of a cystic duct in association with chronic inflammation of the gallbladder may result in calcification of the organ's wall (porcelain gallbladder) or in deposition of calcium in the lumen (milk of calcium or limy bile). Abdominal radiographs reveal irregular calcification conforming to the shape of the gallbladder if there is a porcelain gallbladder, while a right upper quadrant calcification may represent limy bile.

Acute inflammation of the gallbladder may cause spasm, edema, and deformity of the hepatic flexure of the colon or contiguous portion of the duodenum, and these changes may be detected on a barium study of the upper gastrointestinal

tract. Marked dilatation of the common duct may compress and displace the duodenum. Additionally, on a barium study, edema of the ampullary region due to an
impacted gallstone may cause a smooth, radiolucent defect in the lumen of the duodenum at the ampulla.

Ultrasound may be helpful in diagnosing acute cholecystitis or cholangitis, especially when gallstones are present. The stones can be detected, as can dilatation
of the bile ducts proximal to an impacted stone. An enlarged gallbladder also can
be noted by ultrasound. Intravenous cholangiography is useful in evaluating patients with possible acute cholecystitis. If the bile ducts but not the gallbladder
opacify, acute cholecystitis is supported, whereas if the bile ducts and gallbladder
both opacify, acute cholecystitis is unlikely. Nonopacification of the ducts and
gallbladder are nonspecific findings. Until recently, cholescintigraphy was limited
to ^{131}I rose bengal in evaluating patients for acute cholecystitis. Radionuclide
gallbladder imaging with technetium 99m N-substituted iminodiacetic acid derivatives is a relatively new method for assessing the flow of bile in the biliary tract.
The main application of this procedure is to exclude cholecystitis by demonstrating
gallbladder filling and therefore, it is an alternative to intravenous cholangiography.

Differential Diagnosis

The principal conditions that one should consider in the differential diagnosis of
acute cholecystitis are acute intermittent porphyria, acute pancreatitis, appendicitis, pyelonephritis or renal calculus, peptic ulcer with or without perforation,
acute hepatitis, pneumonitis, hepatic abscess or tumor, gonococcal perihepatitis,
or cardiac disease. Acute appendicitis most often is confused with acute cholecystitis; however, fever, leukocytosis, and abdominal tenderness usually progress
more inexorably in appendicitis. Pancreatitis may occur in conjunction with acute
cholecystitis. Hepatitis may cause right upper-quadrant abdominal pain and tenderness, fever, leukocytosis, and elevations in liver function tests and may be difficult to distinguish from acute cholecystitis. Gonococcal perihepatitis (Fitz-Hugh-
Curtis syndrome) may produce symptoms localized to the right upper quadrant but
usually adnexal tenderness also will be present. If one suspects pyogenic or amebic hepatic abscesses, a history of antecedent abdominal or amebic infection may
be helpful. ^{99m}Technetium liver scan, ultrasound examination, computerized axial tomography, or hepatic angiography, may be necessary to differentiate liver
from gallbladder disease.

Treatment

Patients with acute cholecystitis usually require hospitalization for combined medical and surgical therapy. Specific medical modalities include analgesics, nasogastric suction, and intravenous fluids. These maneuvers minimize pancreatic secretion and the mechanical and chemical stimuli causing cholecystokinin-induced
gallbladder contraction and also favorably influence ileus. In the patient who is
responding to medical management, the optimal time for cholecystectomy remains unknown. It would be reasonable to postpone surgery until the patient is
clinically stable and has had adequate fluid and electrolyte replacement and correction of other medical problems. Parenteral antibiotics and urgent surgery are
indicated for empyema or perforation of the gallbladder, emphysematous cholecystitis, or progressive signs of peritonitis and sepsis. Since a polymicrobial flora including facultative and obligate anaerobes is involved with these complications of
acute cholecystitis, ampicillin or penicillin plus gentamicin or tobramycin are the

preferred antimicrobial agents. Chloramphenicol is a reasonable alternative agent. Even though certain antimicrobial agents are excreted in high concentration in the bile in experimental animals and in the normal human biliary tract, the concentration of these agents is markedly decreased in the presence of biliary tract obstruction. Additionally, a high bile level of an antibiotic may not correspond to clinical efficacy. The role of antibiotics in uncomplicated acute or chronic cholecystitis with respect to alleviation of symptoms or prevention of complications is unknown.

Acute cholangitis is a serious disease and should be aggressively treated both with measures designed to restore circulatory homeostasis and with systemic antibiotics effective against enteric organisms. Consequently, the same antibiotic regimens as described previously for the complications of acute cholecystitis are appropriate. Since episodic cholangitis is a symptom of mechanical obstruction, radiographic studies and biliary tract surgery are necessary. The timing of surgery is dependent upon the clinical presentation, i.e., acute suppurative obstructive cholangitis usually requires immediate surgery.

Prognosis and Complications

The overall mortality of acute cholecystitis is approximately 5%; however, morbidity and mortality increase with age. Most deaths are due to sepsis, pneumonitis, or cardiovascular complications. Acute cholecystitis is associated with suppurative complications including emphysematous cholecystitis and gangrene or perforation of the gallbladder, especially in patients with diabetes mellitus, and has a mortality of about 20%. Consequently, elective cholecystectomy has been advocated in diabetics with asymptomatic cholelithiasis. If acute cholecystitis is accompanied by jaundice and cholangitis or pancreatitis secondary to concomitant choledocholithiasis, morbidity increases significantly. Additionally, empyema or gangrene of the gallbladder and localized or diffuse peritonitis decrease the operative survival rate. The mortality in suppurative cholangitis is about 50% and is due to septic shock and hepatic or renal failure.

Selected Bibliography

Andrew, D. J. and Johnson, S. E.: Acute suppurative cholangitis, a medical and surgical emergency. A review of ten years experience emphasizing early recognition. *Am J Gastroenterol* 54:141-154, 1970.

Bourgault, A-M., England, D. M., Rosenblatt, J. E., Forgacs, P., and Bieger, R. C.: Clinical characteristics of anaerobic bactibilia. *Arch Intern Med* 139: 1346-1349, 1979.

Cheung, L. Y. and Chang, F. C.: Intravenous cholangiography in the diagnosis of acute cholecystitis. *Arch Surg* 113:568-570, 1978.

Dye, M., MacDonald, A., and Smith, G.: The bacterial flora of the biliary tract and liver in man. *Br J Surg* 65:285-287, 1978.

England, D. M. and Rosenblatt, J. E.: Anaerobes in human biliary tracts. *J Clin Microbiol* 6:494-498, 1977.

Finegold, S. M.: Anaerobes in biliary tract infection. *Arch Intern Med* 139:1338–1339, 1979.

Glenn, F.: Acute acalculous cholecystitis. *Ann Surg* 189:458–465, 1979.

Goodhart, G. L., Levison, M. E., Trotman, B. W., and Soloway, R. D.: Pigment vs. cholesterol cholelithiasis. Bacteriology of gallbladder stone, bile, and tissue correlated with biliary lipid analysis. *Am J Dig Dis* 23:877–882, 1978.

Goswitz, J. T.: Bacteria and biliary tract disease. *Am J Surg* 128:644–646, 1974.

Huck, W. and Britt, M. R.: *Haemophilus aphrophilus* cholecystitis. *Am J Clin Pathol* 69:361–363, 1978.

Jacob, H., Appelman, R., and Stein, H. D.: Emphysematous cholecystitis. *Am J Gastroenterol* 71:325–330, 1979.

Keighley, M. R. B., McLeish, A. R., Bishop, H. M., Burdon, D. W., Quoraishi, A. H., Oates, G. D., Dorricott, N. J., and Alexander-Williams, J.: Identification of the presence and type of biliary microflora by immediate Gram stains. *Surgery* 81:469–472, 1977.

Lam, S. K., Wong, K. P., Chan, P. K. W., Ngan, H., and Ong, G. B.: Recurrent pyogenic cholangitis. A study by endoscopic retrograde cholangiography. *Gastroenterology* 74:1196–1203, 1978.

Lou, M. A., Mandal, A. K., Alexander, J. L., and Thadepalli, H.: Bacteriology of the human biliary tract and the duodenum. *Arch Surg* 112:965–967, 1977.

McLeish, A. R., Keighley, M. R. B., Bishop, H. M., Burdon, D. W., Quoraishi, A. H., Dorricott, N. J., Oates, G. D., and Alexander-Williams, J.: Selecting patients requiring antibiotics in biliary surgery by immediate Gram stains of bile at operation. *Surgery* 81:473–477, 1977.

Mentzer, R. M., Jr., Golden, G. T., Chandler, J. G., and Horsley, J. S., III: A comparative appraisal of emphysematous cholecystitis. *Am J Surg* 129:10–15, 1975.

Miller, D. D.: Postoperative acalculous cholecystitis due to *Torulopsis glabrata*. *Arch Surg* 111:1404–1405, 1976.

Morris, S. J., Greenwald, R. A., Turner, R. L., and Tedesco, F. J.: Brucella-induced cholecystitis. *Am J Gastroenterol* 71:481–484, 1979.

Salk, R. P., Greenburg, A. G., Farris, J. M., and Peskin, G. W.: Spectrum of cholangitis. *Am J Surg* 130:143–150, 1975.

Shimada, K., Inamatsu, T., and Yamashiro, M.: Anaerobic bacteria in biliary disease in elderly patients. *J Infect Dis* 135:850–854, 1977.

Sjodahl, R., Tagesson, C., and Wetterfors, J.: On the pathogenesis of acute cholecystitis. *Surg Gynecol Obstet* 146:199–202, 1978.

Soto, J. M. and Dreiling, D. A.: *Giardia lamblia*. A case presentation of chronic cholecystitis and duodenitis. *Am J Gastroenterol* 67:265–269, 1977.

29

PANCREATIC INFECTIONS
David L. Hoover, M.D.

Infective Pancreatitis

Pancreatitis usually is associated with noninfectious conditions including alcoholism, biliary tract disease, hyperlipidemia, and the administration of various drugs. Certain viruses, however, including mumps and coxsackievirus B, have been clearly implicated in causing acute pancreatitis in adults and children. Several strains of coxsackievirus B likewise can cause acute pancreatic acinar inflammation in mice. Pancreatitis in association with infectious mononucleosis, cytomegalovirus infection, and mycoplasmal pneumonia also has been described in humans. Glucose intolerance may develop in the course of infective pancreatitis. Conservative management as in noninfective forms of the disease is indicated. Pancreatitis associated with mycoplasmal infection might reasonably be treated with erythromycin. Otherwise, antibiotics have no role in management. There is at present no conclusive proof of a viral etiology for juvenile- or adult-onset diabetes mellitus, although several animal models are consistent with such a hypothesis.

Pancreatic Abscess

Pancreatic abscess, a collection of infected pus associated with the pancreas, occurs in about 4% of the cases of acute pancreatitis. Surgical procedures involving structures in the upper abdominal cavity, especially the biliary tract or pancreas, or performed in the presence of pancreatitis, also predispose to abscess formation. Cultures commonly show mixed organisms, with a preponderance of gram-negative bacilli; staphylococci are occasionally seen. Anaerobes have not been reported commonly, but 20% of cultures in some series have been "sterile."

Two patterns of pancreatic abscess development are observed. In the first, fulminant pancreatitis may be present from the start, with prominent signs of sepsis. More commonly, however, a patient with pancreatitis appears to respond initially to conservative management, then relapses in several days to weeks. Recurrence of epigastric pain, local tenderness, and fever (usually $\geq 38.5°C$) should prompt further investigation for the possibility of pancreatic abscess. A palpable epigastric mass or fullness occurs in about 50% of the patients. Leukocytosis with polymorphonuclear leukocyte predominance is usual; elevated serum amylase is found in approximately one-fourth and positive blood cultures in less than half of the cases.

Radiography is helpful in establishing the diagnosis in almost all instances. Chest x-ray, abnormal in the majority, may show an elevated hemidiaphragm, pleural effusion, or atelectasis. Abdominal films may show a localized ileus. A "soap bubble" sign due to loculated extraintestinal air in the abscess cavity is diagnostic, but is seen in fewer than 10% of the cases. Barium contrast studies may reveal mass effects, with displacement of stomach, duodenum, or colon. Ultrasound is often valuable, especially if a cystic mass with multiple internal echoes is observed. Pancreatic pseudocyst and local inflammation of the pancreas presenting as a mass may cause difficulties in diagnosis. This differentiation is of significance because surgery is necessary in the case of abscess and best avoided in the other two conditions.

Successful therapy requires adequate drainage, generally through an anterior abdominal approach. One-third of cases may require repeated drainage procedures. Antibiotic coverage with an aminoglycoside and clindamycin or chloramphenicol should be started immediately before surgery and continued for 7-10 days. Postoperatively, hospital stays of 4-6 weeks are common, and may be complicated by fistula formation, recurrent abscess, intraabdominal or gastrointestinal hemorrhage, pleural effusion, empyema, pneumonia, and atelectasis. Renal insufficiency commonly occurs. Nutritional support may be difficult during this period. Placement of a feeding tube via jejunostomy at the time of initial operation has therefore been advocated. In most series, the case fatality rate is 100% without surgery and 30-40% with surgery. Hemorrhage and pulmonary complications are the most common causes of death. Among survivors, significant sequelae are unusual. There is no evidence that routine treatment of pancreatitis with prophylactic antibiotics prevents the development of an abscess.

Selected Bibliography

Infective Pancreatitis

Craighead, J. E.: The role of viruses in the pathogenesis of pancreatic disease and diabetes mellitus. *Prog Med Virol* 19:161-214, 1975.

Freeman, R. and McMahon, M. J.: Acute pancreatitis and serological evidence of infection with *Mycoplasma pneumoniae. Gut* 19:367-370, 1978.

Hedstrom, S. A. and Belfrage, I.: Acute pancreatitis in two cases of infectious mononucleosis. *Scand J Infect Dis* 8:124-126, 1976.

Imrie, C. W., Ferguson, J. C., and Sommerville, R. G.: Coxsackie and mumpsvirus infection in a prospective study of acute pancreatitis. *Gut* 18:53-56, 1977.

March, P. A. and Ursing, B.: The occurrence of acute pancreatitis in *Mycoplasma pneumoniae* infection. *Scand J Infect Dis* 6:167-171, 1974.

Pancreatic Abscess

Altmeier, W. V. and Alexander, J. W.: Pancreatic abscess: A study of 32 cases. *Arch Surg* 87:80-89, 1963.

Bolooki, H., Jaffe, B., and Gliedman, M. L.: Pancreatic abscesses and lesser omental sac collections. *Surg Gynecol Obstet* 126:1301-1308, 1968.

Camer, S. J., Tan, E. G. C., Warren, K. W., and Braasch, J. W.: Pancreatic abscess. *Am J Surg* 129:426-431, 1975.

Miller, T. A., Lindenauer, S. M., Frey, C. F., and Stanley, J. C.: Pancreatic abscess. *Arch Surg* 108:545-550, 1974.

Ranson, J. H. and Spencer, F. C.: Prevention, diagnosis and treatment of pancreatic abscess. *Surgery* 82:99-106, 1977.

Warshaw, A. L.: Pancreatic abscesses. *N Engl J Med* 287:1234-1236, 1972.

30

ABDOMINAL ABSCESS
Ronica M. Kluge, M.D.

Intraabdominal abscesses can develop following primary or secondary peritonitis. The problem is usually manifested acutely but may take a more indolent course.

Etiology

These abscesses are almost always polymicrobial since they result from spillage of intestinal contents or pelvic secretions into the abdominal cavity. When good anaerobic techniques are applied to abdominal abscess material, an extremely high yield of anaerobes is found (80%). *Bacteroides fragilis,* anaerobic streptococci, and *Clostridium* spp are the most common anaerobic isolates (Table 30.1). Aerobic organisms include *Escherichia coli, Klebsiella, Enterobacter, Proteus, Pseudomonas,* staphylococci, and streptococci including enterococci. Mixed anaerobes and aerobes are recovered about five times as often as either alone.

Epidemiology

Patients of any age can develop abdominal abscesses. The exact origin and location of the abscess will be related to the disease that preceded the abscess. For example, an abscess following a perforated diverticulum is more likely to be seen in an older patient and to occur in the left lower quadrant; a lesser sac abscess most often follows pancreatitis or posterior penetrating peptic ulcer. The most common sources of abdominal abscess are listed in Table 30.2. The miscellaneous group includes septicemia, osteomyelitis of the spine, amebiasis, and inflammatory bowel disease. Surgical procedures and trauma usually are the predisposing factors to

TABLE 30.1   Common Organisms Isolated from Abdominal Abscess*

	Organisms	Percentage
Anaerobes		
	B. fragilis	80-95
	Streptococci	50
	Clostridium spp	50
	Fusobacterium	40
Aerobes		
	E. coli	80-95
	Enterococci	60
	Proteus spp	38

*Usually present as mixed flora

TABLE 30.2   Sources of Abdominal Abscess

Source	Percentage
Appendicitis	10-20
Genitourinary tract	10
Pancreatitis	12
Biliary tract	8
Diverticulitis	7
Trauma	3
Perforating tumors	3
Peptic ulcer	2
Leaking suture line	2
Miscellaneous	15-30
Unknown	10

the development of intraabdominal abscesses. It is well known that emergency surgical procedures carry a greater risk of subsequent abdominal abscesses than do elective procedures.

Pathogenesis

Intraperitoneal abscesses represent areas of localized peritonitis in which the infection is progressive yet is contained ("walled-off") by the inflammatory reaction. There are two general patterns of intraperitoneal abscess development. One is the result of diffuse peritonitis in which loculations of purulent material occur in anatomically dependent areas (pelvis, kidney pouch, subphrenic, paracolic "gutter"). The second is the result of a localized focus of peritonitis related to some contiguous disease process or injury in which the inflammatory defenses prevented diffuse peritonitis. Retroperitoneal abscesses can form in the potential space between the peritoneum and transversalis fascia lining the posterior aspect of the abdominal cavity.

Visceral abscesses (liver, pancreas, kidney) are discussed in other chapters.

Diagnostic Features (Table 30.3)

Clinical

The most characteristic picture is that of an acute illness with fever, chills, and abdominal pain seen following trauma or abdominal surgery. Most abdominal abscesses are recognized within 2-4 weeks postoperatively, but some cases are more indolent and may present 6-12 months later. The fever can be low grade, hectic, or continuously high. It is not uncommon for the patient to have a persistent draining wound or sinus tract. Signs of atelectasis and/or effusion are found on examination in many cases. The patient may have a palpable abdominal mass.

TABLE 30.3   Diagnostic Features of Abdominal Abscess

Feature	Percentage
Fever	82
Abdominal pain	38
Persistent drainage	18
Chest dullness	12
Abdominal mass by palpation	7
Abnormal chest x-ray	61
Abnormal plain film, abdomen	14

Laboratory

The peripheral white blood cell count is usually elevated (15-30,000/mm^3) and shifted markedly to the left. Plain films of the abdomen are suggestive of abscess in a minority of cases: look for collection of gas outside the intestinal lumen, or for a mass. Chest x-rays are abnormal in patients with subphrenic collections: elevated diaphragm, atelectasis, pleural effusion. Gastrointestinal barium studies may show displacement of organs by a mass; an IVP may show similar findings. A combination radionuclide scan of the liver and lungs is frequently of value in outlining a right-sided subphrenic abscess. Gallium scan will detect abdominal abscess in about 80% of the cases. Ultrasound and CT scan are even more helpful in diagnosing intraabdominal collections of pus. Arteriography is rarely needed since gallium, ultrasound and CT have become widely available (Table 30.4).

Differential Diagnosis

The differential diagnosis may include pneumonia, pancreatitis, cholecystitis, diverticulitis, tumor, inflammatory bowel disease, peptic ulcer disease, and genitourinary tract disease. In fact, many of these processes can become complicated by the development of intraabdominal abscess, either directly, or following surgery.

Complications

Diffuse peritonitis, bacteremia, metastatic abscesses, shock and development of fistulae, can complicate intraabdominal abscesses. Almost every abscess of this sort is associated with a prolonged convalescence.

Therapy

Treatment includes supportive measures directed toward nutrition, fluid and electrolyte balance, pulmonary toilet, and good nursing care. The major thrust must

TABLE 30.4   Radiologic Diagnosis of Abdominal Abscess

Test	Percentage
Abnormal chest film	61
Abnormal abdomen film	14
Liver-lung scan	98 (subphrenic)
Gallium scan	82
Ultrasound	96
CT scan	98

be adequate drainage whether by surgery or by catheter placement, in combination with appropriate antimicrobials. Initial antibiotics should be chosen to give coverage of usual enteric flora: gram-negative bacilli and anaerobes. This might be an aminoglycoside, such as gentamicin or tobramycin, plus clindamycin or chloramphenicol. The drugs should be given parenterally in full therapeutic doses. Once culture results are available it is appropriate to modify the antibiotic treatment. Some authorities would add high-dose penicillin to the initial therapy to include coverage against the enterococcus.

Prevention

Careful attention to surgical technique can decrease the incidence of postoperative abscesses. Recent information indicates that patients who are lymphocytopenic and/or anergic before surgery have a greater number of infections following their procedures. Thus the patient who is anergic from malnutrition might well benefit from several days of hyperalimentation.

Prognosis

Mortality averages 30%. It is higher (60-90%) in the patient whose abscess is undiagnosed or undrained, and in the elderly or debilitated patient. Patients who develop their abscesses following emergency surgery have a higher mortality than those following elective procedures (35 vs 26%). Multiple abscesses carry a higher mortality than single ones. Of special note is the prolonged hospital stay that is to be expected in patients with intraabdominal abscesses (20-80 days).

Selected Bibliography

Altemeier, W. A., Culbertson, W. R., Fullen, W. D., and Shook, C. D.: Intraabdominal abscesses. *Am J Surg* 125:70-79, 1973.

Bradley, E. L., III and Isaacs, J.: Appendiceal abscess revisited. *Arch Surg* 113: 130-132, 1978.

Coleman, R. E., Black, R. E., Welch, D. M., and Maxwell, J. G.: Indium-III labeled leukocytes in the evaluation of suspected abdominal abscesses. *Am J Surg* 139:99-104, 1980.

DeCrosse, J. J., Poulin, T. L., Fox, P. S. and Condon, R. E.: Subphrenic abscess. *Surg Gynecol Obstet* 138:841-846, 1974.

Dineen, P.: Management of post-traumatic intra-abdominal abscesses. *Bull N Y Acad Med* 55:266-271, 1979.

Dineen, P. and Shires, G. T.: Tetracycline in abdominal trauma and abdominal infections. *Bull N Y Acad Med* 54:177-195, 1978.

Elyaderani, M. K., Skolnick, M. L., and Weinstein, B. J.: Ultrasonic detection and aspiration confirmation of intra-abdominal collection of fluid. *Surg Gynecol Obstet* 149:529-533, 1979.

Gerzof, S. G., Robbins, A. H., Johnson, W. C., Birkett, D. H., and Nabseth, D. C.: Percutaneous catheter drainage of abdominal abscesses: A five-year experience. *N Engl J Med* 305:653-657, 1981.

Korobkin, M., Callen, F. W., Filly, R. A., Hoffer, P. B., Shimshak, R. R., and Kressel, H. Y.: Comparison of computed tomography, ultrasonography, and gallium-67 scanning in the evaluation of suspected abdominal abscess. *Radiology* 129:89-93, 1978.

Lewis, R. T. and Klein, H.: Risk factors in postoperative sepsis: Significance of preoperative lymphocytopenia. *J Surg Res* 26:365-371, 1979.

Milligan, S. L., Luft, F. C., McMurray, S. D., and Kleit, S. A.: Intra-abdominal infection and acute renal failure. *Arch Surg* 113:467-472, 1978.

Nagler, S. M. and Poticha, S. M.: Intraabdominal abscess in regional enteritis. *Am J Surg* 137:350-354, 1979.

Pietsch, J. B. and Meakins, J. L.: Predicting infection in surgical patients. *Surg Clin N Am* 59:185-197, 1979.

Wang, S. M. A. and Wilson, S. E.: Subphrenic abscess - the new epidemiology. *Arch Surg* 112:934-936, 1977.

Weinstein, W. M., Onderdonk, A. B., Bartlett, J. G., Louie, T. J., and Gorbach, S. L.: Antimicrobial therapy of experimental intra-abdominal sepsis. *J Infect Dis* 132:282-286, 1975.

White, P. H., Hayes, M., and Benfield, J. R.: Combined liver-lung scanning in the management of subdiaphragmatic abscess. *Am J Surg* 124:143-148, 1972.

31

PERITONITIS
Ronica M. Kluge, M.D.

Inflammation of the peritoneum caused by microbial organisms is usually divided into primary and secondary for ease of discussion. The primary form is also called spontaneous or idiopathic, reflecting the fact that no primary focus of infection is obvious. Secondary peritonitis results from some injury to the abdominal organs. Both forms will be considered in this chapter.

Etiology

Organisms known to cause peritonitis are listed in Table 31.1. Patients who develop primary peritonitis most often have ascites secondary to cirrhosis or nephrotic syndrome as a predisposing factor. These patients usually are infected with a single organism. In contrast, secondary peritonitis can develop in anyone and almost always is polymicrobial in nature. Patients requiring peritoneal dialysis are at risk from skin and enteric flora. Tuberculous peritonitis is discussed in Chapter 104.

Epidemiology

Peritonitis is a fairly common infection. Most cases are secondary, related to intraabdominal pathology. The microbes usually gain access to the peritoneum from the gastrointestinal or genitourinary tracts, although direct introduction from outside can occur with surgery, trauma, or peritoneal dialysis. Rupture of a hollow viscus, injury or infection of biliary tract or pancreas, and lesions of the gastrointestinal or genitourinary tract can cause contamination of the peritoneum. Primary peritonitis is less frequently seen. Rarely, the gonococcus or pneumococcus causes primary peritonitis in the absence of preexisting ascites.

296

TABLE 31.1 Microbial Causes of Peritonitis

Primary Peritonitis

Pneumococcus	Gram-negative bacilli
Streptococcus	Enteric anaerobes
Staphylococcus	*M. tuberculosis*

Gonococcus

Secondary Peritonitis

Enteric anaerobes	*Streptococcus,* including enterococcus
E. coli	*Candida*
Other gram-negative bacilli	Amoeba
	Strongyloides

Peritonitis During Peritoneal Dialysis

Candida	Gram-negative bacilli, including *Pseudomonas*
Staphylococcus	

TABLE 31.2   Intraabdominal Processes Causing Secondary Peritonitis

Obstruction	Neoplasm
Infarction	Foreign body
Perforation	Inflammatory bowel disease

Pathogenesis

As mentioned previously, the source of primary peritonitis is not obvious. It is presumed that the organisms reach the peritoneum through the blood stream, lymphatic channels, across the intact intestinal wall, or via the fallopian tubes. Numerous intraabdominal processes may give rise to secondary peritonitis (Table 31.2). Perforated peptic ulcer and perforated appendix are the most common. In peritoneal dialysis patients, the organisms may reach the peritoneum across the gut wall, or from the outside along the catheter tract, or in the dialysis fluid.

Once in the peritoneal cavity, microbes seem to have enhanced virulence in the presence of mucus, enzymes, or free hemoglobin. A synergistic effect also occurs when certain organisms are present as a mixed infection. The microbes provoke an inflammatory response consisting mainly of high-protein fluid and polymorphonuclear leukocytes. Fibrinogen present in the fluid polymerizes causing exudates to form on the inflamed surfaces. The process may be contained by the host's defenses resulting in resolution or abscess formation, or may continue unchecked causing widespread sepsis. The systemic manifestations can be profound, and hypovolemic shock is not uncommon in this setting.

Diagnostic Features

Clinical

Primary peritonitis in patients with cirrhosis and ascites is usually heralded by abdominal pain, fever, and rebound tenderness. These patients frequently have hypotension, decreased or absent bowel sounds, and may show signs of hepatic encephalopathy. In children with the nephrotic syndrome, primary peritonitis presents with similar symptoms plus nausea, vomiting, and occasionally diarrhea. Uncommonly, primary peritonitis may have a more gradual onset and be seen in the absence of abdominal pain or much fever. Gonococcal perihepatitis, seen almost exclusively in women, presents with sudden right upper-quadrant abdominal pain and low-grade fever. The pain may be referred to the shoulder and accompanied by abdominal guarding.

Secondary peritonitis usually presents first with the manifestations of the underlying disease process. Abdominal pain is present and may be quite severe. Nausea, vomiting, and abdominal distension may be present. The temperature varies from hypothermia to levels of 105-106°F. Tachycardia, tachypnea, and hypotension are frequent. The abdomen is markedly tender to palpation and may be rigid; there is guarding and rebound tenderness as well. Bowel sounds are hypoactive or absent.

Peritoneal dialysis patients who develop peritonitis usually present with fever, abdominal pain, and some rebound tenderness. Rarely, the peritonitis is asymptomatic.

Laboratory

Peripheral leukocytosis with a left shift is usually present. The peritoneal fluid has an increased protein level and leukocytosis; the Gram stain will reveal the organism(s) in most instances. Cultures of peritoneal fluid will confirm the identity and antimicrobial susceptibilities of the microbe(s). The fluid should be cultured aerobically and anaerobically. Blood cultures will be positive in up to 75% of patients. Elevated hematocrit and blood urea nitrogen reflect the degree of hemoconcentration and dehydration of the patient. Serum amylase may be high even in the absence of pancreatitis. Acidosis, both metabolic and respiratory, are present in severe peritonitis. Plain films of the abdomen can confirm the presence of ascites and ileus, and may suggest the diagnoses of obstruction, volvulus, intussusception, or vascular occlusion. Free air is present following perforation of the gastrointestinal tract and may be best demonstrated on chest x-ray.

Differential Diagnosis

The differential includes pulmonary infections, sickle cell crisis, herpes zoster, ketoacidosis, tabes dorsalis, porphyria, familial Mediterranean fever, drug poisoning, lead toxicity, renal disease, and orchitis. Complete historic information, physical examination, and baseline laboratory data will assist in ruling out these entities.

Complications

Intraabdominal abscess formation, metastatic infection, septicemia, shock, and death can complicate the course of peritonitis.

Therapy

Peritonitis requires aggressive management including major supportive measures: (1) fluid and electrolyte replacement with colloids (plasma, blood) if indicated; (2) reduction of abdominal distension by drainage, and the patient should receive nothing by mouth; (3) appropriate antimicrobials in adequate dosages (Table 31.3); (4) operation to halt continuing contamination and to provide drainage; (5) ventilatory support. Patients with peritonitis related to peritoneal dialysis are treated without surgical intervention in most instances. Primary and secondary peritonitis can be treated satisfactorily with parenteral antibiotics; intraperitoneal injections are not necessary.

Prevention

Preventive measures are limited to secondary peritonitis and to dialysis-related peritonitis. Good surgical technique and mechanical plus antimicrobial "cleansing" of the bowel are known to decrease the risk of secondary peritonitis. Maintenance of a closed drainage system will help prevent the occurrence of peritonitis in patients undergoing peritoneal dialysis.

Prognosis

The prognosis of peritonitis is directly related to the causative organism, and the age and underlying medical condition of the patient (Table 31.4). Peritonitis due to gram-positive organisms generally responds well to therapy and even in patients with nephrotic syndrome the survival rate is greater than 90%. Primary peritonitis in cirrhotics is less successfully treated; mortality ranges between 50 and 90%.

TABLE 31.3   Antimicrobial Therapy for Peritonitis

Primary

    Pneumococcus

    Streptococcus   Penicillin
                                        100,000 U/kg/day
    Gonococcus

    Staphylococcus   Penicillinase-resistant penicillin[1]
                                        150-200 mg/kg/day

Secondary

    Mixed aerobes and anaerobes   Gentamicin or tobramycin[2]
                                        5 mg/kg/day

                                            plus
                                      Clindamycin 30 mg/kg/day
                                            or
                                      Chloramphenicol 50-100 mg/kg/day

Peritoneal Dialysis

    Staphylococcus   Vancomycin[3]
                                        1 g q wk

    Gram-negative bacilli   Gentamicin or tobramycin, give
                                        loading dose of 2 mg/kg, then give
                                        1.5 mg/kg after each dialysis; alter-
                                        native is to add aminoglycoside to
                                        dialysate, 5 µg/ml in dialysate

    Candida   Amphotericin B 20 mg/day IV plus
                                        2-4 µg/ml in dialysate

[1]If using methicillin, dosage is up to 300 mg/kg/day
[2]In newborns, give up to 7 mg/kg/day
[3]In infants and children, give 25 mg/kg/day

TABLE 31.4   Poor Prognostic Indicators in Patients with Peritonitis

Primary (cirrhosis)	Secondary
Worsening encephalopathy	Extremes of age
Temperature < 100.4°F	Delayed surgery
Shock, hepatorenal syndrome	Gross contamination
Absence of fever and abdominal pain	Shock
Enteric organisms	Acidosis
WBC > 85% polys	Underlying abdominal process or medical condition
Bilirubin > 8 mg/dl	
Albumin < 2.5 mg/dl	

Selected Bibliography

Bayer, A. S., Blumenkrentz, M. J., Montgomerie, J. Z., Galpin, J. E., Coburn, J. W., and Guze, L. B.: Candida peritonitis. Report of 22 cases and review of the English literature. *Am J Med* 61:832-840, 1976.

Conn, H. O. and Fessel, J. M.: Spontaneous bacterial peritonitis in cirrhosis: Variations on a theme. *Medicine* 50:161-197, 1971.

Epstein, M., Calia, F. M., and Gabuzda, G. J.: Pneumococcal peritonitis in patients with post-necrotic cirrhosis. *N Engl J Med* 278:69-73, 1968.

Golden, G. T. and Shaw, A.: Primary peritonitis. *Surg Gynecol Obstet* 135:513-516, 1973.

Hau, T., Ahrenholz, D. H., and Simmons, R. L.: Secondary bacterial peritonitis. *Curr Prob Surg* 16:1-65, 1979.

Jennings, M. M., Jennings, S. A., Robson, M. C., and Heggers, J. P.: Mechanisms of host defense and quantitative comparisons of bacterial populations in experimental peritonitis. *Can J Microbiol* 26:175-178, 1980.

Kopelson, G., Silva-Hutner, M., and Brown, J.: Fungal peritonitis and malignancy. *Med Pediatr Oncol* 6:15-22, 1979.

Mandell, I. N., Ahern, M. J., Kliger, A. S., and Andriole, V. T.: Candida peritonitis complicating peritoneal dialysis: Successful treatment with low dose amphotericin B therapy. *Clin Nephrol* 6:492-496, 1976.

Onderdonk, A. B., Weinstein, W. M., Sullivan, N. M., Bartlett, J. G., and Gorbach, S. L.: Experimental intraabdominal abscesses in rats: Quantitative bacteriology of infected animals. *Infect Immun* 10:1256-1259, 1974.

Oreopoulos, D. G.: Chronic peritoneal dialysis. *Clin Nephrol* 9:165-173, 1978.

Rubin, J., Rogers, W. A., Taylor, H. M., Everett, E. D., Prowant, B. F., Fruto, L. V., and Nolph, K. D.: Peritonitis during continuous ambulatory peritoneal dialysis. *Ann Intern Med* 92:7-13, 1980.

Speck, W. T., Dresdale, S. S., and McMillan, R. W.: Primary peritonitis and the nephrotic syndrome. *Am J Surg* 127:267-269, 1974.

Stephen, M. and Loewenthal, J.: Generalized infective peritonitis. *Surg Gynecol Obstet* 147:231-234, 1978.

Targan, S. R., Chow, A. W., and Guze, L. B.: Role of anaerobic bacteria in spontaneous peritonitis of cirrhosis. *Am J Med* 62:397-403, 1977.

Weinstein, M. P., Iannini, P. B., Stratton, C. W., and Eickhoff, T. C.: Spontaneous bacterial peritonitis. *Am J Med* 64:592-598, 1978.

Weinstein, W. M., Onderdonk, A. B., Bartlett, J. G., and Gorbach, S. L.: Experimental intra-abdominal abscesses in rats: Development of an experimental model. *Infect Immun* 10:1250-1255, 1974.

Weinstein, W. M., Onderdonk, A. B., Bartlett, J. G., Louie, T. J., and Gorbach, S. L.: Antimicrobial therapy of experimental intraabdominal sepsis. *J Infect Dis* 132:282-286, 1975.

32

INFECTIONS OF THE URINARY TRACT
Enayatollah Osanloo, M.D.

The general term *urinary tract infection* (UTI) encompasses the presence of pathogenic microorganisms anywhere between the vesicular outlet and the kidney.
This term is used here instead of traditional ones such as pyelonephritis or cystitis, because it is easy to define and simple to understand. In addition, there are
few clinical and laboratory techniques which aid in recognizing the exact site of
the infectious process. The presence of bacteria in the urine may mean contamination or infection. When bacteriuria is due to infection, usually more than
100,000 microorganisms per milliliter are present in a clean midstream urine specimen. This is called significant bacteriuria.
    Urinary tract infection is one of the most common forms of infection. It is
estimated that, at any given time, at least 8 million Americans have a UTI. Moreover, it is the most common hospital-acquired infection and is the most common
identifiable source of bacteremia due to gram-negative rods.

Microbiology

A wide variety of microorganisms (Table 32.1) can cause a urinary tract infection;
with only a few exceptions, the source of these organisms is the intestinal flora.
The frequency with which a given species has been isolated from the urine varies
with the patient population and clinical circumstances.
    Escherichia coli is the most prevalent cause of uncomplicated urinary tract in-
fection. Other organisms such as *Klebsiella, Proteus, Pseudomonas,* enterococcus,
and staphylococci are seen much less frequently.
    The proportion of *E. coli*-induced infection decreases considerably, whereas in-
fection due to other gram-negative organisms increases dramatically in patients who

TABLE 32.1   Etiologic Agents in Urinary Tract Infections

Bacterial Species	Outpatients (%)	Inpatients (%)
E. coli	90	55
P. mirabilis	3	15
K. pneumoniae	2	10
S. fecalis	2	7
P. aeruginosa	< 1	6
E. aerogenes	< 1	4

experience nosocomial infections, have had prior antibiotic therapy, or have had urethral instrumentation. *Pseudomonas aeruginosa,* for example, is almost exclusively seen in the latter group. These organisms are often resistant to most of the currently used antibiotics and therefore pose a therapeutic dilemma.

Proteus spp are urea splitters, thereby forming ammonia and alkalinizing the urine. This environment favors the formation of renal stones which, in turn, may cause renal damage, making it more difficult to eradicate infection. *Proteus* spp also are the predominant microorganisms causing urinary tract infections in male children.

A small percentage of urinary tract infections are caused by staphylococci. Old age, prior urinary tract surgery, catheterization, or other invasive procedures are predisposing factors for staphylococcal bacteriuria. In the absence of the above predisposing factors, *Staphylococcus aureus* bacteriuria is largely hematogenous and the primary focus of infection should be sought.

Coagulase-negative staphylococci are usually contaminants in urine. However, one variety of this species, the "novobiocin-resistant subgroup 3 micrococci," can cause symptomatic urinary tract infection with a high incidence of pyuria and hematuria. Micrococci are considered one of the most frequent pathogens in young women between the ages of 18 and 24, second only to *E. coli.* This pattern of age distribution suggests a probable connection between micrococci bacteriuria and sexual intercourse. The rarity of micrococci in the male urethra or prepuce suggests that the infection is not sexually transmitted. On the basis of available evidence it seems that, similar to other bacteria associated with urinary tract infections, micrococci also are a constituent of the bowel flora.

Urinary tract infection due to viruses is rather rare. Recent reports, however, implicate adenovirus type 11 as causing hemorrhagic cystitis in children.

Finally, yeast, particularly *Candida* spp, are recovered from diabetics and patients treated with broad-spectrum antibiotics. Unusual gram-negative organisms such as *Serratia* and indole-positive *Proteus* spp are generally hospital-acquired organisms, occurring in patients with prolonged indwelling catheters.

Epidemiology

Because of difficulties in obtaining urine samples it has been difficult to estimate the prevalence of UTI in the neonate. Available data suggest that 1-2% of infants have significant bacteriuria and its incidence is much greater in boys than girls.

TABLE 32.2   Prevalence of Urinary Tract Infections by Age and Sex

Age Group	Approximate Prevalence (% of Total Group)	Male/Female Ratio
< 6 mo	1	1.5:1
1-6 yr	2	1:10
6-16 yr	1	1:30
16-50 yr	3	1:50
> 50	15	1:1

Except for the neonatal period, UTI is more common in females than males (Table 32.2). In males, the sterility of the proximal two thirds of the urethra, its longer length, and the bactericidal effect of prostatic secretions, constitute an excellent defense against bacterial invasion. On the other hand, the shorter length of the urethra, its proximity to the gastrointestinal tract, and the trauma from sexual intercourse in young women, make females more susceptible to bladder contamination.

In preschool children, 1.2% of girls and boys have significant bacteriuria, and its incidence rises steadily in girls from age 6 to 12 at an annual rate of 0.32%; thus 3% of girls have a UTI before age 11. About 4% of females and fewer than 0.5% of males between the ages of 16 and 65 show significant bacteriuria. Sexual activity, childbearing, and relaxation of the pelvic floor account for the increasing rates with age among women. Since spontaneous remission and new infection occur at a rate of about 1%, at any given time the prevalence of UTI in adults remains constant. The incidence of UTI in pregnant women is about 6-7%. Only 1% of these acquire bacteriuria during the pregnancy and most have bacteriuria prenatally. About 40% of the group with bacteriuria will have evidence of acute pyelonephritis (implying infection of the kidney, manifested by loin pain, flank tenderness, in addition to high temperature, shaking chills, and significant bacteriuria) at some time during the pregnancy. This can be decreased by successful treatment to 5-10%.

In contrast to nonpregnant women and schoolgirls, spontaneous remission in other groups is extremely rare. In general, the incidence of UTI increases with age and parity, is not dependent on race, and follows no particular geographic distribution.

Pathogenesis and Pathology

An indwelling bladder catheter is a major source of infection in hospitalized patients. The incidence of bacteriuria after catheterization with an open drainage system is 50% after 24 hr and 95% after 4 days. A closed system of drainage with good care will delay infection significantly, e.g., up to 50% at 10 days. If the catheter is left in place over a long enough period, however, virtually all patients will become infected.

Obstruction to the flow of urine is an important predisposing infective factor. A stone, congenital abnormality, tumor, prostatic enlargement, stricture, and retroperitoneal fibrosis are important causes of obstruction. Functional obstruction secondary to neurogenic bladder in patients with spinal cord injury, stroke, or diabetes also predisposes. How obstruction increases susceptibility is not entirely clear. Multiplication of microorganisms in a stagnated environment is a significant factor. The frequent use of an indwelling catheter and urologic investigations are additional factors initiating infection in patients with urinary tract obstruction.

Primary vesicoureteral reflux begins at an early age, usually under 3 years, and seems to be a major factor predisposing to infection and renal damage in this age group. Thirty to fifty percent of children 5 years old with UTI have reflux and about 20-30% of children undergoing dialysis and transplant have reflux. Data are inconclusive regarding whether or not infection causes reflux.

It is widely believed that diabetic patients have a higher rate of UTI. Careful studies in adults, and more specifically in pregnant women, have not shown a difference between diabetics and nondiabetics. Although the incidence of UTI is the same, diabetic patients are more liable to serious life-threatening complications of UTI, such as papillary necrosis, sepsis, etc. Therefore, the use of an indwelling catheter as a standard procedure in caring for the diabetic with ketoacidosis or hyperosmolar coma should be abandoned.

Other conditions in which urinary tract infection are more common are listed in Table 32.3.

Diagnostic Features

Clinical

The hallmark of UTI is the presence of significant bacteriuria. Common symptoms are dysuria, urinary frequency, lower abdominal pain, loin pain, fever, and hematuria. However, not all patients with these symptoms have significant bacteriuria. A sterile urine culture or insignificant bacteriuria is present in up to 40% of patients who present with symptoms of UTI. These patients have a poorly understood condition called *acute urethral syndrome.* This syndrome is thought to be due to infection confined to the urethra and surrounding glands or to an infection caused by a microorganism other than the classic bacteria, such as viral agents, chlamydiae, or cell-wall defective bacteria.

The patient with pyelonephritis usually presents with the sudden onset of fever, chills, flank pain, frequency, and dysuria. In addition, the patient may have cloudy and offensive urine. The major finding on physical examination is excruciating tenderness over the kidneys. Pain is frequently located in the lumbar region, although it may be felt in the epigastrium or the lower-abdominal quadrants. This is a common problem in children in whom it becomes difficult to differentiate UTI from acute appendicitis. Children may present with urinary incontinence or enuresis, or "failure to thrive."

Laboratory

Laboratory findings may include leukocytosis although in uncomplicated UTI the white cell count is usually normal. Abundant bacteria and leukocytes in clumps are usually seen in the urine. White cell casts may be seen, and their presence usually indicates pyelonephritis. Hematuria is often present, and sometimes the urine is grossly bloody. Mild proteinuria and low urine specific gravity also may be present.

TABLE 32.3   Predisposing Factors

Obstruction	Strictures
	Calculi
	Neoplasms
	Aberrant vessels
	Periureteral fibrosis
	Foreign bodies
	Prostatic hypertrophy
	Congenital valves
Renal disease	Chronic renal failure of any cause
	Acute tubular necrosis
	Analgesic abuse
	Cystic disease
	Hypoplasia
	Renal scars
Trauma	Injury
	Catheter
	Instrumentation
	Surgery
Metabolic disorders	Hypokalemia
	Gout
	Nephrocalcinosis
	Diabetes mellitus
	Agammaglobulinemia
	Vitamin A deficiency
Miscellaneous	Sickle cell disease and trait
	Pregnancy
	Reflux

Acute renal failure is rarely a result of acute pyelonephritis and must always raise the possibility of necrotizing papillitis (papillary necrosis).

The question of when to perform radiographic examination of a patient is a difficult one. It is generally agreed that all male patients with bacteriuria, regardless of presenting syndrome or age, and all females with evidence of acute pyelonephritis regardless of age, should be referred for an intravenous pyelogram (IVP). An IVP may be postponed until a second episode of infection in a woman who has a lower urinary tract infection such as "honeymoon cystitis" or asymptomatic bacteriuria. After a single episode all infants and children should have an IVP performed. Because of the high incidence of vesicoureteral reflux, a voiding cystoureterogram also should be included if the child is under 5 years of age. After this age, some renal damage from gross vesicoureteral reflux would have occurred; thus if the IVP is completely normal and kidney size is normal for the child, a voiding cystoureterogram can safely be omitted.

There have been a number of methods devised to pinpoint the site of infection in the urinary tract. Tests that are recommended for this purpose include ureteral catheterization, bladder wash out, renal biopsy, presence of leukocyte casts in the urine, specific serum antibodies, renal concentrating ability, presence of glitter cells, etc., but none of these tests are considered to be tremendously accurate. Bacteria from the kidney appear to become coated with antibody, which can be detected by fluorescent antibody techniques. Thus the presence of antibody-coated bacteria in the urine indicates infection of the kidneys. The problems with this technique are the delay in appearance of antibody after infection and that false-positive test results may be found with prostatic infection.

Differential Diagnosis

The patient who complains of dysuria may not have a urinary tract infection. The patient may have suffered trauma to the urethra secondary to a jolting ride in a truck or on a motorcycle, or have irritation due to vaginal tampons. Trauma is easily ruled out by an adequate history. Intermittent discomfort may be due to a spastic bladder. In older women estrogen deficiencies lead to urethritis and vaginitis which may present as dysuria. Obstruction due to stone, stricture, or prostatic hypertrophy can cause dysuria even when infection is not present. Rarer causes of dysuria are carcinoma of the bladder, psychosexual disorders, and cyclophosphamide therapy.

Treatment

The goal of therapy is to eradicate existing infection, to prevent further symptomatic and asymptomatic infection, and to forestall renal function impairment. A simple course of antibiotic therapy may not be effective in all cases. Relief of obstruction or removal of an indwelling catheter or an infected stone sometimes can be the most important therapeutic or preventive measure. In general, the outcome of therapy depends upon the type of organism, its sensitivity to antibiotics, and the clinical condition and status of the host. For purposes of therapy, UTI may be divided into the following groups:

1. Asymptomatic bacteriuria
2. Symptomatic but uncomplicated UTI
3. Complicated UTI
4. UTI with indwelling catheter
5. Infection in renal failure
6. Recurrent or persistent infection

Asymptomatic Bacteriuria

Because of a high risk of acute pyelonephritis, pregnant women should be screened and treated for asymptomatic bacteriuria. A 7-day course of antibiotic therapy is recommended; ampicillin is appropriate in most cases. A longer duration and/or continuous therapy throughout pregnancy may be required in some cases. Screening and treatment of asymptomatic bacteriuria in patients other than pregnant women are of doubtful value.

Symptomatic But Uncomplicated UTI

The patient, usually a woman, in the childbearing age group, presents with symptoms such as dysuria, frequency, and urgency. *Escherichia coli* is the most common cause of infection, and it readily responds to a wide variety of antimicrobial agents. Symptoms usually disappear within 72 hr with or without therapy, and bacteriuria disappears spontaneously. When seen by a physician for the first time, based on the urinalysis, therapy with an antimicrobial agent such as sulfonamide or ampicillin should be started. Recent studies suggest that a shorter duration of therapy, e.g., 3 days, or even a single dose may be as effective as a 10-day course. Unnecessary instrumentation should be avoided. A follow-up urinalysis within 2 weeks of cessation of antibiotics is advised.

Complicated UTI

The patient with suspected upper-tract disease or with complications, such as bacteremia or stones, should receive parenteral therapy initially with an amino-glycoside. When the organism and its sensitivities are known, therapy may be continued with the most effective, least toxic antibiotic. Treatment for 2-3 weeks is recommended.

With Indwelling Catheter

It is impossible to eradicate a UTI in the presence of a bladder catheter. The acute infection can be treated as for complicated UTI.

UTI in Patients with Renal Failure

This poses some difficulty in management. Antimicrobial agents may not reach the urinary tract. Ampicillin or trimethoprim-sulfamethoxazole (TMP-SMX) in a standard dose, if renal failure is mild, or a reduced dose in far-advanced renal failure, for 2 weeks is usually effective. A rising serum creatinine level following therapy with TMP-SMX should not be interpreted as a decline in renal failure. Trimethoprim competes with the excretion of creatinine thus raising the serum creatinine. Since there is no change in glomerular filtration rate with TMP-SMX therapy, to withhold its use in renal failure is not warranted.

Recurrent/Persistent UTI

See the prevention section.

Prevention

The indications for prophylactic antibiotics are uncertain. Beneficial effects have been seen in the following circumstances:

1. In children with vesicoureteral reflux, prophylactic antibiotics seem to halt progression of symptoms and renal scarring.
2. In young women with frequent symptomatic UTIs, the infection is generally related to sexual activity and a single dose of an antibiotic after intercourse reduces the number of infections. Another successful treatment is one-half tablet TMP-SMX at bedtime. Trimethoprim-sulfamethoxazole is the drug of choice for prophylactic use since these drugs do not alter the sensitivity of organisms in the bowel or periurethral flora.

Intermittent catheterization in the management of patients with a neurogenic bladder seems to be an effective measure to prevent UTI, especially in patients with spinal cord injury. Preventing UTI in patients with an indwelling catheter is a difficult task. Three-way drainage used with antibiotics such as neomycin, polymyxin, or other bladder rinse such as acetic acid, probably is no better than a simple closed drainage system. In addition, suppressive therapy with bacteriostatic agents such as methanamine in these patients with chronic indwelling catheters is useless.

Complications and Prognosis

The survival rate for untreated patients with bilateral acute pyelonephritis is 95 and 86% at 5 and 10 years, respectively. Patients with unilateral disease have 100% survival at 10 years. Bacteremia is a frequent complication of UTI. Metastatic infections are common, with about 75% of all metastatic infections arising from UTI. Urinary tract manipulation and impaired host defenses are the most important predisposing factors for metastasis.

The relationship between UTI and hypertension has not been clarified. It appears, however, that women with UTI have higher blood pressures than controls, that hypertensive patients are more susceptible to UTI, that hypertension can be aggravated by UTI, that controlling infection with antibiotics may be associated with reduction of hypertension, and that morbidity and mortality from hypertension may increase with UTI.

Acute pyelonephritis in pregnancy is associated with increased prematurity, preeclampsia, fetal mortality, and congenital defects. Whereas, the risk from the development of acute pyelonephritis in pregnant women is beyond question, the adverse effect of asymptomatic bacteriuria on the fetus and mother has been highly controversial. Current evidence favors the notion that the frequency of premature delivery, prenatal mortality, and infection of amniotic fluid is much higher in pregnant women with bacteriuria than in nonbacteriuric persons. In addition, gestational hypertension is significantly more frequent in infected than in uninfected mothers. The prevention of these complications and of acute pyelonephritis is a strong argument in favor of screening pregnant women for asymptomatic bacteriuria and for its eradication with suitable antibiotics.

There is continuing debate regarding the evidence that chronic pyelonephritis is a cause of end-stage renal failure. The risk of chronic renal failure appears to be great in children with UTI, particularly during infancy and the preschool period when infection is frequently associated with vesicoureteral reflux. Outside this age group, most recent evidence supports the view that chronic, persistent bacteriuria in an otherwise normal urinary tract does not result in a deterioration of renal function.

Selected Bibliography

Abbot, G. D.: Neonatal bacteriuria. A prospective study in 1,460 infants. *Br Med J* 1:267-269, 1972.

Dupont, H. L. and Spink, W. W.: Infections due to gram-negative organisms: An analysis of 860 patients with bacteremia at the University of Minnesota Medical Center 1954-1966. *Medicine* 48:307-332, 1969.

Fang, L. S. T., Tolkoff-Rubin, N. E., and Rubin, R. H.: Efficacy of single-dose and conventional amoxicillin therapy in urinary tract infection localized by the antibody-coated bacteria technique. *N Engl J Med* 298:413, 1978.

Freeman, R. B. and Smith, W. M.: Long-term therapy of chronic bacteriuria in man: U. S. Public Health Science Corporation Study. *Ann Intern Med* 83:133-147, 1975.

Gillenwater, J.: Diagnosis of urinary tract infection. Appraisal of diagnostic procedures. *Kidney Int* 8:S3-S11, 1975.

Gower, P. E.: A prospective study of patients with radiological pyelonephritis, papillary necrosis and obstructive atrophy. *Am J Med* 45:315-349, 1976.

Jones, S. R.: Prostatitis as cause of antibody coated bacteria in urine (Letter to editor). *N Engl J Med* 291:365, 1974.

Kass, E. H.: Bacteriuria and pyelonephritis of pregnancy. *Arch Intern Med* 105:194-198, 1960.

Kass, E. H., Miall, W. E., and Stuart, K. L.: Relationship of bacteriuria to hypertension. Abstract #12. Annual Meeting, Am Soc Clin Invest, 1961. *J Clin Invest* 40:1053, 1961.

Kleeman, C. R., Hewitt, W. L., and Guze, L. B.: Pyelonephritis. *Medicine* 39:3-116, 1960.

Linculm, K. and Winber, J.: Studies of urinary tract infections in infancy and childhood. II. Quantitative estimation of bacteriuria in unselected neonates with special reference to the occurrence of asymptomatic infection. *Acta Paediatr* 53:307-310, 1964.

Martin, C. M. and Bookrajian, E. N.: Bacteriuria prevention after indwelling urinary catheterization: A controlled study. *Arch Intern Med* 110:703-711, 1962.

McCabe, W. R. and Jackson, G. G.: Gram-negative bacteremia: I. Etiology and ecology. *Arch Intern Med* 110:847-864, 1962.

McGowan, J. E., Jr. and Finland, M.: Infection and antibiotic usage at Boston City Hospital. Changes in prevalence during the decade, 1964-1973. *J Infect Dis* 129:421-428, 1974.

Naeye, R. L.: Causes of the excessive rates of perinatal mortality and prematurity in pregnancies complicated by maternal urinary-tract infections. *N Engl J Med* 300:819-823, 1979.

Ronald, A. R., Boutros, P., and Mourtada, H.: Bacteriuria localization and response to single-dose therapy in women. *JAMA* 235:1854, 1976.

Shapiro, A. P.: Experimental pyelonephritis and hypertension: Implication for the clinical problem. *Ann Intern Med* 59:37-52, 1963.

Siroky, M. G., Moyland, R., and Austen, G., Jr.: Metastatic infection secondary to genitourinary tract sepsis. *Am J Med* 61:351-360, 1976.

Smith, J. W., Jones, S. R., and Kaijser, B.: Significance of antibody coated bacteria in urinary sediment in experimental pyelonephritis. *J Infect Dis* 135:577-581, 1977.

Stamm, W. E., Wagner, K. F., Amsel, R., Alexander, E. R., Turck, M., Counts, G. W., and Holmes, K. K.: Causes of the acute urethral syndrome in women. *N Engl J Med* 303:409, 1980.

Zinner, S. H. and Kass, E. H.: Long-term (10-14 years) follow-up of bacteriuria of pregnancy. *N Engl J Med* 285:820-824, 1971.

33

PERINEPHRIC ABSCESS AND RENAL CARBUNCLE
Rashida A. Khakoo, M.D.

Perinephric Abscess

Definition

As is the case with most types of intraabdominal abscesses, the diagnosis of a perinephric abscess is extremely difficult and may be missed, especially if there is a low index of suspicion. This is because of its protean manifestations, including variable length of time the patient has been ill before presenting to a physician. The disease is not uncommonly diagnosed only very late in the course of illness, or at autopsy.

Perinephric abscess is a collection of pus in the perinephric space – an area anatomically defined between the kidney and Gerota's fascia (perirenal). Anterior and posterior leaves of Gerota's fascia fuse superiorly with the diaphragm, pass downward enveloping the kidney and perirenal fat, and are open inferiorly so that the perirenal fat is continuous with the pelvic fat. Laterally the fascial layers fuse with the transversalis fascia. The abscess is usually confined to the anatomic boundaries of Gerota's fascia but may extend in several directions.

Etiology

In the older series, *Staphylococcus aureus* as a result of hematogenous spread, usually from a cutaneous focus of infection, was the most common causative agent of perinephric abscess, and *Mycobacterium tuberculosis* and *Actinomyces* spp were occasionally reported. Recent studies have emphasized the role of gram-negative bacteria, particularly *Escherichia coli* and *Proteus* spp. Occasionally, more than one bacterial species is cultured from the abscess. In one recent report,

67% of those perinephric abscesses cultured revealed gram-negative bacteria, and 76% of the abscesses were directly attributed to renal causes.

Epidemiology

The incidence appears to be rising slightly from 0.9 cases per 10,000 admissions in 1950 to 1.3 cases per 10,000 admissions from 1970 to 1974. This may reflect more clinical awareness and better diagnostic tools. Patients of all ages are affected. There is a very slight preponderance of females, most likely reflecting the higher prevalence of urinary tract infections in women.

Pathogenesis and Pathology

It is believed that the initiating event almost always is the rupture of an abscess within the renal parenchyma into the perinephric space. The original lesion in the kidney may heal, thus by the time the perinephric abscess is drained and the kidney examined, evidence of the preceding lesion may have disappeared. Occasionally a perinephric abscess arises via the hematogenous route from a primary focus of infection. Perinephric abscesses secondary to ascending infection are associated most often with hydronephrosis or with renal or ureteric calculi which lead to damaged and infected kidneys. Rare cases are associated with prostatic abscess or polycystic kidney disease with infected cysts. Diabetes mellitus is associated with perinephric abscess in 15-35% of cases.

Diagnostic Features

Clinical

Almost all patients present with fever. Flank pain is a common symptom present in about 75% of the cases. With an anteriorly located abscess, anterior upper- and lower-quadrant abdominal pain may be found. Occasionally the pain is felt in the hip, thigh, or knee during extension of the corresponding thigh during walking and assuming a position in bed with the ipsilateral thigh flexed. Pain may be referred to the testes. The duration of symptoms before presentation ranges from 1 to 4 weeks, and 50% of patients present with symptoms of less than 2 weeks. Physical examination reveals unilateral flank tenderness in about 50% of the cases, and a flank mass in about one-fourth, with another one-fourth presenting with an abdominal mass.

Laboratory

As would be expected, the leukocyte count and erythrocyte sedimentation rate are elevated. The urinalysis is usually abnormal, with pyuria in one-third of the patients, proteinuria in one-third, and occasional hematuria.

Blood cultures are positive in 20-40% of patients, and urine cultures are positive in approximately two-thirds. In some patients, urine cultures demonstrate bacteria other than those isolated from the abscess.

Abdominal x-rays demonstrate abnormalities in 50% of patients. These include a poorly defined renal outline, poorly visualized iliopsoas shadow, thoracolumbar scoliosis with concavity towards the side of the lesion because of spasm of paraspinal muscles, and renal calculi. Occasionally gas may be present in the retroperitoneal space. Rarely, ribs and lumbar transverse processes may be obscured on the side of the lesion when the abscess is of sufficient size to overlie these structures and obscure the bone detail by the density of the purulent collection. A chest roentgenogram may reveal pleural effusion, lower-lobe infiltrate, or elevated hemidiaphragm. Intravenous pyelogram is abnormal in 85% of the patients. The changes include poor to nonvisualization and caliectasis. A mass in the region of the kidney is manifest by an increased homogeneous density in the area. Anterior displacement of the kidney is present if the abscess is mainly posterior to the kidney, a common site for the pus collection.

Some authorities feel that renal mobility is a very useful test. This can be evaluated by fluoroscopy, inspiration-expiration films, or by supine and upright films (either plain abdominal or intravenous pyelogram). When a perinephric abscess is present, the involved kidney is fixed to the surrounding tissues. Other processes that may impair renal mobility from perirenal adhesions include prior infection, surgery, or tumor. Diaphragmatic immobility from paralysis, pulmonary or pleural pathologic changes, or subphrenic abscess, can result in limited movement of the kidney on the side of the fixed hemidiaphragm.

Ultrasonography is a useful noninvasive technique for the detection of perinephric abscess. Conventional radiologic techniques described earlier generally yield inferential data regarding the presence of a retroperitoneal inflammatory process. Ultrasonography allows direct visualization of abnormal fluid collections. However, it does not differentiate between the various forms of fluid, e.g., pus, blood, urine. The gallium scan is another useful technique. As more experience is gained with computerized tomography in examination of the retroperitoneal space, this could become a useful noninvasive technique for delineation of perinephric abscess. The anatomic detail provided by this technique is very good and could demonstrate the extent of the abscess. Arteriography has been reported to be useful on occasion with some patients. However, it is an invasive technique with attendant morbidity and is of limited usefulness now that newer noninvasive techniques are available.

Differential Diagnosis

From the clinical presentation, the most common diagnosis considered in most cases is pyelonephritis, unless the patient presents with an obvious mass in the costovertebral area. Patients with perinephric abscesses are, on the average, older than those with pyelonephritis, but there is a lot of overlap, making age a useless clinical criterion. Diabetes mellitus is more often an associated problem in patients with perinephric abscesses. However, the major discriminatory feature is the duration of symptoms before hospitalization – 90% of patients with acute uncomplicated urinary tract infection have been symptomatic for less than 5 days when first seen. Eighty percent of patients with perinephric abscess have been symptomatic for longer than 5 days. After institution of antimicrobial therapy patients with acute urinary tract infection are rarely febrile for longer than 4 days. Patients with perinephric abscess remain febrile for much longer than that, most remaining febrile until surgical drainage.

Another differential diagnostic group of patients present with fever of undetermined origin or with "sepsis." The diagnosis of perinephric abscess often can be missed if patients do not present with symptoms and signs pointing to the urinary tract. The various causes of fever of undetermined origin may be considered. Some patients present with pain referred to the hip, and attention may be directed away from the perinephric abscess. Occasionally the pain may be felt more in the upper or lower quadrants of the abdomen, making considerations of intraabdominal pathology, e.g., cholecystitis, hepatic abscess, diverticulitis, and appendicitis likely, as opposed to retroperitoneal pathology. The differential on radiologic examination may be varied. Pneumonia or pleural effusion/empyema may be considered on chest roentgenogram. Intrarenal or intraabdominal pathology may be considered on a flat plate of the abdomen or on intravenous pyelogram. From the results of ultrasonography, hematoma or urinoma would have to be differentiated. From the gallium scan, a tumor would have to be ruled out. When retroperitoneal gas is demonstrated on an abdominal film, traumatic duodenal perforation and pancreatic or lesser sac abscess have to be considered.

Treatment

As with abscesses elsewhere, treatment consists of the combination of surgery and antimicrobial therapy. Most patients require only simple drainage, but nephrectomy may be necessary when there is extensive destruction of the kidney. The choice of antimicrobial agent will depend on the causative organism. With infections caused by aerobic gram-negative bacteria, depending on the sensitivity pattern, ampicillin or an aminoglycoside initially could be used parenterally. Before the availability of culture data in a perinephric abscess resulting from ascending infection, an aminoglycoside (gentamicin or tobramycin) would be appropriate. When *S. aureus* is suspected or isolated as the causal agent, parenteral penicillinase-resistant penicillin should be used. It is difficult to comment on the duration of therapy because of lack of firm data, but 2-3 weeks or longer of therapy may be needed. This will depend upon the response during follow-up of each patient. The parenteral therapy could be changed to oral whenever possible after 7-10 days if the patient is doing well. Serum "cidal" levels could be obtained as a guide to the adequacy of therapy. If fever persists with appropriate antimicrobial therapy, one of the major considerations must be undrained pus. A redrainage procedure may be necessary.

Complications and Prognosis

Extension into the subphrenic or pleural spaces, or onto the skin forming a sinus tract has been reported but is an unusual complication. Thrombosis of the renal vessels or bronchial fistula is even more uncommon.

The mortality continues to be high, about 45%. In those patients who present without symptoms or signs referable to the urinary tract the mortality is 65%, reflecting underlying factors and probably delayed diagnosis because of the presentation. Those presenting with findings clearly pointing to the perinephric abscess have a mortality of about 25%, reflecting early diagnosis. A poor prognosis is associated with a history of previous urinary tract infections, urinary outflow obstruction, admission diagnosis of acute pyelonephritis, diabetic ketoacidosis, "sepsis," and maximum temperature of 104°F or higher.

Renal Carbuncle

Definition

Renal carbuncle is an intracortical collection of pus first described by Israel in 1905. It is an uncommon condition which usually presents a difficult diagnostic problem.

Etiology

Staphylococcus aureus and gram-negative rods (*E. coli, Proteus* spp, *Klebsiella pneumoniae*) are the commonly isolated organisms from renal carbuncles. Carbuncles occurring as a result of hematogenous spread of bacteria from a primary site (usually skin, sometimes bone, endocardium, or lung) are caused by *S. aureus*. Carbuncles caused by gram-negative bacilli are commonly associated with obstructive uropathy.

Epidemiology

Renal carbuncles have been reported in many different age groups, ranging from 6 to 60 years. A recent study, however, reported mostly young adults, probably a result of, to some extent, the higher incidence of drug abuse in this age. Renal carbuncle may be more common in men than women.

Pathogenesis and Pathology

Renal carbuncle can arise either as a result of hematogenous spread of bacteria to the renal cortex or extension of infection to the cortex, usually from an obstructed renal pelvis. The process may be diffuse, involving the entire cortex or kidney, or remain localized. The carbuncle usually arises from coalescence of multiple cortical microabscesses.

Diagnostic Features

Clinical

The patient usually presents with fever, chills, malaise, and other systemic or nonspecific complaints. Symptoms and signs pertaining to the primary focus of infection in cases of hematogenously derived carbuncles may occasionally be present at the time of presentation. Symptoms referring to the urinary tract may be present if the renal carbuncle arose as a result of ascending infection from the renal medulla, or if a carbuncle that was initially localized to the cortex has ruptured through the medulla. Localized tenderness in the costovertebral angle usually is present. Swelling, or appearance of a mass, in the region of the kidney is an uncommon and most likely a late presentation.

The diagnosis should be suspected in the appropriate clinical setting. Renal carbuncle is a consideration when a patient with staphylococcal bacteremia, receiving appropriate antimicrobial therapy has continued fever or develops loin pain, or when a patient who has had a staphylococcal infection elsewhere in the previous 1-8 weeks presents with loin pain. Renal carbuncle is also a possibility when a patient with pyelonephritis receiving appropriate antimicrobial therapy does not respond or becomes febrile again after discontinuation of antibiotics. Obstruction is one of the most common associations and needs to be ruled out.

Laboratory

Urinalysis is not usually diagnostic. When the carbuncle is a result of the hematogenous route of infection, the urinalysis results are often normal. Occasionally, leukocytes may be demonstrated. Cultures will show no growth unless the abscess has ruptured into the medulla. When the carbuncle is a complication of ascending infection, urinalysis may reveal findings suggestive of a urinary tract infection with leukocytes and bacteria, or it may be normal. Culture may show gram-negative bacteria.

Polymorphonuclear leukocytosis is common, but occasionally the leukocyte count is normal. Usually the BUN and creatinine levels are normal unless preexisting renal damage is present or gross renal destruction has occurred from the abscess. Blood cultures may be positive. The rate of positivity varies since bacteremia from the primary source may be transient.

The abdominal roentgenogram may be totally normal or may demonstrate diffuse or local enlargement of the kidney. If a perinephric abscess is also present, the psoas margin may be obliterated. The intravenous pyelogram may be totally normal when the abscess is small and confined to the cortex. Depending on the extent of the abscess, the findings may vary from partial or poor to nonvisualization of the collecting systems. The calyces may appear amputated, distorted or stretched, and draped around a suggested mass. Nephrotomography has been used for better delineation of a mass. The need for retrograde pyelography in the diagnosis of renal carbuncle is limited. It is necessary, however, to exclude the presence of ureteric obstruction when the collecting system is not visualized.

As more experience is gained with the use of ultrasonography for detection of renal carbuncles, it will probably be one of the most useful noninvasive techniques for diagnosis. Early on, internal echos may be present giving the appearance of a solid or semisolid mass. After coalescence, an abscess can be identified ultrasonographically as a fluid-filled, thick-walled mass. The presence of an abscess can be confirmed by aspiration under ultrasound guidance if the lesion does not appear solid. Experience in this area is limited. The advantages of ultrasonography include: easy availability, rapid results, no need for nuclide injection, and abscess aspiration can be done. The study is of less value in the presence of distended loops of bowel. Ultrasonography can be used in following the size of the abscess if a nonsurgical mode of therapy is employed. Gallium accumulates in inflammatory lesions and neoplastic tissue and has been a useful technique for detecting abscesses. The limitations of the gallium scan are that it will be positive posttrauma or postsurgery and there is a delay of 24-72 hr in obtaining a final reading. Early scanning has been done at 6 hr. Either or both techniques can be used in the diagnosis of renal carbuncle, and when the two techniques are compared, there is no significant difference in the true positivity rate.

Computerized tomography could become a useful noninvasive technique in the detection of renal carbuncle, but there has been insufficient experience to evaluate its value.

Since arteriography is an invasive technique with attendant morbidity, its use is restricted to confirming findings in certain cases, e.g., those with an abnormal intravenous pyelogram, ultrasound, or gallium scan. Arteriography, when used in conjunction with the clinical picture, intravenous pyelography, and ultrasonography, permits a high degree of accuracy in the diagnosis. Angiographically, a renal carbuncle presents as a mass that produces stretching and attenuation of adjacent arteries. The rim around the carbuncle may be poorly visualized very early, but later on a dense rim is seen.

Differential Diagnosis

On the basis of the clinical presentation of fever, chills, and malaise, the differential is essentially that of any systemic febrile illness. Findings pointing to the urinary tract, such as abnormal urinalysis and costovertebral angle tenderness, suggest pyelonephritis or perinephric abscess (which is occasionally a complication of renal carbuncle). The differential from various radiographic tests would be neoplasm or cyst. A cyst usually can be differentiated based on clinical presentation. Aspiration under ultrasound guidance is of help. A neoplasm can occasionally be confused with renal carbuncle from ultrasound studies because of the early appearance of semisolid or solid mass. Renal cell carcinoma may occasionally present with fever. Renal carbuncle can usually be distinguished arteriographically from neoplasms because the major portion of an abscess is avascular while the wall is hypervascular. Renal carcinoma may be hypervascular or hypovascular but rarely both. Carcinoma will often demonstrate neovascularity.

Treatment

The treatment of renal carbuncle, until recently, has consisted of surgical intervention and appropriate antimicrobial therapy. It now appears that antibiotics alone may be curative in selected patients. The etiologic diagnosis can be confirmed in such cases by aspiration of the abscess under ultrasound guidance before institution of antimicrobial therapy. Ultrasound also can be used for following the size of the abscess. When *S. aureus* is the causative microorganism, therapy can be switched to oral penicillinase-resistant penicillins after a week or two of parenteral therapy. Serum "cidal" levels may be obtained for judging adequacy of therapy. The duration of therapy can be guided by the size of the abscess on repeat ultrasound examination. Drainage will be required if there is no change in size of the abscess while the patient is receiving appropriate antimicrobial therapy. The patient who has renal carbuncle associated with ascending infection will need, in almost all instances, surgical intervention in addition to antimicrobial therapy because of associated obstruction. Surgery usually consists of incision and drainage, or very rarely nephrectomy if there is extensive destruction. The choice of antimicrobial therapy will depend on the organisms isolated from intraoperative cultures. Before surgery the therapy should be directed to cover aerobic gram-negative rods: a parenteral aminoglycoside, e.g., gentamicin or tobramycin, would cover nearly all of the usually identified organisms. The therapy can be modified after cultural data are available. The duration of therapy will vary depending on the extent of involvement and the type of surgical intervention. The response can be assessed clinically. The abscess size can be followed by ultrasound if it is suspected that drainage has been inadequate, or that there is a lack of clinical response or deterioration.

Complications and Prognosis

The main complications are perforation through the renal capsule to form a perinephric abscess or perforation into the collecting system.
The mortality in some studies has been high, reflecting delayed diagnoses. The lowered mortality is ascribed mainly to early surgical intervention. The prognosis depends on the extent of renal involvement, underlying diseases, and time of diagnosis.

Selected Bibliography

Perinephric Abscess

Altemeir, W. A. and Alexander, J. W.: Retroperitoneal abscess. *Arch Surg* 83: 512-524, 1961.

Atcheson, D. W.: Perinephric abscess with a review of 117 cases. *J Urol* 46:201-208, 1941.

Bruce Hopkins, G. B., Hall, R. L., and Mende, C. W.: Gallium 67 scintigraphy for the diagnosis and localization of perinephric abscesses. *J Urol* 115:126-128, 1976.

Campbell, M. F.: Perinephric abscess. *Surg Gynecol Obstet* 51:674-682, 1930.

Hotchkiss, R. S.: Perinephric abscess. *Am J Surg* 85:471-485, 1953.

Laing, F. C. and Jacobs, R. P.: Value of ultrasonography in the detection of retroperitoneal inflammatory masses. *Radiology* 123:169-172, 1977.

Leopold, G. R. and Asher, W. M.: Diagnosis of extraorgan retroperitoneal space lesions by B-scan ultrasonography. *Radiology* 104:133-138, 1972.

Obrant, O.: Perirenal abscess. *Acta Chir Scand* 97:338-353, 1949.

Parks, R. E.: The radiographic diagnosis of perinephric abscess. *J Urol* 64:555-563, 1950.

Plevin, S. N., Balodimos, M. C., and Bradley, R. F.: Perinephric abscess in diabetic patients. *J Urol* 103:539-543, 1970.

Salvatierra, O., Bucklew, W. B. , and Morrow, J. W.: Perinephric abscess: A report of 71 cases. *J Urol* 98:296-302, 1967.

Thorley, J. D., Jones, S. R., and Sanford, J. P.: Perinephric abscess. *Medicine* 53:441-451, 1974.

Truesdale, B. H., Rous, S. N., and Nelson, R. P.: Perinephric abscess: A review of 26 cases. *J Urol* 118:910-911, 1977.

Renal Carbuncle

Caplan, L. H., Siegelman, S. S., and Bosniak, M. A.: Angiography in inflammatory space occupying lesions of the kidney. *Radiology* 88:14-23, 1967.

Colby, F. M., Baker, M. P., and St. Goar, W. T.: Renal carbuncle - report of a response to modern treatment. *N Engl J Med* 256:1147-1148, 1957.

Fair, W. R. and Higgins, M. H.: Renal abscess. *J Urol* 104:179-183, 1970.

Gadrinab, N. M., Lome, L. G., and Presman, D.: Renal abscess: Role of renal arteriography. *Urology* 2:39, 1973.

Gelman, M. L. and Stone, L. B.: Renal carbuncle: Early diagnosis by retroperitoneal ultrasound. *Urology* 7:103-107, 1976.

Graves, R. C. and Parkins, L. E.: Carbuncle of the kidney. *J Urol* 35:1-13, 1936.

Lyons, R. W., Long, J. M., Lytton, B., and Andriole, V. T.: Arteriography and antibiotic therapy of a renal carbuncle. *J Urol* 107:524-526, 1972.

Moore, C. A. and Gangai, M. P.: Renal cortical abscess. *J Urol* 98:303-306, 1967.

Pederson, J. F., Hancke, S., and Kvist Kristensen, J.: Renal carbuncle: Antibiotic therapy governed by ultrasonically guided aspiration. *J Urol* 109:777-778, 1973.

Rabinowitz, J. G., Kinkhabwala, M. N., Robinson, J., Spyropoulos, E., and Becker, J. A.: Acute renal carbuncle. The roentgenographic clarification of a medical enigma. *Am J Roentgenol Radium Ther Nucl Med* 116:740-748, 1972.

Schiff, M., Glickman, M., Weiss, R. M., Ahern, M. J., Touloukian, R. J., Lytton, B., and Andriole, V. T.: Antibiotic treatment of renal carbuncle. *Ann Intern Med* 87:305-308, 1977.

Spence, H. M. and Johnston, L. W.: Renal carbuncle - case report and comparative review. *Ann Surg* 109:99-108, 1939.

34

PROSTATITIS, EPIDIDYMITIS, AND ORCHITIS
Melanie A. Fisher, M.D. and William F. Tarry, M.D.

Prostatitis

Prostatitis encompasses several disease states that vary in etiology, presentation, clinical course, and therapy. Bacterial prostatitis may be acute or chronic. Non-bacterial prostatitis is characterized by clinical symptoms and leukocytosis of the expressed prostatic fluid, similar to the findings in chronic bacterial prostatitis; however, urine and prostate fluid cultures are negative. Both tuberculous and fungal prostatitis are rare today but can occur in conjunction with systemic involvement.

Pathogenesis and Epidemiology

The pathogenesis of bacterial prostatitis remains unclear. Proposed routes of infection include: (1) ascending urethral infection; (2) reflux of infected urine into prostatic ducts which empty into the urethra; (3) invasion by rectal bacteria by direct extension or lymphatics; (4) hematogenous spread. Some evidence suggests that bacterial prostatitis may occasionally be sexually transmitted. Although gonococcal prostatitis is uncommon, it almost always occurs in men with a history of gonococcal urethritis. Identical strains of coliform bacteria have been found in prostatic fluid cultures of men with chronic bacterial prostatitis and vaginal cultures of their sexual partners.

Both acute and chronic bacterial prostatitis are caused mainly by the gram-negative organisms responsible for urinary tract infections. *Escherichia coli* strains are most common, but species of *Proteus, Klebsiella, Pseudomonas, Enterobacter,* and *Serratia* are isolated frequently. In acute prostatitis a single bacterium is usually responsible, while mixed infections are sometimes found in the chronic form. The only gram-positive organism that has been shown consistently to cause bacterial prostatitis is *Streptococcus faecalis.* This bacterium can persist in the prostate and is an important cause of relapsing urinary tract infections in men.

Diagnosis

Acute bacterial prostatitis is usually diagnosed readily by the clinical presentation of a toxic, febrile man with perineal pain. In addition, urinalysis and urine culture generally indicate acute cystitis which tends to accompany the acute prostatic infection. The major problem lies in the diagnosis of chronic bacterial prostatitis and the nonbacterial syndromes. Clinical symptoms and signs are extremely variable and unreliable. The most helpful methods of diagnosis of chronic prostatitis are examinations of the expressed prostatic fluid and quantitative bacteriologic localization cultures of the urine.

Prostatic fluid normally may contain a small number of leukocytes. Although the precise limit of normal is controversial, the presence of greater than ten white blood cells per high-power field is often considered suggestive of prostatic infection. If greater than 15-20 leukocytes per high-power field are present, the probability of true infection rises significantly. The microscopic analysis of prostatic fluid, however, always must be compared with that of the first voided 10 ml of urine (urethral specimen), as well as the midstream urine (bladder specimen). Leukocytes found in prostatic secretions actually may be a result of urethral or bladder inflammation with white cells entering prostatic fluid as it passes through the urethra. Thus examination of prostatic fluid alone may be misleading.

The most precise method for definitively diagnosing bacterial prostatitis requires quantitative bacteriologic cultures of the urethral and bladder urine and expressed prostatic secretions. The following specimens are obtained in order: (1) the first voided 10 ml of urine (termed VB1, voided bladder 1); (2) the midstream sample (VB2); (3) expressed prostatic secretions obtained by prostatic massage (EPS); and (4) the first voided 10 ml immediately after prostatic massage (VB3). All specimens are cultured quantitatively onto blood and MacConkey agar. True prostatic infection is confirmed when the quantitative bacterial colony counts of the prostatic specimens (EPS and VB3) exceed the VB1 count by at least tenfold. Although cumbersome, this method affords the greatest likelihood of making an accurate diagnosis of chronic bacterial prostatitis. Isolated cultures of either prostatic expressate or ejaculate may be very misleading because of urethral contamination. Cultures taken from prostatic biopsy specimens are likewise easily contaminated and are not recommended.

Recent measurements of humoral immune response in prostatitis are intriguing but thus far have not been helpful in diagnosis. In several studies, serum antibody titers against the particular offending strain of *E. coli* have been elevated in patients with chronic prostatitis. The titers returned to normal following successful treatment of the disease and remained at low titers in normal, noninfected men. Chronic bacterial prostatitis has been shown to produce antibody-coated bacteria with a positive direct immunofluorescent test; however, antibody-coating also occurs in pyelonephritis and possibly epididymitis. Significant elevations in immunoglobulins, particularly IgA, have been found in the prostatic fluid of men with chronic bacterial prostatitis but again, are highly nonspecific and are not helpful in making the diagnosis.

Acute Bacterial Prostatitis

Clinical Features and Pathology

Acute bacterial prostatitis is characterized by sudden chills, fever, malaise, low-back and perineal pain, dysuria, and occasionally severe obstructive voiding symptoms. It is a disease of adults, occurring in both young and elderly men. No definite predisposing factor has been demonstrated. Pathologically, marked inflammation occurs focally or throughout the prostate gland with heavy infiltration by polymorphonuclear leukocytes, lymphocytes, and macrophages. Large abscesses may occur as a late complication.

On gentle rectal examination, the prostate is extremely tender, often swollen, and warm. Because of patient discomfort and the high risk of producing bacteremia, prostatic massage is actually contraindicated in acute prostatitis. The bacterial pathogen usually causes concomitant acute cystitis and can be identified by culturing the clean-voided urine.

Treatment

The toxic condition of patients usually warrants hospitalization. Bed rest, analgesics, sufficient fluids, and stool softeners are important. If significant urinary retention occurs, indwelling urethral catheters should be avoided by placement of a suprapubic tube.

The intense inflammation that accompanies acute bacterial prostatitis allows many drugs to diffuse well into the prostatic fluid. Initial antibiotic therapy may include moderately high doses of gentamicin or tobramycin plus parenteral ampicillin. An alternative regimen is parenteral trimethoprim-sulfamethoxazole, pending culture results. The parenteral drug should be continued several days to a week. An appropriate oral antibiotic then should be continued for at least 30 days to minimize the risk of developing chronic prostatitis and microabscess formation.

Chronic Bacterial Prostatitis

Clinical Features

Chronic bacterial prostatitis is usually characterized by irritative voiding symptoms and pain located in the suprapubic region, perineum, low-back, or scrotum. Fever is generally absent; in fact, the infection sometimes is asymptomatic and only suspected because of unexplained bacteriuria. Pain following ejaculation or hematospermia may occur. Prostatic examination is nonspecific and often normal. Chronic bacterial prostatitis is one of the most common causes of relapsing urinary tract infection in men. Because the clinical picture is confusing, the best method of establishing the diagnosis is by performing bacteriologic localization cultures as previously described.

Pathology

Small prostatic calculi can be found in many men and are usually asymptomatic. On the other hand, in some men with prostatic calculi, relapsing urinary tract infection and chronic prostatitis, the calculi also have been infected. Prostatic calculi therefore have been proposed as one cause for the many treatment failures in chronic bacterial prostatitis.

The pH of prostatic fluid from patients with chronic bacterial prostatitis is usually 7. Theoretically, the alkaline pH of chronically infected prostatic fluid should impair the prostatic concentration of antibiotics that are ionized at acid pH. It is clear, however, that pH alone does not determine the amount of drug that diffuses into the prostate. A defect in prostatic function has been suggested and may be partly responsible for the relative difficulty of antibiotic penetration into the prostate in chronic infection. Numerous alterations in the secretory products of the prostate have been found in patients with chronic bacterial prostatitis, including decreased zinc, magnesium, acid phosphatase, lysozyme, and calcium.

Because most antibiotics diffuse poorly into the chronically infected prostate, medical therapy is difficult. One of the most effective antibiotic regimens is the combination of trimethoprim-sulfamethoxazole which has been shown to cure 30-70% of cases. Other successful antibiotics include carbenicillin and minocycline. The relapse rate is lowest when the antibiotic is administered continuously for 2-6 months.

Total suprapubic prostatectomy can cure chronic bacterial prostatitis; however, the high prevalence of postoperative urinary incontinence and sexual impotence makes this surgery too hazardous an alternative. Transurethral prostatectomy can be curative only if all infected tissue can be removed, a difficult procedure at best. Surgery therefore has been used for only the most serious and disabling cases.

Nonbacterial Prostatitis

The most common inflammatory condition of the prostate is nonbacterial prostatitis. Patients have voiding symptoms, perineal pain, a normal prostate on palpation, and prostatic expressate containing a large number of leukocytes. Unlike many patients with true chronic bacterial prostatitis, however, these patients have no history of documented urinary tract infection. In addition, bacteriologic localization cultures of urine and prostatic expressates are negative for the usual bacteria.

The causal agent of this ill-defined entity is unclear. The following organisms have been suggested as pathogens in nonbacterial prostatitis with little or no supporting evidence: fungi, obligate anaerobic bacteria, trichomonads, and viruses. Conflicting evidence exists regarding the possible roles of both *Ureaplasma urealyticum* and *Chlamydia trachomatis* in nonbacterial prostatitis.

Because the causative agent (if any) is unknown in nonbacterial prostatitis, treatment is frustating. A clinical trial with a tetracycline or erythromycin may be warranted. If the clinical response is not favorable, the use of other antibiotics is not beneficial. Symptomatic therapy including sitz baths and antiinflammatory drugs may be useful.

Other Types of Prostatitis

Tuberculous prostatitis has been found in a number of patients who usually have evidence of urinary tract tuberculosis. Needle biopsy of the prostate may reveal noncaseating granulomata as often as caseation, emphasizing the importance of cultures. X-ray evidence of pulmonary disease need not be present.

Rare cases of granulomatous prostatitis have been reported with systemic fungal infections including coccidioidomycosis, cryptococcosis, blastomycosis, and histoplasmosis. Occasionally granulomatous prostatitis has been found in the absence of any identifiable agent.

Epididymitis

Epididymitis is the most common intrascrotal inflammation. Isolated orchitis, on the other hand, is exceedingly rare. Nevertheless, we shall consider the two entities separately first, then look at the combination known as epididymo-orchitis. Epididymitis is a disease of adults, being rare in prepubertal boys and never documented in a child less than 6 years of age. It may be viral, bacterial (including chlamydial and tuberculous), fungal, traumatic, or chemical in origin. Orchitis may have a similar spectrum of etiologies.

Pathogenesis

The usual urinary pathogens are the most common bacterial causes of epididymitis. In addition, staphylococci, streptococci, and even meningococci may be present. *Chlamydia* is the most common agent in patients between the ages of sexual maturity and 35 years, comprising about two-thirds of nonbacterial epididymal infections (documented by aspiration cultures). Brucellosis may present with epididymitis before the systemic signs of undulant fever. Blastomycosis has affected the epididymis both with and without documented systemic disease. The pathology in these less common cases varies from mild inflammation to abscess formation, with or without involvement of the ipsilateral testis.

Organisms most commonly reach the epididymis via the lumen of the vas deferens as evidenced by the frequency with which the same microbes are recovered from the urine and aspiration cultures. In some cases the temporal relationship of the colonization (urine first) has been documented. Hematogenous spread of organisms is less common but appears to occur in cases of epididymitis associated with pneumococcal meningitis. This mode seems to operate as well in viral orchitis, some fungal infections, and in cases of orchitis in the newborn. The existence of infection spread in retrograde fashion via lymphatics remains hypothetical; similarly, direct extension from preexisting orchitis could occur.

Epididymitis has been divided into classes etiologically and clinically. The first classification separates nonspecific, traumatic, and specific infections. The system is old, and "nonspecific" is a misnomer since these infections are usually bacterial or chlamydial and identifiable. "Specific" infections include rarer, systemic agents such as the gonococcus, *Treponema pallidum,* tuberculosis, and fungi. A more useful, clinical classification separates acute, subacute, chronic, and recurrent infections.

Subacute epididymitis is a relatively asymptomatic lesion characterized by swelling and induration or nodularity of a portion of the epididymis, usually the tail or globus minor. It should not be ignored as it may represent secondary syphilis or be a harbinger of urinary infection or systemic fungal infection. Chronic epididymitis is a painful, disabling entity unresponsive to antimicrobials and anti-inflammatory drugs, usually requiring epididymectomy. It also may occur as the sequel of urinary tuberculosis. Recurrent epididymitis frequently accompanies recurrent urinary tract infection, chronic bacterial prostatitis, or seminal vesiculitis, and may require vasectomy if the associated problem cannot be resolved.

Treatment and Complications

The treatment of acute epididymitis consists of general supportive measures and specific antibiotics. Bed rest, elevation of the scrotum, and ice applied to the affected side should be prescribed. In younger patients (< 35 years) where the incidence of chlamydial infection is high, a course of tetracycline should be begun after urine culture is obtained and gonococcal infection ruled out. In older men, any broad-spectrum antibiotic suitable for urinary antisepsis may be employed. The culture results may dictate antibiotic modifications. Aspiration of the epididymis for culture is indicated only when (1) indwelling catheter causes multiple organisms in the urine; (2) infection is refractory; (3) surgical exploration for torsion is undertaken; or (4) recurrent infection due to an unknown agent occurs. In general, 10 days of antibiotics suffice.

There are four complications of bacterial epididymitis: abscess formation, reactive hydrocele, persistent infection leading to chronic epididymitis, and fibrosis causing sterility. Fungal, tuberculous, and gonococcal infections can lead to granuloma formation and sinus tracts. Gram-negative sepsis has been described in a few cases. The abscess must be drained surgically and usually necessitates removal of the involved epididymis and testis. Hydrocele may be drained and excised electively at a later date or left alone if it is not large. Occasionally percutaneous aspiration will relieve the pressure on the testis, thus reducing pain, but the hydrocele will recur. After several courses of rest, ice, and antibiotics, chronic epididymitis usually is managed by epididymectomy. Only if the opposite testis is abnormal, or the infection is bilateral does infertility ensue. Surgical relief of any obstruction is not warranted, even if it were technically feasible, because the epididymis is so damaged that sperm maturation will not occur. Some studies have shown benefit from administration of steroids or nonsteroidal anti-inflammatory agents for 2-3 days during the acute phase. While this may provide some measure of symptomatic relief, it does nothing more. Additional comments will be made in the section on orchitis.

Traumatic Epididymo-Orchitis

The term epididymo-orchitis is reserved by some to describe traumatic lesions; others use it to refer to presumed extension of epididymal infection into the testis itself. Such extension probably occurs only rarely as in the case of abscess formation where all the tissues in the hemiscrotum are involved to a varying degree. Here the traumatic lesion only will be considered.

There is no widespread agreement as to whether the trauma leads to infection of damaged tissues or activates preexisting infection. What is known is that blunt trauma to the scrotum and contents leads to an inflammatory response with swelling, tenderness, redness, and perhaps fever, and that these are often unilateral and associated with reactive hydrocele. Sometimes bacterial infection can be demonstrated. Once rupture of the testis is ruled out, the treatment is the same as that described earlier. Gonococcal epididymitis occurred in 5-10% of cases of male gonorrheal infection in the preantibiotic era, but recently the prevalence has been reduced to about 2%. It is an ascending infection via the vas deferens, results in typical painful inflammation of the globus minor, may be unilateral or bilateral, and may be associated with prostatitis or seminal vesiculitis. Infertility often results from bilateral cases. In contrast, syphilitic epididymitis nearly always involves the globus major and is more common than is generally thought. It can arise from retrograde infection or by extension from gummatous orchitis and occurs early or late in the secondary stage of syphilis (up to 8 years after initial infection). Chronic gummatous epididymitis is a very rare tertiary lesion. The treatment is antibiotics.

Tuberculous epididymitis occurs only subsequently to infection of the prostate and seminal vesicles by organisms present in the urine. The infection rarely presents with an acutely enlarged, tender epididymis; rather a "cold" abscess in the globus minor is found. Orchitis almost never occurs, although a few cases of invasion of the testis have been noted. Epididymectomy with preservation of the testis is the treatment of choice.

Orchitis

Primary orchitis without epididymitis is a rare event. Orchitis may occur by blood or lymphatic spread but more often occurs as an extension of ascending infection via the epididymis. It may be divided into the categories of pyogenic, viral, spirochetal, traumatic, chemical, mycotic, parasitic, and idiopathic. Any blood-borne infection may result in orchitis; the most common bacterial causes are *E. coli, Klebsiella,* streptococci, staphylococci, and *Pseudomonas.*

Pathologically the testis is swollen by edema and infiltration of polymorphonuclear cells. The swelling results in ischemic damage to the seminiferous epithelium, punctate hemorrhage on the tunica albuginea, and sometimes focal necrosis. Trauma, including vas ligation and other surgical manipulations, may result in granulomatous orchitis which is thought to be due to extravasated sperm proteins. The tissue reaction includes giant cells and has been confused with tuberculous orchitis. Chemical substances such as iodine, thallium, lead, carbon disulfide, and alcohol are alleged to cause destruction of the seminiferous tubules.

Orchitis is accompanied by fever, pain in the involved testis that radiates up the inguinal canal, nausea, and vomiting. The testis is swollen, tense, tender, and sometimes fluctuant. An associated hydrocele may be present. The treatment is generally the same as that for epididymitis, i.e., rest, scrotal elevation, ice, and antibiotics. Only if the differentiation from torsion or incarcerated hernia cannot be made, or frank abscess develops, should surgery be employed. Finally, the presence of a tumor must be excluded with certainty on follow-up examination, particularly in cases of trauma and granuloma formation. If the hydrocele makes the testis not palpable or there is doubt for any other reason, the testis must be explored via an inguinal incision.

In addition to the systemic diseases that may cause orchitis, several distant entities may be associated such as sinusitis, tonsillitis, furunculosis, osteomyelitis, endocarditis, and acute rheumatic fever. Often no bacteria can be demonstrated in the testis. Infections with coxsackievirus, varicella, variola, dengue, Epstein-Barr, and mumps viruses may cause orchitis. An acute orchitis may accompany secondary syphilis, and a chronic form occurs with tertiary syphilis.

Mumps orchitis has received much attention because of its frequency. It arises about 4-6 days after the parotitis in about 20% of cases; it has been reported rarely without parotitis. It is unilateral in 70% of the cases with some resultant testicular atrophy in 50% of the patients. The signs and symptoms and the treatment are as outlined above. Gamma globulin, convalescent serum, and diethylstilbestrol have been advocated to reduce the incidence of orchitis; gamma globulin may slightly reduce the frequency; DES provides only symptomatic relief. Likewise, steroids and ACTH have been administered with mixed results, but any benefit is slight and probably offset by the undesirable side effects of the hormones; a significant number of bacterial superinfections have occurred. Surgery (tapping the hydrocele) should be reserved for the most severe cases.

Selected Bibliography

Anderson, R. U. and Weller, C.: Prostatic secretion leukocyte studies in nonbacterial prostatitis (prostatosis). *J Urol* 121:292, 1979.

Berger, R. E., Alexander, E. R., Harnisch, J. P., Paulsen, C. A., Monda, G. D., Ansell, J., and Holmes, K. K.: Etiology, manifestations and therapy of acute epididymitis: Prospective study of 50 cases. *J Urol* 121:750, 1979.

Berger, R. E., Alexander, E. R., Monda, G. D., Ansell, J., McCormack, G., and Holmes, K. K.: *Chlamydia trachomatis* as a cause of acute "idiopathic" epididymitis. *N Engl J Med* 298:301, 1978.

Berger, R. E., Holmes, K. K., Mayo, M. E., and Reed, R.: The clinical use of epididymal aspiration cultures in the management of selected patients with acute epididymitis. *J Urol* 124:60, 1980.

Blacklock, N. J.: Anatomical factors in prostatitis. *Br J Urol* 46:47, 1974.

Drach, G. W.: In vitro antibiotic susceptibility of bacteria isolated from prostatic fluid. *Urology* 14:237, 1979.

Eykyn, S., Bultitude, M. I., Mayo, M. E., and Lloyd-Davies, R. W.: Prostatic calculi as a source of recurrent bacteriuria in the male. *Br J Urol* 46:527, 1974.

Fair, W. R. and Cordonnier, J. J.: The pH of prostatic fluid: A reappraisal and therapeutic implications. *J Urol* 120:695, 1978.

Fauer, R. B., Goldstein, A. M. B., Green, J. C., and Onofrio, R.: Clinical aspects of granulomatous orchitis. *Urology* 12:416, 1978.

Gislason, T., Noronha, R. F. X., and Gregory, J. G.: Acute epididymitis in boys: A 5-year retrospective study. *J Urol* 124:533, 1980.

Gleckman, R. and Crowley, M.: Epididymitis as cause of antibody-coated bacteria in urine. *Urology* 14:241, 1979.

Graves, R. S. and Engel, W. J.: Experimental production of epididymitis with sterile urine; clinical implications. *J Urol* 64:601, 1950.

Hermansen, M. C., Chusid, M. J., and Sty, J. R.: Bacterial epididymo-orchitis in children and adolescents. *Clin Pediatr* 19:812, 1980.

Meares, E. M.: Serum antibody titers in treatment with trimethoprim-sulfamethoxazole for chronic prostatitis. *Urology* 11:142, 1978.

Meares, E. M.: Prostatitis syndromes: New perspectives about old woes. *J Urol* 123:141, 1980.

O'Dea, M. J., Moore, S. B., and Greene, L. F.: Tuberculous prostatitis. *Urology* 11:483, 1978.

Oliveri, R. A., Sachs, R. M., and Caste, P. G.: Clinical experience with geocillin in the treatment of bacterial prostatitis. *Curr Ther Res* 25:415, 1979.

Paulson, D. F., and deVere White, R.: Trimethoprim-sulfamethoxazole and minocycline-hydrochloride in the treatment of culture-proved bacterial prostatitis. *J Urol* 120:184, 1978.

Schwarz, J.: Mycotic prostatitis. *Urology* 19:1, 1982.

Smith, J. W., Jones, S. R., Reed, W. P., Tice, A. D., Deupree, R. H., and Kaijser, B.: Recurrent urinary tract infections in men: Characteristics and response to therapy. *Ann Intern Med* 91:544, 1979.

Stamey, T. A., Meares, E. M., and Winningham, D. G.: Chronic bacterial prostatitis and the diffusion of drugs into prostatic fluid. *J Urol* 103:187. 1970.

Stankova, L., Drach, G. W., Hicks, T., Zukoski, C. F., and Chvapil, M.: Regulation of some functions of granulocytes by zinc of the prostatic fluid and prostate tissue. *J Lab Clin Med* 88:640, 1976.

Williams, C. B., Litvak, A. S., and McRoberts, J. W.: Epididymitis in infancy. *J Urol* 121:125, 1979.

35

VAGINITIS, CERVICITIS, AND
BARTHOLIN'S GLAND ABSCESS
Robert M. D'Alessandri, M.D.

Vulvovaginitis

Vulvovaginitis is perhaps the most common of all female genital infections. Inflammation of the vulva and vagina usually occurs concomitantly, hence the term vulvovaginitis. Specific etiologies are often obscure, and treatment is often unsatisfactory. Therefore, vulvovaginitis represents a difficult clinical problem.

Epidemiology

The normal adult vagina under estrogen control maintains a pH of 3.5-4.5. Lactobacilli predominate in the flora and are responsible for lactic acid production and vaginal acidity. Under these conditions the vagina is resistant to most infections. During the prepubertal and postmenopausal years, and during pregnancy, the pH rises and the flora changes. As a result, the vagina is less resistant to pathogens and more prone to infection. Antibiotics alter the intestinal and vaginal flora and may permit mycotic overgrowth and predispose to vaginal infections. Postmenopausal and pregnant patients taking antibiotics are particularly predisposed to the development of vulvovaginitis. Other factors that appear to predispose to vaginal infections include poor personal hygiene, sexual activity, diabetes mellitus, corticosteroids, and birth control pills. The role of birth control pills in the development of vulvovaginitis is somewhat controversial. It is believed that oral contraceptives increase the glycogen content of vaginal secretions and decrease the thickness of the vaginal wall resulting in increased susceptibility to mycotic infections. Oral contraceptives frequently modify sexual behavior, and it is this factor that may play a significant role in the development of vulvovaginitis. Certainly, trichomonal vaginal infections are sexually transmitted diseases and are more common in sexually active females.

Etiology

In recent years, *Candida* has replaced *Trichomonas* as the most common cause of vaginal infections. *Candida* may be isolated in over 50% of symptomatic patients. The most commonly isolated species is *C. albicans*. *Torulopsis glabrata* and *C. tropicalis* account for most of the remaining isolates. Other yeasts are less commonly associated with vaginal infections.

Trichomonal vaginitis accounts for 10-20% of the cases of vulvovaginitis. This pear-shaped protozoan is 8-30 mm in length and has a short undulating membrane, three to five anterior flagellae and no posterior flagellae. These organisms grow well in a proteolyzed liver-horse serum media adjusted to a pH of 6.5.

The other infectious causes of vulvovaginitis include a small pleomorphic gram-negative rod called *Gardnerella vaginalis* or *Corynebacterium vaginale*. This organism frequently is isolated in cases of "nonspecific" vaginitis. When inoculated into vaginas of healthy volunteers symptoms and signs of vaginitis occur. The organisms are fastidious and are difficult to isolate from vaginal cultures. *Mycoplasma* and *Chlamydia* spp have been commonly isolated in patients with cervicitis and vaginitis. These organisms are often found with other organisms more commonly associated with genital infections. The exact relationship between the presence of these organisms and genital infection has yet to be determined.

Pinworm is also a common cause of vulvovaginitis especially in young children. It may or may not be associated with rectal itching. On occasion older children and adults also may develop vaginitis as a result of pinworm infestation. Amebic vulvovaginitis also occurs and results from the mechanical spread of infected feces. Most persons have associated gastrointestinal symptoms of amebic dysentery.

Pathogenesis

The pathogenesis of both candidal and trichomonal vulvovaginitis is poorly understood. *Candida* is commonly a harmless saprophyte in the vagina. The initiation of symptomatic disease appears to depend upon a variety of systemic and local alterations, some of which have already been mentioned. It is interesting that the discharge associated with candidal vaginitis is relatively free of leukocytes. It is composed of clumps of epithelial cells and fungal organisms. Candidal growth is unaffected by vaginal pH, and may be favored by a slightly lower pH. The intense inflammatory appearance of the vagina and the pruritus have been attributed to the production of mycotoxins by the organism. Others have suggested that the inflammation and pruritus are caused by acidic products of carbohydrate metabolism.

The pathogenetic mechanism of disease caused by *Trichomonas* organisms is similarly obscure. This organism appears to have little or no cytotoxicity in human cell tissue cultures and appears not to produce a toxin. Several predisposing factors, the foremost of which is an elevated vaginal pH, are necessary for initiation of symptomatic illness. The discharge has many polymorphonuclear leukocytes and motile trichomonads. If there is any disruption of the cervical or vaginal epithelium, organisms may gain access and cause an intense inflammatory response.

The presence of clue cells (epithelial cells covered with bacteria) in smears of vaginal secretions and the relative absence of PMNs, is characteristic of infection caused by *G. vaginalis*. Vaginal wall necrosis and friable ulcerations are most commonly found in patients with amebic vulvovaginitis. Also ulceration of the cervix, and in severe cases involvement of the endometrium, may occur.

Manifestations

The symptoms of vulvovaginitis are nonspecific and consist of vaginal discharge, pruritus, burning, dyspareunia, dysuria, urinary frequency, and low-back pain. Classically the discharge is described as "cheesy" in cases caused by *Candida* spp, greenish and malodorous in cases caused by *Trichomonas,* and grey in cases caused by *Gardnerella*. If the pruritus is intense and occurs only at night, infestation with *Enterobius* is likely. Systemic signs of infection are absent. Fever is distinctly unusual and if present another cause must be sought. Except for inflammation of the vulva and vagina, the remainder of the pelvic examination is usually unremarkable. In severe cases of vaginitis, inguinal adenopathy may be present, but that is rare.

Diagnosis

In most cases the diagnosis of vulvovaginitis is made based upon the history and physical examination. In all cases the search for an etiologic agent is essential to determine specific therapy. Samples of vaginal secretions should be examined microscopically as wet (NaCl) preparations, KOH preparation, and Gram-stained specimen. The presence of motile trichomonads, on wet preparations, yeast and hyphae on KOH preparation, or clue cells on Gram stain assists in the diagnosis.

Papanicolaou's smears may be useful in diagnosing causes of infectious vulvovaginitis but many false-positive and false-negative results occur. Atypical cells are commonly seen in patients with inflammation and when present a repeat Pap smear is indicated 6 weeks after therapy. Cultures for *Neisseria gonorrhoeae* should be performed when indicated. If the wet mount fails to reveal trichomonads, culture for these organisms should be performed on suitable media; a commercially available trypticase serum culture media should be used. Young children should be examined by the Scotch-Tape method for pinworms. Suspicious lesions of the vulva or vagina should be biopsied. Follow-up examination after therapy is necessary because many vaginal pathogens coexist and treatment of one unmasks another.

Differential Diagnosis

The differential diagnosis of leukorrhea is extensive (Table 35.1). Physiologic leukorrhea as seen in newborns and during pregnancy and sexual excitement can often be excluded by history alone. Other noninfectious leukorrheas include atrophic vaginitis, chemical- or foreign-body-induced vaginitis, neoplasia, and cervical lesions. In addition to the infectious causes discussed previously, gonorrhea, syphilis, and herpesvirus infection may be associated with leukorrhea. Careful physical examination of the vagina, microscopic examination and appropriate cultures of vaginal secretions, and biopsy of any specific lesions will yield a diagnosis in almost all cases.

Treatment

If a specific etiology and precipitating factors can be identified treatment is often successful. After a complete history and physical examination to identify the problem and the precipitating factors, appropriate studies as outlined earlier should be performed to determine the responsible agent. Therapy aimed specifically at the causative organism should be employed. In the case of candidal infection, many agents have been employed. Nystatin vaginal tablets or cream, 100,000 U, twice daily for 2 weeks or miconazole nitrate cream daily for 5-7 days are effective

TABLE 35.1   Differential Diagnosis of Vaginal Discharge

Disease	Consistency	Color	Odor	Pruritus	Inflammation	Diagnosis
Candida	Thick, cheesy	White	None	Intense	Intense	Wet prep or Gram stain
Trichomonas	Frothy	Yellow-green-grey	Foul	Mild	Yes	Wet prep
Nonspecific	Thin	Gray-white-yellow	Foul	None or minimal	No	Vaginal epithelial cells covered by many gram-negative rods; no PMNs
Atrophic	Thin	Colorless-white	No	No	Minimal	Clinical
Foreign body	Thin	Colorless, serosanguirous	Foul	No	Minimal	Clinical
Physiologic	Thin	Colorless	No	No	No	–

antifungal agents. Clotrimazole, fatty-acid gels, rosanilin and acridine dyes, iodine compounds, and a host of other agents all have been used to treat candidal vulvovaginitis. Eliminating the precipitating cause, e.g., discontinuing systemic antibiotics, improves the likelihood of a successful therapeutic outcome. Intercourse should be interdicted or a condom used during the course of treatment.

Metronidazole is the mainstay of treatment for trichomonal vulvovaginitis. While intravaginal metronidazole is effective in 60% of patients, systemic therapy achieves success in 85-95% of patients. The single 2-g oral dose of metronidazole appears to be highly effective and is the preferred method of administration. Metronidazole should not be administered to pregnant females. Male consorts need not be treated since the disease is self-limited and of short duration in males. Male sexual partners should refrain from intercourse for 4 weeks or use condoms. The major side effects of the single 2-g dose of metronidazole are gastrointestinal upset and the appearance of dark urine. The patient should be warned not to drink alcoholic beverages while taking metronidazole.

Metronidazole is effective treatment of *G. vaginalis* vaginal infections. However, the potential toxicity of this agent limits its usefulness in the treatment of this mild infection. The widespread use of sulfonamide cream is inappropriate. The organism is frequently isolated in asymptomatic male patients. However, treatment with metronidazole is similarly unnecessary. The use of the condom provides adequate protection from reinfection of female partners.

The possibility of chemical vaginitis secondary to any of the vaginal douches and sprays sold over-the-counter must be considered. Patients should be advised to discontinue use of these preparations. In children with pinworm infestation a single dose of mebendazole 100 mg is sufficient treatment.

In all cases of vulvovaginitis local measures such as sitz baths and gentle cleansing of the vulva will reduce the symptoms of pruritus and burning.

Immunology Prevention

There is evidence that the female genital tract is part of the secretory immunologic system. Secretory IgA has been detected in vaginal secretions. However, the role of vaginal secretory immunoglobulins and the site of their production has yet to be determined. Local vaginal immunization in animals against *Brucella abortus* produces very high titers of antibody in vaginal secretions. Presumably immunization could proceed via this route to prevent local vaginal infections and other venereally transmitted infections.

Prognosis

Specific treatment in conjunction with the elimination of inciting or predisposing factors often results in improvement or cure. Recurrence, however, is the rule. Complications including secondary infection and sepsis are rare. In the presence of secondary bacterial infections specific parenteral antibiotics may be necessary.

Cervicitis

Infection of the endocervix may occur in the absence of infection elsewhere in the female genital tract. Recognition of endocervical infection may be difficult because of lack of symptoms and because physiologically, cervical mucus may be profuse and may contain polymorphonuclear neutrophils.

Cervicitis occurs most commonly during the sexually active period of life. There are many different etiologic agents and the epidemiological picture is more typical of the responsible infecting agent than a specific syndrome. The micro-flora of the endocervix is quite diverse and includes the bacteria found in the vagina.

Acute gonococcal cervicitis is a well-recognized entity. Gonococci are more frequently isolated from the endocervix than any other site in women. *Chlamydia* may be isolated in over two-thirds of sexual partners of men with chlamydial ure-thritis. Herpetic cervicitis occurs and may or may not be associated with lesions of the external genitalia. Herpetic cervicitis is important because of its associa-tion with cervical carcinoma and because, if present at the time of delivery, there is considerable risk of transmission to the newborn. Other etiologies include adeno-virus and enterobiasis.

Unlike the vaginal epithelium which cornifies under the influence of estrogens, the lining of the endocervix is columnar epithelium. As a result, the endocervix remains relatively more susceptible to a variety of infectious agents. The cervix or ectocervix is lined with stratified squamous epithelium similar to the vaginal walls.

Acute bacterial cervicitis involves the endocervix and the squamous columnar junctions, with polymorphonuclear leukocyte infiltration of the subepithelial tis-sue. The mucosa becomes erythematous, hypertrophic, and may desquamate. There are increased cervical secretions which may be grossly purulent. Occlusion of the endocervical glands may lead to Nabothian cyst formation.

Salpingo-oophoritis is an important complication of bacterial cervicitis. Gono-cocci spread by way of the endometrium, while other pyogenic bacteria, especially streptococci, spread by way of the lymphatics.

Vaginal discharge is the most common symptom associated with cervical in-fection. Pelvic pain is uncommon, although dyspareunia may occur. In patients with herpetic cervicitis, abdominal pain may occur, although most cases are asymp-tomatic. On physical examination, the area around the cervical os may be ery-thematous. There may be ulcerations or frank necrosis. Tenderness on palpation of the cervix may or may not be present.

Because most patients with cervical infections have minimal or no symptoms, the pelvic examination is an essential element in diagnosing cervicitis. All cases of purulent cervicitis should be cultured for gonococci and a Pap smear performed. In addition, a wet mount, Gram stain, and KOH preparation of cervical secretions should be performed. Patients with suspected herpetic cervicitis should have con-firmatory viral cultures and require at least yearly cytologic examinations. The diagnosis of chlamydial cervicitis may be made on clinical and epidemiologic grounds, or may require special culture techniques.

The treatment of gonococcal or chlamydial cervicitis is the recommended treatment for these infections, as outlined in Chapter 36. There is no specific treatment for herpetic cervicitis, although a variety of agents, including acyclo-vir, may prove to be efficacious. It is important to emphasize that cytologic ex-amination (Pap smear) should be part of the evaluation of cervicitis. In cases of suspicious cytologic results, a repeat smear after appropriate treatment may be necessary.

Control of sexually transmitted diseases would result in fewer cases of cer-vicitis. Other preventive measures must await a clearer understanding of the causes of chronic cervicitis.

The most important complication of acute purulent cervicitis is spread via the lymphatics or the uterine cavity to the fallopian tubes and ovary. It is unclear what effect chronic cervical infections may have on fertility and/or the develop-ment of cervical carcinoma. There is a significant epidemiologic correlation be-tween herpetic infections and cervical carcinoma. Herpetic and chlamydial cer-vical infections present at the time of delivery may lead to serious neonatal infec-tion.

Bartholin's Gland Abscess

Definition

Bartholin's or vulvovaginal glands secrete mucus for lubrication of the vaginal orifice and canal during intercourse. These glands are frequently the site of infection.

Etiology

The gonococcus is isolated from about 10% of infected Bartholin's glands, and anaerobes in nearly 75% of the cases. Anaerobic streptococci and *Bacteroides* spp are the most commonly isolated anaerobes. Other less common isolates are *E. coli, Staphylococcus* and *Streptococcus pyogenes.* On occasion, *Trichomonas* is isolated from infected glands.

Epidemiology

Infected Bartholin's glands occur most commonly during the reproductive years. In diabetics gland abscess may extend to necrotizing fasciitis and several anaerobes are frequently isolated.

Pathogenesis

Bartholin's glands are lobulated racemose glands placed deeply in perineal structures on either side of the vaginal orifice. Infected vaginal secretions gain access to the transitional ductular epithelium and induce inflammation with resultant obstruction and abscess formation. With continued mucous secretion the gland may enlarge and the swelling involve the entire labium of the affected side. Surrounding edema and inflammatory skin changes are common accompaniments. Ultimately the abscess may drain through the lower vaginal wall. Persistence of infection leads to a chronic form with eventual fibrosis, duct closure, and cyst formation.

Diagnosis

Initially there is painless swelling and cyst formation. The gland enlarges slowly and may interfere with walking and coitus. When pain, erythema, and tenderness develop, infection is present. A suppurative exudate may be expressed from the gland. Fever and other systemic manifestations of infection are usually absent. In diabetics the abscess may extend to necrotizing fasciitis and involve the subcutaneous tissues of the abdomen with extensive undermining of the skin.

Differential Diagnosis

The clinical diagnosis of an infected Bartholin's gland offers little difficulty. Infection is almost always secondary to cyst formation and therefore, enlargement generally precedes signs of local infection. Rarely, neoplasia of the gland may cause enlargement with secondary infection.

Treatment

The treatment of acute bartholinitis is surgical drainage. Recurrence is common following simple incision and drainage. Excision of the gland is useful in patients with chronic recurrent disease but should not be performed as treatment of acute infection. Marsupialization is a simple procedure designed to reestablish the mucocutaneous function of the duct with the labia. Since this procedure preserves the function of the gland, and recurrence is rare, this is the recommended surgical procedure.

Limitation of activity, sitz baths, and analgesics are helpful for pain relief. Antibiotics are not indicated in uncomplicated cases.

Gram stains and culture (aerobic and anaerobic) of infected material should be performed in all cases. The presence of gram-negative diplococci on smear or *N. gonorrhoeae* on culture requires appropriate antibiotic treatment. In cases of extending infection or necrotizing fasciitis, wide surgical excision of necrotic and infected tissues may be lifesaving. Antibiotic therapy should be instituted to cover anaerobes and Enterobacteriaceae. Clindamycin and tobramycin or chloramphenicol in full therapeutic doses are the initial drugs of choice.

Immunology and Prevention

Marsupialization of Bartholin's gland cysts should be performed before infection especially in diabetics. Excision of the gland may be necessary in patients with recurrent infection.

Complications and Prognosis

In most cases marsupialization is curative. Recurrences are not common. Extension of infection is rare and has been reported most commonly in diabetics. In these patients the mortality is high, approaching 50%. Extensive surgical debridement and antibiotic coverage of aerobic and anaerobic gram-negative rods are the treatments of choice.

Selected Bibliography

Azzan, B. B.: Bartholin's cyst and abscess. A review of treatment of 53 cases. *Br J Clin Pract* 32:101-102, 1978.

Gorbach, S. L. and Bartlett, J. G.: Anaerobic infections. *N Engl J Med* 290:1177-1184, 1237-1245, 1289-1294, 1974.

Lee, Y. H., Rankin, J. S., Alpert, S., Daly, A. K., and McCormack, W. M.: Microbiological investigation of Bartholin's gland abscesses and cysts. *Am J Obstet Gynecol* 129:150-153, 1977.

Pheiffer, T. A., Forsyth, P. S., Durfee, M. A., Pollack, H. M., and Holmes, K. K.: Nonspecific vaginitis, role of hemophilis vaginitis and treatment with metronidazole. *N Engl J Med* 298:1429-1434, 1978.

Roberts, D. B. and Hester, L. L., Jr.: Progressive synergistic bacterial gangrene arising from abscesses of the vulva and Bartholin's gland duct. *Am J Obstet Gynecol* 114:285-291, 1972.

36

SEXUALLY TRANSMITTED DISEASES
Robert M. D'Alessandri, M.D.

In recent years, sexually transmitted diseases (STDs) have posed an increasingly greater public health problem. This problem is only partly reflected in the increasing incidence and prevalence of these diseases. In addition, there is evidence that there are more diseases that are occasionally sexually transmitted (Table 36.1). As a result it has become apparent that these diseases have primarily social and behavioral connotations and only secondarily represent important medical problems. Table 36.2 lists the causative agents for some of these diseases.

The physician has a dual role: first to diagnose and treat these diseases and their complications, and second to be conscious of the threat to the community posed by these diseases (Tables 36.3-36.5). All physicians must recognize that control of STDs will require their full support and cooperation.

Gonorrhea

Gonorrhea is the most frequently reported sexually transmitted disease in the United States. As a result of this and the often severe complications associated with gonococcal infections, it represents the most important of all the STDs.

Gonorrhea is caused by a gram-negative diplococcus, *Neisseria gonorrhoeae*. This organism is a strict aerobe that requires relatively high humidity and ambient CO_2 for growth. Gonococci are very sensitive to drying, an important fact to remember when attempting clinical isolation.

In 1979 there were 1,003,958 reported cases and an additional 1-2 million unreported cases of gonorrhea in the United States. In 1957 reported cases of gonorrhea reached a low of 214,496. From 1966 until 1973 reported cases increased at a rate of 2%/yr. Since 1975 more than 1 million cases have been reported each year. Age-specific case rates show that the 20- to 24-year group accounts for

TABLE 36.1 Incidence of Sexually Transmitted Diseases (STDs)

	Incidence	
STDs	Reported	Estimated
Gonorrhea	1.004×10^6	$1.6-2.0 \times 10^6$
NGU	$-^1$	3.0
Trichomoniasis	–	1.5
Genital herpes	–	0.2-0.5
Condyloma accuminatum	–	Unknown
Syphilis	0.067	0.085
Occasionally STD [2]		Unknown

[1]Not reportable
[2]CMV, hepatitis B, amebiasis, giardiasis, shigellosis prevalence as sexually transmitted diseases is unknown

TABLE 36.2 Etiologies of Sexually Transmitted Syndromes

Male urethritis	*N. gonorrhoeae, C. trachomatis,* herpes simplex virus, ? *U. urealyticum*
Vulvitis	*C. albicans,* herpes simplex virus
Vaginitis	*T. vaginalis, C. albicans*
Cervicitis	*N. gonorrhoeae, C. trachomatis,* herpes simplex virus
Female urethritis	*N. gonorrhoeae, C. trachomatis*
Genital ulceration	Herpes simplex virus, *T. pallidum, H. ducreyi, C. granulomatis, C. trachomatis*
Pelvic inflammatory disease	*N. gonorrhoeae, C. trachomatis*
Proctitis	*N. gonorrhoeae,* herpes simplex virus, ? *C. trachomatis*
"TORCHES" syndrome	Cytomegalovirus, herpes simplex virus, *T. pallidum*

TABLE 36.3   Public Health Aspects of Some Common Sexually
Transmitted Diseases

Disease	Relative Incidence	Specific Diagnosis	Treatment	Prevention Method
Gonorrhea	High	Inexpensive, available	Very good	Proved
Chlamydia	High	Expensive, limited	Good	Possible
Herpes	High	Expensive, limited	Limited	Questionable
Syphilis	Moderate	Inexpensive, available	Excellent	Proved

TABLE 36.4   Sexually Transmitted Diseases in Homosexuals

Disease	% by History
Pediculosis	65
Gonorrhea	40
Nonspecific urethritis	25
Venereal warts	20
Syphilis	15
Hepatitis	10
Herpes simplex	10

Significant correlates with infection:

Number of different lifetime sexual partners

Anonymous contacts

Years as practicing homosexual

Anal intercourse

TABLE 36.5   Physicians' Office Visits for Genital Herpes Infection

Years	Rate/100,000 Visits
1966–1969	~ 4
1970–1973	10
1974–1977	25
1978–1981	30

nearly 40% and the 15- to 19-year group 25% of all reported cases. Urban areas report significantly higher case rates.

During 1979 nearly 9 million women were screened and culture tested for gonorrhea. Nearly 400,000 (4.5%) were positive for gonorrhea. Of the 1 million reported cases of gonorrhea, over 350,000 contacts were identified, 215,000 interviewed, and 175,000 treated for gonorrhea.

It is estimated that half of the 413,000 cases of gonorrhea in women result in pelvic inflammatory disease, and 25-30,000 cases of Bartholin's gland abscess. Approximately 3000 cases of ectopic pregnancy complicated gonorrhea in 1979. Most of the 6000 cases of disseminated infection occur in women.

Columnar and transitional cell epithelia are the primary sites of gonococcal infections. In males purulent urethritis develops first. Prostatitis and epididymitis may develop by direct spread of the infection. On rare occasions the seminal vesicles may become involved. It is estimated that 35% of males with a single exposure to gonorrhea develop infection and that 95% of infected males become symptomatic. Pharyngitis and proctitis may develop in the male, but these symptoms are almost always associated with homosexual activity.

If untreated, 95% of the patients with urethritis will be asymptomatic within 6 months. A small percentage of individuals will continue to have a small amount of mucoid urethral discharge or "gleet" with little or no discomfort.

In the female, urethritis, when present, is usually mild and transient. Bartholin's or Skene's glands may be infected, and abscess formation is common. Spread to these areas is caused by infected cervical secretions. The cervix may be infected and with contiguous spread to the fallopian tubes, salpingitis may occur. Tubo-ovarian abscess may form and infection with other organisms is frequent. The spread of infection occurs in association with menstruation and may be related to disruption of local immune mechanisms. With healing, fibrosis and scarring occurs which may lead to obstruction of the fallopian tubes and sterility.

The adult vagina is remarkably resistant to gonococcal infection because of its squamous epithelium. Gonococcal vaginitis does occur in prepubertal children and frequently results from molestation.

During childbirth gonococci may infect the conjunctiva, pharynx, respiratory tract, or anus of the newborn. Conjunctivitis, the most common site of neonatal infection, was a frequent cause of blindness in the preantibiotic era.

Social factors and life-styles have played an important part in the changing character of gonococcal disease. Gonococcal pharyngitis has been reported with greater frequency in homosexuals and in women practicing fellatio. It is believed that the only mode of transmission of pharyngeal gonococcal infection is by oral-penile contact of the "deep throat" type. This is often associated with erythema of the hard palate.

Disseminated gonococcal disease occurs twice as frequently in women than in men. This is thought to be related to the greater frequency of asymptomatic or mildly symptomatic infections in females. The source of disseminated infection may be the genital tract, pharynx, or rectum. The frequency of dissemination is greater during pregnancy and, in the nonpregnant state, appears to be associated with menstruation. It is interesting that the strains of N. *gonorrhoeae* that disseminate tend to be very sensitive to penicillin and require arginine, hypoxanthine, and uracil for growth. In addition, dissemination occurs in individuals deficient in certain components of complement, especially C6 or C8.

The manifestations of gonococcal infection appear to depend mostly upon the sexual behavior and gender of the patient. Gonococcal infections in heterosexual men almost always involve the urethra with presenting complaints of purulent urethral discharge, dysuria, urinary frequency, and the absence of systemic signs.

The incubation period is 2-8 days. The symptoms are usually severe enough for the patient to seek treatment; following treatment the disease subsides promptly. In about 10% of untreated males complications of epididymitis, prostatitis, and seminal vesiculitis develop. Urethral stricture, once a common sequel of gonococcal urethritis, is now much less frequently seen.

In homosexual men, pharyngitis and proctitis occur more frequently. Pharyngeal involvement presents in several different ways. The infection may be asymptomatic without signs of infection; asymptomatic with tonsilar edema and erythema; or symptomatic with sore throat and erythema, edema, and vesicles on the tonsils and pharynx. Anorectal involvement too is usually asymptomatic but may be associated with anal discharge, blood in the stools, and tenesmus. On proctosigmoidoscopic examination, the mucosa may be erythematous, friable, and covered with a purulent exudate. Rarely perirectal abscess or fistula formation occurs.

In females, the cervix, urethra, anorectal area, and pharynx may be involved, in that order of frequency. Cervicitis is associated with a mucopurulent yellow vaginal discharge. On examination the cervical os may be erythematous, friable, and seen to exude pus. Compression of the cervix yields a yellowish, thick discharge. The cervix is nontender in uncomplicated infections.

Unilateral swelling of Bartholin's gland and abscess formation may occur. Often the gland is quite tender and an erythematous halo about the duct is noted. With involvement of the urethra and Skene's glands, pus may be expressed from these sites by urethral compression. Endometritis may occur as a result of extension of infection from the cervix and is associated with abnormal menstrual bleeding, abdominal pain, and tenderness on examination. Salpingitis occurs in approximately 20% of infected women. It is manifested by signs of pelvic peritonitis, fever, nausea, and vomiting. On examination there is lower abdominal tenderness, pain on movement of the cervix, adnexal tenderness, and occasionally a palpable adnexal mass. Repeated episodes of pelvic infections are associated with a very high incidence of ectopic pregnancy and sterility. Bacteremia and pelvic thrombophlebitis develop less frequently. Spread of gonococci into the upper abdomen may cause perihepatitis and be associated with right upper-quadrant abdominal pain. A friction rub may be heard over the liver.

Disseminated gonococcal infection occurs in 3% of women and 1% of men with gonorrhea. Local symptoms are often absent and the incubation period appears to be longer than in those patients with local urogenital symptoms. Dissemination in women is usually associated with menses.

Fever, arthralgias, arthritis, tenosynovitis, and skin lesions characterize disseminated gonococcal infections (Table 36.6). The skin lesions may be papular, pustular, or hemorrhagic, are present on distal extremities, and number less than 30 (generally 3-10). Gram-negative diplococci may be seen on stained or immunofluorescent preparations of material from skin lesions. Tenosynovitis of the extensor tendons of the wrists, fingers, ankles, or knees is nearly pathognomonic for gonococcal infection. It is believed that circulating immune complexes are responsible for the arthralgias and tenosynovitis.

Arthritis, often without prior symptoms of bacteremia, may occur and may involve more than one joint. Joint fluid is purulent and may yield gonococci on culture. Gonococcal arthritis is the most common form of disseminated gonococcal infection and the most common type of septic arthritis.

In the male patient with a purulent urethral discharge and dysuria, the diagnosis of gonococcal urethritis may be made by Gram-stained examination of the discharge. The presence of gram-negative diplococci within leukocytes is very strong presumptive evidence of gonococcal infection. Male urethral exudate cultures should be obtained whenever the Gram stain fails to reveal gonococci, in

TABLE 36.6   Major Manifestations of Disseminated Gonococcal Infection*

Manifestation	% of Patients
Arthritis	85
Meningitis	5
Endocarditis	5
Bacteremia without arthritis	5
Pericarditis	2

*Ann Intern Med 74:979, 1971

contacts of patients with gonorrhea, in areas where penicillinase-producing gono-cocci are prevalent, and in the presence of equivocal smears. The Gram stain al-lows for rapid identification of gonococcal infections and treatment without de-lay. In homosexual males, cultures of the pharynx and rectum should be obtained.

In female patients diagnosis of gonococcal infection is more difficult because of the frequency of asymptomatic patients. Additionally, the Gram stain of cer-vical secretions is considerably less reliable because of the presence of bacteria which may be confused with gonococci. Cervical and rectal cultures should be ob-tained in all symptomatic female patients, in contacts of patients with gonorrhea, and in patients suspected of having disseminated gonococcal disease. In addition pharyngeal cultures in female patients should be obtained in cases of suspected disseminated disease and in patients who practice fellatio.

In patients with skin lesions, Gram stains and culture of material from these lesions should be performed in addition to blood cultures. Gonococci are very sen-sitive to drying and all cultures should be quickly inoculated on Thayer–Martin medium or a suitable transport medium. Calcium alginate or synthetic fiber swabs should be used to avoid the bactericidal properties of cotton fibers.

In 1976 strains of gonococci were identified which were resistant to penicillin. These strains, shown to produce penicillinase, originated in Southeast Asia and have now disseminated throughout the world. In the first 9 months of 1981 in the United States, there were 1910 reported cases of penicillinase-producing N. gon-orrhoeae (PPNG). In 1979 there were only 328 reported cases in the United States (Table 36.7). It is believed that about 50% of the strains from Southeast Asia are PPNG. Many of these strains are resistant to tetracycline as well. Spectinomycin is the mainstay of therapy for PPNG.

The CDC treatment schedule for uncomplicated gonococcal infections in men and women calls for aqueous procaine penicillin G (AAPG) 4.8 million U intramus-cularly with 1 g of oral probenecid (Table 36.8). Tetracycline 2 g/day for 7 days (total dosage 14 g) or spectinomycin hydrochloride, 2 g intramuscularly, may be used for patients allergic to penicillin. Ampicillin 3.5 g or amoxicillin 3.0 g, with 1 g probenecid orally, are alternative treatments.

Intramuscular penicillin is the preferred treatment for several reasons: treat-ment can be administered in one dose at the time of diagnosis, eliminating prob-lems of compliance; this regimen is recommended for pharyngeal and anorectal gonorrhea and incubating syphilis and can be used in pregnant patients.

TABLE 36.7   Cases of Penicillinase-Producing *N. Gonorrhoeae* (PPNG)

Year	Approximate Number of Cases
1976	< 100
1977	200
1978	250
1979	300
1980	1000
1981	2500
1982	4000

TABLE 36.8   Gonococcal Treatment

1. Uncomplicated infection

    A. Aqueous procaine penicillin G 4.8 million U IM, at two sites with 1 g of probenecid by mouth or;

    B. Amoxicillin 3.0 g or ampicillin 3.5 g with probenecid 1 g by mouth or;

    C. Tetracycline HCl 500 mg four times daily by mouth for 7 days or doxycycline, 100 mg twice daily for 7 days,

    D. A and C alone are preferred for pharyngeal gonococcal infection.

2. Disseminated gonococcal infection

    A. Aqueous crystalline penicillin G, 10 million U IV daily until improvement followed by ampicillin or amoxicillin, 500 mg four times a day for a total of 7 days or;

    B. Ampicillin 3.5 g or amoxicillin 3.0 g with probenecid 1 g by mouth followed by 500 mg four times a day of ampicillin or amoxicillin for 7 days or;

    C. Tetracycline, 500 mg by mouth, four times daily for 7 days or;

    D. Erythromycin, 500 mg by mouth, four times daily for 7 days or;

    E. Cefoxitin 1 g IV four times daily for 7 days. Recommended for disseminated PPNG infections.

3. Acute PID

    A. Doxycycline IV 100 mg twice daily plus cefoxitin 2 g IV four times daily. Continue for at least 4 days and at least 48 hr after defervescence.

    B. Clindamycin 600 mg IV four times daily plus gentamicin (tobramycin) 2 mg/kg IV followed by 1.5 mg/kg IV three times daily in patients with normal renal function.

Tetracycline has the advantage of reducing the occurrence of postgonococcal urethritis. However, compliance is a major factor in the effectiveness of this treatment.

In pregnant patients allergic to penicillin, tetracycline should not be used. Instead cefazolin 2 g intramuscularly with probenecid or spectinomycin 2 g intramuscularly are recommended. If cefazolin is used caution must be observed because of cross-allergenicity with penicillin.

All men and women exposed to gonorrhea should be examined, cultures taken, and treated as above. Follow-up cultures should be obtained in 3-7 days and again at 4-8 weeks, the latter because of the high recurrent infection rate. Treatment failures should be re-treated with spectinomycin (2 g intramuscularly). All patients should have a serologic test for syphilis performed initially. If treated with spectinomycin a repeat test in 8-12 weeks is recommended.

Acute salpingitis or pelvic inflammatory disease (PID) generally requires hospitalization and parenteral therapy. Combination regimens recommended are as follows: doxycycline 100 mg IV, twice a day plus cefoxitin 2 g IV four times daily, or clindamycin 600 mg four times a day plus gentamicin (or tobramycin) 2 mg/kg IV followed by 1.5 mg/kg IV three times a day in patients with normal renal function. Continue IV drugs for at least 4 days or 48 hr after defervescence. Doxycycline or clindamycin may be continued orally to complete a 10- to 14-day course of treatment. Outpatient treatment may be accomplished by using APPG 4.8 million U intramuscularly, or ampicillin 3.5 g, or amoxicillin 3 g, whichever choice plus 1 g of probenecid, followed by doxycycline 100 mg twice daily or tetracycline HCl 2 g/day in divided doses, both for 10-14 days. Table 36.9 reviews the cost of various treatment schedules for uncomplicated genital gonorrhea.

The treatment for disseminated gonococcal infection is penicillin G IV 10 million U/day until improvement, followed by ampicillin or amoxicillin 2 g/day for at least 7 days. Tetracycline 2 g/day orally for at least 7 days may also be used.

Spectinomycin is the treatment of choice for uncomplicated infections caused by PPNG (Table 36.10). In patients with PPNG-associated PID, 2 g of spectinomycin intramuscularly daily for 5-10 days, or cefoxitin, 2 g intramuscularly or intravenously every 8 hr for 5-10 days should be administered. For PPNG pharyngeal infections, sulfamethoxazole (400 mg)/trimethoprim (80 mg), nine tablets daily for 5 days is recommended.

TABLE 36.9   Cost of Various Treatment Schedules for Uncomplicated Genital Gonorrhea

Schedule	Wholesale Price
Ampicillin 3.5 g + probenecid	$0.86
Tetracycline 500 mg q.i.d. x 5 days	0.87
Procaine penicillin G 4.8×10^6 U + probenecid	1.32
Amoxicillin 3.0 g + probenecid	1.37
Doxycycline 100 mg b.i.d. x 5 days	7.05
Minocycline 100 mg b.i.d. x 5 days	7.94

TABLE 36.10   Management of Patients with Penicillinase-Producing
              N. Gonorrhoeae (PPNG)

Culture all patients suspected of gonorrhea, including all orifices that are exposed to the organism during sexual contact; culturing is the only way to prove
patient has PPNG.

Patients with positive smear on initial visit should be treated with procaine penicillin G or ampicillin (either one plus probenecid) in accordance with recommended treatment schedules.

Patients with history of recent travel (past 30 days) to high-incidence area should
be monitored particularly closely.

Alert patients regarding existence of PPNG strains and stress importance of returning for their "test-of-cure" culture 5-7 days later.

Patients with uncomplicated anogenital PPNG infections should be given spectinomycin HCl, 2 g IM.

Patients with positive test-of-cure culture should also be given spectinomycin.

Sexual contacts of PPNG-infected patients should be cultured and treated with
spectinomycin.

Test of-cure cultures should be done 1 week after treatment with spectinomycin;
those who are positive should be treated with cefoxitin, 2 g IM, plus probenecid,
1 g p.o.

Patients with PPNG pharyngeal infection should be treated with trimethoprim-
sulfamethoxazole, nine tablets daily, for 5 days, because spectinomycin and
cefoxitin are ineffective against pharyngeal gonococcal infection.

Females with PPNG PID, males with PPNG epididymitis, and patients with disseminated PPNG infection should be treated with spectinomycin, 2 g IM for
5-10 days, or cefoxitin 2 g q8h IM or IV.

   With treatment, patients usually improve within 2-3 days. In patients with
septic arthritis, repeated arthrocentesis usually is adequate, and open drainage is
unnecessary.
   Prevention begins with the education of the public concerning all aspects of
gonorrhea, and other STDs. To reduce the incidence of STDs contacts must be
identified and treated. The patient is often best able to notify contacts and urge
them to seek treatment.
   At present there is no vaccine for gonorrhea. Antibiotic prophylaxis has had
limited success in preventing disease and is not recommended. Condom use is
probably the best single method (short of abstinence from sexual activity) of preventing gonorrhea, both in terms of acquisition and transmission.

Nongonococcal Urethritis (NGU)

It is estimated that over 3 million cases of NGU occur annually in the United States, making it the most common STD. Symptoms occur most commonly in males. It is generally believed that a causative agent of NGU is *Chlamydia trachomatis,* an intracellular bacterial pathogen that requires tissue culture techniques for isolation. This organism has been isolated from the urethral discharge of men with NGU and from the cervical secretions of their contacts. Isolation has been associated with an appropriate antibody response in symptomatic individuals. Additionally *C. trachomatis* has been isolated from cervical secretions in patients with PID and postpartum endometritis.

It is believed that *C. trachomatis* is responsible for at least 50% of the cases of NGU and most of the cases of postgonococcal urethritis. The simultaneous acquisition of gonorrhea and NGU occurs in nearly 30% of males and 50% of women with gonorrhea.

Ureaplasma urealyticum (T strain mycoplasm) is another agent responsible for NGU. This organism is frequently isolated from asymptomatic patients as well as patients with symptoms of urethritis. Another agent responsible for NGU is *Trichomonas vaginalis.* All of these agents produce a similar clinical syndrome.

It is believed that the annual incidence of NGU is at least double that of gonorrhea. The difficulty in isolating these organisms and because NGU is not a reportable disease necessitate only rough incidence estimates. The syndrome occurs in the same age group as gonorrhea, has a higher prevalence in whites and higher socioeconomic groups, and tends to recur. Because of the very high prevalence of positive cultures in partners and because partners are rarely treated, public health measures to control NGU have not been successful.

Chlamydia trachomatis gains access to the male urethra at the time of intercourse and causes epithelial cell damage in the form of "cobblestoning" of the urethra. The incubation period is 2-3 weeks, much longer than that of gonorrhea.

Dysuria and a scant, watery, urethral discharge are the major manifestations of NGU in the male. The discharge may be noticeable only upon awakening and the dysuria is often more an annoyance than a true burning. Systemic signs and symptoms are absent and if untreated the symptoms will disappear in 2 or 3 months. In a proportion of patients, prostatitis or epididymitis develops. The association between Reiter's syndrome and NGU has been suggested but is unproved.

The diagnosis is strongly suggested by findings of mild dysuria and scant discharge. Gram stains of the uretheral discharge reveal polymorphonuclear leukocytes but no organism. Cultures for gonococci should be obtained. The special culture techniques required for isolation of *C. trachomatis* are rarely available, and in the light of an appropriate history and Gram stain findings they are clinically unnecessary.

In addition the genitalia should be carefully examined for ulceration or chancre, the presence of epididymitis or prostatitis. In females with cervicitis culture for gonorrhea should be obtained as well as a Gram stain, wet mount, and KOH preparation of the vaginal discharge to identify possible causes of cervical infection.

The treatment of choice for NGU is tetracycline, 2 g/day for at least 7 days. Alternatively, erythromycin 2 g/day for at least 7 days may be used. If the patient continues to have symptoms a reevaluation which includes repeating the previously mentioned stains and culture should be made. A trial of erythromycin may be instituted if no other specific agent is identified. Sexual contacts also should be treated.

Lymphogranuloma Venereum (LGV)

Lymphogranuloma venereum is a STD also caused by *C. trachomatis* but by different serotypes than those causing NGU (see Chapter 79). These organisms are also called LGV-TRIC agents. They are important as a potential cause of multisystem disease. The LGV organism has all of the characteristics of the chlamydiae, including intracellular parasitism, intracytoplasmic inclusions, and the chlamydial group-reactive antigen. The chlamydia immunotypes most often responsible for LGV are L_1, L_2, and L_3.

Lymphogranuloma venereum occurs most commonly in tropical and subtropical climates and only occasionally is reported in the United States with fewer than 1000 cases reported annually. Most cases occur in homosexuals, prostitutes, travelers, and military personnel. The disease occurs more commonly in males. The peak incidence, like other STDs, occurs in the second and third decades of life.

The LGV organisms gain access through abrasions in the skin and lead to a dermal granuloma. The usual site of the primary lesions is the coronal sulcus or the posterior vaginal wall (Tables 36.11 and 36.12). Superficially vesiculation or ulceration occurs and heals without scarring within a few days. The primary lesion develops within 1-4 weeks of inoculation.

From the primary site, LGV organisms are carried by macrophages to regional lymph nodes and cause extensive lymphadenitis. During the early stage of active lymphadenitis, systemic spread may occur, leading to involvement of joints, heart, and (rarely) the central nervous system. During the later stages of regional lymphatic involvement fibrosis, stricture, and obstruction occur. Histologically, lymph nodes show acute and chronic inflammation with multiple stellate abscesses. These abscesses may coalesce, rupture, and form sinus tracts. Suppuration occurs in most cases. This resolves with time, but often an indurated inguinal mass persists for life. Obstruction of the lymphatics may lead to elephantiasis of the external genitalia. With anorectal involvement, proctocolitis and rectal stricture formation may occur.

TABLE 36.11   Differential Diagnosis of Penile Ulcer

Disease	Characteristics
Syphilis	Painless Positive dark-field examination
Herpes	Painful, multiple Recurrent Positive Tzanck's smear
Chancroid	Painful Small gram-negative rods
Lymphogranuloma venereum	Systemic symptoms Culture of *C. trachomatis*

TABLE 36.12   Diagnosis and Treatment of Vaginitis

Etiology	Diagnostic Features	Therapy
T. vaginalis	Motile trichomonads ph 5.5-6.0 Amine odor with 10% KOH	Metronidazole 2.0 g single oral dose, or 250 mg t.i.d. x 10 days
C. albicans	Yeast, pseudomycelia pH < 4.5 Culture of organism	Nystatin vaginal tablet b.i.d. x 7 days Clotrimazole or miconazole intravaginally q.d. x 7 days
G. vaginalis	Clue cells pH > 4.5 Amine odor with 10% KOH Culture of organism	Metronidazole 500 mg b.i.d. x 7 days
Normal	pH < 4.5 No odor with 10% KOH	-

Following exposure a primary lesion develops on the external genitalia. The incubation period is from a few days to several weeks. The lesion is a small papule or vesicle which may ulcerate or may go unnoticed. Healing occurs in several days. Soon thereafter, the inguinal nodes enlarge, become tender and matted. Nonspecific systemic symptoms occur and include fever, chills, malaise, and weight loss. Physical findings may include meningismus, splenomegaly, and conjunctivitis. In males, the nodes above and below Poupart's ligament are enlarged and the ligament is seen to form the "groove sign." Suppuration of nodes is common.

In 25% of the patients anorectal involvement occurs and is marked by a bloody, purulent, rectal discharge. Rectal abscesses, fistulas, and strictures occur. Systemic signs are usually absent.

Other clinical manifestations include acute meningitis, pneumonia, generalized adenopathy, lymphedema of the eyelids, and a polyarthritis. Associated skin eruptions include erythema multiforme and erythema nodosum.

Definitive diagnosis can be made only by isolation of LGV organisms from appropriate specimens. Since this requires special techniques not generally available, a presumptive diagnosis is made based on clinical manifestations and serologic tests. The most useful diagnostic tests include the complement-fixation (CF) and microimmunofluorescent (MIF) tests. The heat-stable antigen used in the CF test is group-specific for all Chlamydia spp. Although a sensitive test it is not specific for LGV. The MIF test is more sensitive and specific because it utilizes multiple chlamydial antigens.

The Frei skin test has been used to diagnose LGV since 1925. The antigen is prepared from organisms grown in vitro and administered by intradermal injection. Erythema and induration within 48-72 hr signals a positive test. Once positive, the skin test remains positive for life. The Frei test is considered the least specific and sensitive of the three tests.

Tetracycline in dosages of 2-3 g/day for 3-4 weeks is the treatment of choice. Sulfonamides in dosages of 4-6 g/day also have been used successfully to reduce symptoms and prevent recurrences. Several courses of therapy may be required in some patients. Doxycycline 100 mg twice daily or erythromycin 500 mg four times daily for at least 2 weeks are alternative regimens. Additionally, aspiration of fluctuant nodes and surgical correction of fistulas may be required.

Granuloma Inguinale

Granuloma inguinale is an indolent granulomatous and ulcerative disease of the skin and mucous membranes of the genitalia and perineal regions. The disease is transmitted by sexual contact and has a low-degree of communicability.

Calymmatobacterium granulomatis are nonmotile encapsulated gram-negative bacilli. When intracellular, the organisms are unencapsulated and are found in the vacuoles of monocytes and neutrophils. The capsule forms as the organism matures and when the organisms are released, the encapsulated bacteria are infectious.

Granuloma inguinale occurs most commonly in the tropical and semitropical climates of India, South America, the islands of the South Pacific, and the west coast of Africa. In the United States most cases are reported from the southeastern states in blacks. The disease is often of a low order of communicability and may not occur in spouses of grossly infected partners. In homosexuals the disease may be transmitted by anal intercourse.

Organisms gain entrance via a break in the skin and at that site a papule develops and forms an irregularly shaped ulcer. These are nontender, 1-4 cm in diameter with firm edges and a beefy red base. The lesion spreads by direct extension and heals by leaving behind fibrous atrophic scar tissue. Rarely hematogenous dissemination occurs with involvement of bones, joints, or liver. Pseudobuboes develop following lymphatic spread to inguinal nodes.

In male lesions are first noted on the glans or prepuce. In women, papules most frequently appear on the labia. Ulcers may have at the same time an active edge and depigmented scar tissue. Coalescence occurs and extension to the abdominal wall occasionally occurs. Systemic symptoms are absent.

The diagnosis of granuloma inguinale can be made by obtaining a biopsy or scraping of an ulcer and staining for intracellular organisms (Donovan's bodies). Dark-field examination should be performed as well as serologic tests to rule out syphilis. Biopsies of chronic ulcers should be taken to eliminate the possibility of concurrent skin cancer.

Tetracycline, ampicillin, chloramphenicol, and gentamicin all have been reported to successfully treat granuloma inguinale. Tetracycline or ampicillin, 2 g/day orally, should be used first and should be continued until the lesions are healed, for a minimum of 3 weeks. Chloramphenicol 1.5 g/day, or gentamicin 1 mg/kg twice daily, may be used for treatment failures or resistant cases.

Syphilis

Syphilis is an infectious disease of humans, usually acquired by sexual contact. It is of both historical and clinical significance. Because of its protean clinical manifestations it has been called the great imitator.

The causative agent of syphilis is a spirochete *Treponema pallidum.* The organism is related to other spirochetes including those that cause pinta and yaws. *Treponema pallidum* has not been cultured in vitro but can be propagated in certain animal models. Nonpathogenic strains have been cultivated in vitro. *Treponema pallidum* is sensitive to drying, heat, soap and water, and a variety of heavy metals.

Direct contact is the usual mode of transmission. One exception to this is congenital syphilis, which is transmitted from mother to fetus in utero. Transfusion of blood from a syphilitic donor also has been reported to cause syphilis.

As in other STDs, the peak incidence occurs between 15 and 30 years of age. In 1979 there were 67,049 cases reported and another estimated 20,000 cases of recent acquisition unreported. Clinical syphilis may be divided into several stages: primary, secondary, latent, and late syphilis. There were 24,874 reported cases of primary and secondary syphilis in 1979. Men accounted for over three-fourths of the reported cases, reflecting the increasing prevalence of syphilis in the homosexual population. Late and latent syphilis cases numbered more than 41,000 in 1979. Most reported cases are from urban areas. It is believed that many cases of syphilis are undetected.

Following penetration of mucous membranes, skin, or hair follicles, *T. pallidum* disseminates throughout the body via the bloodstream or lymphatics. This appears to occur within hours of infection, long before the first clinical manifestations of primary syphilis are noted. Blood from individuals at this stage is infectious.

The incubation period is from 3 to 90 days (usually 3 weeks). The development of the primary lesion of syphilis, the chancre, marks the onset of the primary stage. Chancres are usually single, painless, and heal within 3 weeks. The borders of the chancre are raised, firm, and indurated, and the base is smooth. Multiple chancres are common and the appearance is often atypical. In women, chancres are less commonly observed because of their cervical location. In homosexuals, rectal chancres may occur and may be mistaken for rectal carcinoma.

Regional lymphadenopathy may accompany *primary syphilis.* The inguinal adenopathy may be unilateral or bilateral and painless unless there is secondary infection. Extragenital chancres may occur on any part of the body. The anus, oropharyngeal area, eyelids, breasts, or fingers are among the most common sites of extragenital infection. Healing without treatment occurs in 3-6 weeks and is usually complete before the onset of secondary manifestations.

Six weeks following contact (2-12 weeks) a generalized disorder develops, marked by constitutional and mucocutaneous manifestations (*secondary syphilis)* (Table 36.13). Patients frequently complain of fever, malaise, headache, sore throat, anorexia, and arthralgias. Most patients have generalized lymphadenopathy; nodes are large, nontender and firm.

Cutaneous manifestations occur in almost all patients with secondary syphilis. The skin lesions are nonpruritic and painless, and may vary greatly. The skin lesions include macules, papules, or nodular lesions, are similar in size and often symmetric, usually on the torso, palms, soles, and mucous membranes. Papular lesions are often dark-field positive. Patchy alopecia may occur and is reversible. Other manifestations include a mild meningitis, hepatitis, osteolytic lesions, nephritis, or nephrotic syndrome. An absolute lymphocytosis and an elevated erythrocyte sedimentation rate are common.

Latent syphilis begins with the passing of the first attack of secondary syphilis and lasts until the onset of late syphilis. Latent syphilis is marked by positive serology in the absence of clinical signs or symptoms of disease.

There may or may not be a history of antecedent infection and/or treatment. False-positive serology, congenital syphilis, and asymptomatic neurosyphilis must be ruled out. Positive serology on several occasions, a normal CSF, a positive, specific treponemal test, and the absence of disease known to cause false-positive serology are necessary before one can make the diagnosis of latent syphilis. Latent syphilis is arbitrarily divided into early and late periods. *Early latent syphilis*

TABLE 36.13   Signs and Symptoms of Secondary Syphilis

Constitutional symptoms	Headache Fever Arthralgias Sore throat Rhinitis Tearing	∿ 70%

Lymphadenopathy
  Inguinal
  Cervical
  Occipital
  Axillary
  Epitrochlear
	Diffuse
	Rubbery
	Symmetric
	Painless
	Small
		∿ 85%

Skin and mucous membranes	Macular, papular or maculopapular Mucous patches Condylomata lata Pustular	∿ 90%
CNS	Meningismus Aseptic meningitis Cranial nerve involvement Anterior uveitis	
Uncommon	Glomerulonephritis Hepatitis Arthritis Intestinal involvement	

is infection of less than 4-years duration and *late latent,* greater than 4-years duration. During early latency, recurrent mucocutaneous manifestations may occur in approximately 25% of the patients. After 1 year recurrence is much less common. During late latency, the patient is considered to be noninfectious except in pregnancy. Approximately one-third of the patients with late latent syphilis will go on to develop the complications of late or tertiary syphilis.

Late syphilis is the destructive phase of untreated early syphilis. Any organ of the body may be involved (Table 36.14). The manifestations of late syphilis do not occur until years after the initial infection. The disease progresses slowly, is noninfectious, and includes three major presentations; *late benign* or *gummatous syphilis, cardiovascular syphilis,* and *neurosyphilis.*

Late benign syphilis develops 1-20 years after the initial infection in approximately 15% of untreated syphilitics. In the penicillin era, gummas are distinctly unusual. Gummas may be found in any organ but preponderantly in skin and bones. Gummas are usually solitary, asymmetric, indolent, and slowly progressive. They may start as an indurated nodule, which may ulcerate centrally. The margins may be curved or polycyclic. Gummas respond dramatically to appropriate antimicrobial therapy.

TABLE 36.14   Late (Tertiary) Syphilis

		Approximate % of Untreated Patients
Neurosyphilis		

Asymptomatic	CSF abnormalities
	    Elevated protein
	    Pleiocytosis
	    Positive serology
		25

Symptomatic	Meningovascular 5-10 yr
	    Seizures
	    Stroke
	    Transverse myelitis
	Parenchymatous
	    General paresis 15-20 yr
	    Tabes dorsalis 25-30 yr
		6

Cardiovascular	Aortic insufficiency Aortic ectasia, particularly ascending aorta Coronary artery stenosis	10

Gumma	Skin: Painless nodule or ulcer
	Bone pain, pathologic fractures,
	    joint destruction
	Upper respiratory: nasal septal
	    and/or palatal perforation
	Hepatitis
		Uncommon

Cardiovascular manifestations of late syphilis occur in approximately 10% of untreated patients, beginning 5-10 years after the initial infection. The major cardiovascular complications are aortic insufficiency and aneurysm of the ascending aorta. Other large arteries are less commonly involved. Obstruction of the coronary ostia may lead to coronary insufficiency. The underlying lesion is an obliterative endarteritis of the vasa vasorum resulting in intimal and medial necrosis, usually of the ascending aorta. This results in aneurysmal dilatation of the aorta, a widened and thickened aortic ring and valve leaflets, with resultant aortic regurgitation. Radiographically, linear calcification of the ascending aorta is seen. Rarely, the descending aorta may be involved.

Neurosyphilis occurs in four major clinical categories, although overlap is common. These categories are: asymptomatic, meningovascular, tabes dorsalis, and general paresis. In asymptomatic neurosyphilis, there are no clinical signs or symptoms of CNS disease. The diagnosis is established in the presence of a positive cerebrospinal fluid VDRL in an asymptomatic individual. A false-positive cerebrospinal fluid VDRL in the absence of a traumatic tap does not occur. Early neurosyphilis is assumed in individuals with a positive serology and negative spinal fluid VDRL but with an increased cerebrospinal fluid protein and lymphocytosis in the absence of other neurologic causes. Treatment prevents progression to symptomatic neurosyphilis.

Meningovascular syphilis is an aseptic meningitis which usually occurs within the first year of infection but may occur anytime after the primary stage in a small percentage of patients. Meningovascular syphilis coincides with the onset of the cutaneous manifestations of secondary syphilis. The clinical manifestations are similar to other forms of meningitis. In addition, there may be cranial nerve palsies resulting from vascular occlusion and infarction of the base of the brain. There is a CSF lymphocytosis, an increased protein and a normal CSF glucose. Although very few cerebrovascular accidents are caused by syphilis, such an event in a young person with a history of syphilis must raise the question of meningovascular syphilis.

A second form of neurosyphilis is tabes dorsalis which is a slowly progressive degenerative disease of the posterior columns and posterior roots of the spinal cord. This results in ataxia, impairment of position and vibratory sense, and loss of peripheral reflexes. Incontinence, impotence, and severe "lightning-like" pains of the extremities triggered by cold or other stresses are common.

Ocular involvement in the form of optic atrophy and pupillary disturbances is common. The Argyll-Robertson pupil is characteristic of syphilis and involves a failure to constrict to light with normal pupillary constriction to accommodation.

Progressive loss of cortical function, or general paresis, is a chronic meningoencephalitis. There are personality changes, focal neurologic signs, and seizures. In the brain, there is perivascular and meningeal inflammation, with degenerative changes in the cortex. Altered mental status, irritability, headaches, memory loss, and confusion are characteristics of the paretic patient. The CSF has a lymphocytosis, increased protein content, and positive VDRL.

Congenital syphilis results from the transplacental spread of syphilis from mother to fetus. In untreated patients, fetal wastage occurs in 25%, another 30% of infected neonates die shortly after birth, and nearly half of those who survive develop symptomatic disease (Table 36.15). This may be divided into early and late congenital syphilis.

Early syphilis develops after birth and resembles secondary syphilis in the adult. There is rhinitis, hemolytic anemia, hepatosplenomegaly, and paralysis of an extremity due to painful osteochondritis. The cutaneous lesions may be vesicular and bullous, frequently on the palms and soles. Papular lesions occur somewhat later. An immune-complex nephritis also may be seen.

Late congenital syphilis is characterized by positive serology and evidence of healed early and late lesions involving periostitis of the bridge of the nose (saddle nose), screwdriver-shaped incisors (Hutchinson's teeth), interstitial keratitis, eighth nerve deafness, and other manifestations.

The diagnosis of primary syphilis can best be made by finding typical spirochetes on dark-field examination of early lesions. A negative dark-field does not exclude the diagnosis of primary syphilis. Two successive dark-field examinations on different days should be made on all suspected lesions in addition to serologic testing for syphilis. Chancres, condylomata, and lesions of secondary syphilis, as well as mucous patches of congenital syphilis, are most likely to be dark-field positive. Experienced observers are required to accurately interpret dark-field specimens.

Lesions should be carefully cleaned with saline and gauze to avoid bleeding. Serous fluid may be obtained by gently squeezing suspected lesions and either applying it directly to a glass slide or into a sterile capillary tube and then transferred to a slide.

Nontreponemal serologic tests are used to determine the presence of anticardiolipin antibodies. Among the more common nontreponemal tests, the VDRL

TABLE 36.15   Congenital Syphilis

Mucocutaneous	Rhinitis (snuffles) Bullae and vesicles Diffuse papulosquamous desquamative rash Mucous patches, condylomata lata

Skeletal	Osteochondritis
	Periostitis
	    Saddle nose
	    Saber shin

Hepatosplenomegaly, jaundice	
Hematologic	Thrombocytopenia Leukocytosis Anemia Paroxysmal cold hemoglobinuria
Glomerulonephritis	
Later manifestations	Interstitial keratitis (aged 5-25) Deafness Recurrent arthropathy (Clutton's joints) Hutchinson's teeth, Moon's molar Frontal bossa Poor maxillary development Rhagades Neurosyphilis Gumma
Abortion or stillborn	

and the RPR tests (rapid reagin) are inexpensive, well standardized, and easy to perform. If any degree of positivity is noted, quantitation by serial dilutions should be performed.

The test becomes positive 1-3 weeks after the chancre appears, peaks during the secondary stage, and falls thereafter. The test often remains positive for life. It is estimated that 75% of primary cases, more than 95% of secondary and early latent, and only 70% of late latent and late cases have positive nontreponemal tests.

False-positive nontreponemal tests occur in direct proportion to the number of positive tests in a population. False-positive reactions (FPR) may be characterized as acute false-positive reactions of less than 6-months duration or chronic false-positive reactions of more than 6 months. An acute FPR is often associated with viral infections. Other associated conditions include malaria, pregnancy, and of course laboratory error. Chronic FPR may be associated with connective tissue disease, especially SLE, narcotic addiction, leprosy, and malignancy. Occasionally healthy individuals will have FPR. However, all individuals with FPR require thorough evaluation and observation to rule out serious underlying disease.

Occasionally, a false-negative reaction occurs as a result of a prozone reaction in the presence of antibody excess. This may be expected in patients with secondary syphilis and very high titers of reagin. In these cases serially diluting the serum will overcome this effect.

There are many different varieties of treponemal tests that utilize *T. pallidum* as the antigen to detect specific antitreponemal antibodies. These tests are specific, more difficult to perform, and more costly. As a result, these tests are used as confirmatory tests.

The *Treponema pallidum* immobilization test (TPI) was the first acceptable treponemal test. The TPI utilizes live *T. pallidum* (Nichols strain) as the antigen. The fluorescent treponemal antibody-absorption (FTA) test is one of the most widely used treponemal tests. Dessicated *T. pallidum* (Nichols strain) is used as the antigen to which is added the patient's serum. Before mixing, the serum is absorbed with various nonpathogenic treponemal strains to remove cross-reacting antibodies. An IgM-FTA-ABS test is used to identify the presence of congenital syphilis in neonates of seropositive mothers, since IgM antibody does not cross the placenta.

Other treponemal tests include the *T. pallidum* hemagglutination and micro-hemagglutination assay utilizing erythrocytes sensitized with components of *T. pallidum*. The hemagglutination tests are less difficult to perform and less expensive. In general, these tests are probably as specific as the FTA; however, there is less experience using them.

Comparative sensitivities show that the FTA is probably the most sensitive test for syphilis. More than 50% of patients with primary syphilis, nearly 100% of patients with secondary, and more than 95% of patients with late or latent disease have positive FTA tests. False-positive FTA reactions occur in less than 1% of the patients. A false-positive FTA-ABS should lead one to search for SLE or to reconsider the possibility of syphilis. A major drawback of the FTA-ABS test is that it is not reliably performed on CSF and is not as sensitive as the cerebrospinal fluid VDRL.

The treatment of choice for all stages of syphilis is parenteral penicillin. In patients with primary, secondary, or latent syphilis of less than 1-year duration, benzathine penicillin G, 2.4 million U IM, at one time, is the recommended treatment. In penicillin-allergic patients, tetracycline HCl, 2 g/day by mouth in divided doses for 15 days is recommended.

All patients should be encouraged to return for repeat quantitative nontreponemal tests at least 3, 6, and 12 months following treatment. The titer should fall to a low level or become nonreactive within this time.

Syphilis of greater than 1-year duration (latent and late stages) requires three IM injections, a week apart, of benzathine penicillin G, 2.4 million U. This routine has been shown to be effective for most patients with neurosyphilis, despite the fact that these doses of penicillin fail to produce treponemicidal levels of penicillin in the CSF. As a result, some have recommended that 12-24 million U of IV aqueous penicillin G per day be administered to patients with neurosyphilis. An alternative regimen is aqueous procaine penicillin G, 2.4 million U IM, daily plus probenecid 500 mg by mouth, four times daily, both for 10 days. This is followed by the three weekly benzathine penicillin G injections.

Penicillin-allergic patients with latent or late disease other than neurosyphilis may be treated with tetracycline HCl, 2 g in divided doses for 30 days. In penicillin-allergic patients with neurosyphilis, specialty consultation is required to confirm the presence of penicillin allergy. Tetracycline may be used in the proven penicillin-allergic patients with neurosyphilis. Close follow-up is required in these patients and desensitization to penicillin may be required if patients fail to respond to tetracycline.

Cerebrospinal fluid examination is required for all patients with syphilis of longer than 1-year duration or of indeterminate duration to exclude the presence of asymptomatic neurosyphilis. All treated cases of neurosyphilis require repeat quantitative nontreponemal serology and clinical evaluation at 3, 6, 12, 18, 24, 30, and 36 months after treatment. Repeat CSF examination is recommended at 6-month intervals for at least 3 years. All patients with early syphilis should return for repeat quantitative nontreponemal tests at 3, 6, and 12 months after treatment. Patients with syphilis of longer than 1-year duration should also have repeat testing 24 months after treatment.

Response to adequate treatment is nearly always followed by cure in patients with early disease. In fact, treatment of incubating syphilis will completely abort the disease before lesions develop and serology becomes positive (Table 36.16). Unfortunately, once destructive cardiovascular or neurologic lesions have occurred, response to treatment is incomplete and the lesions do not regress. Thus, it becomes very important to recognize and treat syphilis early, before the late stages of the disease occur.

Although treatment is extremely effective, particularly in early disease, this has done little to eradicate the disease particularly in certain populations such as homosexuals. Since a vaccine is not immediately on the horizon, effective control programs are the major means of preventing disease. Unfortunately, underreporting and often ineffective and poorly staffed control programs, have stymied efforts to eradicate syphilis.

The ability to culture pathogenic strains in vitro and the understanding of the immunologic response to infection are important steps leading to the development of a safe, effective vaccine. In the meantime, it is important that physicians recognize their responsibility not only to treat but also to report and aid in the identification of contacts.

TABLE 36.16   Preventing Syphilis by Treatment After Exposure*

Treatment	% Developing Syphilis
Penicillin (2.4-4.8 x 10^6U)	0
Tetracycline (3.0 g)	13
Tetracycline (1.5 g)	22
No treatment	30

*Exposure within 30 days of treatment. *JAMA* 218:711, 1971

Chancroid

Chancroid, a relatively uncommon disease in the United States, is caused by *Haemophilus ducreyi* a gram-negative bacillus. The organism grows on blood-enriched media and positive cultures are noted in over three-fourths of patients with chancroid. Bacterial contamination reduces the likelihood of positive cultures.

The organism gains entrance through a break in the skin or mucous membrane. A small papule or vesicle develops 3-5 days after contact and gradually ulcerates. The base of the ulcer has a dirty gray exudate composed of polymorphonuclear and mononuclear cells. There is a reddened overhanging edge. The ulcer is tender and painful and frequently solitary. It is often on the prepuce or on the edge of the foreskin. Ulcers enlarge and may produce multiple ulcerations by autoinoculation. In the female, ulcers may occur on the labia or at the introitus.

Typically, within a week, lymphadenopathy develops. It is often a unilateral, unilocular enlargement which may go on to suppuration.

Scrapings should be obtained from the ulcer's edges for microscopic examination and culture. Repeated dark-field examinations are necessary to rule out syphilis. Pus aspirated from an intact node also may be cultured and stained. The finding of typical organisms in these specimens is adequate for a strong presumptive diagnosis of chancroid.

The drug of choice for the treatment of chancroid is erythromycin, 500 mg given orally four times daily for at least 10 days or until the lesions have healed. Trimethoprim-sulfamethoxazole (160/800 mg) twice daily may be substituted. Sexual partners require similar therapy. In patients that fail to respond, sensitivity testing may provide useful information for further treatment.

Selected Bibliography

Brooks, G. F., Darrow, W. W., and Day, J. A.: Repeated gonorrhea: An analysis of importance and risk factors. *J Infect Dis* 137:161-169, 1978.

Dunlap, E. M. C., Al-Egaily, S. S., and Honang, E. T.: Penicillin levels in blood and CSF achieved by treatment of syphilis. *JAMA* 241:2538-2540, 1979.

Eisenstein, B. I. and Mosi, A. T.: Disseminated gonococcal infection and gonococcal arthritis: I. Bacteriology, epidemiology, host factors, pathogen factors and pathology. *Sem Arthritis Rheum* 10:155-172, 1981.

Gjestland, T.: The Oslo study of untreated syphilis. *Acta Derm-Venereol* 35:1-368, 1955.

Goodrich, J. T.: Pelvic inflammatory disease: Considerations related to therapy. *Rev Infect Dis* 4:S778-S787, 1982.

Gump, D. W., Dichstein, S., and Gibson, M.: Endometritis related to *Chlamydia trachomatis* infection. *Ann Intern Med* 95:61-63, 1981.

Hammond, G. W., Slutchuk, M., Satliff, J., Sherman, E., Well, W. C., and Ronald, A. R.: Epidemiology, clinical, laboratory and therapeutic: Traits of an urban outbreak of chancroid in North America. *Rev Infect Dis* 2:867-879, 1980.

Handsfield, H. H., Wiesner, P. J., and Holmes, K. K.: Treatment of the gonococcal arthritis-dermatitis syndrome. *Ann Intern Med* 84:661-667, 1976.

Holmes, K. K., Counts, G. W., and Beaty, H. N.: Disseminated gonococcal infection. *Ann Intern Med* 74:979-993, 1971.

Jaffe, H. W.: Non-gonococcal urethritis: Treatment of men and their sexual partners. *Rev Infect Dis* 4:S772-S777, 1982.

Jaffe, H. W. and Kabins, S. A.: Examination of cerebrospinal fluid in patients with syphilis. *Rev Infect Dis* 4:S842-S847, 1982.

Kearns, D. H., Seibert, G. B., O'Reilly, R., Lee, L., and Logan, L.: Paradox of the immune response to uncomplicated gonococcal urethritis. *N Engl J Med* 289: 1170-1174, 1973.

Kraus, S. J., Kaufman, H. W., Albritton, W. L., Thornsberry, C., and Biddle, J. W.: Chancroid therapy: A review of cases confirmed by culture. *Rev Infect Dis* 4:S848-S856, 1982.

Madiedo, G., Ho, K. C., and Walsh, P.: False positive VDRL and FTA in cerebrospinal fluid. *JAMA* 244:688-689, 1980.

McGee, Z. A., Johnson, A. P., and Taylor-Robinson, D.: Pathogenic mechanisms of *Neisseria gonorrhoeae:* Observations on damage to human fallopian tubes in organ culture by gonococci of colony type 1 or 4. *J Infect Dis* 143:413-421, 1981.

Moore, J. E. and Mohr, C. F.: Biologically false positive serologic tests for syphilis. Type, incidence and cause. *JAMA* 150:467-473, 1952.

Owens, W. F., Jr.: Sexually transmitted diseases and traumatic problems in homosexual men. *Ann Intern Med* 92:805-808, 1980.

Quinn, T. C., Corey, L., Chaffee, R. G., Schuffler, M. D., Brancato, F. P., and Holmes, K. K.: The etiology of anorectal infections in homosexual men. *Am J Med* 71:395-406, 1981.

Sexually transmitted diseases, treatment guidelines. *Morbid Mortal Wk Rep Suppl* Vol. 31, No. 25, 8/20/82.

STD   Fact Sheet, ed. 35. U. S. Dept. Health and Human Services, HHS Public No (IDC) 81-8195.

Thompson, S. E., III and Pretter, R. H.: Epidemiology and treatment of chlamydial infections in pregnant women and infants. *Rev Infect Dis* 4:S747-S757, 1982.

37

INFECTIOUS ARTHRITIS

Bruce A. Wallin, M.D., Rashida A. Khakoo, M.D. and
Ronica M. Kluge, M.D.

Infection within a joint is curable if effective therapy against the invading organism is given early and if the pus is drained effectively. Despite the availability of potent chemotherapeutic agents, infectious arthritis continues to be one of the most damaging and prevalent forms of arthritis. Failure to establish an early diagnosis may lead to loss of joint function or death of the patient. The patient that presents with single or multiple warm, swollen joint(s) will have an extensive differential diagnosis, but infectious etiologies must always be a consideration. Infectious causes include bacteria (including mycobacteria), viruses, and fungi.

Microbiology

The most common causes of infectious arthritis in the adult are shown in Table 37.1, and those for children in Table 37.2. Recently, there has been an increase in the prevalence of infectious arthritis caused by gram-negative bacilli. This is seen predominantly in two populations: intravenous drug abusers and immunosuppressed patients.

Host factors that predispose to infectious arthritis are age (the very young and the very old seem to be more susceptible), chronic illnesses (such as rheumatoid arthritis, diabetes mellitus, cirrhosis, uremia, and malignancy), prior immunosuppressive therapy with corticosteroids or cytotoxic agents, intravenous drug abuse, and a previously damaged joint. Rheumatoid arthritis is the most common predisposing local anatomic derangement, but almost every underlying joint disease has been implicated including osteoarthrosis, systemic lupus erythematosus, gout, pseudogout, trauma, and Charcot's arthropathy.

TABLE 37.1   Bacterial Causes of Infectious Arthritis in Adults

Organism	% of Cases
N. gonorrhoeae	50
S. aureus	25
S. pyogenes	15
Gram-negative bacilli	10

TABLE 37.2   Bacterial Causes of Infectious Arthritis in Children

Age	Organism(s)
Neonates	S. aureus, gram-negative bacilli
1-18 mo	H. influenzae, S. aureus
18 mo	S. aureus

Pathogenesis

Organisms reach the synovium and joint space by one of three different routes. The most frequent route is hematogenous dissemination from a primarily infected site such as pneumonia or meningitis. Direct penetration of the organism into the joint space may occur following trauma, an operative procedure, or an intraarticular injection. Local extension may occur from an adjacent infected soft tissue or as a result of spread from contiguous osteomyelitis.

Once a virulent organism establishes an infectious process in a joint, joint destruction will ensue unless the organism is quickly eradicated. The joint reaction to infection varies markedly, depending upon the number and type of organisms, virulence of the organism, and status of the host's defense mechanisms. The inflammatory response that occurs in the joint also is related to substances produced by the organism, such as exotoxins, endotoxins, and chemotactic factors. Bacterial debris also participates in the reaction. Three stages of articular cartilage destruction have been identified. In the first stage, activated polymorphonuclear leukocytes release proteolytic enzymes, which are augmented by synovial lysosomal enzymes. This results in rapid removal of proteoglycan from the cartilage. This stage is reversible as long as the chondrocytes have not been destroyed. During the second stage, the biomechanical properties of the cartilage are altered. As the proteoglycans are removed, cartilage loses its compressive strength and the chondrocytes receive increased mechanical stresses. Also, there is altered diffusion of nutrients into the cartilage, leading to impairment of the chondrocytes, which causes an impaired capacity for cartilage matrix reconstitution.

The final stage is characterized by proliferating synovium at the periphery of the joint space, and the release of collagenase, elastase, and cathepsins. Collagen and the residual proteoglycans of the cartilage are destroyed. With destruction of the cartilage superstructure, gross deformation of the cartilage occurs.

Diagnostic Features

Clinical (Table 37.3)

Acute infectious arthritis is manifested by an abrupt onset of monoarticular swelling and pain, associated with fever. On examination, the patient frequently will not allow either active or passive movement of the involved joint. The most commonly involved joint is the knee, followed by the other large weightbearing joints of the lower extremity. The sternoclavicular joint and the sacroiliac joints are commonly infected in intravenous drug abusers. In children, the hip is frequently involved. Except for gonococcal arthritis, males are more frequently affected than females. In those patients who have previously damaged joints, and especially in patients with rheumatoid arthritis in which the patient routinely has some inflammatory joint findings, the clue is a joint that is inflamed out of proportion to the general level of disease found in the other joints, with or without a low-grade fever.

Laboratory

The diagnosis of acute infectious arthritis is confirmed by synovial fluid analysis and culture (Table 37.4). In general, one-half to two-thirds of patients will have mild to moderate peripheral leukocytosis and an elevated erythrocyte sedimentation rate. But, the synovial fluid analysis is the critical test. The typical findings are a white blood cell count greater than 50,000/mm^3 with > 90% polymorphonuclear leukocytes. On occasion, a white blood cell count as low as 10,000 may be seen, especially in patients infected with low-virulence organisms or in patients who have been partially treated. Synovial fluid glucose levels are low, usually

TABLE 37.3   Clinical Characteristics of Septic Arthritis

Mono- or oligoarticular

Lower > upper extremity

Fever

Local inflammation

Pain with motion

Leukocytosis

↑ Erythrocyte sedimentation rate

TABLE 37.4   Laboratory Diagnosis of Infectious Arthritis

Elevated peripheral white blood cell count

Elevated erythrocyte sedimentation rate

Synovial fluid analysis

    White blood cell count $\geq$ 50,000 mm^3
    Percent PMNs $\geq$ 90
    Glucose concentration decreased
    Poor mucin clot
    Gram-stain positive in 50-75%
    Culture positive

Blood culture

---

40 mg/dl less than the simultaneous plasma glucose. There is a poor mucin clot. Polarizing microscopy should also be performed as the differential diagnosis may include crystal-induced arthritis and in fact, both these processes may be present.

When infectious arthritis is suspected, it is mandatory to obtain a culture and Gram stain of the synovial fluid. The Gram stain is positive in one-half to two-thirds of the patients who are subsequently proved to have infectious arthritis. This procedure can provide a basis for prompt and appropriate institution of antibiotics. However, the joint fluid culture is the definitive test and provides the basis for specific antibiotic treatment. As the usual cause of infectious arthritis is hematogenous dissemination, other foci of infection should be sought and routine cultures of blood, sputum, urine, and wound(s) should be done before instituting antibiotic therapy. Blood cultures are positive in three-quarters of the patients. In patients suspected of having gonococcal infection, additional cultures should be obtained from the cervix, rectum, urethra, throat, and skin pustules. If mycobacteria or fungi are suspected, acid-fast stains, fungal stains, appropriate cultures, and synovial biopsy should be performed.

Radiographic studies usually are not helpful. Early in the course, the x-rays reveal only soft-tissue swelling or synovial effusion. After 7-10 days, juxtaarticular osteopenia may be detected. Later joint space narrowing will develop, followed by subchondral bone destruction. In the infant with infectious arthritis of the hip, the only early radiographic finding may be subluxation of the hip. An unusual radiographic manifestation is gas in the joint or periarticular tissues which can be caused by *Escherichia coli* or anaerobes. Radionuclide imaging may provide localization of unsuspected involvement and may help to differentiate overlying cellulitis from synovitis or osteomyelitis. Computerized axial tomography may demonstrate abnormalities before conventional radiographs, especially in evaluating infectious arthritis of the sacroiliac joints.

Special diagnostic techniques have been studied as possible means of detecting acute infectious arthritis when cultures are negative owing to partial treatment, inadequate bacteriologic techniques, or for unknown reasons. Counterimmunoelectrophoresis is a rapid, specific, and sensitive technique for detecting bacterial antigens in synovial fluid. It has been successfully employed in pneumococcal, meningococcal, and *Haemophilus influenzae* infections. This test may be positive in the absence of viable organisms by culture. Other tests that have been used but remain experimental are gas-liquid chromatography, the nitroblue tetrazolium test, the limulus lysate test, and synovial fluid lysozyme and lactoferrin levels.

Differential Diagnosis

The differential diagnosis of acute monoarticular arthritis includes crystal-induced arthritis (gout, pseudogout, or hydroxyapatite), traumatic arthritis, and acute hemarthrosis. Monoarticular rheumatoid arthritis, a peripheral manifestation of ankylosing spondylitis, Reiter's syndrome, adult Still's disease, or in children monoarticular juvenile rheumatoid arthritis might be considered, but generally these entities do not have as abrupt an onset or are characterized by other manifestations that would lead to the appropriate diagnosis. If the presentation is polyarticular, the differential diagnosis includes gout, acute rheumatic fever, serum sickness, rheumatoid arthritis and the seronegative spondyloarthropathies (Table 37.5).

Treatment

The management of infectious arthritis should begin immediately after reasonable suspicion of the diagnosis or, certainly, following confirmation of that diagnosis. Early treatment leads to the best long-term results. The treatment consists of appropriate antibiotic therapy and adequate drainage. Closed drainage or needle aspiration must be repeated as often as the effusion(s) reaccumulate to prevent cartilage destruction. Open drainage is indicated for all hip joint infections and when adequate drainage cannot be done by closed drainage. Other indications for surgical drainage (Table 37.6) are a persistent febrile course, a clinical response not occurring within 72 hr of institution of appropriate antibiotic therapy, purulent accumulation in spite of frequent aspirations and effective serum levels of antibiotics, unsuccessful complete aspiration of viscous pus through a large bore needle, and inaccessibility to the joint (Table 37.7).

Antibiotic therapy should be administered parenterally to provide the maximum serum and synovial fluid concentrations. The initial choice of antibiotic should be based upon the findings on Gram stain, the results of culture, and the sensitivities, or on the basis of the greatest clinical likelihood (Table 37.8). If the Gram stain is negative, antibiotic treatment is chosen on the basis of the most likely possibility on clinical grounds, which takes into account the age of the patient, the clinical presentation, and the presence of any underlying disease.

With adequate blood levels of an antibiotic that penetrates the synovial membrane, intraarticular instillation of antibiotics is unnecessary and indeed, may cause a chemical synovitis which may confuse the issue. In patients with gram-negative bacillary infections, the antibacterial activity of the synovial fluid should be monitored by a tube dilution procedure.

The acute infected joint should be immobilized to reduce pain and trauma to the cartilage. After 72 hr passive range-of-motion exercises may be initiated, as long as these exercises do not produce excessive pain. As inflammation subsides, active range-of-motion exercises should be initiated to regain mobility and increase strength.

TABLE 37.5   Usual Synovial Fluid Findings in Various Diseases

Type of Arthritis	Appearance	Leukocytes	% PMNs	Fibrin Clot	Glucose Difference[1]	Mucin Clot
Septic	Turbid	70,000[2]	80	2–4+	60	Poor
Tuberculous	Turbid	20,000	60	2–3+	60	Poor
Rheumatoid	Clear to turbid	14,000	70	2–4+	30	Poor
Gouty	Turbid	13,000	70	2–4+	20	Poor
Rheumatic fever	Slightly turbid	18,000	50	1–2+	10	Good
Degenerative joint disease	Clear	700	10	0–+	5	Good
Traumatic	Clear	1,200	10	0–+	10	Good
Normals	Clear	60	10	0	5	Good

[1]Difference between blood and synovial fluid glucose
[2]Average number/mm^3

TABLE 37.6   Indications for Surgical Drainage of Infected Joints

All hip joint infections

Inadequate closed drainage

Persistent febrile course

Inaccessible joint

TABLE 37.7   Comparison of Needle vs Open Drainage of Septic Arthritis*

Results	Needle	Open
Complete recovery	80%	47%
Patients with chronic underlying diseases	More	–
Patients on corticosteroids	More	–

*Goldenberg and Cohen, *Am J Med* 60:369, 1976

Prognosis

The prognosis depends on the duration of symptoms before treatment, the infecting organism, and the underlying disease. The prognosis is poorer in those patients with symptoms present for more than 1 week before institution of appropriate antibiotic therapy and in those patients with infections due to gram-negative bacilli.

Individual Organisms

Many infectious agents produce a distinctive clinical picture which aids in their recognition (Table 37.9).

Neisseria Gonorrhoeae

Gonococcal arthritis begins as a migratory polyarthralgia/arthritis associated with characteristic skin lesions, and tenosynovitis of the wrist, dorsum of the hands or feet, and/or Achilles' tendon. Synovial fluid analysis reveals a mild to moderate inflammatory state. The typical skin lesion consists of vesicopustular lesions on an erythematous base, hemorrhagic papules, or hemorrhagic bullae. Similar skin lesions have been seen in association with *N. meningitidis* and *H. influenzae* infections. An asymptomatic genital, pharyngeal, or rectal infection is the usual source. Cultures should be obtained from joint fluid, blood (50% are positive), pharynx, cervix or urethra, and rectum. Gram stains should be performed on joint fluid, urethral material, and fresh skin lesions. As the gonococcus is a very

TABLE 37.8   Initial Antibiotic Choices for Infectious Arthritis

Gram Stain	Most Likely Organism	Initial Treatment	Duration
Gram-negative cocci (in adult)	N. gonorrhoeae	Penicillin G 100–150,000 U/kg/day IV	3–7 days
Gram-positive cocci	S. aureus	Methicillin 200–300 mg/kg/day	4 wk
Gram-positive in pairs	S. pneumoniae	Penicillin G 100–150,000 U/kg/day IV	10–14 days
Gram-positive in chains	S. pyogenes		
Gram-negative bacilli or cocci (in children)	H. influenzae	Ampicillin 150 mg/kg/day IV	10–14 days
Gram-negative bacilli	E. coli, P. aeruginosa or S. marcescens	Gentamicin or tobramycin 5 mg/kg/day IV + carbenicillin in immunocompromised host	4–6 wk

TABLE 37.9   Distinctive Features of Certain Types of Infectious Arthritis

Organism	Features
Bacterial	
N. gonorrhoeae	Previously healthy adult Predominates in young women Often within 1 week of onset of menses or last trimester pregnancy Initial migratory polyarthritis Tenosynovitis (wrist, dorsum of hands or feet, Achilles' tendon) Typical skin lesions Knee or wrist most common
S. aureus	Neonates; children over age 2 years Adult with chronic underlying disease, especially diabetes and rheumatoid arthritis
S. pyogenes	Hematogenous spread from respiratory or skin infection
S. pneumoniae	Primary focus in lung, middle ear Associated meningitis, endocarditis Alcohol abusers
H. influenzae	Infants, young children Debilitated adults
Gram-negative bacilli	Chronic debilitating diseases (diabetes, malignancy, immunosuppressive drugs) Urinary tract infection may precede IV drug abusers, especially P. aeruginosa and S. marcescens, may involve sternoclavicular or sacroiliac joints Neonates; alcoholics
N. meningitidis	2-10% of meningococcal meningitis cases Oligoarticular; appears as meningitis is resolving
M. tuberculosis	Reactivation of latent disease Chronic, insidious, monoarticular Knee most common Most do not have concomitant active pulmonary tuberculosis PPD almost always positive Synovial fluid: acid-fast stain + in 20%, cultures + in 80%, biopsy + in 95%

TABLE 37.9 (Cont'd)

Organism	Features
Fungal	Insidious onset, indolent course May occur in debilitated patients Males > females; usually 40s-50s
Viral	Arthralgias common Usually transient Most common: hepatitis B (10-30% of patients) usually preicteric Rubella: usually adult women - fingers, wrists, and knees Arboviruses: rash, encephalitis, nephritis, and hemorrhage

fastidious organism, extra care should be maintained to obtain effective cultures. In the absence of positive cultures, the syndrome in a young, sexually active female may be so highly suspected that a therapeutic trial is justified. The response to penicillin is brisk, occurring within 2 days, and in the culture-negative situation, this rapid response to penicillin, without associated use of antiinflammatory agents, is diagnostic. Penicillin G given in high doses intravenously for 3 days is probably adequate treatment, but some authorities recommend completing a 10-day course of therapy with oral ampicillin, 2 g/day. Appropriate drainage must be carried out as well.

Gram-Negative Bacilli

The gram-negative bacilli cause approximately 10-15% of acute nongonoccal infectious arthritis. The increasing incidence of infections due to these organisms appears to be related primarily to host factors. Organisms are commonly cultured from extraarticular sites such as blood and/or urine. Other gram-negative bacilli reported to produce infectious arthritis include: salmonellae, *Aeromonas hydrophila, Arizona hinshawii, Vibrio fetus, Yersinia enterocolitica,* and anaerobic organisms. *Aeromonas hydrophila* appears to be uniquely associated with acute myelogenous leukemia.

Mycobacterium Tuberculosis

Tuberculous spondylitis (Pott's disease) occurs most often in the thoracolumbar spine. Any part of the vertebral body may be involved, but it usually occurs at the anterior border, with associated disc involvement leading to disc-space narrowing and anterior vertebral body collapse. A hump or gibbus deformity of the spine may result. There are no unique radiographic features of Pott's disease and therefore histologic and cultural examination of involved tissue must be obtained to distinguish this lesion from atypical mycobacterial or fungal infections, or from malignancy.

Atypical Mycobacteria

Since the atypical mycobacteria undergo systemic dissemination less often than does *M. tuberculosis,* skeletal disease is rare. The disease produced by these organisms is generally indistinguishable from tuberculosis on clinical, radiologic, or histologic grounds and therefore, diagnosis depends on isolation of the organism by culture. Most of these patients have periarticular involvement. The most common sites are about the wrists, fingers, and bursae. Knees and digital joints are the most common articular sites. The disease process is insidious. Treatment has consisted of synovectomy and antituberculous agents, depending on in vitro susceptibility studies.

Fungi

The most frequent fungal diseases causing arthritis are coccidioidomycosis, blastomycosis, and sporotrichosis. Recently there has been an increasing incidence of reports of candidal arthritis. Fungal arthritis is relatively rare. During acute primary coccidioidomycosis, transient arthralgias occur in about one-third of the patients. In a much smaller number of patients with disseminated disease, joint involvement secondary to contiguous osteomyelitis may occur. The knee is most commonly involved. Synovial fluid smear and culture are usually negative. The diagnosis is made on the basis of synovial tissue culture or synovial tissue pathology. *Blastomyces dermititidis* causes pulmonary or cutaneous manifestations, but in one-third of disseminated blastomycosis cases, osteomyelitis with secondary joint involvement occurs. The knee or ankle is most commonly involved. Diagnosis can be made by synovial fluid smear and/or culture. With hematogenous dissemination in sporotrichosis, 80% of the patients will have arthritis or bone involvement. It most commonly affects the knee, ankle, wrist, or elbow. Synovial fluid and synovial tissue culture demonstrate the diagnosis. Amphotericin B, either intravenously or in combination with intraarticular injection, with/without surgery is the therapy of choice. Candidal arthritis develops during the course of hematogenous dissemination. All patients have significant underlying diseases such as carcinoma, rheumatoid arthritis, SLE, and often have intravenous or urinary catheters. Neonates with candidal arthritis have had low birth weights, bacterial sepsis, pulmonary disease, or have required prolonged insertion of intravenous catheters. The most commonly involved joint is the knee. Diagnosis depends on synovial fluid culture. The treatment of choice is intravenous amphotericin B, although intraarticular amphotericin B or surgery has also been helpful.

Other

Arthralgias and arthritis are associated with a number of viral infections. The arthritis of hepatitis B begins suddenly and involves the small joints of the hands, usually in a symmetric pattern. About 50% of these patients will have an associated rash. The arthritis usually lasts less than 4 weeks. Hepatitis B surface antigen usually is present. Complement levels may be low. Rubella arthritis usually resolves within 30 days. Arthritis has also been seen in association with mumps, smallpox, varicella, infectious mononucleosis, and erythema infectiosum.

Lyme disease is of presumed spirochetal etiology and is so-named because of its close geographic clustering in a small community, Lyme, Connecticut. It is presumably tick-transmitted. The arthritis usually begins suddenly in the large joints, the knees being the most common site. Attacks are usually brief but can be recurrent. Approximately 75% of patients will have a typical skin eruption that begins as a red macule or papule on the proximal extremity or trunk that often expands with central clearing. This has been labeled erythema chronicum migrans and usually lasts for a few weeks. Patients also may have fever, chills, headache, malaise, fatigue, meningoencephalitis, and myocardial conduction defects. Laboratory findings are nonspecific but cryoprecipitates are often seen early in the course of the disease. Treatment consists of salicylates although recent evidence seems to indicate that oral penicillin G, 250,000 U, q.i.d. for 7-10 days may shorten the duration of erythema chronicum migrans and may attenuate the subsequent arthritis.

Selected Bibliography

Argen, R. J., Wilson, C. H., Jr., and Wood, P.: Suppurative arthritis. Clinical features of 42 cases. *Arch Intern Med* 117:661-666, 1966.

Bayer, A. S., Chow, A. W., Louie, J. S., Nies, K. M., and Guze, L. B.: Gram-negative bacillary septic arthritis: Clinical, radiographic, therapeutic, and prognostic features. *Sem Arthritis Rheum* 7:123-132, 1977.

Chartier, Y., Martin, W. J., and Kelly, P. J.: Bacterial arthritis: Experiences in the treatment of 77 patients. *Ann Intern Med* 50:1462-1472, 1959.

Eisenstein, B. I. and Masi, A. T.: Disseminated gonococcal infection and gonococcal arthritis: I. Bacteriology, epidemiology, host factors, pathogen factors, and pathology. *Sem Arthritis Rheum* 10:155-172, 1981.

Goldenberg, D. L., Brandt, K. D., Cathcart, E. S., and Cohen, A. S.: Acute arthritis caused by gram-negative bacilli: A clinical characterization. *Medicine* 53:197-208, 1974.

Goldenberg, D. L., Brandt, K. D., Cohen, A. S., and Cathcart, E. S.: Treatment of septic arthritis. Comparison of needle aspiration and surgery as initial modes of joint drainage. *Arthritis Rheum* 18:83-90, 1975.

Goldenberg, D. L. and Cohen, A. S.: Acute infectious arthritis. A review of patients with nongonococcal joint infections. *Am J Med* 60:369-373, 1976.

Goldenberg, D. L. and Cohen, A. S.: Arthritis due to tuberculous and fungal microorganisms. *Clin Rheum Dis* 4:211-224, 1978.

Handsfield, H. H., Wiesner, P. J., and Holmes, K. K.: Treatment of the gonococcal arthritis-dermatitis syndrome. *Ann Intern Med* 84:661-667, 1976.

Holmes, K. K., Counts, G. W., and Beaty, H. N.: Disseminated gonococcal infection. *Ann Intern Med* 74:979-993, 1971.

Masi, A. T. and Eisenstein, B. I.: Disseminated gonococcal infection and gonococcal arthritis: II. Clinical manifestation, diagnosis, complications, treatment and prevention. *Sem Arthritis Rheum* 10:173-197, 1981.

Mitchell, W. S., Brooks, P. M., Stevenson, R. D., Buchanan, W. W.: Septic arthritis in patients with rheumatoid disease: A still undiagnosed complication. *J Rheumatol* 3:124-133, 1976.

Murray, H. W., Fialk, M. A., and Roberts, R. B.: Candida arthritis: A manifestation of disseminated candidiasis. *Am J Med* 60:587–595, 1976.

Rytel, M. W.: Microbial antigen detection in infectious arthritis. *Clin Rheum Dis* 4:83, 1978.

Sauter, S. V. H. and Utsinger, P. D.: Viral arthritis. *Clin Rheum Dis* 4:225, 1978.

Sharp, J. T., Lidsky, M. D., Duffy, J., and Duncan, M. W.: Infectious arthritis. *Arch Intern Med* 139:1125–1130, 1979.

Steere, A. C., Malawista, S. E., Hardin, J. A., Ruddy, S., Askenase, P. W., and Andimore, W. A.: Erythema chronicum migrans and Lyme arthritis. *Ann Intern Med* 86:685–698, 1977.

Steere, A. C., Malawista, S. E., Newman, J. H., Spieler, P. N., and Bartenbagen, N. H.: Antibiotic therapy in Lyme disease. *Ann Intern Med* 93(Part 1):1–8, 1980.

Wallace, R. and Cohen, A. S.: Tuberculous arthritis. A report of two cases with review of biopsy and synovial findings. *Am J Med* 61:277–282, 1976.

Ward, J., Cohen, A. S., and Bauer, W.: The diagnosis and therapy of acaute suppurative arthritis. *Arthritis Rheum* 3:522, 1960.

Ward, J. R. and Atcheson, S. G.: Infectious arthritis. *Med Clin N Am* 61:313–329, 1977.

38

OSTEOMYELITIS
Robert H. Waldman, M.D.

Osteomyelitis is a bacterial or fungal infection of the bone, leading to suppuration. It is a difficult disease therapeutically, because relapses are common and there is a tendency to develop the chronic form of the disease. Understanding the disease is complex, because of the large number of variables, including the differences with respect to the causative organism (e.g., *Staphylococcus aureus* versus *Mycobacterium tuberculosis*), the age of the patient, the bone involved, and the underlying health of the patient.

Microbiology

The microbiology of osteomyelitis has changed in recent years. There has been a relative decrease in the occurrence of cases caused by *S. aureus,* although this organism still accounts for two-thirds to three-quarters of the total, and even a higher percentage in previously healthy children (Tables 38.1 and 38.2). There has been an increased number of cases caused by gram-negative enteric organisms and mixed flora, especially in vertebral osteomyelitis in adults and following trauma. The cause of this change in the bacterial etiology of osteomyelitis is unclear but probably is related to the changes in flora secondary to widespread antibiotic use.

Another change in bacterial etiology of osteomyelitis has been the emergence of group B streptococci as a frequent pathogen in neonatal osteomyelitis. Other unusual organisms of increasing prevalence are *Salmonella* in sickle cell hemoglobinopathies, *Pseudomonas* as the organism in most cases of osteomyelitis in drug addicts (Table 38.3), and fungal osteomyelitis, nearly always in patients with compromised host defenses receiving prolonged intravenous therapy. The fungi most commonly seen are *Candida, Aspergillus,* and *Rhizopus.*

TABLE 38.1   Culture Results in Children with Osteomyelitis

Culture	Approximate % of Patients
Staphylococcus	60
Streptococcus	10
Gram-negative rods	2
Anaerobes	1
Pneumococcus	< 1
Negative	25

TABLE 38.2   Organisms Responsible for Osteomyelitis Secondary
             to Contiguous Focus*

S. aureus

Pseudomonas

Proteus

Streptococcus (non-group A)

E. coli

Klebsiella

Streptococcus (group A)

(∿50% caused by mixed flora)

*Listed in order of frequency

TABLE 38.3   Gram-Negative Osteomyelitis

Increasing prevalence

Salmonella: associated with hemoglobinopathies particularly
            sickle cell disease

Pseudomonas: in heroin addicts

Common cause of vertebral osteomyelitis: via avalvular
            paravertebral lumbar plexus from intestines or genito-
            urinary tract

It is of interest that *Haemophilus influenzae* is a fairly common cause of septic arthritis in children but is exceedingly rare as a cause of osteomyelitis. The reason for this is unknown. Tuberculous osteomyelitis is unusual but not terribly rare and usually involves the vertebrae or phalanges (Table 38.4).

Pathogenesis

Osteomyelitis can be categorized in many different ways, but from a pathogenetic point of view, one of the most helpful is to classify the disease as acute hematogenous osteomyelitis, osteomyelitis secondary to contiguous spread, and osteomyelitis secondary to direct inoculation (Table 38.5).

TABLE 38.4   Tuberculous Osteomyelitis

Site

      Vertebral: lower thoracic

      Proximal femur

      Distal femur, proximal tibia

      Ankle

Surgery indicated for radical debridement

      Progression despite chemotherapy

      Instability of involved spine

      Paravertebral abscess

TABLE 38.5   Miscellaneous Categories of Osteomyelitis

Secondary to adjacent infection	Includes overlying abscesses or burns
Traumatic	Animal bites, iatrogenic heel puncture in children, other puncture wounds of heel (pseudomonal most common)
Postoperative	
Multifocal	Typical in neonatal infants, drug addicts, recurrent multifocal osteomyelitis with pustularis palmoplantaris

Acute hematogenous osteomyelitis occurs at the extremes of life and is usually due to *S. aureus*. In children it usually involves rapidly growing bone, i.e., the femur, tibia, and humerus (Table 38.6). The metaphysis of the bone is usually involved, and this is believed to be because of stasis of blood in the venous sinusoids. The peak incidence is between the ages of 5 and 14. In infants, there are vascular connections through the epiphyseal plate, so septic arthritis frequently accompanies acute hematogenous osteomyelitis. Brodie's abscess is a pyogenic abscess of the bone, almost always caused by *S. aureus*. Table 38.7 indicates some features of various sites involved in osteomyelitis.

TABLE 38.6   Osteomyelitis: Incidence by Site

Site	Approximate % of Total
Femur	30
Tibia	25
Vertebra	15
Humerus	10
Pelvis	5
Fibula	5
Tarsal	5
Radius	2
Rib	1

TABLE 38.7   Features of Various Sites Involved in Osteomyelitis

Long bones	Femur or tibia involved in most cases of childhood hematogenous osteomyelitis
Vertebrae	Adults; less acute; surgery usually not necessary
Pelvis	Fever; abnormal gait; point tenderness over involved bone
Clavicle	IV drug abusers; subacute onset
Fingers	Common complication of fingertip abscess (felon)
Feet	From puncture wound; *P. aeruginosa* common

In adults, the vertebral body is usually involved, most commonly the lower thoracic or lumbar areas (Table 38.8). The peak incidence is over the age of 60, and the patient is often debilitated. The infection begins in the highly vascular subchondral region and frequently involves two adjacent bone plates and the intervertebral disk. In drug addicts the most frequently involved areas are the vertebrae, pelvis, and clavicle.

TABLE 38.8   Features of Pyogenic Vertebral Osteomyelitis*

Feature	Approximate % of Patients
Location	
Cervical	10
Thoracic	35
Thoracolumbar	10
Lumbar	45
Lumbosacral	10
Organism	
Staphylococcus	30
Gram-negative rod	15
Streptococcus	3
Predisposing infection	
Genitourinary	30
Skin	5
Respiratory	5
Complication	
Death	5
Paraplegia	10

*N Engl J Med 303:360, 1980

Neonatal hematogenous osteomyelitis is commonly multifocal, commonly involves the facial bones, is subacute in onset, and is usually seen following high-risk pregnancies and/or in sick infants. It is commonly iatrogenic, i.e., following umbilical or scalp vein cannulation (Tables 38.9-38.11).

TABLE 38.9   Neonatal Osteomyelitis

40% occurrence of multiple bone involvement

Increasing occurrence of *E. coli*

Often secondary to complications during pregnancy or delivery: preeclampsia, premature rupture of membranes, etc.

Iatrogenic: heel or scalp resulting from infected heel-stick or phlebitis

TABLE 38.10   Neonatal Osteomyelitis[3]

	Etiology	
	Group B *Streptococcus*	*Staphylococcus*
	Approximate %	
Multiple bone involvement	0	40
Septic arthritis	35	70
Fever (> 100.6°F)	0	40
Leukocytosis (> 20,000/mm^3)	10	40
% of total cases		
1949-1957[1]	0	60
1965-1972[2]	0	55
1967-1977[3]	40	30

[1]*Lancet* 1:544, 1957
[2]*Pediatrics* 53:505, 1974
[3]*J Pediatr* 93:578, 1978

TABLE 38.11   Presenting Signs of Neonatal Osteomyelitis*

Sign	Approximate % of Patients
Swelling	75
Fever	65
Decreased movement	55
Erythema	30
Tenderness	15

*J Pediatr 92:485, 1978

TABLE 38.12   Osteomyelitis Commonly Caused by Mixed Anaerobic
and Aerobic Flora

Skull or facial bones, secondary to ENT
procedures

Long-bone compound fractures

Pelvic bone, secondary to intraabdominal sepsis

Hand, secondary to bites, particularly human

Foot, associated with vascular insufficiency
and/or diabetes

Cervical spine, secondary to retropharyngeal
abscess

Osteomyelitis secondary to contiguous spread is also preponderantly caused by
S. aureus, but many cases are from gram-negative enteric organisms, or of mixed
flora (Table 38.12). It commonly involves the lower extremity and is secondary to
vascular insufficiency. Osteomyelitis secondary to direct inoculation, which has
also been called primary osteomyelitis, is seen following trauma or surgery.
    Osteomyelitis tends to become chronic because the nonanastomosing blood
supply and the tendency for vascular thrombosis to occur, leads to necrosis of the
bone. It is therefore difficult to obtain adequate antibiotic levels at the site of
infection, and the dead bone fragments serve as foreign bodies (sequestra).

Diagnosis

The diagnosis of osteomyelitis is clinical (Table 38.13). This is extremely important; if one waits until the laboratory studies, particularly the bone scan or x-ray, become positive, there will be delay in beginning treatment. This is undesirable because early diagnosis and institution of treatment result in significant improvement in prognosis; which is especially true of osteomyelitis in children. Acute hematogenous osteomyelitis in children usually presents as a septic disease with fever, chills, and considerable toxicity. There is tenderness, erythema, soft-tissue edema, decreased limb usage (pseudoparalysis), and joint effusion near the involved bone (Tables 38.14 and 38.15). There is a history of trauma in about one-third of the children. Neonates are usually not as toxic as older children.

Adults rarely present with a toxic picture. About one-third are afebrile. Much more likely is a picture of aching pain accentuated by movement. The symptoms are vague and evanescent. This is especially true with osteomyelitis in illicit drug users.

Chronic osteomyelitis presents as an ulcer or boil that intermittently opens and drains. One may only see a hyperpigmented, scarred area over the bone. Chronic osteomyelitis is common underlying decubitus ulcers. It is extremely important always to consider the possibility of underlying osteomyelitis when a chronic soft-tissue infection of any form exists.

Laboratory studies, as mentioned previously, are not helpful in the early diagnosis of osteomyelitis. Leukocytosis parallels the symptoms and signs. Anemia is common, particularly in chronic osteomyelitis.

TABLE 38.13 Differential Diagnosis of Osteomyelitis

Cellulitis	Multiple myeloma
Bone infarction	Primary or metastatic malignancy
Subperiostial hematoma (traumatic periostitis)	Congenital syphilis
	Pyomyositis
Bone cyst	Wound infection
Eosinophilic granuloma	
	Soft-tissue abscess
Osteitis deformans	Acute rheumatic fever
Neurofibromatosis	
	Septic arthritis
Monoarticular rheumatoid arthritis	
Osteodystrophy in patients on long-term dialysis	
Recurrent multifocal osteomyelitis with pustularis palmoplantaris (very rare, apparently noninfectious)	

TABLE 38.14   Presenting Complaint in Children with Osteomyelitis*

Complaint	Approximate % of Patients
Bone pain, limp, or disuse	100
Fever	85
Joint pain	65
History of injury	45

*N Y State J Med 78:910, 1978

TABLE 38.15   Site of Childhood Osteomyelitis

Site	Approximate % of Patients
Femur	30
Proximal	(60)
Middle	(10)
Distal	(30)
Tibia	30
Proximal	(45)
Middle	(5)
Distal	(50)
Pelvis	10
Humerus	10
Fibula	10
Radius	3

Radionuclide scanning is very valuable, but may not differentiate osteomyelitis from Paget's disease, neoplasms, bone infarcts, and sickle cell anemia, or surrounding soft-tissue infection. Radionuclide scanning, however, is usually abnormal earlier than changes in the bone x-rays can be detected. Radionuclide scanning is *not* a very accurate method for following patients; clinical evaluation of a patient is much more accurate, and certainly less expensive.

Roentgenographic changes cannot be depended upon for at least 10–14 days, although changes may be seen as early as 5–6 days in some children. Periosteal elevation due to a subperiosteal abscess is an early finding, seen in children but rarely in adults because the periosteum is firmly attached to the bone. To reiterate, treatment should be begun before definite changes are seen by x-ray.

Isolation of the offending organism has become more important as the relative frequency of *S. aureus* as the causative organism in acute osteomyelitis has decreased, and as a prerequisite for determining optimal antibiotic treatment in cases which do not respond to initial antibiotic therapy. Blood cultures are positive in about one-third of the patients with a slightly higher percentage in those who appear septic. Culture of a sinus tract is of little value since the tract is nearly always contaminated by irrelevant bacteria, except in cases where *S. aureus* is isolated as the sole or predominant organism. Aspiration of a subperiosteal abscess is helpful but as mentioned earlier, is usually only present in children, and it may be difficult to obtain material. Culture of material obtained at surgery is very important, particularly in patients with chronic osteomyelitis.

Treatment

Prompt and appropriate treatment is much more likely to eradicate the infection without residua. The principles of therapy are high-dose, parenteral (at least at first), and prolonged antibiotic therapy. The duration of the treatment has been controversial. There are no control studies that answer the question as to whether or not 6 weeks is better than 4. Clinical observations suggest that the relapse rate is greatly reduced if therapy continues beyond 3 weeks. A word of caution regarding evaluation of clinical trials in osteomyelitis: relapses may occur several years after the initial disease, so studies indicating a low relapse rate in patients followed for only 1 or 2 years may be overly optimistic. A general conclusion is that therapy should continue for at least 4 weeks, and that beyond that the duration should be individualized depending upon the clinical response of the patient, such as the general feeling of well-being, the appetite, and the erythrocyte sedimentation rate returning to normal or nearly so.

In the septic patient one should assume that the offending organism is *S. aureus*. Blood cultures should be obtained and there is no need to undertake invasive or surgical procedures (Table 38.16). The patient should be started on a regimen of high-dose oxacillin, or clindamycin if the patient is allergic to penicillin. A definite clinical response should occur within 72 hr. If there is no definite response, and the blood cultures are negative, more aggressive techniques for obtaining culture material and drainage should be undertaken. In neonates, gentamicin should

TABLE 38.16   Indications for Surgery in Acute Osteomyelitis

Biopsy for diagnosis in atypical or unresponsive cases

Drainage of collections of pus

Debridement of necrotic bone (sequestrum)

Development of neurologic abnormalities in vertebral or cranial osteomyelitis

Spread to hip joint in child

be added to the oxacillin regimen. In blacks, ampicillin should be added to the oxacillin, because of the possibility of salmonella osteomyelitis in the patient with sickle cell anemia. If the osteomyelitis is secondary to direct extension or inoculation from trauma or surgery, the patient should be treated with oxacillin and gentamicin.

After the patient has shown a definite response to intravenous antibiotics, treatment can be switched to oral antibiotics. Guidelines for oral treatment of osteomyelitis are that the peak serum bactericidal level, when tested against the patient's own organism, must be 1:8 or greater. This can usually be obtained with high-dose oral dicloxacillin (100 mg/kg/day), possibly necessitating the addition of probenecid (25-40 mg/kg/day). If the patient cannot tolerate dicloxacillin, i.e., development of diarrhea, cephalexin may be tried. Following establishment of the oral regimen, the patient may be followed as an outpatient, but serum bactericidal levels should be obtained about once a week to assure that adequate blood levels are maintained, and as a test of the patient's compliance. If adequate blood levels are not maintained, the patient should be restarted on parenteral therapy.

Closed irrigation of the infected area with an antibiotic solution is commonly used, but there are no controlled studies to show its effectiveness. Immobilization of the involved bone gives good symptomatic relief early in the course of treatment.

Conditions for prophylactic use of antibiotics in orthopedic reconstructive surgery are summarized in Table 38.17.

Prognosis

In the preantibiotic era the fatality rate from osteomyelitis was about 25%. Today it is less than 2%. Delay in the institution of appropriate treatment leads to bone necrosis, difficulty in eradication, and the development of chronic osteomyelitis. Relapse is much less likely to occur if treatment is begun within 72 hr of the onset of symptoms. An unusual but important complication of chronic osteomyelitis is the development of amyloidosis.

TABLE 38.17   Prophylactic Antibiotics in Orthopedic Reconstructive Surgery

Should be used in high-risk patients

Aged over 60

Severe underlying cardiovascular, respiratory or gastrointestinal disease

Prolonged operating time

Compound fractures

Infection elsewhere

Previous surgery in same area

TABLE 38.18   Complications and Sequelae of Childhood Osteomyelitis*

Complication	Approximate % of Patients
Septic arthritis	20
Growth disturbance	20
Restricted motion	15
Deformity	15
Draining sinus	15
Recurrence	10
Chronicity	5
Pathologic fracture	5
Death	1

*Orthop Clin N Am 6:935, 1975

A serious complication of vertebral osteomyelitis is posterior extension leading to epidural abscess and paraplegia. In infants, epiphyseal growth centers may be damaged leading to shortening of the involved limb (Table 38.18).

Selected Bibliography

Bryson, Y. J., Connor, J. D., LeClerc, M., and Giammona, S. T.: High dose oral dicloxacillin treatment of acute staphylococcal osteomyelitis in children. *J Pediatr* 94:673, 1979.

Edwards, M. S., Baker, C. J., Wagner, M. L., Tabor, L. H., and Barrett, F. F.: An etiologic shift in infantile osteomyelitis: The emergence of the group B streptococcus. *J Pediatr* 93:578, 1978.

Fitzgerald, R. H. and Kelly, P. J.: Penetration of methicillin, oxacillin and cephalothin into bone and synovial tissue. *Antimicrob Agents Chemother* 14:723, 1978.

Fox, L. and Sprunt, K.: Neonatal osteomyelitis. *Pediatrics* 62:535, 1978.

Greenstone, J. and Greensides, R.: Osteomyelitis of the pelvis, a diagnostic problem. *Am J Dis Child* 132:581, 1978.

Hedstrom, S. A.: The prognosis of chronic staphylococcal osteomyelitis after long-term antibiotic treatment. *Scand J Infect Dis* 6:33, 1974.

Jara, F. A., Yap, A., Toledo-Pereyra, L. H., et al.: The role of surgery in primary osteomyelitis of the chest wall. *J Thorac Cardiovasc Surg* 77:147, 1979.

Kelly, P. J.: Osteomyeliltis in the adult. *Orthop Clin N. Am* 6:983, 1975.

Mackowiak, P. A., Jones, S. R., and Smith, J. W.: Diagnostic value of sinus-tract cultures in chronic osteomyelitis. *JAMA* 239:2772, 1978.

Manzella, J. P., Van Voris, L. P., and Hruska, J. F.: Isolated calcaneal tuberculous osteomyelitis. *J Bone Joint Surg* 61:946, 1979.

Medoff, G.: Current concepts in the treatment of osteomyelitis. *Postgrad Med* 58:157, 1975.

Morrey, B. F. and Peterson, H. A.: Hematogenous pyogenic osteomyelitis in children. *Orthop Clin N Am* 6:935, 1975.

Musher, D. M., Thorsteinsson, S. B., Minuth, J. N., and Luchi, R. J.: Vertebral osteomyelitis. Still a diagnostic pitfall. *Arch Intern Med* 136:105, 1976.

Prober, O. J.: Oral antibiotic therapy for bone and joint infections. *Pediatr Infect Dis* 1:8, 1982.

Sapico, F. L. and Montgomerie, J. Z.: Pyogenic vertebral osteomyelitis: Report of nine cases and review of the literature. *Rev Infect Dis* 1:754, 1979.

Sapico, F. L. and Montgomerie, J. Z.: Vertebral osteomyelitis in intravenous drug abusers: Report of three cases and review of the literature. *Rev Infect Dis* 2:196, 1980.

Septimus, E. J. and Musher, D. M.: Osteomyelitis: Recent clinical and laboratory aspects. *Orthop Clin N Am* 10:347, 1979.

Simpson, M. B., Jr., Merz, W. G., Kurlinski, J. P., and Solomon, M. H.: Opportunistic mycotic osteomyelitis: Bone infections due to *Aspergillus* and *Candida* species. *Medicine* 56:475, 1977.

Stone, D. B. and Bonfiglio, M.: Pyogenic vertebral osteomyelitis. A diagnostic pitfall for the internist. *Arch Intern Med* 112:491, 1963.

Tetzlaff, T. R., Howard, J. B., McCracken, G. H., Calderon, E., and Larrondo, J.: Antibiotic concentrations in pus and bone of children with osteomyelitis. *J Pediatr* 92:135, 1978.

Ugino, M. R. and Evarts, C. M.: Osteomyelitis: A review of the basic principles. *Contemp Orthop* 4:543, 1982.

Waldvogel, F. A. and Vasey, H.: Osteomyelitis: The past decade. *N Engl J Med* 303:360, 1980.

39

IMPETIGO AND CELLULITIS
Ronica M. Kluge, M.D.

This chapter will consider superficial skin infections and cellulitis caused by bacteria. Viral and mycotic skin infections are covered in other chapters.

Impetigo

Impetigo, a superficial skin infection which occurs most commonly in children, is usually caused by group A streptococci. Not infrequently, the lesions may also be colonized by *Staphylococcus aureus*. The disease occurs sporadically as well as in epidemic form, the latter primarily in "closed" populations such as military recruits. Impetigo cases peak in the warm and humid months.

The presence of group A streptococci on the skin plus minor trauma result in the characteristic lesions: first, an erythematous papule, then rapid evolution through a vesicular phase to a crusted one. The lesions vary in size from a few millimeters to 1 or 2 cm and are initially discrete. Coalescence of lesions occurs primarily on the scalp. Cellulitis surrounding the lesions and regional lymphadenitis are prominent features. Patients are usually afebrile and do not appear systemically ill. Diagnosis is made on clinical grounds alone in most cases, but can be confirmed by exudate Gram stain and culture. Possible complications of impetigo include superinfections and poststreptococcal glomerulonephritis (see Chapter 83).

The therapy of choice for impetigo is parenteral penicillin or erythromycin; clindamycin may be substituted in the penicillin-allergic patient.

Bullous Impetigo

This disease, characterized by superficial skin blebs, occurs mostly in newborns and young children, and is caused by *S. aureus* strains which produce epidermolytic toxin. This form of impetigo also occurs in both sporadic and epidemic forms, the latter frequently in newborn nurseries.

The lesions begin as vesicles which develop into larger, flaccid, thin-walled bullae and range in size from 0.5 to 3.0 cm. The bullous fluid may appear watery or turbid. There is little erythema surrounding the bullae and no regional adenopathy in the average patient. Nikolsky's sign is *not* present.

Differential diagnosis includes thermal injury in limited cases and the bullous dermatoses in more extensive cases (Table 39.1). A specific diagnosis can be made by Gram stain and culture of the bullous fluid. In more severe cases, a skin biopsy is recommended to rule out other bullous dermatoses. Bullous impetigo has the cleavage plane located in the upper epidermis; polymorphonuclear leukocytes and staphylococci can be seen in the bullae.

A penicillinase-resistant penicillin administered orally is the appropriate treatment. Erythromycin or clindamycin is an acceptable alternative in the penicillin-allergic patient.

Erysipelas

Group A streptococci cause a distinctive form of cellulitis, which is called erysipelas and involves the dermis, lymphatics, and uppermost subcutaneous tissue. The disease tends to occur in the very young and the very old. Factors predisposing to erysipelas are listed in Table 39.2. Erysipelas can occur as a result of surgical

TABLE 39.1   Differential Diagnosis of Bullous Impetigo

Limited

    Thermal injury

Extensive

    Bullous pemphigoid
    Dermatitis herpetiformis
    Pemphigus
    Stevens-Johnson syndrome

TABLE 39.2   Factors Predisposing to Erysipelas

Age: newborn, elderly
Nephrotic syndrome
Preexisting lymphatic obstruction or edema
Prior episode of erysipelas
Any break in the skin

wounds or other trauma, but often the inciting event is trivial or not even apparent. The characteristic lesion has a sharply demarcated, slightly raised border surrounding a deeply erythematous, indurated, and painful plaque. Erysipelas commonly involves the cheeks and nose or occurs in a circumferential pattern on the extremities. The patient will be febrile and appear toxic in most instances. The diagnosis can be made on the basis of the appearance of the lesion and confirmed by Gram stain and culture of material aspirated from the leading margin. Possible complications include deeper cellulitis and bacteremia. The differential diagnosis is listed in Table 39.3.

Penicillin is the antimicrobial of choice for erysipelas. Many authorities recommend the intravenous route for at least 24-48 hr, followed by the oral route to complete the course (10 days total). Erythromycin would be an appropriate alternative in the penicillin-allergic patient.

Staphylococcal Scalded Skin Syndrome (SSSS)

Called "dermatitis exfoliative neonatorum" by Ritter, SSSS is now known to be caused by an epidermolytic toxin produced by certain strains of S. aureus in phage groups 1, 2, or 3. The disease occurs in sporadic form or in outbreaks particularly in newborn nurseries (nosocomial). Affecting primarily infants and young children, SSSS has been reported rarely in adults.

Presence of a toxin-producing strain of S. aureus in conjunctivae or broken skin (e.g., abrasion, circumcision site) sets the stage. The disease begins abruptly with fever and diffusely tender erythroderma, which is followed shortly by the appearance of large, flaccid, thin-walled bullae. Nikolsky's sign is present. The bullae rupture spontaneously and large sheets of the epidermis separate and slough revealing bright red skin underneath. The denuded areas dry quickly, undergo another desquamation, and then heal without scarring. The appearance of the typical lesions in a febrile child suggests the clinical diagnosis. The diagnosis can be confirmed by the recovery of an isolate of S. aureus which is a producer of the epidermolytic toxin.

Cellulitis

Cellulitis is an inflammatory process of the skin and subcutaneous tissues which can affect patients of any age. The most common causative organisms are S. aureus, group A streptococci, and in children under 3 years of age, Haemophilus influenzae. Gram-negative enteric bacilli and Erysipelothrix rhusiopathiae are uncommon causes of cellulitis.

TABLE 39.3   Differential Diagnosis of Erysipelas

Early herpes zoster

Contact dermatitis

Giant urticaria

Inflammatory carcinoma

Breaks in the skin, whether due to trauma or to surgery, predispose to the development of cellulitis. This is an illness which occurs sporadically and without seasonal variation. The usual incubation period is 1-3 days after which local tenderness, warmth, edema, and erythema develop. Most patients have chills, fever, and general malaise. The margins of the lesions of cellulitis are distinct, in contrast to those of erysipelas. Regional lymph node enlargement and tenderness is a frequent finding. Bacteremia may be present.

Diagnosis is made on clinical grounds, and the causative agent is confirmed by culture of material aspirated from the leading edge of the cellulitis or by blood culture. Certain clinical features may provide clues to the etiologic organism (Table 39.4). Streptococcal cellulitis frequently occurs as a surgical wound complication. The lesion spreads extremely rapidly (within hours) and has prominent lymphangitis. Patients with streptococcal cellulitis often appear acutely toxic. In contrast, staphylococcal cellulitis tends to be a more indolent process. The lesion is more localized and may have fluctuant areas. Cellulitis caused by *H. influenzae* occurs primarily in children between the ages of 3 months and 3 years, but cases in adults have been reported. The lesion frequently appears on the face, has a bluish tinge, and usually follows an upper respiratory infection. Patients are almost always bacteremic at the time of presentation. In an immunocompromised host with cellulitis, enteric gram-negative bacilli are likely pathogens. *Erysipelothrix rhusiopathiae* is a small, gram-positive bacillus found as a commensal in many animals including fish and birds. It is the cause of erysipeloid which almost always occurs on the hands in those exposed to fish, shellfish, or poultry. Systemic symptoms are uncommon, but a joint adjacent to the cellulitis may be involved.

Complications of cellulitis include bacteremia and seeding of distant sites.

Antimicrobial therapy should be chosen to cover the specific organism (Table 39.5).

TABLE 39.4   Distinguishing Features of Cellulitis

Streptococcal: extremely rapid spread; patient appears toxic; lymphangitis prominent

Staphylococcal: more indolent; central fluctuance

Haemophilus: primarily in children ages 3 months to 3 years; bluish tinge; frequently facial

Gram-negative bacilli: immunocompromised host

E. rhusiopathiae: summer peak; exposure to fish, shellfish; erysipeloid; joint involvement common

TABLE 39.5 Initial Antimicrobial Therapy for Cellulitis

Organism	Antimicrobial
Group A streptococci	Penicillin
S. aureus	Antistaphylococcal penicillin
H. influenzae	Chloramphenicol
Gram-negative bacilli	Aminoglycoside
E. rhusiopathiae	Penicillin

Selected Bibliography

Blake, P. A., Merson, M. H., Weaver, R. E., et al.: Disease caused by a marine *Vibrio*. *N Engl J Med* 300:1-5, 1979.

Dajani, A. S., Asmar, B. I., and Thirnmoorthi, M. C.: Systemic *Haemophilus influenzae* disease: an overview. *J Pediatr* 94:355 364, 1979.

Davis, W. A., Kane, J. G., and Garagusi, V. F.: Human *Aeromonas* infections. *Medicine* 57:267-277, 1978.

Drapkin, M. S., Wilson, M. E., Shrager, S. M., et al.: Bacteremic *Hemophilus influenzae* type B cellulitis in the adult. *Am J Med* 63:449-452, 1977.

Elias, P. M., Fritsch, P., Epstein, E. H., Jr.: Staphylococcal scalded skin syndrome. *Arch Dermatol* 113:207-219, 1977.

Fleisher, G., Ludwig, S., and Campos, J.: Cellulitis: Bacterial etiology, clinical features, and laboratory findings. *J Pediatr* 97:591-593, 1980.

Florman, A. L. and Holzman, R. S.: Nosocomial scalded skin syndrome. *Am J Dis Child* 134:1043-1045, 1980.

Koblenzer, P. J.: Toxic epidermal necrolysis (TEN; Ritter's disease) and staphylococcal skin syndrome (SSSS), a description and review. *Clin Pediatr* 15:724-730, 1976.

Peter, G. and Smith, A. E.: Group A streptococcal infections of the skin and pharynx. *N Engl J Med* 297:311-317, 365-370, 1977.

Prystowsky, S. D., Vogelstein, B., Ettinger, D. S., et al.: Invasive aspergillosis. *N Engl J Med* 295:655-658, 1976.

Selwyn, S.: Microbiology and ecology of human skin. *Practitioner* 224:1059-1062, 1980.

Solem, L. D., Zaske, D., and Strate, R. G.: Ecthyma gangrenosum: Survival with individualized antibiotic therapy. *Arch Surg* 114:580–583, 1979.

Wannamaker, L. W.: Changes and changing concepts in the biology of group A streptococci and in the epidemiology of streptococcal infections. *Rev Infect Dis* 1:967–975, 1979.

40

FURUNCLES AND CARBUNCLES
Ronica M. Kluge, M.D.

Furuncles and carbuncles evolve most commonly from folliculitis, a limited infection of the hair follicle. Furuncles represent deep inflammatory nodules surrounded by an exuberant tissue reaction. Carbuncles are more extensive than furuncles and frequently composed of a number of interconnecting deep abscesses.

Microbiology

Staphylococcus aureus is almost always the causative microorganism. This is related in part to the nature of the organism, and perhaps to the fact that it is a normal skin inhabitant. On rare occasions, *Pseudomonas aeruginosa* has been documented to cause folliculitis, and could conceivably result in furuncle formation; this has resulted from heavily contaminated swimming pools or whirlpools.

Epidemiology

Staphylococcus aureus is a normal inhabitant of skin, anterior nares, and even the colon in most humans. What is not clear is why it causes disease in some individuals and not in others. Personal hygiene may be a factor. Certain age groups seem more susceptible; i.e., infancy and adolescence.

Pathogenesis

Since folliculitis is usually the predisposing lesion to the development of a furuncle, it is not surprising that furuncles usually occur in hair-bearing areas such

TABLE 40.1   Factors Predisposing to Development of Furuncle or Carbuncle

Folliculitis	Blood dyscrasias
Friction	Corticosteroid therapy
Perspiration	Defective neutrophils
Obesity	Diabetes

as axilla, groin, and extremities. Other predisposing factors are listed in Table 40.1

Furuncles are thick-walled abscesses with necrotic, purulent centers. Carbuncles result from a more extensive process which reaches into the subcutaneous fat.

Recurrent staphylococcal infections are known to be associated with some diseases such as Chediak-Higashi and hyperimmunoglobulinemia E syndromes, in which decreased neutrophil chemotaxis has been demonstrated. However, in patients with active furunculosis, there is a significant increase in neutrophil chemotactic response to a specific staphylococcal chemotaxin when compared with either normal controls or patients with inactive furunculosis.

Diagnostic Features

Clinical

Furuncles present as firm, tender, and erythematous nodules which soon become fluctuant and pustular. They are often quite painful during their evolution. A carbuncle is a larger lesion, frequently located on the back of the neck. It is deeper, more extensive, indurated, and may present with one or more draining areas around hairs. Patients may be febrile and complain of general malaise; an occasional patient may appear acutely toxic.

Laboratory

An elevated white blood cell count, shifted to immature forms, is common. A blood culture may be positive in the toxic-looking patient. Material aspirated from the lesion shows gram-positive cocci on stain and yields S. aureus on culture.

Differential Diagnosis

Sporotrichosis, leukemia, or other neoplastic disease may present rarely as a furuncle. The Gram stain is of great help in differentiating these diseases from furuncles. A draining carbuncle could be confused with actinomycosis or atypical tuberculosis of the skin. Stains and cultures are helpful, and a carbuncle should be warm, whereas the other lesions are frequently cold or normal in temperature.

TABLE 40.2   Appropriate Antimicrobial Therapy for Furuncle or Carbuncle

Penicillinase-resistant penicillin

Penicillin, if organism susceptible

Clindamycin

Erythromycin   } in the penicillin-allergic patient

Cephalosporin

Complications

Bacteremia resulting in metastatic spread of infection to distant organs is the most serious complication. Furuncles on the face may spread to the cavernous sinus.

Therapy

Early furuncles may be treated with warm soaks to encourage spontaneous drainage. Larger lesions will require surgical incision and drainage. The patient with extensive disease (carbuncles), cellulitis around the lesion, or fever should also be treated with a specific antistaphylococcal antimicrobial for 7-10 days (Table 40.2).

Prevention

Prophylaxis against recurrent furunculosis is less than satisfactory, but these measures may prove of benefit to some individuals. Strong emphasis must be placed on good personal hygiene: daily showers, hexachlorophene soap, daily change of wash cloth, towel, and clothes. Use of bacitracin ointment applied to the anterior nares results in temporary disappearance of staphylococci.

Prognosis

In the absence of complications, the prognosis with appropriate therapy is good for the individual episode.

Selected Bibliography

Blume, R. S. and Wolff, S. M.: The Chediak-Higashi syndrome: Studies in four patients and a review of the literature. *Medicine* 51:247-280, 1972.

Cates, K. L. and Quie, P. G.: Neutrophil chemotaxis in patients with *Staphylococcus aureus* furunculosis. *Infect Immun* 26:1004-1008, 1979.

Hill, H. R. and Quie, P. G.: Defective neutrophil chemotaxis associated with hyperimmunoglobulinemia E, In: J. A. Bellanti and D. H. Dayton (eds.): *The Phagocytic Cell in Host Resistance.* Raven Press, New York, 1975, pp. 249-266.

Pinkus, H.: Furuncle. *J Cutaneous Pathol* 6:517-518, 1979.

Washburn, J., Jacobson, J. A., Marston, E., and Thorsen, B.: *Pseudomonas aeruginosa* rash associated with a whirlpool. *JAMA* 235:2205-2207, 1976.

41

OTHER DERMATOLOGIC INFECTIONS
Ronica M. Kluge, M.D.

This chapter will consider ectoparasites and certain viral infections of the skin. Superficial fungal infections are covered in Chapter 108, and bacterial infections are found in Chapters 39 and 40.

Scabies

A burrowing mite, *Sarcoptes scabiei*, is the cause of human scabies. The disease affects all ages and is found throughout the world. Scabies appears to have an increased incidence in 15-year cycles, but in the past few years has occurred in epidemic proportions. Transmission generally requires intimate person-to-person contact, although fomites such as combs and clothing have been incriminated. Outbreaks have been related to unsanitary conditions, overcrowding, poor nutrition, and sexual promiscuity.

The life cycle of *S. scabiei* is short. Eggs hatch 3-3-1/2 days after being deposited in a superficial burrow in human skin and mature within 10-14 days. The adults mate; the males soon die, and the gravid females excavate new tunnels. The histology includes perivascular infiltrates of lymphocytes, histiocytes, plasma cells, and eosinophils. Papillary edema is a prominent feature. Immunofluorescent studies reveal the presence of IgM, IgA, IgG, C3, and fibrin in the cornified layer of the epidermis, in the papillary dermal vessels, and at the dermoepidermal junction.

Scabies is characterized by moderate to severe pruritus, particularly marked at night. After the initial infestation, symptoms do not occur for about 1 month; following subsequent exposures, the symptoms become manifest within 1-2 days suggesting previous sensitization of the host. The lesions, often obscured by excoriations, are distributed between fingers, on the hands, wrists, elbows, female breasts, periumbilical area, penis, buttocks, knees, ankles, and feet. Other areas, such as palms, soles, face, and scalp may be involved in infants and young children. Look for linear burrows in a typical case. Pruritic, erythematous nodules occur often in adults, and children may manifest eczematous or bullous lesions. In the immunodeficient/compromised individual a severe variant of scabies may be seen consisting of extensive crusting and plaques. Pruritus is minimal in these cases, but thousands of mites can be seen in skin scrapings.

The diagnosis can be confirmed by applying mineral oil to the skin over a burrow then examining the scrapings under the microscope looking for mites and eggs. *Sarcoptes scabiei* is 0.3-0.4 mm in length, rounded, with three pairs of very short legs.

Gamma-benzene hexachloride in a lotion or cream preparation is recommended for most infestations. This compound may not be safe for infants, so sulfur in petroleum ointment may be substituted. Personal items such as clothes, towels, and bed linens should be washed in hot water at the end of therapy. Since the infestation is so highly contagious, all family/household members should receive therapy simultaneously.

The clinical evolution of recurrent episodes of scabies strongly suggests that the host becomes sensitized to the organism. This is supported by the finding of immunoglobulins deposited in affected tissues and by the demonstration of immediate skin test reactions to an extract of *S. scabiei* in patients infested less than 1 year before testing. There is evidence that scabies is more likely to affect patients of a specific HLA type (HLA-A11).

Pediculosis

Two variants of the ectoparasite *Pediculus humanus* cause infestations of humans: the body louse and the head louse. A related ectoparasite, *Phthirus pubis,* the pubic ("crab") louse, also infests humans. As is true of scabies, pediculosis affects all ages and is worldwide in distribution. Transmission is most likely to occur under conditions of crowding and poor personal hygiene, or is related to sexual promiscuity. Fomites, including personal items, can transfer the parasites.

Pediculus humanus has a life cycle of about 1.5 months. The eggs attached to body hairs hatch in 7-10 days and mature 2 weeks later. The adults mate, and the fertilized female produces eggs for the remaining 20-30 days of its life. Histologic examination of the papule resulting from louse bites reveals edema, lymphocytic infiltration, and extravasation of red blood cells.

The common names of these members of the family, Pediculidae, reflect their usual human habitats. The head louse is confined to the scalp, the body louse to seams of clothing, and the pubic louse to the genital area. Pubic lice may occasionally be found in other places including facial hair, axillae, or even the eyelashes. The louse bite causes an intense pruritus. The lesions develop into erythematous papules and may appear slightly hemorrhagic. Bacterial superinfections are not uncommon. The diagnosis is made by observation of the ectoparasite and/or its eggs (nits). The head louse and body louse have a similar appearance. They are 2-4 mm in length, wingless, oval, and gray to red. The pubic louse is much more rounded.

In addition to the nuisance factor, the body louse serves as a vector for certain epidemic infections (Table 41.1). The causative organisms are not injected directly by the louse but gain entrance to the host through louse feces contamination of bite sites.

Therapy for lice is the same as that for scabies; gamma-benzene hexachloride and sulfur in petroleum ointment are effective. In cases of body lice, clothing

TABLE 41.1   Epidemic Infectious Diseases Carried by
P. humanus var corporis

Typhus fever, caused by *Rickettsia prowazekii*

Trench fever, caused by *R. quintana*

Relapsing fever, caused by *Borrelia recurrentis*

---

should be boiled or discarded. All members of the household should be treated at the same time.

Molluscum Contagiosum

This is a benign and self-limited disease caused by the largest member of the pox-virus group known to infect humans. The disease is probably transmitted from person to person through direct contact; epidemics have been reported in closed populations. Molluscum contagiosum is found throughout the world and primarily affects children, adolescents, and young adults.

Histologically, the lesion is a pseudotumor composed of hypertrophied epidermis extending into the dermis. The basement membrane is not breached. Intracytoplasmic inclusion bodies are seen in the malpighian cell layer and enlarge as the infected cells near the skin surface. A central umbilication is characteristic. There is little surrounding inflammatory reaction present.

The clinical appearance of molluscum contagiosum is that of discrete, 1-5 mm in diameter, pearlized papules with umbilicated centers. Only a few lesions are present in the typical case, but the immunosuppressed patient has large numbers of lesions. Examination of material expressed from the lesions will reveal the intracytoplasmic inclusions.

No specific antiviral therapy is available. Lesions can be easily removed by curettage, electrocautery, or cryocautery. Left untreated, the lesions will resolve in months to years.

Warts

Probably the most common skin problem, warts are caused by viruses of the papo-vavirus group. Warts are found in all age groups, though more commonly in children, and are seen in all areas of the world. Transmission is from person to person; fomites may be involved. Outbreaks in closed populations have been reported.

The histopathology of warts is characteristic: large vacuolated cells with basophilic nuclei are located in the upper malpighian and granular cell layers. Acanthosis and hyperkeratosis are seen in some forms. There is no inflammatory reaction present.

At least four clinical forms of warts are recognized (Table 41.2). Common warts are found mostly on the face, neck, and hands. Plantar warts occur only on the sole of the foot. Venereal warts are found in the anogenital regions. The diagnosis is usually clinically evident, but a biopsy may be performed in confusing cases. In the case of venereal warts, the diagnosis of condyloma lata due to syphilis must be ruled out.

TABLE 41.2   Clinical Forms of Warts

Common: verruca vulgaris; solid, circumscribed, elevated
tumor with multiple, horny projections

Flat: verruca plana juvenilis; smooth, slightly raised,
occurring in large numbers

Plantar: verruca plantaris; conical, bulging from skin
surface on sole of foot

Venereal: condyloma acuminatum; clusters of soft,
fleshy lesions

Left untreated, most warts will resolve in 1-2 years. There is no antiviral antimicrobial agent for the therapy of warts. When indicated, cryotherapy, electrodessication, or applications of cantharidin or salicylic acid preparations may be tried. Retinoic acid has been successful in many cases of flat warts. Plantar warts are particularly resistant to therapeutic measures, and surgery may be required. Podophyllin has been useful in treating veneral warts. Experimental therapies include contact allergins, bleomycin injections, levamisole, and vaccines.

Selected Bibliography

Briggarman, R. A. and Wheeler, C. E., Jr.: Immunology of human warts. *J Am Acad Dermatol* 1:297-304, 1979.

Bunney, M. H., Nolan, M. W., and Williams, D. A.: An assessment of methods of treating viral warts by comparative treatment trials based on a standard design. *Br J Dermatol* 94:667- 679, 1976.

Falk, E. S. and Bolle, R.: In vitro demonstration of specific immunological hypersensitivity to scabies mite. *Br J Dermatol* 103:367-373, 1980.

Falk, E. S. and Thorsby, E.: HLA antigens in patients with scabies. *Br J Dermatol* 104:317-320, 1981.

Felman, Y. M., Phil, M., and Nikitas, J. A.: Scabies. *Cutis* 25:32-42, 1980.

Hoefling, K. K. and Schroeter, A. L.: Dermatoimmunopathology of scabies. *Am Acad Dermatol* 3:237-240, 1980.

Hubler, W. R., Jr. and Clabaugh, W.: Epidemic Norwegian scabies. *Arch Dermatol* 112:179, 1976.

Medical Letter: Kwell and other drugs in treatment of lice and scabies. *Med Lett* 19:18-19, 1977.

Orkin, M., Epstein, E., Sr., and Maibach, H. I.: Treatment of today's scabies and pediculosis. *JAMA* 236:1136-1139, 1976.

Orth, G., Jablonska, S., Favre, M., Croissant, O., Obalek, S., Jarzabek-Chorzelska, M., and Jibard, N.: Identification of Papillomaviruses in Butchers' Warts. *J Invest Dermatol* 76:97-102, 1981.

Sher, A. M.: Viral infections of the skin. *Compr Ther* 7:35-43, 1981.

Solomon, L. M., Fahrner, L., and West, D. P.: Gammabenzene hexachloride toxicity: A review. *Arch Dermatol* 113:353, 1977.

Youshock, E. and Glazer, S. D.: Norwegian scabies in a renal transplant patient. *JAMA* 246:2608, 1981.

G. Central Nervous System

42

MENINGITIS
Robert H. Waldman, M.D.

Meningitis, the most common of all central nervous system infections, can be caused by a variety of protozoa, fungi, bacteria, and viruses (Tables 42.1-42.4). The most important form of meningitis because of the combination of its commonness and seriousness, especially if unrecognized and not treated promptly, is acute or pyogenic bacterial meningitis. It is also this type of meningitis that has been most impressively impacted upon by the antibiotic breakthroughs which have occurred in the last 40 years. The mortality from this serious illness has been cut to almost one-tenth the level that occurred before antibiotics were available.

Because of differing etiologies, clinical course, and laboratory findings, it is convenient to divide meningitis into four categories: viral, neonatal, acute bacterial (in the non-neonate), and chronic. This differentiation is far from perfect, as exemplified by the fact that some of the so-called chronic meningitides can present in a very acute manner, as will be discussed in more detail later. This chapter will mainly be oriented toward discussing acute bacterial meningitis, with the other forms being contrasted.

Microbiology

Haemophilus influenzae type b occurs almost exclusively in young children between the ages of 3 months and 2 years. It is the most common cause of meningitis in young children with 8000 cases yearly. It is believed that children less than 3 months of age have a much lower incidence of the disease because of the protective effect of transplacentally acquired maternal antibody.

Streptococcus pneumoniae (the pneumococcus) is the most common cause of meningitis in the adult. On the basis of the capsular polysaccharide, more than

TABLE 42.1   Major Pathogens in Acute Bacterial Meningitis

S. pneumoniae

H. influenzae b

N. meningitidis A, B, and C

S. pyogenes

E. coli K1

TABLE 42.2   Most Common Pathogens Causing Chronic Meningitis

M. tuberculosis

C. neoformans

C. immitis

H. capsulatum

Naegleria

TABLE 42.3   Uncommon Causes of Chronic Meningitis

Fungi	Candidiasis
	Blastomycosis
	Sporotrichosis
Bacteria	Brucellosis
	Syphilis
	Actinomycosis
	Nocardiosis
Noninfectious	Cancer
	Sarcoidosis
	Behcet's disease
	Mollaret's meningitis

TABLE 42.4   Frequency of Various Etiologic Agents as Causes of
Viral Infections of CNS

Agent	Approximate % of Total	
	Encephalitis or Meningoencephalitis	Meningitis
Enteroviruses	20	35
Herpes simplex	10	5
"Arboviruses"	5	2
Influenza A	3	3
Mumps	3	2
Measles	3	2
Adenoviruses	3	1

80 serotypes can be identified. The meningococcus is also divided into serotypes on the basis of the capsular polysaccharide; however, there are many fewer types. The meningococcus type B is the most common isolate in the United States today, with type C being the next most common.

Listeria monocytogenes, a gram-positive, motile bacillus which looks like diphtheroids on Gram stain, is a common cause of acute bacterial meningitis in immunosuppressed patients. It is very rare in people who have normal host defense mechanisms.

Acute bacterial meningitis related to trauma usually is caused by gram-negative rods if penetration of the skull has occurred. Following neurosurgical procedures, Staphylococcus aureus, S. epidermidis, or gram-negative rods, in that order, are most common. Recurrent meningitis following head trauma, in patients in whom there is a communication of cerebrospinal fluid with the outside, is usually caused by S. pneumoniae.

Neonatal meningitis is most commonly caused by either a group B streptococci, or one of the Enterobacteriaceae. These organisms are normal flora of the female genital tract, and the group B streptococci increase in frequency during pregnancy, so that 30% of women have this organism in their genital tract at term.

The most common viruses causing meningitis are the enteroviruses, mumps virus, herpes simplex virus, and lymphocytic choriomeningitis virus. The enteroviruses, i.e., coxsackievirus B and echovirus, are more common in the late summer. Herpes simplex virus infection of the central nervous system appears to be increasing in frequency.

Mycobacterium tuberculosis and various fungi are relatively uncommon causes of meningitis and usually present as chronic meningitis. Most patients with tuberculous meningitis have disseminated tuberculosis. Fungal meningitis is seen most commonly in cryptococcosis and coccidioidomycosis, less commonly in disseminated histoplasmosis, and rarely in sporotrichosis, blastomycosis, and candidiasis. Meningitis associated with histoplasmosis is an exceedingly difficult diagnosis to make because there are very few organisms in the cerebrospinal fluid, and the skin test is not helpful.

Brief mention should be made of amebic meningitis, caused by *Naegleria* and *Acanthamoeba*. These are normally free-living (i.e., nonparasitic) amebas. *Naegleria* gains access to the central nervous system by being forced under pressure through the nasal mucosa covering the cribiform plate in patients who have been swimming or diving in brackish water, particularly in the southern United States, Australia, Czechoslovakia, and Britain. The organism produces an acute meningitis. Spinal fluid shows motile cells when a wet-mount examination is performed. Olfactory signs and symptoms may be a distinguishing feature of this type of acute meningitis. The infection has a short incubation period and a fulminant course lasting 10-14 days, appearing to be uniformly fatal if untreated. Treatment is very unsatisfactory, but the organism appears to show some response to amphotericin B, miconazole, and rifampin. Acanthamoeba infection is extremely rare, has no known mode of transmission, runs a more chronic course, is probably associated with immunosuppression, and may resolve spontaneously. Treatment with sulfonamides, clotrimazole, and/or pentamidine appears to be somewhat effective.

Epidemiology

The risk of meningitis is greatest in the newborn with an incidence of 1-2 cases per 1000 children less than 2 months of age. The peak incidence of *H. influenzae* and meningococcal meningitis is at about 1 year, and three-fourths of the cases of *H. influenzae* meningitis occur in children under 2 years of age (Tables 42.5 and 42.6). Pneumococcal meningitis has two peaks of incidence, one at slightly less than 1 year of age, and another in people over age 50. Viewing all cases of acute bacterial meningitis there are two peaks of incidence, one in neonates under 1 month of age, and the other in children 6-8 months of age. Seventy percent of all cases occur in children under 5 years of age. Prematurity is a predisposing factor among newborns, as are premature rupture of membranes, prolonged labor, omphalitis, and neonatal skin infections.

TABLE 42.5   Acute Bacterial Meningitis - Incidence and Fatality Rate

Organism	% of Total Cases	Cases Per 100,000 Population	Fatality Rate (%)
H. *influenzae*	46	1.2	7
N. *meningitidis*	27	0.7	14
S. *pneumoniae*	11	0.3	28
Group B *Streptococcus*	3	0.1	22

TABLE 42.6   Incidence by Age (Per 100,000 Population)

Age	H. influenzae	N. meningitidis	S. pneumoniae	Group B Streptococcus
< 1 mo	6	4	3	42
1–2 mo	17	8	5	8
3–5 mo	46	13	8	2
6–8 mo	59	13	4	< 1
9–11 mo	41	12	3	< 1
1–2 yr	16	5	1	< 1
3–4 yr	3	2	< 1	< 1
5–9 yr	< 1	< 1	< 1	< 1

The seasonal incidence is winter for meningococcal and pneumococcal meningitis, and spring and fall for *H. influenzae*. *Haemophilus influenzae* is primarily a disease of the poor with the prevalence being inversely proportional to family income. Blacks have a higher prevalence than whites even when family income is controlled for. Meningococcal meningitis is related to crowded living conditions and therefore, is somewhat related to socioeconomic status, but it also occurs classically in crowded situations such as army barracks (Table 42.7).

Pathogenesis and Pathology

Acute bacterial meningitis certainly seems to be caused frequently by organisms that have a capsule which is antiphagocytic. The source of the pneumococcus and *H. influenzae* most commonly appears to be infection of the middle ear and sinuses. Meningitis does not appear to result from asymptomatic carriage which may be protective by stimulating an immune response in the absence of causing infection. Meningitis caused by *H. influenzae* occasionally results from facial cellulitis, but interestingly enough, almost never from epiglottitis (Table 42.8). Pneumonia is found in about one-third of patients with pneumococcal meningitis. Other factors related to the development of pneumococcal meningitis are sickle cell anemia (9:1000 children, which is 36 times the prevalence for black children without sickle cell anemia) and splenectomy.

In contradistinction to the pneumococcus and *H. influenzae,* it cannot be said that asymptomatic carriage of the meningococcus does not lead to meningitis. Meningococci are found in the nasopharynx of 5–10% of normal people. This increases to 20% during epidemics, but it is unknown whether this change in asymptomatic carriage rate is a cause or an effect of the prevalence of meningococcal disease.

TABLE 42.7   Special Epidemiologic Factors Related to Specific
Organisms Causing Meningitis

Organism	Factors
S. aureus	Foreign body; parameningeal or brain abscess
Gram-negative bacilli	Neonate; adult with sepsis (urinary tract infection or pneumonia); immunosuppressed; head trauma; or neurosurgical procedure
Pneumococcus	From pulmonary focus; otitis media, sinusitis; or cranial defect (previous head trauma); more common in infants, elderly, alcoholics
L. monocytogenes	Newborns; immunosuppressed
C. immitis	Travel to San Joaquin Valley
Meningococcus	Epidemics; prior pharyngitis is common
H. influenzae	Prior otitis media

TABLE 42.8   Findings That Are Relatively Specific for Certain
Etiologic Agents Causing Meningitis

Agent	Finding
Meningococcus	Hemorrhagic skin lesions
H. influenzae	Septic arthritis; cellulitis of face or upper extremity
Tuberculosis	Ophthalmoplegia or facial paralysis

In addition to *Escherichia coli* and group B streptococci which cause neonatal sepsis, herpes simplex virus may be acquired by the neonate during passage through the birth canal.

Pathologically pneumococcal and haemophilus meningitides tend to be pancerebral and basal. Meningococcal and mycobacterial meningitides tend to be more basal in nature, thereby explaining the more frequent involvement leading to palsy of the third, fourth, sixth, seventh, and eighth cranial nerves. In pneumococcal and mycobacterial meningitides one frequently finds vasculitis which leads to infarcts, transverse myelitis, and cerebral edema. Involvement of the anterior pituitary area leads to the syndrome of inappropriate antidiuretic hormone secretion. It has been hypothesized that a low glucose level in the central nervous system (secondary to the metabolism of glucose by the organisms and the phagocytic inflammatory cells) may contribute to the neurologic defect. This has led to the recommendation of glucose infusions as part of the therapy of patients with hypoglycorrhachia.

Diagnosis

Early diagnosis is nowhere more important than in the management of patients with acute bacterial meningitis since a delay in institution of therapy of even a very few hours worsens the prognosis. The first step is to make the diagnosis of meningitis, the second step is to distinguish viral from bacterial, and the third step is to determine the bacterial etiology so therapy with proper antibacterial agents may be administered.

The most common symptom is headache, often the worst that the patient has ever had. It usually is abrupt in onset particularly in patients with pneumococcal meningitis. Obscuring the presence of headache may be the presence of an altered state of consciousness, which is the most reliable sign of central nervous system infection. This altered state of consciousness can range from mild confusion to deep coma. Occasionally, particularly in cryptococcal or coccidioidal meningitis, patients may develop psychiatric disorders in the prodromal state of the disease. Seizures occur in about 30% of children with meningitis and can be focal or generalized. Fever is an unreliable indicator of meningitis especially in immunosuppressed patients, the very young, or the very old. Papilledema is unusual in meningitis and when present suggests the occurrence of a space-occupying lesion such as a brain abscess.

Stiff neck is caused by nerve root irritation and is usually not found in infants under 6-12 months of age. Two important physical findings for which patients should be tested are spontaneous flexion of knees upon flexion of the neck (Brudzinsky's sign) and pain and neck flexion upon 90° flexion of the knee and hip joints (Kernig's sign). As with the physical finding of stiff neck, these signs are unreliable in very young children, and they also are unreliable in older patients with lumbar disc disease or other diseases which cause neck rigidity, such as Parkinson's disease. Meningismus, i.e., pain upon passive flexion of the neck, is commonly found in patients with meningitis, but it is less specific since it is found in a number of less serious conditions.

Focal neurologic findings may be present, but should make one think of a more focal process than meningitis.

Diagnosis of neonatal meningitis is particularly difficult but important because time is even more of a factor in terms of morbidity and mortality being increased with delay in starting therapy. The presenting signs are extremely nonspecific including findings as minimal as a change in feeding habits. An important rule should be that virtually any abnormality of change in a neonate's behavior or

activities must evoke suspicion of meningitis and therefore lead to the performance of a lumbar puncture.

Tuberculous meningitis is very variable in presentation: some patients have a
clinical picture similar to that of acute bacterial meningitis, or the picture may
be very chronic, with an initial diagnosis of viral meningitis being made, only to
have the patient relapse months later at which time the correct diagnosis reveals
itself. Although most patients have evidence for tuberculosis elsewhere, 20% do
not, and a similar percentage have a completely normal chest x-ray.

Cryptococcal meningitis may be present either in a subacute or chronic form
with progressive lethargy and confusion typically being present. Focal neurologic
signs and papilledema are more common with cryptococcal meningitis than with
other forms.

The most important laboratory test is obviously the lumbar puncture. One
polymorphonuclear leukocyte or more than four lymphocytes are abnormal. A lumbar puncture should be performed in any suspected case, the only exception being
patients in whom a lumbar epidural abscess is suspected. A recent study demonstrated the risk of performing a lumbar puncture during bacteremia in children
(Table 42.9). The lumbar puncture should be performed with care in patients with
increased intracranial pressure caused by a mass lesion, in patients with a bleeding diathesis, or in those in whom a spinal cord tumor may be present. The spinal
fluid must be examined immediately. In viral meningitis, polymorphonuclear leukocytes may be predominant initially but are rapidly replaced by lymphocytes
(Table 42.10). In chronic meningitis, either tuberculous or cryptococcal, lymphocytes also predominate, but there usually are some polymorphonuclear leukocytes
(up to 30%) even well into the course of the disease which differentiates the cellular findings from those in patients with viral meningitis (Table 42.11).

Although the spinal fluid glucose is usually greater than half of the blood glucose in patients with viral meningitis, mild hypoglycorrhachia may be seen in meningitis caused by lymphocytic choriomeningitis virus or mumps virus. Tuberculous
meningitis typically causes an extremely low spinal fluid glucose, and progressive
hypoglycorrhachia is very suggestive of a mycobacterial etiology. Hypoglycorrhachia also can be seen in carcinomatous meningitis. It should be remembered
that a comparison of spinal fluid and blood glucose may be misleading if the blood
glucose is changing rapidly, since the spinal fluid glucose reflects the blood glucose
2 hr previously.

**TABLE 42.9   Meningitis Associated with Lumbar Puncture Performed
During Bacteremia***

	Approximate % Developing Meningitis	
Group	LP	No LP
All children	15	1
Age < 1 yr	30	2
< 1 yr, not receiving antibiotic at time of LP	85	2

*N Engl J Med 305:1079, 1981

TABLE 42.10   Usual CSF Findings in CNS Infections

Disease	Cells/mm^3	Protein (mg/dl)	Glucose (mg/dl)
Viral meningitis	25–500 lymphocytes, PMNs early in illness	50–100	Normal
Pyogenic (acute bac- terial meningitis)	≧ 1000 PMNs	100–1000	< 1/3 of blood
Tuberculous meningitis	25–200, lymphocytes usually predominate	100–1000	Normal to extremely low
Cryptococcal (and other fungal) meningitis	25–500, lymphocytes usually predominate	50–200	Normal to slightly low
Brain and epidural abscess	10–100, lymphocytes usually predominate	50–250	Normal
Syphilis	10–500, lymphocytes predominate	75–150 (IgG increased)	Normal

TABLE 42.11   Diseases That May Be Confused with Chronic Meningitis

Viral meningitis

Partially treated bacterial meningitis

Brain abscess

Parameningeal focus of infection

Subdural hematoma

Subarachnoid hemorrhage

Brain tumor

Multiple sclerosis

Malignant hypertension

Thrombotic thrombocytopenic purpura

Systemic lupus erythematosus

Temporal arteritis

Carcinomatous meningitis

With respect to spinal fluid culture, the more fluid available, the more likely one is to isolate an organism. With repeated lumbar punctures and culture of the obtained spinal fluid, the yield also increases. If tuberculous or cryptococcal disease is suspected, fluid should be centrifuged and the pellet stained for fungi and acid-fast organisms. One of the more recent advances is the use of fluorescent stains employing rhodamine conjugates for screening spinal fluid for mycobacteria. The Ziehl-Neelson stain is positive in only 10-15% of patients with tuberculous meningitis. The fluorescent stain should double the yield. If spinal fluid is allowed to stand, a caseous, fatty pellicle often forms in patients with tuberculous meningitis. Organisms are often difficult to find on Gram stain, particularly in patients with *H. influenzae* meningitis. Despite a very large number of phagocytic cells, organisms often are not intracellular, an interesting finding demonstrating the antiphagocytic properties of the organisms. Cultures for mycobacteria are positive in 40-90% of cases.

Another very important recent advance is the measurement of antigen from the organism causing the meningitis. The antigen determinations are particularly helpful in *H. influenzae* and cryptococcal meningitis. In the near future, it is probable that antigen determinations for pneumococcal, meningococcal, and group B streptococcal meningitis will also be generally available. The usual method, with the exception of that for determination of cryptococcal antigen, is counterimmunoelectrophoresis. The advantages of this technique are that it is unaffected by previous antibiotic usage and it is very rapid with a result obtainable within 30 min. It also may be possible to detect antigen in blood or urine. Another method for detecting antigen which is being investigated is gas-liquid chromatography.

Other tests on spinal fluid, which may be helpful, are a reduced chloride in tuberculous meningitis, cytologic examination to investigate the possibility of carcinomatous meningitis, and measurement of spinal fluid lactic acid. With respect to the latter, it has been reported that a level of greater than 30 mg/dl is diagnostic of bacterial meningitis with an accuracy of greater than 95%. The level falls to normal within 48-72 hr with appropriate antibiotic therapy. Similar levels are seen in tuberculous meningitis, with a fall to normal levels in 1-2 weeks with appropriate therapy. In patients suspected of having coccidioidal meningitis, antibody to the organism should be determined.

As mentioned earlier, repeat lumbar punctures can be very helpful. This is not only because of an increased chance of isolating a bacterial or fungal organism, but also because follow-up cell counts and glucose determinations are important aids in diagnosis. In cases of viral meningitis, a repeat spinal fluid examination in 8-24 hr will show a fall in number of polymorphonuclear leukocytes in the fluid in 95% of the cases. In tuberculous meningitis, a progressive worsening of the spinal fluid findings, particularly the glucose, is seen. In patients who are being treated, a repeat spinal fluid examination in 24-48 hr may be helpful in determining the appropriateness of the therapy. In that period, the glucose should be returning toward normal and the Gram stain and culture should be negative. However, the cell count usually does not change dramatically within that brief period. On the other hand, in patients who have received inappropriate or inadequate antibiotic therapy before arrival at a tertiary care center, there is surprisingly little effect on the spinal fluid. Very little change in glucose, protein, or cell count is usually found. There may be a slight decrease in the rate of positive cultures in pneumococcal or meningococcal meningitis, but there is no effect on the ability to isolate *H. influenzae*.

Culture of other sites should not be overlooked. Blood cultures are positive in 70% of patients with haemophilus or pneumococcal meningitis and only slightly less in meningococcal. A positive throat culture may be found in patients with meningococcal meningitis. Throat and/or rectal swabs for virus isolation may be positive. Penile or vaginal cultures for herpes simplex virus also may be useful. Urine cultures for mycobacteria, even if the urinalysis is normal, should be performed. In meningococcal meningitis, cultures of skin lesions should be performed, although the yield is low. Fungal cultures of urine also should be obtained. Bone marrow should be cultured in patients who are suspected of having tuberculosis or histoplasmosis. A liver biopsy may be helpful in tuberculosis, even if the liver function tests are normal.

Treatment (Tables 42.12-42.16)

The most important aspect of treatment is that it must be started immediately. A problem of recent vintage is *H. influenzae's* resistance to ampicillin. Recent data indicate that nearly 20% of organisms causing meningitis in the United States are β-lactamase producers. Therefore, patients should be started on both ampicillin and chloramphenicol until sensitivities can be determined. There have been a few reports of organisms resistant to both of these antibiotics; these patients should be treated with the combination of trimethoprim and sulfamethoxazole. A few strains of pneumococcus resistant to penicillin have been isolated in Canada and South Africa.

Because of the relatively low yield from staining spinal fluid for mycobacteria and the slow growth of the organism, one cannot wait for confirmatory evidence before starting treatment for tuberculous meningitis. If the data base is consistent with the diagnosis, in terms of history, predisposing factors, chest x-ray, and spinal fluid examination, and the patient has a positive tuberculin skin test, therapy should be started along with obtaining appropriate cultures. If the skin test is negative, or the clinical picture is obscure, a short observation period is

TABLE 42.12 Diagnostic–Therapy Algorithm

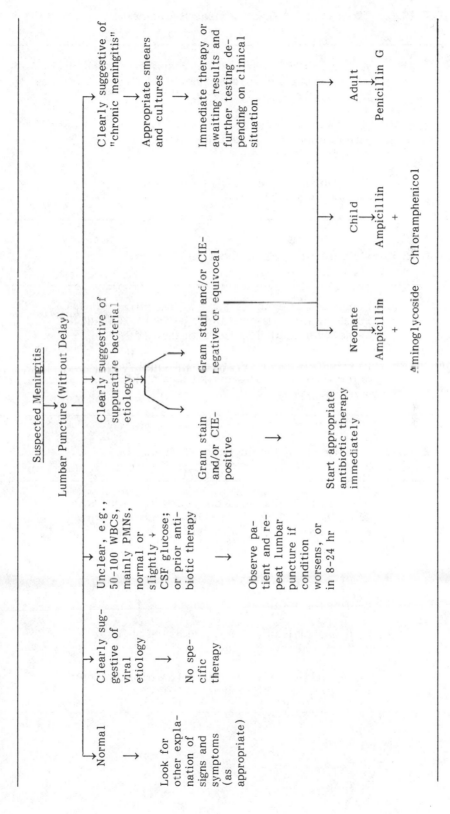

Suspected Meningitis

Lumbar Puncture (Without Delay)

- Normal → Look for other explanation of signs and symptoms (as appropriate)
- Clearly suggestive of viral etiology → No specific therapy
- Unclear, e.g., 50–100 WBCs, mainly PMNs, normal or slightly ↓ CSF glucose; or prior antibiotic therapy → Observe patient and repeat lumbar puncture if condition worsens, or in 8–24 hr
- Clearly suggestive of suppurative bacterial etiology →
  - Gram stain and/or CIE-positive → Start appropriate antibiotic therapy immediately
  - Gram stain and/or CIE-negative or equivocal →
    - Neonate: Ampicillin + Aminoglycoside
    - Child: Ampicillin + Chloramphenicol
    - Adult: Penicillin G
- Clearly suggestive of "chronic meningitis" → Appropriate smears and cultures → Immediate therapy or awaiting results and further testing depending on clinical situation

TABLE 42.13   Treatment of *H. influenzae* B Meningitis

Ampicillin, 400 mg/kg/day, divided into 6 daily doses, IV, *plus* chloramphenicol, 100 mg/kg/day, divided into 4 daily doses, IV

If organism is ampicillin-sensitive, discontinue chloramphenicol, continue ampicillin for 10-14 days

If organism is ampicillin-resistant, continue chloramphenicol only

---

TABLE 42.14   Treatment of Pneumococcal Meningitis

Penicillin, begun as soon as possible, adults, 10-20 million U/day and children, 250,000 U/kg/day, divided into 8-12 doses, IV

In penicillin-allergic: chloramphenicol or erythromycin 100 mg/kg/day divided into 4 doses, IV

TABLE 42.15   Treatment of Meningococcal Meningitis

Penicillin 10-20 million U/day for adults, 250,000 U/kg/day for children, divided into 8-12 doses, IV for 2 weeks

IV heparin

Prophylaxis of *close* contacts with minocycline or rifampin

IV hydrocortisone if any evidence of Waterhouse-Friderichsen syndrome

In penicillin-allergic patient, chloramphenicol 100 mg/kg/day divided into 4 doses, IV

TABLE 42.16   Meningitis in Immunocompromised Host

Common Etiologies	Initial Therapy (Pending Sensitivities)
L. monocytogenes	Ampicillin 200 mg/kg/day x 4 wk (± gentamicin)
Gram-negative bacilli	Carbenicillin 500 mg/kg/day + gentamicin 5 mg/kg/day IV and 2-4 mg intrathecally; or moxalactam 12 g/day IV
Gram-positive cocci	Oxacillin 200 mg/kg/day
Fungal	Amphotericin B

relatively safe, probably because doubtful cases are earlier and/or less severe. Therapeutic trials for tuberculous meningitis should be continued for 2-3 months. If the patient improves or definite proof of the etiology is obtained, then a full course of antituberculous therapy should be given. In unproven cases, steroids must not be administered, because of the possibility that the patient may have fungal meningitis. Therapy should include isoniazid, at a dosage of 600 mg/day (or 10 mg/kg) and rifampin, both of which cross the blood-brain barrier well. The use of corticosteroids in tuberculous meningitis is unproved, but should be considered when the patient is critically ill.

There are a number of other aspects of therapy that are less commonly important. Intravenous gamma globulin has been suggested but not proved effective in acute bacterial meningitis, particularly pneumococcal because of the observed phagocytic defect. In acute bacterial meningitis, steroids have not been shown to be beneficial and in fact, there is a suggestion that they may be harmful. Heparin has been used for the disseminated intravascular coagulopathy seen in meningococcal disease. In suspected or proven gram-negative meningitis in non-neonates, if *Pseudomonas* is not the likely organism, moxalactam or cefotaxime, 12 g/day IV, should be used. Although "first" and "second generation" cephalosporins cross the blood-brain barrier extremely poorly, "third generation" cephalosporins cross moderately well. An alternative treatment, depending on the organism and susceptibility, is the combination of trimethoprim and sulfamethoxazole. If *Pseudomonas* is suspected, intrathecal aminoglycosides usually are indicated since this class of antibiotics crosses the blood-brain barrier extremely poorly. Intrathecal gentamicin may be given in a dose of 4 mg every 12-24 hr. In the newborn, intrathecal aminoglycosides may not be necessary in the treatment of gram-negative meningitis.

Treatment should be continued for a minimum of 2 weeks, or longer if spinal fluid values have not returned to normal or very near normal.

Immunity and Prevention

With respect to the bacteria which cause acute meningitis, antibody to capsular polysaccharide antigens appears to be protective. Unfortunately, these antigens are not very immunogenic. This is especially true in young children, the group for whom a vaccine would be most valuable. Maternal antibody appears to be protective, but it also inhibits the antibody response if immunization is attempted in the neonate.

An approach to vaccine development, which is somewhat promising, is based on the fact that there are shared antigens found on the surface of other bacteria, which when administered, may lead to a rise in protective antibody. For example, it may be possible to immunize orally with strains of E. coli which have capsular antigens which cross-react with bacterial species that cause meningitis, particularly H. influenzae. Another potential advantage to the oral administration of living bacteria is that this approach may also stimulate secretory IgA antibody in addition to serum antibody. Oral immunization probably stimulates both gastrointestinal secretory antibody and respiratory secretion antibody.

The best-studied vaccine has been the purified meningococcal capsular polysaccharide. Vaccines are available for groups A and C. The current recommendation is that the vaccine should be used for control of epidemics, for travelers to countries experiencing epidemic disease, and for household contacts. Disease has been controlled in armed forces recruits since the vaccine has been used routinely for the past several years. Routine use is not recommended in children. However, the group A vaccine stimulates supposedly protective levels of antibody (although the data defining this protective level are not firm) when administered early in childhood, and it is conceivable that it would be effective if used routinely in areas of the world where group A meningococcal epidemics frequently occur. The group C vaccine stimulates low levels of antibody that persist for only a short period. The vaccines are of value in epidemic situations because half of the secondary cases occur more than 5 days after the primary case.

The second approach to prevention of meningitis is the use of prophylactic antibiotics for the patient's contacts. The justification for prophylactic antibiotics is that the secondary attack rates, i.e., infection in people who have contact with primary cases, is much higher than that for the general population. For example, in meningococcal meningitis, the secondary attack rate is 700–1000 times the primary attack rate, and in some epidemics the secondary attack rate has been as high as 15,000 times the primary rate. The other advantage of prophylactic antibiotics is that after 24 hr of prophylaxis, close surveillance of a family for the development of disease can be discontinued, thereby providing a great savings in personnel costs. For meningococcal infection, antibiotic prophylaxis is recommended for family members and nursery school or day-care center classmates. Although the organisms are sensitive to penicillin, this antibiotic is not effective in eradicating the carrier state and therefore should not be used for prophylaxis. The drug of choice is rifampin, 600 mg (or 5–10 mg/kg) every 12 hr for 4 doses. Good levels of the antibiotic are found in oral secretions, which probably explains its effectiveness and penicillin's ineffectiveness. The main side effect of rifampin therapy is a harmless orange discoloration of urine and sweat. An alternative is minocycline, but it has the serious side effect of causing vestibular abnormalities. Sulfonamides are excellent for prophylaxis and should be used if the epidemic strain is susceptible; however, serogroup C organisms are usually resistant to sulfonamides. The use of prophylactic antibiotics in H. influenzae meningitis is more controversial. Secondary cases appear to be about 600 times more common in household contacts than in controls but only in households that have children under 6 years of age. Therefore some authorities suggest chemoprophylaxis in households in which there are children under 6 years old.

With respect to neonatal meningitis, studies are underway to evaluate the effectiveness of routine cultures for group B streptococci and of administration of penicillin to women carrying this organism just before delivery. Similarly, it has been suggested that pregnant women be examined for the typical lesions of herpes simplex, and if this is confirmed by virus culture or histopathology, that a cesarean section be performed.

TABLE 42.17   Factors Correlating with Poor Prognoses

Coma

Delay in starting therapy

CSF glucose < 10 mg/dl, protein > 300 mg/dl

Advanced age

Bacteremia (found in nearly all fatal cases)

Coexisting illness

Prognosis and Complications (Table 42.17)

Acute bacterial meningitis had a mortality of 85% in the preantibiotic era. The mortality now is about 15%. Serious sequelae occur in over one-third of patients and are inversely related to the age of the patient when infected. The sequelae include mental retardation, hydrocephalus, inappropriate secretion of antidiuretic hormone, blindness, deafness, brain abscess, convulsive states, strabismus, and learning disabilities. With respect to the latter, postmeningitic children function at a significantly lower psychologic intelligence level than nonmeningitic peers, one study showing an 11-point lower mean intelligence quotient. With pneumococcal meningitis, the prognosis is worse in older, debilitated patients, especially those who are immunosuppressed. Type III pneumococcal meningitis has a mortality of nearly 50%. Recurrent pneumococcal meningitis should make one suspect that a traumatic injury has led to a cerebrospinal fluid leak, although recurrences also occur in patients who have undergone a splenectomy, patients with sickle cell anemia, and those with chronic otitis media. In meningococcal meningitis the prognosis is extremely poor if the patient develops the Waterhouse-Friderichson syndrome, with disseminated intravascular coagulation, renal failure, and shock lung.

Viral meningitis usually has a better prognosis, with few fatalities. However, mental retardation is not rare following viral meningitis in infants. The exception to the good prognosis of viral meningitis is that caused by herpes simplex virus, which has a very high mortality and rate of sequelae. The various causes of chronic meningitis had a mortality of 100% before the appearance of effective antimicrobial therapy. Today, if the patient is mentally alert when therapy begins, tuberculous meningitis has only a 10% mortality. The prognosis is worse in younger patients. Sequelae are common, however, with cranial nerve palsies found in 15-20% of patients, deafness being the most common. Other sequelae are mental retardation, hydrocephalus, and hemiparesis. In patients with tuberculous meningitis, or any other form of chronic meningitis, it is extremely important to be cognizant of the potential for development of hydrocephalus, since it is such a devastating complication if unrecognized, but it is treatable. The diagnosis must be considered in any patient who deteriorates during or after therapy, even in patients who have received full courses and have done very well.

Selected Bibliography

Applebaum, P. C. Bhamjee, A., Scragg, J. N., Hallett, A. F., Bowen, A. J., and Cooper, R. C.: *Streptococcus pneumoniae* resistant to penicillin and chloramphenicol. *Lancet* 2:995-997, 1977.

Artenstein, M. S., Winter, P. E., Gold, R., and Smith, C. D.: Immunoprophylaxis of meningococcal infection. *Mil Med* 139:91-95, 1974.

Austrian, R.: Random gleanings from a life with the pneumococcus. *J Infect Dis* 131:474-484, 1975.

Duma, R. J. and Finley, R.: In vitro susceptibility of pathogenic *Naegleria acanthamoeba* species to a variety of therapeutic agents. *Antimicrob Agents Chemother* 10:370-376, 1976.

Ellner, J. J. and Bennett, J. E.: Chronic meningitis. *Medicine* 55:341, 1976.

Finland, M. and Barnes, M. W.: Acute bacterial meningitis at Boston City Hospital during 12 selected years, 1935-1972. *J Infect Dis* 136:400-415, 1977.

Gold, R., Lepow, M. L., Goldschneider, I., Draper, T. F., and Gotschlich, E. C.: Kinetics of antibody production to group A and group C meningococcal polysaccharide vaccines administered during the first six years of life: Prospects for routine immunization of infants and children. *J Infect Dis* 140:690-697, 1979.

Goldacre, M. J.: Acute bacterial meningitis in childhood: Incidence and mortality in a defined population. *Lancet* 1:28-31, 1976.

Hodges, G. R. and Perkins, R. L.: Acute bacterial meningitis: An analysis of factors influencing prognosis. *Am J Med Sci* 270:427-440, 1975.

Idriss, Z. H., Sinno, A. A., and Kronfol, N. M.: Tuberculous meningitis in childhood. *Am J Dis Child* 130:364-367, 1976.

Lavetter, A., Leedom, J. M., Mathies, A. W., Jr., Ivler, D., and Wehrle, P. F.: Meningitis due to *Listeria monocytogenes*. A review of 25 cases. *N Engl J Med* 285:598-603, 1971.

Maguire, G. F. and Myers, M. G.: Antimicrobial selection for meningitis in young infants. *Am J Dis Child* 133:1132-1133, 1979.

Mangi, R. J., Kundargi, R. S., Quintiliani, R., and Andriole, V. T.: Development of meningitis during cephalothin therapy. *Ann Intern Med* 78:347-351, 1973.

McCormick, J. B. and Bennett, J. V.: Public health considerations in the management of meningococcal disease. *Ann Intern Med* 83:883-886, 1975.

McCracken, G. H., Jr.: Neonatal septicemia and meningitis. *Hosp Prac* 11:89-97, 1976.

Menkes, J. H.: Improving the long-term outlook in bacterial meningitis. *Lancet* 2:559-560, 1979.

Sawyer, T. K., Visvesvara, G. S., and Harke, B. A.: Pathogenic amoebas from brackish and ocean sediments, with a description of *Acanthamoeba hatchetti* n. sp. *Science* 196:1324-1325, 1977.

Sell, S. H. W., Webb, W. W., Pate, J. E., and Doyne, E. O.: Psychological sequelae of bacterial meningitis: Two controlled studies. *Pediatrics* 49:212-217, 1972.

Sells, C. J., Carpenter, R. L., and Ray, C. G.: Sequelae of central-nervous system enterovirus infection. *N Engl J Med* 293:1-4, 1975.

Varki, A. P. and Puthuran, P.: Value of second lumbar puncture in confirming a diagnosis of aseptic meningitis. A prospective study. *Arch Neurol* 36:581-582, 1979.

Wahdan, M. H., Rizk, F., El-Akkad, A. M., El Ghoroury, A. A., Hablas, R., Girgis, N. I., Amer, A., Boctar, W., Sippel, J. E., Gotschlich, E. C., Triau, R., Sanborn, W. R., and Cvjetanovic, B.: A controlled field trial of serogroup A meningococcal polysaccharide vaccine. *Bull WHO* 48:667-673, 1973.

Ward, J. I., Fraser, D. W., Baraff, L. J., and Plikaytis, B. D.: *Haemophilus influenzae* meningitis: A national study of secondary spread in household contacts. *N Engl J Med* 301:122-126, 1979.

Wehrle, P. F., Mathies, A. W., Leedom, J. M., and Ivler, D.: Bacterial meningitis. *Ann N Y Acad Sci* 145:488-498, 1967.

43

ENCEPHALITIS
Gary R. Plotkin, M.D.

Encephalitis is inflammation of the brain, and alterations in state of awareness,
responsiveness, or behavior are the prevailing clinical characteristics. If the inflammatory process extends from the brain into either the meninges or spinal cord,
then the terms meningoencephalitis or encephalomyelitis are employed. Acute
disseminated encephalomyelitis, including postinfectious and postvaccinal encephalomyelitis, is an acute or subacute disease of the central nervous system (CNS)
which occurs after certain viral infections or as a complication of immunizations
and is characterized by symptoms indicating damage mainly to the white matter
of the brain or spinal cord. Reye's syndrome refers to an acute and often fatal
encephalopathy that predominantly affects children and is characterized by brain
edema associated with fatty infiltration and dysfunction of the liver.

Etiology

The etiologic agents of encephalitis with representative examples are shown in
Tables 43.1 and 43.2. The arboviruses or arthropod-borne animal viruses which
cause encephalitis in the United States have been classified into the families
Togaviridae and Bunyaviridae based upon morphologic and serologic relationships,
dependent upon complement fixation, hemagglutination inhibition, and infectivity
neutralization tests. Viruses causing Eastern, Western, and Venezuelan equine
encephalitis are members of the genus *Alphavirus* (family Togaviridae) while the
agents of St. Louis and Powassan encephalitis are within the genus *Flavivirus*
(family Togaviridae). California encephalitis virus is a member of the family
Bunyaviridae. Measles virus belongs to the family Paramyxoviridae, genus *Morbillivirus,* and contains a single-stranded RNA genoma. Mumps virus is also a member of the family Paramyxoviridae (genus *Paramyxovirus*). Rubella virus is a

TABLE 43.1   Encephalitis – Etiologic Agents

Virus	Lassavirus
	Bunyaviruses
	Herpesviruses
	Polyomavirus
	Enteroviruses
	Measles
	Rubella
	Mumps
	Slow infections
	Cytomegalovirus
	Rabies
Bacteria	Rickettsiae
	Mycoplasmas
	Chlamydiae
	Those associated with brain abscess and meningitis
	Spirochetes
	Mycobacteria
Fungi	*C. neoformans*
	C. immitis
	Candidiasis
	H. capsulatum
	Aspergillosis
	Phycomycosis
Protozoa	Plasmodia
	Naegleria
	Trypanasoma
	Toxoplasmosis
Helminths	*Echinococcus*
	T. solium
	Trichinosis
	Schistosomiasis
	Cysticercosis

togavirus (genus *Rubivirus*). As opposed to the above RNA viruses, varicella-zoster is a DNA virus (family Herpesviridae, subdivision *Alphaherpesviruses*). Herpes simplex virus types 1 and 2 are also *Alphaherpesviruses,* and the two distinct serotypes can be differentiated by serologic, biologic, and biochemical means.

Since the description of the syndrome of encephalopathy and fatty liver by Reye in 1963, an increasing number of cases have been reported. Reports have been published of isolation of viruses from the brain or cerebrospinal fluid of patients with a confirmed or probable diagnosis of Reye's syndrome. Such isolates

TABLE 43.2   Center for Disease Control Classification

Arboviral

Enteroviral

Associated with childhood infections (measles, mumps, varicella, rubella)

Associated with respiratory infections

Other infectious agents

Indeterminate

---

have included herpes simplex, coxsackievirus B4 or B5, coxsackievirus A9, echo-virus type 8, untyped echovirus, reovirus type 1, cytomegalovirus, influenza A or B, and vaccine-like poliovirus type 1. In other patients with Reye's syndrome, viruses isolated from throat swabs, feces, urine, or other organs outside the central nervous system included influenza A or B, parainfluenza type 2 or 3, adenovirus type 3, untyped coxsackievirus A, coxsackievirus B1 or B4, echovirus type 11, reovirus type 2, untyped reovirus, and respiratory syncytial virus. Serum antibody measurements in patients with Reye's syndrome have demonstrated recent infections with varicella-zoster virus, Epstein-Barr virus, parainfluenza 1, and respiratory syncytial virus.

The term slow-virus diseases was first used in 1954 by Björn Sigurdsson when he studied slow-evolving diseases of sheep in Iceland. Slow-virus infections of the nervous system in humans include subacute spongiform virus encephalopathies (kuru and Creutzfeldt-Jakob disease), subacute sclerosing panencephalitis, progressive multifocal leukoencephalopathy, and progressive rubella panencephalitis. The infectious origin of kuru has been demonstrated by transmitting the disease to chimpanzees, monkeys, mink, and ferrets by intracerebral inoculation of suspensions of brain from human cases. The agent responsible for kuru, however, has not been visualized with the electron microscope and does not evoke an apparent immune response in either the natural or experimental host. Creutzfeldt-Jakob disease has similarly been transmitted to monkeys, cats, guinea pigs, and chimpanzees, but neutralizing antibodies to the agent have not yet been demonstrated in the sera of humans or animals with the disease. The Creutzfeldt-Jakob agent has not yet been characterized. A virus very similar to the measles virus has been isolated from brain tissue from patients with subacute sclerosing panencephalitis (SSPE). However, differences between the viruses of measles and subacute sclerosing panencephalitis can be detected in tissue culture. These differences probably indicate that the SSPE virus is a variant of measles virus rather than a separate virus. Two and perhaps three papovaviruses (family Papovaviridae, genus *Polyomavirus)* have been isolated from brain tissue of patients with progressive multifocal leukoencephalopathy.

Free-living amebae from two genera, *Naegleria* and *Acanthamoeba* spp, are now known to cause central nervous system infections in humans. The pathogenic free-living amebae share a relatively simple life-style consisting of a vegetative trophozoite which feeds mostly on bacteria, and a resistant cyst phase. Additionally, *Naegleria* may exist in a transient flagellate phase.

Epidemiology

In 1977, 1536 cases of encephalitis were reported to the Center for Disease Control, 70% of which were of indeterminate etiology, and 16% were due to arboviruses. The latter figure was higher than usual due to the late season outbreak of St. Louis encephalitis in Florida. The various etiologies of encephalitis as reported to the CDC in 1977 are summarized in Table 43.3, and their mortality in the United States is summarized in Table 43.4. About half of all cases were reported from six states: California, Ohio, Florida, Illinois, Indiana, and Mississippi.

A summary of the epidemiological characteristics is given in Table 43.5.

TABLE 43.3   Incidence of Encephalitis in the United States

Etiology	% of Total
Arboviral	16
Western equine	(3)
Eastern equine	(<1)
St. Louis	(9)
California	(4)
Enteroviral	1
Associated with childhood infections	8
Measles	(2)
Mumps	(3)
Chickenpox	(3)
Rubella	(<1)
Associated with respiratory illness	<1
Associated with other known etiologies	5
Herpes simplex	(4)
Herpes zoster	(1)
Infectious mononucleosis	(<1)
Indeterminate	70

TABLE 43.4   Mortality, USA

Etiology	% of Total Encephalitis Deaths	Death/Case Ratio
Arboviral	6	4%
Western equine	(0)	(0/41)
Eastern equine	(<1)	(1/1)
St. Louis	(5)	(7%)
California	(0)	(0/65)
Enteroviral	<1	6%
Associated with childhood infections	5	8%
Associated with respiratory illness	0	0/5
Associated with other known etiologies	19	41%
Herpes simplex	(15)	(40%)
Herpes zoster	(4)	(50%)
Infectious mono-nucleosis	(<1)	(1/3)
Indeterminate	69	11%
Total	100%	11%

Herpes simplex encephalitis is the most common sporadic or nonepidemic form of encephalitis in the United States. Estimates of prevalence range from 2-19% of all cases of encephalitis to 20-75% of sporadic necrotizing encephalitis. Herpes simplex type 1 is the usual cause of adult herpes encephalitis, while type 2 primarily causes nervous system infections of neonates and meningitis in adults. The major mode of spread is by close personal contact, and the source of virus is an individual with a subclinical or clinically inapparent primary or recurrent infection.

Kuru is restricted to a small population of Melanesian natives living in a well-defined geographic area in the eastern highlands of Papua New Guinea. Kuru accounted for the death of approximately 1% of the population annually during its peak incidence in the 1950s. Adult females have a marked tendency for this disease, but during the past 10 years, the incidence of kuru has been declining concomitantly with the decline in cannibalism. The infectious agent responsible for kuru may be introduced by conjunctival, nasal, or skin contamination at the time of practicing cannibalism.

TABLE 43.5   Epidemiologic Characteristics of Encephalitides

	Geographic	Reservoir	Human Vector
Eastern equine (EEE)	Eastern U.S., Central America, Caribbean Islands, Brazil, Guyana, Argentina	Horses, birds	*Aedes* mosquitoes
Western equine (WEE)	All of U.S., Canada, Central America, Guyana, Brazil, Argentina	Birds, horses	*Culex tarsalis* mosquito
Venezuelan equine (VEE)	Florida, Texas, Central America, northern S. America	Horse, rodents, dogs, bats, birds	*Culex* mainly, also *Aedes* and *Deinoceritca* mosquitoes
St. Louis (SLE)	U.S., Central America, Caribbean Islands, Colombia, Brazil, Argentina	Birds, bats	*Culex* mosquitoes
Powassan	Canada, northern U.S.	Rodents	Tick
California encephalitis	North-Central U.S.	Rabbits, squirrels, mice	*Aedes* and *Culex* mosquitoes
Measles	Worldwide	Humans	Aerosolized droplets

Creutzfeldt-Jakob disease occurs throughout the world and has a rate of one or two cases per million. Libyan Jews and individuals residing in the area of central Slovakia and adjacent Hungary have an increased incidence. Many patients with Creutzfeldt-Jakob disease have had a history of brain or eye operations during the previous 2 years. Cases of transmission by corneal graft and by contaminated stereotactic electroencephalographic electrodes have been reported.

Subacute sclerosing panencephalitis (SSPE) is more common in males than females and occurs mainly between ages of 5 and 12 years. The incubation period following clinical measles is usually 6 years, and the disease is more frequent in the southeastern United States. It occurs with a prevalence of approximately 1:1 million.

Progressive multifocal leukoencephalopathy (PML) usually occurs in patients who are on immunosuppressive therapy or who have leukemia, lymphoma, or carcinomatosis. However, PML has been reported in individuals without apparent defects in either cellular or humoral immunity. The disease affects both sexes, and its duration from onset of symptoms to death is 1-4 months. Although PML is a rare disease, antibody to the papovaviruses thought to cause the disease is quite common. In one study 27.5% of children between the ages of 5 and 9 years had antibody, and by the age of 15 this figure had reached 65%.

The free-living amebae are distributed widely in nature, and the overwhelming majority of recorded cases of meningoencephalitis due to these organisms have been caused by species of *Naegleria*. However, since there have been few ultrastructural studies of human tissue from cases of primary amebic meningoencephalitis, morphologic criteria enabling one to differentiate *Naegleria* from *Acanthamoeba* in human tissues are limited. *Naegleria* meningoencephalitis is contracted by swimming in pools or lakes. Besides having been reported in the United States, it occurs in Czechoslovakia, New Zealand, Great Britain, and Belgium. The distribution of cases of *Naegleria* meningoencephalitis has demonstrated a strong cluster effect.

Pathogenesis and Pathology

By definition, arboviruses are transmitted by arthropod vectors in which there is virus multiplication. The biologic transmission may be supplemented by mechanical transmission, i.e., the virus may be passively carried externally on the vector or excreted. The duration of virus multiplication within the arthropod host before it becomes infectious is dependent upon such factors as specific virus, vector, and temperature. For most arboviruses under average summer temperatures, the extrinsic incubation period varies from 7 to 14 days. Arboviruses are transmitted by the bite of the appropriate vector, and thus the skin represents the primary portal of entry. Several togaviruses, notably Venezuelan equine encephalitis virus, are infectious by aerosol and have caused numerous infections in laboratory workers. Arboviruses probably multiply in the vascular epithelium and within lymph nodes, liver and spleen. Liberation of virus from these organs constitutes the systemic phase of viremia. The role of immunologic injury remains unknown; however, antigen-antibody complexes may be important in the pathogenesis of certain clinical manifestations, e.g., the dengue shock syndrome. Cell-mediated immunity also may be important in controlling virus persistence and in determining the immunopathologic lesions.

The response of the central nervous system to arbovirus infections consists of cellular infiltration, microglial hyperplasia and proliferation, and neuronal degeneration. In the acute stages, cellular infiltration is composed mainly of polymorphonuclear leukocytes; however, later the exudate contains lymphocytes, monocytes, and plasma cells. Perivascular localization of these inflammatory cells is a characteristic finding. Microglial proliferation may be diffuse or focal, and glial reaction may occur in both gray and white matter. Neuronal changes may range from slight swelling and hyalinization to total destruction, and neuronophagia is often observed. The meninges and blood vessels may show inflammatory changes, and brain edema is present in severe cases.

In measles encephalitis there is patchy demyelination, scattered petechial hemorrhages, and lymphocytic cell infiltration. Either direct viral invasion or an autoimmune reaction may explain the pathogenesis of measles encephalitis. The neurons may be altered by the virus and thus rendered susceptible to destruction by immunocompetent cells. Measles virus has only rarely been isolated from brain tissue.

After being inoculated by direct contact into a break in the skin or mucous membrane, herpes simplex virus spreads to local lymph nodes thus resulting in further viral multiplication. This initial infection ordinarily occurs in the second year of age and is inapparent. The route by which herpes simplex virus may reach the nervous system is unknown; however, since portions of the brain subserving olfactory functions are involved in the encephalitic process, it has been proposed that the virus travels along the olfactory tract to reach the brain. Additionally, the virus may spread hematogenously, and because of a special affinity for neurons in the limbic system it may remain localized to this area. Pathologically both gray and white matter are affected by an inflammatory process characterized by marked infiltration with phagocytic cells. Perivascular accumulations of lymphocytes and plasma cells are commonly found, and cell necrosis involves all elements of the nervous system. Frequently there is also destruction of walls of the small blood vessels with resulting microhemorrhages. Cowdry's type A intranuclear inclusion bodies may be demonstrated in both the neural and glial elements. Cortical involvement is most prominent especially in the temporal and basal frontal regions.

Such factors as viral infection, congenital metabolic defects, and exogenous or endogenous toxins have been implicated in the etiology of Reye's syndrome. Epidemics of this syndrome have occurred in association with epidemics of influenza type B infection; however, isolation of virus from the liver or brain has been rare. Numerous toxins have been proposed as possible causes of this syndrome. Clinically, the illness resembles the vomiting sickness of Jamaica which is caused by ingesting the toxin hypoglycin found in the unripe fruit of the akee tree. Hypoglycin is metabolized to methylene cyclopropylacetic acid (MCPA). The toxicity of MCPA is related to inhibition of fatty acid oxidation, increased glucose utilization, and defective mobilization of glucose. Microscopically, the liver in Reye's syndrome reveals the accumulation of small droplets of fat within the hepatocytes. The cells are swollen and compress the sinusoids. Inflammatory changes are not present initially and hepatocyte necrosis is uncommon. In biopsy specimens obtained after day 4 of clinical illness, portal triaditis may be present. Fatty infiltration may also occur in other organs including the myocardium and kidney. Ultrastructurally, hepatocyte mitochondria are enlarged, assume bizarre ameboid forms with rarefaction of the matrix and loss of the dense body. Other changes include progressive loss of hepatocyte glycogen and increased numbers of peroxisomes. The encephalopathy of Reye's syndrome may be related to the elevation of blood ammonia, fatty acids, short-chain fatty acids, and other substances. The light microscopic examination of brain tissue obtained at autopsy reveals swollen or shrunken neurons and swollen astrocytes and oligodendrogliocytes. Inflammatory changes usually are not observed and in several patients electron microscopy showed alteration of neuronal mitochondria similar to that seen in the liver.

Kuru is an invariably fatal disease among the Fore people in the eastern highlands of Papua New Guinea. Pathologically, the brain usually appears grossly normal. Microscopically, widespread neuronal degeneration and gliosis, swollen and vacuolated degenerating neurons, and argentophilic axonal enlargement of degenerating Purkinje cells have been described. These changes are present throughout the gray matter and involve most consistently the cerebellum, pons, thalamus, and basal ganglia.

Except for slight atrophy, the gross appearance of the brain from patients with Creutzfeldt-Jakob disease is unremarkable. Widespread status spongiosus in the gray matter and intense gliosis are characteristic light microscopic findings. Astrocytic proliferation may be seen in areas which do not exhibit marked neuronal degeneration. Loss of granule cells and degenerating Purkinje cells with axonal swellings are noted in the cerebellum. Gliosis, occasional swollen or vacuolated nerve cells, and microglial clusters are present in the basal ganglia, brain stem, and spinal cord.

In subacute sclerosing panencephalitis, inflammatory changes are found in the brain, and measles virus antigens have been demonstrated in lymph nodes, spleen, liver, renal glomeruli, and mononuclear cells from cerebrospinal fluid. Macroscopically, signs of congestion or atrophy may be seen in the brain, but it can appear normal depending upon the stage of the disease. Microscopically, the changes are widespread throughout the gray and white matter. Nonspecific changes of subacute inflammation are present. Intranuclear and intracytoplasmic inclusion bodies are variably present in neurons, astrocytes, and oligodendroglial cells. Electron microscopy of the inclusions shows filamentous structures consisting of fine tubules 17-23 nm in outer diameter but which can measure up to 400-500 nm. Immunofluorescence reveals measles antigen in the inclusion bodies and in nuclei and cytoplasm of neurons and glial cells.

Progressive multifocal leukoencephalopathy (PML) may result from the activation of a polyomavirus which has been latent in brain tissue. Alternatively, certain individuals may have failed to acquire immunity in childhood and thus may be exposed to the viral agents during a vulnerable period in adulthood. This disease has a distinctive neuropathology. The lesions may be widespread in the central nervous system and consist of numerous foci of demyelination of varying size. The characteristic features of PML are observed microscopically at the periphery of the early demyelinative lesions. At these sites there is enlargement of the oligodendrocytes with marked nuclear changes, and the nuclei become basophilic and may contain inclusions. Toward the center of the lesions, oligodendrocytes are generally absent, and the astrocytes are often enlarged and multinucleated. During the course of the illness new foci of demyelination are continually developing.

Progressive rubella panencephalitis is a chronic, inflammatory, and progressive central nervous system disorder which appears as a delayed reaction of either congenital rubella or a postnatal rubella infection. The neuropathologic investigations have shown meningeal and perivascular plasma cells and lymphocytes, gliosis, glial nodules, and diffuse neuronal loss. Inclusion bodies have not been detected, and amorphous deposits have been seen in blood vessel walls throughout the white matter and within the cerebral hemispheres, basal ganglia, and cerebellum. Rubella virus has been isolated from brain tissue cultures.

Diagnostic Features (Clinical and Laboratory), Complications and Prognosis

The clinical features of the various arboviral encephalitides that occur in the United States are similar. There are, however, variations in severity of symptoms during different epidemics involving even the same virus. Arboviruses may also be responsible for asymptomatic infections. Eastern equine encephalitis (EEE) characteristically has an abrupt onset with few prodromal symptoms. Typically, the patient develops high fever, headache, nuchal rigidity, and vomiting. Drowsiness or coma and focal or generalized convulsions commonly occur within 24-48 hr. Cranial nerve palsies, hemiplegia, and other focal neurologic signs are often noted. Even though the ratio of inapparent infection to overt encephalitis may be 25:1, as many as three-fourths of patients with symptomatic Eastern equine encephalitis die within 3-5 days. Patients, especially infants, who survive usually have severe neurologic deficits including mental deficiency, hemiplegia, convulsive disorders, aphasia, and cranial nerve palsies.

The patient with EEE has a peripheral blood leukocytosis and a cerebrospinal fluid which is cloudy in appearance. The fluid is under increased pressure and has elevated protein and normal glucose levels and a white cell count ranging from 500 to 3000/mm^3 with a polymorphonuclear predominance. As the acute phase of

illness subsides, the CSF cell count falls and lymphocytes predominate. The serologic diagnosis of illness caused by most of the arboviruses depends upon demonstrating a significant rise in the titer of specific antibodies measured by hemagglutination-inhibition, complement-fixation, neutralization, or radioimmunoassay.

Western equine encephalitis (WEE) is typically less severe than EEE, and occurs more commonly as an inapparent infection. Patients of all ages may exhibit
fever and drowsiness; however, convulsions occur frequently in infants and children under 4 years of age but rarely in adults. Occipital headaches, nuchal rigidity, and mental confusion may also be present. In approximately one-third of the
patients, obtundation progresses to stupor or coma. Clinical improvement is usually precipitous and occurs from 5 to 10 days after the onset of illness. Severe and
permanent sequelae are rare in adults but are seen with increased frequency in
younger groups. More than half of the infants less than 1 month of age have recurrent seizures or marked motor or behavioral deficits. The average mortality
is 10%; however, infants and the elderly constitute the high-risk groups. Cerebrospinal fluid abnormalities are less marked than those observed in EEE, the pressure is normal, and the cell count usually does not exceed $200/mm^3$ with mononuclear forms predominating.

Clinically apparent disease due to Venezuelan equine encephalitis (VEE) virus
can be categorized into three forms: (1) "influenzal" as manifested by constitutional symptoms, pharyngitis, and a febrile course of 1-4 days; (2) fulminant as
manifested by a short febrile course with rapid progression to shock, coma, and
convulsions; and (3) encephalitic as evidenced by a febrile course of 2 weeks or
longer with central nervous system manifestations beginning after several days to
a week of prodromal illness. Fatalities are rare and occur most commonly in children. Virus can be isolated from blood and pharyngeal swab specimens.

Infection with St. Louis encephalitis virus is often clinically inapparent, but
when symptoms are present, they are similar to those produced by other arboviruses. Adults are affected more commonly than children, and the central nervous
system symptoms may be preceded by prodromal illness of 3-4 days duration. The
spectrum of encephalitis ranges from very mild neurologic signs to extremely severe illness which leads to death within days after onset. Although 20% of the
cases may be fatal, remissions can occur with complete recovery. Among those
who survive, significant permanent neurologic sequelae are uncommon. Cerebrospinal fluid findings are similar to those of other arbovirus encephalitides.

Only a limited number of cases of Powassan virus encephalitis have been reported. Most have occurred in children in Canada and New York State during late
summer or early fall. The illness is characterized by moderate to severe encephalitic signs including headache, fever, convulsions, disturbance in consciousness,
and occasionally focal deficits. Most patients recover but neurologic deficits can
persist.

Most cases of California encephalitis have been in children and relatively few
cases have been among infants under 1 year of age, in contrast to the Western and
Eastern equine encephalitis viruses, which have predilection for this age group.
Adults who become infected may remain asymptomatic. The clinical illness varies in severity with the minority of patients presenting with mild symptoms including malaise, headache, and gastrointestinal complaints. Most cases follow a
constant pattern consisting of a 2- or 3-day prodrome of fever and nonspecific
systemic signs. These are followed by a severe illness lasting 7-10 days but from
which most patients recover. Seizures are common in California encephalitis, and
other signs include tremulousness, rigidity of neck and limbs, and hyperreflexia.
Despite the severity of the acute encephalitic manifestations, major neurologic
sequelae are uncommon; however, a small percentage of children will suffer recurrent convulsions. Cerebrospinal fluid cellular response varies from no leukocytes

to more than $600/mm^3$ with most patients having a cell count of $50-200/mm^3$. The glucose content is normal, and the protein content may be normal or elevated.

Abnormal electroencephalographic patterns and cerebrospinal fluid pleocytosis may be present in patients with measles who clinically lack apparent central nervous system involvement. Clinically, encephalitis occurs in approximately 1:1000 cases of measles. It usually develops between the second and sixth day after the rash but rarely may commence in the prodromal period. Patients may have fever, vomiting, headache, somnolence, convulsions, and coma, and nuchal rigidity and positive Kernig's and Brudzinski's signs commonly are present. Mortality is approximately 10%, and the incidence of residual damage varies between 20 and 65%. The cerebrospinal fluid may be normal but often contains cell counts of $25-500/mm^3$ with lymphocytes predominating, and the protein content may be increased moderately.

Rubella encephalitis is rare, estimated to occur in 1:6000 cases; it is more common in adults than children, has an abrupt onset, and occurs a few days after the rash. Headache, drowsiness and coma may follow in rapid succession. Mortality may be as high as 20%, but if the patient survives, residual damage is uncommon even after prolonged coma. The cerebrospinal fluid may be normal or show a slight mononuclear pleocytosis and modest elevation of the protein. The diagnosis is made serologically.

Mumps encephalitis which is less frequent but more severe than meningitis usually begins with fever and meningeal signs but is promptly complicated by mental confusion, disorientation, drowsiness, and convulsions. Various cerebral, brain stem, or spinal cord signs may be present. This illness is often prolonged and can be followed by lasting sequelae including nerve deafness. Fatalities have been rare. Mumps encephalitis may occur in the absence of clinical parotitis; however, it usually appears 7-9 days following salivary gland enlargement. Cerebrospinal fluid findings include pleocytosis with cell counts ranging from 10 to $20,000/mm^3$ with a predominance of lymphocytes. Polymorphonuclear leukocytes are more prevalent during the first or second day of the illness. The protein content is normal or moderately increased, and the glucose concentration is normal in the majority of cases, although occasionally it may be depressed. During the acute stage of mumps infection, the serum contains complement-fixing antibodies against the S antigen and negligible or low titers against the V antigen. Both rise during convalescence, and subsequently the anti-S antibody declines more rapidly than does the anti-V antibody titer.

Encephalitic manifestations complicating varicella commonly appear on the fourth to sixth posteruptive day; however, neurologic signs can occur before development of vesicles. Headache, vomiting, fever, convulsions, and declining consciousness are the initial manifestations. Some patients exhibit focal deficits such as hemiparesis, ataxia, localized seizures, or cranial nerve abnormalities. The severity of varicella encephalitis is variable, and the mortality varies from 5 to 35%. Cerebrospinal fluid examination reveals clear fluid under moderately increased pressure. Pleocytosis varies cell counts from 10 to $150/mm^3$ with polymorphonuclear cells predominating initially. The glucose and protein content may be normal or increased. The diagnosis of varicella remains a clinical one. Laboratory assistance is usually not necessary; however, examination of cells from scraping of cutaneous lesions may reveal multinucleated giant cells containing eosinophilic intranuclear inclusions (Cowdry's type A), which are indicative of a herpesvirus infection. Virus may be isolated from vesicular fluid; however, a variety of serologic techniques are available for demonstrating antibody to the varicella-zoster virus. Table 43.6 summarizes the criteria for use of varicella-zoster immune globulin for prophylaxis of varicella.

TABLE 43.6   Criteria for Varicella–Zoster Immune Globulin for Prophylaxis of Varicella

One of the following underlying conditions

    Leukemia or lymphoma
    Congenital or acquired immunodeficiency
    Immunosuppressive medication
    Newborn of mother with varicella

One of the following types of exposure to varicella or zoster patient

    Household contact
    Playmate contact (> 1 hr play indoors)
    Hospital contact (in same two- to four-room bedroom or adjacent beds in a large ward)
    Newborn contact (newborn whose mother contracted varicella less than 5 days before delivery or within 48 hours after delivery

Negative or unknown prior disease history

Age less than 15 years

Request for treatment initiated within 72 hr of exposure

Herpes simplex encephalitis may occur at any age, but more than 50% of the cases are in persons over 15 years. In adults and older infants, herpes simplex virus type 1 is more common, whereas in neonates antigenic strain type 2 virus predominates. Prodromal symptoms such as fever, malaise, and upper respiratory complaints often precede the onset of neurologic symptoms by 1–3 days. Signs and symptoms of cerebral involvement include headache and focal or generalized motor seizures. Other neurologic signs include paresis of cranial nerves, hemiparesis, conjugate eye deviation, aphasia, and temporal lobe localizing signs. The latter include bizarre behavior, confusional state, gustatory and olfactory hallucinations, and loss of smell, taste, and recent memory. The overall mortality of herpes simplex encephalitis is not known; however, it probably ranges from about 30 to 70%. Coma is a grave prognostic sign and when present, the mortality is about 70%. Many patients recover completely, but severe sequelae are common, including prominent impairment of memory and either focal or generalized neurologic deficits.

The cerebrospinal fluid in patients with herpes simplex encephalitis is usually abnormal. Pleocytosis with counts ranging from less than 100 to more than 1000/mm^3 has been recorded; normal cell counts are found in a minority of patients at the time of initial examination. Polymorphonuclear cells may predominate during the first 24 hr, but thereafter lymphocytes represent the majority of cells. Spinal fluid glucose concentration generally is normal, but hypoglycorrhachia may occur in later phases of herpes simplex encephalitis. The protein content is elevated, and red blood cells, as many as several thousand per cubic millimeter, indicative of the hemorrhagic necrotic nature of the encephalitic process, may appear in the spinal fluid. Virus can only rarely be isolated from cerebrospinal fluid, but herpes simplex antigens can be detected frequently in CSF lymphocytes by immunofluorescence. Serum antibody determinations are of limited value; however, ratios of serum to CSF antibody titers have been employed in diagnosing encephalitis.

Electroencephalographic recordings are usually markedly abnormal in herpes simplex encephalitis. Widespread arrhythmic slow-wave activity, which often has a unilateral or regional predominance, may be present. In certain cases, herpes simplex virus selectively involves the basomedial portions of the frontal and temporal lobes, and the encephalitic picture may be that of a temporal lobe space-occupying lesion. Under these conditions, the technetium brain scan configuration and angiographic pattern may be indicative of an intracranial mass lesion (Table 43.7). The earliest and most frequent abnormality observed by computed axial tomography is a poorly marginated area of diminished attenuation in the temporal lobe or insular area. Serial CT scans reveal progressive enlargement of this abnormal area and more marked diminution of cerebral attenuation. Areas of abnormal contrast enhancement may be present, and the most characteristic appearance of such enhancement is a gyriform pattern involving the region of the Sylvian cistern. Unfortunately, various radiologic studies may not become abnormal for days.

Definitive diagnosis of herpes simplex encephalitis involves obtaining a biopsy of brain tissue for culture and microscopy. Light microscopy may reveal Lipschutz inclusions, and intracellular herpesvirus capsids may be present on electron microscopy. Immunoperoxidase and direct, indirect, and anticomplement immunofluorescence have been used to locate herpes simplex antigen in biopsy tissue. Virus

TABLE 43.7   Features of Herpes Simplex Encephalitis

Feature	Approximate %
Clinical	
Fever	80-95
Focal neurologic signs	85-95
Headache	55-70
Stiff neck	45-55
Herpes labialis	15-20
Laboratory	
CSF: abnormal	85-100
Leukocytosis (10-1000/mm^3)	80-100
Elevated protein	55-90
Blood (> 10 RBC/mm^3)	65-75
Hypoglycorrhachia	0-25
Localized findings on EEG, brain scan or arteriogram, usually localized to temporoparietal lobes	60-95
Fatality	65

culture, by inoculating brain homogenate onto sensitive cells, remains the optimal means for diagnosing herpes encephalitis, but in some cases, co-culture of intact brain cells may be necessary. In some instances, virus can be isolated from ventricular fluid.

Typically a child with Reye's syndrome initially develops a mild prodromal illness which lasts 5-7 days. The condition abruptly worsens, vomiting begins, and neurologic symptoms appear. Hepatomegaly is present in about half of the patients; however, jaundice is minimal and the spleen is usually not enlarged. Reye's syndrome can be a rapid, fulminating disease with a mortality of 35% or greater. Severe neurologic sequelae, including mental impairment, seizures or hemiplegia, occur in some survivors.

Blood ammonia elevation occurs early in the course of Reye's syndrome, and initial levels correlate with the severity of the encephalopathy but not with the course of the disease. Increased levels of serum free fatty acids also have been reported in patients with Reye's syndrome. These elevations may be secondary to abnormal mitochondrial metabolism of fatty acids. Serum prebetalipoprotein levels are reduced and transaminase levels are elevated. Prothrombin time is usually prolonged, and the serum bilirubin is elevated above 2 mg/100 ml in 20% of patients. Approximately 20% of patients will have hypoglycemia. The cerebrospinal fluid is under increased pressure, and the cell count, protein, and glucose are normal.

Kuru affects primarily adult females, but children may also develop the illness. The disease begins insidiously with titubations of the head and mild truncal ataxia. Symmetric cerebral ataxia progresses until the patient cannot walk. Aphonia, abnormalities of extraocular movements, and mental changes appear later. Fever, convulsions, and sensory abnormalities usually are not present, but the disease terminates fatally in 3-6 months. The results of spinal fluid examination are unremarkable. Clinical diagnosis is dependent upon characteristic neurologic findings in individuals living in the eastern highlands of New Guinea. Creutzfeldt-Jakob disease usually occurs during the fifth or sixth decade although patients in their 20s and 70s have been reported. Dementia is rapid with deterioration of intellect occurring within weeks. Myoclonus is present and may be precipitated by visual or auditory stimuli. A variety of neurologic signs are present including spasticity, extrapyramidal movement disorders, cerebellar ataxia, sensory abnormalities, visual loss, and lower motor disease with muscle atrophy and fasciculations. The disease commonly terminates in death within a year, but occasionally patients after initial deterioration stabilize and survive for extended periods. The spinal fluid is usually normal. The electroencephalogram may show diffuse slowing and often periodic sharp-wave complexes.

Subacute sclerosing panencephalitis (SSPE), a disease of children, occurs in 5-10:1 million cases of measles and is classified with the slow-virus infections since it develops months or years after acute measles. The primary infection is usually mild and occurs before the second birthday. Clinically, SSPE begins slowly with intellectual impairment, personality and behavioral abnormalities, and motor changes affecting locomotion. Neurologic deterioration is progressive ending with profound intellectual deficits, myoclonic seizures, blindness, and decerebrate rigidity. Death occurs within 6 months. The diagnosis is confirmed serologically by demonstrating high titers of measles antibody in serum and spinal fluid. Variants of measles virus have been recovered from brain cells of patients with SSPE by co-cultivation. Characteristic electroencephalographic patterns consist of periodic, high-voltage, polyphasic slow-wave complexes which recur at 3.5- to 20-sec intervals in all leads. They are present during sleep and occur in synchrony with myoclonic jerks. Background activity in the EEG becomes slower as the disease progresses.

Progressive multifocal leukoencephalopathy (PML) is a chronic noninflammatory demyelinating disease which occurs primarily in patients with lymphoproliferative diseases, solid neoplasms, sarcoid, and tuberculosis, or in individuals who are being treated with immunosuppressive agents. Characteristic signs are paralysis, mental deterioration, visual loss, sensory abnormalities, and ataxia. Brain stem and spinal cord dysfunctions are less common. The course of PML usually is progressive leading to death in less than 1 year. The electroencephalogram typically shows nonspecific focal or diffuse slowing, and the cerebrospinal fluid contains no cells and a normal protein concentration. Determination of serum papovavirus antibodies is not helpful since such antibodies are found in normal persons. Although recovery of papovavirus in tissue cultures has proved difficult, diagnosis can be made by fluorescent antibody staining or by immune electron microscopic agglutination of particles extracted directly from brain tissue obtained by cerebral biopsy.

Patients with progressive rubella panencephalitis have variable stigmata of congenital rubella infection but have remained clinically stable until intellectual deterioration begins at age 11 or 12 years. Seizures, myoclonus, cerebellar ataxia, and corticospinal tract signs develop over a period of several years. The cerebrospinal fluid has an increased cell count, and the protein and IgG levels are elevated. Serum and cerebrospinal fluid contain high titer of antibody to rubella virus. Rubella virus has been recovered from brain by the co-cultivation technique.

The majority of patients with meningoencephalitis due to *Naegleria* are children and young adults. Illness often develops 2-7 days after swimming in pools or lakes, with the sudden onset of symptoms suggestive of an upper respiratory infection, followed rapidly by symptoms and signs of meningitis, coma, and death within 3-11 days. Cerebrospinal fluid findings consist of an increased protein content, low or normal glucose, polymorphonuclear pleocytosis, and the presence of red blood cells. *Naegleria* can be observed microscopically in wet specimens of cerebrospinal fluid. Central nervous system disease due to *Acanthamoeba* may present as a subacute illness characterized by impairment of consciousness, high fever, and multiple, focal neurologic signs. Cerebrospinal fluid protein levels are usually elevated, the glucose content is normal to low, and the cell count is elevated with a predominance of lymphocytes.

Differential Diagnosis

More than 50% of cases of encephalitis reported to the Center for Disease Control are of unknown etiology. Since there is a large number of potential pathogens, epidemiology becomes important in evaluating a patient with encephalitis. The physical findings are usually not pathognomonic. Arthropod-borne encephalitides prevail during the summer months, and St. Louis encephalitis is more frequent in adults than in children. The converse applies to California and Western equine encephalitis. As compared with the arboviral encephalitides, central nervous system infections associated with measles, mumps, rubella, and varicella are more common during the winter months.

Patients with herpes simplex encephalitis frequently present with signs of a temporal lobe mass lesion, and consequently the differential diagnosis must include a pyogenic cerebral abscess. The presence of another site of bacterial infection especially in the sinuses or mastoids should suggest a pyogenic rather than viral process. Distinction between herpes simplex encephalitis, cerebral neoplasms, and other acute viral encephalitides can be difficult, and craniotomy may be necessary to establish a herpesvirus etiology. Table 43.8 summarizes the etiologies of viral diseases of the central nervous system.

TABLE 43.8   Viral Diseases of CNS

Syndrome	Etiology	
	Common	Occasional

Aseptic meningitis	Mumps
	Coxsackievirus
	   (B1-6, A9)
	Echovirus (4,6,
	   9,11,14,18,30)
		Other enterovi-
		   ruses
		Poliovirus
		Herpes simplex
		Lymphocytic cho-
		   riomeningitis

Paralysis	Polio	Coxsackievirus A7
Encephalitis	"Arboviruses" Herpes simplex	Mumps Rabies Adenovirus 7 Herpes B (Herpes- virus simiae)
Postinfectious encephalomyelitis	Measles	Varicella Mumps Influenza Rubella
Reye's syndrome	Influenza Varicella-zoster	
SSPE	Measles	

Progressive
   multifocal
   leukoencephalopathy
	Papovavirus	

Others
   Kuru
   Creutzfeldt-Jakob disease
   Guillain-Barré syndrome
   Transverse myelitis
   Bell's palsy		

Treatment

Supportive measures including maintenance of nutrition and fluid and electrolyte balance, prevention of secondary infections, and utilization of anticonvulsants, are the main therapeutic modalities in the treatment of encephalitis. Modes of therapy for Reye's syndrome also have included intravenous hypertonic glucose and insulin (to lower free fatty acid levels), peritoneal dialysis, exchange transfusions, and decompressive craniotomy. Since most children who die from Reye's syndrome have cerebral edema, various therapeutic regimens are directed against this complication, e.g., mannitol, corticosteroids, and controlled hyperventilation.

In a NIAID collaborative study, intravenous adenine arabinoside, 15 mg/kg/day infused over 12 hr for 10 days, reduced the mortality of herpes simplex type 1 encephalitis from 70 to 28%; however, it was not efficacious in comatose patients. Additionally, there was a reduction in moderately debilitating neurologic sequelae among the survivors treated with ara-A as compared with placebo-treated patients. Adverse reactions have included nausea, vomiting, diarrhea, anemia, neutropenia, thrombocytopenia, erythroid megaloblastosis, thrombophlebitis at intravenous site, tremors, ataxia, confusion, hallucinations, psychosis, and cutaneous eruptions.

Even though primary amebic meningoencephalitis is associated with a high mortality, central nervous system infections due to *N. fowleri* apparently have been treated successfully with amphotericin B administered both parenterally and intrathecally, and occasionally intraventricularly as well. One patient also recovered while receiving miconazole, rifampin, and intravenous and intrathecal amphotericin B. In vitro, *N. fowleri* is very susceptible to amphotericin B and miconazole, and synergism has been demonstrated by adding either tetracycline or minocycline to amphotericin. *Acanthamoeba* is sensitive in vitro to sulfonamides, clotrimazole, pentamidine, flucytosine, polymyxin B, and paromomycin; sulfonamides are effective against *Acanthamoeba* infections in experimental animals. Clinical experience has been too limited to make a recommendation regarding treating human infections due to *Acanthamoeba*.

Immunology

Immunity conferred by natural infections with the arboviruses encountered in the United States apparently is long lasting, and reinfections manifested by clinical symptoms probably do not occur. Immunity rates to California encephalitis virus are especially high in population groups with extensive forest exposure. The specific factors involved in arbovirus immunity are not entirely known.

A recently described form of neurologic involvement by measles virus that preponderantly affects children with acute lymphoblastic leukemia and other neoplasms has been termed immunosuppressive measles encephalopathy or encephalitis. This neurologic syndrome is presumably due to defects of cellular immunity that result from a neoplastic disease and/or its treatment. The diagnosis of immunosuppressive measles encephalopathy may be established by the following: isolation of measles virus from brain tissue, presence of inclusion bodies microscopically and ultrastructurally indistinguishable from those found in subacute sclerosing panencephalitis (SSPE), presence of measles antigen by immunofluorescent studies and immunodiffusion techniques, and demonstration of a measurable measles virus complement-fixation titer in the cerebrospinal fluid. Typically, 2-5 months after apparently recovering from measles, an acute or subacute neurologic illness develops, characterized by confusion, lethargy progressing to coma, focal and generalized seizures, athetosis, myoclonus, hemiparesis, and other focal signs. Patients die within a week to 5 months. A few patients have survived with severe neurologic impairment. Immunosuppressive measles encephalitis differs from SSPE since it occurs in a setting of neoplasia, has a short interval between primary measles infection and onset of encephalitis, has a rapid clinical course, and lacks both a characteristic EEG pattern and consistent elevation of measles antibody in the serum and cerebrospinal fluid. The CSF may only reveal an elevated protein content. Brain tissue from patients with immunosuppressive measles encephalitis, in contrast to SSPE, contains abundant intranuclear inclusions in neurons and glial cells and only a mild inflammatory response.

There are elevated levels of antibodies to various measles antigens in patients with SSPE, and these antibodies neutralize measles virus and are capable of lysing measles-infected target cells in the presence of complement. The blastogenic and lymphokine responses are unimpaired after stimulation with mitogens unrelated to measles virus. Skin tests with measles antigen often are negative whereas primary sensitization with dinitrochlorobenzene is positive. Varying results have been obtained in in vitro assays for cell-mediated immunity to measles virus depending upon the test system and potency and purity of virus antigens. There is a blocking factor in the serum and cerebrospinal fluid of some patients with SSPE that is able to inhibit lymphocyte transformation, lymphocyte cytotoxicity, and production of lymphotoxin and migration inhibitory factor. This blocking factor probably is an immune complex consisting of measles antigen, antibody, and complement.

The viral agents associated with progressive multifocal leukoencephalopathy (PML) produce widespread subclinical human infection. Seroepidemiologic studies show that by age 14 years, 65% of individuals have acquired antibody. Most patients with PML have underlying diseases associated with abnormalities involving humoral and/or cell-mediated immunity; however, there have been several cases in which neither predisposing disease nor immunologic defects were detectable.

Immunologic studies of the humoral and cell-mediated immune responses had been conducted in a few patients with progressive rubella panencephalitis, but no consistent defect has been detected, nor have these patients had underlying diseases.

Prevention

Prevention of illnesses mediated by the arboviruses is dependent upon controlling the arthropod vector either by eliminating breeding sites or by employing insecticides. Avoiding vector bites by use of protective clothing, application of insect repellents, or screening of houses is also important. Vaccines have been used experimentally for protection against Eastern, Western, and Venezuelan equine encephalitis.

Since the decrease of ritual cannibalism in Papua New Guinea, the incidence of kuru has declined dramatically. Measles immunization significantly reduces the chances of developing subacute sclerosing panencephalitis. Several precautions for individuals caring for patients with Creutzfeldt-Jakob disease have been formulated since evidence suggests that this slow-virus disease may be communicable. The etiologic agent of Creutzfeldt-Jakob disease which resists inactivation by boiling, ultraviolet irradiation, 70% alcohol, and formaldehyde vapor may remain active in pathologic specimens fixed in 4% formaldehyde. Five percent hypochlorite, 0.03% permanganate, phenolics, and iodine solutions are adequate disinfectants. Autoclaving for 1 hr at 121°C and 20 psi also inactivates the Creutzfeldt-Jakob agent. It is recommended that workers exposed to infected saliva, nasopharyngeal secretions, urine, or feces wash their hands thoroughly with soap. One should avoid accidental percutaneous exposure to blood, cerebrospinal fluid, or brain tissue. If accidental puncture occurs, the wound should be cleaned with an iodine or phenolic antiseptic, 0.5% sodium hypochlorite solution, or with a 1:3000 solution of potassium permanganate. Equipment or instruments that have come into direct contact with blood or tissues of Creutzfeldt-Jakob patients should either be autoclaved for 1 hr or immersed in 5% sodium hypochlorite for 2 hr. Needle electrodes used in electroencephalography and electromyography probably should be discarded or at least autoclaved for 1 hr. One should also autoclave lumbar puncture needles and discard them. Various instruments, clothing, and linens exposed to cerebrospinal fluid from demented patients should be appropriately decontaminated. Tonometers and other ocular instruments should be handled in the same manner as other surgical instruments. Demented patients should not donate blood or other tissues even though non-nervous tissues are probably less infectious than brain.

Selected Bibliography

Agamanolis, D. P., Tan, J. S., and Parker, D. L.: Immunosuppressive measles encephalitis in a patient with a renal transplant. *Arch Neurol* 36:686-690, 1979.

Aicardi, J., Goutieres, F., Arsenio-Numes, M-L., et al.: Acute measles encephalitis in children with immunosuppression. *Pediatrics* 59:232-239, 1977.

Appelbaum, E., Kreps, S., and Sunshine, A.: Herpes zoster encephalitis. *Am J Med* 32:25-31, 1962.

Carter, R. F.: Primary amoebic meningo-encephalitis. An appraisal of present knowledge. *Trans R Soc Trop Med Hyg* 66:193-213, 1972.

Dolin, R., Reichman, R. C., Mazur, M. H., et al.: Herpes zoster-varicella infections in immunosuppressed patients. *Ann Intern Med* 89:375-388, 1978.

Duma, R. J., Helwig, W. B., and Martinez, A. J.: Meningoencephalitis and brain abscess due to a free-living amoeba. *Ann Intern Med* 88:468-473, 1978.

Ehrenkranz, N. J., Sinclair, M. C., Buff, E., et al.: The natural occurrence of Venezuelan equine encephalitis in the United States. First case and epidemiologic investigations. *N Engl J Med* 282:298-302, 1970.

Ehrenkranz, N. J. and Ventura, A. K.: Venezuelan equine encephalitis virus infection in man. *Ann Rev Med* 25:9-14, 1974.

Gajdusek, D. C., Gibbs, C. J., Jr., Asher, D. M., et al.: Precautions in medical care of, and in handling materials from, patients with transmissible virus dementia (Creutzfeldt-Jakob disease). *N Engl J Med* 297:1253-1258, 1977.

Griffin, N., Keeling, J. W., and Tomlinson, A. H.: Reye's syndrome associated with respiratory syncytial virus infection. *Arch Dis Child* 54:74-76, 1979.

Horstmann, D. M.: Problems in measles and rubella. *Disease-A-Month* 24(6):1-52, Mar 1978.

Johannes, R. S. and Sever, J. L.: Subacute sclerosing panencephalitis. *Ann Rev Med* 26:589-601, 1975.

Johnson, K. M. and Martin, D. H.: Venezuelan equine encephalitis. *Adv Vet Sci Comp Med* 18:79-116, 1974.

Johnson, R. T. and ter Meulen, V.: Slow infections of the nervous system. *Adv Intern Med* 23:353-383, 1978.

Lampert, P. W., Gajdusek, C., and Gibbs, C. J., Jr.: Subacute spongiform virus encephalopathies. Scrapie, kuru and Creutzfeldt-Jakob disease: A review. *Am J Pathol* 68:626-652, 1972.

Leclair, J. M., Zaia, J. A., Levin, M. J., et al.: Airborne transmission of chickenpox in a hospital. *N Engl J Med* 302:450-453, 1980.

Lee, K. K., Karr, S. L., Jr., Wong, M. M., et al.: In vitro susceptibilities of *Naegleria fowleri* strain HB-1 to selected antimicrobial agents, singly and in combination. *Antimicrob Agents Chemother* 16:217-220, 1979.

Levine, D. P., Lauter, C. B., and Lerner, A. M.: Simultaneous serum and CSF antibodies in herpes simplex virus encephalitis. *JAMA* 240:356-360, 1978.

Linnemann, C. C. Jr., Shea, L., Kauffman, C. A., et al.: Association of Reye's syndrome with viral infection. *Lancet* 2:179-182, 1974.

Luby, J. P.: St. Louis encephalitis. *Epidemiol Rev* 1:55-73, 1979.

Martin, D. B., Weiner, L. B., Nieburg, P. I., et al.: Atypical measles in adolescents and young adults. *Ann Intern Med* 90:877-881, 1979.

Mazur, M. H., Whitley, R. F., and Dolin, R.: Serum antibody levels as risk factors in the dissemination of herpes zoster. *Arch Intern Med* 139:1341-1345, 1979.

McConnell, S.: Venezuelan equine encephalomyelitis: Past, present, and future. *J Am Vet Med Assoc* 161:1579-1583, 1972.

Miller, J. R. and Harter, D. H.: Acute viral encephalitis. *Med Clin N Am* 56: 1393-1404, 1972

Morgan, E. M. and Rapp, F.: Measles virus and its associated diseases. *Bacteriol Rev* 41:636-666, 1977.

Nahmias, A. J. and Norrild, B.: Herpes simplex viruses 1 and 2 - basic and clinical aspects. *Disease-A-Month* 25(10):1-49, July 1979.

Pedersen, F. K., Schitz, P. O., Valerius, N. H., et al.: Immunosuppressive measles encephalopathy. *Acta Paediatr Scand* 67:109-112, 1978.

Powell, K. E. and Kappus, K. D.: Epidemiology of St. Louis encephalitis and other acute encephalitides. *Adv Neurol* 19:197-215, 1978.

Price, R., Chernik, N. L., Horta-Barbosa, L., et al.: Herpes simplex encephalitis in an anergic patient. *Am J Med* 54:222-228, 1973.

Robert, V. B. and Rorke, L. B.: Primary amebic encephalitis, probably from *Acanthamoeba*. *Ann Intern Med* 79:174-179, 1973.

Rockwell, D., Ruben, F. L., Winkelstein, A., et al.: Absence of immune deficiencies in a case of progressive multifocal leukoencephalopathy. *Am J Med* 61: 433-436, 1976.

Schiff, G. M.: Reye's syndrome. *Ann Rev Med* 27:447–452, 1976.

Schubert, W. K., Bobo, R. C., Partin, J. C., et al.: Reye's syndrome. *Disease-A-Month* 22(12):1–55, 1975.

Sutton, A. L., Smithwick, E. M., Seligman, S. J., et al.: Fatal disseminated herpesvirus hominis type 2 infection in an adult with associated thymic dysplasia. *Am J Med* 56:545–553, 1974.

ter Meulen, V. and Hall, W. W.: Slow virus infections of the nervous system: Virological, immunological and pathogenetic considerations. *J Gen Virol* 41: 1–25, 1978.

Townsend, J. J., Baringer, J. R., Wolinsky, J. S., et al.: Progressive rubella panencephalitis. Late onset after congenital rubella. *N Engl J Med* 292:990–993, 1975.

Weil, M. L., Itabashi, H. H., Cremer, N. E., et al.: Chronic progressive panencephalitis due to rubella virus simulating subacute sclerosing panencephalitis. *N Engl J Med* 292:994–998, 1975.

Whitley, R. J., Soong S-J., Dolin, R., et al.: Adenine arabinoside therapy of biopsy-proved herpes simplex encephalitis. National Institute of Allergy and Infectious Diseases collaborative antiviral study. *N Engl J Med* 297:289–294, 1977.

Whittle, H. C., Dossetor, J., Oduloju, A., et al.: Cell-mediated immunity during natural measles infection. *J Clin Invest* 62:678–684, 1978.

44

BRAIN ABSCESS
Rashida A. Khakoo, M.D.

Definition

Brain abscess results from a collection of pus within the brain substance. It is a potentially curable problem if recognized early and managed appropriately. Despite the advent of effective antimicrobial therapy, improvements in radiographic and neurosurgical techniques, the mortality continues to be high.

Etiology

There have been few careful studies of the bacteriology of brain abscess. Anaerobes are the most common isolates with peptostreptococci being most frequently cultured, either alone or in combination with different species of *Bacteroides*. In many reports the incidence of "sterile" brain abscesses ranges from 9 to 63%. It is likely that a significant percentage of these were caused by anaerobes, since the series with the lowest percentage of sterile cultures reported the highest percentage of anaerobes. Staphylococci or gram-negative aerobes are reported from abscesses caused by penetrating injury or neurosurgery. With sinusitis and involvement usually of the frontal lobe, aerobic streptococci are most common. With chronic otitis media and temporal lobe abscess, mixed flora including gram-negative aerobes and anaerobes are present. With cryptogenic or metastatic infection, aerobic streptococci or mixed flora are present. Other organisms causing brain abscesses include *Nocardia, Actinomyces, Candida,* and *Entamoeba histolytica.*

Epidemiology

Most series report no significant change in incidence of brain abscess in the past several years, despite the presumably better control of common infectious diseases. Studies show that brain abscess accounts for about 3/10,000 general hospital admissions. The disease has been reported at almost any age, but the incidence is greatest between 10 and 30 and between 50 and 70 years. Almost all series report a male preponderance of about 2:1.

Pathogenesis and Pathology

Brain abscesses are usually secondary to infection elsewhere, except when they are related to penetrating skull injury or surgery. The most common predisposing factors are otitis media and sinusitis, despite the fact that the percentage of cases secondary to these two conditions has been decreasing since the introduction of antibiotics. In the last 10 years or so more patients have had a source of infection elsewhere, particularly the lungs. Patients with cyanotic congenital heart disease have an increased predisposition to the development of cerebral abscess, presumably because bacteria bypass the pulmonary clearing mechanism and are shunted directly into the systemic circulation. As with abscesses elsewhere, it has been questioned whether or not organisms alone can produce an abscess without previous trauma or local ischemia or infarction. Cerebral infarction occasionally has been noted to precede brain abscess. Brain abscesses may occur secondary to infective endocarditis; in these patients there usually are multiple abscesses. Other sources of metastatic brain abscess include dental and facial infection, and rarely bacteremia from other sources.

Infection extends into the brain parenchyma by different routes. The infection may be spread via septic thrombophlebitis of emissary veins communicating with the cortical veins. This is the usual mode of spread from an adjacent focus of infection, e.g., sinusitis, otitis media, or mastoiditis. Less frequently bacteria gain access to the brain by direct extension with osteitis of the adjacent bone progressing to dural necrosis with the formation of a fistulous tract. About one-fourth of patients with subdural empyema have cerebral abscess. The bacteria may be directly implanted into the brain in cases of penetrating trauma or neurosurgery. Infection may be hematogenously spread from a distant focus.

The initial stage of infection in the brain is a focal area of cerebritis with infiltration by polymorphonuclear leukocytes, lymphocytes, and activated microglia. There is hyperemia and evidence of vasculitis. Central necrosis and liquefaction develop at a later stage. An abscess capsule forms following proliferation of fibroblasts, inflammatory cells, and capillaries adjacent to the pus. The capsule usually thickens in the first 2-3 weeks and an astroglial layer is added to the outside of the capsule. The brain surrounding an abscess is extremely edematous.

Most abscesses are solitary. Multiple abscesses have been reported in 5-20% of the patients. The most common sites of brain abscesses vary in different series depending on preponderance of particular predisposing factors. Abscesses secondary to frontal sinusitis are often located in the frontal lobe or occasionally in the temporal or parietal lobes. When the predisposing factor is chronic otitis media the abscess is most commonly located in the middle or basal portion of the temporal lobe or in the lateral cerebellar hemisphere. More rarely the abscess may be in the occipital lobe. Abscesses secondary to pleuropulmonary disease are often multiple, affecting the frontal, parietal, and occipital lobes with equal frequency.

Diagnostic Features

Clinical (Table 44.1)

The clinical presentation varies depending on the site of the abscess, the duration of illness, and predisposing factors. The clinical course in almost all cases is less than 2 months, and many patients have symptoms for less than 2 weeks. Headache may be intermittent initially but usually becomes constant later and may be localized to the area of the abscess or generalized. Fever, if present, is usually low-grade, although occasional patients present with a high fever. The most common focal neurologic deficits are hemiparesis, sensory disturbances of a cortical nature, visual field defects, and dysphasias. Patients with cerebellar lesions may present with ataxia, dysdiadochokinesia, dysarthria, vertigo, and nystagmus. Evidence of predisposing factors such as sinusitis, otitis, skull trauma, pleuropulmonary infection, cyanotic congenital heart disease, or endocarditis may be present.

Laboratory

Most of the usual laboratory tests are nonspecific for the diagnosis of brain abscess. About 40% of patients have a leukocytosis of 10-15,000/mm^3. The erythrocyte sedimentation rate is elevated in most patients, averaging about 45-50 mm/hr. The sedimentation rate is usually low in patients with cyanotic congenital heart disease.

If a brain abscess is suspected, a spinal tap should be avoided, since deaths have been reported immediately following that procedure. When spinal taps have been done, the fluid usually shows abnormal but nondiagnostic findings: elevated pressure and leukocyte count (but usually < 200/mm^3 and predominantly mononuclear cells); elevated protein (usually < 200 mg/100 ml) and normal glucose levels; Gram stains and culture results are normal or negative unless concomitant meningitis is present as a result of rupture of the abscess into the ventricle.

TABLE 44.1   Signs and Symptoms in Patients with Brain Abscess

Sign or Symptom	Approximate Frequency (%)
Headache	70
Fever	50
Altered consciousness	50
Papilledema	50
Focal neurologic defects	40
Seizures	25
Nuchal rigidity	Rare

With raised intracranial pressure, a shift of a calcified pineal may be evident from the skull roentgenogram. Other findings might be: osteomyelitis of the skull resulting from sinusitis, otitis, penetrating skull trauma, or surgery; a foreign body introduced as a result of penetrating trauma; or evidence of sinusitis.

The electroencephalogram is abnormal in about half of the patients, showing high-amplitude delta waves.

The radionuclide brain scan is a noninvasive, highly sensitive technique for detection of brain abscess and is positive in nearly all patients. It becomes positive much earlier than angiography. The brain scan is also very useful in cases of multiple abscesses. Although the brain scan is very sensitive, it is not specific. Increased uptake may be secondary to overlying osteomyelitis, thrombophlebitis, or tumor. Even the classic "doughnut" sign is not pathognomonic of abscess since tumor with necrosis may have a similar appearance.

Computerized tomography has been very useful for detection of brain abscesses. Diagnosis and localization of the lesion is made by CT in over 90% of the cases, but the diagnosis has been missed in cases in which no contrast enhancement was used. The typical appearance of an abscess on CT is an area of ill-defined low density, surrounded by a high-density ring enhanced by contrast material, around which is an area of edema (low density). The administration of steroids (which the patients are often taking because of increased intracranial pressure) can markedly reduce the contrast enhancement of an abscess capsule. This is thought to be due to the stabilizing effect of steroids upon the capillary endothelium, resulting in reduced extravascular diffusion of circulating contrast medium. If positive, the CT is very helpful for follow-up after appropriate management.

Prior to the advent of CT, angiography was used to document the findings of the radionuclide brain scan. Arteriography unlike radionuclide scans may take longer to become "positive." Findings on angiography include an avascular radiolucent area, segmental arterial constriction, displaced arteries, displaced veins, occlusion of small arterial branches, early venous filling, and an abscess capsule. With newer diagnostic techniques ventriculography is seldom used.

Differential Diagnosis

On the basis of clinical presentation, particularly in the absence of fever, a neoplasm or other space-occupying lesion is often considered. When fever is present meningitis, encephalitis, and subdural empyema should be considered. Meningitis may be present simultaneously if rupture into the ventricle has occurred. Early on, with minimal central nervous system manifestations, the attention may be directed only to the primary site of infection, e.g., sinusitis. On the basis of spinal fluid findings, viral, tuberculous, or fungal meningitis may be considered. The major differentials on CT or brain scan are neoplasm or infarction. On enhancement the capsule surrounding a neoplasm is usually irregular and less uniform in thickness.

Treatment

The treatment of brain abscess consists of a combination of antimicrobials and surgery. The choice of antimicrobials depends upon the most common bacterial isolates. A combination of high-dose aqueous penicillin (20 million U/day) and chloramphenicol (75-100 mg/kg intravenously) is a good regimen. If staphylococci are suspected, a penicillinase-resistant penicillin should be used. The antimicrobial therapy should be modified once the cultural data are available. Occasionally, aerobic gram-negative bacteria are demonstrated. These are difficult to treat if they are sensitive only to aminoglycosides; adequate levels of aminoglycosides may not be attained after systemic administration. Other routes (intrathecal or intraventricular) may have to be employed in addition to systemic route. Other antibiotics with better central nervous system penetration, such as "third generation" cephalosporins, may prove effective. For nocardial brain abscess, sulfonamides, or a combination of sulfonamides with cycloserine, or the combination trimethoprim-sulfamethoxazole is employed. Serum levels of sulfonamides of 12-15 mg/100 ml are recommended. Amphotericin B is used for the treatment of brain abscess caused by *Candida* spp or *Aspergillus* spp. Metronidazole is effective for *E. histolytica* brain abscess and in anaerobic brain abscess. The duration of antimicrobial therapy depends upon the predisposing factors: if associated with endocarditis, the treatment will be essentially that of endocarditis. The response can be judged clinically by CT scans following surgical intervention.

The nature, timing, and extent of a surgical approach to brain abscess remains controversial. At present the surgical approach to brain abscess is mostly for its mass effect rather than for control of the central nervous system infection, which is different from the situation before antimicrobial therapy. Whenever possible, complete excision of the abscess cavity and capsule should be done. When excision is not possible, purulent material should be evacuated from the abscess cavity and piecemeal removal of the capsule is then performed.

Early on, during the cerebritis stage, antimicrobial treatment alone may be adequate. If patients are treated expectantly by medical therapy alone, they must be observed closely for signs of deterioration or relapse with surgical intervention initiated when necessary.

Other therapy of patients with brain abscess is supportive: anticonvulsants and steroids whenever indicated. Drainage of other foci of infection, e.g., sinusitis, may be required.

Complications and Prognosis

Mortality continues to range near 40%. The outcome relates more to the complications of a space-occupying lesion than to uncontrolled infection. Certain factors seem to correlate with increased mortality, e.g., coma, rupture into the ventricle, multiple abscesses (Table 44.2). The higher mortality in patients with a distant source for the infection can be explained in part by the fact that multiple abscesses form as a consequence of bacteremia. Lack of early recognition also adds to the mortality.

Sequelae depend upon the localization of the abscess, the condition of the patient at the time he presents, rapidity of diagnosis, and the therapeutic approach. Hemiparesis, visual field defects, cerebellar dysfunction, or seizures may be persistent.

TABLE 44.2   Effect of Various Factors on the Mortality in Brain Abscesses

Factor	Associated Mortality (%)
Level of consciousness	
Alert	20
Comatose	90
Rupture into ventricle	80–90
Number of abscesses	
Single	45
Multiple	70–100
Source of infection	
Contiguous	50
Distant	100

Selected Bibliography

Black, P., Graybill, R., and Charache, P.: Penetration of brain abscess by systemically administered antibiotics. *J Neurosurg* 38:705–709, 1973.

Brewer, N. S., MacCarty, C. S., and Wellman, W. E.: Brain abscess: A review of recent experience. *Ann Intern Med* 82:571–576, 1975.

Claveria, L. E., du Boulay, G. H., and Moseley, I. F.: Intracranial infections. Investigation by computerized axial tomography. *Neuroradiology* 12:59–71, 1976.

Davis, D. O. and Potchen, E. J.: Brain scanning and intracranial inflammatory disease. *Radiology* 95:345–346, 1970.

deLouvois, J., Gortvai, J., and Hurley, R.: Bacteriology of abscesses of the central nervous system, a multicentric prospective study. *Br Med J* 2:981–987, 1977.

French, L. A. and Chou, S. N.: Treatment of brain abscess. *Adv Neurol* 6:269–275, 1974.

Garfield, J.: Management of supratentorial intracranial abscess. A review of 200 cases. *Br Med J* 2:7–11, 1969.

Heineman, H. S. and Braude, A. I.: Anaerobic infection of the brain. Observations on eighteen consecutive cases of brain abscess. *Am J Med* 35:682–697, 1963.

Heineman, H. S., Braude, A. I., and Osterholin, J. L.: Intracranial suppurative disease. Early presumptive diagnosis and successful treatment without surgery. *JAMA* 218:1542-1546, 1971.

Jordon, C. E., James, A., and Hodges, F. J.: Comparison of the cerebral angiogram and the brain radionuclide image in brain abscess. *Radiology* 104:327-331, 1972.

Joubert, M. J. and Stephanov, S.: Computerized tomography and surgical treatment in intracranial suppuration. Report of 30 consecutive unselected cases of brain abscess and subdural empyema. *J Neurosurg* 47:73-78, 1977.

Kaplan, R. J.: Neurologic complications of head and neck. *Otolaryngol Clin N Am* 9:729-749, 1976.

Karadanis, D. and Shulman, J.: Factors associated with mortality in brain abscess. *Arch Intern Med* 135:1145-1150, 1975.

Liske, E. and Weikers, N. J.: Changing aspects of brain abscesses, review of cases in Wisconsin 1940 through 1962. *Neurology* 14:294-300, 1964.

Paul, F. J., Davis, K. R., and Ballantine, H. T.: Computed tomography in cerebral abscess. *Radiology* 121:641-646, 1976.

Samson, D. S. and Clark, K.: A current review of brain abscess. *Am J Med* 54:201-210, 1973.

45

**SPINAL EPIDURAL, EXTRADURAL, SUBDURAL
ABSCESSES, AND SUBDURAL EMPYEMA**
Rashida A. Khakoo, M.D.

Spinal Epidural Abscess

Definition

Spinal epidural abscess results from a purulent collection in the epidural space.
The consequences of an unrecognized spinal epidural abscess can be devastating.
In a high percentage of cases, delayed diagnosis results in irreversible cord damage.

Etiology

Staphylococcus aureus is the most frequently reported isolate. Streptococci, including non-group A streptococci, are the second most common group of organisms. Anaerobes and aerobic gram-negative rods also have been reported. Occasionally, multiple organisms are isolated.

Epidemiology

The incidence ranges from 0.2 to 1.2/10,000 hospital admissions each year. Any age group can be affected. Females predominate at a ratio of 2:1.

Pathogenesis and Pathology

The epidural space is largest posteriorly over the lower thoracic and lumbar areas and is the most common location for an epidural abscess. The space is very small or almost nonexistent in the cervical and upper thoracic area. Bacteria may spread to the epidural space by the hematogenous route from a primary site of

448

infection, e.g., skin, furuncle, respiratory or dental infection, perinephric abscess, or pyelonephritis. Vertebral osteomyelitis is a fairly common source of infection (about 40%). Vertebral osteomyelitis may be hematogenous or caused by spread from other contiguous sources, e.g., a psoas abscess, decubitus ulcer, or operative wound.

The basis for destructive changes in the cord is thought to be twofold: pressure from the pus and vascular thrombosis as a result of inflammation.

Other possible associated factors for epidural abscess include trauma to the back, diabetes mellitus, and parenteral drug abuse.

The inflammatory reaction varies from acute to chronic. In most cases, vascular granulation tissue containing pockets of pus is found. In more chronic cases, dense adherent granulation tissue is noted. Pathologic changes in the spinal cord consist of liquefaction and vacuolation in the cord substance and the disappearance of nerve cells and disintegration of fiber tracts.

Diagnostic Features

Clinical

The clinical presentation of spinal epidural abscess may be either acute or chronic. A basic clinical pattern or presentation appears common to all cases: in phase I the patients complain of "spinal ache" and if untreated they can progress to phase II, III, and IV with root pain, weakness of voluntary muscles and loss of sphincter control, and sensory deficit and paralysis, respectively. In patients presenting acutely, the time span from occurrence of back pain to root symptoms averages 3 days; from root pain to weakness, 4.5 days; progression to paraplegia within 24 hr from the third stage (weakness). Patients with the acute syndrome present with very high fever; a few complain of headache and many are disoriented. Neck stiffness is fairly common. Examination of the spine reveals local tenderness in all patients. The presentation of the chronic form of spinal epidural abscess differs from the acute form in three respects: the various phases occur over weeks or months instead of occurring over days or hours, patients usually do not present with high fever, and tenderness over the spine is much less pronounced.

Laboratory

The leukocyte count is usually elevated in the "acute" group but normal in patients presenting with the chronic form. The erythrocyte sedimentation rate generally is elevated. Blood cultures are positive in about one-fourth to one-half of patients.

Spinal fluid gives useful information, but a lumbar puncture should be performed with caution. Aspiration should be carried out intermittently while the spinal needle is advanced. Once the needle enters the epidural space and pus is encountered, penetration of the subarachnoid space must be avoided. Usually the spinal fluid findings are suggestive of a parameningeal infection. Increased pressure suggests a block. The protein level is usually markedly elevated. The spinal fluid leukocyte count is elevated with the differential usually showing approximately equal numbers of neutrophils and mononuclear cells, although neutrophils may predominate. If the abscess is directly aspirated, extremely high numbers of neutrophils will be demonstrated. The spinal fluid may be normal in some patients.

Vertebral osteomyelitis, if present, will be demonstrated on roentgenograms of the spine when the illness has been present for 2–3 weeks. A radionuclide bone scan will demonstrate the presence of osteomyelitis much earlier. The myelogram is abnormal in all patients. A complete or partial block suggestive of extradural compression is present.

Differential Diagnosis

The diagnosis is based on the clinical presentation, supported by laboratory findings, and confirmed by a myelogram. The clinical presentation of acute spinal epidural abscess is fairly characteristic later, but can be confusing when the patient is seen early in his illness. Chronic spinal epidural abscess can be mistaken for other entities.

Early on, the spinal epidural abscess, particularly in children, may be mistaken for any systemic illness. Specific considerations are:

1. Vertebral osteomyelitis, which can coexist with spinal epidural abscess, and in which the spinal fluid findings should be normal
2. Disc space infection in young children in which there are no neurologic deficits, spinal fluid findings are normal, and bone scan and later roentgenograms will demonstrate the characteristic findings
3. Meningitis is often considered because of neck stiffness, but headache is uncommon in spinal epidural abscess, and spinal fluid findings of meningitis are fairly characteristic, although occasionally the two may coexist
4. With the development of root signs, a prolapsed disc or spinal cord tumor is often considered, particularly in the chronic form of spinal epidural abscess
5. With the presence of paralysis, a transverse myelopathy is considered, although this is usually more rapid in onset, back pain is absent, and the myelogram is usually normal
6. Epidural hematoma may present in a manner similar to epidural abscess

Treatment

Spinal epidural abscess, particularly the acute type, is a surgical emergency since cord damage occurs very rapidly. At surgery the average extent of the abscess is four to five vertebral segments, but may be much more extensive. Surgery consists of drainage of pus or removal of granulation tissue and decompression of the dura. In the acute cases, the wound is partially closed with a drain or packed open. The wound is closed in most cases of chronic spinal epidural abscess. Antimicrobial therapy should be directed against the most likely organisms, *S. aureus* and gram-negative bacteria, and a combination of parenteral penicillinase-resistant penicillin and an aminoglycoside (gentamicin or tobramycin) should be given. The antimicrobial therapy should be modified once the cultural data are available. The optimal duration of antimicrobial therapy is 3-4 weeks, although a more prolonged course of 6 weeks is required if osteomyelitis is also present.

Complications and Prognosis

Recovery of neurologic function is dependent upon the extent of the deficit before surgery. Most patients with root weakness and mild paraparesis improve. Patients with paraplegia, in most instances, are left with the deficits. The mortality has been decreasing: in a series of patients with acute spinal epidural abscess before 1927, the mortality was 92%. The mortality in a recent series is 21%.

Cranial Extradural Abscess

Definition

Extradural abscess is a collection of pus on the external layer of the dura and between the dura and the bone. This complication of sinusitis and otitis media is much rarer now, probably as a result of early diagnosis and therapy of sinusitis and otitis media. A significant number of patients with subdural empyema also have extradural abscess.

Etiology

No systematic studies on the bacteriology of extradural abscess have been reported. Most of the older series reported streptococci, *Streptococcus pneumoniae* or staphylococci. Since both extradural abscess and subdural empyema are associated with sinusitis, and since extradural abscess may be complicated by subdural empyema, the bacteriology may be similar.

Pathogenesis and Pathology

The infection may spread from the sinuses or middle ear cavity to the extradural space by retrograde thrombophlebitis or by direct extension, or the bacteria may be implanted in the extradural space during surgery. Osteomyelitis of the skull is commonly associated with extradural abscess. Osteomyelitis may be a result of direct extension of infection from the sinuses or spread of infection via veins. Frontal, parietal, and temporal bones are most frequently involved: the frontal bone as a result of the spread of infection from frontal or maxillary sinuses, and the parietal and temporal bones as a result of the spread of infection from otitis and mastoiditis. Extension through the outer table of the skull produces a pericranial abscess described as "Pott's puffy tumor," while extension through the inner table produces an extradural abscess. The extension of infection from the middle ear to the extradural space is usually by osteitis, cholesteatomatous erosion, or via veins. Rupture through the tegmen tympani to the outside of the dura will form a middle cranial fossa extradural abscess. Since the dura is lightly attached to the skull, an extradural abscess in the middle cranial fossa may become very large. Extradural abscess in the posterior fossa is limited in size by the firm attachment of the dura in the subarcuate fossa, the internal auditory meatus medially, and along the groove for the lateral sinus.

Infection from the extradural space may extend through areas of necrosis in the dura, or via thrombophlebitis to the subdural space, to cause subdural empyema. The infection may extend from the subdural space or from extradural space to form a brain abscess. Dural sinus thrombosis may also occur.

Diagnostic Features

Clinical

Symptoms and signs will depend upon the underlying conditions, speed of formation, duration, and extension of the abscess. Headache is very common, severe, continuous, and with periodic exacerbations. Headache may be generalized later, but early on it usually is localized to the area of the abscess. Fever usually is present, occasionally with chills, especially with frontal sinusitis, osteomyelitis, and extradural abscess in the anterior cranial fossa. With extradural abscess resulting from middle ear infection, fever may or may not be present. If the pus is present near the tip of the petrous portion of the temporal bone, unilateral peri-orbital pain may be present. Paresis of the sixth cranial nerve on the side of oti-tis and severe trigeminal pain may occur. Extradural abscesses associated with middle ear diseases have been described as "open" or "closed" depending upon whether or not there is drainage through the tegmen. Patients usually report im-provement of symptoms with increased drainage. In patients with osteomyelitis, localized tenderness of the skull may be present. Swelling of the forehead is usu-ally present in patients with subperiosteal abscess, i.e., Potts' puffy tumor. More than one scalp abscess may be present. Swelling of the eye is often present when rupture of the frontal sinus has occurred. The rupture may occur through the floor into the orbit or through the anterior wall.

Occasionally neck stiffness is present. If alteration of level of consciousness or focal neurologic signs occur, presence of other intracranial suppurative compli-cations such as subdural abscess, intracerebral abscess, meningitis, or dural sinus thrombosis is likely. Very rarely, with large or long-standing extradural abscess, signs of raised intracranial pressure have been reported.

Laboratory

Most of the usual laboratory tests are nonspecific, such as leukocytosis and/or a left shift.   The cerebrospinal fluid is usually normal, although cells or increased protein may occasionally be found. Smears and cultures are negative unless con-comitant meningitis is present. Skull and sinus roentgenograms may show evidence of sinusitis, mastoiditis, and osteomyelitis. The presence of "epidural gas" has been reported. Computerized tomography is a useful noninvasive technique for making the diagnosis. Subdural empyema and brain abscess may coexist with an extradural abscess and may be demonstrated by computerized tomography or an-giography.

Differential Diagnosis

The major differential is that of the underlying condition alone without extradural abscess, e.g., frontal sinusitis with osteomyelitis, or chronic otitis media with mas-toiditis. The presence of certain clinical features, as mentioned previously, in pa-tients with these underlying conditions, is helpful in making the diagnosis. When neck stiffness, headache, and fever are present, meningitis should be considered. Spinal fluid findings should help in distinguishing meningitis from extradural ab-scess. Subdural empyema and cerebral abscess are also considered in the differen-tial diagnosis and may be suspected on clinical grounds. These can coexist with an extradural abscess.

Treatment

A combined medical and surgical approach is usually essential. Drainage is car-ried out by burr holes or craniotomy. The choice of antimicrobial therapy will de-pend upon the most likely organism. A combination of chloramphenicol and high-dose penicillin is a common, effective regimen. When extradural abscess is a com-plication of trauma or neurosurgery, staphylococci and aerobic gram-negative or-ganisms are found more often and therefore, antimicrobial therapy should be di-rected against these. In the absence of osteomyelitis, 2-3 weeks of therapy are adequate. The duration may be judged on clinical progress and presence or ab-sence of other intracranial suppurative processes. When osteomyelitis is present, at least 6 weeks of therapy are required. In the older literature, wide excision of all infected bone was suggested. However, with appropriate antimicrobial therapy, in most patients this is not necessary. Surgery is required for the drainage of abscesses and removal of sequestra. Drainage of sinuses or mastoidectomy may be required.

Complications and Prognosis

Major complications are osteomyelitis, subdural empyema, and brain abscess. In the preantimicrobial era when osteomyelitis of the skull became very extensive and other concomitant intracranial suppurative processes were present, the morbidity and mortality were high. Patients who have been reported recently have done well. If extradural abscess is present without other intracranial suppurative foci and is recognized early and treated appropriately the prognosis should be good.

Spinal Subdural Abscess

Definition

A collection of pus confined to the spinal subdural space, a subdural spinal abscess is even rarer than a spinal epidural abscess.

Etiology

Staphylococcus aureus is the most frequently isolated organism, followed by hemolytic streptococci.

Pathogenesis and Pathology

As in epidural abscess, distant foci of infection such as furuncles, hand infection, pneumonitis, and cellulitis have been associated. The spread to the spinal subdural space is most likely via the bloodstream. Since the spinal subdural space is not circumscribed by any major anatomic barrier, a suppurative process may easily extend in a longitudinal manner.

Diagnostic Features

Clinical

The clinical presentation is similar in some respects to spinal epidural abscess in that both present with fever, backache, and root pain. However, spinal subdural abscess is not usually associated with spine tenderness or osteomyelitis.

Laboratory

Cerebrospinal fluid findings are similar to those reported with spinal epidural abscess. A myelogram will reveal a block as well as defects characteristic of arachnoiditis. In the appropriate clinical setting, when the myelogram reveals defects at several levels, subdural abscess is likely.

Differential Diagnosis

The major differential is from spinal epidural abscess.

Treatment

A combined surgical-medical approach is required: surgical drainage plus adjunctive antimicrobial therapy. Antibiotics are chosen on the basis of the expected organisms until culture results are available.

Complications and Prognosis

The most significant complication is residual neurologic deficits. The mortality approaches 50%, probably due to delays encountered in the diagnosis and the institution of appropriate therapy.

Subdural Empyema

Definition

Subdural empyema is a collection of pus between the dura and the arachnoid. Various other names have been used synonymously in the past, including pachymeningitis interna, intrapia-arachnoid abscess, and phlegmonous meningitis. Subdural empyema is an uncommon but not a rare problem, accounting for 20% of intracranial suppurative disease. The mortality remains high mainly because of delayed or missed diagnosis.

Etiology

Aerobic streptococci and staphylococci have been the most common organisms recovered, with anaerobic or microaerophilic streptococci and pneumococci isolated less frequently. Although anaerobes have been isolated in only about 12% of reported cases, this is probably an underestimation. About one-fourth of the cases have been "sterile," and might represent situations in which conditions were not appropriate for isolation of anaerobes. When anaerobic techniques have been employed, a variety of anaerobic bacteria, primarily anaerobic and microaerophilic streptococci, comprise 25-35% of isolates. Since frontal sinusitis is a common predisposing factor and since anaerobes have been isolated in about half of cultures from chronically infected sinuses, the presence of anaerobes in subdural empyema is not surprising. In children in whom subdural empyema is a sequel to meningitis, the same bacterium that causes meningitis is isolated from the subdural space. In posttraumatic and postsurgical patients, other bacterial isolates, e.g., staphylococci or aerobic gram-negative bacilli may be found.

Epidemiology

Subdural empyema is seen in all age groups, but most commonly in young adults. It is more common in males in a ratio of about 3:1.

Pathogenesis and Pathology

As a result of the more intimate relationship of the base of the brain with the fossae of the skull, as well as the firm attachment to the cranial base, the subdural space in this region is very small. However, over the dorsolateral surfaces of the cerebral hemispheres the space extends widely without anatomic interruption, which favors the accumulation of large amounts of pus. Thus this is the most common location of a subdural empyema.

The most common predisposing factor is frontal sinusitis, with otitis media being another predisposing factor. Sinusitis may lead to osteomyelitis, epidural abscess, and then by either erosion through the dura or by thrombophlebitis, to subdural empyema. Or, the bacteria may be introduced directly either by trauma or surgery. Subdural empyema in children may be a rare sequel to bacterial meningitis. Very rarely, a chronic subdural hematoma may become secondarily infected during an episode of bacteremia.

Pus usually has been found to be most abundant in the lower lateral frontal region anterior to the motor cortex with extension to the medial and orbital surfaces to the temporal lobe as far back as the parietal or posterior parietal region. In some cases there is extension beneath the falx to the opposite hemisphere. Beneath the exudate the surface of the brain appears depressed. A purulent subarachnoid exudate limited to the area covered by the subdural exudate is found. Thrombosis of the subarachnoid veins is common. Microscopically, there is a layer of fibrinous polymorphonuclear exudate on the inner surface of the dura but a pronounced basilar meningitis is not usual. Necrosis, mild or severe, of the underlying cerebral cortex and subcortical white matter is common.

Subdural empyema is bilateral in about 30% of the patients. In some cases there may be a parafalcine collection. With a contiguous site of infection, the empyema usually is located primarily in the adjacent subdural space.

Diagnostic Features

Clinical

The symptomatology can be thought of in terms of associated conditions, most often sinusitis; systemic symptoms from infection; meningeal symptoms; and symptoms of increased intracranial pressure and a space-occupying lesion.

The patient may have acute or chronic sinusitis or evidence of otitis media and/or mastoiditis. High fever and headache are early symptoms and almost always present. Neck stiffness is a very common finding. Symptoms usually progress rapidly. Focal neurologic deficits are common and include hemiparesis, aphasia, homonymous hemianopsia, cranial nerve palsies, and focal seizures. Generalized seizures may also occur. Signs of raised intracranial pressure may be present, with papilledema noted in up to half of the patients.

Laboratory

Most of the usual laboratory tests are nonspecific, e.g., leukocytosis with a shift to the left is commonly found. Evidence of frontal sinusitis, involvement of other sinuses or mastoiditis, signs of raised intracranial pressure, or osteomyelitis of the skull may be seen with a skull roentgenogram.

A lumbar puncture should be avoided when subdural empyema is suspected, especially when signs of raised intracranial pressure are present. Spinal fluid findings are nondiagnostic. The opening pressure is often elevated, and the fluid in almost all patients demonstrates abnormalities. Pleocytosis is often present, with cell counts as high as $23,000/mm^3$, but the usual range is from 50 to $400/mm^3$. The protein level is usually elevated, ranging from 60 to 220 mg/100 ml. The glucose level is usually normal. Cultures are sterile unless subdural empyema is secondary to meningitis.

The diagnostic usefulness of the radionuclide brain scan is limited because the increased uptake of the isotope around the subdural empyema blends into the normally increased uptake of the vascular rim. Scans are also not sensitive enough to visualize small, bilateral, or parafalcine collections.

Although the experience in the use of computerized tomography (CT) for cerebral abscess is wide, it is limited regarding subdural empyema. It may demonstrate the collection of pus and signs of raised intracranial pressure with a shift of midline structures.

Arteriography in the past has been the most reliable method for detecting a subdural empyema, demonstrating the avascular subdural area in nearly all patients studied. Bilateral and parafalcine collections also can be demonstrated. Small subdural collections, however, have been missed by arteriography. The electroencephalogram may show slow frequency delta activity, but is nonspecific and rarely of localizing value.

Differential Diagnosis

The differential diagnosis includes intracerebral abscess, which may coexist with subdural empyema. Both are associated with sinusitis. The usual clinical picture of subdural empyema evolves much more rapidly, and focal neurologic signs are more frequently present. However, in a particular patient it may be difficult to separate the two on clinical grounds alone. Meningitis is another major differential because headache, fever, and neck stiffness are frequent. Meningitis in adults, however, is usually not associated with focal seizures, hemiparesis, or papilledema. Spinal fluid findings may also be confusing in some patients, especially those who have received antimicrobials and may have partially treated bacterial meningitis. Extradural abscess is associated with sinusitis but is not usually associated with focal neurologic findings. Viral encephalitis may be confused because of the mononuclear pleocytosis in the spinal fluid. However, there is no associated sinusitis and focal neurologic findings are unusual. Tuberculous or fungal meningitis may be confused, but the course in these is usually prolonged, there is no sinusitis, and the cerebrospinal fluid glucose may be depressed.

Treatment

A combined surgical and medical approach is optimal. Surgery usually consists of unilateral or bilateral burr holes with drainage of pus. In children with subdural empyema secondary to meningitis, needle aspiration of the pus may be sufficient. Appropriate Gram stains and cultures of pus should be carried out. Sinus drainage also may be required. High-dose intravenous antimicrobial therapy is necessary - a combination of aqueous penicillin and chloramphenicol is recommended for subdural empyema associated with a contiguous source of infection, e.g., sinusitis. For subdural empyema secondary to trauma, coverage against staphylococci and aerobic gram-negative bacteria is necessary. In children with meningitis and subdural empyema, since the organisms are the same as those causing meningitis, the therapy should be directed against these. Initial antimicrobial management should be modified once the cultural data are available. The duration of therapy should be 4 weeks from the time of drainage. Longer treatment may be necessary when osteomyelitis is present. The patient should be followed closely after surgery for any evidence of reaccumulation of undrained pus. Intracerebral abscess is found in about one-fourth of the patients with subdural empyema. Other supportive treatment in these patients may be necessary, e.g., anticonvulsants and temporary measures for increased intracranial pressure.

Complications and Prognosis

Cerebral edema with tentorial herniation is the most dreaded complication. Cortical venous thrombosis with infarction and abscess formation also may occur. Thrombosis of dural sinuses has been reported. Mortality remains high, about 35%. Increased mortality is related to abnormal neurologic status before surgery, massive parafalx collections, severe meningitis, ventriculitis, and venous sinus thromboses. About 50% of patients are left with neurologic deficits: hemiparesis, hemianopia, and facial weakness.

Selected Bibliography

Spinal Epidural Abscess

Baker, A. S., Ojemann, R. G., Swartz, M. N., and Richardson, E. P.: Spinal epidural abscess. *N Engl J Med* 293:463-468, 1975.

Baker, C. J.: Primary spinal epidural abscess. *Am J Dis Child* 121:337-339, 1971.

Browder, J. and Meyers, R.: Pyogenic infections of the spinal epidural space. A consideration of the anatomic and physiologic pathology. *Surgery* 10:296-308, 1941.

Campbell, M. M.: Pyogenic infections within the vertebral canal. *Bull Neurol Inst N Y* 6:574-591, 1937.

Dandy, W. E.: Abscesses and inflammatory tumors in the spinal epidural space (so-called pachymeningitis externa). *Arch Surg* 13:477-494, 1926.

Heusner, A. P.: Nontuberculous spinal epidural infections. *N Engl J Med* 239:845-854, 1940.

Hulme, A. and Dott, N. M.: Spinal epidural abscess. *Br Med J* 1:64-68, 1954.

Extradural Abscess

Dawes, J. D. K.: The management of frontal sinusitis and its complications. *J Laryngol Otol* 75:297-344, 1961.

French, L. A. and Chou, S. N.: Osteomyelitis of the skull and epidural abscess, In: E. S. Gurdjian (ed): *Cranial and Intracranial Suppuration.* Charles C Thomas Publisher, Springfield, Ill, 1969, pp. 59-72.

Handel, S. F., Klein, W. C., and Kim, Y. W.: Intracranial epidural abscess. *Radiology* 111:117-120, 1974.

Lott, T., El Gammal, T., DaSilva, R., Hanks, D., and Reynolds, J.: Evaluation of brain and epidural abscesses by computed tomography. *Radiology* 122:371-376, 1977.

Skillerin, H.: Extradural abscess complicating frontal sinusitis: Report of a case. *Trans Am Laryngol Assoc* 44:56-77, 1922.

Thomas, J. N. and Nel, J. R.: Acute spreading osteomyelitis of the skull complicating frontal sinusitis. *J Laryngol Otol* 91:55-62, 1977.

Spinal Subdural Abscess

Fraser, R. A. R., Ratzan, K., Wolpert, S. M., and Weinstein, L.: Spinal subdural empyema. *Arch Neurol* 28:235-238, 1973.

Negrin, J. and Clark, R. A.: Pyogenic subdural abscess of the spinal meninges. Report of two cases. *J Neurosurg* 9:95-100, 1952.

Schiller, F. and Shadle, O. W.: Extrathecal and intrathecal suppuration. Report of two cases and discussion of the spinal subdural space. *Arch Neurol* 7:33-36, 1962.

Subdural Empyema

Bhandari, Y. S. and Sarkari, N. B. S.: Subdural empyema. A review of 37 cases. *J Neurosurg* 32:35-39, 1970.

Coonrod, J. D. and Dans, P. E.: Subdural empyema. *Am J Med* 53:85-91, 1972.

Courville, C. B.: Subdural empyema secondary to purulent frontal sinusitis. A clinicopathologic study of forty-two cases verified at autopsy. *Arch Otolaryngol* 39:211-230, 1944.

Farmer, T. W. and Wise, G. R.: Subdural empyema in infants, children and adults. *Neurology* 23:254-261, 1973.

Kaufman, D. M., Miller, M. H., and Steigbigel, N. H.: Subdural empyema: Analysis of 17 recent cases and review of the literature. *Medicine* 54:485-498, 1975.

Kubik, C. S. and Adams, R. D.: Subdural empyema. *Brain* 66:18-42, 1943.

List, C. F.: Diagnosis and treatment of acute subdural empyema. *Neurology* 5:663-670, 1955.

Yoshikawa, T. T., Chow, A. W., and Guze, L. B.: Role of anaerobic bacteria in subdural empyema. Report of four cases and review of 327 cases from the English literature. *Am J Med* 58:99-104, 1975.

46

OPHTHALMOLOGIC INFECTIONS
Ronica M. Kluge, M.D.

Infections of the eye can be aggravating (conjunctivitis) or serious (endophthalmi-tis), but generally are sufficiently uncomfortable and/or frightening that the patient seeks medical care early. Any part of the eye can be involved by infection: lids, lacrimal glands, conjunctivae, cornea, uvea, lens, and periorbital/orbital soft tissues. Each area and its common infections will be considered separately. The microbiology of these infections is summarized in Table 46.1.

Lids

Inflammation of the eyelids is termed blepharitis; it is usually bilateral and often chronic in nature. Infections of the eyelids are particularly common in children, and in patients with seborrhea, diabetes mellitus, or other debilitating illnesses. The lids appear edematous and erythematous with a crusting exudate. When seborrhea is the underlying factor, greasy scales also are present. The diagnosis is made on the basis of clinical appearance, and appropriate cultures may yield the causative bacterial or fungal organism. Contact dermatitis and parasitic infestations should be part of the differential. Blepharitis benefits from gentle removal of exudates and application of warm compresses. Topical antimicrobials may be helpful. When viruses are the etiologic agents cold compresses provide relief of symptoms; specific antivirals have not been shown to be beneficial.

Hordeolum (sty) is an acute infection of the glands of the lid margin. Usually caused by staphylococci, a hordeolum can be directed externally or internally, and frequently accompanies seborrheic or bacterial blepharitis. It appears as a painful, erythematous swelling along the lid margin and rapidly evolves into a pustular lesion. Culture of the purulent material usually yields *Staphylococcus aureus*. Initial therapy consists of warm compresses and topical antibiotics. A hordeolum may drain spontaneously but occasionally requires incision.

TABLE 46.1   The Microbiology of Eye Infections

Infection	Most Common Organisms
Blepharitis	Staphylococci Gram-negative bacilli Viruses Fungi
Hordeolum	Staphylococci
Dacrocystitis/adenitis	Staphylococci *S. pneumoniae* Viruses *Chlamydia*
Conjunctivitis	Staphylococci Streptococci *S. pneumoniae* *N. gonorrhoeae* *Haemophilus* spp Gram-negative bacilli Adenovirus *Chlamydia*
Keratitis	Staphylococci Streptococci *P. aeruginosa* Herpes simplex Fungi
Endophthalmitis	Staphylococci Gram-negative bacilli *Candida* Other fungi Viruses
Uveitis	Toxoplasmosis Herpes simplex Histoplasmosis *T. canis*
Cellulitis < 3 years of age	*H. influenzae*
All others	Staphylococci *S. pyogenes* *S. pneumoniae* Anaerobes Mucormycosis *Aspergillus*

Chalazion is a chronic, granulomatous condition of the meibomian glands, located away from the lid margin. The process is indolent and often without signs of active inflammation. Topical antibiotics are without benefit. Although a small chalazion may regress spontaneously, surgical curettage is usually required.

Inflammation of the lacrimal sac, dacrocystitis, is a common condition in the pediatric age group. It usually occurs as a complication of lacrimal duct obstruction and is due to staphylococci or *Streptococcus pneumoniae*. It appears as an acute, painful swelling, often with purulent ductal discharge. Treatment consists of warm compresses and local or systemic antibiotics depending upon the severity of the infection. Relief of the obstruction is a necessary part of therapy. Dacroadenitis, inflammation of the lacrimal gland, may be seen in infectious mononucleosis or as part of chlamydial infection. Pain and swelling are common presenting complaints, and there may be conjunctivitis as well. Therapy with warm compresses is advised; systemic antibiotics are indicated if the infection is caused by bacteria or chlamydia.

Conjunctivae

Conjunctivitis is the most common eye infection in the United States and is caused by a variety of organisms. The two prominent features common to all forms of conjunctivitis are hyperemia and exudate formation. Viral or chlamydial conjunctivitis frequently results in follicle formation (lymphoid hyperplasia). The first important differentiation is between the relatively benign inflammation of the conjunctivae and the more serious keratitis or iritis (Table 46.2). Next, it is helpful to differentiate between bacterial and viral conjunctivitis in the child or adult (Table 46.3). In the newborn period, inflammation of the conjunctivae can be caused by the gonococcus or chlamydia, or it can result from chemical reaction to silver nitrate instillation (Table 46.4).

TABLE 46.2   Distinguishing Features of Inflammatory Processes of the Conjunctiva and Cornea or Iris

Feature	Conjunctivitis	Keratitis/Iritis
Vision	Intact	May be compromised
Pain	Mild	Severe
Injection	Diffuse	Localized to iris ("ciliary flush")
Exudate	Present	Absent
Photophobia	Absent	Present
Lacrimation	Normal	Increased
Pupil	Normal	Contracted

TABLE 46.3   Distinguishing Features of Bacterial and Viral Conjunctivitis in the Child or Adult

Feature	Bacterial	Viral
Injection	Moderate	Mild
Exudate	Moderate to profuse	Minimal
Follicles	Absent	Present
Preauricular lymph node enlargement	No	Yes

TABLE 46.4   Distinguishing Features of Conjunctivitis in the Newborn

Feature	Gonococcal	Chlamydial	Chemical
Age at onset	2–4 days	7–10 days	12–24 hr
Extent	Bilateral	Uni-/bilateral	Bilateral
Edema	Marked	Moderate	Minimal
Purulent discharge	Copious	Copious	Minimal
Smear	PMNs, gram-negative diplococci	PMNs, intracyto-plasmic inclusions on Giemsa stain	Few polys

Bacterial conjunctivitis can be diagnosed by Gram stain and subsequent culture of the exudate. Topical, specific antibiotic therapy is usually curative, although systemic agents are advised for gonococcal infections. Conjunctivitis due to adenovirus requires only supportive treatment with cold compresses; attempts to abort epidemics require excellent hygiene. Herpes simplex conjunctivitis should be treated with specific antivirals (Table 46.5), preferably under the direction of an ophthalmologist. Chlamydial conjunctivitis in the older child (> 8 years) or adult is effectively treated by a 3-week course of tetracycline; erythromycin is an appropriate alternative.

Therapy of conjunctivitis in the newborn is outlined in Table 46.6. Although the value of topical antibiotics in gonococcal conjunctivitis is questionable, most authorities recommend that some form of antibiotic drops/ointment be administered every 2–3 hr. For the infant with chlamydial conjunctivitis, some suggest concomitant systemic treatment with a sulfonamide to prevent pneumonia or other organ involvement; data are not available to support or disprove this approach.

TABLE 46.5   Treatment of Viral Conjunctivitis/Keratitis

Herpes simplex: idoxuridine
vidarabine
trifluridine

Herpes zoster: local steroids

TABLE 46.6   Treatment of Conjunctivitis in the Newborn

Gonococcal - treat 5-7 days

Topical: penicillin 10,000 U/ml
or
tetracycline, erythromycin,
or chloramphenicol

Systemic: aqueous penicillin 50,000 U/kg/day
in divided doses

Chlamydial - treat 2-3 wk

Topical: 1% tetracycline
or
10% sulfacetamide

Chemical

None advised, will resolve spontaneously

Cornea

A large number of bacteria, viruses, and fungi can cause inflammation of the cornea (keratitis). Trauma or chronic corneal disease usually precedes keratitis. This process is extremely serious and must be diagnosed and treated rapidly to prevent scarring or perforation. Consultation with an ophthalmologist is strongly advised.

Patients usually present with considerable eye pain and may have decreased visual activity; although exudate is not a feature, increased lacrimation is often present (see Table 46.2). Dilation of the limbal blood vessels is responsible for a pericorneal injection ("ciliary flush").

Bacterial or fungal keratitis usually causes localized oval to round ulcerations. This is in contrast to the dendritic ulcers seen with herpes simplex keratitis. Sometimes visible with the naked eye, the ulcers can be detected easily by fluorescein dye or slit-lamp examination. If there is any question about the etiology of the ulceration, corneal scrapings should be obtained for cytologic examination, Gram,

acid-fast, and Giemsa stains, and appropriate cultures. Scrapings of corneal ulcerations should be performed only by an ophthalmologist.

Keratitis should be considered a medical emergency and should be managed by,
or in conjunction with, an ophthalmologist. Bacterial keratitis is usually treated
with topical and subconjunctival antibiotics directed specifically against the causative organism; systemic antimicrobials are not required unless endophthalmitis
is present. The antivirals useful in treating herpes simplex keratitis are listed in
Table 46.5. Although local steroids are contraindicated in herpes simplex keratitis, they are of benefit in cases of herpes zoster keratitis. Fungal keratitis is generally treated with topical and subconjunctival agents: nystatin, amphotericin, or
natamycin. Supportive measures include cycloplegics and avoidance of light.

Lens

The lens is frequently affected by intrauterine infection which leads to cataract formation. The most common cause is rubella; others include cytomegalovirus, toxoplasmosis, and syphilis. Neonatal herpes simplex infection can also result in cataracts. The appropriate treatment is surgical removal of the cataract.

Intraocular Tissues

Infectious endophthalmitis can result from exogenous or endogenous sources. In
postoperative or posttrauma cases (exogenous), the patient has the abrupt onset of
pain and hyperemia. Other symptoms include blurred vision, chemosis, lid and
corneal edema, and inflammatory cells in the anterior chamber and/or vitreous.
In endogenous cases the process may be more indolent. Candidal infection presents
with focal white lesions in the retina and choroid with an overlying vitreous haze.

Staphylococci and gram-negative bacilli are etiologic in 75% of bacterial endophthalmitis cases; Candida is the most frequent fungal pathogen. Herpes (simplex or zoster) keratitis occasionally progresses to endophthalmitis. Conjunctival
cultures cannot be relied upon; material from the anterior chamber and vitreous
cavity will yield the organism in most instances. Blood cultures may be positive
in patients with endogenous endophthalmitis.

Endophthalmitis must be considered an emergency with the need for rapid diagnosis and institution of appropriate treatment if vision is to be preserved. Again,
an ophthalmologist should assist in, or direct the care. Initial treatment can be
guided by stains and specific antimicrobial agents are administered topically, sub-
conjunctivally, and systemically to achieve high concentrations in the affected
tissues. Even with the best therapy, many patients will have severe visual loss and
some will require enucleation.

Uvea and Retina

Uveitis refers to inflammatory processes of the iris, ciliary body, and choroid.
Retinal infections will be included here since the choroid and retina often are simultaneously involved. Patients with uveitis may present with eye pain, photophobia, increased lacrimation, and decreased visual acuity; systemic complaints
are rare. Chorioretinitis may be discovered on a routine examination.

Most toxoplasmosis of the eye is acquired in utero; symptomatic disease is
believed to represent a relapse of the original infection. The parasites are lodged
in the retina and when the lesions are "active," granulomatous inflammation with

exuberant vitreous exudate occurs. It is not clear whether this "relapse" is a response to recurrent parasitemia or represents a hypersensitivity reaction to released antigen. However, specific antiparasitic therapy (pyrimethamine and sulfonamide) is usually recommended only when extensive and very active inflammation is present near the macula. Steroids, both topical and systemic, are administered to decrease the inflammatory response.

Toxocara canis is a common cause of ocular disease in children. The lesion appears as an elevated, white mass in the posterior pole of the globe; histologically this is a granuloma. Occasionally a diffuse endophthalmitis can result. Most authorities recommend topical and systemic steroids for this condition. Although thiabendazole is effective against visceral larva migrans, there are no data to confirm effectiveness against ocular toxocara.

Histoplasmosis appears on most lists of the causes of uveitis. However, it is more appropriate to use the term presumed ocular histoplasmosis. The syndrome, seen in association with skin reactivity to histoplasmin, is benign and results in round, yellow choroidal lesions. The changes are usually detected on routine examination and do not require treatment.

Preseptal Soft Tissue

Preseptal (periorbital) cellulitis is confined to the soft tissues anterior to the eyelid septum. This condition must be differentiated from the more serious orbital cellulitis (Table 46.7). The patient with preseptal cellulitis presents with moderate to marked lid edema, mild chemosis, fever, and leukocytosis. However, there is no proptosis, no pain on eye movement, and vision and eye mobility are normal.

Preseptal cellulitis most commonly follows trauma or is related to contiguous spread from nearby skin infection; staphylococci and streptococci are the expected organisms. In the child under 3 years of age, preseptal cellulitis is likely to result from *Haemophilus influenzae* bacteremia; the involved skin will have a bluish hue. Sinusitis or osteomyelitis can be accompanied by preseptal cellulitis; staphylococci, streptococci, and anaerobes are etiologic. Cultures of conjunctivae, nearby skin lesions, sinus drainage, or blood (in the case of *H. influenzae*) will yield the causative organism. Mild cases may be treated with oral antibiotics, but moderate to severe preseptal cellulitis should be treated with high-dose parenteral antibiotics directed specifically against the causative microbe. Patients should be observed closely for spread of the process to the orbital soft tissues.

TABLE 46.7   Distinguishing Features of Preseptal and Orbital Cellulitis

Feature	Preseptal	Orbital
Proptosis	Absent	Present
Chemosis	Mild	Marked
Pain on eye movement	Absent	Present
Eye mobility	Normal	Compromised

Orbital Soft Tissue

Orbital cellulitis involves the soft tissue behind the eyelid septum within the bony orbit. This condition differs from preseptal cellulitis in pathogenesis, clinical presentation (see Table 46.7), therapeutic management, and prognosis. The patient with orbital cellulitis has marked lid edema and chemosis, fever, leukocytosis, pain, and limitation of eye movement, and may develop decreased vision and/or proptosis. Consultation with an ophthalmologist is strongly recommended.

The condition frequently results from contiguous spread from the sinuses, but also follows endophthalmitis, facial osteomyelitis, and dental abscess. In addition to those organisms causing preseptal cellulitis, orbital cellulitis may be caused by anaerobes and certain fungi. Fungal cellulitis of the orbit is accompanied by a necrotizing vasculitis, is rapidly progressive, and is seen almost exclusively in patients with diabetes or malignancy. The responsible organism can be recovered in many instances from conjunctivae, sinus drainage, blood, or tissue cultures. Specific antimicrobial therapy should be administered in high doses by parenteral routes. Surgical drainage of sinuses or orbital abscess collections may be necessary. Complications include central nervous system involvement, cavernous sinus thrombosis and loss of vision.

Selected Bibliography

Amos, C. S.: Posterior segment involvement in selected pediatric infectious diseases. *J Am Optom Assoc* 50:1211-1220. 1979.

Armstrong, J. H., Zacarias, F., and Rein, M. F.: Ophthalmia neonatorum: A chart review. *Pediatrics* 57:884-892, 1976.

Barkin, R. M., Todd, J. K., and Amer, J.: Periorbital cellulitis in children. *Pediatrics* 62:390-392, 1978.

Baum, J. L.: The treatment of bacterial endophthalmitis. *Ophthalmology* 85:350-356, 1978.

Baum, J. L.: Ocular infections. *N Engl J Med* 299:28-31, 1978.

Corwin, J. M. and Weiter, J. J.: Immunology of chorioretinal disorders. *Surv Ophthalmol* 25:287-305, 1981.

Dawson, C. R., Hanna, L., Wood, T. R., et al.: Adenovirus type 8 keratoconjunctivitis in the United States. Epidemiologic, chemical, and microbiologic features. *Am J Ophthalmol* 69:473-480, 1970.

Fishman, L. S., Griffin, J. R., Sapico, F. L., and Hecht, R.: Hematogenous candida endophthalmitis – a complication of candidemia. *N Engl J Med* 268:675-681, 1972.

Forester, R. K. and Rebell, G.: The diagnosis and management of keratomycoses. I and II. *Arch Ophthalmol* 93:975-978, 1134-1136, 1975.

Frerichs, J., Chiang, J., and Meek, E. S.: Types and sensitivity patterns of ocular pathogens. *Ann Ophthalmol* 11:421-423, 1979.

Furgiuele, F. P.: Eye and eyelid infections: Treatment and prevention. *Drugs* 15: 310-316, 1978.

Ganley, J. P., Smith, R. E., Knox, K. L., et al.: Presumed ocular histoplasmosis. *Arch Ophthalmol* 89:116, 1973.

Gellady, A. M., Shulman, S. T., and Ayoub, E. M.: Periorbital and orbital cellulitis in children. *Pediatrics* 62:272-277, 1978.

Grayston, J. T. and Wang, S.: New knowledge of *Chlamydia* and the diseases they cause. *J Infect Dis* 132:87-105, 1975.

Jackson, W. B. and Gilmore, N. J.: Ocular immunology: A review. *Can J Ophthalmol* 16:3-9, 59-65, 1981.

Jones, D. B.: Therapy of postsurgical fungal endophthalmitis. *Ophthalmology* 85: 357-373, 1978.

McMeel, J. W., Naegele, D. F., Pollalis, S., Badrinath, S. S., and Murphy, P. L.: Acute and subacute infections following scleral buckling operations. *Ophthalmology* 85:341-349, 1978.

Nishida, H. and Risemberg, H. M.: Silver nitrate ophthalmic solution and chemical conjunctivitis. *Pediatrics* 56:368-373, 1975.

O'Connor, G. R.: The uvea. *Arch Ophthalmol* 93:675-691, 1975.

O'Connor, G. R.: Uveitis and the immunologically compromised host. *N Engl J Med* 299:130-132, 1978.

Ostler, H. B., Thygeson, P., Okumoto, M., and Weddell, J.: Opportunistic ocular infections. *Am Fam Physician* 17:134-140, 1978.

Pavan-Langston, D.: Chemical evaluation of adenine arabinoside and idoxuridine in the treatment of ocular herpes simplex. *Am J Ophthalmol* 80:495-502, 1975.

Perkins, E. S.: Ocular toxoplasmosis. *Br J Ophthalmol* 57:1-17, 1973.

Sabiston, D. W.: The use of antibiotics in ophthalmology. *Drugs* 14:207-212, 1977.

Thoft, R. A.: Corneal disease. *N Engl J Med* 298:1239-1241, 1978.

Wander, A. H., Centifanto, Y. M., and Kaufman, H. E.: Strain specificity of clinical isolates of herpes simplex virus. *Arch Ophthalmol* 98:1458-1461, 1980.

Weinstein, G. S., Mondino, B. J., Weinberg, R. J., and Biglan, A. W.: Endophthalmitis in a pediatric population. *Ann Ophthalmol* 11:935-943, 1979.

Wilkinson, C. P. and Welch, R. B.: Intraocular toxocara. *Am J Ophthalmol* 71: 921-930, 1971.

I. Systemic System

47

BACTEREMIA
Ronica M. Kluge, M.D.

Literally translated, bacteremia means bacteria are present in the blood. The average individual has transient, asymptomatic bacteremia almost every day as a result of such activities as chewing, brushing teeth, manipulation of skin infections, and straining at stool. This chapter, however, will discuss bacteremia as a syndrome accompanied by systemic signs and symptoms of illness. Primary emphasis will be on gram-negative rod bacteremia and neonatal bacteremia. Bacteremia caused by gram-positive organisms and gram-negative cocci is discussed in detail in chapters dealing with the specific microbe.

Gram-Negative Bacteremia

Etiology

In most reports of gram-negative bacteremia, whether collected in community or university hospitals, *Escherichia coli* is the most common organism. Other frequent causes of gram-negative bacteremia are listed in Table 47.1. Polymicrobial bacteremia suggests certain underlying problems (perforated viscus, carcinoma) and carries a worse prognosis.

Epidemiology

The prevalence of gram-negative bacteremia appears to be slowly increasing, and estimates vary depending on the methods used for collection of data and the populations studied. The higher prevalence in university hospitals (Table 47.2) may be related to the fact that the more compromised patients who require more invasive procedures are clustered in these tertiary care facilities. A disproportionate

468

TABLE 47.1   Organisms Causing Gram-Negative Bacteremia

Organism	Approximate %
E. coli	30
Klebsiella-Enterobacter-Serratia group	20
Pseudomonas spp	10
Other gram-negatives	15
Bacteroides spp	8
Polymicrobial	17

TABLE 47.2   Incidence of Gram-Negative Bacteremia/10,000 Hospital Admissions

Hospital	
Community	18-20
University	100-130
Age	
< 30 yr	50
> 60 yr	130-150

number of bacteremias occur in the patient over age 60 years. It is estimated by various sources that 100,000-500,000 cases of bacteremia occur each year with mortality ranging between 20 and 50%.

The gastrointestinal tract, which normally harbors millions of gram-negative organisms, serves as the reservoir for these infections. However, the most common portal of entry for gram-negative bacteremia is the urinary tract; this probably reflects the frequency with which the genitourinary tract is instrumented. Other sources of gram-negative bacteremia are listed in Table 47.3. The 30% unknown source in the more recent studies by Kreger and colleagues may be explained by the ever-increasing number of immunocompromised patients in whom a source frequently is not identified.

The hospitalized patient undergoes multiple diagnostic procedures and receives various therapies. Many of these have been documented as producing a transient bacteremia, which can be cleared quickly by the normal host but not by one predisposed to infection (Tables 47.4 and 47.5).

TABLE 47.3   Sources of Gram-Negative Bacteremia

Source	Approximate %	
	Kreger, et al.	Dupont and Spink
Genitourinary	34	45
Gastrointestinal	14	10
Respiratory	9	7
Skin and soft tissue	7	10
Biliary tract	2	6
Other	3	10
Unknown	30	12

TABLE 47.4   Predisposing Factors in Gram-Negative Bacteremia

Increasing age
Underlying medical condition
Surgery or trauma
Invasive diagnostic procedures
Mechanical ventilatory support
Antibiotic treatment
Immunosuppressive agents
Indwelling catheters, vascular or bladder

Pathogenesis

The combination of an organism with some virulence factors and a susceptible host are needed before the gram-negative bacteremia syndrome is produced. Certain properties of gram-negative bacilli have been implicated: ability to adhere to cell surfaces; resistance to human serum; capsules or other surfaces which prevent phagocytosis; presence of endotoxin; and the ability to survive within cells. Much investigative effort has been put into attempts to prove that endotoxin is responsible for the clinical syndrome of bacteremia (Table 47.6). The accumulated evidence for the role of endotoxin is suggestive, but exotoxins and various other factors produced by some gram-negative bacilli cause similar changes. In

TABLE 47.5   Procedures Known to Produce Transient
Gram-Negative Bacteremia

Respiratory

Nasotracheal suction
Nasal packing
Rigid bronchoscopy

Gastrointestinal

Rectal examination
Sigmoidoscopy, colonoscopy
Barium enema

Genitourinary

Transrectal prostatic biopsy
Prostatectomy, any approach
Urethral dilatation

Vascular

Angiography
Umbilical catheterization

TABLE 47.6   Evidence That Endotoxin Is Responsible for the Clinical
Manifestations of Gram-Negative Bacteremia

Some similarities between clinical, biochemical, and
hematologic changes and gram-negative bacteremia
when lipopolysaccharide (endotoxin) is administered
to animals or man.

The presence of antibodies against the core portion of
endotoxin is protective in animals and man against the
sequelae of gram-negative bacteremia, i.e., shock and
death.

addition, it is almost impossible to differentiate gram-negative bacteremia from that in some patients caused by *Staphylococcus aureus, Streptococcus pneumoniae,* or *Candida,* organisms which do not contain endotoxin.

Using endotoxin and its effects, one can construct a model of the syndrome of gram-negative bacteremia. Endotoxin activates the complement system leading to inflammation and increases vascular permeability. Endotoxin also activates the Hageman factor setting off both clotting and fibrinolysis mechanisms. And, endotoxin triggers the release of bradykinin which causes hypotension.

Septic shock occurs when cardiac output can no longer compensate for the falling blood pressure. Then cellular hypoxia ensues with a shift to anaerobic metabolism; acidosis, liposomal injury, and cell death follow. Microthrombosis of blood vessels, tissue necrosis, and hemorrhage are the changes seen histologically.

Diagnostic Features

Clinical (Table 47.7)

The classic picture of fever, rigors, and falling blood pressure makes one strongly consider the diagnosis of gram-negative bacteremia. Unfortunately, these symptoms may also accompany bacteremia due to gram-positive bacteria and even fungi. The patient might be hypothermic instead of febrile, and changes in sensorium may be the first clue to the diagnosis, especially in the elderly. Very early in the disease the patient begins to hyperventilate causing a respiratory alkalosis. Only later does acidosis become evident. A variety of skin lesions can be seen: ecthyma gangrenosum, vesicular or bullous lesions, diffuse erythema, and petechiae. Hemorrhagic lesions (purpura fulminans) and oozing from needle punctures are seen when disseminated intravascular coagulation occurs.

TABLE 47.7   Clinical Features of Gram-Negative Bacteremia

Feature	Approximate %
Fever	90-95
Hypothermia	5-10
Chills	50
Increased respiratory rate	50-60
Change in mental status	60-70
Skin lesions	5-10
Hypotension	40-60
Oliguria	30-50
Bleeding from needle-sticks or mucosal surfaces	7-10

Laboratory (Table 47.8)

Leukocytosis is the general rule, but 10-15% of patients will have leukopenia. At least half of the time thrombocytopenia will occur; less frequently decreased fibrinogen and increased fibrin split products herald the presence of disseminated intravascular coagulation. Hypoxia and acidosis often correlate with hypotension as do abnormalities of liver and kidney function. However, it is possible to see depressed renal function in gram-negative bacteremia in the absence of documented hypotension. Blood cultures will be positive; two cultures obtained during the time the patient is being admitted and evaluated are sufficient in most cases. Cultures of material from other likely portals of entry (urine, skin lesions, respiratory tract) also should be obtained.

Differential Diagnosis

Bacteremia due to *S. aureus, S. pneumoniae,* and *Candida* may present in exactly the same manner as that due to gram-negative bacilli. Presence of these organisms (stain and culture) in other sites such as sputum, urine, or skin may be helpful. Only blood cultures can differentiate definitively. Shock due to blood loss or myocardial infarction can be differentiated by use of the history, electrocardiogram, and hemodynamic studies (Table 47.9).

TABLE 47.8   Laboratory Features of Gram-Negative Bacteremia

Feature	Approximate %
Leukocytosis	85-90
Leukopenia	10-15
Thrombocytopenia	50-60
Acidosis	50-80
Elevated BUN, creatinine	50-80
Abnormal liver function tests	20-30
Positive blood cultures	100

TABLE 47.9   Hemodynamics in Various Types of Shock

Shock Type	Cardiac Output	Vascular Resistance
Septic	High	Low
Cardiogenic	Low	Normal to high
Hemorrhagic	Low	High

Complications

The most feared complication of gram-negative bacteremia is shock. This occurs more frequently among the elderly and in patients with underlying medical conditions which are ultimately or rapidly fatal. Other interrelated complications include disseminated intravascular coagulation, adult respiratory distress syndrome, and metastatic infection.

Therapy

Gram-negative bacteremia should be considered a medical emergency. As soon as the diagnosis is suspected, appropriate specimens for culture should be obtained and therapy instituted. General measures (Table 47.10) include aggressive fluid replacement, oxygenation, monitoring of hemodynamic status (Swan-Ganz pressures, urine output), judicious use of a vasoactive amine such as dopamine or dobutamine, and digitalization. Much controversy surrounds the adjunctive use of corticosteroids in bacteremia, but few would refuse to administer them when shock is also present. Suprapharmacologic doses are recommended for 24 hr. Initial antimicrobial therapy should be chosen on the basis of the most likely source and taking into consideration various host factors (Table 47.11). Once the etiologic organism has been identified and antibiotic susceptibilities are known, the antibiotic which is the most effective, least toxic, and least costly should be continued or substituted. Therapy duration is 7-10 days in most instances. A number of new cephalosporin and modified penicillin compounds are under study and may prove useful as single agents for initial therapy of gram-negative bacteremia; sufficient data are not available at present to allow this recommendation.

Prevention

Avoidance of indwelling catheters, sparing use of ventilatory equipment, judicious administration of antibiotics for the shortest effective time, and prompt relief of obstruction in the gastrointestinal or genitourinary tracts will help prevent gram-negative bacteremia. Prophylactic antimicrobials are of benefit in carefully selected instances when used in the appropriate manner, i.e., just before the procedure, and for no longer than 48 hr after the procedure.

TABLE 47.10   General Measures in the Treatment of
Gram-Negative Bacteremia

Fluids, including colloids

Oxygen

Vasoactive amines

Corticosteroids

TABLE 47.11   Antibiotic Treatment of Gram-Negative Bacteremia

Genitourinary tract source

Gentamicin or tobramycin, 5 mg/kg/day

Intraabdominal or pelvic source

Aminoglycoside 5 mg/kg/day *plus*
    clindamycin 2400 mg/day or
    chloramphenicol 50-100 mg/kg/day

Unidentified source

Aminoglycoside 5 mg/kg/day *plus*
    penicillinase-resistant penicillin
    (e.g., oxacillin 12 g/day)

Neutropenic patient

Aminoglycoside 5 mg/day *plus*
    carbenicillin 30 g/day or
    ticarcillin 18 g/day *plus*
    penicillinase-resistant penicillin

Prognosis

Factors adversely affecting the outcome in gram-negative bacteremia are listed in Table 47.12. Mortality is directly related to the presence/severity of the underlying disease and to the development of shock. Appropriate antibiotic therapy, even when instituted after shock has developed, can decrease the mortality by half.

Neonatal Bacteremia

Etiology

Escherichia coli and group B streptococci cause most neonatal bacteremias. Other causative organisms are listed in Table 47.13. Rarely, *Neisseria meningitidis* or anaerobes will be recovered.

Epidemiology

The two most common causes of neonatal bacteremia are found routinely in the gastrointestinal tract. In addition, group B streptococci frequently colonize the vagina/rectum of pregnant women. Vertical transmission from mother to infant during vaginal delivery has been documented. Spread of infection within nurseries also occurs. In these cases, the hands of personnel, ventilatory support equipment, and intravascular monitoring devices have been implicated as transmitters. The prevalence of neonatal bacteremia is variously estimated at 1-4/1000 live births.

TABLE 47.12   Poor Prognostic Signs in Gram-Negative Bacteremia

Age > 60 years
Persistent lack of fever
Ultimately or rapidly fatal underlying disease
Granulocytopenia
Coagulation abnormalities
Hospital-acquired bacteremia
Antecedent treatment with antibiotics or
    immunosuppressive agents
Shock
Adult respiratory distress syndrome
Polymicrobial bacteremia

TABLE 47.13   Organisms Causing Neonatal Bacteremia

E. coli
Group B streptococci
Other gram-negative bacilli
Other streptococci
L. monocytogenes
S. aureus
S. pneumoniae
H. influenzae

Pathogenesis

A number of factors act in concert to predispose the newborn to bacteremia (Table 47.14). When the mother develops amnionitis, the infant has up to a 5% chance of becoming infected; this risk is even greater when the membranes have been ruptured 24 hr before delivery. Specific antibody against group B streptococci has been proved protective against subsequent disease; the data for other organisms are not known. Neonatal bacteremia is accompanied by meningitis in 25-30% of cases.

Diagnostic Features (Table 47.15)

Clinical

Many of the signs and symptoms of neonatal bacteremia are nonspecific and the clinician must maintain a high index of suspicion. Difficulty regulating body temperature, tachypnea, poor feeding, or just "not looking well" may be the initial clue and should cause the physician to consider the diagnosis of bacteremia. The infant may present with purulent conjunctivitis, otitis, omphalitis, skin or joint involvement, or even a bulging fontanelle.

TABLE 47.14   Predisposing Factors in Neonatal Bacteremia

Infant
  Absence of specific antibodies
  Polymorphonuclear leukocyte dysfunction
  Decreased complement
  Prematurity

Mother
  Prolonged rupture of membranes
  Complicated delivery
  Infection

Environment
  Ventilatory support equipment
  Intravascular monitoring devices
  Bladder catheters

TABLE 47.15   Diagnostic Features of Neonatal Bacteremia

Clinical
  Temperature may be normal or low; ele-
    vated in only 40%
  Evidence of respiratory distress, including
    apnea
  Poor feeding
  Jaundice

Laboratory
  Leukopenia with increased percentage band
    forms
  Positive cultures

Laboratory

Recovery of the pathogen from blood or other involved site is the only certain way to make a diagnosis. Most of the infants will have depressed white blood cell counts and a shift toward immature forms. Some have increased erythrocyte sedimentation rates or C-reactive proteins, but these tests cannot be relied upon. A lumbar puncture should be performed in all infants suspected to have bacteremia since the incidence of meningitis is particularly high. Detection of bacterial antigen in body fluids by latex-particle agglutination or by counterimmunoelectrophoresis is useful for rapid diagnosis but is not generally available.

TABLE 47.16   Initial Antibiotic Treatment for Neonatal Bacteremia

Antibiotic and Dosage	Age of Infant	
	< 1 wk	> 1 wk
Ampicillin 25 mg/kg/dose *plus* Gentamicin 2.5 mg/kg/dose	q 12 h	q 8 h

Differential Diagnosis

Because the signs and symptoms of neonatal bacteremia are so nonspecific, a number of other diagnoses must be considered: hypoglycemia, hypocalcemia, hypoxemia, and hemolysis.

Complications

Complications include meningitis, respiratory distress syndrome, metastatic infection, coagulation abnormalities, and shock.

Therapy

Bacteremia in the newborn should be considered cause for urgent therapy. When the diagnosis is suspected, appropriate material for culture should be obtained (blood, urine, exudates, spinal fluid, gastric aspirate, ear canal), and antimicrobials quickly instituted. Initial therapy, as outlined in Table 47.16, will provide adequate coverage for *E. coli,* group B streptococci, *Listeria,* enterococci, *Klebsiella-Enterobacter, Proteus, Pseudomonas,* and staphylococci. When the causative organism and its susceptibilities have been determined, it is appropriate to modify the antibiotic treatment. Therapy is usually continued for 7-10 days. Supportive therapy with fluids, nutrition, oxygen, etc., are equally important. Exchange transfusion is an experimental therapy which may prove to be of some benefit.

Prevention

Vaccines against group B streptococci and gram-negative bacilli are under investigation. Administration of the streptococcal vaccine to women produces a good antibody response; theoretically, these antibodies could pass across the placenta to afford protection in the newborn. Antibiotic prophylaxis has prevented group B streptococcal disease in infants, but resulted in an increase in other infections.

Prognosis

The mortality of neonatal bacteremia ranges between 25 and 75% in various reports. Those who survive frequently have significant morbidity.

Selected Bibliography

Aber, R. C., Allen, N., Howell, J. T., Wilkenson, H. W., Facklam, R. R.: Nosocomial transmission of group B streptococci. *Pediatrics* 58:346-353, 1976.

Ablow, R. C., Driscoll, S. G., Effmann, E. L., Gross, I., Jolles, C. J., Vauy, R., and Warshaw, J. B.: A comparison of early-onset group B streptococcal neonatal infection and the respiratory-distress syndrome of the newborn. *N Engl J Med* 294:65-70, 1976.

Alexander, J. B. and Giacoia, G. P.: Early-onset nonenterococcal group D streptococcal infection in the newborn infant. *J Pediatr* 93:489-490, 1978.

Anderson, E. T., Young, L. S., and Hewitt, W. L.: Simultaneous antibiotic levels in "breakthrough" gram-negative rod bacteremia. *Am J Med* 61:493-497, 1976.

Baker, C. J. and Kasper, D. L.: Correlation of maternal antibody deficiency with susceptibility to neonatal group B streptococcal infection. *N Engl J Med* 294: 753-756, 1976.

Baker, C. J. and Kasper, D. L.: Immunological investigation of infants with septicemia or meningitis due to group B streptococcus. *J Infect Dis* 136(suppl): 98-103, 1977.

Butt, J., Hentges, D., Pelican, G., Henstorf, H., Haag, T., Rolfe, R., and Hutchinson, D.: Bacteremia during barium enema study. *Am J Roentgenol* 130:715-718, 1978.

Christy, J. H.: Treatment of gram-negative shock. *Am J Med* 50:77-88, 1971.

Dobkin, J. F., Miller, M. H., and Steigbigel, N. H.: Septicemia in patients on chronic hemodialysis. *Ann Intern Med* 88:28-33, 1978.

DuPont, H. L. and Spink, W. W.: Infections due to gram-negative organisms: An analysis of 860 patients with bacteremia at the University of Minnesota Medical Center, 1958-1966. *Medicine* 48:307-332, 1969.

Edson, R. S., VanScoy, R. E., and Leary, F. J.: Gram-negative bacteremia after transrectal needle biopsy of the prostate. *Mayo Clin Proc* 55:489-491, 1980.

Everett, E. D. and Hirschmann, J. V.: Transient bacteremia and endocarditis prophylaxis. A review. *Medicine* 56:61-77, 1977.

Fearson, D. T., Ruddy, S., Schur, P. H., and McCabe, W. R.: Activation of the properidin pathway of complement in patients with gram-negative bacteremia. *N Engl J Med* 292:937-940, 1975.

Fenton, L. J. and Strunk, R. C.: Complement activation and group B streptococcal infection in the newborn: Similarities to endotoxin shock. *Pediatrics* 60: 901-907, 1977.

Freid, M. A. and Vosti, K. L.: The importance of underlying disease in patients with gram-negative bacteremia. *Arch Intern Med* 121:418-423, 1968.

Harris, L. F., Jackson, R. T., Breslin, J. A., Jr., and Alford, R. H.: Anaerobic septicemia after transrectal prostatic biopsy. *Arch Intern Med* 138:393-395, 1978.

Hermans, P. E. and Washington, J. A., II.: Polymicrobial bacteremia. *Ann Intern Med* 73:387-392, 1970.

Hoffman, B. I., Kobasa, W., and Kaye, D.: Bacteremia after rectal examination. *Ann Intern Med* 88:658-659, 1978.

Hopkins, R. W. and Damewood, C. A.: Septic shock: Hemodynamics of endotoxin and inflammation. *Am J Surg* 127:476-483, 1974.

Kaplan, R. L., Sahn, S. A., and Petty, T. L.: Incidence and outcome of the respiratory distress syndrome in gram-negative sepsis. *Arch Intern Med* 139:867-869, 1979.

Kasper, D. L. and Seiler, M. W.: Immunochemical characterization of the outer membrane complex of *Bacteroides fragilis* subspecies *fragilis*. *J Infect Dis* 132:440, 1975.

Kiani, D., Quinn, E. L., Burch, K. H., Madhavan, T., Saravolatz, L. D., and Neblett, T. R.: The increasing importance of polymicrobial bacteremia. *JAMA* 242:1044-1047, 1979.

Kluge, R. M. and DuPont, H. L.: Factors affecting mortality of patients with bacteremia. *Surg Gynecol Obstet* 137:267-269, 1973.

Kreger, B. E., Craven, D. E., Carling, P. C., and McCabe, W. R.: Gram-negative bacteremia. III. and IV. *Am J Med* 68:332-343, 344-355, 1980.

Levin, J., Poore, T. E., Zauber, N. P., and Oser, R. S.: Detection of endotoxin in the blood of patients with sepsis due to gram-negative organisms. *N Engl J Med* 283:1313-1316, 1970.

Lilien, L. D., Yeh, T. F., Novack, G. M., and Jacobs, N. M. : Early-onset *Haemophilus* sepsis in newborn infants: Clinical, roentgenographic, and pathological features. *Pediatrics* 62:299-303, 1978.

McCabe, W. R., Kreger, B. E., and Johns, M.: Type-specific and cross-reactive antibodies in gram-negative bacteremia. *N Engl J Med* 287:261-267, 1972.

McGowan, J. E., Jr., Bratton, L., Klein, J. O., and Finland, M.: Bacteremia in febrile children seen in a "walk-in" pediatric clinic. *N Engl J Med* 288:1309-1312, 1973.

McGowan, J. E., Jr., Barnes, M. W., and Finland, M.: Bacteremia at Boston City Hospital: Occurrence and mortality during 12 selected years (1935-1972) with special reference to hospital-acquired cases. *J Infect Dis* 132:316-335, 1975.

Moriarity, R. R. and Finer, N. N.: Pneumococcal sepsis and pneumonia in the neonate. *Am J Dis Child* 133:601-602, 1979.

Noone, P., Parsons, T. M. C., Pattison, J. R., Slack, R. C. B., Garfield-Davies, D., and Hughes, K.: Experience in monitoring gentamicin therapy during treatment of serious gram-negative sepsis. *Br Med J* 1:477-481, 1974.

Nsouli, K. A., Lazarus, J. M., Schoenbaum, S. C., Gotteleib, M. N., Lowrie, E. G., and Shocair, M.: Bacteremic infection in hemodialysis. *Arch Intern Med* 139: 1255-1258, 1979.

Quintiliani, R., Klimek, J., Cunha, B. A., and Maderazo, E. G.: Bacteremia after manipulation of the urinary tract. The importance of pre-existing urinary tract disease and compromised host defenses. *Postgrad Med J* 54:668-671, 1978.

Robinson, J. A., Klodnycky, M. L., Loeb, H. S., Racic, M. R., and Gunnar, R. M.: Endotoxin, prekallikrein, complement and systemic vascular resistance. *Am J Med* 59:61-67, 1975.

Rowley, O.: Endotoxins and bacterial virulence. *J Infect Dis* 123:317, 1971.

Salit, I. E. and Gotschlich, E. C.: Type 1 *Escherichia coli* pili: Characterization of binding to monkey kidney cells. *J Exp Med* 146:1182, 1977.

Scheckler, W. E.: Septicemia in a community hospital 1970 through 1973. *JAMA* 237:1938-1941, 1977.

Schumer, W.: Steroids in the treatment of clinical septic shock. *Ann Surg* 184: 333-341, 1976.

Sheagren, J. N.: Editorial: Septic shock and corticosteroids. *N Engl J Med* 305: 456-458, 1981.

Shine, K. I., Kuhn, M., Young, L. S., and Tillisch, J. H.: Aspects of the management of shock. *Ann Intern Med* 93:723 734, 1980.

Shubin, H. and Weil, M. H.: Bacterial shock. *JAMA* 235:421-424, 1976.

Siber, G. R.: Bacteremias due to *Haemophilus influenzae* and *Streptococcus pneumoniae*. Their occurrence and course in children with cancer. *Am J Dis Child* 134:668-672, 1980.

Siegel, J. D. and McCracken, G. H.: Sepsis neonatorum. *N Engl J Med* 304:642-647, 1981.

Siegel, J. D., McCracken, G. H., Jr., Threlkeld, N., Milvenan, B., and Rosenfeld, C. R.: Single-dose penicillin prophylaxis against neonatal group B streptococcal infections. *N Engl J Med* 303:769-775, 1980.

Teele, D. W., Marshall, R., and Klein, J. O.: Unsuspected bacteremia in young children. *Pediatr Clin N Am* 26:773-784, 1979.

Vain, N. E., Mazlumian, J. R., Swarner, O. W., and Cha, C. C.: Role of exchange transfusion in the treatment of severe septicemia. *Pediatrics* 66:693-697, 1980.

Washington, J. A. II: Blood cultures: Principles and techniques. *Mayo Clin Proc* 50:91, 1975.

Winslow, E. J., Loeb, H. S., Rahimtoola, S. H., Kamath, S., and Gunnar, R. M.: Hemodynamic studies and results of therapy in 50 patients with bacteremic shock.   *Am J Med* 54:421–432, 1973.

Wolff, S.:   Biological effects of bacterial endotoxins in man. *J Infect Dis* 128 (suppl):259, 1973.

Young, L. S., Martin, W. J., Meyer, R. D., Weinstein, R. J., and Anderson, E. T.: Gram-negative rod bacteremia: Microbiologic, immunologic, and therapeutic considerations. *Ann Intern Med* 86:456–471, 1977.

Part 4

ORGANISMS

A. RNA Viruses

48

INFLUENZA VIRUS
Robert H. Waldman, M.D.

Influenza virus causes the principal infectious disease which has defied measures to prevent its becoming pandemic. This is attributable to at least three factors: (1) variable antigenicity among viral strains responsible for pandemics; (2) difficulty in preparation of effective vaccines for mass immunization of nonimmune populations at risk of infection; and (3) unavailability of a chemotherapeutic agent which will reliably and safely prevent or treat infection. The term influenza should be reserved for that illness caused by influenza virus. This is unfortunately not the case with respect to most of the lay public and many in the health industry. Such terms as "intestinal flu" are particularly misleading and inaccurate because one of the characteristics of influenza epidemics is the very small percentage of patients who have intestinal symptoms.

Influenza is an acute febrile illness, worldwide in distribution. There are three major serotypes of influenza which infect humans, influenza A, B, and C. Type A is the most common and is responsible for most of the morbidity and mortality associated with influenza. Type B occurs less frequently, while type C has never been associated with epidemic influenza.

Influenza virus causes a small percentage of what the lay public calls the "flu," by which is usually meant respiratory infection accompanied by some or all of the following: headache, fever, myalgias, and cough. Of all the viruses which may cause this syndrome, influenza viruses are unique in their ability to cause periodic widespread outbreaks (pandemics) of febrile respiratory disease in both adults and children. These outbreaks are associated with deaths in excess of the number normally expected during the period the pandemic or epidemic is occurring. Even with the skills of modern medicine, it is estimated that 12-15,000 "excess" deaths occur in the United States each year as a result of influenza virus infection.

The illness is characterized by a very abrupt onset, followed by 3 days of fe-brile illness, with moderately severe systemic symptoms and cough, followed by several days of respiratory symptoms, often with a prolonged convalescence in which asthenia is a prominent symptom. However, the clinical picture may be extremely variable, and influenza infection may result in no apparent illness, mild afebrile respiratory symptoms (the common cold), or fatal influenza pneumonia.

Microbiology (Tables 48.1 and 48.2)

Influenza virus is an RNA virus having two virus-coded protein antigens on its surface, hemagglutinin and neuraminidase (Figure 48.1). The hemagglutinin is re-sponsible for virus attachment to cells (including erythrocytes from many species) which have specific receptors for the hemagglutinin on their surface. The enzyme neuraminidase facilitates release of newly formed virus particles from infected cells. These proteins are antigenic, and antibodies to both are involved in develop-ment of acquired immunity.

The nucleoprotein antigen of influenza virus enables separation of strains into the three main types mentioned previously. Influenza virus has a lipid membrane which forms during the process of budding of the virus from the host cell, and therefore contains host-derived lipid and carbohydrate from the cell's plasma membrane.

Structure of Influenza Viruses

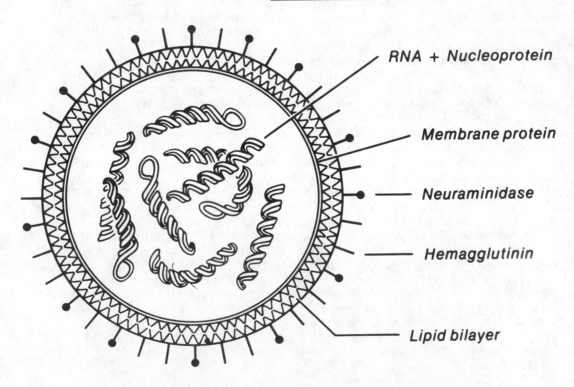

- RNA + Nucleoprotein
- Membrane protein
- Neuraminidase
- Hemagglutinin
- Lipid bilayer

FIGURE 48.1   Structure of influenza viruses.

TABLE 48.1   Influenza Virus Nomenclature

Type/place isolated/strain number/year isolated (hemagglutinin and neuraminidase types)

Example

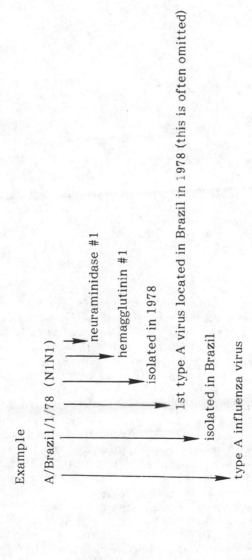

A/Brazil/1/78 (N1N1)

→ neuraminidase #1

→ hemagglutinin #1

→ isolated in 1978

→ 1st type A virus located in Brazil in 1978 (this is often omitted)

→ isolated in Brazil

→ type A influenza virus

TABLE 48.2   Major Influenza A Viruses

Pandemic	Antigenic Designation	Common Name	Prevalence
1890–1892	H2N2[1]	–	1890–1901
1902–1903	H3N2[1]	–	1902–1917
1918–1919	HswNsw[1]	Swine-like	1918–1928
1929	HON1[1,2]	–	1929–1943
1947	H1N1	A-prime	1947–1957
1957	H2N2	Asian	1957–1968
1968	H3N2	Hong Kong	1968–
1976[3]	HswHsw	Swine	1976–
1977	H1N1	Russian	1977–

[1]Identified by serologic cross-reaction between sera of people who had lived during those pandemics and modern influenza A virus isolates

[2]First influenza isolated, 1933

[3]No epidemic

The most important characteristic of influenza virus is its remarkable capability to undergo antigenic change, thereby enabling it to "outwit" the host's immune system. The capability of the various types to cause illness in epidemics is directly related to its capability to undergo antigenic change, i.e., type C is not known to undergo antigenic variation, type B only to a small extent, and type A to a very great extent. These strain changes result from mutations or genetic rearrangement or *recombinations* in hemagglutinin, neuraminidase, or both. Changes in the hemagglutinin are more important than changes in the neuraminidase, indicating that the immune response to the hemagglutinin is more protective than that to the neuraminidase. These genetic changes are, at least to a large extent, made possible because the genome of influenza A is in eight separate single-stranded pieces which separate independently in the infected cell. If a cell is doubly infected, production of recombinants or hybrids results.

More specifically, the term *antigenic drift* is used to describe the results of a point mutation, leading to one amino acid change in the hemagglutinin. This slight change is probably selected out as a result of immunologic pressure. *Antigenic shift* is not a mutation, but a recombination and results in epidemics or pandemics, since a new virus is introduced into a relatively immunologically "virgin" population.

Also of importance in this process of recombination is that type A viruses not only infect humans, but also infect many animals; the influenza A viruses do not appear to be species specific. Therefore, there is an opportunity for double infection and recombination of a wide variety of different type A influenza viruses in a variety of animal species, followed by transmission into other species, including humans. It is postulated that influenza type B does not show antigenic shift because there are no type B influenza viruses known to infect nonhuman animals.

Epidemiology

Influenza occurs in sporadic outbursts which begin abruptly and spread rapidly through a region. Morbidity is high, but mortality is usually low. During the 1918–1919 pandemic, 20-40% of the population of most countries were ill, with a mortality of about 4.8%. This was, by far, the highest mortality for any influenza pandemic. There were about 10 million deaths during a single year of that pandemic. By comparison, in the most severe recent pandemic, that of 1957-1958, approximately 40% of the United States population became ill, while mortality was only 0.1%, or about 40 excess deaths per 100,000 population. There has been a further decrease in the "excess mortality" with recent epidemics. It is too early to determine if indeed this is a significant trend, and even more difficult to explain it if it is real (Table 48.3).

Influenza A is characterized by three distinct periodicities. The most supraordinate of these is the pandemic cycle, which, since 1946, has occurred at approximately 11-year intervals. Each of these periods begins when a *new* variant of influenza A virus appears. Since the population is immunologically inexperienced with the new virus, it spreads rapidly and it is typically worldwide within 1 year (hence pandemic). Before the 1940s, pandemics apparently occurred less frequently, being separated by 15-20 years in the early twentieth century, and perhaps by 30 years before that. It has been hypothesized that this shortening of the pandemic interval is due to modern travel increasing the rate of spread of new influenza variants. This exhausts the number of susceptible individuals more rapidly and shortens the interval in which one virus variant may remain dominant.

The epidemic period is characterized by heavy regional outbursts of influenza, generally 2-3 years apart and lasting from 1 to 2 months. While pandemic years are identified by the high worldwide incidence of a new viral variant, the situation within one particular region may not differ from other epidemic years. A region

TABLE 48.3   Estimated Excess Mortality Associated with
Influenza Epidemics

Dates	Total Excess Deaths	Type of Influenza
Oct 1957–March 1958	69,800	A/Japan/57
Dec 1968–Jan 1969	33,800	A/Hong Kong/68
Jan–Feb 1973	24,800	A/England/72
Jan–Feb 1976	26,700	A/Victoria/75

skipped by the initial pandemic wave may suffer very high morbidity in an epidemic the following year. A very small number of influenza cases are occurring every year, throughout the year, and this endemic influenza infection accounts for persistence of the virus until another epidemic occurs.

The third, and most subordinate periodicity, is the seasonal pattern of influenza. Epidemics occur almost exclusively during the winter months in temperate regions. In tropical climates, influenza outbreaks are most often associated with the rainy season, but morbidity seldom reaches the levels observed in temperate climates. These seasonal and geographic variations could be due to several factors: (1) influenza virus is very sensitive to heat and ultraviolet light, (2) more crowded conditions exist during the winter months, and (3) our social and behavioral habits (many influenza outbreaks correspond to the time schools open or people return to school or work after winter holidays).

During a pandemic, disease incidence is highest in persons aged 5-14, and in parents of this age group. This age distribution does not hold for succeeding epidemics since the individuals afflicted are generally persons who did not have influenza during the antecedent pandemic or epidemic. From this, it is clear that children play an important role as vectors of the disease, as well as being victims.

Many pandemics of influenza have begun in the Far East, although this is not invariably so. The Asian origin has been explained by the fact that humans and animals live in greater density with much closer contact in that part of the world. Horses, swine, and birds have all been shown to be infected naturally by influenza viruses which are very similar to human influenza A. In addition, cattle, goats, and yak have been shown to be susceptible to influenza A viruses, and antibodies to influenza viruses have been found in sheep, rat, bear, dog, monkey, and whale.

The most recent pandemic, the "Russian flu" outbreak, was a very mild one, since the responsible strain is very similar to one which fairly recently circulated throughout the world. Therefore, most people who were living in the 1947-1957 era had had experience with the H1N1 antigens and were at least partially immune. The A/Russia/77(H1N1) virus was first noted in Northern China in May 1977. It spread south, causing a major epidemic in September. It spread into the eastern part of the USSR in November. Because of air travel, there was rapid spread, so that the first isolate was detected in Britain by December. Nearly all illnesses occurred in people under 26 years of age, and there was no measurable excess mortality. This epidemic was also unusual in that there was simultaneous occurrence of both the H1N1 and H3N2 strains. While not thought to have occurred before, this difference between previous pandemics and the Russian pandemic may be more apparent than real, since surveillance is much more intense, and laboratory techniques are better today than ever before.

Transmission of influenza virus from one person to another is by close contact or by inhalation of droplets. In small-particle aerosols (droplet nuclei) the virus does not retain its viability for long. During an epidemic, since there are five or six infected but asymptomatic people for every symptomatic person, it is probable that the former are as important in the spread of infection as are the ill. This points out the difficulty in stopping an epidemic, or protecting oneself since it is obviously extremely difficult to identify the asymptomatic but infected individual.

As alluded to earlier, a major problem in the control of influenza is confusing "clinical influenza" with "virologic or expertly defined influenza." The latter makes up a small percentage of the former with respect to total illness. Control therefore, such as with vaccines or chemotherapeutic agents, would be expected to have a minor impact on total morbidity, although it should have a great impact on excess mortality, which is almost entirely due to the latter entity.

Pathogenesis and Pathology

Necrosis and denudation of the ciliated epithelium of the respiratory tract is the primary lesion of influenza. The trachea is the most severely affected, but the upper respiratory tract also may be involved. Reepithelization begins after the third day of infection, and ciliated cells appear after 2 weeks. There are no residual lesions in uncomplicated influenza. In influenza virus involvement of the lung parenchyma, there is hemorrhagic edema of alveolar walls, infiltration of mononuclear cells and neutrophils, and hyaline membrane formation.

Viremia does not occur commonly in influenza nor does infection of other organ systems outside of the respiratory tract. Fever, myalgia, and the occurrence of other symptoms indicative of a systemic illness are thought to be a result of release of pyrogenic and toxic substances from affected cells and of hypoxemia from lung involvement.

Diagnosis

The diagnosis of influenza virus infection is a clinical and epidemiologic one. Asymptomatic infection is the most common form. Most persons who become sick, however, experience an acute febrile illness with myalgia, frontal or orbital headache, dry harassing cough, and substernal aching. The disease is characteristically of abrupt onset, with many patients being able to remember the exact time that they became ill. Rhinitis and pharyngitis, common manifestations of rhinovirus and adenovirus infection, are relatively uncommon in influenza. Diarrhea and vomiting are not characteristic. Scattered rales or rhonchi in the chest, even without abnormal roentgenographic findings, often are observed in influenza. Fever persists for only 3–4 days, unless there are complications such as pneumonia or sinusitis. Weakness, fatigability, anorexia, and malaise, however, may disappear within 1 week or persist for 3 weeks or more. When uncomplicated, delay in recovery from these symptoms is seen mostly in patients who are more aware of illness and who frequently report minor complaints to physicians.

The laboratory is of no help in diagnosing or managing an uncomplicated influenza patient. Virus isolation and serologic studies are of help epidemiologically.

Complications (Table 48.4)

Influenza virus pneumonia (primary influenzal pneumonia) is a devastating, usually fatal, form of influenza, which develops 1–3 days after the onset of the original influenzal symptoms. Nearly all patients developing this complication of influenza have underlying heart disease, usually rheumatic valvular disease. Patients develop high fever, dyspnea, and cyanosis. The chest roentgenogram reveals diffuse reticulonodular infiltrates, usually in the midlung fields. Most go on to respiratory failure and vascular collapse. The manifestations of influenzal pneumonia may be confused with pulmonary congestion in heart failure, but the central venous pressure is normal, which allows differentiation.

Bacterial pneumonia is a much more common complication, developing 3–6 days after the onset of the first influenzal symptoms. It is characterized by deteriorating clinical status and a cough productive of purulent sputum. The chest roentgenogram shows consolidation and confluent pneumonitis rather than a diffuse pulmonary infiltrate. Hypoxemia is usually less severe and cyanosis absent. Most patients developing secondary bacterial pneumonia are elderly, have preexisting chronic pulmonary disease, or are pregnant. Less commonly, patients with

TABLE 48.4   Individuals at Increased Risk from Influenza Virus Infection*

Heart disease, either acquired or congenital, with impaired
or potentially impaired hemodynamics

Chronic lung disease with compromised pulmonary function

Chronic renal disease

Diabetes mellitus

Chronic anemia

Immunosuppressed

---

*Should be immunized each year, 1-2 months before expected epidemic,
usually during months of September to November

valvular heart disease develop this complication. The most common organisms causing secondary bacterial pneumonia are *Streptococcus pneumoniae,
Staphylococcus aureus* and *Haemophilus influenzae*. In all respects, pneumonia
secondary to influenza is not different from noninfluenza-related pneumonias,
i.e., the same case-fatality rate, same age distribution, and the same organisms.
The highest case/fatality ratio occurs with *S. aureus* pneumonia. Secondary bacterial pneumonia is very uncommon in children with influenza.

Next to secondary bacterial pneumonia, the most common cause of death in
patients with influenza is a deterioration in the tenuous condition of patients with
severe cardiovascular disease. These patients die with no evidence of pneumonia,
either viral or bacterial. An important question for which there is no definite answer at the present time is whether or not healthy elderly persons have an increased risk for complications of influenza. There is no solid evidence that the
increased mortality from influenza with advanced age is related to anything other
than the increased incidence of underlying diseases. A similar question is with
respect to increased risk to pregnant women. Again, the data are only suggestive
of any increased maternal or fetal mortality from influenza.

A very severe complication of influenza, particularly influenza B infection, as
well as some other viral infections, is Reye's syndrome (Table 48.5). This is a noninflammatory encephalopathy, associated with hepatic dysfunction. Usually within a few days of a young patient improving from influenza or varicella virus infection, the acute onset of vomiting will occur. This is fairly rapidly followed by
changes in mentation. The mean age of patients is 8, but 4% of the cases occur
in young adults over 16. Liver biopsy findings are pathognomonic; however, the
diagnosis can be made on clinical grounds. Treatment is supportive, with dexamethasone or mannitol used to treat the increased intracranial pressure, and exchange transfusions as another common mode of therapy. However, there is no
convincing evidence of the efficacy of any particular type of treatment. The fatality rate is currently estimated at about 20%. Some survivors are left with neurologic sequelae, such as mental impairment or seizures. The overall incidence of
Reye's syndrome is about 1:200,000 in the susceptible (i.e., under 17 years old)
population.

TABLE 48.5   Diagnosis of Reye's Syndrome in Absence of Liver Biopsy*

Required	History of viral infection
	Vomiting
	Change in sensorium (combativeness,
	    confusion, coma)
	Absence of spinal fluid pleocytosis
	No evidence of drug intoxication
	Slightly elevated or normal serum
	    bilirubin

Plus two or more of	Elevated transaminase Prolonged prothrombin time Elevated serum ammonia Hypoglycemia (only in children < 5 years old)

*Criteria of Atkins and Haponik

Other less common complications are obstructive laryngotracheitis in children, polyneuritis, radiculitis, Guillain-Barré syndrome, and myocarditis. A form of parkinsonism probably occurred as a complication of the 1918-1919 influenza pandemic, but apparently has not occurred following subsequent pandemics.

Therapy

Chemotherapy will be discussed in the section on Immunity and Prevention, since there are more data with respect to prophylaxis than to treatment of influenza. Suffice it to say that chemotherapy, at the present time, is not very effective. Therefore symptomatic care is all that can be done to treat patients with uncomplicated influenza. For this, the treatment is no different than that for other viral respiratory infections, as covered in Chapter 11. However, antipyretics are more likely to be used, since the fever is higher and the symptoms more severe. If aspirin is given, it should be taken regularly and not prescribed only when the temperature exceeds a specified level or irregularly when the patient feels particularly bad. The irregular use of aspirin often results in marked swings in temperature, with intense sweating and chills, which may exhaust the patient and cause dehydration. Bed rest ordinarily need not be prescribed because the patient will voluntarily restrict activities according to his symptoms. Patients having cough without sputum production and having associated substernal aching with tracheitis may be given codeine as a cough suppressant. Occasionally, inhalation of steam will also produce significant relief of cough and the tracheitis. If the cough is productive of much sputum, codeine should not be used or should be given with caution.

The management of influenza virus pneumonia is directed largely toward alleviation of hypoxemia by oxygen administration. Antimicrobial therapy is required if bacterial pneumonia supervenes, but administration of antibiotics prophylactically will not reduce the likelihood of bacterial pneumonia and will increase the probability of infection by antibiotic-resistant bacteria. If the Gram stain of sputum reveals neutrophils and clusters of gram-positive cocci, a penicillinase-resistant antibiotic, such as oxacillin, should be used until further bacteriologic data are available. Careful examination for gram-negative bacilli should be carried out because *H. influenzae* is often difficult to see on a Gram stain of sputum, since it is a small organism and tends to blend into the background. Corticosteroids have never been shown to be of benefit in influenza viral pneumonia.

Immunity and Prevention

After the first infection with influenza A virus in a given individual, the serum antibody produced is highly strain-specific. Repeated infection results in production of specific antibody as well as "recall" of antibody to earlier strains. Because antibody to the first virus strain experienced tends to remain particularly robust throughout life it is called "original antigenic sin" and is the basis for the "sero-archeology" which has identified the predominant strains of the late nineteenth and early twentieth centuries.

The translation of changes in antibody titer into protection from infection is not direct. In addition to a serum antibody response, there are also local and cell-mediated immune responses. Presence of serum antibody does not absolutely guarantee protection from infection, although there is a general correlation. The relative contributions of systemic, local, and cell-mediated immunity are not yet firmly established. It is known, however, that immunity decreases with time in the absence of reexposure to influenza virus. Reinfection does occur, and is probably determined by the extent of antigenic drift undergone by the virus, and the solidity of immunity, as determined by host factors and the extent of virus replication with the preceding infection.

Inactivated influenza virus vaccines have been used for over 35 years and their effectiveness has been demonstrated to vary from insignificant to 90% protection, depending on the amount of antigen administered, the similarities between the virus strain in the vaccine and the epidemic strain, the age and immunologic status of the recipient, etc. The overall average protection rate is about 70%. Vaccine formulation is reviewed annually by the Public Health Service. There are several problems, however: production of sufficient vaccine quickly enough when a new strain appears, the 30% incidence of vaccine failure, the low but significant incidence of side effects of the vaccine, the fact that children usually respond less well to immunization, the fairly short-lived nature of vaccine-induced immunity, and the low public and physician acceptance of the vaccine. The latter is largely due to confusion between clinical influenza and virologic or expertly defined influenza, leading to a great overestimation of vaccine failures by the public and many physicians; and because up until the last 15 years, the side effects of immunization, due to contamination of vaccine with much extraneous material, were much higher. Also, there is the problem that the inactivated influenza virus vaccine given parenterally does not stimulate local immunity, which may be of some importance.

A live, attenuated vaccine given intranasally would obviate many of the problems associated with the parenteral inactivated vaccine. Because of replication, a small amount of virus is used with each vaccine dose, and therefore a single egg can produce at least 10 times as much more vaccine. There are several candidate attenuated vaccines being studied, and one or more should be generally available within a few years.

Another approach to improve influenza immunization has been the use of adjuvants. The most commonly tested ones have been emulsified oil and mineral (aluminum hydroxide and aluminum phosphate) adjuvants. At the present time, no adjuvant appears to be safe and effective enough to warrant use.

Influenza is not a very hardy virus, and its ability to be contagious is dependent upon rapid transmission from one host to the next. A key factor in the rapidity of spread of virus is the ratio of the number of susceptible persons to the number of immune persons. "Herd immunity" refers to the effect of changes in this ratio in favor of the number of immune persons, and the effect this has on spread of disease. The more contagious the infectious disease, the more the ratio must be in favor of immune persons for effective herd immunity to occur. It has been suggested that when approximately 80% of the population is immune, influenza virus is no longer able to spread actively enough to infect the remaining numbers of susceptible persons.

Current influenza vaccine use is recommended for "high-risk" individuals. These are people who are at risk for increased morbidity or mortality with influenza virus infection (Tables 48.6 and 48.7). It is disturbing that only 20-25% of people who fall in the high-risk group receive the influenza vaccine each year. Individuals other than those in the high-risk group may receive the influenza vaccine, as long as there is adequate material to immunize the high-risk group.

TABLE 48.6   Protective Effect of Influenza Immunization in the
High-Risk Elderly*

1972-1973 Epidemic	Vaccinated	Nonvaccinated
Hospitalizations/10,000 persons	18	65
Deaths/10,000	0	35

*JAMA 244:2547, 1980

TABLE 48.7   Two Studies of Influenza Vaccine Effectiveness

	A/Victoria Epidemic	
	% Illness	% Deaths
Nursing home		
Vaccine	28	1.3
Control	31	0.0
Geriatric patients		
Vaccine	20	1.9
Control	19	1.6

Current vaccines are available as either whole virus preparations or "split virus." The latter is produced by chemically disrupting the virus, and the resulting vaccine has somewhat fewer side effects, particularly in children, but it is also somewhat less immunogenic, especially in antibody-negative people. This necessitates giving two doses of split virus vaccine to people who have not been primed (Tables 48.8 and 48.9).

It is very difficult to obtain an accurate measure of the prevalence of vaccine side effects. Different studies have shown rates ranging from 5 to 65%. The most common type of systemic reaction involves fever, myalgia, malaise, and headache, usually commencing 6-12 hr after immunization, and lasting from 24 to 48 hr. The reaction is worse in children, in antibody-negative individuals, and in those receiving the whole virus vaccine. Some individuals experience a local wheal-and-flair reaction, which is thought to be a result of an allergic reaction, possibly to minute amounts of residual egg protein. This reaction is rarely accompanied by wheezing, but leads to the recommendation that the vaccine not be given to people with known egg hypersensitivity.

The Guillain-Barré syndrome, as a complication of influenza immunization, has received a great deal of recent attention. It is usually a self-limited, reversible paralysis, starting within 8 weeks of immunization. It occurred in approximately 1:100,000 recipients of the "swine" influenza vaccine given in 1976. The risk of death from Guillain-Barré syndrome is probably less than the risk of death from influenza in healthy unimmunized adults during an average influenza epidemic, and therefore is far less than the risk of mortality in high-risk patients. There has been no evidence of an increased risk to develop the Guillain-Barré syndrome with influenza vaccines other than the swine influenza vaccine.

TABLE 48.8   Influenza Virus Immunization, 1982-1983

Age (yr)	Product[1]	Dose	Number of Doses
≥ 13	Whole or split virus	0.5 ml	1
3-12	Split virus	0.5 ml	2[2]
1/2-3	Split virus	0.25 ml	2
< 1/2	Not recommended[3]		

[1]Contains 15μg each of A/Brazil/78 (H1N1), A/Bangkok/79 (H3N2) and B/Singapore/79 per 0.5 ml

[2]≥ 4 wk between doses; if individual received ≥ 1 dose of vaccine in 1978-1981, only one dose is required this year

[3]In general, risk > benefit

TABLE 48.9   Vaccine Side Effects and Immune Response in Various
High-Risk Groups

Disease	Side Effects	Response
Normals	Low rate	90% seroconversion[1]
Malignancy	Same	70% if on therapy; 90% if not
Chronic renal failure	Same	80%
Renal transplantation	Same	30-70%[2] (better if not azotemic)
Systemic lupus erythematosus	? Increased	70%
Asthma (children)	Increased	90%
Multiple sclerosis	Same (no new neurologic defects)	Not studied
Rheumatic diseases receiving corticosteroids	Same	Decreased[2]

[1] $\geq$ Fourfold rise in serum antibody titer

[2] Should consider giving these patients a second dose of vaccine

Pregnancy is neither an increased nor decreased indication for immunization and therefore, pregnant women should be treated the same as other non-high-risk individuals.

With respect to chemoprophylaxis, the most widely tested, and only available drug, is amantadine (Table 48.10), which definitely has some effectiveness, but which also causes significant side effects (Table 48.11). Since the attack rate during an influenza epidemic is usually only 10-20%, of 100 people placed on amantadine, at most, 10-15 influenza illnesses would be prevented. On the other hand, as much illness may be caused in those 100 people from the side effects of the amantadine. Other findings with respect to the use of amantadine are: it may be most effective, or possibly only effective, in people with preexisting antibody, thereby reducing its effectiveness during pandemics; the benefit of the drug ends very quickly after it is discontinued, usually within 48 hr; and resistant strains of influenza have been detected in vitro.

An analog of amantadine, rimantadine has been tested, and appears to be similar in effectiveness, but probably better tolerated. Another novel approach to influenza chemoprophylaxis, which is being studied experimentally, is the use of aerosolized amantadine, the reasoning behind this approach being that systemic side effects might be avoided.

Another drug which has been tested experimentally is inosiplex (Isoprinosine). This drug probably exerts its beneficial effect by being an immunoenhancer. In several challenge studies, Isoprinosine appears to be at least as effective as amantadine in prevention, possibly better as a therapeutic agent, and undoubtedly has fewer side effects.

TABLE 48.10   Amantadine in Prevention and/or Treatment of
Influenza Virus Infection

Mechanism of action	Probably blocks uncoating of virus
Spectrum	Influenza A only
Effectiveness	
Prophylactically	30-70% reduction in infection and illness; ↓ duration and quantity of virus shedding
Treatment	Less effective, but probably somewhat beneficial
Side effects	Incidence: 5-25%
	CNS: nervousness, headache, difficulty in concentration, dizziness or light-headedness, slurred speech, ataxia, depression, lethargy, insomnia, anxiety and psychosis
	Other: livedo reticularis, ankle edema, urinary retention, skin rash, vomiting, leukopenia, congestive heart failure
	Side effects have been reported to require cessation of use in 10%
Recommended use	1. Major antigenic shift, insufficient time for vaccine preparation
	2. Persons allergic to eggs
	3. Unimmunized high-risk patient
	4. Hospitalized patients and personnel
	5. Institutionalized individuals, particularly elderly
	Started when influenza outbreak has begun in the community. Give with vaccine, if available
Precautions	Psychiatric illness, epilepsy, elderly with cerebral atherosclerosis, recurrent eczema, cardiovascular disease

TABLE 48.11   Side Effects of Amantadine*

Side Effects	% of Subjects	
	Amantadine	Placebo
Total	33	10
Insomnia	33	8
Nervousness	30	6
Dizziness	18	2

*Adapted from *J Infect Dis* 141:543, 1980

A final drug to be mentioned is ribavirin; however, toxicity (anemia, teratogenic effects in experimental animals) precludes its widespread use, even if it were shown to be effective.

Selected Bibliography

Atkins, J. N. and Haponik, E. F.: Reye's syndrome in the adult patient. *Am J Med* 67:672, 1979.

Choppin, P. W., Kilbourne, E. D., Dowdle, W., Hirst, G. K., Joklik, W. K., Simpson, R. W., and Wright, D. O.: Genetics, replication and inhibition of replication of influenza virus; summary of Influenza Workshop VII. *J Infect Dis* 132:713, 1975.

Easterday, B. C. and Couch, R. B.: Animal influenza, its significance in human infections; summary of Influenza Workshop VI. *J Infect Dis* 131:602, 1975.

Editorial: Metabolic abnormalities in Reye's syndrome. *Lancet* 2:183-184, 1976.

Foy, H. M., Cooney, M. K., Allan, I., and Kenny, G. E.: Rates of pneumonia during influenza epidemics in Seattle, 1964-1975. *JAMA* 241:253-258, 1975.

Gregg, M. B., Hinman, A. R., and Craven, R. B.: The Russian flu - its history and implications for this year's influenza season. *JAMA* 240:2260-2263, 1978.

Herron, A., Dettleff, G., Hixon, B., Brandwin, L., Ortbals, D., Hornick, R., and Hahn, B.: Influenza vaccination in patients with rheumatic diseases. Safety and efficacy. *JAMA* 242:53-59, 1979.

Hoskins, T. W., Davies, J. R., Smith, A. J., Miller, C. L., and Allchin, A.: Assessment of inactivated influenza A vaccine after 3 outbreaks of influenza A at Christ's hospital. *Lancet* 1:33-35, 1979.

Huttenlocher, P. R. and Trauner, D.: Reye's syndrome in infancy. *Pediatrics* 62: 84-90, 1978.

Kasel, J. A., Fulk, R. V., and Cough, R. B.: Antigenic relationship between equine and the Hong Kong human variant of influenza type A virus. *J Immunol* 102: 530, 1969.

Louria, D. B., Blumenfeld, H. J., Ellis, J. T., Kilbourne, E. D., and Rogers, D. E.: Studies on influenza in the pandemic of 1957-1958; II. Pulmonary complications of influenza. *J Clin Invest* 38:231, 1959.

Parkman, P. D., Galasso, G. H., Top, F. H., and Noble, G. R.: Summary of clinical trials of influenza vaccines. *J Infect Dis* 134:100-107, 1976.

Richman, D. D.: Use of temperature-sensitive mutants for live, attenuated influenza-virus vaccine. *N Engl J Med* 300:137-138, 1979.

Schwartzmann, S. W., Adler, J. L., Sullivan, R. J., Jr., and Marine, W. M.: Bacterial pneumonia during the Hong Kong influenza epidemic of 1968-1969. *Arch Intern Med* 127:1037, 1971.

Spencer, M. J., Cherry, J. D., Powell, K. R., Sumaya, C. V., and Garakian, A. J.: Clinical trials with Alice strain, live, attenuated serum inhibitor-resistant intranasal influenza A vaccine. *J Infect Dis* 132:415, 1975.

Varma, R. R., Riedel, D. R., Komorowski, R. A., Harrington, G. J., and Norwak, T. V.: Reye's syndrome in non-pediatric age groups. *JAMA* 242:1373-1375, 1979.

Waldman, R. H., Bond, J. O., Levitt, L. D., Hartwig, E. C., Prather, E. C., Baratta, R. L., Neill, J. S., and Small, P. A., Jr.: An evaluation of influenza immunization. *Bull WHO* 41:543, 1969.

Waldman, R. H., Mann, J. J., and Small, P. A., Jr.: Immunization against influenza. *JAMA* 207:520, 1969.

Wright, P. F., Dolin, R., and LaMontagne, J. R.: Summary of clinical trials of influenza vaccines II. *J Infect Dis* 134:633-638, 1976.

49

MUMPS
Robert H. Waldman, M.D.

Mumps virus causes a generalized infection which is most commonly manifested by parotid gland involvement. It is almost always a benign illness, can be prevented by an effective vaccine, and could potentially be eradicated, since humans are the only known host.

Microbiology

Mumps virus is a paramyxovirus, related to parainfluenza and Newcastle disease viruses. The latter is an agent which is important to the poultry industry, but which only rarely causes human disease and then only very mild illness. There is only one known serotype of mumps virus.

Epidemiology

The virus most commonly infects schoolchildren, ages 5-14. Before the mumps virus vaccine was available, more than 80% of people had been infected by age 20. The disease is rare in newborns because serum antibody is protective, and nearly all neonates have transplacentally acquired maternal antibody. One-third of the people infected with mumps virus will have a subclinical infection, and the disease has a worldwide distribution. Cases may occur year-round, but peak incidence is in the winter and early spring. Virus shedding is most intense just before and early into the illness. Although asymptomatic people may shed virus, there is no chronic carrier state. Transmission requires fairly intimate contact, and virus is acquired through the upper respiratory tract. The incubation period is usually 2-3 weeks.

Pathogenesis

Mumps virus first infects the epithelial cells of the upper respiratory tract. Following replication in these cells, viremia occurs, with secondary seeding of various glands, including the salivary glands, gonads, and pancreas, as well as the central nervous system.

Diagnosis

The diagnosis almost always can be made on the basis of clinical findings (Table 49.1). In about 60% of the cases, there is unilateral or bilateral involvement of the parotids, causing nonsuppurative, tender swelling, following a nonspecific prodrome characterized by low-grade fever and headache. The first indication of parotid involvement is the complaint of an earache. The pain and tenderness are maximal in the first 2 days as the parotid continues to enlarge. Parotid enlargement is usually asymmetric, and this can best be recognized by a posterior inspection of the patient. As every mother knows, the diagnosis can be confirmed by finding an exacerbation of parotid gland pain when the patient tastes something sour, such as citrus fruits. On examination one may also find that the orifice to Stensen's duct may be red and/or edematous. However, in contradistinction to staphylococcal parotitis, no purulent material can be expressed from the duct.

TABLE 49.1   Clinical Manifestations of Mumps

Site	Approximate % Involvement
Salivary gland	70
Parotid	60
Submandibular	10
Submaxillary	5
CNS	10
Symptomatic	5
Encephalitis	0.02
Gonadal	
Prepubertal	1
Postpubertal	
Epididymo-orchitis	25
Oophoritis	5

Other salivary glands are involved much less commonly than the parotid. Involvement of the submandibular glands causes difficulty in differentiating this entity from anterior cervical adenopathy. Unusual manifestations of salivary gland involvement are edema of the tongue and upper anterior chest which results from sublingual and/or submandibular salivary gland enlargement leading to obstruction of lymphatic drainage.

In adults, the illness is usually more severe than in children, and there is more likely to be extrasalivary involvement.

Nearly all patients with mumps have a headache of mild to moderate intensity. It is surprising that, in the absence of signs or symptoms referable to the central nervous system, 20% of these patients will have meningitis as defined by an abnormal collection of cells in the spinal fluid (Table 49.2). The percentage of patients with clinical meningitis depends on how rigidly one defines this entity, but a reasonable figure is less than 10% of mumps cases. The development of meningitis is independent of the development of parotitis, i.e., meningitis develops at the same frequency in patients with or without parotitis, and vice versa; either manifestation may precede the other but almost never by more than 2 weeks. The spinal fluid in mumps patients often has more polymorphonuclear leukocytes and a lower glucose level than is found in other types of viral meningitis.

Encephalitis is rare, but when it does develop, it occurs 7-10 days after the parotitis and is thought to be analogous to other types of postinfectious demyelinating processes. The patient may have convulsions, aphasia, or paresis. Residual

TABLE 49.2   Characteristics of Mumps Meningitis

Age	5-14 yr, same as mumps without meningitis
Sex	Males > females
Season of year	
With parotitis	Spring
Without parotitis	Summer
CSF	
Cells	Up to 2000 WBC/mm^3, usually lymphocyte predominant, but may be polymorphonuclear
Protein	Normal or very mildly increased
Glucose	Normal or mildly decreased
Sequelae	Externally rare
Encephalitis	About 1:5000 cases

neurologic sequelae or death, while unusual, do occur. Therefore, it is unfortunate that the term "mumps meningoencephalitis" is used, since this implies the lumping together of a fairly common and benign process, with a very rare, but potentially dangerous one.

Epididymo-orchitis is usually unilateral and may be the only manifestation of mumps infection, or it may be noted either before or after parotitis. The disease resolves in nearly all cases with no serious residual, other than some degree of perceptible testicular atrophy in about half of the cases. Oophoritis occurs less commonly and manifests itself by nausea, vomiting, and lower abdominal pain.

Pancreatitis is usually mild. Rarer manifestations of mumps infection are migratory polyarthritis, myocarditis, and interstitial nephritis.

Laboratory confirmation of the diagnosis is rarely necessary. The most reliable test is the complement-fixation test, which can be set up to measure antibody to the S and V antigens (Figure 49.1). Anti-S appears early and declines rapidly and if present, is indicative of recent infection. Anti-V, if present in high titers in the absence of anti-S, is indicative of old infection. The skin test is unreliable; there are too many false-positive and false-negative results. In addition, the skin test may cause a rise in serum antibody, thus leading to great difficulty in interpreting the serologic tests.

Treatment, Prognosis, and Complications

Treatment is entirely symptomatic: analgesics and antipyretics if necessary, and avoidance of sour foods or drinks. The prognosis is for virtually 100% complete recovery, and complications are rare. Permanent unilateral deafness occurs in about 1:20,000 cases. Vertigo almost always resolves. Other neurologic syndromes which have been reported, but which are extremely rare, are facial palsy, Guillain-Barré syndrome, and cerebellar ataxia. Gonadal involvement leading to sterility is extremely rare. Impotence, if it occurs following mumps, is never physiologic but is psychologic.

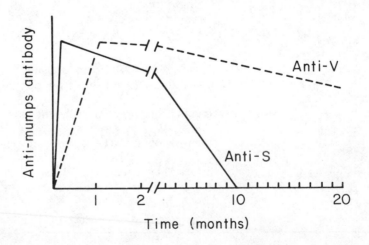

FIGURE 49.1   The time/titer relationship between mumps V and S antibodies.

It is questionable whether mumps occurring in the first trimester of pregnancy has any deleterious effect with respect to an increased incidence of abortion or congenital malformations. Mumps has been suggested as an etiologic agent in diabetes, but evidence for this is scanty.

Immunity and Prevention

Serum IgG antibody is protective as indicated by the fact that newborns with transplacentally acquired maternal antibody are immune for the first few months of life. The disease leads to lifelong immunity. A common belief among the lay public is that unilateral parotitis from mumps does not protect the patient against mumps on the contralateral side. This is obviously false, since serum IgG is the protective mechanism and is stimulated equally well by unilateral or bilateral parotitis. The belief probably has its basis in that other viruses, e.g., parainfluenza virus, can cause parotitis impossible to distinguish from that caused by mumps (Table 49.3).

TABLE 49.3   Other Causes of Parotid Enlargement

Infectious
    Other viruses: parainfluenza, coxsackicviruses
    Suppurative parotitis (usually staphylococcal), myco
        bacterial, actinomycosis

Neoplastic

Cysts

Drugs
    Iodides, bromides
    Phenothiazines
    Propylthiouracil
    Isoproterenol

Obstruction

Metabolic

    Malnutrition
    Gout
    Uremia

Sarcoidosis

Mikulicz's disease

Sjogren's syndrome

Cystic fibrosis

Conditions resembling parotid enlargement
    Lymphadenopathy
    Masseter hypertrophy
    Dental abscess

The live, attenuated mumps vaccine leads to almost 100% protection against naturally occurring disease. It is recommended that the vaccine be given in combination with rubella and rubeola vaccines. The duration of immunity may be lifelong, as is that following natural infection, but this is now difficult to predict because the vaccine has only been available for about 15 years. The mechanism of the very long immunity following either natural mumps or mumps vaccine is unknown, but it is unlikely that a single stimulus, as occurs when one is infected, would be sufficient to cause serum IgG antibody to persist for life. Thus, the explanation may be similar to that which pertains to other systemic viral infections, such as rubeola and rubella, i.e., occasional boosting by subclinical infection, or persistence of viral antigens in the body.

Selected Bibliography

Azimi, P. H., Cramblett, H. G., and Haynes, R. E.: Mumps meningoencephalitis in children. *JAMA* 207:509, 1969.

Brickman, A. and Brunell, P. A.: Susceptibility of medical students to mumps: Comparison of serum neutralizing antibody and skin tests. *Pediatrics* 48:447, 1971.

Brunell, P. A., Brickman, M. B., O'Hare, D., and Steinberg, S.: Ineffectiveness of isolation of patients as a method of preventing the spread of mumps. Failure of the mumps skin-test antigen to predict immune status. *N Engl J Med* 279: 1357–1361, 1968.

Hayden, G. F. Preblud, S. R., Orenstein, W. A., and Conrad, J. L.: Current status of mumps and mumps vaccine in the United States. *Pediatrics* 62:965, 1978.

Johnstone, J. A., Ross, C. A. C., and Dunn, M.: Meningitis and encephalitis associated with mumps infection. A 10-year survey. *Arch Dis Child* 47:647, 1972.

Philip, R. N., Reinhard, K. B., and Lackman, D. B.: Observation on a mumps epidemic in a "virgin" population. *Am J Hyg* 69:91, 1959.

Russell, R. R. and Donald, J. C.: The neurological complications of mumps. *Br Med J* 2:27, 1958.

St. Geme, J. W., Peralta, H., Fariase, E., Davis, C. W. C., and Noren, G. R.: Experimental gestational mumps virus infection and endocardial fibroelastosis. *Pediatrics* 48:821, 1971.

St. Geme, J. W., Jr., Yamauchi, T., Eisenklam, E. J., Noren, G. R., Aase, J. M., Jurmain, R. B., Henn, R. M., Gabel, M. C., Hollister, A. W., and Paumier, R.: Immunologic significance of the mumps virus skin test in infants, children and adults. *Am J Epidemiol* 101:253, 1975.

Sultz, H. A., Hart, B. A., Zielezny, M., and Schlesinger, E.: Is mumps virus an etiologic factor in juvenile diabetes mellitus? *J Pediatr* 86:654, 1975.

Travis, L. W. and Hecht, D. W.: Acute and chronic inflammatory diseases of the salivary glands, diagnosis and management. *Otolaryngol Clin N Am* 10:329, 1977.

50

MEASLES
Rama Ganguly, Ph.D.

Etiology

Measles virus belongs morphologically to the paramyxovirus group and is one of the most infectious agents contracted in childhood. Measles is an acute febrile exanthematous disease having man and monkeys (in captivity) as natural hosts. It is an RNA virus that lacks the enzyme neuraminidase. It agglutinates monkey but not human or chimpanzee erythrocytes. Measles virus receptors on the RBC are not susceptible to neuraminidase. The virus has a single-stranded RNA genome, which probably accounts for the existence of only one serotype and its lack of antigenic variation. From virus-infected tissue cultures various antigenic components can be recovered which exhibit infectivity, hemolysis, complement-fixing, and hemagglutinating properties, the latter corresponding to the virion's surface projections. The hemolytic factor induces fusion of tissue culture cells (thus resulting in the formation of giant cells) probably by alteration of cell surface membranes. The virus is highly labile and is inactivated at acid pH, at $37°C$ by the action of proteolytic enzymes, and by strong light. The virus survives well upon drying in microdroplets, which probably partly explains its contagious nature.

Epidemiology (Table 50.1)

Measles is contracted via the nasopharyngeal route. Virtually all susceptible children develop the disease upon their first contact with the virus. The disease is of worldwide distribution and is endemic in most places. The highest incidence is seen in children of 5-7 years old in the United States with epidemics every 2-3 years. The epidemic occurs every year in developing countries and 90% of the

TABLE 50.1   Measles Incidence, United States

| Year | Reported/100,000 Population | |
	Cases	Deaths
1915	∿ 300	∿ 8.00
1930	300	3.00
1945	300	0.60
1960	300	0.30
1975	10	0.01

population becomes immune by the age of 5 years. Since man is the only natural reservoir of the infection, the disease is much more sporadic, but explosive, in small isolated communities, such as islands in the South Pacific, where epidemics occur only after the introduction of the virus from the outside world.

Diagnosis

Clinical

The characteristic clinical features of measles are the best diagnostic tools (Table 50.2). Koplik's spots, on the buccal mucosa, usually on the inner lip or opposite the lower molars, are bright red, with a small bluish-white dot in the middle. They develop during the prodromal stage and are of diagnostic value 2-3 days before the appearance of the rash. The rash is of typical appearance and is maculopapular. It starts to develop on the head and face and then spreads to the body and extremities.

Laboratory

The formation of giant cells is also characteristic and may be detected in smears of the nasal mucosa. The virus may be isolated in a number of primary and continuous cell lines. Using chicken RBC, hemabsorption tests may detect the presence of virus in the infected cells. Serologic diagnosis may be done using paired sera, with a rise in the hemagglutination-inhibition and complement-fixing antibody titers being seen in the second serum specimen.

Pathogenicity and Pathology

The severity of the clinical disease often is not appreciated. In the United States the disease occurs in a milder form, preponderantly in the 5- to 7-year-old. In adults and younger children the disease may assume a more severe clinical course. The infection is transmitted in the form of aerosol and droplets of nasopharyngeal

TABLE 50.2   Differential Diagnosis of Childhood Exanthems

Disease	Conjunctivitis	Pharyngitis	Rhinitis	Exanthem
Measles	++	0	+	+
Rubella	+/–	+/–	+/–	+/–
Enterovirus infection	0	+/–	+/–	0
Scarlet fever	+/–	++	+/–	0
Infectious mononucleosis	0	+	0	0
Drug rash	0	0	0	0

secretions of infected individuals during the prodromal period. The prodromal period is characterized by symptoms of coryza, conjunctivitis, dry cough, sore throat,
headache, low-grade fever, and formation of Koplik's spots. After implantation
on the respiratory tract, the virus multiplies locally in the epithelium and probably
in the conjunctiva and spreads to the local lymph nodes. This is followed by hematogenous dissemination and subsequent distribution of the virus to the lymphoreticular organs, all of which takes place within about 10-12 days. A more massive
viremic stage follows within 1-2 days and causes more widespread viral dissemination to the lymphoid tissues and the skin. This results in the appearance of the
characteristic rash. The virus may be excreted in the prodromal period in nasopharyngeal secretions, urine, tears, and it may be isolated from lymphocytes. Leukopenia is also evident at this stage. The skin rash is more intense in appearance
but shows pathologic changes similar to the Koplik's spots. Foci of epithelial giant
cells containing viral nucleocapsids, edema, and round cell infiltration are seen.
The virus is transmitted to the skin via the capillaries of the corium which induces
a range of inflammatory changes. These include proliferation of epithelial cells,
serous exudations spreading into the epidermis, and necrosis of the epithelial cells.
The tonsils, adenoids, lymph nodes, spleen, appendix, and the epithelium of the alveoli and bronchi show formation of multinucleated giant cells.

Interstitial pneumonia may develop ("giant cell pneumonia"). Simultaneously
with the appearance of rash, IgM and IgG antibodies appear. Probably both the virus and immunologic reactivities play a part in the formation of rash. Cellular
immunity possibly plays a role in the elimination of the virus, especially from leukocytes.

Treatment

Antibiotics are helpful only if bacterial pneumonia or otitis media is present. Antipyretic drugs may be used for symptomatic relief. In young children severe

laryngotracheitis (croup) may require surgical intervention (tracheostomy). Encephalomyelitis needs excellent supportive care, especially in prolonged coma, and
barbiturates may be employed for the control of seizures.

Immunology and Prevention

The clinical disease results in solid immunity. By the age of 8-9 years, 95% of
children become immune from the clinical infection. Complement-fixing, hemagglutination-inhibition, and neutralizing antibodies are present. Measles virus is of
single antigenic type and the immunity developed from the natural disease persists
throughout life.

    Both formalin-inactivated and live, attenuated virus vaccines have been de-
veloped. The former has been found to be poorly immunogenic and less effective.
Unanticipatedly severe disease has been reported in vaccinees who were subsequently infected naturally or reimmunized with live virus vaccine. The live, attenuated vaccines induce febrile reactions and occasionally rash. These reactions
have been modified by simultaneous administration of pooled human gamma globulin (Edmonston vaccine). Viruses of greater attenuation have been subsequently
developed which produce milder side effects and no neurologic sequelae (Schwartz
strain; "Attenuvax," etc.). Field trials indicate that the live, attenuated vaccine is
highly effective in preventing the clinical disease (95% protection). Effective immunity persists at least 8 years. Antibody titers decline two- to threefold 5 years
after vaccination. Naturally acquired immunity from the clinical disease results
in five- to tenfold higher antibody levels. The clinical significance, if any, of these
lower antibody responses to attenuated, as compared with wild virus strains, is unknown. Mass immunization in the United States has dramatically reduced the prevalence of the disease by 90% and probably has the potential to eradicate the virus
totally. However, there is the rare possibility of development of SSPE from measles vaccine. This would appear to be a justified risk, since the natural disease is
more likely to cause SSPE than is the vaccine (5.2-9.7:1 million cases vs 0.5-1.1:
1 million doses of vaccine). The live, attenuated measles virus vaccine should be
given to all normal children at 15 months of age. Older children immunized before 1 year of age should be revaccinated. The vaccine is contraindicated in immunodeficiency and pregnancy (Table 50.3). Despite the effort of mass immunization programs in the United States, seronegative pockets of the population have

TABLE 50.3   Contraindications to Use of Measles Vaccine

Pregnancy

Leukemia, lymphoma, or other generalized malignancy

Immunosuppressive therapy

Severe febrile illness

Tuberculosis

Marked egg or antibiotic sensitivity (vaccine is produced in chick embryo cell
    culture and contains trace amounts of antibiotics)

Recent human gamma globulin injection (within preceding 3 mo)

---

kept the virus circulating. Recently, there has been an increase in the number of reported cases of measles. Furthermore, in the past few years, there has been a steady increase in attack rates in teenagers and young adults. Various explanations have been given, including use of the killed vaccine, declining antibody titers in vacinees, and failure of optimal response to vaccination because the vaccine was administered before 1 year of age. After natural disease, inapparent infection or a second attack is rare. These are much more common in the vaccinees. Therefore, reinforcement of vaccine-induced immunity by booster dose may be required, depending upon the results of more extensive analysis of this problem.

Complications and Prognosis

Resistance to secondary bacterial infections (e.g., hemolytic streptococcal infection) is reduced in measles. Development of encephalomyelitis may result from measles virus involvement of the CNS and immunologic reactions probably also play a role here. Patchy demyelination in the brain and cord with scattered petechial hemorrhages and infiltration by lymphocytic cells are observed. Encephalomyelitis, however, is a rare complication, more often found in older children, but when it develops, leaves some form of neurologic sequelae in 50% of cases. Subacute sclerosing panencephalitis (SSPE) is another rare complication. It is a slowly progressive neurologic disease of older children with a past history of measles infection or immunization. Probably IgG and IgM antibodies play a role in its development. The virus may be isolated from brain biopsy specimens from these patients. A high incidence of bacterial otitis media is also observed as a secondary complication of measles.

In uncomplicated cases, recovery is rapid with quick disappearance of catarrhal symptoms. Cough, however, may persist for several days.

Selected Bibliography

Adams, J. M.: Clinical pathology of measles encephalitis and sequelae: Conference on Measles Virus and Subacute Sclerosing Panencephalitis. *Neurology* 18 (suppl):52-57, 1968.

Ault, K. A. and Weiner, H. L.: Natural killing of measles-infected cells by human lymphocytes. *J Immunol* 122:2611-2616, 1979.

Bellanti, J. A., Sanga, R. L., Klutinis, B., Brandt, B., and Artenstein, M. S.: Antibody responses in serum and nasal secretion of children immunized with inactivated and attenuated measles-virus vaccines. *N Engl J Med* 280:628-633, 1969.

Center for Disease Control. U. S. Public Health Service: Measles Surveillance Report, No. 10, 1973-1976, issued July 1977.

Enders, J. F.: Measles virus: Historical review, isolation and behavior in various systems. *Am J Dis Child* 103:282-287, 1962.

Fujinami, R. S. and Oldstone, M. B. A.: Antiviral antibody reacting on the plasma membrane alters measles virus expression inside the cell. *Nature* 279:529-530, 1979.

Fulginiti, V.: Commentary: Measles immunization (editorial). *J Pediatr* 94:1019–1020, 1979.

Gallagher, M. and Flanagan, T. D.: Growth of measles in continuous lymphoid cell lines. (Abst. No. 4128). *Fed Proc* 34:948, 1975.

Horstman, D. M.: Problems in measles and rubella. *Disease-a-Month* 24:1–27, 1978.

Krugman, S.: Present status of measles and rubella immunization in the United States. A medical progress report. *J Pediatr* 90:1–12, 1977.

Martin, D. B., Weiner, L. B., Nieburg, P. I., and Blair, D. C.: Atypical measles in adolescents and young adults. *Ann Intern Med* 90:877–881, 1979.

Nichols, E. M.: Atypical measles syndrome: A continuing problem. *Am J Public Health* 69:160–162, 1979.

Paule, C. L., Bean, J. A., Burmeister, L. F., and Isacson, P.: Post vaccine era measles epidemiology. *JAMA* 241:1474–1476, 1979.

Rand, K. H. and Reuman, P. D.: Measles; ready for eradication? *Ann Intern Med* 90:978–980, 1979.

Rosenblatt, S., Gorecki, M., Shure, H., and Privesc, L.: Characterization of measles virus – specific proteins synthesized in vivo and in vitro from acutely and persistently infected cells. *J Virol* 29:1099–1116, 1979.

Weiner, L. B., Corwin, R. M., Nieburg, P. I., and Feldman, H. A.: A measles outbreak among adolescents. *J Pediatr* 90:17–20, 1977.

51

PARAINFLUENZA VIRUS
Robert H. Waldman, M.D.

Parainfluenza viruses are frequent causes of respiratory infection in humans and a variety of lower animals. They are particularly troublesome in young children in whom they are the most common cause of croup, and next to respiratory syncytial virus, the most common cause of pneumonia in infants.

Microbiology

Parainfluenza is the prototype virus for the paramyxoviruses, which along with the orthomyxoviruses (influenza virus) make up the class of viruses known as the myxo-viruses. There are three genera, the *Paramyxovirus* genus itself, which contains parainfluenza virus, Newcastle disease virus, and mumps virus; *Pneumovirus* (respiratory syncytial virus), and *Morbillivirus* (measles virus). These are single-stranded (this is in contradistinction to influenza virus which has segmented genetic material, a prerequisite for its antigenic instability) RNA viruses, containing he-magglutinin and neuraminidase. As indicated from the preceding statement, these viruses are antigenically stable.

There are four parainfluenza serotypes. Types 1 and 2 have similar clinical characteristics (Table 51.1), causing autumn and winter epidemics. Type 1 is more common than type 2. Type 3 parainfluenza virus is clinically more like respiratory syncytial virus, i.e., generally causes more severe illness than types 1 and 2. Type 4 parainfluenza virus causes very mild illness, generally not requiring patients with this infection to seek medical attention, and therefore, much less is known about this serotype.

TABLE 51.1   Characteristics of Various Parainfluenza Virus Strains

Type	Age of Infection	Epidemiology	Usual Clinical Manifestations
1	Nearly all children under 5 yr	Epidemic usually every other year	Croup, tracheobronchitis, febrile nasopharyngitis
2	About half under 5 yr	Same as above	Same
3	About half under 1 yr	Endemic	Pneumonia, bronchiolitis, croup, tracheobronchitis
4	About half under 5 yr	Endemic	Common cold

Epidemiology and Pathogenesis

One of the characteristics of parainfluenza viruses is the wide variety of animal species which are infected, e.g., mice, cattle, sheep, horses, monkeys, cats, and dogs. It is generally believed that, despite this wide distribution among various animal species, there are no cross-infections between species. The viruses have a worldwide distribution and spread quite readily. Transmission is by respiratory secretions, either direct contact or inhalation of large droplets. The incubation period is 3-8 days. For unexplained reasons, infection is more severe in male infants. This sex difference does not appear to be true of other age groups infected.

Another important characteristic of parainfluenza viruses is that reinfection is quite common, even in the presence of high levels of serum antibody (see the Immunology and Prevention section). However, reinfection usually causes less severe disease, with lower respiratory infection, fever, and significant systemic symptoms being unusual as compared with the primary infection. Type 3 virus usually infects children the first time in the infant age group. Types 1 and 2 usually cause their primary infection in the 2- to 6-year-olds.

Like many other viruses that cause respiratory infection, the most common clinical occurrence is asymptomatic infection. Even a large percentage of primary infections are subclinical. Only 2% of primary infections cause illness severe enough to lead parents to seek medical care. On the other hand, parainfluenza virus causes at least one-third of all cases of croup, 10% of childhood pneumonias, and 10-15% of cases of bronchiolitis.

The virus infects the ciliated epithelium, and viremia is extremely rare, if it ever occurs. In children with croup, there is inflammation of the subglottic area which causes varying degrees of inspiratory obstruction.

Persistent infection with parainfluenza virus has been described in patients with chronic lung disease, patients with immunodeficiencies, or elderly individuals.

Diagnosis

A presumptive diagnosis of parainfluenza virus infection can be made on clinical and epidemiologic grounds. An exact virologic diagnosis is of no practical clinical importance, since there is no specific therapy available.

The majority of people will show no signs of illness following infection with parainfluenza virus. Of those who do show symptoms or signs, the most frequent manifestation is a "common cold" syndrome lasting 3-4 days and tending to be more severe in children. Hoarseness and bronchitis are more common with parainfluenza virus common colds, than with those caused by other viruses.

The most characteristic syndrome caused by parainfluenza viruses is acute laryngotracheobronchitis, i.e., croup. Croup is unusual in the first few months of life, but is common in the 1- to 4-year age group. There is usually a fairly acute onset of nasal and pharyngeal symptoms, followed by the development of a harsh cough, hoarseness, and in more severe cases, stridor, dyspnea and chest retraction. After 3-4 days, the symptoms begin to subside. In contradistinction to lower respiratory infection, croup is usually more severe when caused by parainfluenza than when caused by respiratory syncytial virus.

Other clinical manifestations of parainfluenza virus infection are much less common and include pneumonia, otitis media, and acute parotitis. Adults with chronic lung disease may develop an acute exacerbation of their illness when they are infected with parainfluenza virus, as they may following infection with most of the other viruses involved in upper respiratory infections.

The laboratory diagnosis of parainfluenza virus infection is only of real importance for research and epidemiologic purposes. Viral antigen may be demonstrated directly by immunofluorescent examination of respiratory secretions. Serologic diagnosis can be made by showing a four fold or greater rise in antibody, using the complement fixation, hemagglutination-inhibition, or neutralization tests.

Treatment

There is no specific mode of therapy for patients with parainfluenza virus infection. Illness is generally mild and self-limited and therefore requires no intervention. For more severe cases, humidified air and mild sedation may be useful. In the few severe cases, ipecac may be useful for treatment of laryngeal spasm, but it must be used with care to avoid aspiration pneumonia, i.e., one must avoid making the treatment worse than the disease. In very severe cases endotracheal intubation or tracheostomy may be required to maintain oxygenation. Corticosteroids have not been beneficial in controlled studies, and the same can be said for aerosolized adrenergic drugs.

Prognosis

Parainfluenza virus infection, even in its severest form, has a very low mortality and is generally a self-limited infection. Patients nearly always recover with no sequelae. It has been hypothesized that bronchiolitis caused by parainfluenza virus may predispose to subsequent development of chronic obstructive lung disease and/or asthma. However, data supporting this hypothesis are not strong.

Immunology and Prevention

Studies on the immunology of parainfluenza virus infection reveal two very inter-esting and important findings. The first is that reinfection is common, and second that immunity does not seem to be related to levels of serum antibody to the vi-rus. On the other hand, immunity does seem to be related to the levels of respira-tory secretion IgA antibody. It is concluded from these findings that immuniza-tion is unlikely to be extremely successful in eliminating the disease, and that in-activated viral vaccines given parenterally are unlikely to be very effective at all. The finding of frequent reinfection may be related to the fact that secretory anti-body does not generally persist for an extremely long period, i.e., in comparison with serum IgG antibody. Thus, the aim of immunization would be to make the first infection milder, i.e., similar to subsequent reinfections. It would appear that the best chance of accomplishing this would be a live, attenuated vaccine given intranasally. An alternative would be a killed vaccine also given locally, e.g., by a spray into the nasopharynx.

Selected Bibliography

Brandt, C. D., Kim, H. W., Chanock, R. M., et al.: Parainfluenza virus epidemi-ology. *Pediatr Res* 8:422, 1974.

Clarke, S. K. R.: Parainfluenza virus infection. *Postgrad Med J* 49:792, 1973.

Downham, M. A. P. S., McQuillin, J., and Gardner, P. S.: Diagnosis and clinical significance of parainfluenza virus infections in children. *Arch Dis Child* 49: 8-15, 1974.

Glezen, W. P. and Denny, F. W.: Epidemiology of acute lower respiratory disease in children. *N Engl J Med* 288:498, 1973.

Monto, A. S.: Tecumseh study of respiratory illness. V. Patterns of infection with the parainfluenza viruses. *Am J Epidemiol* 97:338, 1973.

Smith, C. B., Purcell, R. H., Bellanti, J. A., et al.: Protective effect of antibody to parainfluenza type 1 virus. *N Engl J Med* 275:1145, 1966.

Wigley, F. M., Fruchtman, M. H., and Waldman, R. H.: Aerosol immunization of humans with inactivated parainfluenza type 2 vaccine. *N Engl J Med* 283: 1250, 1970.

52

RESPIRATORY SYNCYTIAL VIRUS
Robert H. Waldman, M.D.

Respiratory syncytial virus is an important pathogen because of the high degree of morbidity and mortality associated with the infection in very young children, and also because of the growing data indicating its possible relationship to the development of chronic lung disease in later life. It is an interesting infection because it occurs repeatedly throughout life, but there is a strong relationship between the severity of the disease and its occurrence in the first 6 months of life. It is the most common pathogen associated with bronchiolitis and pneumonia in young children.

Microbiology and Epidemiology

Respiratory syncytial virus (RSV) is an enveloped paramyxovirus of medium size. Humans are the only known host. It is very contagious; virtually every child is infected at least once by the age of 3. It causes yearly outbreaks, in the winter or spring. During an outbreak there are usually no other respiratory viruses present in the community. The virus causes lower respiratory tract illness in young children and upper respiratory tract illness and tracheobronchitis in older children and adults. The virus is rarely isolated from children or adults without respiratory disease. Although the infection rate is the same, the severity of illness is worse in males compared with females, and in lower socioeconomic groups. The overall attack rate is about 6% of the population per year. The incubation period is 2–8 days, and inoculation occurs by the nose or eye.

Pathogenesis and Pathology

As mentioned above, the disease is more severe in very young infants, and this is related to lower respiratory tract involvement. The reason for this is undoubtedly related to immune mechanisms, not in the usual sense of an absence of immunity, but actually owing to the presence of the "wrong" type of immunity. The basis for this conclusion is that virtually all newborns have maternally derived IgG antibody to RSV, and this is the age group that has the most severe illness. In addition, trials with a parenterally administered killed RSV vaccine led to more severe illness, not protection against illness. This has resulted in the conclusion that the severe disease is caused by immune complexes, i.e., IgG antibody complexing with viral antigens. The explanation of the observation that the disease becomes less severe as children get older, despite the fact that serum IgG antibody levels remain high, is that with infection, children develop secretory IgA antibody in the respiratory tract, thereby protecting against infection, or binding the viral antigens before they have a chance to complex with the serum IgG antibody. (It is important to note that IgA complexes fix complement very poorly, if at all.)

In patients with bronchiolitis there is a peribronchiolar lymphocytic infiltration and edema, followed by epithelial necrosis. Small airways obstruction results from sloughed epithelium and increased mucous secretion. As in asthma, hyperinflation results from the expiratory obstruction, which is more intense than the inspiratory. With complete obstruction, atelectatic areas develop. In patients with pneumonia, an interstitial mononuclear cell infiltration is seen. Complete histologic recovery from bronchiolitis or pneumonia may take several weeks.

Diagnosis

The diagnosis can be made on the basis of clinical and epidemiologic observations. One can be fairly confident that a patient has respiratory syncytial virus infection if there is a marked increase in bronchiolitis and pediatric pneumonia in the community, or if there is a rise in the number of hospital admissions of young children with acute lower respiratory disease. The typical child develops upper respiratory tract symptoms first, with moderately high fever. Next, cough, usually in paroxysms, develops. The cough is not usually accompanied by the characteristic "whoop" as is seen in pertussis. Croup is also fairly uncommon, occurring in less than 5% of infants. In severe cases, following cough, dyspnea, intercostal retraction, rales, ronchi, and wheezing may develop. Other more unusual manifestations are pleural effusion and otitis media. The latter may be a pure viral infection, with no bacterial superinfection, as is seen with most other viral infections.

In adults and older children, the more common symptom complex is upper respiratory involvement, with nasal congestion and cough being the most common symptoms. Upper respiratory infection with RSV tends to be more severe and of longer duration than that caused by other viruses. The average duration of symptoms is 9 days. Conjunctivitis occasionally is seen with RSV infection.

The differential diagnosis is difficult if one does not take into account the epidemiologic setting, since a similar clinical picture can be seen with other viral respiratory infections, and differentiating RSV pneumonia from bacterial infection can be difficult at times. Laboratory findings are not helpful in the diagnosis of individual patients, although virologic or serologic diagnosis may be of help in identifying the causal agent during an outbreak. Patients usually shed virus for 3-6 days. The only laboratory study which is of help in managing individual patients is determination of arterial blood gases.

Treatment

There is no specific mode of therapy, and therefore the main goal of treatment is general supportive measures, especially sufficient oxygen to correct hypoxemia. Steroids and bronchodilators are not beneficial. In the future, specific antiviral therapy may be available, and an experimental drug, ribavirin, does show some activity in vitro; however, it has not been tested against RSV in the human host.

Prognosis and Complications

The illness usually lasts from 7 to 21 days. Hospitalization, when it is necessary, is for an average of 6 days. Most fatalities occur in infants with underlying disease. Death is usually a result of apnea, respiratory failure or rarely, secondary bacterial infection. Apnea is common, and when looked for carefully, has been found to occur in 20% of hospitalized infants with RSV. It is more common in premature and very young infants and also has been seen at the first symptom of RSV infection. Apnea in RSV infection has been associated with the sudden infant death syndrome. Secondary bacterial infection is surprisingly uncommon, except in patients who have been on broad-spectrum antibiotics. A common epidemiologic complication of RSV infection is hospital spread. Infants are highly infectious, and spread through a pediatric ward is common.

In adults with chronic lung disease, or in the elderly, RSV is also dangerous. People with chronic lung disease are very likely to have a worsening of that condition, and a high percentage of elderly people develop bacterial superinfection following RSV. As has been mentioned previously, there is some epidemiologic evidence of an association between RSV infection as a child and the subsequent development of asthma and chronic obstructive pulmonary disease.

Immunology and Prevention

As mentioned earlier, immunity following infection appears to be incomplete and reinfection is common. All newborns have passively acquired maternal antibody, the titer of which falls over the first 6 months or so of life, or until the infant is infected and develops naturally acquired antibody. However, serum antibody does not correlate with protection, severity of the illness, or recovery from the illness.

Breast-feeding may offer some protection against the infection, possibly on the basis of maternal secretory IgA antibody in the colostrum and breast milk. This secretory IgA antibody probably coats the upper respiratory tract in the newborn, since they do not have a very mature swallowing mechanism, and breast milk almost always finds its way throughout the upper respiratory tract.

Active research is going on with the goal of developing an effective vaccine against RSV. Parenteral vaccines, both inactivated and live, attenuated ones, have been tested and have given no protection. In fact, the parenteral killed vaccine led to more severe illness in vaccinees compared with controls. It would seem most logical that a vaccine, either killed or live, which would stimulate the secretory immune system, would give the best protection.

Nosocomial RSV infections can be decreased in incidence by careful public health measures such as careful hand-washing, segregation of infected infants, and ensuring that personnel with upper respiratory infections not work, or at least not care for, high-risk children.

Selected Bibliography

Bruhn, F. W., Mokrohisky, S. T., and McIntosh, K.: Apnea associated with respiratory syncytial virus infection in young adults. *J Pediatr* 90:382, 1977.

Bruhn, F. W. and Yeager, A. S.: Respiratory syncytial virus in early infancy. *Am J Dis Child* 131:145, 1977.

Burrows, B., Knudson, R. J., and Lebowitz, M. D.: The relationship of childhood respiratory illness to adult obstructive airway disease. *Am Rev Respir Dis* 115:751, 1977.

Denny, F. W., Collier, A. M., Henderson, F. W., et al.: The epidemiology of bronchiolitis. *Pediatr Res* 11:234, 1977.

Downham, M. A. P. S., Gardner, P. S., McQuillin, J., and Ferris, J. A. G.: Role of respiratory viruses in childhood mortality. *Br Med J* 1:235-239, 1975.

Downham, M. A. P. S., Scott, R., Sims, D. G., Webb, J. K. G., and Gardner, P. S.: Breast-feeding protects against respiratory syncytial virus infections. *Br Med J* 2:274-276, 1976.

Evans-Jones, G., Fielding, D. W., Todd, P. J., and Tomlinson, M.: Breast-feeding as protection against respiratory syncytial virus. *Br Med J* 2:1434, 1978.

Glezen, W. P.: Pathogenesis of bronchiolitis - epidemiologic considerations. *Pediatr Res* 11:239, 1977.

Hall, C. B.: The shedding and spreading of respiratory syncytial virus. *Pediatr Res* 11:239, 1977.

Hall, C. B. and Douglas, R. G., Jr.: Respiratory syncytial virus and influenza: Practical community surveillance. *Am J Dis Child* 130:615, 1975.

Hall, C. B., Douglas, R. G., Jr., and Geiman, J. M.: Quantitative shedding patterns of respiratory syncytial virus in infants. *J Infect Dis* 132:151, 1975.

Hall, C. B., Douglas, R. G., Jr., and Geiman, J. M.: Respiratory syncytial virus infections in infants: Quantitation and duration of shedding. *J Pediatr* 89:11, 1976.

Hall, C. B., Douglas, R. G., Jr., Geiman, J. M., and Messner, M. K.: Nosocomial respiratory syncytial virus infections. *N Engl J Med* 293:1343-1346, 1975.

Hall, C. B., Geiman, J. M., Biggar, R., and Messner, M. K.: Respiratory syncytial virus infections within families. *N Engl J Med* 294:414-419, 1976.

Hall, J. W., Hall, C. B., and Speers, D. M.: Respiratory syncytial virus infections in adults: Clinical, virologic and serial pulmonary function studies. *Ann Intern Med* 88:203, 1978.

Kattan, M., Keens, T. G., Lapierre, J. G., Levison, H., Bryan, A. C., and Reilly, B. J.: Pulmonary function abnormalities in symptom-free children after bronchiolitis. *Pediatrics* 59:683-688, 1977.

Kim, H. W., Leikin, S. L., Arrobio, J., Brandt, C. D., Chanock, R. M., and Parrott, R. H.: Cell-mediated immunity to respiratory syncytial virus induced by inactivated vaccine or by infection. *Pediatr Res* 10:75-78, 1976.

Lamprecht, C. L., Krause, H. E., and Mufson, M. A.: Role of maternal antibody in pneumonia and bronchiolitis due to respiratory syncytial virus. *J Infect Dis* 134:211, 1976.

Lebowitz, M. D. and Burrows, B.: The relationship of acute respiratory illness history to the prevalence and incidence of obstructive lung disorders. *Am J Epidemiol* 105:544, 1977.

McIntosh, K., Masters, H., Orr, I., Chao, R. K., and Barkin, R. M.: Secretory antibody following respiratory syncytial virus infection in infants. *Pediatr Res* 10: 389, 1976.

Mellins, R. B.: Bronchiolitis - comments on pathogenesis and treatment. *Pediatr Res* 11:268-269, 1977.

Ogra, P. O., Ogra, S. S., and Coppola, P. R.: Secretory component in sudden infant death syndrome. *Lancet* 2:387, 1975.

Sims, D. G., Downham, M. A. P. S., Gardner, P. S., Webb, J. K. G., and Weightman, D.: Study of 8-year-old children with a history of respiratory syncytial virus bronchiolitis in infancy. *J Epidemiol* 105:544, 1977.

53

RHINOVIRUSES
Rama Ganguly, Ph.D.

Rhinoviruses are the most important causative agents of the "common cold" -
acute afebrile upper respiratory diseases of humans. The genus *Rhinovirus* belongs
to the picornavirus family. It comprises more than 100 different antigenic types,
thus making the possibility of its control extremely difficult.

Etiology

Rhinoviruses resemble other members of the picornaviruses in their icosahedral
symmetry, size, shape, nucleic acid composition, and ether-resistance. They are
different from other groups of the family in being highly susceptible to inactivation at low pH (3-5) and in having a greater buoyant density. M (monkey) strains
grow and produce cytopathic changes in monkey kidney monolayers, or in continuous human malignant cell lines (HeLa). H (human) strains easily grow in human
embryonic kidney cultures and in diploid human embryonic lung cells (WI 38). O
(organ) strains grow only in organ cultures of human embryo respiratory epithelium. Those O strains adapted to grow in human respiratory fibroblasts are designated as O-H strains. H strains appear to be more stable than M strains. Both
M and H strains grow optimally at 33°C at pH 7.0 on revolving drums to maintain
a relatively high oxygen tension. They replicate in the cytoplasm of infected cells.
They do not have hemagglutinating activity. Rhinoviruses possess type-specific
surface antigens, but there is no common group antigen.

Epidemiology

The common cold is the most frequent of all human infections. It is widespread in all parts of the world. The diseases, although not serious, can cause considerable discomfort and in the United States result in the loss of several hundred million person-days of work. The incidence of the common cold is higher in the winter, fall, and early spring. However, experimental exposure of volunteers to wet and chilling has not increased their susceptibility to the disease. The mode of virus spread is not completely understood. Respiratory secretions (by direct contact) and aerosolized droplets of infected individuals could be vehicles of transmission. Preschool and schoolchildren play significant roles in introducing the infection into the home. The virus spreads very well at school and at home, but not well in the work place. Transmission is more likely from people who have fairly severe symptoms, usually on about the third day, at the time when there are the highest viral titers in the nose. Individuals can have repeated episodes of the common cold and multiple serotypes usually circulate in the community at the same time. However, rhinoviruses are not the causative agents of all common colds. Other viruses such as coxsackieviruses and coronaviruses can also cause the syndrome. New recruits in military camps usually contract the infection during the first 4 weeks of training. The rhinovirus infection rate in young children in the United States has been estimated to be 1.5 per person-year. Serologic studies indicate that rhinovirus infections begin in early life and continue into adulthood. Rhinovirus serum antibody usually persists at a stable level for years in an adult.

Pathogenesis

The incubation period is 2-4 days. The infection in humans is limited to the upper respiratory tract. The major site of virus replication is the nasal epithelium. Tissue culture studies suggest that the virus colonizes the ciliated nasal epithelial cells, harming the cells and inactivating the cilia. Phagocytes engulf virus-damaged cells. This, and also bacterial invasion of damaged cells, may be responsible for the purulent nasal discharge that is so typically seen in the later phase of the common cold.

Clinical Manifestations

Sore throat, cough, and sneezing are followed by a clear, watery nasal discharge in the common cold. Hyperemia, edema, and nasal obstruction are also common symptoms. Laryngitis and hoarseness may be seen in adults. Lack of any severe systemic symptoms distinguishes this disease from influenza. Rhinovirus infections may be associated with periods of acute exacerbation in patients with chronic pulmonary disease. Rhinoviruses do not cause lower respiratory disease. This may be due to its growth preference for temperatures lower than 37°C.

Laboratory Diagnosis

Diagnosis of the causal agent is done by inoculating tissue culture (human kidney or diploid cell lines) with nasal or throat swab or washing. The virus isolated may be typed by the neutralization test with standard sera (using pools of several type-specific sera and then using individual sera for final identification). Serologic diagnosis is impractical except in research laboratories because of the lack of a suitable in vitro assay technique.

Immunity

Serum neutralization antibody rises in most cases after infection. A naturally acquired antibody titer of $\geq$ 1:8 is associated with significant resistance to the disease, but this may be a secondary phenomenon. Nasal secretion antibody titers may be of primary importance. Secretory antibody declines fairly rapidly after infection. Interferon may play an important role in recovery from infection.

Treatment, Prevention, and Control

No suitable vaccine is presently available. An experimental intranasal inactivated vaccine has been shown to induce a good secretory antibody response. Many different serotypes circulate concurrently and no certain serotypes have been associated with most of the infections. Therefore, the prospect of developing a composite vaccine seems remote. Interferon, interferon inducers, and other antiviral agents are being studied for chemoprophylaxis of rhinovirus infections. Vitamin C also has been employed to prevent experimental rhinovirus infections, but its efficacy still remains unproved. An immunoenhancing drug inosiplex (Isoprinosine) has shown efficacy in preventing and treating experimental rhinovirus infection, but this also needs to be confirmed with further studies.

There is no question that hand-washing and good personal hygiene are excellent control methods.

Selected Bibliography

Cate, T. R., Couch, R. B., and Johnson, K. M.: Studies with rhinoviruses in volunteers: Production of illness, effect of naturally acquired antibody and demonstration of a protective effect not associated with serum antibody. *J Clin Invest* 43:56-67, 1964.

DeLong, D. C. and Reed, S. E.: Inhibition of rhinovirus replication in organ culture by a potential antiviral drug. *J Infect Dis* 141:87-91, 1980.

Douglas, R. G., Jr.: Pathogenesis of rhinovirus common cold in human volunteers. *Ann Otol Rhinol Laryngol* 79:563-571, 1970.

Gwaltney, J. M. and Hendley, J. O.: Rhinovirus transmission: One if by air, two if by hand. *Trans Am Clin Climatol Assoc* 89:194-200, 1977.

Gwaltney, J. M. Jr., Moskalski, P. B., and Hendley, J. O.: Hand-to-hand transmission of rhinovirus colds. *Ann Intern Med* 88:463-467, 1978.

Gwaltney, J. M. Jr., Moskalski, P. B., and Hendley, J. O.: Interruption of experimental rhinovirus transmission. *J Infect Dis* 142:811-815, 1980.

Hamory, B. H., Hendley, J. O., and Gwaltney, J. M., Jr.: Rhinovirus growth in nasal polyp organ culture. *Proc Soc Exp Biol Med* 155:577-582, 1977.

Hendley, J. O., Mika, L. A., and Gwaltney, J. M.: Evaluation of virucidal compounds for inactivation of rhinovirus on hands. *Antimicrob Agents Chemother* 14:690-694, 1978.

Hughes, J. H., Mitchell, M. , and Hamparian, V. V.: Rhinoviruses: Kinetics of ultraviolet inactivation and effects of UV and heat on immunogenicity. *Arch Virol* 61:313-319, 1979.

Hussain, A. and Mohanty, S. B.: Cell-mediated immunity to bovine rhinovirus type 1 in calves. *Arch Virol* 59:17-24, 1979.

Jackson, G. G. and Muldoon, R. L.: Viruses causing common respiratory infections in man. *J Infect Dis* 127:328-355, 1973.

Knopf, H. L. S., Perkins, J. C., Bertran, D. M., Kapikian, A. Z., and Chanock, R. M.: Analysis of the neutralizing activity in nasal wash and serum following intranasal vaccination with inactivated type 13 rhinovirus. *J Immunol* 104:566-573, 1970.

Rosenbaum, M. J., DeBerry, P., Sullivan, E. J., Pierce, W. E., Mueller, R. E., and Peckinpaugh, R. O.: Epidemiology of the common cold in military recruits with emphasis on infections by rhinovirus type 1A, 2 and two unclassified rhinoviruses. *Am J Epidemiol* 93:183-193, 1971.

Stenhouse, A. C.: Rhinovirus infection in acute exacerbations of chronic bronchitis: A controlled prospective study. *Br Med J* 3:461-463, 1967.

Tyrell, D. A.: Studies of rhinoviruses and coronaviruses at the Common Cold Unit, Salisbury, Wiltshire. *Postgrad Med J* 55:117-121, 1979.

Waldman, R. H. and Ganguly, R.: Effect of CP-20,961, an interferon inducer on upper respiratory tract infections due to rhinovirus type 21 in volunteers. *J Infect Dis* 138:531-535, 1978.

Waldman, R. H. and Ganguly, R.: Therapeutic efficacy of inosiplex (Isoprinosine) in rhinovirus infection. *Ann N Y Acad Sci* 284:153-160, 1977.

54

ECHOVIRUSES
Rama Ganguly, Ph.D.

In the course of epidemiologic studies of poliomyelitis, echoviruses were discovered using tissue culture techniques. They were found to be present in human feces apparently unrelated to any disease. Thus, they were designated as Enteric Cytopathogenic Human Orphan viruses (ECHO). Gradually, however, it has become evident through further studies that they are not entirely "orphan" in that they can indeed produce varieties of human illnesses. The diseases they produce can range from minor respiratory infections to severe neurologic disorders (Table 54.1).

Etiology

Echoviruses resemble poliomyelitis viruses in their structure, replication, size, stability, and resistance to physicochemical agents. They belong to the family Picornaviridae and the genus *Enterovirus*. They are stable at pH 3-11, survive long periods of time at 4°C, are inactivated at 65°C for 30 min, and can be preserved well at -70°C. Echoviruses grow well in a variety of tissue culture cells. Analysis with serum neutralization tests has indicated that echoviruses can be divided into at least 31 serotypes based on type-specific antigens in their capsid. No group antigen has been detected. Echoviruses were distinguished primarily from coxsackieviruses based on their lack of virulence for suckling mice. Some types, however, do produce lesions resembling those of coxsackieviruses in suckling mice. Several can cause neurologic manifestations upon intraspinal or intracerebral inoculation into monkeys. They resemble in most cases coxsackieviruses and polioviruses in the nature of cytopathic changes observed in tissue cultures.

TABLE 54.1   Echovirus Clinical Syndrome

Aseptic meningitis

Common cold

Gastroenteritis

Systemic viral syndrome

Epidemiology

Echoviruses are prevalent in all parts of the world and humans are the only known natural hosts. The predominant sites of their multiplication are the intestinal and respiratory tracts. Likewise, they are transmitted via the fecal-oral route or respiratory contact. Although some types can cause disseminated types of disease, echoviruses can often induce subclinical or inapparent infections. Some echoviruses have not been associated with any human disease. Echovirus infections are more common in children although often they produce more severe illness in adults. Echovirus types 4, 6, 9, 16, 18, 20, 30 have been known to be associated with epidemic outbreaks in various clinical forms (Table 54.2).

Pathogenesis

Generally echoviruses produce mild illnesses. After multiplication in the cytoplasm of epithelial cells echoviruses are released to spread from cell to cell. The infected cells are disrupted. Most echoviruses primarily affect and remain limited to the alimentary and respiratory tract epithelial cells. Occasionally they may produce systemic manifestations and the virus may be isolated from blood and CNS specimens, particularly types 6, 9, 11, 16, and 18. They also infect secondary target organs. This phase of viremia may continue for 4-5 days before the onset of the illness. Twenty-five serotypes have been associated with CNS infection and type 9 with mild transient paralysis. In rare instances of fatal outcome nonspecific CNS changes have been noted in autopsy specimens with cerebral edema and focal destructive and infiltrative lesions. Experimentally inoculated monkeys and chimpanzees have similar neurologic afflictions upon intracerebral or intraspinal inoculation.

Clinical Manifestations

Echovirus infections are usually mild and often go unrecognized in children. The virus is not infrequently carried by healthy children in their alimentary tract as an inapparent infection, resulting in immunity. Echovirus infections usually have a short incubation period (3-5 days). Depending upon the clinical manifestations they produce, echoviruses have been divided into the following four categories of illness: (1) aseptic meningitis, (2) respiratory infections resembling the common cold, (3) gastrointestinal disorder manifested mainly by diarrhea, and (4) systemic infections producing skin rash, fever, and malaise. Echovirus 9 can invade nervous

TABLE 54.2   Association of Various Serotypes of Enteroviruses and Human Disease

Virus	Syndrome	Types
Coxsackievirus		
Group A (types 1-22, 24)	Summer febrile illness	All
	Aseptic meningitis	1,2,4-7,9,10,14,16,22,24
	Paralysis	4,7,9
	Herpangina	1-6,8,10,22
	Common cold	21
	Exanthem	4,5,9,16
	Pneumonitis	9
Group B (types 1-6)	Summer febrile disease, sometimes with respiratory symptoms	All
	Aseptic meningitis	All
	Pleurodynia	All
	Myocarditis, pericarditis, orchitis	1-5
	Generalized disease of newborn infants	1-5
Echoviruses (types 1-7,9, 11-27,29-32)	Summer febrile illness	All
	Aseptic meningitis	1-7,9,11,14-19,23,24,30,31
	Exanthem	2,4,6,9,11,14,16,18
	Paralysis, encephalitis, ataxia	2,4,6,9,11,16,18,30
	Common cold	11,20

tissues to cause transient mild paralysis. In general, patients recover rapidly and completely from echovirus infections. However, the gastroenteritis produced in children can assume a rather severe form, especially in newborns.

Laboratory Diagnosis

The virus can be isolated using monkey or human kidney cells inoculated with throat swabs, stool, or spinal fluid. Since echoviruses occur in stools in the absence of disease, isolation of the virus does not necessarily mean it is the causative agent of a diarrheal illness. Therefore paired serum sample analysis is required for serologic documentation. This can be measured in terms of neutralizing anti-bodies within 2 weeks after alimentary tract infections, and these antibodies persist for several years. Hemagglutination-inhibition and complement-fixing antibodies also develop, but these disappear quickly.

Prevention, Prognosis, Treatment

No effective preventive measures are known for echovirus infections. Treatment is symptomatic. Neonatal aseptic meningitis may cause some form of permanent neurologic damage in 10% of survivors.

No vaccine is available. Echovirus outbreaks are infrequent. Because of this and since there are so many serotypes the prospect of development of a vaccine is not likely.

Selected Bibliography

Adrain, T., Rosenwith, B., and Eggers, H.: Isolation and characterization of temperature-sensitive mutants of echovirus 12. *Virology* 99:329-339, 1979.

Haynes, R. E., Cramblett, H. G., Hilty, M. D., Azimi, P. H., and Crew, J.: ECHO virus type 3 infections in children: Clinical and laboratory studies. *J Pediatr* 80:589-595, 1972.

Hertenstein, J. R., Sarnat, H. B., and O'Connor, D. M.: Acute unilateral oculomotor palsy associated with ECHO 9 viral infection. *J Pediatr* 89:79-81, 1976.

Jackson, G. G. and Muldoon, R. L.: Viruses causing common respiratory infections in man. II. Enteroviruses and paramyxoviruses. *J Infect Dis* 128:387-408, 1973.

LaBelle, R. L. and Gerba, C. P.: Influence of estuarine sediment on virus survival under field conditions. *Appl Environ Microbiol* 39:749-755, 1980.

Philip, A. C. G. and Larson, E. J.: Overwhelming neonatal infection with ECHO 19 virus. *J Pediatr* 82:391-397, 1973.

Steinhoff, M. C.: Viruses and diarrhea - a review. *Am J Dis Child* 132:302-307, 1978.

von Zeipel, G.: Most echoviruses reach higher titers in RD than in GMK-AHI cells regardless of their passage history. *Arch Virol* 63:143-146, 1980.

Webster, A. D. B., Tripp, Hayward, A. R., Dayan, A. D., Doshi, R., McIntyre, E. H., and Tyrrell, A. J.: Echovirus encephalitis and myositis in primary immunoglobulin deficiency. *Arch Dis Child* 53:33-37, 1978.

Weiner, L. S., Howell, J. T., Langford, M. P., Stanton, G. J., Baron, S., Goldblum, R. M., Lord, R. A., and Goldman, A. S.: Effect of specific antibodies on chronic echovirus type 5 encephalitis in a patient with hypogammaglobulinemia. *J Infect Dis* 140:858-863, 1979.

Welliver, R. C. and Cherry, J. D.: Aseptic meningitis and orchitis associated with echovirus 6 infection. *J Pediatr* 92:239-244, 1978.

Wilfert, C. M., Lauer, B. A., Cohen, M., Costenbader, M. L., and Myers, E.: An epidemic of echoviruses 18 meningitis. *J Infect Dis* 131:75-78, 1975.

Ziegler, J. B. and Penny, R.: Fatal echo 30 virus infection and amyloidosis in X-linked hypogammaglobulinemia. *Clin Immunol Immunopathol* 3:347-352, 1975.

55

COXSACKIEVIRUSES
Rama Ganguly, Ph.D.

Dalldorf and Sickles first demonstrated that coxsackieviruses can produce intestinal infections in humans. In 1948, using suckling mouse inoculation, these workers isolated the virus from the feces of two children in Coxsackie, New York. Coxsackieviruses belong to the enterovirus family and can cause diverse types of illness (Table 55.1).

Etiology

Physicochemical analysis of a few coxsackieviruses has shown that they are similar to polioviruses in many respects, e.g., structure, mode of replication, size, shape, stability, molecular weight, and chemical composition. The remarkable feature of coxsackieviruses is their pathogenicity for suckling mice and hamsters. On the basis of this property the viruses are divided into two groups:

1. Group A (23 serotypes) produces a fulminating lethal infection of these animals, leading to total flaccid paralysis and death. They possess type-specific neutralizing and complement-fixing antigens. Several demonstrate cross-reactivities but do not possess a common group A antigen. The lesions in mice involve necrosis and degeneration of skeletal muscles.
2. Group B (six serotypes) causes widespread but less severe lesions in many organs. Localized lesions are found in liver, pancreas, myocardium, brain, brown fat pads, and skeletal muscles. Some studies conclude that they may cause a diabetes-like syndrome in mice. All group B and one group A (A9) share a group antigen detectable by agar-gel diffusion. Types B1, B3, B5, as well as A20, A21, A24, agglutinate human blood group O cells. Coxsackievirus A9 exhibits intermediate antigenic properties between the echo- and coxsackievirus groups.

TABLE 55.1   Association of Various Serotypes of Enteroviruses and
Human Disease

Virus	Syndrome	Types
Coxsackievirus		
Group A (types 1-22, 24)	Summer febrile illness	All
	Aseptic meningitis	1,2,4-7,9,10,14,16,22,24
	Paralysis	4,7,9
	Herpangina	1-6,8,10,22
	Common cold	21
	Exanthem	4,5,9,16
	Pneumonitis	9
Group B (types 1-6)	Summer febrile disease, sometimes with respiratory symptoms	All
	Aseptic meningitis	All
	Pleurodynia	All
	Myocarditis, pericarditis, orchitis	1-5
	Generalized disease of newborn infants	1-5
Echoviruses		
(types 1-7,9, 11-27,29-32	Summer febrile illness	All
	Aseptic meningitis	1-7,9,11,14-19,23,24,30,31
	Exanthem	2,4,6,9,11,14,16,18
	Paralysis, encephalitis, ataxia	2,4,6,9,11,16,18,30
	Common cold	11,20

Epidemiology

The peak incidence occurs in summer and fall. Coxsackieviruses cause infections
in all parts of the world. Humans seem to be the only natural host, although intracerebral inoculation of rhesus monkeys with some group A viruses may produce
neurologic symptoms resembling poliovirus, and mouse inoculation is used to isolate and propagate coxsackieviruses. As an enterovirus, the spread of the disease
in humans occurs by the fecal-oral route in close contacts and probably from
swimming pools. To a lesser extent, respiratory tract viral shedding may play a
part in dissemination of the disease. After growing in the intestinal tract and

oropharynx these viruses are excreted in feces and can be recovered from sewage and flies. Characteristic epidemics or sporadic cases may occur in all clinical forms, including aseptic meningitis, epidemic myalgia, and herpangina. Most infections occur in children and young adults. Coxsackieviruses are easily transmitted and mild or asymptomatic infections are common. A particular serotype of coxsackievirus is found to be prevalent in a locality, but is replaced by another type in a few years, probably due to the development of herd immunity.

Pathogenesis

Because of the lack of a suitable animal model, studies on the pathogenesis mechanism of coxsackievirus infection remain rather limited. Autopsy specimens from cases of fatal myocarditis of the newborn indicate a wide variety of lesions, e.g., widespread areas of focal necrosis, acute myocardial inflammation, focal necrosis, and inflammatory reactions in the liver, adrenal glands, pancreas, and in skeletal muscles, and sometimes meningoencephalitis. Mild interstitial focal myocarditis and occasional valvulitis in infants and children may also be caused by group B viruses. Group B viruses may be transmitted in utero to the fetus, causing myocarditis and congenital heart disease. They can also produce permanent cardiac abnormalities in adults.

Clinical Manifestations

A remarkable variety of illnesses may be produced by coxsackievirus and divergent types of diseases may be caused by the same virus. Some of the more common clinical forms of coxsackievirus infections are shown in Table 55.2. Herpangina is an acute illness of short duration (1–4 days) manifesting fever and lesions on the tonsils, soft palate, and pharynx. Dysphagia, anorexia, vomiting, as well as abdominal pain may be seen. Pleurodynia (Bornholm disease/devil's grip) is caused by group B viruses and the clinical symptoms last for several days to weeks and include fever, headache, severe pleuritic pain, and malaise. Summer grippe is characterized by fever, sore throat, headache, malaise, and vague pains resembling a rather severe common cold. Acute upper respiratory tract syndromes of this type are caused by group A21 and several group B viruses. The duration is usually short. Group A7 virus in particular can cause an illness simulating paralytic poliomyelitis. Painful stomatitis with vesicular rash on the hands and feet characterize hand-foot-and-mouth disease caused by group A (5,16) viruses. Some viruses in each group can cause at least one distinct syndrome on which basis they can be diagnosed clinically. Not all members of group A viruses have been shown to cause human disease. The group B viruses are a frequent cause of viral myocarditis.

Laboratory Diagnosis

Throat washings, spinal fluid, or feces may be used to isolate the virus by using newborn mice or tissue culture inoculation. The virus may be isolated and identified using pooled and type-specific neutralizing antisera. Paired serum samples may be utilized for retrospective diagnosis of the disease, and the serologic diagnosis is more practical when the virus has been isolated. Immunofluorescence, complement-fixation, and hemagglutination-inhibition titrations may be employed for serologic evidence for infections.

TABLE 55.2   Clinical Syndromes Associated With Group A and
             B Coxsackieviruses

Clinical Syndrome	Coxsackievirus Group	
	A Serotypes	B Serotypes
Aseptic meningitis	2,4,7,9,23	1,2,3,4,5,6
Neurologic damage		
Sustained paralysis	4,7,9,23	–
Transient paralysis	2,9	3,4,5
Encephalitis	–	3
Herpangina	2,3,4,5,6,8,10	–
Fever, exanthema	2,4,9,16	4
Acute upper respiratory infection	21	1,2,3,4,5
Epidemic pleurodynia (Bornholm disease)	–	1,2,3,4,5
Myocarditis of the newborn	–	2,3,4,5
Interstitial myocarditis and valvulitis in infants and children	–	2,3,4,5
Pericarditis	–	2,3,4,5
Hand-foot-and-mouth disease	5,16	

Immunity

Long-term immunity has been found to result from infections with some of the viruses but it is not known with certainty if this is the case with all of them.

Treatment, Prevention, and Control

Since the fecal-oral and respiratory routes spread the disease it appears that sanitary measures (such as avoiding swimming pools during epidemics) and contacts with infected individuals may be helpful in control. Because of the presence of several types of the viruses, prevention by immunization with a composite virus vaccine does not appear promising. The infrequency of epidemics also makes the prospect of immunization less attractive.

Selected Bibliography

Couch, R. B., Cate, R. R., Gerone, P. J., Fleet, W. F., Lang, D. J., Griffith, W. R., and Knight, V.: Production of illness with a small particle aerosol of Coxsackie A-21. *J Clin Invest* 44:535-542, 1965.

Dery, P., Marks, M. I., and Shapera, R.: Clinical manifestation of coxsackievirus infections in children. *Am J Dis Child* 128:464-468, 1974.

Green, R. J. and Webb, J. M.: The nature of virus-like particles in the paraxial muscles of idiopathic scoliosis. *J Pathol* 129:9-12, 1979.

Grist, N. R. and Bell, E. J.: A six-year study of coxsackievirus B infections in heart disease. *J Hyg* 73:165-172, 1974.

Khatib, R., Chason, J. L., Silberber, B. K., and Lerner, A. M.: Age-dependent pathogenicity of group B coxsackieviruses in Swiss-Webster mice: Infectivity for myocardium and pancreas. *J Infect Dis* 141:394-403, 1980.

Lake, A. M., Louer, B. A., Clark, J. C., Wasenberg, R. L., and McIntosh, K.: Enterovirus infections in neonates. *J Pediatr* 89:787-791, 1976.

Lindenbaum, J. E., Van Dyck, P. C., and Allen, R. G.: Hand, foot and mouth disease associated with coxsackievirus group B. *Scand J Infect Dis* 7:161-163, 1975.

Marier, R., Rodriguez, W., Chloupek, R. J., Brandt, D. C., Kim, H.W., Baltimore, R. S., Parker, C. L., and Artenstein, M. S.: Coxsackievirus B5 infection and aseptic meningitis in neonates and children. *Am J Dis Child* 129:321-325, 1975.

McGeady, M.L. and Crowell, R. L.: Stabilization of "A" particles of coxsackievirus B3 by a Hela cell plasma membrane extract. *J Virol* 32:790-795, 1979.

Schultz, M. and Crowell, R. L.: Acquisition of susceptibility of coxsackievirus A2 by the rat L8 cell line during myogenic differentiation. *J Gen Virol* 46:39-49, 1980.

Ujevich, M. M. and Jaffe, R.: Pancreatic islet cell damage: Its occurrence in neonatal coxsackievirus encephalomyocarditis. *Arch Pathol Lab Med* 104:438-441, 1980.

Ward, R. L. and Ashley, C. S.: pH modification of the effects of detergents on the stability of enteric viruses. *Appl Environ Microbiol* 38:314-322, 1979.

Webb, S. R. and Madge, G. E.: The role of host genetics in the pathogenesis of coxsackievirus infection in the pancreas of mice. *J Infect Dis* 141:47-54, 1980.

White, R. W.: Virus infections of the myocardium. *Practitioner* 224:245-247, 1980.

Williams, W. R., Hornig, C., Bauer, H. R., and Klingmuller, V.: Orchitis caused by coxsackie A9 (Letter). *Lancet* 2:1350, 1977.

56

POLIOVIRUSES
Edwin L. Anderson, M.D.

The figure of an Egyptian priest with a withered leg, the characteristic deformity of paralytic poliomyelitis, is the earliest record of an illness that became epidemic in the United States early in the twentieth century. The introduction of a killed vaccine in the mid-1950s and an attenuated vaccine in the 1960s dramatically reduced the incidence of paralytic disease.

Microbiology

Poliomyelitis is caused by the polioviruses, of which there are three distinct serotypes. The polioviruses, along with the echoviruses and coxsackieviruses, are classified as enteroviruses. The enteroviruses are composed of single-stranded RNA, do not have a lipid coat, and are resistant to bile, ether, and various detergents. Chlorine, ultraviolet light, and formalin inactivate them.

Other enteroviruses have been implicated in paralytic illness that is clinically and pathologically indistinguishable from that caused by the polioviruses (Table 56.1). These illnesses are generally milder but persistent paralysis and death have been reported.

Epidemiology

Poliomyelitis became epidemic in the United States just after the beginning of the twentieth century. Before this time it was an endemic illness and almost all of the population was exposed to polioviruses in the early years of life. At first the high incidence was thought to occur only in "civilized" countries, with the explanation that improved public health and sanitation eliminated early exposure to

TABLE 56.1   Viruses Linked Etiologically to Clinical Paralytic Poliomyelitis

Poliovirus types	1,2, and 3
Coxsackievirus A	4,7, and 9
Coxsackievirus B	2,3,4, and 5
Echovirus	1,2,4,6,7,9,11,16,18, and 30

immunizing infections and consequently left large numbers of susceptible older individuals. Better reporting subsequently revealed that a high incidence of paralytic disease occurred in many countries. Epidemic poliomyelitis reached its peak incidence in the United States in the 1950s and then declined progressively after the vaccines were developed (Figure 56.1).

Transmission of poliovirus is by the fecal-oral route, and humans are the only reservoir. In the United States epidemics occurred in late summer and fall. The infection is highly communicable, with the majority of susceptible family members being infected when the virus is introduced. Poliovirus remains infectious in water and milk for relatively long periods. The incubation period ranges from 3 to 21 days, with the usual range of 7-12 days. Silent infection is the main source of contagion. The period of highest communicability is the latter part of the incubation period and the first week of illness; however, virus can be recovered from feces for weeks after infection. In early epidemics the age group attacked were children under 5 years of age in whom 90% of the paralytic cases occurred, hence the name infantile paralysis. Eighty percent of the paralytic cases were caused by type 1 virus.

Pathogenesis

After entering the oropharynx, poliovirus replicates in the alimentary system before spreading to the blood. If the viremia is transient, no serious illness occurs, or the infection may remain asymptomatic; CNS invasion follows persistent viremia. Virus may also reach the CNS via nerves. This is supported by the observation that tonsillectomy was associated with the onset of bulbar poliomyelitis, presumably as a result of the virus entering nerves exposed by the surgery. In addition, paralysis was observed to be localized to the infected extremity following injection of incompletely inactivated poliovirus vaccine, as occurred in 1935 and 1954.

Pathology

Neurons are damaged by viral multiplication. Neuronal lesions can be found in the spinal cord (chiefly, in the anterior horn cells), medulla, cerebellum, midbrain, thalamus, hypothalamus, and cerebral motor cortex. Other enteroviruses can produce disease that is clinically and pathologically indistinguishable (see Table 56.1). Pathologic changes outside the CNS are found largely in the lungs and are related to the extent of respiratory impairment.

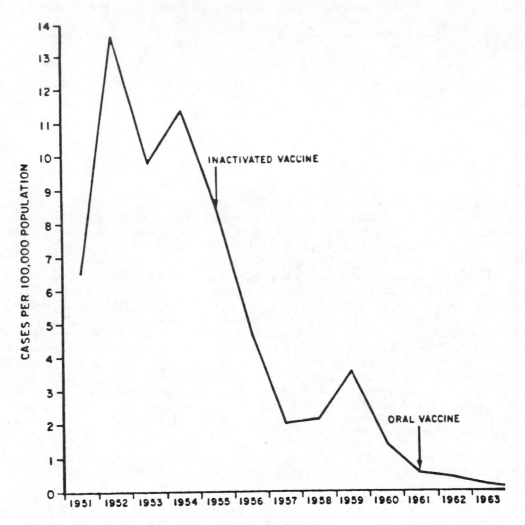

FIGURE 56.1   Paralytic poliomyelitis in the United States, 1951–1963. (From CDC Annual Summary–1980.)

Clinical Manifestations

Ninety to ninety-five percent of poliovirus infections are inapparent, 4–8% are abortive, and 1–2% are frank illnesses, either paralytic or nonparalytic.   Pregnancy, older age, trauma, exertion, and immunodeficiency increase the frequency or severity of paralytic disease. Tonsillectomy before or shortly after exposure can lead to bulbar poliomyelitis.

Abortive poliomyelitis can be identified only during epidemics because the symptoms of fever, malaise, headache, nausea, vomiting, constipation, and abdominal pain are nonspecific. The symptoms of nonparalytic disease are the same as those of abortive poliomyelitis except the headache, nausea, and vomiting are more intense. Stiffness of the neck, back, and hamstrings also occurs. Examination of the CSF at this time shows changes characteristic of aseptic meningitis. If the lumbar puncture is repeated in 2 weeks, the CSF protein concentration is much higher. Muscle weakness may become apparent weeks after the acute infection.

The onset of paralytic disease may develop suddenly or more slowly and be preceded by weakness. Other symptoms are similar to those of nonparalytic disease. The distribution of paralysis is asymmetric, and the legs are more vulnerable than the arms. Difficulty in breathing results from weakness of chest muscles or from involvement of cranial nerve nuclei, or both. Signs of respiratory impairment include an anxious expression, increased respiratory rate, breathless speech, abdominal breathing, retracting, pooling of secretions, and poor cough. Hypertension, arrhythmias, pulmonary edema, renal failure, stress ulcers, and psychosis also may occur.

Diagnosis

During epidemics paralytic poliomyelitis is easily diagnosed clinically. Nonparalytic disease can be suspected on epidemiologic grounds and the diagnosis confirmed either by culturing pharyngeal secretions, CSF, and feces for poliovirus, or serologically with acute and convalescent antibody titers. Interpretation of culture results or antibody titers is made difficult today because vaccine virus is widespread and elevated titers or the presence of poliovirus in body secretions is not necessarily diagnostic of poliomyelitis.

In addition to echoviruses and coxsackieviruses causing paralytic illness identical to poliomyelitis, other diseases can resemble it. Guillain-Barré syndrome in adults is easily confused with paralytic poliomyelitis. Other diseases to consider in the differential diagnosis of poliomyelitis include transverse myelitis, postinfectious myelitis, tick paralysis, tuberculous meningitis, diabetic neuropathy, and pseudoparalysis due to osteomyelitis, fracture, or acute rheumatic fever.

Treatment

The treatment of poliomyelitis is supportive. Relief of muscle pain is the major problem in nonparalytic illness. Patients with paralytic illness require admission to centers experienced in management of respiratory failure. After the acute phase of illness is over, rehabilitation is the principal goal.

Prevention

Vaccination with either the inactivated poliovirus vaccine (IPV) or the live attenuated oral poliovirus vaccine (OPV) will prevent poliomyelitis. The introduction of IPV in 1955 in the United States resulted in a progressive decline in the occurrence of paralytic disease. The OPV was licensed in 1961 and became the recommended method of immunization because it was easy to administer, induced local IgA, and resulted in immunization of some contacts of vaccinated individuals.

The effectiveness of either IPV or OPV is without question. At the peak of epidemic poliomyelitis in the United States there were 21,000 cases of paralytic illness. In 1980 only eight cases of paralytic poliomyelitis were reported to the Centers for Disease Control; four of these cases were classified as vaccine virus associated. The association of vaccine virus with paralytic disease has caused a major controversy, and some authorities have suggested returning to IPV as the primary vaccine. The widespread presence of vaccine virus in the population and the knowledge that other enteroviruses can cause paralytic disease make the question of vaccine-induced disease hard to assess. At the present time in the United States OPV is the principal vaccine, with IPV as an alternative. The IPV is recommended for persons with heightened susceptibility to infection, including immunodeficient children and their siblings, and adults undergoing initial vaccination in preparation for travel to areas with a high prevalence of disease.

Selected Bibliography

Centers for Disease Control: Poliomyelitis prevention. *Morbid Mortal Wk Rep* 31: 22–23, 1982.

Centers for Disease Control: Annual summary – 1980. *Morbid Mortal Wk Rep* 29: 64–65, 1981.

Feigin, R. D., Guggenheim, M. A., and Johnsen, S. D.: Vaccine-related paralytic poliomyelitis in an immunodeficient child. *J Pediatr* 79:642–647, 1971.

Mayer, T. R. and Balfour, H. H.: Prevalence of poliovirus neutralizing antibodies in young adult women. *JAMA* 246:1207–1209, 1981.

Nathanson, N. and Martin, J. R.: The epidemiology of poliomyelitis: Enigmas surrounding its appearance, epidemicity, and disappearance. *Am J Epidemiol* 110:672–692, 1979.

Nightingale, E. O.: Recommendations for a national policy on poliomyelitis vaccination. *N Engl J Med* 297:249–253, 1977.

Ogra, P. L.: Effect of tonsillectomy and adenoidectomy on nasopharyngeal antibody response to poliovirus. *N Engl J Med* 284:59–64, 1971.

Sabin, A. B.: Poliomyelitis vaccination: Evaluation and direction in continuing application. *Am J Clin Pathol* 70:136–140, 1978.

Sabin, A. B.: Paralytic poliomyelitis: Old dogmas and new perspectives. *Rev Infect Dis* 3:543–564, 1981.

Salk, D.: Eradication of poliomyelitis in the United States. I. Live virus vaccine-associated and wild poliovirus disease. *Rev Infect Dis* 2:228–242, 1980.

Salk, D.: Eradication of poliomyelitis in the United States. II. Experience with killed poliovirus vaccine. *Rev Infect Dis* 2:243–257, 1980.

Salk, D.: Eradication of poliomyelitis in the United States. III. Practical considerations. *Rev Infect Dis* 2:258–273, 1980.

57

CORONAVIRUSES
Robert H. Waldman, M.D.

The coronaviruses are relatively recently identified, difficult to isolate viruses which are commonly associated with upper respiratory infection, and possibly with gastrointestinal infection. This group of viruses was given the name "coronavirus" because they have surface projections which look like a crown when seen by electron microscopy.

Microbiology

Coronaviruses are RNA viruses and are composed of several serotypes which cross-react immunologically only slightly. One of this group of viruses was first isolated from nasal wash fluids cultured on organ cultures of human embryonic trachea.

Epidemiology

The virus has a worldwide distribution, causes disease most commonly in winter and spring, and accounts for about 15% of all viral upper respiratory infections. At least half of the infections are subclinical, and half of all children have been infected by about age 3. More than two-thirds of adults have been infected with one of the common coronavirus strains. Reinfection is common. The incubation period is from 2 to 5 days.

Diagnostic Features

The specific etiologic diagnosis can only be made in the laboratory since one cannot differentiate those infections caused by coronavirus from those caused by other viruses commonly infecting the upper respiratory tract. There are slight differences which may be apparent epidemiologically, but which are very unreliable with respect to differentiating the exact viral etiology in an individual patient. As mentioned previously, the infection is most commonly subclinical. When symptoms are present, the patient has a mild upper respiratory infection. The incubation period, on the average, is slightly longer than that for rhinovirus, and the duration of illness is slightly shorter than that for rhinovirus (Table 57.1). Fever is low-grade and is present in only about 20% of patients. In essence, if illness is present, the symptoms are those of a typical common cold. There may be a related gastroenteritis as well, but this has not been definitely shown to be caused by a coronavirus. In infants, coronavirus infection has occasionally caused pneumonia.

In armed forces recruits, a slightly more serious illness than that just described results. It is somewhat similar to that caused by adenovirus in this population.

Treatment and Prognosis

Treatment is supportive and the prognosis is good. Coronaviruses are probably the most benign pathogens of the upper respiratory tract. The only problems are in patients with chronic lung disease in whom coronavirus infection may cause an exacerbation.

Immunology

Little is known about the immunology of coronavirus infection, and vaccine development appears unlikely because the disease is relatively benign, reinfection is common, and there are several serotypes.

TABLE 57.1   Comparison of Common Cold Syndrome Caused by
             Coronavirus and Rhinovirus

Symptom	Coronavirus	Rhinovirus
Incubation period	3.3 days	2.1 days
Duration of illness	6.5 days	9.5 days
Malaise	45%	25%
Fever	20%	15%
Cough	35%	60%

Selected Bibliography

Bradburne, A. F. and Somerset, B. A.: Coronavirus antibody titres in sera of healthy adults and experimentally infected volunteers. *J Hyg* 70:235-244, 1972.

Caul, E. O. and Clarke, S. K. R.: Coronavirus propagated from patient with non-bacterial gastroenteritis. *Lancet* 2:953-954, 1975.

Cavallaro, J. J. and Monto, A. S.: Community wide outbreak of infection with a 229E-like coronavirus in Tecumseh, Michigan. *J Infect Dis* 122:272-279, 1970.

Gump, D. W., Phillips, C. A., Forsyth, B. R., McIntosh, K., Lamborn, K. R., and Stouch, W. H.: Role of infection in chronic bronchitis. *Am Rev Respir Dis* 113:465-474, 1976.

Hendley, J. O., Fishburne, H. B., and Gwaltney, J. M., Jr.: Coronavirus infections in working adults: Eight-year study of 229E OC43. *Am Rev Respir Dis* 105: 805-811, 1972.

McIntosh, K.: Coronaviruses: A comparative review. *Curr Top Microbiol Immunol* 63:85-129, 1974.

McIntosh, K., Chao, R. K., Krause, H. E., Wasil, R., Mocega, H. E., and Mufson, M. A.: Coronavirus infection in acute lower respiratory tract disease of infants. *J Infect Dis* 130:502-507, 1974.

McIntosh, K., Ellis, E. F., Hoffman, L. S., Lybass, T. G., Eller, J. J., and Fulginiti, V. A.: The association of viral and bacterial respiratory infections with exacerbations of wheezing in young asthmatic children. *J Pediatr* 82:578-590, 1973.

McIntosh, K., Kapikian, A. Z., Turner, H. C., Hartley, J. W., Parrott, R. H., and Chanock, R. M.: Seroepidemiologic studies of coronavirus infection in adults and children. *Am J Epidemiol* 91:585-592, 1970.

Wenzel, R. P., Hendley, J. O., Davies, J. A., Gwaltney, J. M., Jr.: Coronavirus infections in military recruits: Three-year study with coronavirus strains OC43 229E. *Am Rev Respir Dis* 109:621-624, 1974.

58

TOGAVIRUSES (ARBOVIRUSES)
Robert H. Waldman, M.D.

This group of viruses was originally classified as arboviruses because they were arthropod-borne. The term arboviruses has been discontinued in the official classification because there are several viruses which are transmitted to humans, but which do not lend themselves to inclusion with the main grouping (Table 58.1). This will be discussed in more detail in this and the succeeding chapters. Togaviruses are enveloped RNA viruses which are assembled in the cytoplasm of infected cells. They have similar epidemiology and clinical findings, and since the latter are not unique for any of these specific diseases, diagnosis is dependent upon laboratory testing. Most of these viruses frequently cause asymptomatic infection, the lowest ratio of inapparent/apparent infection being Eastern equine encephalitis, with a 25:1 ratio. Although greatly feared, these viruses cause relatively little morbidity and mortality, with Japanese B and Eastern equine encephalitis being the most severe (Table 58.2).

Microbiology

The togavirus family is made up of three genera important with respect to human infection, *Alphavirus, Flavivirus,* and *Rubivirus.* The important viruses in the *Alphavirus* genus are Eastern equine encephalitis, Western equine encephalitis, Venezuelan equine encephalitis, and Chikungunya (Table 58.3). The latter virus will not be discussed in detail because of its remote geographic distribution (Africa, India, and Southeast Asia), and because it results in a dengue-like illness which is rarely differentiated clinically from typical dengue. Viruses of the genus exhibit some serologic cross-reactivity.

TABLE 58.1   Modern Classification of Viruses, Many of Which Were
Recently Grouped Together as Arboviruses

Families	Genera	Species	
Arenaviridae		Junin	No arthropod vector
		Machupo	
Togaviridae	*Alphavirus*	EEE	
		VEE	
		WEE	Includes Sindbis
		Semliki	Includes Chikungunya
	Flavivirus	SLE	
		Dengue	
		Yellow Fever	
		Japanese B	

TABLE 58.2   Average Number of Cases (and Deaths) per Year,
Arthropod-Borne Encephalitis

Disease	Cases	Deaths
St. Louis encephalitis	60	4.0
California encephalitis	60	0.2
Western equine encephalitis	35	0.9
Eastern equine encephalitis	3	1.9

The flaviviruses are slightly smaller in size and grow more slowly in tissue culture than the alphaviruses. The important flaviviruses are yellow fever, dengue, St. Louis encephalitis virus, and Powassan encephalitis viruses (Table 58.4).

A third togavirus genus is the *Rubivirus* which contains rubella virus. It is discussed in a separate chapter.

Related to the togavirus family is the bunyavirus family, the most important member being the California encephalitis virus.

The togaviruses have many common histopathologic features of the central nervous system. Infection leads to cellular infiltration by neutrophilic granulocytes, followed by lymphocytes, monocytes, and plasma cells in a perivascular distribution. This is followed by microglial hyperplasia and neuronal degeneration.

TABLE 58.3 Epidemiology and Ecology of Alphaviruses

Virus	Geographic Distribution	Habitat	Reservoir	Mosquito Vector	Season	Incidence	% Fatal
EEE	Atlantic and Gulf coasts	Freshwater swamps	Wild birds	*Culiseta melanura*	Summer and early fall	Average of about 3 cases per year in U.S.	50
WEE	West of Mississippi River	Freshwater swamps and irrigated areas	Wild birds, especially English sparrows	*Culiseta melanura* and *Culex tarsalis*	Summer and early fall	Average of about 20 cases, mainly infants and children	~ 3
VEE	Central and South America, southern U.S.		Rodents and horses	*Culex* spp and others	Variable	Average of < 3 cases per year in U.S.	Rare

TABLE 58.4   Epidemiology and Ecology of More Important Flaviviruses

Virus	Vector	Host	Geographic Distribution	Classical Clinical Manifestation(s)	Control
Yellow fever	Mosquito: *Aedes aegypti* and other *Aedes* spp	Humans and nonhuman primates	South America and Africa	Hepatitis	Immunization and mosquito control
Dengue	*A. aegypti* mosquito	Humans	Worldwide, mainly tropical	Fever, severe myalgias, rash, sometimes hemorrhagic	Mosquito control
St. Louis encephalitis	*Culex* spp of mosquito	Birds, especially English sparrows	Western hemisphere	Encephalitis, more severe in older people	Mosquito control
Tick-borne encephalitis	*Ixodes persulcatus* and *I. ricinus*	Rodents, birds, goats, cattle	NE and Central Europe	Encephalitis (mortality in 20%)	Tick control, inactivated vaccine of unknown efficacy

Eastern Equine Encephalitis (EEE)

Wild birds habitating swamps are the usual host and reservoir for this virus. The insect vectors are several mosquito species, the predominant one being *Culiseta melanura*. The virus is most commonly found along the Atlantic and Gulf coasts in late summer.

Clinical disease is found most commonly in young children and the elderly. There are few nonspecific prodromal symptoms, and usually there is the abrupt onset of high fever, headache, nuchal rigidity, and vomiting which may progress over 24-48 hr to drowsiness, convulsions, and coma. Focal neurologic signs are common but inconsistent.

The spinal fluid obtained early in the course of illness may look like bacterial meningitis, with 500-3000 leukocytes, mainly polymorphonuclear leukocytes. The sugar concentration, however, is nearly always normal. Spinal fluid obtained slightly later shows a shift to predominantly mononuclear leukocytes. The virus is isolated only rarely from spinal fluid.

The prognosis is not good, with a 50-75% mortality, and those who recover usually have severe neurologic sequelae, such as mental deficiency, convulsions, aphasia, or hemiplegia.

Western Equine Encephalitis (WEE)

Epidemiologically and clinically WEE has many similarities to EEE, except that it is usually a more benign illness. As with EEE, the very young and very old are affected more severely. Of those who demonstrate illness, approximately one-third progress to stupor or coma. Patients usually begin to improve rapidly after 5-10 days of illness. Spinal fluid findings are similarly less severe than those of EEE, usually with a cell count less than $200/mm^3$ and with mononuclear cells predominating.

Mortality from WEE is about 10% and sequelae are unusual; however, seizures, motor dysfunction, and behavioral problems are occasionally seen following the illness in young children.

The treatment for WEE, like all of this group of viral infections, is supportive. Prevention is theoretically possible, this again being true of all of this group of viral infections, by vaccine development, but it is not practical because of the low prevalence of disease. Vector control is the only practical measure for prevention of outbreaks of this group of diseases.

Venezuelan Equine Encephalitis (VEE)

This is the mildest of the alphavirus infections, its classic distribution being in South and Central America. However, recently natural occurrence of the disease in the United States has been reported in southern Florida. This represents a trend which has been going on for several years, i.e., the gradual spread of the disease northward. The most common cycle of this disease is the rodent-to-mosquito and back to rodent. Many mosquito species transmit the disease, the most common of which is *Culex melanoconion*. The virus has a broad host range, naturally infecting many mammalian, avian, and reptilian species. In all of the various animal species infected, the asymptomatic host is very common, despite the presence of viremia. This represents an important reservoir for the infection.

Clinically, patients may demonstrate a brief, uneventful febrile illness, a moderately severe systemic viral infection similar to dengue, or the most severe, encephalitis (Table 58.5). The latter represents only about 5% of clinically ill patients.

In those patients who have encephalitis, the mortality is less than 10%, usually children. Sequelae are uncommon, but occasionally a child will show personality changes or motor defects.

Attempts to control the spread of the infection have so far been unsuccessful. A live, attenuated vaccine for use in horses, a reservoir which seems particularly important in human disease, has been quite effective in experimental use.

St. Louis Encephalitis (SLE)

St. Louis encephalitis is the most important arthropod-borne illness in the United States. It causes an average of about 10% of the cases of encephalitis, but in some years this increases significantly, e.g., 1975, when SLE accounted for nearly one-half of the total. The disease occurs in epidemics; however, the factors leading to epidemics and our ability to predict them have eluded discovery. The asymptomatic to symptomatic infection rate is about 200:1. In an average epidemic, the case rate is about 200:100,000 population, but nearly one-half of the population can be shown to have been infected during the epidemic. The disease is more prevalent in warmer climates and epidemics occur in mid- to late summer.

The vector is various mosquito species, usually those of the *Culex* genus. The usual hosts are birds, which are the only animals which have a sustained viremia. Because of its commonness, the English sparrow is the most important reservoir. It is interesting that humans are incidental hosts, i.e., they do not play an important role in sustaining the transmission cycle of the virus, but they are the only host which is known to have clinical illness. Outside the United States, although there is evidence that infection is not uncommon, little or no illness occurs during outbreaks. One can only conclude that this is due to differences in virulence of various strains of virus. Location of one's residence correlates quite well with the attack rate, i.e., there is a greater chance of infection if one lives near an area of high population of infected birds. Socioeconomic class, except as it relates to location of housing, is of no importance.

TABLE 58.5   VEE: Clinical Syndromes

Influenzal	Only constitutional symptoms, febrile course 1-4 days
Fulminant	Short febrile course with rapid progression to shock, coma, and convulsions; DIC; survivors often have sequelae
Encephalitic	Fever for 2 wk or more, sometimes diphasic; CNS symptoms and signs develop during latter phase; usually no sequelae

The incubation period is estimated to be from 4 to 21 days, based on occurrence of illness in travelers coming from an epidemic focus. The disease is much more likely to be symptomatic in elderly individuals.

The illness cannot be differentiated from other forms of encephalitis on the basis of clinical picture. Common symptoms and signs are fever, headache, nausea and vomiting, nuchal rigidity, disorientation, disturbances of consciousness, and tremor. The syndrome of inappropriate antidiuretic hormone secretion, usually mild, occurs in about one-third of the patients. Less common findings are paralyses, ataxia, and seizures. Spinal fluid shows increased protein levels, an increased number of cells, but usually less than $500/mm^3$ with polymorphonuclear leukocytes found early, quickly changing to preponderantly mononuclear cells. Thus, the clinical and laboratory picture is similar to a number of causes of encephalitis and/or aseptic meningitis.

Virus isolation from spinal fluid or blood is so rarely successful that it is not worth attempting. A rise in serum antibody, as determined by hemagglutination inhibition, is the best way to make a definitive diagnosis. Unfortunately, false-positive and false-negative results using the HI test are not rare.

Recovery often occurs precipitously. The mortality is about 10%, but in patients over 60 years of age, this is significantly increased, to about 35%. A prolonged and high fever is a bad prognostic sign. Sequelae are fairly common, but very subjective, including nervousness, headache, and emotional instability. Three years after the illness, about twice as many patients will complain of one or more of these symptoms than would matched controls who have not had the illness. About 10% of patients will be nonfunctional. On the other hand, before the era of advanced life support in critical care units, many of these patients would have died.

Mosquito control is probably effective in decreasing the chance of having an epidemic, but is unproved and probably ineffective once an epidemic has started.

Extensive investigation into prediction of epidemics has been unsuccessful despite careful evaluation of the impact of weather and virus isolation from mosquitoes or birds. There is some recent evidence that an accurate predictor of outbreaks is found by detecting a rise in serum antibody in wild birds.

Dengue

Dengue is known picturesquely as "break-bone fever." Its most severe form is known as dengue hemorrhagic fever (DHF), the manifestations of which are caused by disseminated intravascular coagulation, thought to be a result of circulating immune complexes of antibody and viral antigens. Table 58.6 lists the various hemorrhagic fevers and the viral groups responsible for them. There are at least four serotypes of dengue virus which cross-react immunologically and DHF may be a result of infection in a person who has high titers of cross-reacting antibody as a result of a previous infection with another serotype.

The disease is prevalent in Southeast Asia, Africa, and the Caribbean. Parts of the United States along the Mexican border have great potential for epidemics. Humans are the only known host and the *Aedes aegypti* mosquito is the main vector.

Epidemics in the tropics occur in the rainy season as a result of an increase in the vector density. In more temperate areas outbreaks occur in the summer. In addition to epidemics the disease also is endemic in some areas. During epidemics the attack rate varies from 20 to 80%.

The typical patient develops fever, headache, myalgias and arthralgias, with the low back and thighs commonly the most painful (Tables 58.7 and 58.8). About one-third of patients develop a skin rash which may become hemorrhagic, and which is most common on the extremities and/or torso. A few patients will show evidence of liver involvement with mild jaundice.

TABLE 58.6   Hemorrhagic Fevers

Togaviruses	Yellow Fever
	Dengue
	Crimean hemorrhagic fever (also known as Central Asian hemorrhagic fever)
	Omsk hemorrhagic fever
	Kyasanur Forest disease
Arenaviruses	Bolivian hemorrhagic fever
	Argentine hemorrhagic fever
Unclassified	Marburg disease
	African hemorrhagic fever (Ebola virus)
	Korean hemorrhagic fever

TABLE 58.7   Characteristics of Dengue Hemorrhagic Fever (DHF) and Dengue Shock Syndrome (DSS)

DHF	1. Positive tourniquet test ($\geq$ 20 petechiae/in.^{2})
	2. Hemoconcentration (rise in hematocrit of $\geq$ 20%)
	3. Thrombocytopenia (platelet count < 100,000/mm^3)
DSS	Above, plus hypotension or narrowing of pulse pressure to $\leq$ 20 mmHg
Mortality of DSS	Without rapid volume replacement: 10–20%
	With rapid volume volume replacement: $\leq$ 3%

TABLE 58.8   Symptoms and Signs of Dengue

Symptom	% of Patients
Severe myalgia	100
Arthralgia	90
Retro-ocular pain	75
Nausea	75
Maculopapular rash	30

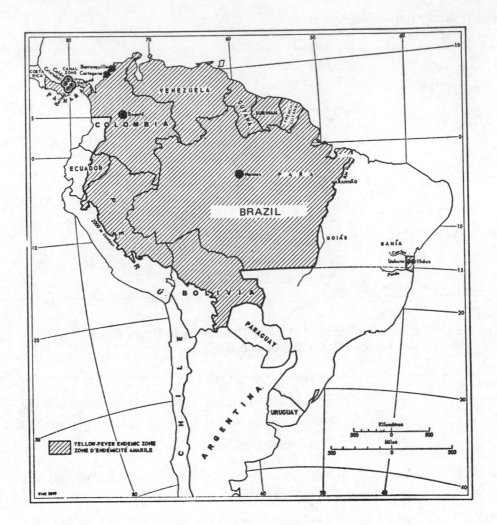

FIGURE 58.1A Yellow fever endemic areas, South America.

Treatment of severe illness involves aggressive fluid replacement and correction of acidosis. In the usual case, after an acute illness of 5-7 days, there is a rather prolonged period of postfebrile asthenia. Patients with DHF have a 5-10% mortality.

Prevention of the disease is by mosquito control with special attention to breeding areas. A live, attenuated vaccine has been tested experimentally, and may be available for general use in endemic and epidemic areas soon.

Yellow Fever (Figure 58.1)

Yellow fever is an important disease historically, being the first viral disease shown to be transmitted by mosquitoes and being the first tropical disease to be brought under control by immunization. It is transmitted from humans or non-human primates by mosquitoes, mainly A. aegypti.

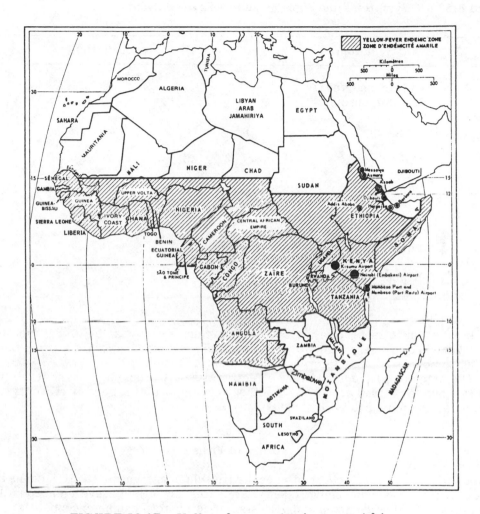

FIGURE 58.1B   Yellow fever endemic areas, Africa.

The histopathology is characteristic, showing coagulative midzonal degeneration of the liver. The liver usually heals completely with little or no scarring. A characteristic finding is the Councilman body, which is hyalinization of the cytoplasm of dead hepatic cells. In addition to liver involvement, patients may have renal damage and coagulopathy.

The incubation period is 3-6 days; therefore, the diagnosis should be suspected in any person returning from an endemic area who becomes ill within this time. Patients characteristically have a relative bradycardia, fever, chills, and headache, all of which come on very suddenly (Table 58.9). Patients have hepatomegaly and jaundice, but no splenomegaly, which helps differentiate the disease from malaria. The clinical course is often biphasic with a period of improvement before further deterioration. Laboratory evaluation shows evidence for disseminated intravascular coagulation. The diagnosis can be confirmed by virus isolation from blood or by showing a rise in serum neutralizing antibody. The diagnosis should be made by means other than liver biopsy because this is a very dangerous procedure in this illness. The differential diagnosis includes malaria, dengue, other causes of viral hepatitis, influenza, leptospirosis, and toxin exposure.

TABLE 58.9   Symptoms and Signs in Yellow Fever Patients

Symptom	% of Patients
Chills and fever (abrupt onset)	96
Headache	90
Myalgias	75
Vomiting	70
Jaundice	100
Palatal petechiae	70
Black vomit	20

In addition to supportive therapy hyperimmune serum may be used. The fatality rate is extremely variable, 10-60%. Bad prognostic signs are a rising pulse, falling temperature, and deterioration of mental status.

The attenuated vaccine is very effective, its only problem being heat lability, and it should be stored at -25°C. Another very important aspect of prevention is control of the mosquito vector.

Powassan Virus

Powassan virus is a rare cause of encephalitis which is transmitted to humans by ticks, with the reservoir being rodents. It causes a relatively severe encephalitis with sequelae being common and very similar to Eastern equine encephalitis.

Selected Bibliography

Bailey, C. L., Eldridge, B. F., Hayes, D. E., Watts, D. M., Tammariello, R. F., and Dalrymple, J. M.: Isolation of St. Louis encephalitis virus from overwintering *Culex pipens* mosquitoes. *Science* 199:1346-1349, 1978.

Bokisch, V. A., Top, F. H., Jr., Russell, P. K., Dixon, F. J., and Muller-Eberhard, H. J.: The potential pathogenic role of complement in dengue hemorrhagic shock syndrome. *N Engl J Med* 289:996-1000, 1973

Creech, W. B.: St. Louis encephalitis in the United States, 1975. *J Infect Dis* 135:1014-1016, 1977.

Ehrenkranz, N. J., Sinclair, M. C., Buff, E., and Lyman, D. O.: The natural occurrence of Venezuelan equine encephalitis in the United States. *N Engl J Med* 282:298-302, 1970.

Ehrenkranz, N. J. and Ventura, A. K.: Venezuelan equine encephalitis virus infection in man. *Ann Rev Med* 25:9, 1974.

Ehrenkranz, N. J., Ventura, A. K., Cuadrado, R. R., Pond, W. L., and Porter, J. E.: Pandemic dengue in Caribbean countries and the Southern United States – past, present and potential problems. *N Engl J Med* 285:1460-1469, 1971.

Elton, N. W., Romero, A., and Trejos, A.: Clinical pathology of yellow fever. *J Clin Pathol* 25:135, 1955.

Luby, J. P.: St. Louis encephalitis. *Epidemiol Rev* 1:55, 1979.

McConnell, S.: Venezuelan equine encephalomyelitis: Past, present, and future. *J Am Vet Med Assoc* 161:1579-1583, 1972.

McGowan, J. E., Jr., Bryan, J. A., and Gregg, M. B.: Surveillance of arboviral encephalitis in the United States, 1955-1971. *Am J Epidemiol* 97:199-207, 1973.

Miller, J. R. and Harter, D. H.: Acute viral encephalitis. *Med Clin N Am* 56: 1393-1404, 1972.

Powell, K. E. and Blakey, D. L.: St. Louis encephalitis. *Epidemiol Rev* 1:55, 1979.

Powell, K. E. and Kappus, K. D.: Epidemiology of St. Louis encephalitis and other acute encephalitides. *Adv Neurol* 19:197-215, 1978.

Smith, R., Woodall, J. P., Whitney, E., Deibel, R., Gross, M. A., Smith, V., and Bast, T. F.: Powassan virus infection. A report of three human cases of encephalitis. *Am J Dis Child* 127:691-693, 1974.

59

BUNYAVIRUSES
Robert H. Waldman, M.D.

California encephalitis virus is the only bunyavirus of importance in the United States (Table 59.1). However, the sand fly fever group viruses which cause acute febrile illnesses in Latin America and the Mediterranean area also belong to this group. The illness caused by the sand fly fever group is known by a variety of names, including Rift Valley fever and Crimean hemorrhagic fever. These are RNA viruses.

California encephalitis is most common in children, especially boys who climb trees. This is because the mosquito vector is commonly found in the lower branches of trees.

Clinically, the disease is similar to other viral encephalitides, and the spectrum of disease ranges from completely asymptomatic persons, to mild nonspecific febrile illness, to fatal encephalitis. Spinal fluid composition is also similar to other encephalitides, and the specific virologic diagnosis can be made by showing a rise in serum antibody titer.

The prognosis is good, with sequelae such as seizures, learning disability, and personality changes being unusual.

TABLE 59.1   California Encephalitis Group of Bunyaviruses Known
to Cause Human Disease

Virus	Mosquito Vector	Principal Vertebrate Host	Geographic Distribution
LaCrosse	*Aedes triseriatus*	Chipmunk, squirrels	Upper Mississippi River valley
California	*A. melanimon*	Ground squirrel	California, Texas, Utah
Tahyna	*Culiseta annulata* and *Aedes* spp	Hares	Europe

Selected Bibliography

Watts, D. M., Thompson, W. H., Yuill, T. M., et al.: Overwintering of LaCrosse
virus in *Aedes triseriatus. Am J Trop Med Hyg* 23:694, 1974.

60

RUBELLA
Rama Ganguly, Ph.D.

Etiology

Rubella virus is the causative agent of German measles and is one of the common childhood exanthems. What makes this disease extraordinary, however, is its teratogenic potential. In the Australian outbreak in 1941, it was recognized that maternal rubella, especially when contracted during the first trimester of pregnancy, was associated with a high occurrence of congenital abnormalities. This observation emphasizes the importance of rubella control and immunization programs. The goal is to protect the future fetus, not the vaccinee per se.

Taxonomically, rubella virus is a togavirus (groups A and B arboviruses), since it is an RNA virus with an envelope (toga). Rubella virus is of a single antigenic type and does not cross-react with other members of the togavirus group. It is an ether-sensitive RNA virus which is unstable at 37 and 56°C but not at -60°C or below. Being an enveloped virus, it is sensitive also to chloroform and to the detergent sodium deoxycholate. The nucleocapsid core of rubella virus contains a single-stranded RNA. Negative-staining techniques show small spikes projecting 50-60 Å from the envelopes of most particles which accounts for the hemagglutinating activities of the virus with fowl and human RBC. Rubella virus is isolated by viral interference assays using green monkey kidney cells. The adapted virus produces significant cytopathic effect in cells in tissue cultures. Human diploid cells, when chronically infected with rubella virus, exhibit many chromosomal breaks. Similar pathogenic mechanisms and impaired cellular division may account for the congenital lesions observed in the infected fetus when the infection has occurred during organogenesis.

Epidemiology

Rubella virus is a highly infectious agent and is spread from person to person by aerosolized nasopharyngeal secretions. Rubella became a nationally reportable disease in 1966 in the United States. The disease is rather mild, hence medical care often is not sought, and cases may therefore go unrecognized. Thus only one in every five to ten clinical cases is reported. Usually several completely inapparent infections occur per case; however, these subclinical cases are epidemiologically significant. Sizable epidemics occur every 6-9 years and major outbreaks occur at up to 30-year intervals. The peak incidence is found in 5- to 9-year-old children. Approximately 80-85% of the population become immune to the disease by the age of 15 years. The 15-20% of the population susceptible to the disease in the childbearing age is the group of concern who need to be protected. The pattern of immunity in isolated communities such as certain islands of Hawaii, northern Japan, and Trinidad is rather low at all ages (25-50%). In these places, rubella occurs repeatedly and is endemic, but sizable epidemics fail to occur. The reason for this variation is not understood. Table 60.1 indicates the percentage distribution of reported rubella cases in the United States during 1977-1978.

Pathogenesis and Pathology

The incubation period of rubella virus infection is 14-25 days after which the rash appears. The mode of virus replication and dissemination is similar to that of smallpox and measles. After implantation of the virus on the respiratory tract, it multiplies locally on the mucous membrane surfaces of the nasopharynx as well as in the local lymph nodes. This is followed by viral dissemination in the blood, and virus shedding from the throat. Seven days before and after the appearance of the rash, the virus can be recovered from the respiratory tract secretions. The rash appears on the face and rapidly spreads to the chest, abdomen, and then to the extremities. Before the onset of the disease the virus is present also in the leukocytes and in synovial and conjunctival fluids. The prodromal period is usually 1-2 days and is accompanied by fever, malaise, mild coryza, and prominent cervical and occipital lymphadenopathy. Cough and conjunctivitis also may occur following viral dissemination in the respiratory tract. Rubella virus can be isolated from blood 1-2 days before and after the rash appears. Rubella basically resembles measles in its clinical picture but is much milder. The virus has been isolated from the genital tract of women, indicating fetal infection by the ascending route may occur in the absence of maternal viremia.

Diagnosis

Clinical

Clinical rubella is a mild disease and variable in symptoms. The most characteristic clinical feature of the disease is the involvement of certain lymph nodes, i.e., postauricular, suboccipital, and posterior cervical. These are usually enlarged and tender for several days before the rash. Transient polyarthralgia and polyarthritis may accompany or follow the illness. Joint symptoms are reported to occur more often in adult women, but they are also observed in adult men and children.

TABLE 60.1   Clinical Manifestations of Congenital Rubella

Intrauterine growth retardation

Failure to thrive

CNS	Psychomotor retardation
	Microcephaly
	Meningoencephalitis
	Chronic progressive panencephalitis (late)
Cardiovascular	Congenital heart disease
	Patent ductus
	Pulmonary artery or valvular stenosis
	VSD
	Fibromuscular proliferation of arterial intima

Interstitial pneumonitis

Auditory	Sensorineural hearing loss
	Vestibular dysfunction
	Otitis media
Ocular	Retinopathy
	Cataract
	Glaucoma
GU	Hypospadias
	Cryptorchidism
	Interstitial nephritis

Diabetes mellitus

Hematologic

Laboratory

The disease may be confused with measles and a number of coxsackie- and echo-virus infections. Virus may be isolated from nasopharyngeal secretions in tissue cultures of primary grivet monkey kidney cells in which the virus is detected by indirect interference assays. Several passages in tissue cultures are often required before the virus can be recovered. Antibodies usually appear very early in the illness. Hemagglutination-inhibition and neutralization antibodies rise promptly. Therefore, serologic testing, looking for rising titers in paired specimens, may be used as a rapid confirmatory diagnostic procedure. The first serum specimen is collected as soon as possible after the rash appears, and the second specimen is collected 4-7 days later. If the serum is not collected until after the patient has recovered, this method of diagnosis is not applicable. This often happens in pregnant women. In such cases, positive determination of a substantial amount of rubella antibody of the IgM class indicates recent infection. Fluorescent antibody techniques, hemolysis in gel, or ELISA (enzyme-linked immunoadsorbent assay) techniques may be used for rubella antibody titration. Complement-fixing antibodies usually rise later than do hemagglutination-inhibition antibodies. Therefore, complement-fixing antibody titers show changes in paired specimens when it may be too late for such changes in hemagglutination-inhibition antibodies.

Treatment

No treatment is required in uncomplicated clinical rubella. Aspirin may be given for relief of discomfort and bed rest is advised for patients with joint involvement. Platelet transfusions and corticosteroids may be useful in thrombocytopenic purpura. Encephalitis requires excellent supportive care as in the case of measles. The usefulness of gamma globulin in pregnant women exposed to rubella is questionable.

Immunology and Prevention

The natural disease induces long-lasting immunity. Three different attenuated vaccine strains have been developed for immunization: HPV$_{77}$ strain which has been passaged through primary green monkey kidney and duck embryo tissue cultures; Cendenhill strain has been isolated in green monkey kidney and passaged in rabbit kidney cells; RA 27/3 has been developed in human diploid WI 38 cells. These three strains are highly effective in providing protection against clinical rubella. The striking feature of the RA 27/3 strain is that it can be administered to recipients by the intranasal route and generates both local and circulating antibodies. This is in distinct contrast to the other two strains which are effective only upon parenteral administration and elicit mainly serum antibodies. Since the nasopharyngeal route is the primary site of infection of the virus, local mucosal immunity is also effective in preventing the subclinical nasopharyngeal carrier state of infection in vaccines, which might play an important role in dissemination of the virus to the susceptible pregnant women.

Rubella vaccine is contraindicated in pregnancy as the vaccine virus strains have teratogenic potential. Vaccine-generated immunity is long lasting, but it is much less pronounced than the immunity acquired from clinical disease. Side effects of immunization are mild and transient. Virus excretion from the throat occurs but is short in duration and does not spread to contacts. Viremia occurs after administration of the vaccines. The serologic response is similar to that in the natural disease. The U. S. Public Health Service Advisory Committee on Immunization Practices recommends rubella immunization of prepubertal schoolchildren. The idea is to develop a high degree of herd immunity to prevent virus circulation. The vaccine is available for use alone or in combination with measles and mumps virus vaccines. An alternative approach is to immunize only susceptible girls in the sixth or seventh grades. This approach has the disadvantage of not significantly decreasing wild virus circulation, but still would eliminate the danger of rubella in a susceptible pregnant woman, and has the advantage of greatly reducing the population which would receive the vaccine and would take advantage of the lifelong immunity induced by natural infection.

Since the licensing of rubella virus vaccine in 1969, both clinical and congenital rubella occurrence has declined. There has been a significant shift in the age of highest prevalence of the disease from the 5- to 9-year-old to the adolescent and young adult. It is too early to determine if vaccine-induced immunity will be capable of providing protection throughout the entire period of childbearing.

Cell-mediated immunity after rubella infection or immunization develops as indicated by delayed hypersensitivity reaction on in vitro tests. Again, the natural disease generates a more durable cellular immune response than that induced by vaccines.

Complications and Prognosis

Postinfection complications are minimal. Encephalitis and thrombocytopenic purpura occur in 1:6000 and 1:3000, respectively.

The most serious complication of rubella is the development of fetal anomalies during maternal infection, especially in the first trimester of pregnancy (15-35% incidence of fetal defects). The virus probably spreads to the fetus by the hematogenous route during maternal viremia. The infection disseminates to every fetal organ resulting in rapid death of some cells and persistent infection in others. Chromosomal aberrations and reduced cell division may result from continued infection. A striking feature of in utero rubella infection is a small-sized baby due to the diminution in the total number of cells. Infected clones of cells die out because they have a shorter life span and may induce serious development defects during the period of organogenesis. The fetus infected during the first trimester of pregnancy is often stillborn. Those who survive may have a wide range of congenital abnormalities: deafness, cataracts, cardiac anomalies, hepatosplenomegaly, thrombocytopenic purpura, icterus, anemia, and low birth weight (rubella syndrome). Virus shedding continues after birth (in the presence of IgG and IgM antibodies to rubella) until the infected cells eventually die.

Selected Bibliography

Bean, J. A., Burmeister, L. F., Paule, C. L., and Isacson, P.: A comparison of national infection and immunization estimates for measles and rubella. *Am J Public Health* 68:1214-1216, 1978.

Chang, T. W.: Rubella reinfection and intrauterine involvement. *J Pediatr* 84: 617-618, 1974.

Dudgeon, J. A.: Measles and rubella vaccines. *Arch Dis Child* 52:907-911, 1977.

Ganguly, R., Ogra, P. L., Regas, S., and Waldman, R. H.: Rubella immunization of volunteers via the respiratory tract. *Infect Immun* 8:497-502, 1973.

Gregg, N. McA.: Congenital cataract following German measles in the mother. *Trans Ophthalmol Soc Aust* 3:35-46, 1942.

Horstman, D. M.: Problems in measles and rubella. *Disease-a-Month* 24:28-52, 1978.

Knox, G. E.: Influence of infection on fetal growth and development. *J Reprod Med* 21:352-358, 1978.

Plotkin, S. A., Farquhar, J. D., and Ogra, P. L.: Immunologic properties of RA 27/3 rubella virus vaccine. *JAMA* 225:585-590, 1973.

Proceedings of the International Congress on Rubella Immunization. *Am J Dis Child* 118:1-410, 1969.

Tingle, A. J., Kettyls, G. D. M., and Ford, D. K.: Studies on vaccine-induced rubella arthritis. Serologic findings before and after immunization. *Arthritis Rheum* 22:400-402, 1979.

Weller, T. H. and Neva, F. A.: Propagation in tissue cultures of cytopathic agents from patients with rubella-like illness. *Proc Soc Exp Biol Med* 111:215-225, 1962.

61

RABIES
Robert H. Waldman, M.D.

Rabies virus causes a highly lethal meningoencephalitis which is usually transmitted to humans by inoculation of saliva from an animal bite. Until recent years it was thought to be uniformly fatal, but with the advent of advanced life-support techniques, there have been a few survivors, most of whom have, after long convalescent periods, apparently recovered completely. The disease is largely preventable by controlling the animal reservoir of the virus. The disease is of great interest, because it is so feared, because the ratio of individuals who receive postexposure immunoprophylaxis to the actual number of cases is so high, and because of the great historic importance of the disease. The original rabies vaccine was prepared by Louis Pasteur.

Microbiology and Epidemiology

Rabies virus is a rhabdovirus, the only virus in this group which is known to be a significant human pathogen. It is a bullet-shaped RNA virus.

Worldwide the most common animal bite leading to rabies in humans is that of dogs. However, in the United States, control of rabies in domestic animals has been relatively successful. Thus most cases result from wild animal bites, particularly those of skunks, bats, raccoons, and foxes (Table 61.1).

The disease is widely distributed throughout the world, and animal cases are reported in every state in the United States except Hawaii (Table 61.2). Although it is theoretically possible for humans to transmit the disease because virus is found in the saliva of human cases just as it is in animals, there have been no documented cases of human transmission, except a single instance of iatrogenic transmission from a patient who died of encephalitis, and whose corneas were transplanted to two recipients. It was only after the recipients developed rabies that it was ascertained that the donor had died of the disease.

TABLE 61.1   Incidence of Rabies in the United States, 1979

	Confirmed Cases	% of Total
Human	5	
Animal	5150[1]	
Wild		88
Skunks		59
Bats		15
Raccoons		10
Foxes[2]		3
Domestic		12
Cattle		4
Dogs		4
Cats		3

[1]67% increase over average number, 1973-1978; in 1980, 6405 cases

[2]Account for 70% of cases in Europe

TABLE 61.2   Areas Known to be Free of Rabies

Bermuda and most of the Caribbean islands

Northern Europe: United Kingdom, Ireland, Norway, Sweden, Finland

Japan, Taiwan, New Zealand, Australia, Fiji, Guam, American Samoa

The incubation period from inoculation to development of the first signs of the disease is extremely variable, from 1 week to 1 year, but in most cases, it is 3-8 weeks. In addition to transmission by inoculation of saliva, usually by a bite, but also by any method by which saliva might traverse the protective barrier of intact skin such as contact of contaminated material with a cut in the skin, the virus can also infect mucosal surfaces, hence transmission has apparently occurred by droplets of virus-containing material landing on the respiratory mucous membrane.

Pathology and Pathogenesis

Rabies virus infects nerves in the skin or mucosal surfaces and travels via the spinal nerves and dorsal root ganglia to the central nervous system. It replicates and spreads back down nerves to various organs in the body, most notably the salivary glands, but also the heart, lungs, kidneys, and eyes.

The pathognomonic finding in the brain is the Negri inclusion body.

Diagnosis

Rabies should be considered in the differential diagnosis of any patient with encephalitis. Obviously, the history of appropriate exposure is of utmost importance.

There is typically a prodrome, but it is not very helpful because it is almost completely nonspecific, i.e., consisting of headache, anorexia, and fever. The only finding that might alert the clinician that the patient has the prodrome of rabies, other than the history, is the finding in about one-half of patients of paresthesias around the site of viral inoculation.

A few days after the prodrome, the diagnosis usually becomes painfully apparent as acute neurologic symptoms and signs develop. The most common are aerophobia, i.e., a severe adverse reaction the patient has to air blowing on his skin, particularly around the face; hydrophobia, which is the result of inability to swallow liquids and handle secretions; hallucinations, confusion, lethargy, and rapid deterioration with seizures, coma, and respiratory arrest. The progression of these symptoms, in the absence of sophisticated life-support methods, is usually a matter of days (Table 61.3).

By supporting the patient and therefore prolonging the course of the disease, other signs develop. Patients usually have an ascending paralysis similar to the Guillain-Barré syndrome, this progresses to complete paralysis. Patients also usually develop evidence of hypothalamic involvement, most commonly troubles with temperature regulation, and either inappropriate secretion of antidiuretic hormone or diabetes insipidus. Patients also frequently develop evidence of myocardial involvement.

TABLE 61.3   Clinical Stages of Rabies

Stage	Duration	Symptoms and Signs
Incubation period	2-8 wk	None
Prodrome	2-10 days	Fever, malaise, anorexia, headache, paresthesias, or pain at site of bite
Acute neurologic	2-7 days	Agitation, hyperventilation, aphasia, paralysis, hydrophobia, pharyngeal spasms, delirium
Coma	Days to weeks	Hypotension, cardiac arrhythmia, hypoventilation, pituitary dysfunction, coma, infection, thromboembolism
Death or recovery	Months	

To confirm the diagnosis, the virus, the viral antigen, or an antibody rise to the virus, must be demonstrated. Virus can be isolated from saliva, brain, or occasionally from urine. Virus can also be identified electron microscopically or by immunofluorescence on tissue obtained from brain biopsy, or less invasively, skin biopsy or corneal touch preparations. The latter technique is the easiest as far as obtaining material, but has a fairly high false-negative rate, with only about 40% of patients having a positive test. A rise in serum antibody is also diagnostic, as long as the patient has not received a rabies vaccine, antiserum, or been transfused with whole blood. A noninfected, nonimmunized, nontransfused individual will have no detectable antibody.

Treatment and Prevention

These two aspects of rabies are discussed together because it is not easy to differentiate treatment from prevention in most situations. It is not well recognized that the most important measure in preventing rabies infection is the immediate and thorough washing of all suspicious wounds with soap and water. The next most important action is to very promptly capture the offending animal, if at all possible. After a suspicious bite or other wound, the next important decision is whether or not to begin postexposure prophylaxis (Table 61.4). Making this decision more difficult is that it must be made immediately because the chance of success is directly related to the speed with which treatment is begun. If the offending animal is a domestic one, i.e., a dog, and if it is acting normally at the time, observe it. If it is acting abnormally, or if it begins to act abnormally during the period of observation, have it killed, and have the head shipped, refrigerated, to a local or state laboratory for examination for rabies virus. If the offending animal is wild, but in your possession, it should be killed and handled in a similar fashion. The standard test currently used for determining if the animal is infected with rabies virus is the fluorescent rabies antibody test. If the animal has escaped and is of a species known to be one at risk of transmitting rabies, and if the attack were not provoked, then treatment should be begun immediately. Casual petting of a strange animal is considered a provocation. No prophylaxis need be given if the biting animal is a rodent (rat, mouse, guinea pig, or squirrel) or rabbit, these species have never been known to transmit rabies to humans. Again, it is important to emphasize that the sooner treatment is begun, the better the chance of preventing disease. Even if begun immediately, it should be recognized that immunotherapy is not 100% effective.

Immunotherapy is of two types, passive and active (Table 61.5). Both should be used in all cases. Active immunization should be carried out using the new human diploid cell rabies vaccine (HDCV). This vaccine is better than the old duck embryo vaccine because it is more immunogenic and has fewer side effects. Rabies virus is grown in human diploid tissue culture and inactivated by tri-n-butyl-phosphate. Passive immunization is carried out using rabies immune globulin (RIG) which is prepared from hyperimmunized human donors and is available in a preparation which contains 150 IU/ml.

Preexposure active immunization should be carried out in high-risk groups, using HDCV. Examples of persons at high risk are animal handlers, persons visiting an endemic area, and spelunkers.

Advice regarding rabies can be obtained from the Centers for Disease Control which can be reached by telephone at (404) 329-3311, or after business hours and on weekends at 329-3644.

TABLE 61.4   Postexposure[1] Rabies Prophylaxis

| Animal | | | |
Type	Condition	Condition of Attack	Treatment
Domestic (dog or cat)	Known to be healthy[2]	Provoked or un-unprovoked	None
	Ill, sacrificed, brain-positive	Provoked or un-provoked	Vaccine and antiserum[3]
	Unknown	Provoked	None
	Unknown	Unprovoked	Vaccine and antiserum
Carnivorous Wild (skunk, raccoon, fox, coyote, bobcat, or bat)	Captured, killed, brain-negative	Provoked or un-provoked	None
	Captured, killed, brain-positive	Provoked or un-provoked	Vaccine and antiserum
	Escaped	Provoked or un-provoked	Vaccine and antiserum

[1]Exposure: bite (penetration of skin by teeth); scratch, abrasion, open wound or mucous membrane contaminated by saliva, urine, or brain tissue. Casual contact such as petting an animal is not considered to be significant

[2]If bite to extremity and not severe, animal can be observed. If bite to head or particularly severe, animal should be sacrificed immediately

[3]HDCV, five to six doses, IM, on days 0, 3, 7, 14, 28 (World Health Organization recommends sixth dose on day 90), and human rabies immune globulin, 20 U/kg IM

TABLE 61.5   Other Aspects of Rabies Immunoprophylaxis

Serum antibody	1. "Protective" titer thought to be $\geq 1:16$ 2. Should be measured on day 28, and if not $\geq 1:16$, another dose of vaccine should be given 3. Titers may be obtained from local or state health departments, or CDC

HDCV	1. Five doses lead to $\geq 1:16$ titer in 100%
	2. > 120 persons bitten by animals known to be rabid, received HDCV (+RIG), and no rabies cases have resulted
	3. Reactions to vaccine
	   a. Pain, swelling at injection site in $\sim$ 25%
	   b. Mild systemic (e.g., headache, dizziness) in $\sim$ 20%
	   c. One reported case of Guillain-Barré syndrome
	4. Once started, immunization should not be stopped or interrupted because of local or mild systemic reaction; treat with aspirin
	5. Pregnancy is *not* a contraindication to immunization

DEV	1. 16-23 doses lead to $\geq 1:16$ titer in 85-90%

RIG	1. Appears to be of benefit if given up to 8 days after exposure
	2. 20 IU/kg
	   a. Half infiltrated into area of wound (after careful and thorough cleansing of wound)
	   b. Half IM
	3. Give no more than recommended dose because may suppress antibody response to HDCV

Previously immunized person	1. If exposed, should receive two doses of HDCV, on day 0 and day 3; no RIG
Live vaccine	1. For use in animals; has caused clinical rabies in animals, but no cases in humans despite several accidental exposures

TABLE 61.6   Complications of Rabies

CNS	Hydrophobia (spasms of pharynx)
	Seizures
	Cerebral edema
	Inappropriate ADH secretion
	Diabetes insipidus
	Hypo- and hyperthermia
Cardiovascular	Arrhythmia
	Congestive heart failure
	Hypotension
Respiratory	Aspiration
	Atelectasis
	Hypoxemia
	Pneumonia
Gastrointestinal hemorrhage	

With respect to supportive care of the patient, hypoxemia, cardiac arrhythmias, fluid imbalance, hypotension, and cerebral edema should be watched for and treated in the usual fashion (Table 61.6). Although there has never been a documented human-to-human transmission of rabies, care should be taken in handling body fluids. Virus is not found in blood, therefore no special precautions need to be taken with respect to that body fluid.

There is no evidence that interferon or other antiviral drugs are of any benefit, although they have been tried. Patients should be immunized against tetanus if their immunizations are not up to date, and measures should be taken to prevent or treat bacterial infection of the wound.

Selected Bibliography

Aok, F. S., Tyrrell, D. A., Nicholson, K. E., and Mill, L. E.: Human diploid cell strain rabies vaccine. *Lancet* 1:1379, 1976.

Bahmanyar, M., Fayza, A., Nour-Salehi, S., Mohammadi, M., and Koprowski, H.: Successful protection of humans exposed to rabies infection. Postexposure treatment with the new human diploid cell rabies vaccine and antirabies serum. *JAMA* 236:2751, 1976.

Bhatt, D. R., Hattwick, M. A. W., Gerdsen, R., Emmond, R. W., and Johnson, H. N.: Human rabies: Diagnosis, complications and management. *Am J Dis Child* 127:862, 1974.

Bryceson, A. D. M., Greenwood, B. M., Warrell, D. A., Davidson, N., Pope, H. M., Lawrie, J. H., Barnes, H. J., Bailie, W. E., and Wilcox, G. E.: Demonstration during life of rabies antigen in humans. *J Infect Dis* 131:71, 1975.

Corey, L. and Hattwick, M. A. W.: Serum neutralizing antibodies after rabies post-exposure prophylaxis. *Ann Intern Med* 85:170, 1976.

Gode, G. R., Raju, A. V., Jayalakshmi, T. S., Kaul, H. L., and Bhide, N. K.: Intensive care in rabies therapy. *Lancet* 2:6, 1976.

Hafkin, B., Hattwick, M. A. W., Smith, J. S., Alls, M. E., Yager, P. A., Corey, L., Hoke, C. H., and Baer, G. M.: A comparison of a WI-38 vaccine and duck embryo vaccine for pre-exposure rabies prophylaxis. *Am J Epidemiol* 107:439, 1978.

Hattwick, M. A. W.: Human rabies. *Public Health Rev* 3:229, 1974.

Hattwick, M. A. W., Corey, L., and Creech, W. B.: Clinical use of human globulin immune to rabies virus. *J Infect Dis* 133(suppl):A266, 1976.

Kappus, K.: Canine rabies in the United States, 1971-1973. *Am J Epidemiol* 103: 242, 1976.

Plotkin, S. A., Wiktor, T. J., Kaprowski, H., Rosanoff, E. I., and Tint, II.: Immunization schedules for the new human diploid cell vaccine against rabies. *Am J Epidemiol* 103:75, 1976.

Porras, C., Barboza, J., Fuenzalida, E., Adaros, H. L., Ovideo, A. M., and Furst, J.: Recovery from rabies in man. *Ann Intern Med* 85:44, 1976.

62

MARBURG AND EBOLA VIRUSES
Robert H. Waldman, M.D.

Two related viruses have been identified recently, but are very rarely recovered; humans appear to be accidental hosts. The viruses have not been identified taxonomically, but by electron microscope seem to be similar to rhabdoviruses.

Ebola virus was isolated from human blood during an epidemic of hemorrhagic fever in Central Africa several years ago. It is thought to be transmitted by intravenous fluid contamination because when more care was taken in medical facilities, the epidemic ceased. The fatality rate in Ebola virus infection is 50-80%. At autopsy the liver shows eosinophilic inclusions.

Marburg virus is serologically related and was first identified in Europe in 1967 in laboratory workers who had handled African monkeys or their tissues. These workers also developed a hemorrhagic fever, with a fatality rate of 20-25%.

Selected Bibliography

Johnson, K. M., Webb, P. A., Lange, J. V., and Murphy, F. A.: Isolation and partial characterization of a new virus causing haemorrhagic fever in Zaire. *Lancet* 1:569, 1977.

Kissling, R. E.: Marburg virus. *Ann NY Acad Sci* 174:932, 1970.

Pattyn, S., Jacob, W., van der Groen, G., Piot, P., and Courtceille, G.: Isolation of Marburg-like virus from a case of hemorrhagic fever in Zaire. *Lancet* 1: 573, 1977.

Zlotnik, I., Simpson, D. I. H., and Howard, D. M. R.: Structure of the vervet-monkey-disease agent. *Lancet* 2:26, 1968.

63

REOVIRUSES
Ronica M. Kluge, M.D.

The term reovirus is derived from respiratory enteric orphan virus and refers to the fact that these viruses infect both respiratory and gastrointestinal tracts. The Reoviridae family includes the genera *Orthoreovirus, Orbivirus,* and *Rotavirus*. Rotavirus is the best known member of this family and will be discussed in detail here. The clinical aspects of rotavirus infections are found in Chapter 23.

Microbiology

Members of the *Reoviridae* group of viruses have two capsid shells both of which are icosahedral (Table 63.1). The complete rotavirus particle is 70 nm in diameter and has 32 capsomeres radiating from the central core. The genome of rotavirus is composed of 11 segments of double-stranded RNA; reovirus and orbivirus each have 10 segments. The Reoviridae are stable after exposure to ether, heat, cold, and to pH of $\geq$ 3. Early efforts to cultivate rotavirus in cell lines or organ cultures proved unsuccessful. Recently, a human strain, first passed serially in piglets, has become adapted to in vitro culture techniques.

Epidemiology

Reoviruses have been recovered from healthy animals and humans and from those with respiratory and gastrointestinal tract illnesses. Rotaviruses have been identified as the etiologic agents causing diarrhea in humans and a number of animal species (Table 63.2). Rotavirus causes 40–55% of the diarrheal episodes in humans aged 6 months to 2 years. The virus is found worldwide and causes a peak

TABLE 63.1   Biologic Properties of Rotavirus

Size	70 nm
Shape	Icosahedral with double-shelled capsid
Density (CsCl)	1.35-1.37 g/cm^3
Stability	
Fluorocarbon	5 min at 37°C
Acid	pH ≧ 3 for 1 hr at 37°C
Heat	56°C for 1 hr
Cold	-20° C for years

TABLE 63.2   Species in Which Rotaviruses Cause Diarrhea

Infant mice	Foals
Calves	Infant rabbits
Piglets	Newborn deer
Lambs	Monkeys
Dogs	Goats
Guinea pigs	

occurrence of disease during the cooler months. Transmission of the agent is primarily by the fecal-oral route and nosocomial outbreaks have been documented. The incubation period is 1-3 days.

Serologic and virus isolation studies suggest that asymptomatic infections of adults exposed to children with rotavirus diarrhea do occur. Infrequently, symptomatic disease is seen in adults, and rotavirus is one cause of traveler's diarrhea. By 18-24 months of age, 85% of children have detectable serum antibody.

Pathogenesis

Illness caused by rotavirus is first manifested in humans by nausea and vomiting and then by diarrhea. The pathogenesis of the vomiting has not been elucidated. However, the histologic changes caused by rotavirus in the small intestine have been well described in various animals and in humans. As is the case in Norwalk-like agent diseases, the stomach and colon mucosae are spared. In the duodenum and upper jejunum the following alterations are seen: shortening and blunting of villus projections, mononuclear cell infiltration of the lamina propria, mitochondrial swelling, and irregularity of the microvillae. The virus particles can be demonstrated by electron microscopy within the intestinal epithelial cells and free in intestinal contents. The histologic changes have been noted to resolve as quickly as 3 days from the onset of symptoms. During the acute illness, maltase, sucrase, and lactase levels in the small intestine are decreased; these revert to normal rapidly in most instances.

Laboratory Diagnosis

Detection of rotavirus is more easily accomplished than detection of the Norwalk-like agents. The standard reference method for rotavirus is still electron microscopy using negative-staining with phosphotungstic acid. Large numbers of virus particles can be demonstrated in stool samples obtained in the first 3 or 4 days of the illness. Counterimmunoelectrophoresis to detect rotavirus antigen has the sensitivity and specificity of electron microscopy but lends itself to more rapid screening with less complex equipment. Radioimmunoassays and an enzyme-linked immunosorbent assay (ELISA) also offer sensitivity, specificity, and convenience in the detection of rotavirus antigens. Isolation of the virus in cell culture is possible but is laborious and expensive.

Antibodies to rotaviruses can be detected by a number of different techniques: complement-fixation, neutralization, immune electron microscopy, indirect immunofluorescence, radioimmunoassay, and ELISA. The latter two tests are available commercially and are particularly easy to use.

Immunology

While there are no demonstrable serologic cross-reactions between human rotaviruses and the other Reoviridae members (reoviruses, orbiviruses), human rotaviruses are related to rotaviruses known to cause diarrhea in other animals. Experimentally, human rotaviruses cause disease in calves, piglets, lambs, and infant monkeys. There are three, perhaps four, serotypes of human rotavirus. Studies of infants and children document that serotype 2 causes most rotavirus disease ($\sim$ 75%) and suggest that this serotype 2 is associated with more severe disease. Eighty-five percent of persons over 3 years of age have antirotavirus antibodies, but the mere presence of serum antibodies against rotavirus does not guarantee protection from reinfection. It is suspected that the second infection is most often due to a different serotype. There is experimental evidence from adult volunteers to suggest that intestinally produced IgA antibody is important in immunity to reinfection. Secretory IgA antibody to rotavirus present in breast milk may offer protection to newborns; this has proved true in animal models.

An effective vaccine against rotavirus probably will require the stimulation of local production of antibody in the intestine. The vaccine will need to include at least the two most common serotypes of human rotavirus and be effective in infants under 6 months of age. Alternatively, the vaccine could be given to women of childbearing age to ensure the presence of antibody in breast milk.

Selected Bibliography

Albrey, M. B. and Murphy, A. M.: Rotavirus and acute gastroenteritis of infants and children. *Med J Aust* 1:82-85, 1976.

Barnes, G. L. and Townley, R. R. W.: Duodenal mucosal damage in 31 infants with gastroenteritis. *Arch Dis Child* 48:343-349, 1973.

Bishop, R. F., Davidson, G. P., Holmes, I. H., and Ruck, B. J.: Virus particles in epithelial cells of duodenal mucosa from children with acute nonbacterial gastroenteritis. *Lancet* 2:1281-1283, 1973.

Blacklow, N. R. and Cukor, G.: Viral gastroenteritis. *N Engl J Med* 304:397-406, 1981.

Flewett, T. H., Bryden, A. S., and Davies, H.: Diagnostic electron microscopy of faeces. 1. The viral flora of the faeces as seen by electron microscopy. *J Clin Pathol* 27:603-614, 1974.

Holmes, I. H.: Viral gastroenteritis. *Prog Med Virol* 25:1-36, 1979.

Holmes, I. H., Ruck, B. J., Bishop, R. F., and Davidson, G. P.: Infantile enteritis viruses: Morphogenesis and morphology. *J Virol* 16:937-943, 1975.

Kapikian, A. Z., Kalica, A. R., Shih, J. W., Cline, W. L., Thornhill, T. S., Wyatt, R. G., Chanock, R. M., Kim, H. W., and Gerin, J. L.: Buoyant density in cesium chloride of the human reovirus-like agent of infantile gastroenteritis by ultracentrifugation, electron microscopy, and complement fixation. *Virology* 70:564-569, 1976.

Kapikian, A. Z., Kim, H. W., Wyatt, R. G., Cline, W. L., Arrobio, J. O., Brandt, C. D., Rodriguez, W. J., Sack, D. A., Chanock, R. M., and Parrott, R. H.: Human reovirus-like agent as the major pathogen associated with "winter" gastroenteritis in hospitalized infants and young children. *N Engl J Med* 294:965-972, 1976.

Kapikian, A. Z., Kim, H. W., Wyatt, R. G., Rodriguez, W. J., Ross, S., Cline, W. L., Parrott, R. H., and Chanock, R. M.: Reovirus-like agent in stools: Association with infantile diarrhea and development of serologic tests. *Science* 185:1049-1053, 1974.

Martin, M. L., Palmer, E. L., and Middleton, P. J.: Ultrastructure of infantile gastroenteritis virus. *Virology* 68:146-153, 1975.

Middleton, P. J., Petric, M., Hewitt, C. M., Szymanski, M. T., and Tam, J. S.: Counter-immunoelectro-osmophoresis for the detection of infantile gastroenteritis virus (orbi-group) antigen and antibody. *J Clin Pathol* 29:191-197, 1976.

Palmer, E. L., Martin, M. L., and Murphy, F. A.: Morphology and stability of infantile gastroenteritis virus: Comparison with reovirus and bluetongue virus. *J Gen Virol* 35:403-414, 1977.

Rodger, S. M., Schnagel, R. D., and Holmes, I. H.: Biochemical and biophysical characteristics of diarrhea viruses of human and calf origin. *J Virol* 16:1229–1235, 1975.

Schreiber, D. S., Blacklow, N. R., and Trier, J. S.: The mucosal lesion of the proximal small intestine in acute infectious nonbacterial gastroenteritis. *N Engl J Med* 288:1318–1323, 1973.

Schreiber, D. S., Trier, J. S., and Blacklow, N. R.: Recent advances in viral gastroenteritis. *Gastroenterology* 73:174–183, 1977.

Wyatt, R. G., Gill, V. W., Sereno, M. M., Kalica, A. R., Van Kirk, D. H., Chanock, R. M., and Kapikian, A. Z.: Probable in-vitro cultivation of human reovirus-like agent of infantile diarrhoea. *Lancet* 1:98–99, 1976.

64

ARENAVIRUSES
Robert H. Waldman, M.D.

The important human pathogens in the arenavirus group are lymphocytic choriomeningitis and various hemorrhagic fevers. The hemorrhagic fevers have in common a very high mortality.

 This group of viruses was so named from the Latin for "sandy" because of the
electron-dense granules seen in the virus by electron microscopy. For most of the
arenaviruses, rodents are the natural host and human infection is an accidental
event.

Lymphocytic Choriomeningitis

Lymphocytic choriomeningitis (LCM) is a rare cause of meningitis but is of great
interest because it is a naturally occurring model of a chronic virus infection in
which the disease has been shown to be caused not by the virus damaging the host
directly, but rather by damage caused by the immune response of the host.

 Chronically infected rodents excrete the virus and are the source of human
disease. The disease is found throughout the United States, and the incidence is
highest in cooler weather in young adults. The mode of transmission is thought to
be inhalation of aerosolized rodent urine or from rodent bites. There is no person-
to-person transmission. It is instructive to briefly mention the various patterns
of disease in rodents. Adults who become infected develop an acute illness from
which they either recover or die. Fetal or neonatal infection leads to chronic
asymptomatic viremia and viruria, with eventual development in many animals of
immune complex disease glomerulonephritis. Adult rodents which have been experimentally infected with a lethal dose of virus, when treated with corticosteroids or other immunosuppressants, develop asymptomatic chronic infection rather
than an acute illness.

Typically LCM in humans causes an influenza-like illness, but often with additional symptoms or signs such as rash, vomiting, arthritis, and less commonly, parotitis, orchitis, or myocarditis. The illness may last as long as 2 weeks and may be biphasic, with aseptic meningitis developing during the second phase. In the most severe cases an encephalomyelitis may develop. The central nervous system symptoms and signs appear about 3 weeks following the initial exposure.

The classic spinal fluid finding is a marked increase in lymphocytes, up to $1000/mm^3$. About one-fourth of patients have hypoglycorrhachia. A definitive virologic diagnosis can be made by isolating virus from blood or spinal fluid, or by demonstrating a rise in serum antibody, with the indirect fluorescent antibody technique being the preferred test.

The prognosis is very good, with nearly all patients showing complete recovery.

Lassa Fever

Lassa fever is the only arenavirus infection in which person-to-person spread occurs, although the disease may also be acquired from rodents in a similar fashion to LCM. Although there is person-to-person spread, for some reason tertiary cases, i.e., disease in people who have had contact with patients to whom the virus was transmitted by the index case, are rare. The disease is more common in pregnant women and health-care workers. The geographic distribution of the disease is in West Africa.

Histopathologically, the predominant finding is liver necrosis, with Councilman-like bodies. The disease may be differentiated pathologically from yellow fever by the absence in the liver of zonal necrosis.

The incubation period is 3-16 days. The disease is severe, and it was, until recently, thought that the case-fatality rate was extremely high. However, as vigorous search for the disease is being carried out, milder cases are being found. The onset of the disease is very nonspecific, but the pharyngitis which is seen in most cases becomes very intense, and the patient develops abdominal and chest pain tenderness. Patients then usually develop conjunctival suffusion and a rash on the face, trunk, and arms. An electrocardiogram usually shows evidence of myocarditis. In severe cases during the second week, patients develop evidence of increased capillary permeability with resultant hypovolemia.

Virologic diagnosis may be made by virus isolation, but this is not recommended because of the associated danger to laboratory personnel. The best way to make the diagnosis is serologically, using an indirect fluorescent antibody or complement-fixation test. Treatment involves support, including dialysis if necessary, the avoidance of aspirin, and the administration of immune serum. Unfortunately, because of the relative rarity of the disease, there are no controlled studies which document the effectiveness of immune serum.

Nearly half of the patients die, and of those who live, nearly half are deaf. Other less serious sequelae of the disease are vertigo and hair loss.

Argentine Hemorrhagic Fever

Argentine hemorrhagic fever is caused by the Junin virus. The disease is seen in the spring, mainly in farmers who become inoculated through cuts in the skin following contact with infected rodent urine. Patients show evidence of myocarditis, renal failure, disseminated intravascular coagulation, and neurologic deficits. The mortality is 10-20%.

Bolivian Hemorrhagic Fever

Bolivian hemorrhagic fever is caused by the Machupo virus. It is clinically similar to Argentine hemorrhagic fever.

Selected Bibliography

Biggar, R. J., Woodall, J. P., Walter, P. D., and Haughie, G. E.: Lymphocytic choriomeningitis outbreak associated with pet hamsters. Fifty-seven cases from New York state. *JAMA* 232:494-500, 1975.

Bowen, G. S., Calisher, C. H., Winkler, W. G., Kraus, A. L., Fowler, E. H., Garman, R. H., Fraser, D. W., and Hinman, A. R.: Laboratory studies of a lymphocytic choriomeningitis virus outbreak in man and laboratory animals. *Am J Epidemiol* 102:233-240, 1975.

Casals, J., Buckley, S. M., and Cedeno, R.: Antigenic properties of the arenaviruses. *Bull WHO* 52:421-427, 1975.

Clayton, A. J.: Lassa immune serum. *Bull WHO* 55:435-439, 1977.

Frame, J. D., Baldwin, J. M., Jr., Gocke, D. J., and Troup, J. M.: Lassa fever, a new virus disease of man from West Africa. I. Clinical description and pathological findings. *Am J Trop Med Hyg* 19:670-676, 1970.

Hinman, A. R., Fraser, D. W., Douglas, R. G., Bowen, G. S., Kraus, A. L., Winkler, W. G., and Rhodes, W. W.: Outbreak of lymphocytic choriomeningitis virus infections in medical center personnel. *Am J Epidemiol* 101:103-110, 1975.

Keane, E. and Gilles, H. M.: Lassa fever in Panguma Hospital, Sierra Leone, 1973-1976. *Br Med J* 1:1399-1402, 1977.

Leifer, E., Gocke, D. J., and Bourne, H.: Lassa fever, a new virus disease of man from West Africa. II. Report of a laboratory-acquired infection treated with plasma from a person recently recovered from the disease. *Am J Trop Med Hyg* 19:677-679, 1970.

Maiztegui, J. I., Fernandez, N. J., and de Damilano, A. J.: Efficacy of immune plasma in treatment of Argentine haemorrhagic fever and association between treatment and a late neurological syndrome. *Lancet* 2:1216-1217, 1979.

Monath, T. P.: Lassa fever: Review of epidemiology and epizootiology. *Bull WHO* 52:577-592, 1975.

Wulff, H. and Lange, J. V.: Indirect immunofluorescence for the diagnosis of Lassa fever infection. *Bull WHO* 52:429-436, 1975.

Zweighaft, R. M., Fraser, D. W., Hattwick, M. A. W., Winkler, W. G., Jordan, W. C., Alter, M., Wolfe, M., Wulff, H., and Johnson, K. M.: Lassa fever: Response to an imported case. *N Engl J Med* 297:803-807, 1977.

65

CYTOMEGALOVIRUS
David L. Hoover, M.D.

Microbiology

Cytomegalovirus belongs to the herpes group. Like other members of the group, the virion contains DNA in its core, a capsid with 162 capsomeres and icosahedral symmetry. The group properties of latency and formation of intranuclear inclusions are also shared by cytomegalovirus. In tissue culture the virus is recognized by its ability to cause a focal cytopathic effect with giant cell formation. Confirmation of the specificity of cytopathic effect is obtained via direct immunofluorescence. Suitable cell lines for culture of human cytomegalovirus (CMV) include those derived from human fibroblasts and myometrium. Human and animal CMV strains generally exhibit species specificity both in vivo and in vitro. Animal cell lines therefore are not suitable for human CMV culture. Human CMV exhibits some antigenic variability, but the number of distinct strains remains in doubt. The complement-fixation (CF) test is the most widely used for detection of antibody to CMV. Indirect immunofluorescent techniques to detect IgG or IgM antibodies and complement are more sensitive and also commonly employed.

Pathology

Histologic manifestations of CMV infection in vivo include the formation of giant cells with intranuclear and often intracytoplasmic inclusions. The host response, with acute and chronic inflammatory cells, is otherwise nonspecific.

Epidemiology

By late adulthood, 80% of people have been infected. In less-developed countries, infection occurs early in life, a situation analogous to that of polio and Epstein-Barr virus (EBV). In the United States, however, only about 8% of children are infected by 1 year of age. Another peak of virus acquisition occurs during late adolescence. Transmission appears generally related to contact with secretions, either natally, or later sexually, except in the iatrogenic instances noted below. Whether virus is acquired orally or parenterally the incubation period before viremia is similar, about 1-2 months. Although most infection is asymptomatic, the long-term consequences of latent virus infection remain unknown. Cytomegalovirus may be cultured from a number of sites in asymptomatic individuals (Table 65.1).

As with other viruses of the herpes group, effective immunity to CMV appears to be cell mediated; clinical disease may occur despite the presence of serum antibody. Both reactivation of infection and persistent viruria have been correlated with depression of CMV-specific cellular immunity. Similarly, the administration of agents such as antithymocyte globulin, which profoundly interfere with T-cell mediated defenses, is associated with increased susceptibility to CMV disease.

Clinical Manifestations

The known clinical manifestations of CMV infection are legion and everincreasing. Tables 65.2-65.4 illustrate congenital infection with CMV. Primary maternal infections occur in approximately 1% of pregnancies. The associated risk of fetal infection is approximately 50%. Offspring may develop a congenital syndrome of microcephaly with major motor and mental retardation and seizures, intracranial periventricular calcifications, chorioretinitis, hepatosplenomegaly with jaundice, and thrombocytopenia with purpura. The case-fatality rate in such instances is high and major neurologic sequelae are common in survivors (Table 65.5). Congenitally infected infants are more likely to appear normal at birth but may continue to excrete virus for up to 4 years. Such a result is more likely in infants of mothers with reactivation of CMV. Even these "asymptomatic" infected infants, however, have a substantially increased risk of deafness, mental retardation, and behavioral disorders in early childhood when compared with control groups (Table 65.6). Congenital infection with CMV may thus represent a major cause of childhood deafness and learning disability.

TABLE 65.1   Site of Positive CMV Culture in Asymptomatic Persons

Saliva	Mostly children
Blood	Rare
Semen	1% (normal)
Breast milk	25% of seropositive women
Cervical secretions	15% of first trimester pregnancies

TABLE 65.2   Congenital CMV Infection

Congenital

Multisystem involvement (cytomegalic inclusion disease)

Usually a sequel of primary maternal infection

Manifestations
Central nervous system
Microcephaly
Seizures
Mental retardation
Periventricular calcification
Deafness (inner ear involvement)
Chorioretinitis
Hepatosplenomegaly
Jaundice
Thrombocytopenia
Petechial rash

TABLE 65.3   Frequency of Clinical Signs in Infants with
Congenital Cytomegalovirus Disease

Feature	Approximate Frequency (%)
Hepatomegaly	100
Splenomegaly	100
Mental retardation	80
Microcephaly	80
Motor disability	75
Jaundice	65
Petechiae	55
Chorioretinitis	30
Cerebral calcification	25

TABLE 65.4   Laboratory Abnormalities in Congenital CMV Infection

Abnormality	Approximate % of Patients
↑ Cord serum IgM	85
Atypical lymphocytosis	80
↑ SGOT	80
Thrombocytopenia	60
↑ Bilirubin	60
↑ CSF protein	45

TABLE 65.5   Sequelae in Survivors of Clinically Apparent Congenital CMV

	Approximate %
Apparently normal	10
Microcephaly	70
Mental retardation	60
Hearing loss	30
Spasticity	25
Seizures	20
Chorioretinitis	15
Optic atrophy	15

TABLE 65.6   Abnormalities 4 Years After Asymptomatic Congenital CMV Infection

Abnormality	Percent
Microcephaly	16
Bilateral hearing loss	12
IQ < 90	29
IQ < 80	16
Chorioretinitis	2

In the first 4 months after birth, one-fifth of infants born to seropositive mothers may develop viruria. Recent evidence suggests that peripartum infection is acquired by passage through an infected birth canal, or by ingestion of infected breast milk (Table 65.7). Although many infected mothers shed virus in urine or saliva, they are unlikely to infect infants by these routes. Most infants so infected appear normal. As with congenitally infected infants, however, active infection manifested only by viruria may persist for months to years, with unknown long-term consequences. Some, however, particularly premature infants, may develop pneumonia, a "peculiar gray pallor," respiratory distress, hepatosplenomegaly, atypical lymphocytes, and widespread involvement by CMV (Table 65.8). The relative role of multiple blood transfusions versus natal acquisition in this setting is obscure. Usually, the disease is self-limited with appropriate supportive care but may be fatal. Full-term as well as premature infants have also been reported to develop CMV-related pneumonitis in early infancy. Diagnosis may be made by finding CMV viruria and a rising CF antibody titer.

TABLE 65.7   Maternal Excretion of CMV and Subsequent Infection of Newborn

Site of Maternal Excretion	% Infected Newborns
Breast milk	
Breast fed	60
Bottle fed	0
Cervix	
Third trimester and postpartum	55
Third trimester	25
First and second trimester	10
Urine	0
Saliva	0

Generally, little further symptomatic disease attributable to CMV occurs until young adulthood, when primary infection may be evidenced by a mononucleosis syndrome, probably acquired by salivary exchange with kissing, as in infectious mononucleosis due to EBV (Table 65.9). Patients usually present with fever, often of 3 or more weeks duration. In contrast to EBV-induced disease, sore throat, adenopathy, and splenomegaly are unusual. Marked malaise and myalgia also are

TABLE 65.8   Syndromes Associated with Perinatal CMV Infection

Asymptomatic viruria
   20% of infants of seropositive mothers
   30% of third trimester viruric mothers
   57% of postpartum and third trimester viruric mothers
   Viruria delayed for 6 weeks

Pneumonia
   Premature or (uncommonly) full-term infants
   Manifestations
      "Gray pallor"
      Hepatosplenomegaly
      Respiratory distress
      Viruria

uncommon. A fine macular or maculopapular rash may occur spontaneously or in association with the administration of ampicillin. Biochemical evidence of hepatitis is characteristic, but jaundice is not. The appearance of atypical lymphocytes and absolute lymphocytosis may be delayed for 1-2 weeks after onset of symptoms. A number of serologic abnormalities including cold agglutinins, cryoglobulins, rheumatoid factor and antinuclear antibodies may occur. Complications are uncommon but include meningoencephalitis, pneumonia, thrombocytopenia and hemolytic anemia. Viruria and a rising CF titer establish the diagnosis. The CF antibody rise may not occur until the third week of illness. Epstein-Barr virus infection may falsely elevate the CMV CF titer and must be excluded by appropriate serologic tests. Mononucleosis caused by CMV may also occur following open-heart surgery (postperfusion syndrome) or blood transfusion for any reason. The risk of CMV infection is in the order of 3% per unit of blood transfused. It may be substantially reduced by the use of frozen RBC or blood from antibody-negative donors.

A number of other syndromes have been associated with CMV infection, often without fever or atypical lymphocytosis. These are listed in Table 65.9. The virus has also been associated with various ulcerative lesions of the gastrointestinal tract, but its etiologic role in such instances remains obscure.

Active CMV infections in recipients of allografts of bone marrow, kidney or heart are highly associated with evidence of graft rejection. Most renal transplant patients develop primary or reactivation CMV infection, usually 1-3 months after immunosuppression and transplantation. The seronegative individual who receives a kidney from a seropositive donor develops a primary infection in about 80% of cases (Table 65.10). Seronegative recipients of kidneys from seronegative donors,

TABLE 65.9   Manifestations of Cytomegalovirus Infection in
Adolescents and Adults

Mononucleosis syndrome
  Fever
  Splenomegaly
  Lymphadenopathy
  Hepatitis
  Atypical lymphocytosis
  Nonspecific serologic findings
    Antinuclear antibodies
    Rheumatoid factor
    Cold agglutinins

CNS
  Encephalitis
  Chorioretinitis
  Guillain-Barré syndrome

Gastrointestinal
  Hepatitis
  Intestinal ulceration
  Pancreatitis

Myocarditis

Pneumonia

Hematologic
  Thrombocytopenic purpura
  Hemolytic anemia

however, develop CMV infection only about 10% of the time. The kidney thus appears to be the source of CMV acquisition. Attempts to directly demonstrate the virus in normal donor kidneys have been unsuccessful, however. The risk of renal allograft rejection associated with primary infection appears to be nearly 40%. Reactivation of CMV occurs in about 80% of seropositive recipients. Clinical manifestations may be milder and the relationship to graft rejection less obvious in the latter group.

Diagnosis of CMV infection in transplant patients can be exceedingly difficult. Symptoms which can be caused by CMV are often present in the absence of demonstrable CMV infection (see Table 65.10). Presumptive diagnosis is made by documenting virus excretion or rising antibody titer in association with compatible clinical symptoms.

TABLE 65.10   Clinical Findings and Presence or Absence of CMV Infection in Renal Transplant Patients

Clinical Manifestation	CMV	
	Present (%)	Absent (%)
Fever	45	10
Leukopenia	30	10
Abnormal liver function	15	20
Pulmonary infiltrate or respiratory symptoms	15	20
Hepatomegaly	15	5
Splenomegaly	10	0
Arthralgia	5	0

Interstitial pneumonia occurs in approximately 50% of bone marrow allograft recipients, especially in those who develop graft-vs-host disease. Nearly half of interstitial pneumonia is related to pulmonary CMV infection, alone or with other agents such as *Pneumocystis carinii*. The case-fatality rate is 80%. The source of virus in this setting and the pathophysiologic relationship between active CMV infection and graft-vs-host disease are unknown.

Cytomegalovirus also represents a threat to patients who are immunosuppressed iatrogenically or because of underlying disease. Disseminated disease with various combinations of atypical lymphocytosis, fever, interstitial pneumonia, hepatitis, arthralgia and leukopenia, hemolytic anemia and meningoencephalitis may appear. A distinct entity, that of acquired CMV retinitis, occurs almost exclusively in immunosuppressed patients. Painless progressive, visual loss is associated with retinal exudates, vascular sheathing, and eventual retinal atrophy. The disease may often be the first sign of disseminated CMV infection.

Therapy

Treatment of CMV infections has been disappointing. Trials of idoxuridine, cytosine arabinoside, adenine arabinoside, interferon, and transfer factor have, at best, shown reduction in viremia or viruria but no improvement in clinical result.

Prevention

A live, attenuated vaccine has been shown to be immunogenic with an acceptable level of adverse reactions in renal transplant patients. Its efficacy in altering the course of CMV infection in immunosuppressed hosts, however, is still under investigation. Another problem is the potential relationship between the herpes group of viruses and the later development of malignancy. Although CMV can transform fibroblasts in tissue culture, no evidence now exists for in vivo oncogenicity. Moreover, the ubiquity of the virus among healthy people suggests that any additional risk (and perhaps benefit) from vaccination would be minimal.

Selected Bibliography

Ballard, R. A., Drew, W. L., Hufnagle, K. G., et al.: Acquired cytomegalovirus infection of preterm infants. *Am J Dis Child* 133:482–485, 1979.

Chatterjee, S. N., Fila, M., Weiner, J., et al.: Primary cytomegalovirus and opportunistic infections. Incidence in renal transplant recipients. *JAMA* 240: 2446–2449, 1978.

Cheeseman, S. H., Rubin, R. H., Stewart, J. A., et al.: Controlled clinical trial of prophylactic human-leukocyte interferon in renal transplantation. *N Engl J Med* 300:1345–1349, 1979.

Fiala, M., Payne, J. E., Berne, T. V., et al.: Epidemiology of cytomegalovirus infection after transplantation and immunosuppression. *J Infect Dis* 132:421–433, 1975.

Gehrz, R. C., Knorr, S. O., Macker, S. C., et al.: Specific cell-mediated immune defect in active cytomegalovirus infection of young children and their mothers. *Lancet* 1:844–847, 1977.

Glazer, J. P., Friedman, H. M., Grossman, R. A., et al.: Live cytomegalovirus vaccination of renal transplant candidates: A preliminary trial. *Ann Intern Med* 91:676–683, 1979.

Hanshaw, J. B.: Congenital cytomegalovirus infection: A fifteen-year perspective. *J Infect Dis* 123:555–561, 1971.

Hanshaw, J. B., Scheiner, A. P., Moxley, A. W., et al.: School failure and deafness after "silent" congenital cytomegalovirus infection. *N Engl J Med* 295:468–470, 1976.

Ho, M.: Virus infections after transplantation in man. *Arch Virol* 55:1–24, 1977.

Jordan, M. C., Rousseau, W. E., Stewart, J. A., et al.: Spontaneous cytomegalovirus mononucleosis. Clinical and laboratory observations in nine cases. *Ann Intern Med* 79:153–160, 1973.

Kantor, G. L., Goldberg, L. S., Johnson, B. L., et al.: Immunologic abnormalities induced by post-perfusion cytomegalovirus infection. *Ann Intern Med* 73:553–558, 1970.

Klemola, E., Van Essen, R., Wager, O., et al.: Cytomegalovirus mononucleosis in previously healthy individuals. *Ann Intern Med* 71:11–19, 1969.

Leinikki, P., Grantrom, M. L., Santavuori, P., et al.: Epidemiology of cytomegalovirus infections during pregnancy and infancy. A prospective study. *Scand J Infect Dis* 10:165–171, 1978.

May, A. G., Betts, R. F., Freeman, R. B., et al.: An analysis of cytomegalovirus infection and HLA antigen matching on the outcome of renal transplantation. *Ann Surg* 187:110–117, 1978.

Murray, H. W., Knox, D. L., Green, W. R., et al.: Cytomegalovirus retinitis in adults. A manifestation of disseminated viral infection. *Am J Med* 63:574-584, 1977.

Neiman, P. E., Reeves, W., Ray, G., Flournoy, N., et al.: A prospective analysis of interstitial pneumonia and opportunistic viral infection among recipients of allogeneic bone marrow grafts. *J Infect Dis* 136:754-767, 1977.

Reynolds, D. W., Stagno, S., Hosty, T. S., et al.: Maternal cytomegalovirus excretion and perinatal infections. *N Engl J Med* 289:1-5, 1973.

Simmons, R. L., Matas, A. J., Rattazi, L. C., et al.: Clinical characteristics of the lethal cytomegalovirus infection following renal transplantation. *Surgery* 82:537-546, 1977.

Stagno, S., Reynolds, D. W., Huang, E-S., et al.: Congenital cytomegalovirus infection. Occurrence in an immune population. *N Engl J Med* 296:1254-1258, 1977.

Tolkoff-Rubin, N. E., Rubin, R. H., et al.: Cytomegalovirus infection in dialysis patients and personnel. *Ann Intern Med* 89:625-628, 1978.

Weller, T. H.: The cytomegaloviruses: Ubiquitous agents with protean clinical manifestations. *N Engl J Med* 285:203-214, 267-274, 1971.

66

HERPES SIMPLEX VIRUS
John J. Barry, M.D.

Herpes simplex virus (HSV) has a wide variety of clinical manifestations causing great morbidity and occasional mortality. The advent of more accessible diagnostic techniques and effective antiviral agents has increased the necessity of recognizing these features.

There are two antigenic types of HSV: type 1 is generally associated with orofacial lesions while type 2 usually causes genital infections. The spectrum of disease varies from mucocutaneous lesions, to keratitis, to mild or fulminant CNS involvement. Neonatal HSV infection can present with any or all of these. The immunosuppressed patient is susceptible to more invasive disease and may develop esophagitis, pneumonia, extensive skin involvement, or dissemination.

Microbiology

Herpes simplex virus belongs to the family Herpesviridae, all of which contain a double-stranded DNA genome surrounded by a capsid manufactured in the nucleus of the infected cell. This structure is in turn enveloped in a lipid-containing membrane originating from the nuclear membrane of the host cell. One of the major features of the Herpesviridae is the ability to remain latent, reactivating to a wide variety of stimuli.

Herpes simplex virus types 1 and 2 share 50% DNA homology. Separation can be made presumptively on the basis of clinical presentation. This can be achieved biologically by the appearance of pock size, plaque formation in tissue culture, or sensitivity to heparin. Serologic techniques are also useful, especially the immunofluorescent or microneutralization tests. In addition, different strains of HSV-1 and HSV-2 can be identified by enzymatic cleavage of HSV DNA. This method is useful epidemiologically, confirming that different strains of HSV-2 can infect the same host.

Epidemiology

Infected secretions are the principal mode of transmission of herpes simplex virus. The HSV-1 is usually spread by contact with oral fluids; HSV-2 is most frequently a sexually transmitted disease. There is no anatomic specificity of infection. With changing sexual practices, oral and pharyngeal HSV-2 and genital HSV-1 infections have been documented. Exogenous reinfection occurs, as does autoinoculation to other body sites. Health care personnel in potential contact with HSV-infected secretions are at a particular risk.

Antibody to HSV-1 develops at an early age in the lower socioeconomic groups. In contrast, only half of adults in the higher socioeconomic groups have antibody (Tables 66.1-66.3). It is also estimated that 20% of Americans have antibody to HSV-2. Recurrences of both labial and genital infections are extremely variable and usually are due to reactivation. Inciting factors of particular importance include anxiety, fever, sunlight, menstruation, and trauma.

Pathogenesis

With cutaneous infection HSV enters epithelial cells causing degeneration. Vesicles are formed in which multinucleated giant cells with intranuclear Cowdry's type A inclusions are found. These changes, however, are not specific for HSV. If the infection is primary, lymphatics become involved and lymphadenopathy is prominent. Centripetal spread occurs via sensory nerves and the virus remains latent in the affected ganglion. However, with immunodeficiency widespread dissemination may occur.

Reactivation occurs with the centrifugal migration of the virus. It passes from its latent site along the nerve to a mucocutaneous area where replication in epithelial cells is established and cell lysis begins once again. The factors that allow

TABLE 66.1   Epidemiologic Trends in HSV Infection

HSV-1

    Generally decreased in incidence (40% of young adults serologically in 1965, 30% in 1975)

    Increased proportion of genital (37% of total in a recent study)

HSV-2 Increased incidence

Socioeconomic effect

    Lower incidence of primary disease in higher socioeconomic groups

    Paradoxically higher incidence of recurrent disease in higher socioeconomic groups

---

TABLE 66.2   Rates of Patient Visits for HSV Infections

| Year | Approximate No. of Visits for HSV Infection/ 100,000 Patient Visits | | |
	Genital	Oral	Ocular
1966	3.5	20	15
1968	4	15	15
1970	6	30	20
1972	8	20	20
1974	15	25	25
1976	20	25	20
1978	25	25	25

TABLE 66.3   Relationship of Age and Site of Involvement by Herpes Simplex Virus

| Site | Age (yr) | | | | |
	< 1	1-4	5-14	15-29	$\geq$ 30
Gingivostomatitis	+	4+	2+	-	-
Labialis	-	-	+	2+	3+
Keratitis	-	+	+	2+	3+
Genital	-	-	-	3+	2+
Encephalitis	+	+	+	+	2+
Dermatitis	+	+	+	2+	2+

and/or stimulate this sequence of events are not clear; however, cell-mediated immunity seems to be of importance since its transient depression has been associated with the invasiveness of primary disease and reactivation. High humoral antibody levels, on the other hand, seem to correlate with more *frequent* occurrence of HSV. This may only represent a response to infection and not reflect a causal role.

Diagnosis

Laboratory

There are a variety of methods available for the detection of an HSV infection. A Tzanck smear is made from material obtained from scraping the base of a fresh vesicular lesion and staining with Wright or Giemsa stain. Multinucleated giant cells are seen, and with a Papanicolaou smear, viral inclusions may be detected. The Papanicolaou smear is a reliable diagnostic procedure but only two-thirds as sensitive as viral culture. Immunofluorescent or immunoperoxidase tests detect viral antigens, but tissue culture is presently more reliable.

A characteristic cytopathologic effect (CPE) can be seen in infected tissue cultures. If vesicular fluid from a new lesion is used for culture, diagnostic CPE is usually seen within 24 hr. Storage of specimens before inoculation into tissue culture is best done at -70°C.

Typing of HSV can be accomplished by the immunofluorescent or microneutralization techniques. Strain differences can be determined by restriction enzyme cleavage of viral DNA.

Serology is helpful in primary infections. The acute-phase serum has no detectable antibody and a fourfold or greater increase is seen in the convalescent specimen.

Newer techniques such as the enzyme-linked immunosorbent assay (ELISA) and radioimmunoassay are becoming available. The detection of specific viral enzymes such as the thymidine kinase of HSV, as well as specific products of the infected cell, may become useful. In addition, electron microscopy can be used to detect viral particles.

Clinical Syndromes

Mucocutaneous Infections

It has been estimated that herpes labialis affects 40% of the United States population. New episodes of herpes genitalis range from 400,000 to 600,000 a year and overall, 5-25 million Americans are affected (Table 66.4). Mucocutaneous disease is therefore the most common manifestation of HSV infection.

Herpetic gingivostomatitis is almost always caused by HSV-1. Ulcerations appear in the gingiva and oral mucosa after an average incubation period of 6 days. Localized lymphadenopathy, pharyngitis, and fever are also seen. Pharyngotonsillitis has been reported with HSV-2 infections acquired sexually. A recurrence of herpes labialis may be seen with pneumococcal and meningococcal infection.

Herpetic whitlow or paronychia is usually located on a finger or hand. The lesion is extremely painful with erythema and vesicular formation occasionally associated with systemic complaints of headache and malaise and regional lymphadenopathy. Recognition is important to avoid unnecessary surgical drainage. Pain usually resolves in several days and healing occurs in about 3 weeks. The HSV-1 has been implicated in herpetic whitlow in medical personnel; HSV-2 whitlow is frequently associated with herpetic genital lesions. Recurrence is common, often with a prodrome of dysethesias in the affected area.

TABLE 66.4   Clinical Types of Herpes Simplex Infection

Age	Disease	Source	Usual Serotype
Neonatal	Disseminated	Exogenous	2
Childhood	Gingivostomatitis	Exogenous	1
	Recurrent orofacial	Endogenous	1
	Disseminated associated with atopic eczema	Exogenous	1
Adult	Recurrent orofacial	Endogenous	1
	Primary genital	Exogenous	2
	Recurrent genital	Endogenous	2
	Encephalitis	Endogenous or exogenous	1
	Meningitis	Exogenous	2

Genital herpes simplex is epidemic, in many areas more frequent than gonorrhea. The usual agent is HSV-2, but approximately 10-15% are caused by HSV-1. Primary infection is more severe than is recurrent infection, with fever, dysuria, viremia, regional lymphadenopathy, and extreme pain. Aseptic meningitis has also been associated with HSV-2 genital infections. It is fortunately a relatively benign disease with complete recovery in nearly all cases. In addition, herpetic proctitis may be seen in homosexual men. Lesions associated with a primary infection have a more prolonged course with maculopapular to vesicular crops which ulcerate, crust, and heal (Table 66.5). Infrequent manifestations are intravaginal lesions and acute urinary retention associated with signs of a lumbosacral radiculopathy.

Just as herpes simplex has been found in a latent state in the trigeminal ganglion associated with reactivating oral lesions, it has been found in sacral ganglia as well. Approximately two-thirds of individuals will suffer recurrences of genital herpes. Those patients with primary HSV-1 genital infection, however, have less frequent recurrences, about 15% vs 60% for HSV-2. In general, recurrences decrease with time, are frequently incited by emotional stress and the onset of menses, and are heralded by paresthesias. During asymptomatic periods, cervical shedding of viruses occurs in only 4% and in very low titers.

The evidence associating squamous cervical carcinoma with HSV-2 genital infections has been accumulating rapidly. It is because of this potentially increased risk that Papanicolaou smears are recommended every 6-12 months in women with genital herpes.

Neonatal Herpes (Table 66.6)

Herpetic infections are seen in 1:1000-30,000 live deliveries. The infected birth canal is usually the source of the disease, either ascending via ruptured membranes or by direct contact during vaginal delivery. Transplacental infection is rare but may be seen with the viremia of primary herpes.

TABLE 66.5   Comparison of Primary and Recurrent Genital Herpes

Feature	Primary	Recurrent
Time from onset of lesions to healing	14-18 days	8-10 days
Virus shedding	8 days	4 days
Virus isolated from the cervix	90%	30%

TABLE 66.6   Neonatal Herpes Simplex

Increased risk	Maternal primary infection Premature rupture of membranes Delayed delivery
Types 1 and 2	Both of equal severity Latter more common
Incidence	∿ 1:7500 deliveries
Source of infection	Maternal genital in ≥ 75% also, maternal nongenital Nonmaternal, e.g., indirect transmission from another infant in nursery ∿ 10% of symptomless hospital staff excrete HSV in saliva; prevention - good hygiene, soap and water inactivates HSV
Prognosis	Mortality 50% Half of survivors have severe sequelae

The risk of developing a herpetic infection in an infant delivered at the time of active genital herpetic disease is about 50%. Cesarean section in the actively infected female at term may prevent the spread of disease if membranes are intact. Cesarean section within 4-6 hr of membrane rupture may still minimize risk. Therefore it is important to monitor the pregnant patient with a history of, or contact with, herpes genitalis (Table 66.7). This can be done by culturing the cervix and/or area of frequent recurrence. If direct viral isolation is not available, then Papanicolaou smears can be utilized.

TABLE 66.7   Prevention of Neonatal Herpes Simplex Infection

Monitor

    Patients with history of herpes genitalis

    Patients with a history of sexual contact with an HSV-infected partner

Culture cervix and any recurrence site

    At 32, 34, and 36 wk and once a week subsequently

    Patient should report any prodrome to her physician

Cesarean section

    Patient with active disease, i.e., lesion visible

    Patient with a positive culture should have elective C section before membrane rupture

Vaginal delivery permitted

    Culture-negative, no active lesions seen

Neonatal herpes is seen 2-12 days after delivery. Both HSV-1 and 2 are implicated but more commonly the latter. Immunoglobulin M HSV antibodies appear around 2-3 weeks and help confirm a neonatal infection. The child presents with vesicles in 70% of the cases with the remaining 30% manifesting CNS or visceral disease. Seventy percent will progress and the efficacy of adenine arabinoside therapy is directly related to the extent of the disease. The use of hyperimmune globulin prophylactically or therapeutically is still under study.

Herpes CNS Infection

Herpes simplex virus type 2 has been associated with a rapidly resolving aseptic meningitis, rarely with ascending myelitis and a fulminant encephalitis in the newborn. In the United States, the most prevalent cause of sporadic encephalitis in the adult is HSV-1 (Table 66.8). Just as in neonatal disease prompt diagnosis and therapy are mandatory.

The patient with herpes encephalitis will usually present with headaches, fever, occasionally a stiff neck, and frequently focal neurologic findings (Table 66.9). These findings include motor or sensory loss, aphasia, and in over half, seizures. Most characteristic of the disease, however, is a change in mental status, including olfactory and auditory hallucinations. Aphasia, memory deficits, unusual behavior, irritability, and dementia with frontal lobe signs also may be prominent. Progression from onset to coma usually occurs in 6 days with death in 11 days without therapy.

Herpes simplex encephalitis causes hemorrhagic necrosis with a preference for the frontal lobes. The lack of associated dissemination and inability to culture HSV-1 from blood or CSF suggest neural spread from a latent ganglionic source.

TABLE 66.8   Herpes Simplex Encephalitis

Most common cause of sporadic fatal encephalitis in U.S.

All age groups, but usually children and young adults

Whites > blacks

No seasonal predominance

Pathogenesis: usually reactivation

Pathology
    Hemorrhagic, necrotic, inflammatory lesions
    Most commonly temporal lobe
    Intranuclear eosinophilic inclusion bodies: Cowdry's type A

Brain biopsy
    Positive in ∿ 90%
    May discover another treatable cause - cryptococcal meningoencephalitis,
        tuberculosis, brain abscess, brain tumor

Treatment: vidarabine, possibly acyclovir, effective

TABLE 66.9   Features of Herpes Simplex Encephalitis

Feature	Approximate %
Clinical	
Fever	80-95
Focal neurologic signs	85-95
Headache	55-70
Stiff neck	45-55
Herpes labialis	15-20
Laboratory	
CSF - abnormal	85-100
Leukocytosis ($10-1000/mm^3$)	80-100
Elevated protein	55-90
Blood (> 10 RBC/mm^3)	65-75
Hypoglycorrhachia	0-25
Localized findings on EEG, brain scan, or arteriogram, usually localized to temporo-parietal lobes	60-95
Fatality	65

A presumptive diagnosis can be made looking for focal defects on the CAT scan, brain scan, or EEG, where localized spiking activity may be seen in the involved area. Cerebral spinal fluid abnormalities are detected in about 85% of patients at presentation.

A brain biopsy remains the only definitive diagnostic method, with about 5% false-negative results and few complications. The specimen may be cultured, but fluorescent stains or electron microscopy yield rapid results. Just over half of the patients with compatible clinical and laboratory symptoms will have a positive biopsy. In the biopsy-negative group, one-fourth will have another diagnosis made which requires alternative therapy (tuberculosis, tumor, abscess, cryptococcosis).

The outcome of therapy with adenine arabinoside is directly related to the level of consciousness on admission. In addition, age is a factor, with patients under 30 years of age showing an improved response.

Herpetic Ocular Infections

Infectious blindness in the United States is most commonly caused by herpes simplex - usually HSV-1. For the neonate, HSV-2 is most frequently implicated. The incidence of herpetic ocular disease is probably less than 1% in HSV-infected patients.

Primary disease presents as a keratoconjunctivitis. An ulcerative blepharitis also is seen. Corneal lesions present as elevations that eventually ulcerate. The erosions stain with fluorescein dye in a branching fashion termed dendritic keratitis. Periauricular adenopathy also may be helpful diagnostically. The recurrence rate is around 20% and increases to 50% in 2 years if two or more recurrences have taken place. Uveitis and retinitis may occur as well as deep corneal stromal disease. Diagnosis can be made from corneal scrapings or viral culture. With healing, scar formation may impede or obliterate vision in the involved eye.

Visceral Infections in the Compromised Host

The immunocompromised host, especially with depressed T-cell function, is at increased risk for developing viscerally disseminated HSV infections. Patients with leukemia or lymphoma are particularly susceptible. Herpetic esophagitis is the most common manifestation and is usually asymptomatic. Secondary infection of these herpetic lesions may be associated with disseminated bacterial and/or fungal disease. Transplant recipients, because of iatrogenic immunosuppression, may develop deep cutaneous ulcers and keratitis due to HSV. Visceral HSV spread also may occur.

Patients with extensive burns may develop severe HSV infections, occasionally with hepatic, adrenal, and pulmonic dissemination. Other ailments characterized by interruption in the integument may result in widespread disease, especially Kaposi's varicelliform eruption in the eczematoid patient.

Therapy

Because HSV infections usually run a waxing-and-waning course, confusion frequently arises over the validity of any new antiviral agent. Only under strictly controlled circumstances can treatment be accurately evaluated.

Idoxuridine (5-iodo-2-deoxyuridine, IDU) has been effective topically for the treatment of herpetic keratitis. It has been associated, however, with a toxicity in about 10%. In addition, the emergence of viral resistance has been seen. The systemic use of IDU is toxic and has been ineffective for HSV infections.

Vidarabine (adenine arabinoside, 9-β-D-arabinofuranosyladenine, Ara-A) was originally developed as an anticancer agent (Table 66.10). Vidarabine functions by competitively inhibiting HSV DNA polymerase. It is excreted in the urine and penetrates tissues well, including CSF where levels one-third to one-half of those in the serum are obtained. Toxicity at dosages used for encephalitis is minimal, but gastrointestinal toxicity and neurologic abnormalities can be seen, i.e., tremors, ataxia, hallucinations, psychosis, and EEG changes. Because of its route of elimination, it should be avoided or used with caution in those with renal failure.

Vidarabine has been found effective for HSV keratitis, is less toxic than IDU, and effective for strains resistant to IDU. Both compounds, because of relative insolubility, are poor for deep stromal disease. As noted previously, vidarabine has been found to reduce mortality and morbidity in patients with HSV encephalitis and neonatal disseminated or CNS disease (Table 66.11). It is administered in a dosage of 15 mg/kg/day and in a concentration not exceeding 0.7 mg/ml for 10 days.

TABLE 66.10   Vidarabine Treatment of Herpes Simplex Encephalitis

	Mortality (%)	Morbidity (%)		
		Severe	Moderate	Mild
Placebo	70	10	15	5
Vidarabine (Ara-A)	40	10	15	35

TABLE 66.11   Effect of Vidarabine on Serious Herpes Simplex Infection in Newborns*

	Mortality (%)		% normal at 1 yr	
	Placebo	Vidarabine	Placebo	Vidarabine
CNS	50	10	15	50
CNS and dissemination	75	40	10	30
Disseminated disease without CNS involvement	85	55	8	15
Localized skin, eye, or mouth	0	0	60	75

*Adapted from *Pediatrics* 66:495, 1980

TABLE 66.12   Evidence of Association of Genital Herpes Simplex Virus Infection and Carcinoma of Cervix

Epidemiologic

High incidence in same groups
Lower socioeconomic
Early coitus
Multiple sexual partners

Low incidence in same groups
Nuns
Children

Pathologic

Virus usually infects squamocolumnar junction, same location from which most cervical carcinomas originate

Women with genital HSV infection have greater incidence of cervical precancerous and cancerous lesions

Immunovirologic

Women with cervical precancerous and cancerous lesions have greater incidence antibodies to HSV-2

HSV antigens have been demonstrated in cervical cancer cells

HSV genome has been demonstrated in some precancerous and cancerous lesions

Animal studies

Mice: cervical cancer following genital inoculation

Newborn hamsters: sarcomas following inoculation

Rodent cell tissue culture cells transformed by HSV-2, forming tumors after injection into animals

---

Adenine arabinoside 5-monophosphate (Ara-Amp) is a more soluble derivative of Ara-A and in the future may help to decrease the fluid load necessary in the administration of its parent compound. Cutaneous therapy of herpes labialis or genitalis with Ara-A or Ara-Amp has been ineffective.

Acyclovir, 9-[(2-hydroxyethoxy)-methyl] guanine, is a new potent antiviral of low toxicity. It is phosphorylated by herpesvirus-specific thymidine kinase to its monophosphate and ultimately its triphosphate derivative by other enzymes. This compound stops virus replication by inhibiting HSV DNA polymerase. The interaction is fairly specific, with cellular DNA polymerase affected only by much higher concentrations of the drug.

Acyclovir has been shown to have some effect on mucocutaneous HSV infections. Used topically, acyclovir decreases the duration of viral shedding in genital herpes. In the immunocompromised host, IV acyclovir has had a similar effect but also accelerates healing and decreases the duration of pain. In bone marrow transplant recipients it has been used effectively for prophylaxis against reactivation of HSV. Further studies are being conducted to evaluate acyclovir as an antiviral for herpes simplex labialis, keratitis, and encephalitis.

Interferon has been used effectively as prophylaxis against reactivation of herpes labialis in patients undergoing trigeminal nerve root decompression. Interferon also has been used for HSV keratitis with debridement resulting in increased healing and prevention of recurrences.

Trifluorothymidine is a topically applied antiviral which has been found to be more potent and soluble than IDU, and in some situations more effective than Ara-A for herpetic keratitis. Corticosteroids are considered contraindicated in ocular infection caused by HSV, potentially exacerbating the disease. Steroids, however, may be of use in stromal disease when used in association with an antiviral agent. 2-Deoxy-D-glucose and inosiplex (Isoprinosine) are also under study. Levamisole, lysine, ether, and photoinactivation have been ineffective.

Impeding the development of a herpes simplex vaccine is the danger of oncogenesis, since the virus may be associated with carcinoma of the cervix (Table 66.12).

Selected Bibliography

Adams, G., Stover, B. H., Keenlyside, R. A., Hooton, T. M., Buchman, T. G., Roizman, B., and Stewart, J. A.: Nosocomial herpetic infections in a pediatric intensive care unit. *Am J Epidemiol* 113:126, 1981.

Baringer, J. R.: Recovery of herpes simplex virus from human sacral ganglions. *N Engl J Med* 291:828, 1974.

Barr, R. J., Herten, R. J., and Graham, J. H.: Rapid method for Tzanck preparations. *JAMA* 237:1119, 1977 .

Barza, M. and Pauker, S. G.: The decision to biopsy, treat, or wait in suspected herpes encephalitis. *Ann Intern Med* 92:641, 1980.

Binder, P. S.: Herpes simplex keratitis. *Surv Ophthalmol* 21:313, 1977.

Burns, W. H., Saral, R., Santos, G. W., Laskin, O. L., Lietman, P. S., McLaren, C., and Barry, D. W.: Isolation and characterisation of resistant herpes simplex virus after acyclovir therapy. *Lancet* 1:421, 1982.

Buss, D. H. and Scharyj, M.: Herpesvirus infection of the esophagus and other visceral organs in adults. Incidence and clinical significance. *Am J Med* 66:457, 1979.

Caplan, L. R., Kleeman, F. J., and Berg, S.: Urinary retention probably secondary to herpes genitalis. *N Engl J Med* 297:920, 1977.

Cheeseman, S. H., Rubin, R. H., Stewart, J. A., Tolkoff-Rubin, N. E., Cosimi, A. B., Cantell, K., Gilbert, J., Winkle, S., Herrin, J. T., Black, P. H., Russell, P. S., and Hirsch, M. S.: Controlled clinical trial of prophylactic human-leukocyte interferon in renal transplantation. *N Engl J Med* 300:1345, 1979.

Chou, S., Gallagher, J. G., and Merigan, T. C.: Controlled clinical trials of intravenous acyclovir in heart-transplant patients with mucocutaneous herpes simplex infections. *Lancet* 1:1392, 1981.

Corey, L. and Holmes, K. K.: The use of 2-deoxy-D-glucose for genital herpes. *JAMA* 243:29, 1980.

Craig, C. P. and Nahmias, A. J.: Different patterns of neurologic involvement with herpes simplex virus type 1 and 2: Isolation of herpes simplex virus type 2 from the buffy coat of two adults with meningitis. *J Infect Dis* 127:365, 1973.

Eron, L., Kosinski, K., and Hirsch, M. S.: Hepatitis in an adult caused by herpes simplex virus type 1. *Gastroenterology* 71:500, 1976.

Foley, F. D., Greenawald, K. A., Nash, G., and Pruitt, B. A., Jr.: Herpesvirus infection in burned patients. *N Engl J Med* 282:652, 1970.

Glogau, R., Hanna, L., and Jawetz, E.: Herpetic whitlow as part of genital virus infection. *J Infect Dis* 136:689, 1977.

Hanna, L., Keshishyan, H., Jawetz, E., and Coleman, V. R.: Diagnosis of herpesvirus hominis infections in a general hospital laboratory. *J Clin Microbiol* 1: 318, 1975.

Hensleigh, P. A., Glover, D. B., and Cannon, M.: Systemic herpesvirus hominis in pregnancy. *J Reprod Med* 22:171, 1979.

Hirsch, M. S. and Swartz, M. N.: Antiviral agents. *N Engl J Med* 302:903, 1980.

Hirsch, M. S. and Swartz, M. N.: Brain biopsy in herpes simplex encephalitis. *N Engl J Med* 303:700, 1980.

Kalinyak, J. E., Fleagle, G., and Docherty, J. J.: Incidence and distribution of herpes simplex virus -1 and -2 from genital lesions in college women. *J Med Virol* 1:175, 1977.

Kaufman, H. E.: Ocular antiviral therapy in perspective. *J Infect Dis* 133:A96, 1976.

Kibrick, S.: Herpes simplex infection at term. *JAMA* 243:157, 1980.

Klapper, P. E., Laing, I., and Longson, M.: Rapid non-invasive diagnosis of herpes encephalitis. *Lancet* 2:607, 1981.

Lehrich, J. R.: Case 44-1979: Presentation of case. *N Engl J Med* 301:987, 1979.

Levine, D. P., Lauter, C. B., and Lerner, A. M.: Simultaneous serum and CSF antibodies in herpes simplex virus encephalitis. *JAMA* 240:356, 1978.

Linneman, C. C., Buchman, T. G., Light, I. J., and Ballard, J. L.: Transmission of herpes-simplex virus type 1 in a nursery for the newborn. Identification of viral isolates by DNA "fingerprinting." *Lancet* 1:964, 1978.

Marks-Hellman, S. and Ho, M.: Use of biological characteristics to type herpesvirus hominis types 1 and 2 in diagnostic laboratories. *J Clin Microbiol* 3:277, 1976.

Melnick, J. L., Adam, E., and Rawls, W. E.: The causative role of herpesvirus type 2 in cervical cancer. *Cancer* 34:1375, 1974.

Mitchell, C. D., Gentry, S. R., Boen, J. R., Bean, B., Groth, K. E., and Balfour, H. H., Jr.: Acyclovir therapy for mucocutaneous herpes simplex infections in immunocompromised patients. *Lancet* 1:1389, 1981.

Muller, S. A., Herrmann, E. C., Jr., and Winkelmann, R. K.: Herpes simplex infections in hematologic malignancies. *Am J Med* 52:102, 1972.

Naraqi, S., Jonasson, O., Jackson, G. G., and Yamashiroya, H. M.: Clinical manifestations of infections with herpesviruses after kidney transplantation. *Ann Surg* 188:234, 1978.

Pazin, G. J., Armstrong, J. A., Lam, M. T., Tarr, G. C., Jannetta, P. J., and Ho, M.: Prevention of reactivated herpes simplex infection by human leukocyte interferon after operation on the trigeminal root. *N Engl J Med* 301:225, 1979.

Reeves, W. C., Corey, L., Adams, A. G., Vontver, L. A., and Holmes, K. K.: Risk of recurrence after first episodes of genital herpes. *N Engl J Med* 305:315, 1981.

Russell, A. S., Brisson, E., and Grace, M.: A double-blind controlled trial of levamisole in the treatment of recurrent herpes labialis. *J Infect Dis* 137:597, 1978.

Saral, R., Burns, W. H., Laskin, D. L., Santos, G. W., and Lietman, P. S.: Acyclovir prophylaxis of herpes-simplex-virus infections. A randomized, double-blind, controlled trial in bone-marrow-transplant recipients. *N Engl J Med* 305:63, 1981.

Spruance, S. L., Crumpacker, C. S., Haines, H., Bader, C., Mehr, K., MacCalman, J., Schnipper, L. E., Klauber, M. R., Overall, J. C., Jr., and the collaborative study group: Ineffectiveness of topical adenine arabinoside 5'-monophosphate in the treatment of recurrent herpes simplex labialis. *N Engl J Med* 300:1180, 1979.

Vellar, I. D., Goldwasser, N., and Morrison, W.: Herpetic whitlow. *Med J Aust* 1:349, 1979.

Whitley, R. J., Soong, S., Dolin, R., Galasso, G. J., Ch'ien, L. T., Alford, C. A., and the collaborative study group: Adenine arabinoside therapy of biopsy-proved herpes simplex encephalitis. *N Engl J Med* 297:289, 1977.

Wise, T. G., Pavan, P. R., and Ennis, F. A.: Herpes simplex virus vaccines. *J Infect Dis* 136:706, 1977.

Wolontis, S. and Jeansson, S.: Correlation of herpes simplex virus type 1 and 2 with clinical features of infection. *J Infect Dis* 135:28, 1977.

Young, E. J., Vainrub, B., Musher, D. M., Kumpuris, A. G., Uribe, G., Gyorkey, P., Min, K., and Gyorkey, F.: Acute pharyngotonsillitis caused by herpesvirus type 2. *JAMA* 239:1885, 1978.

67

VARICELLA-ZOSTER VIRUS
Robert H. Waldman, M.D.

In recent years the evidence has been accumulating, and is now compelling, that what were once thought to be two diseases, varicella (chickenpox) and herpes zoster, are caused by the same virus. This evidence will be considered in more detail below. The relationship between chickenpox and zoster might be thought of as the viral equivalent of tuberculosis, i.e., the primary infection leads to the former, and the latter represents reactivation of the dormant or latent organism.

Chickenpox is generally considered to be a benign childhood disease, but it can be fatal, especially in people who are immunologically compromised. Zoster, commonly known as shingles, is best described by examination of the derivation of its names. Zoster is Greek, and shingles is Latin, for "belt." The virus which causes chickenpox and zoster, now known as varicella-zoster virus, is a DNA virus similar to herpes simplex virus. It was first suspected that the two clinical syndromes were caused by the same virus when susceptible children exposed to a grandparent with zoster would occasionally develop chickenpox. Experimental studies showed that material from a zoster lesion injected into a susceptible individual resulted in chickenpox. Persons with a history of either disease, when inoculated with material from a skin lesion from either, are completely protected against the disease. Immunologically, viruses isolated from either, are identical.

Epidemiology

With respect to varicella, the peak occurrence in temperate climates is between 2 and 8 years of age. Thirty percent of the population has had chickenpox by age 4, 90% by age 9. There are an estimated 200,000 cases each year in the United States. In the tropics there are areas in which the disease is more common in

adults than in children. The disease is worldwide in distribution and occurs throughout the year but with a somewhat increased incidence in winter and spring.

Chickenpox is a highly contagious disease, stated to be even more so than
measles. With household exposure, infection will occur in 90-95% of susceptibles.
A patient is known to be infectious from 1 day before to 6 days after the first appearance of the rash. Because patients are known to be infectious before the appearance of the rash, it is believed that, in addition to direct contact, the disease
is spread via respiratory secretions, but it has been surprisingly hard to isolate virus from the respiratory tract, possibly because it is present only during the incubation period, before the rash is present. The vesicle fluid contains readily detectable virus, but scabs usually do not. There are no large epidemics of varicella, but
small epidemics commonly occur in schools, neighborhoods, etc.

With respect to zoster, there is no seasonal predominance, and two-thirds of
the cases occur in people over 45 years of age. There are slightly more males affected than females.

Pathogenesis and Pathology

Varicella-zoster virus causes injury and death of cells in the deeper layers of the
epidermis and an outpouring of extracellular fluids. Histopathologically one sees
giant cells, some of which are multinucleated, in the base of lesions. There are
intranuclear inclusion bodies (in contrast to smallpox, in which inclusions are cytoplasmic). Although virus is presumed to persist in the posterior root ganglia or
cranial nerve roots, it has been impossible to isolate or identify virus or viral antigens. Involved nerves may show axonal degeneration and demyelination.

Zoster reflects reactivation of latent virus. The definite cause of reactivation
is unknown, but factors include exposure to cold, trauma, age, and altered immunity, more specifically cell-mediated immunity. In adults, there seems to be a particular relation of reactivation to occult neoplasm, particularly Hodgkin's disease
and non-Hodgkin's lymphoma (Table 67.1). This raises the controversial question

TABLE 67.1 Herpes Zoster in Hodgkin's Disease

	Approximate % of Patients With Hodgkin's Disease Developing Herpes Zoster
Initial therapy	
Chemotherapy	7
Radiation	20
Radiation + chemotherapy	35
Sex	
Male	7
Female	35
Overall	25

of how hard the clinician should pursue the search for a malignancy in an elderly patient who develops zoster. It is hard to justify the expensive and uncomfortable search unless there is some other suggestive symptom, sign, or abnormality in the basic laboratory tests (such as anemia). Zoster is much less common in normal children, but it does occur; however, it is common in children with leukemia or Hodgkin's disease (Table 67.2).

There is evidence that after reactivation, the virus moves down the sensory nerves to the skin. Most commonly involved are the thoracic nerves; the most frequent cranial nerve is the trigeminal. This distribution corresponds to the location of the most severe rash in chickenpox.

Diagnosis

The diagnosis of chickenpox or shingles is made clinically. With respect to the former, it is no longer a problem for clinicians in endemic areas to have to differentiate varicella from smallpox.

The incubation period of chickenpox is 14-18 days. In children, there is usually no prodrome, but there may be mild fever, headache, and malaise. In adults, the prodrome is usually more noticeable. The rash is the cardinal feature of the disease, and first appears as a brief scarlatiniform eruption. Then crops of pox appear, first on the trunk and then on the face. The rash spreads to the extremities, but is much less intense. The rash evolves from macules, to papules, to vesicles. The vesicles are surrounded by erythema, and they evolve to pustules, and then they crust. In contrast to smallpox lesions, the pox are superficial and soft. Pruritus is usually marked. The rash may be present on the scalp but is unusual on the palms and soles. Since new crops appear for up to a week, lesions are seen in various stages, again in contrast to smallpox. The mucous membranes are often involved, and lesions may be seen on the nasal, pharyngeal, oral, conjunctival, and genital mucosae. These lesions are usually quite painful. Rare, but ominous, is involvement of the esophagus, larynx, or bronchi. The rash is more severe in adults, and may be hemorrhagic and bullous.

In children, systemic symptoms are mild to moderate, with low-grade fever, respiratory symptoms, and lymphadenopathy. These symptoms are much more intense in the adult, and pneumonia is fairly common and may be severe. There may also be secondary bacterial pneumonia (Table 67.3). Adults rarely may develop hepatitis. Children or adults may develop encephalitis, which appears before, during, or after the eruption.

TABLE 67.2   Development of Herpes Zoster in Cancer Patients Exposed to VZV

	Approximate % Developing Zoster after Exposure
Solid tumors	3
Hodgkin's disease	25

TABLE 67.3   Differentiation of Primary Varicella Pneumonia and Secondary Bacterial Pneumonia in Varicella

Primary Varicella Pneumonia	Secondary Bacterial Pneumonia
Adults	Usually children < 7 yr
Early in disease	Late
White count normal or only slightly elevated	White count elevated with left shift
Cultures normal	Positive sputum and (occasionally) blood cultures
Diffuse nodular infiltrate	Segmented or lobar infiltrate or consolidation

The differential diagnosis of chickenpox no longer includes smallpox or vaccinia, but does include erythema multiforme, Stevens-Johnson syndrome, impetigo, acne, enterovirus infection, drug rash, and insect bites.

In zoster, in contrast to chickenpox, the rash is preceded, and often accompanied, by pain. Typically, patients describe a drawing, burning, or piercing feeling for 3-4 days before the appearance of the skin lesions. This leads to the fairly common mistaken diagnosis of such diseases as pleurisy, myocardial infarction, or ureteral colic, depending on the dermatome involved. One helpful finding is the presence of regional lymphadenopathy with zoster, but not with the other diseases mentioned. Once the rash appears, the main differential diagnosis is with herpes simplex.

The rash of zoster looks like chickenpox, but persists longer and has a distribution which is strictly dermatomal and usually unilateral.

Cranial nerve involvement may lead to uveitis if the ophthalmic branch of the trigeminal nerve is involved. Involvement of the mandibular branch causes vesicles in the mouth and on the tongue. Involvement of the maxillary branch leads to vesicles on the uvula and tonsil. Involvement of the geniculate ganglion causes ear pain, facial paralysis, and vesicles in the external auditory canal, known as the Ramsay-Hunt syndrome. The latter can be caused also by herpes simplex virus infection.

Laboratory confirmation of varicella-zoster virus infection can be made from vesicle fluid, scrapings from the base of a lesion, and serologically. Giemsa stain of scrapings, known as the Tzanck test, reveals intranuclear inclusion bodies and multinucleate cells. This does not differentiate herpes simplex virus from VZV, and it is also positive in cytomegalovirus infection and with some adenoviruses. The inclusions are classified as Cowdry's type A, and are round, homogeneous, eosinophilic, fill the nucleus, and have been described as "owls' eyes."

Virus can be isolated in primary human amnion tissue culture. Material from a lesion is usually positive for the first 3 days in chickenpox but for several days longer in zoster. Spinal fluid has been reported to be positive for virus in zoster if the rash is in the distribution of the trigeminal or a cervical nerve. The cytopathic effect in tissue culture is the same as that of herpes simplex virus, and the two can be differentiated using immunofluorescence on the tissue culture. Diagnosis of varicella-zoster virus can also be made by direct immunofluorescence of material from a lesion.

The complement-fixation test also can be used to make the diagnosis. In zoster, one must obtain the acute-phase specimen very early, since the antibody rise is an anamnestic one and therefore extremely rapid, i.e., within 1 week.

The only other laboratory study which is usually of note is the peripheral white count, which shows a neutropenia and lymphocytosis, with immature lymphocytes and plasma cells accounting for up to 8% of the total white count.

Prognosis and Complications

Chickenpox is generally a benign, self-limited disease, but may be fatal, especially in immunocompromised children. But even in leukemic children, the mortality is only about 7%, with the worst prognosis being in those who are lymphopenic. In normals, the most common complication is secondary bacterial infection of the skin, usually with *Staphylococcus aureus* or *Streptococcus pyogenes*. This occasionally is very severe, resulting in venous thrombosis and/or gangrene.

Pneumonia occasionally complicates chickenpox, especially in adults, who have chest roentgenographic evidence of pulmonary involvement in about 15% of the cases. Invariably these lesions calcify resulting in a distinctive x-ray picture. Even in adults, recovery is the rule, usually in 6-10 days.

The most threatening complication of varicella is central nervous system involvement, which may occur before, during, or after the rash. Encephalitis occurs in about 0.1% of cases, and although most survive without sequelae, there is approximately 10% mortality, and about 20% of the survivors have permanent central nervous system defects. Reye's syndrome is seen after chickenpox (Table 67.4), and will not be discussed in detail here, since it is covered in more detail in Chapters 43 and 48. Other complications are arthritis, glomerulonephritis, and purpura fulminans.

Infection during pregnancy is a problem with respect to chickenpox. Virus crosses the placenta, infecting the fetus, and if this occurs early in pregnancy, can lead to congenital abnormalities. If the mother is infected just before delivery, the baby may develop chickenpox at birth, or shortly thereafter. This leads to severe infection, with significant mortality. If the baby develops chickenpox after 10 days of age, the disease was not acquired congenitally, and the illness is usually mild, probably because of the presence of maternal antibody.

The prognosis in zoster is very good, but there is the significant complication of persistent neuralgia, more common in the elderly, which may persist for months to years. There is some evidence that postzoster neuralgia is less frequent if patients with zoster are treated with corticosteroids, and this is probably justified in the elderly or those with severe disease. The use of corticosteroids is paradoxical, because of the fear of disseminated disease in patients who are immunosuppressed. However, it appears to be safe to use steroids for relatively short periods, and it is only in patients who are receiving very high doses for more prolonged periods that dissemination has occurred. Zoster may involve motor roots, leading to paresis. Other complications are a result of involvement of the trigeminal nerve, such as conjunctivitis or keratitis.

TABLE 67.4   Characteristics of Reye's Syndrome (1980-81)

Characteristic	Approximate %
Age	
≤ 4 yr	35
5-14	60
Race	
Caucasian	94
Black	4
Oriental	2
Antecedent illness	
Respiratory	55
Varicella	25
Diarrhea	10
None reported	10
Mortality	30
Use of salicylates during antecedent illness	
Reye's syndrome patients*	100
Controls	41

*Only 12 patients studied, but highly statistically significant

Treatment

Treatment is mainly symptomatic, with control of fever and itching in children with chickenpox and control of pain in zoster. In patients with encephalitis, hemorrhagic chickenpox, or pneumonia, steroids have been used, with no evidence of either efficacy or harm. Passive administration of antibody is of no value once the disease is present. Antiviral treatment with vidarabine has accelerated healing in disseminated zoster. Other modalities that have been used in disseminated disease are transfer factor and interferon, with suggestive benefit, but without proof by controlled studies. The new antiviral drug acyclovir is promising. This drug acts by inhibiting viral DNA polymerase, and is 10-30 times more active against the viral as compared with the human cellular enzyme. The side effects of acyclovir are rare, and include delirium, abnormal liver function tests, and nephrotoxicity.

Immunology and Prevention

It has been suggested that antibody plays some role in protection, since neonates who are infected postpartum have relatively mild disease. The presumption is that this occurs because of the presence of maternal antibody. There is some experimental evidence, however, that maternal T-cell activity may be transferred to the newborn, thus this could be playing a role. Certainly after the neonatal period, cell-mediated immunity appears to play more of a part in protection than does antibody since agammaglobulinemic patients have no increased problem with varicella-zoster infection which is not the case with patients with abnormal T-cell activity.

The role of antibody, however, is also emphasized by the prophylactic effect of passive antibody administration. While it has been shown that there is no protection afforded by pooled gamma globulin, high-titered antibody preparations, when given within 72 hr of exposure, are protective. Varicella-zoster immune globulin (VZIG) prepared from outdated blood bank plasma of normal persons selected for high titers is administered in a dose of 2-5 ml. The VZIG should be used in high-risk patients who are known or suspected to be nonimmune (Table 67.5). In

TABLE 67.5   Varicella–Zoster Immune Globulin (VZIG) for Prophylaxis of Chickenpox (Varicella)

Administration limited to

   Patients with one of following:
      Leukemia or lymphoma
      Congenital or acquired immunodeficiency
      Immunosuppressive therapy
      Newborn whose mother had onset of chickenpox within a period of 5 days
         before and 2 days after delivery

   And one of the following types of exposure to a chickenpox or herpes zoster
   patient
      Household contact
      Playmate contact (of a fairly close nature)
      Hospital contact (adjacent beds)
      Newborn contact

   With negative or unknown prior history of chickenpox (except patients who
   have bone marrow transplant)

   Age < 15 years, with some exceptions (adult with good evidence of *not* having
   been infected previously)

   < 96 hr after exposure

Supplies are limited

Give 1 vial/10 kg body weight up to maximum of 5 vials

No evidence of beneficial effect against established infection or fetal infection
(i.e., exposure of women in early pregnancy)

Immunodeficient patients, especially children, with a negative or unknown history of chickenpox, should be tested for serum antibody to VZ virus, thus avoiding unnecessary VZIG administration in the future

---

TABLE 67.6   Experimental Live, Attenuated Varicella-Zoster Vaccine in Patients with Malignancies

	Seroconversion	Fever and/or Rash
	Approximate %	
Malignancy, chemotherapy discontinued	98	15
Chemotherapy continued	93	45

several hundred high-risk patients treated with VZIG, the mortality from chicken-pox has been < 1%. The problems with VZIG are that it is not always available, it is investigational, the exposure to varicella is often unrecognized or not reported to the physician, and the recommendation is usually made that chemotherapy be interrupted until the danger of severe varicella infection has passed.

There has been significant work done on the development of a VZV vaccine, especially in Japan. A live, attenuated vaccine has been developed, which would not be for general use, but for high-risk patients (Table 67.6). The vaccine stim-ulates a seroconversion rate of 98%, and side effects are relatively mild, with fe-ver and rash being most common. The unresolved questions regarding the vaccine are the duration of immunity, the possibility of latency with subsequent reactiva-tion, and the possibility that the vaccine would be more poorly tolerated in Ameri-can than in Japanese children since the former are usually more immunosuppressed because of more intensive chemotherapy.

Isolation of patients with chickenpox is not indicated, except in the hospital setting.

Selected Bibliography

Baba, K., Yabuuchi, H., Okuni, H., and Takahashi, M.: Studies with live varicella vaccine and inactivated skin test antigen: Protective effect of the vaccine and clinical application to the skin test. *Pediatrics* 61:550, 1978.

Feldman, S. and Epp, E.: Detection of viremia duration incubation of varicella. *J Pediatr* 94:746, 1979.

Gershon, A. A.: Live attenuated varicella-zoster vaccine. *Rev Infect Dis* 2:393, 1980.

Gershon, A. A. and Steinberg, S. P.: Cellular and humoral immune response to varicella-zoster virus in immunocompromised patients during and after vari-cella-zoster infections. *Infect Immun* 25:170, 1979.

Grose, C., Edmond, B. J., and Brunell, P. A.: Complement-enhanced neutralizing antibody response to varicella-zoster. *J Infect Dis* 139:432, 1979.

Myers, M. G.: Viremia caused by varicella–zoster virus: Association with malignant progressive varicella. *J Infect Dis* 140:229, 1979.

Peterslund, N. A., Ipsen, J., Schonheyder, H., Seyer-Hansen, K., Esmann, V., and Juhl, H.: Acyclovir in herpes zoster. *Lancet* 2:827, 1981.

Preblud, S. R. and D'Angelo, L. J.: Chickenpox in the United States, 1972–1977. *J Infect Dis* 140:257, 1979.

Priest, J. R., Urick, J. J., Groth, K. E., and Balfour, H. H.: Varicella arthritis documented by isolation of virus from joint fluid. *J Pediatr* 93:990, 1978.

Raker, R. K., Steinberg, S., Drusin, L. M., and Gershon, A.: Antibody to varicella zoster virus in low-birthweight newborn infants. *J Pediatr* 93:505, 1978.

Zaia, J. A., Levin, M. J., Wright, G. G., and Grady, G. F.: A practical method for preparation of varicella–zoster immune globulin. *J Infect Dis* 137:601, 1978.

68

EPSTEIN-BARR VIRUS
David L. Hoover, M.D.

Epstein-Barr virus (EBV) is a ubiquitous agent associated with a number of human diseases including infectious mononucleosis (IM), X-linked proliferative immuno-deficiency disease, Burkitt's lymphoma, and nasopharyngeal carcinoma. Like other herpes group viruses, it produces latent infection.

Microbiology

The double-stranded DNA of EBV resides in infected cells both integrated into the host cell genome and as a separate, circular episome-like particle. In vitro cultivation is usually achieved using fetal blood lymphocytes which are transformed to lymphoblasts by the virus. Only B lymphocytes possess surface receptors for EBV, and all established EBV-infected lymphocytic cell lines are of B-cell origin. After EBV penetration into the cell, a series of events ensue, which are marked by the formation of various antigens shown in Table 68.1. Lymphocyte-determined membrane antigen (LYDMA), EBV nuclear antigen (EBNA), and early membrane antigen (EMA) are produced in latently infected cells. Early antigen (EA) may represent a virus-coded inhibitor of cellular synthetic processes; it is seen only when virion production begins, and marks inevitable cell death. With the production of mature virus particles, virus capsid antigen (VCA) and late membrane antigen (LMA) appear.

TABLE 68.1   Cellular Antigens Associated with EBV Infection

Antigen	Abbreviation
Lymphocyte-determined membrane antigen	LYDMA
Epstein-Barr nuclear antigen	EBNA
Early membrane antigen	EMA
Early antigen	EA
Virus capsid antigen	VCA
Late membrane antigen	LMA

Immunology and Pathogenesis

Antibody responses reflect not only the timing of EBV-coded antigen expression by host cells but also the interaction of host immune responses with infected cells. An understanding of the response sequence is critical for interpretation of EBV-specific serologic tests (Table 68.2). Anti-VCA antibodies of both IgM and IgG class rise first. They are usually of significant titer at the time patients first have symptoms. Immunoglobulin G anti-VCA antibodies persist for life; thus their presence simply indicates past infection of unknown duration. Immunoglobulin M directed against VCA, however, is useful diagnostically since its titers disappear over a several month period following initial infection. Antibody titers to EA rise during the first few weeks of illness in 80% of the patients. Anti-EBNA titers rise late, usually after weeks to months, but persist for life. Of these EBV-specific diagnostic tests, IgG anti-VCA is most readily available and easiest to perform, but it is of little use to diagnose acute disease. The IgM-VCA has the advantage of defining acute disease on the basis of a single blood sample and is probably the single specific test of choice. Unfortunately, it is available in only a few research laboratories.

In addition to EBV-specific antibodies, the infected individual may produce immunoglobulins directed against many other autologous, homologous, and heterologous antigens. Of these, the heterophil antibody, which agglutinates the red blood cells of sheep and other hoofed animals, forms the basis for clinically useful non-EBV-specific diagnostic tests. The sheep cell agglutination test, originally described by Paul and Bunnell in 1932, and modified by Davidsohn in 1938 using differential adsorption of serum with guinea pig kidney and beef red blood cells, is positive in 80% of the cases of acute IM by the third week of illness. Substitution of beef or horse for sheep cells increases both sensitivity and specificity. A number of quicker, easier, commercially available slide tests have now largely replaced the older tube methods.

Although antibody production is easily quantified in EBV infections, termination of acute clinical illness is probably largely cell-mediated. The atypical lymphocytes seen on the peripheral blood smear during acute IM are mostly T cells. T cells in the blood of seropositive individuals increase under in vitro culture conditions and cause regression of EBV-induced B-cell proliferation. Immunosuppressive agents increase salivary excretion of virus approximately threefold, but

TABLE 68.2   EBV-Specific Antibodies of Clinical Significance

Antibody	Appearance	Duration
Anti-VCA (IgM)	1-2 wk	3 mo
Anti-VCA (IgG)	1-2 wk	Life
Anti-EA	1-4 wk	6 mo
Anti-EBNA	2-52 wk	Life

they do not alter antibody titers. Some measures of cell-mediated immunity to non-EBV-specific stimuli are depressed early in the course of disease but return to normal with convalescence. Antibody production is likewise suppressed during acute clinical illness, perhaps due to an increase in a suppressor T-cell population.

Following a variably symptomatic period, host defenses generally suppress disease manifestations. Persistence of the virus, however, is lifelong. It may be isolated from lymph nodes, saliva, or peripheral blood lymphocytes from a variable proportion of asymptomatic adults depending upon the recency of primary infection, the site of tissue sampled, the volume assayed, and the host's state of immune competence.

Epidemiology

Infants acquiring EBV in the first 2 years of life are generally asymptomatic; such acquisition occurs with increased frequency (up to 50%) in children from the lower socioeconomic groups. Symptomatic primary EBV infection almost always takes the form of infectious mononucleosis in children and young adults (Table 68.3). The development of symptoms may be related to three factors: exposure to the virus, seronegativity, and enough maturation of the immune system to cause clinical disease. Epstein-Barr virus may be rarely transmitted via blood, causing a postperfusion syndrome. More commonly, however, virus is probably acquired after salivary exchange with kissing, accounting for its frequency in adolescence. The attack rate in exposed susceptibles is 30-60%, with an incubation period of 1-2 months. In prospective studies of seronegative college freshmen, 13% seroconverted each year. Clinical disease occurred in 90% of seroconverters.

Diagnosis

The majority of patients present a typical picture including fever, fatigue, sore throat, and adenopathy, particularly of the posterior and anterior cervical chains (Table 68.4). Pharyngeal hyperemia and tonsillar enlargement are common. Whitish or greenish pharyngeal or tonsillar exudate is seen in one-third of the cases. Lymph nodes usually are only slightly tender, in contrast to those of streptococcal pharyngitis. An enanthem at the junction of hard and soft palate is seen in one-third of the cases, splenomegaly in one-half, and hepatomegaly in 10%. Periorbital edema is seen in 10-20%. Uncommon findings (less than 5%) include macular or maculopapular rash and jaundice. Administration of ampicillin to patients with IM results in a rash in 90%.

TABLE 68.3   Effect of Age on Clinical and Laboratory Findings in Symptomatic Patients with E–B Virus Infection

	Approximate % of Patients	
	Age < 8 yr	Age 15–30 yr
More common in children		
Hepatomegaly	45	10
More common in adolescents and adults		
Lymphadenopathy	50	95
Abnormal liver function tests	45	95
Heterophil antibody	5	90
Lymphocytosis (> 50% of WBCs)	40	90
Exudative pharyngitis	40	80
Sore throat	45	80
Autoantibodies	0	25
About equal		
Fever	90	85
Splenomegaly	60	55
> 25% atypical lymphocytes	55	45

TABLE 68.4   Comparison of Clinical Features of Mononucleosis Syndromes

Feature	EBV	CMV	Toxo
Fever	+	+	±
Rash	+	–	+
Pharyngitis	+	–	–
Atypical lymphs	+	+	+
Adenopathy	+	–	+
Splenomegaly	+	+	+

Laboratory findings include leukocytosis in the first 2 weeks, followed by a normal or decreased white cell count. Mononuclear cells are increased, usually to 50% or more; more than 10% of leukocytes are atypical lymphocytes. A mildly depressed platelet count is common. Diagnosis is based on a consistent clinical presentation, atypical lymphocytosis, and positive serology.

Therapy

Treatment of IM is mainly supportive. Avoidance of vigorous exertion is usually prescribed in an attempt to prevent splenic rupture. Otherwise, activity should be tailored to the patient's sense of well-being. Corticosteroids may be useful in treatment of impending respiratory obstruction, hemolytic anemia, and thrombocytopenic purpura. The long-term effects of steroid-induced acute suppression of cellular immunity are unknown, however, and the indiscriminate use of these agents in IM is inadvisable.

Prognosis

Infectious mononucleosis is rarely fatal except in certain cases of hereditary immunodeficiency discussed later. Splenic rupture is the most common cause of death. Respiratory obstruction from greatly enlarged tonsils, and liver or central nervous system involvement also may be fatal. Almost all cases, however, recover completely in several weeks. Fatigue occasionally may persist for months. Rarely, reactivation or persistence of infection has been described.

Complications of IM, some of which are listed in Table 68.5, are uncommon but amazingly diverse. Hemolytic anemia is usually due to anti-i antibodies and severe thrombocytopenia to antiplatelet antibodies. Severe neutropenia, another rare complication, may be due to opsonic antibodies directed against granulocytes. Neurologic diseases have been reported either as complications of acute IM or as appearing de novo. The EBV has been isolated from cerebrospinal fluid in a case of meningoencephalitis. In cases not associated with IM, diagnosis is usually made by demonstrating EBV-specific antibody rises. Pneumonia has been reported in 3-5% of cases of IM, although other infectious causes have not been rigorously excluded. Pleural effusion rarely may be present.

Other Diseases Associated With EBV

The EBV has also been related to an X-linked lymphoproliferative disease characterized by diverse disorders ranging from lymphoma to agammaglobulinemia which become apparent following IM. More than 60 cases in several kindreds have been described. The EBV infection in these individuals is frequently fatal.

Nasopharyngeal carcinoma also is associated intimately with EBV. The virus is present in the genome of all malignant epithelial cells in this disorder and is likely the causative agent or a necessary cofactor.

Burkitt's lymphoma may develop in approximately 1:2000 EBV-infected children in areas of Africa marked by high malaria prevalence. The neoplastic B cells in this disease contain the EBV genome integrated into host DNA and express LYDMA and EBNA. In prospective studies, sera obtained before onset of Burkitt's lymphoma have higher EBV-specific antibody titers than do sera from cohort controls. The interactions among host defenses, environmental agents, and EBV that result in development of this malignancy have not yet been clarified.

TABLE 68.5   Complications of IM

Hematologic
Hemolytic anemia
Aplastic anemia
Thrombocytopenia
Neutropenia
Disseminated intravascular coagulation

Cardiorespiratory
Airway obstruction
Pneumonia
Pleural effusion
Myocarditis
Pericarditis

Neurologic
Aseptic meningitis
Meningoencephalitis
Encephalitis
Transverse myelitis
Peripheral neuritis
Facial nerve palsy
Optic neuritis
Guillain–Barré syndrome

Miscellaneous
Hepatic necrosis
Reye's syndrome
Splenic rupture

Selected Bibliography

Carter, J. W., Edson, R. S., and Kennedy, C. C.: Infectious mononucleosis in the older patient. *Mayo Clin Proc* 53:146–150, 1978.

Chang, R. S., Lewis, J. P., and Abilgaard, C. F.: Prevalence of oropharyngeal ex- creters of leukocyte – transforming agents among a human population. *N Engl J Med* 289:1325–1329, 1973.

Epstein, M. A. and Achong, B. G.: Recent progress in Epstein–Barr virus research. *Ann Rev Microbiol* 31:421–445, 1977.

Evans, A. S.: Infectious mononucleosis in University of Wisconsin students. Re- port of a five-year investigation. *Am J Hyg* 71:342–362, 1960.

Fleisher, G., Henle, W., Henle, G., et al.: Primary infection with Epstein–Barr virus in infants in the United States: Clinical and serologic observations. *J Infect Dis* 139:553–558, 1979.

Fleisher, G., Lennette, E. T., Henle, G., et al.: Incidence of heterophil antibody re- sponses in children with infectious mononucleosis. *J Pediatr* 94:723–728, 1979.

Grose, C., Henle, W., Henle, G., et al.: Primary Epstein-Barr virus infections in neurologic diseases. *N Engl J Med* 292:392-395, 1975.

Haller, T. J., Evans, A. S., Niederman, J. C., et al.: Infectious mononucleosis at the United States Military Academy. A prospective study of a single class over four years. *Yale J Biol Med* 3:182-195, 1974.

Henle, W., Henle, G. E., and Horwitz, C. A.: Epstein-Barr virus specific diagnostic tests in infectious mononucleosis. *Human Pathol* 5:551-565, 1974.

Karzon, D. T.: Infectious mononucleosis. *Adv Pediatr* 22:231-265, 1976.

Mangi, R. J., Neiderman, J. C., Kelleher, J. E., et al.: Depression of cell-mediated immunity during acute infectious mononucleosis. *N Engl J Med* 291: 1149-1153, 1974.

Nikoskelainen, J., Ablashi, D. V., and Genberg, R. A.: Cellular immunity in infectious mononucleosis. II. Specific reactivity to Epstein-Barr virus antigens and correlation with clinical and hematologic parameters. *J Immunol* 121: 1239-1244, 1978.

Pattengale, P. K., Smith, R. W., and Perlin, E.: Atypical lymphocytes in acute infectious mononucleosis. Identification by multiple T and B lymphocyte markers. *N Engl J Med* 291:1145-1148, 1974.

Pejme, J.: Infectious mononucleosis. A clinical and haematological study of patients and contacts, and a comparison with healthy subjects. *Acta Med Scand* 413(Suppl):5-83, 1964.

Purtilo, D. T., DeFlorio, D., Jr., Hutt, L. M., et al.: Variable phenotypic expression of an X-linked recessive lymphoproliferative syndrome. *N Engl J Med* 297: 1077-1081, 1977.

Sawyer, R. N., Evans, A. S., Niederman, J. C., et al.: Prospective studies of a group of Yale University freshmen. I. Occurrence of infectious mononucleosis. *J Infect Dis* 123:263-270, 1971.

Silverstern, A., Steinberg, G., and Nathanson, M.: Nervous system involvement in infectious mononucleosis. *Arch Neurol* 26:353-358, 1972.

Strauch, B., Siegal, N., Andrews, L., et al.: Oropharyngeal excretion of Epstein-Barr virus by renal transplant recipients and other patients treated with immunosuppressive drugs. *Lancet* 1:234-237, 1974.

Sutton, R. N. P., Edmond, R. T. D., Thomas, D. B., et al.: The occurrence of auto-antibodies in infectious mononucleosis. *Clin Exp Immunol* 17:427-436, 1974.

Thorley-Lawson, D. A., Chess, L., and Strominger, J. L.: Suppression of in vitro Epstein-Barr virus infection. A new role for adult human T lymphocytes. *J Exp Med* 146·495-508, 1977.

Tosato, G., Magrath, I., and Koski, I.: Activation of suppressor T cells during Epstein-Barr virus-induced infectious mononucleosis. *N Engl J Med* 301: 1133-1137, 1975.

Wechsler, H. F., Rosenblum, A. H., and Sills, C. T.: Infectious mononucleosis report of an epidemic in an army post. *Ann Intern Med* 25:113-135, 236-265, 1946.

Woodruff, A. J., Row, P. G., Meadoros, R., et al.: Nephritis in infectious mononucleosis. *Quart J Med* 43:451-460, 1974.

Ziegler, J. L., Magrath, I. T., Gerber, P., et al.: Epstein-Barr virus and human malignancy. *Ann Intern Med* 86:323-326, 1977.

69

SMALLPOX AND RELATED VIRUSES
Patrick A. Robinson, M.D.

Smallpox is an infection of humans caused by variola virus, a member of the genus *Orthopoxvirus*. Two forms of the disease are recognized and appear to be virus strain-specific: variola major and variola minor (alastrim). Several other human illnesses of minor importance are caused by other viruses of the family Poxviridae, such as molluscum contagiosum, vaccinia, and monkeypox.

The conquest of smallpox by a worldwide cooperative effort has relegated this disease to history and represents one of the greatest achievements of public health and medicine. The history of smallpox is at least thousands of years old, having been recorded in ancient China, India, and Egypt. Smallpox may have first become epidemic when agricultural developments advanced sufficiently to allow villages of 500 or more persons, sufficient to support an outbreak. The mummified remains of Pharoah Ramses V (c. 1160 B.C.) suggests that he was a victim of smallpox. Epidemics swept through Europe during the Middle Ages resulting in appalling mortality: 20-40% of those infected. Perhaps as much as 80% of the European population experienced illness. Sixty million Europeans were estimated to be infected with smallpox in the 1700s alone. Early sixteenth century Spanish explorers carried smallpox to the Western Hemisphere where it rapidly became an important cause of mortality in native Americans.

Immunity to smallpox from prior infection has been recognized for many years. Inoculation was originally recognized as effective in the Orient. "Pock-sowing" was practiced in 1000 B.C. in China and eventually found its way to Europe and Africa in the 1600s. Variolation, the inoculation of pustular material into a scratch or nostril of a susceptible person, was practiced in Turkey. Here it was witnessed by Lady Mary Wortley Montagu who proselytized its use in England, resulting in its widespread acceptance. Although several other individuals recognized the protection conferred by cowpox against smallpox, Edward Jenner was the first to experiment with and publish the success of vaccination with cowpox (1798).

Epidemiology

Despite widespread use of vaccination, epidemics continued to occur in the nineteenth and twentieth centuries. Between 10 and 15 million cases of smallpox were estimated to have occurred in 1967 and 33 countries were recognized as having endemic foci. Countries with particularly high rates included Brazil, India, Bangladesh, and much of Central and Southern Africa. In 1967 the World Health Organization (WHO) instituted a program of worldwide eradication. This was possible for several reasons: (1) humans are the only natural hosts for variola virus, (2) virtually all infections are symptomatic and there is no chronic carrier state, (3) immunization is safe and easily performed, and (4) vaccination provides satisfactory and long-term protection from infection. The program carried out was one of containment and immunization. Outbreaks and cases were identified and health workers were dispatched to areas of involvement. Susceptible contacts were immunized, and in areas of widespread outbreaks, population immunization was carried out. In 10 years time naturally occurring smallpox was eradicated. The last case of variola occurred as variola minor in a 23-year-old from Somalia. Two subsequent cases resulted from a laboratory accident in England in 1978, but no other cases have been identified. On December 9, 1979, the WHO Global Commission for Certification of Smallpox Eradication concluded that eradication had been achieved. Now, only a handful of closely controlled laboratories maintain variola virus for research and archival purposes.

Virology

Variola is a member of the Orthopoxvirus genus, a group of closely related viruses which infect mammals. Variola and vaccinia, the virus currently used for vaccination, are large double-stranded DNA viruses (Table 69.1). Although humans are the only natural hosts for variola, animal models and tissue culture techniques have been developed for virus cultivation. Viral antigens of the orthopoxviruses are very similar and infection with one virus usually confers immunity to the others. Previously, it was impossible to distinguish many of the viruses antigenically. Endonuclease reduction has allowed species and virus strain differentiation to be made. However, there does not seem to be any remarkable differences between the variola major and variola minor virus strains.

Pathophysiology

Smallpox is most highly communicable in the first week of illness. Variola virus infections can be transmitted by direct contact with respiratory secretions. Infected individuals are capable of transmitting illness several days before the first onset of rash. Once lesions appear, they contain infectious virus which can transmit illness until all scabs have dropped off. Fomites may play a role in virus transmission, because of the long-term stability of the virus. Airborne spread is probably an unusual occurrence.

The pathogenesis of variola major and variola minor infections is identical. During an incubation period of approximately 12 days, the virus multiplies in the upper respiratory mucosa and in nearby lymph nodes. An initial viremia results in dissemination of virus to parenchymal organs. Following intensive viral multiplication, a subsequent viremia occurs which marks the beginning of symptomatic illness. The early cutaneous lesions result from mononuclear and plasma cell infiltration, edema, and congestion. Epithelial cells balloon and there is perinuclear

TABLE 69.1   Smallpox/Vaccinia Virus Characteristics

Genus	Orthopoxvirus
Nucleic acid	DNA (double-stranded)
Morphology	Brick-shaped to ovoid
Size	250-390 nm x 200-260 nm
Enzyme for early mRNA production	DNA-dependent RNA polymerase
Stability	Lipid solvent inactivated – resists inactivation by heat, cold, drying, or disinfectants
Site of infection	Epidermal cells
Site of multiplication	Cell cytoplasm
Natural host range	Man
Laboratory cultivation	Animals – especially rabbit, calf, sheep Chick embryo Cell cultures – especially human embryonic kidney, monkey kidney, Hela

clearing. Acidophilic Guarnieri bodies, 10 μm in diameter, are inclusions surrounded by a pale halo found within the infected cells' cytoplasm. Epithelial cell degeneration, necrosis, and interstitial fluid collection lead to papule formation followed by vesicles. Nonspecific reticuloendothelial hyperplasia is seen and small foci of fatty degeneration, petechial hemorrhage, and mononuclear cell infiltrations have been noted in parenchymal organs. Similar changes are seen in noncutaneous organs.

Both cell-mediated immunity and antibody response appear to play a role in the formation of the eruptive smallpox lesions. Resolution of disease appears to depend upon the adequacy of antibody and cell-mediated immune response. Immunocompromised individuals are less likely to develop cutaneous lesions, but they have a higher mortality.

Immunity following infection is generally complete and permanent. Although vaccinated individuals can acquire modified smallpox as immunity wanes, vaccination provides essentially complete immunity for at least 3 years. All unexposed, unvaccinated persons are susceptible.

Clinical Manifestations

Smallpox has an incubation period of 7-17 days. Most patients experience a typical course of illness. The prodrome lasts 2-4 days and is marked by a sudden onset of febrile illness with accompanying headache, malaise, prostration, backache, and abdominal discomfort. Fever diminishes as the eruptions begin to appear. The rash begins as macules which progress to papules, vesicles, and then pustules, which finally form scabs. Although the eruptions may occur in waves, they usually progress through these stages simultaneously. Lesions are initially seen on the face and scalp, and subsequently will appear in a centrifugal distribution over the back, chest, arms, and legs. Lesions are most dense over bony prominences, trauma or pressure areas, and over the distal extremities. Vesicles develop over a 24- to 48-hr period and scabs form by the second week of illness. Ten days later, the scabs fall off leaving pitted scars. The total course of uncomplicated illness is generally 2-3 weeks.

Ordinary or typical smallpox may occur as variola major (classic smallpox), having a mortality of 20-50%, or variola minor (alastrim), frequently having < 1% mortality in outbreaks. Intermediate forms of smallpox have been described in Africa and Indonesia, and fall between variola major and variola minor in severity and in fatality rates (5-15%). The clinical presentation of each form is similar but is distinguishable by the severity of disease, the mortality, and the epidemiology.

Approximately 10% of the patients may have one of four other presentations. Hemorrhagic smallpox is rapidly fatal and often misdiagnosed. Typical lesions are not seen, but petechiae, purpura, and ecchymoses are prominent. Flat smallpox is somewhat less severe, but often fatal. The patient is very toxic and a dusky facial erythema may be present. Macular eruptions are widespread, and soft, velvety, atypical papules are seen. The papules develop slowly and do not progress to pustules. Partially immune patients may present with a modified smallpox. The clinical picture is variable, but the disease is often mild with few fatalities. Lesions are often less dense, the rash may evolve more quickly, and the illness may superficially resemble chickenpox. Variola sine eruptione is essentially a subclinical infection. A febrile prodrome occurs, but existing immunity interrupts the course of illness and skin lesions do not occur.

Diagnosis

Although typical smallpox can be diagnosed clinically, unusual presentations may suggest chickenpox, meningococcemia, hemorrhagic diatheses, and herpesvirus infections. Chickenpox generally lacks the pronounced febrile prodrome of smallpox, and chickenpox lesions are generally uniformly distributed over the entire body. Chickenpox lesions develop in several crops over 2-4 days and progress to scabbed lesions more quickly. Absence of exposure history or presence of a vaccination scar makes the diagnosis of smallpox very unlikely.

Laboratory diagnosis can be made by virus isolation on chorioallantoic membrane or tissue culture from vesicular or pustular fluid or lesion scrapings. Virus can be isolated also from blood and throat cultures during the prodrome. Electron microscopy and gel precipitation can identify poxvirus, but cannot distinguish smallpox from others. Serology is useful for retrospective diagnosis.

Prevention

Smallpox vaccination is no longer recommended in the United States except for those individuals who may have laboratory exposure to variola. As of 1981, only two countries required smallpox vaccination for entering travelers.

Freeze-dried vaccinia virus is the best preparation for vaccination when indicated. The vaccine may be delivered by airjet injection or by scarification. A bifurcation needle is dipped into vaccine and five (for primary inoculation) or 15 (for revaccination) small stab wounds are made. A typical skin reaction will be seen in all successful primary or revaccinations. Primary vaccination lesions evolve over 2 weeks, and revaccination lesions evolve more quickly.

Vaccination results in local virus replication, but local delayed hypersensitivity reactions, which do not necessarily indicate vaccine potency, may occur in revaccinees 24-72 hr after inoculation. Primary vaccination confers 3-5 years of protective immunity, although partial immunity may persist for up to 20 years. Individuals at risk of exposure should be revaccinated triannually.

Serious complications of smallpox vaccination are infrequent but may result in death. A morbidity of 74/1 million and a mortality of 1/1 million primary vaccinations has been estimated in the United States and 4.7 complications per million revaccinations have been noted. Another study indicated a complication rate of 100,253/1 million primary vaccinations and of 108,000/1 million revaccinations. Infants under 1 year of age are at highest risk. Accidental implantation and infection, generalized vaccinia, and eczema vaccinatum are the most commonly seen complications. Vaccinia necrosum and central nervous system illness, such as postvaccinial encephalitis, myelitis, and Guillain-Barré syndrome, are the most severe complications. Vaccinia infections may occur in contacts of vaccinates. Vaccination should be avoided in individuals with hematopoietic or lymphoreticular malignancies, immunologic disorders or immune suppression, eczema or eczema history in patient or household members, acute febrile illness, and pregnancy. Smallpox vaccination should not be used for prevention of herpes simplex recurrences because there is no evidence of its usefulness, and severe complications as a result of this therapy have occurred.

Treatment

Passive immunization with hyperimmune vaccinial gamma globulin (VIG) may reduce the incidence and severity of illness in close contacts of the patient with smallpox. Methisazone has been used to treat vaccinia gangrenosa and for prophylaxis of intimate contacts of smallpox patients. However, treatment of symptomatic patients has not been effective.

Other Significant Poxviruses

Other members of the poxviruses are important for their potential infectivity of man and their close resemblance to variola virus (Table 69.2). Molluscum contagiosum virus produces an uncommon skin infection of children and young adults. The virus produces proliferative lesions and stimulates division in neighboring uninfected cells. This virus, which is indistinguishable by electron microscopy from other poxviruses, may be intermediate between viruses causing acute infection and those producing tumors.

TABLE 69.2   Other Important Poxviruses

Virus	Manifestations
Vaccinia	Artificially propagated virus used for human vaccination; no natural animal hosts; may have evolved from cowpox
Molluscum contagiosum	Chronic, proliferative epithelial lesions
Cowpox[1]	Self-limited localized vesicular lesions; source: cattle
Paravaccinia[1]	Milker's nodules - smooth or warty painless lesions and mild systemic complaints; source: cattle
Orf[1]	Contagious pustular dermatitis - solitary painless, vesicular lesion on finger which progresses to pustule, crust, and heals spontaneously (rare in man); source: sheep
Tanapox	Outbreaks of febrile illness with rare upperbody pock lesions - Kenya, Africa
Monkeypox	Rare human infections which resemble smallpox, but very limited spread
Whitepox	Probably variant of monkeypox virus; resembles smallpox virus; no recognized human cases
Other animal poxviruses[2]	Elephantpox, carnivorepox, buffalopox, camelpox, mousepox, pox in American raccoon, avian and other poxviruses

[1]Occupational illness in livestock workers

[2]No human infections recognized

Cowpox, milker's nodules (paravaccinia), and contagious pustular dermatitis (orf) are self-limited occupational infections. These lesions are usually transmitted from livestock to workers' hands by direct contact. Dissemination or man-to-man transmission rarely occurs. Tanapox virus has been recently recognized as a cause of two outbreaks among Kenya tribesmen. Infection results in a febrile illness with one or two pock-like lesions on the upper body. The origins of vaccinia virus are unclear, but it may have derived from Jenner's original cowpox strain. Illness caused by vaccinia is generally related to vaccination. There is no apparent animal reservoir.

Monkeypox virus has been isolated from simians and humans in West Africa. Human illness and its mortality (15%) are similar to smallpox in that region, leading to concern that it might represent a new epidemic strain. However, monkeypox does not appear to be adapted for propagation of human illness since secondary transmission occurred in only 3.6% of contacts.

Whitepox virus may be a variant of monkeypox but it cannot be distinguished from smallpox by the usual laboratory means. Embryonated egg inoculation with monkeypox produces hemorrhagic pox on the chorioallantoic membrane, while whitepox may appear from the same inoculation as nonhemorrhagic (white) pox. Some investigators have suggested that this is evidence for the evolution of variola from monkeypox. It has been isolated from apparently normal monkeys, but no human illness has been recognized, despite concerted surveillance in areas of monkeypox endemicity.

Selected Bibliography

Angulo, J. J.: Variola minor in Bragana Paulista County, 1956: Overall description of the epidemic and its study. *Internat J Epidemiol* 5:359-365, 1976.

Arita, I.: Virological evidence for the success of the smallpox eradication program. *Nature* 279:293-298, 1979.

Bauer, D. J.: Antiviral chemotherapy: The first decade. *Br Med J* 3:275-279, 1973.

Baxby, D.: Identification and interrelationships of the variola/vaccinia subgroups of poxvirus. *Prog Med Virol* 19:215-246, 1975.

Baxby, D.: Poxvirus hosts and reservoirs - brief review. *Arch Virol* 55:169-179, 1977.

Breman, J. G. and Arita, I.: The confirmation and maintenance of smallpox eradication. *N Engl J Med* 303:1263-1273, 1980.

Breman, J. G., Bernadon, J., and Nakano, J. H.: Poxvirus in West African nonhuman primates: Serological survey results. *Bull WHO* 55:605-612, 1977.

Breman, J. G., Kalisa-Ruti, Steniowski, M. V., Zanotto, E., Gromyko, A. L., and Arita, L.: Human monkeypox 1970-1979. *Bull WHO* 58:165-182, 1980.

Breman, J. G., Nakano, J. H., Coffi, E., et al.: Human poxvirus disease after smallpox eradication. *Am J Trop Med Hyg* 26:273-281, 1977.

Brilliant, L. B. and Hodakevic, L. N.: Certification of smallpox eradication. *Bull WHO* 56:723-733, 1978.

Costa, E. A. and Morris, L.: Smallpox epidemics in a Brazilian community. *Am J Epidemiol* 101:552-561, 1975.

Downie, A. W., Taylor-Robinson, C. H., Caunt, A. E., Nelson, G. S., Manson-Bahr, P. E. C., and Matthews, T. C. H.: Tanapox: A new disease caused by a pox virus. *Br Med J* 1:363-368, 1971.

Dumbell, K. R. and Archard, L. C.: Comparison of white pock (h) mutants of monkeypox viruses with parental monkeypox and with variola-like viruses isolated from animals. *Nature* 286:29-32, 1980.

Du Mont, G. C. L. and Beach, R. C.: Continuing mortality and morbidity from smallpox vaccination. *Br Med J* 1:1398-1399, 1979.

Esposito, J. J., Obijeski, J. F., and Nakano, J. H.: Orthopoxvirus DNA: Strain differentiation by electrophoresis of restriction endonuclease fragmented virion DNA. *Virology* 89:53-66, 1978.

Foege, W. H. and Eddins, D. L.: Mass vaccination in developing countries. *Prog Med Virol* 15:205-243, 1973.

Foege, W. H., Millar, J. D., and Henderson, D. A.: Smallpox eradication in West and Central Africa. *Bull WHO* 52:209-222, 1975.

Foster, S. O., Brink, E. W., Hutchins, D. L., et al.: Human monkeypox. *Bull WHO* 46:569-576, 1972.

Foster, S. O., El Sid, A. G. H., and Deria, A.: Spread of smallpox among a Somali nomadic group. *Lancet* 2:831 833, 1978.

Hawker, N.: Smallpox death in Britain challenges presumption of laboratory safety. *Science* 203:855-856, 1979.

Hughes, K., Foster, S. O., Tarantola, D., Mehta, H., Tulloch, J. L., and Joarder, A. K.: Smallpox surveillance in Bangladesh: II. Smallpox facial scar survey assessment of surveillance effectiveness. *Internat J Epidemiol* 9:335-340, 1980.

Lane, J. M., Ruben, F. L., Neff, J. M., and Millar, J. D.: Complications of smallpox vaccination, 1968. National surveillance in the United States. *N Engl J Med* 281:1201-1208, 1969.

Lane, J. M., Ruben, F. L., Neff, J. M., and Millar, J. D.: Complications of smallpox vaccination, 1968: Results of ten statewide surveys. *J Infect Dis* 122: 303-309, 1970.

Mack, T. M.: Smallpox in Europe, 1959-1971. *J Infect Dis* 125:161-169, 1972.

Marennikova, S. S. and Shelukhina, E. M.: Whitepox virus isolated from hamsters inoculated with monkeypox virus. *Nature* 276:291-292, 1978.

Marennikova, S. S., Shelukhina, E. M., Maltseva, N. N., and Matsevich, G. R.: Monkeypox virus as a source of whitepox virus. *Intervirology* 11:333-340, 1979.

Marsden, J. P.: Variola minor: A personal analysis of 13,686 cases. *Bull Hyg* 23: 735-746, 1948.

Mazumder, D. N. G., De, S., Mitra, A. C., and Mukherjee, M. K.: Clinical observations on smallpox: A study of 1233 patients admitted to the Infectious Diseases Hospital, Calcutta, during 1973. *Bull WHO* 52:301-306, 1975.

Rao, A. R.: Some epidemiological and clinical features of smallpox and its diagnosis. *Bull Indian Soc Malar Commun Dis* 3:96–112, 1966.

Sarkar, J. K., Mitra, A. C., and Mukherjee, M. K.: The minimum protective levels of antibodies in smallpox. *Bull WHO* 52:307–311, 1975.

Wenner, H. A.: Virus diseases associated with cutaneous eruptions. *Prog Med Virol* 16:269–336, 1973.

Zuckerman, A. and Rondle, C.: The enigma of poxviruses. *Nature* 276:212–213, 1976.

70

PAPILLOMAVIRUSES
Robert H. Waldman, M.D.

Papillomaviruses are the group of viruses that cause human warts. They are related to similar groups of viruses that cause infection in other mammalian species. They are double-stranded DNA viruses, and six serotypes have been identified.

They usually infect children or young adults and cause benign tumors of the skin and mucous membranes. In almost all cases the tumors undergo spontaneous resolution, apparently as a result of the body's immune response, i.e., tumor immunity. The virus gains access to the skin through very small breaks, and proceeds to infect epithelial cells, which are then stimulated to more rapid mitosis. The time between infection and clinical appearance of the tumor is 1-6 months. Histopathologically the lesions show large vacuolated cells in the upper stratum malpighi and granular layer. This differentiates warts from nonviral papillomas. The virus is found mainly in the superficial layers of the epidermis which is relatively protected from the immune system. This explains why almost any treatment which tends to disrupt the integrity of the wart leads to the usual cure.

The different types of warts are shown in Table 70.1. Plantar warts grow inward, are more painful, and are more resistant to therapy. They should be differentiated from corns and calluses by cutting away the keratotic surface, which should reveal dark brown dots that are small, thrombosed vessels.

Condyloma acuminata are genital or perineal soft, pinkish-brown cauliflower-like masses. They may be premalignant. They should be easily differentiated from condyloma lata, a manifestation of secondary syphilis, which are gray and sessile.

It is very important to keep in mind that warts clear spontaneously in almost all cases and therefore, the keystone to therapy is patience and reassurance of the patient, keeping in mind that throughout history more people have been harmed by the treatment for warts than by the warts themselves. If treatment is deemed necessary, it should be as mild as possible, and the aim of treatment, as mentioned earlier, is to expose the virus-infected cells to the body's immune system, especially

TABLE 70.1   Various Types of Warts

Common and flat (most common)

Plantar

Condyloma acuminata

Laryngeal papillomas

---

cell-mediated immunity. This can be accomplished by a variety of physical or chemical destructive procedures, including electro- and cryotherapy, and salicyclic acid. Condyloma acuminata are very effectively treated with topical podophyllum.

Member(s) of this group of viruses, the papovaviruses, have been isolated from patients with progressive multifocal leukoencephalopathy (see Chapter 78).

Selected Bibliography

Bunney, M. H.: The treatment of viral warts. *Drugs* 13:445, 1977.

Hursthouse, M. W.: A controlled trial on the use of topical 5-fluorouracil on viral warts. *Br J Dermatol* 92:93, 1975.

Kovi, J., Tillman, R. L., and Lee, S. M.: Malignant transformation of condyloma acuminatum. *J Clin Pathol* 61:702, 1974.

71

ADENOVIRUSES
Patrick A. Robinson, M.D.

Introduction

In the early 1930s it became apparent that respiratory illness was not entirely attributable to influenza. The development of tissue culture techniques in the early 1950s led to further elucidation of noninfluenza viruses causing respiratory disease. Adenovirus was first isolated from surgically removed human adenoids in 1953 by Rowe et al. and was subsequently isolated during a respiratory epidemic from army recruits. Adenoviruses are part of a large spectrum of noninfluenza viruses causing significant upper and lower respiratory disease.

Microbiology

Adenoviruses (AV) are nonenveloped icosahedral DNA viruses with a surrounding capsid and a dense nucleoid core. They contain a single chain of double-stranded DNA and a nucleoprotein core which maintains the DNA integrity. More than 35 antigenically different human serotypes have been recognized. The virus is 60-90 nm in size, although intracellular virions may be smaller (50 nm). Rod-like fibers project from the penton base, and play a role in the hemagglutination of AV groups. The hexon protein antigens are common to all human AV, but fiber antigens are type-specific.

Adenoviruses are remarkably resistant to environmental inactivation, which probably aids in their transmission. They remain viable between temperatures of 4 and 36°C and can be frozen with little loss of infectivity. They retain infectivity in homogenates of infected cells for several weeks (at 4°C) or months (at -25°C). Since they lack a lipid envelope, they are not inactivated by ether and will survive at a pH of 5-9.

Most steps of viral replication occur in the nucleus of the infected cell. The virus adsorbs slowly to the host cell and then enters the cytoplasm where viral DNA is uncoated. The penton-related fibers block the host cell's synthesis of macromolecules. Infection of the host cell shuts off its cellular DNA production, subsequent RNA production, and mitosis. The protein-naked viral DNA enters the host cell's nucleoplasm through nuclear membrane pores and early messenger RNA is constructed before viral DNA replication. The double-stranded DNA replicates 6-24 hr after infection. Late mRNA synthesis then takes place, using the new DNA as templates. Viral proteins are formed in the cytoplasm, enter the nucleus, and take part in virion assembly.

Human adenoviruses have been divided into three groups, based on their hemagglutination characteristics. Group I viruses agglutinate rhesus monkey erythrocytes, group II agglutinate rat erythrocytes, and group III partially agglutinate rat but do not agglutinate monkey red cells (Table 71.1). Each serotype within these three groups is distinct from other adenovirus serotypes. Although human adenoviruses can infect animals and animal tissue culture in the laboratory, humans are the only known natural host. Adenoviruses of other mammals and birds share some group antigens with human virus, but they do not cause human infection. Some will transform hamster cells in tissue culture and cause tumors in newborn hamsters; however, there is no evidence of human oncogenicity.

Adenovirus-associated viruses are small defective viruses (20-25 nm), members of the Parvoviridae family, which are unrelated to adenoviruses, but are adenovirus-dependent: they cannot replicate in the absence of adenovirus. They probably take part in dual infections in humans.

Pathogenesis

The clinical presentation of adenovirus disease is dependent upon the complex interactions of viral transmission, the site of virus localization, the viral serotype, and the host response to infection (Table 71.2). Human adenoviruses are transmitted by several routes. Fecal-oral transmission is the most important mechanism among children and families. Adenoviruses are commonly shed in the stool for extended periods. Aerosolized respiratory secretions transmit virus. This is especially important in acute respiratory disease outbreaks in military camps and in acute pharyngeal conjunctival fever. Direct inoculation of nasopharyngeal secretions induces illness less efficiently but is another important means of spread. Direct inoculation of the conjunctiva with the appropriate virus serotypes can produce conjunctivitis; swimming pools and lakes have been implicated in this mode of transmission. Conjunctivitis following direct eye contact with infected ointments or ophthalmologic instruments has been described, as has nosocomial transmission. Virus may be present in inapparently infected respiratory tissues, thus pharyngeal carriage in the absence of symptoms may be high during outbreaks in closed populations, resulting in ample opportunity for transmission. There are no natural animal sources for human adenovirus, and vector transmission has not been described.

Since good animal models are not available, most data on pathogenesis come from clinical observations or human volunteer studies. The incubation period is 6-9 days for naturally occurring infections, but it may be shorter with a large experimental inoculum.

Adenovirus infection may result in two outcomes. Acute symptomatic illness results from lysis of host cells. The virus undergoes the entire replication cycle and infected cells die releasing 10^4-10^6 virions per cell, 1-5% of which are infectious. However, infection often results in latent or chronic infection of tonsils and

TABLE 71.1   Hemagglutination Adenovirus Subgroups

Subgroup	Serotype	RBC Agglutination		Oncogenic Potential	Some Associated Human Illnesses
		Rat	Rhesus		
I	3,7,11,14,16,20, 21,25,28	0	+	Moderate	Upper and lower respiratory illness, ARD, PCF, AHC
II	8,9*,10,13*,15*, 17,19,22,23,24, 26,27	+	0 or +*	Low	EKC, conjunctivitis, trachoma
III	1,2,4,5,6	Partial	0	Low	Respiratory infection
IV	12,18,21	0	0	High	ARD, trachoma

*Agglutinate at lower titers than rat RBCs

TABLE 71.2   Clinical Findings in Several Typical Adenoviral Outbreaks

	Pneumonia		Respiratory	
	Children Type 7 (%)	Adults (%)	Children Type 3 (%)	Adults Type 4 (%)
Cough	97	100		44[1]
Fever	97	100	87	89
Vomiting	63	58	26	*
Dyspnea	55	*	*	*
Diarrhea	45	25	35	*
Heart failure	48	*	*	*
Deaths	10	*	*	*
Meningismus	38	*	*	*
Pharyngitis	*	92	91	56
Rhinorrhea/rhinitis	*	75	30	44
Nausea	*	75	48	*
Adenopathy	*	50	*	*
Conjunctivitis	*	33	*	*
Myalgia	*	33	*	78[2]
Headache	*	33	74	78[2]
Chest x-ray infiltrates	100	100	*	22
Bilateral	65	33		0/2
≥ 2 lobes or segments	79	17		0/2

*None or not reported

[1]Reported as tracheobronchitis

[2]Reported as part of "systemic symptoms"

mesenteric lymph nodes. The host cell's integrity is preserved and incomplete
virions are produced. The early stages of replication take place, and the virion
genome is inserted into the host cell's DNA. Infective virus can be isolated subsequently when latently infected cells are placed in tissue culture. Reactivation
of latent virus may occur as a result of another infection, including other respiratory viruses or mycoplasma.

   Although upper respiratory tract tissue usually is involved, alveolar cell infection can result in severe or fatal pneumonia. Lower respiratory tract involvement
results in mononuclear cell infiltrates, focal areas of parenchymal necrosis and
hemorrhage, and consolidation. Other pulmonary findings are typical of nonbacterial pneumonia. As subvirion components accumulate in the host cell's nuclei
they form characteristic eosinophilic rosette-shaped inclusions visible by light microscopy. Infections of other tissue exhibit similar findings.

   Most infections do not result in detectable viremia, but dissemination may occur in immunocompromised individuals and following measles, rubella, and possibly Epstein-Barr virus infections. Renal infections have been described. Adenovirus often causes latent tonsillar infections as indicated by 50-80% isolation rates
from apparently normal tonsils. Neurotropism may result in encephalitis and meningeal infection, particularly with type 7.

   Adenovirus infection results in formation of three demonstrable antibody
types. Neutralizing antibodies directed against penton fiber antigens are serotype
specific and appear to confer lifelong immunity. Hemagglutination-inhibiting
(HAI) antibodies are also type-specific. Complement-fixing (CF) antibodies are
group-specific, cross-reacting antibodies and, since they are relatively short-lived,
are useful for detecting acute infection. The antibody response appears to be important in limiting adenovirus infection. Individuals with a poor IgA response tend
to have a more severe course of infection and immunocompromised persons may
occasionally develop severe or fatal infections. Maternal antibodies offer protection in children under 6 months of age.

Epidemiology

Adenoviruses are ubiquitous, but serotypes may vary geographically. Type 8 and
higher-numbered serotypes are found more commonly in underdeveloped countries,
whereas lower-numbered serotypes usually cause disease in both developed and
underdeveloped areas. Certain serotypes tend to cause different clinical illness
patterns, but there is substantial overlap. Serotypes 1, 2, 5, and 6 are more likely
to cause endemic disease, while serotypes 4, 7, 14, and 21 may result in respiratory epidemics. Type 3 may result in either endemic or epidemic illness and nosocomial infections have been described with types 3 and 4. Although infections occur all seasons of the year, adenoviruses are isolated most often in late winter,
spring, and early summer. Outbreaks of acute respiratory disease (ARD) are usually seen at these times, independent of geography or climate, but swimming-
associated pharyngeal conjunctival fever (PCF) generally occurs in the summer.
A 4-year-long nationwide outbreak of AV type 7 with mixed clinical presentation
had no seasonal variation in England. Adenovirus causes up to 40% of all "atypical" pneumonias in the military, it causes approximately 5% of civilian respiratory
disease, and 10% of respiratory illness in children. Although infants generally are
protected by maternal antibody up to the age of 6 months, primary infection often
occurs in the first year of life. Adenovirus shedding is commonly present in asymptomatic children, with as many as 50% of children who shed virus being asymptomatic. Approximately 5-20% of childhood upper respiratory illness, pharyngitis,
and pneumonia and 1-5% in adults may be caused by adenovirus.

The epidemic behavior of ARD in military populations is substantially different from that occurring in civilians. Acute respiratory disease-associated pneumonia can be attributed to adenovirus in as many as 44% of recruits early in their training period and about 50% of all recruits experience adenovirus infection. Epidemic virus types may vary from one country to another, but the United States military generally experiences infections with types 4 and 7. Outbreaks with types 3, 11, 14, and 21 also may occur. Vaccination with adenovirus type 4 and type 4/7 vaccines has resulted in a decreased prevalence of these serotypes, but other serotypes may take their place. The ARD-associated immunity appears to be acquired early in military life since outbreaks are uncommon in seasoned troops. Because crowding is a major factor in transmission, changes in recruit environments, such as decreasing the size of groups sharing sleeping quarters and diminishing the number of new recruits, can change ARD's epidemic nature. Outbreaks of ARD are unusual in college students despite the age and environmental similarity to military recruits.

Adenovirus respiratory illness is often seen within family settings, where serotypes 1, 2, 3, and 5 are usually encountered. Institutions and day-care settings are important areas of AV transmission, and swimming pool water may be a vehicle.

Pharyngeal conjunctival fever (PCF) may occur sporadically, or result from outbreaks within family or other closely associated groups. Direct contact with infected secretions and contaminated lake and swimming pool water appear to be the important means of transmission. Secondary transmission is common following infection of a family member from such a source. Serotypes 3 and 7 are the major AV pathogens causing PCF, but occasionally types 1, 4, and 14 may be seen. Adenovirus has also caused nosocomial conjunctivitis or PCF.

Epidemic keratoconjunctivitis (EKC) may be seen in three important settings: factories and ship-building industries, ophthalmology offices, and in circumstances where crowding and decreased hygiene occur, such as refugee camps. This illness has been described also in community and hospital epidemics. Outbreaks usually occur in late summer and fall, but may be seen at other seasons. Serotype 8 was recognized as the almost exclusive cause of EKC until 1973, when type 19 was discovered in European and North American outbreaks. Institutions and day-care settings are important areas of AV transmission and outbreaks. Occasionally serotypes 4, 10, 11, and 14 cause EKC.

Acute hemorrhagic cystitis (AHC) caused by AV has been described in Japanese and United States children and occasionally in Japanese adults. Thus far, only serotypes 11 and 21 have been associated with AHC.

Clinical Illness

Adenovirus infection usually results in mild upper or lower respiratory illness or conjunctivitis, but gastrointestinal illness, acute hemorrhagic cystitis, central nervous system infection, and rarely, dissemination also can occur. Symptomatic infection is usually mild; as many as half of all AV infections may be asymptomatic. Occasionally fulminant infections may occur requiring hospitalization and even resulting in death.

Respiratory Illness

Acute respiratory disease has been associated most often with military personnel, but it can be seen in civilians as well. Four to five days following viral exposure, ARD begins most typically with cough, fever, sore throat, and rhinorrhea. Illness

lasts 3-5 days and is usually self-limited. However, up to 20% of military personnel may require hospitalization, and approximately 10% of military-associated
ARD results in pneumonia. Fever, cough, and systemic symptoms are prominent,
and rhinitis, tracheobronchitis, and pharyngitis are often seen with ARD pneumonia. Chest roentgenograms demonstrate lower-lobe patchy infiltrates, which resolve over about 3 weeks. Severe respiratory infection is more common in infants
and young children, especially with AV type 7, and the infection may be fatal.
Pneumonia, wheezing associated with respiratory illness, and bronchiolitis are the
most severe presentations seen in children. Adenovirus may be isolated from about
10% of children with wheezing, and up to 40% of lower respiratory infections result in bronchospasm. Children under 5 years of age are most often affected. The
severity of illness may approach that of respiratory syncytial virus infections in
hospitalized infants. Bronchiectasis, obliterative bronchitis, and hyperlucent lung
syndrome may follow pediatric adenovirus respiratory infections. Upper respiratory illness may also present with the pertussis syndrome. Infection due to adenovirus has been associated rarely with chronic interstitial fibrosing pneumonitis.

Conjunctivitis

Pharyngeal conjunctival fever is seen most often in school-aged children. Following an incubation of 6-9 days (as short as 2 days in experimental models) PCF has
an acute onset and generally lasts 3-5 days. Illness is marked by malaise, headache, mild to moderate pharyngitis, rhinitis, and preauricular and cervical lymphadenopathy. Fever to 39°C or higher is common. Approximately 50-70% of patients develop unilateral conjunctivitis which may become bilateral. The conjunctivae are injected and the palpebral conjunctivae may be granular in appearance.
The cornea is rarely affected and no permanent damage ensues. Tonsillar exudate
is often present. Occasionally diarrhea, coryza, or otitis may accompany PCF.
    Epidemic keratoconjunctivitis usually occurs as outbreaks in industrial set-
tings, ophthalmologic practices, communities, or refugee camps, but may result in
solitary infections. Four to twelve days following exposure, a mild bilateral follicular conjunctivitis insidiously develops. Periauricular lymphadenopathy and occasional upper respiratory illness accompanies acute conjunctivitis which lasts 1-
4 weeks. Palpebral edema, pain, photophobia, and lacrimation are present during
acute illness. Fever and systemic symptoms are usually lacking, and mucopurulent
discharge is unusual. As the acute conjunctivitis resolves, keratitis begins. Superficial corneal erosions are followed by 0.2- to 1.5 mm round, subepithelial corneal
infiltrates, which are centrally located. Temporary visual impairment occurs in
one- to two-thirds of the patients and keratitis usually persists for 2-6 months but
may last up to 16 months.

Gastrointestinal Disease

Both cultivable and noncultivable adenoviruses have been associated with infant
diarrhea. Although some studies have shown adenoviruses in 10-20% of diarrhea
stools, they are probably an uncommon cause of diarrhea. They are often shed
asymptomatically in the stool following symptomatic or asymptomatic respiratory
infections, and their presence may represent prolonged shedding or reactivation of
a latent respiratory focus rather than as a cause of diarrhea.
    Intussusception in children has been linked with adenovirus infection by serol-
ogy and by virus isolation. Mesenteric adenitis and enlarged Peyer's patches may
serve as a focal point for beginning "idiopathic" intussusception. Serotypes 1-7
are the more commonly recognized serotypes associated with intussusception.

Acute Hemorrhagic Cystitis

Adenovirus types 11 and 21 are important agents causing AHC in children. Adenoviruria continues through the approximately 4-14 days of gross hematuria, dysuria, and increased urinary frequency. Suprapubic pain, enuresis, and fever are less commonly seen. Cystitis resolves spontaneously without any apparent residual urinary tract damage.

Other Illness

Other unusual adenovirus infections have been described. Encephalitis has been associated with adenovirus epidemics. Renal and liver infections, rhabdomyolysis, and disseminated infection occur, but they are limited usually to neonates or immunocompromised patients. Adenovirus has been isolated from patients with a rubelliform rash but this may reflect viral reactivation or asymptomatic shedding concomitant with another viral infection.

Laboratory Diagnosis

Tentative diagnosis of adenovirus infection may be made on epidemiologic and clinical presentation. However, three laboratory techniques most useful in diagnosis are: (1) serology, (2) virus culture, and (3) virus antigen detection. Serologic confirmation of infection is based on a fourfold or greater rise of complement-fixing (CF), neutralizing, or hemagglutination-inhibiting (HAI) virus antibodies, each of which begins to appear approximately 1 week following onset of infection and peaks at 2-3 weeks. Antibodies are directed against the three main viral antigen components. Complement-fixing and neutralizing antibodies are produced against the hexon protein, while penton antigens elicit CF antibodies. Complement-fixation tests are the convenient methods of making a diagnosis of acute illness but their sensitivity depends on the CF antigen used and the population studied. Complement-fixing antibodies rise promptly in acute infection but will be gone by 1 year following infection. They are group-specific, since they combine with cross-reacting family antigens and thus cannot be used for serotyping. Neutralizing antibodies and hemagglutination-inhibiting antibodies are homotypic and are used to serotype adenovirus. Neutralizing antibodies may persist for more than 10 years and a subsequent infection with a heterotypic adenovirus will boost the titers. The HAI is a simpler test, and it is almost as sensitive as neutralization, especially when hemagglutination enhancement is used. The HAI titers will remain high for many years following infection and appear to be boosted by subsequent infections. Both HAI and neutralizing antibodies are useful for seroepidemiology. An enzyme-linked immunosorbent assay (ELISA) has recently been described for detection of adenovirus antibodies. This system shows great future promise for serodiagnosis.

Virus isolation on tissue culture is a specific method of identifying adenovirus-caused infection. Virus can be easily recovered from the respiratory tract, conjunctiva, nasopharynx, or feces. Isolation does not necessarily indicate symptomatic infection, since adenovirus may be obtained from asymptomatic individuals. Isolations from the respiratory tract are more suggestive of AV illness than fecal isolations since asymptomatic stool shedding may persist for months. A cytopathologic effect can usually be seen 2-14 days following inoculation of AV into human epithelial cells, such as Hep-2, HeLa, KB cells, or human embryonic kidney.

When virus culture and serology are compared, culture yields the higher detection rate. Combining culture and serologic methods gives the best diagnostic yield.

In recent years, indirect fluorescence (IFA), countercurrent immunoelectro-phoresis (CIE), and enzyme-linked immunosorbent assay (ELISA) have been used for rapid detection of adenovirus antigen. The IFA has successfully identified virus antigen in EKC, PCF, and hemorrhagic cystitis as well as detected it early in tissue culture. The ELISA can detect adenovirus-infected nasopharyngeal cells and stool, and CIE has been used to identify virus in stool.

Treatment and Prevention

Currently, there is no specific therapy available for adenovirus infection. Anti-viral agents, interferon, and interferon producers have not proved effective in al-tering the course of disease. Severe adenovirus illness is uncommon. Individuals with severe infections, such as pneumonia and dissemination, should be treated supportively.

Variable success in limiting outbreaks of disease has been obtained by modify-ing the environment of closed population groups such as military recruits. Dust control and changing sleeping arrangements have offered only modest success in limiting outbreaks. Ultraviolet light and virucidal sprays have proved of little value. Swimming pool chlorination appears to prevent PCF transmission and heat sterilization and hygienic methods appear to prevent spread of EKC in ophthal-mologists' offices. The avoidance of sharing possible fomites, such as towels, may limit intrafamilial transmission, and proper isolation techniques and hand-washing should be emphasized in nosocomial outbreaks.

Epidemics of AV infection in recruits prompted development of vaccines in the early 1960s. The first vaccines developed were formalin inactivated and di-rected against serotypes 3, 4, and 7. However, the potency of these vaccines was variable, and contamination with SV40 virus made them less than satisfactory. Vaccines derived from highly purified subunit protein were very effective, but some vaccine production difficulties remained.

Subsequently, live virus vaccines were developed, and testing in mililtary and adult civilian populations demonstrated satisfactory immunogenicity and safety of the type-specific live virus vaccines. These vaccines were nonattenuated and de-livered to the gastrointestinal tract in an enteric-coated capsule which bypassed the respiratory tract and produced no symptoms. Serotype 4 and serotypes 4/7 virus vaccines proved useful in preventing illness. However, when type 4 was used in a monovalent vaccine, type 7 disease replaced type 4 disease in recruits, and type 21 emerged as a pathogen when bivalent (type 4/7) vaccine was used. Suc-cessful immunization of civilian adults has been obtained using type 1/2/5 trivalent vaccine. Intranasal administration vaccination has also been an effective means of producing antibody. There appears to be no interference with induction of adeno-virus immunity from concomitant infection with several viruses.

Although adenovirus vaccines appear to be an important preventive and cost-saving measure in the military, and possibly of significance in other closed popula-tions, concern over potential oncogenic properties of type 3 and type 7 in animals and the usually benign course of infection has limited general vaccine use. Addi-tionally, children and spouses who have been vaccinated gastrointestinally can in-fect other household members.

Selected Bibliography

Baraff, L. J., Wilkins, J., and Wehrle, P. F.: The role of antibiotics, immunizations, and adenoviruses in pertussis. *Pediatrics* 61:224-230, 1978.

D'Angelo, L. J., Hierholzer, J. C., Holman, R. C., and Smith, J. D.: Epidemic keratoconjunctivitis caused by adenovirus type 8: Epidemiologic and laboratory aspects of a large outbreak. *Am J Epidemiol* 113:44-49, 1981.

D'Angelo, L. J., Hierholzer, J. C., Keenlyside, R. A., Anderson, L. J., and Martone, W. J.: Pharyngeal conjunctival fever caused by adenovirus type 4: Report of a swimming pool-related outbreak with recovery of virus from pool water. *J Infect Dis* 140:42-47, 1979.

Dowling, J. M. and Wynne, H.: Role of enteric adenoviruses and rotaviruses in infantile gastroenteritis. *Lancet* 2:305-306, 1981.

Fox, J. P., Hall, C. E., and Cooney, M. K.: The Seattle virus watch. II. Observations of adenovirus infections. *Am J Epidemiol* 105:362-386, 1977.

Gary, G. W., Hierholzer, J. C., and Black, R. E.: Characteristics of noncultivable adenovirus associated diarrhea in infants: A new subgroup of human adenoviruses. *J Clin Microbiol* 10:96-103, 1979.

Henderson, F. W., Clyde, W. A., Collier, A. M., et al.: The etiologic and epidemiologic spectrum of bronchiolitis in pediatric practice. *J Pediatr* 95:183-190, 1979.

Hierholzer, J. C. and Sprague, J. B.: Five-year analysis of adenovirus 8 antibody levels in an industrial community following an outbreak of keratoconjunctivitis. *Am J Epidemiol* 110:132-140, 1979.

Hilleman, M. R. and Werner, J. H.: Recovery of new agent from patients with acute respiratory illness. *Proc Exp Biol Med* 85:183-188, 1954.

Johansson, M. E., Unkoo, I., Kidal, A. H., Madeleg, C. R., and Wadell, G.: Direct identification of enteric adenovirus, a candidate new serotype associated with infantile gastroenteritis. *J Clin Microbiol* 12:95-100, 1980.

Kelsey, D. S.: Adenovirus meningitis. *Pediatrics* 61:291-293, 1978.

Kim, S. and Gohd, R. S.: Fatal pneumonia caused by adenovirus type 35. *Am J Dis Child* 135:473-475, 1981.

Levandowski, R. A. and Rubenis, M.: Nosocomial conjunctivitis caused by adenovirus type 4. *J Infect Dis* 143:28-31, 1981.

Martone, W. J., Hierholzer, J. C., Keenlyside, R. A., Fraser, D. W., D'Angelo, L. J., and Winkler, W. G.: An outbreak of adenovirus type 3 disease at a private recreation center swimming pool. *Am J Epidemiol* 111:229-237, 1980.

Meshkinpour, H. and Vazir, N. D.: Acute rhabdomyolysis associated with adenovirus infection. *J Infect Dis* 143:133, 1981.

Pearson, R. D., Hall, W. J., Menegus, M. A., and Douglas, R. G.: Diffuse pneumonitis due to adenovirus type 21 in a civilian. *Chest* 78:107-109, 1980.

Pingleton, S. K., Pingleton, W. W., Hill, R. H., Dixon, A., Sobonya, R. E., and Gertzen, J.: Type 3 adenoviral pneumonia occurring in a respiratory intensive care unit. *Chest* 73:554-555, 1978.

Rowe, W. P., Huebuer, R. J., Gilmore, L. K., Parrott, R. H., and Ward, T. G.: Isolation of a cytopathogenic agent from human adenoids undergoing spontaneous degeneration in tissue culture. *Proc Soc Exp Biol Med* 84:570-573, 1953.

Schmidt, O. W., Cooney, M. K., and Foy, H. M.: Adenovirus-associated virus in type 3 conjunctivitis. *Infect Immun* 11:1362-1370, 1975.

Siegal, F. P., Dikman, S. H., Arayata, R. B., and Bottone, E. J.: Fatal disseminated adenovirus II pneumonia in an agammaglobulinemic patient. *Am J Med* 71: 1062-1067, 1981.

Smith, R. H.: Fatal adenovirus infection with misleading positive scrology for infectious mononucleosis. *Lancet* 1:294-300, 1979.

Stadler, H., Hierholzer, J. C., and Oxman, M. N.: New human adenovirus (candidate adenovirus type 35) causing fatal dissemination in renal transplant recipient. *J Clin Microbiol* 6:257-265, 1977.

Takafuji, E. T., Gaydos, J. C., Allen, R. G., and Top, F. H.: Simultaneous administration of live, enteric-coated adenovirus type 4, 7, and 21 vaccines: Safety and immunogenicity. *J Infect Dis* 140:48-53, 1979.

Vesikari, T., Maki, M., Sarkkininen, H. K., Arstila, P. P., and Halonen, P. E.: Rotavirus, adenovirus, and non-viral enteropathogens in diarrhoea. *Arch Dis Child* 56:264-270, 1981.

Wigand, R., Gelderblom, H., and Waddell, G.: A new human adenovirus (candidate adenovirus 36), a novel member of subgroup D. *Arch Virol* 64:225-233, 1980.

Zakradnik, J. M., Spencer, M. J., and Porter, D. D.: Adenovirus infection in the immunocompromised patient. *Am J Med* 68:725-732, 1980.

C. Viruses of Uncertain Nucleic Acid Content and
   Diseases Possibly Caused by Viruses

72

HEPATITIS VIRUSES
H. Preston Holley, Jr., M.D.

There have been a number of viruses which have been associated with hepatitis (Table 72.1). Viruses which primarily infect the liver causing hepatic inflammation and necrosis have been named the hepatitis viruses, e.g., hepatitis A virus (HAV) and hepatitis B virus (HBV). There is now good evidence that one or more other hepatitis viruses exist which have not yet been characterized. These viruses are presently called non-A, non-B hepatitis viruses (NANBHV) until the viruses are isolated or specific serologic markers are found that would enable specific diagnosis. The hepatitis viruses generally cause similar clinical illnesses (see Chapter 26) and therefore, certain diagnosis is usually dependent on serologic testing.

Hepatitis A Virus

Hepatitis A was known long before the virus was identified. Epidemics have been recognized for centuries (Table 72.2). Work by Krugman et al. demonstrated the difference in incubation period of the MS-1 (infectious hepatitis) strain from the MS-2 (serum hepatitis) strain. In 1973 Feinstone et al. reported the use of immune electron microscopy to detect 27-nm virus-like particles in the stools of volunteers who developed acute hepatitis following inoculation with MS-1 strain hepatitis A virus. Specific antibody was found in the volunteers during convalescence which was not present before infection and which did not react with hepatitis B surface antigen. Gravelle et al. confirmed these observations by recovering identical-appearing virus-like particles from the stools of patients infected during a foodborne epidemic of hepatitis A. In addition, they demonstrated transmission of the hepatitis to chimpanzees by inoculation with concentrated stool specimens and later recovered virus-like particles from the feces of the animals.

TABLE 72.1   Viruses Associated with Hepatitis

The hepatitis viruses

Hepatitis A virus
Hepatitis B virus
Non-A, non-B hepatitis viruses

Cytomegalovirus

Epstein-Barr virus

Herpes simplex virus

Yellow fever virus

Lassa virus

TABLE 72.2   Antibody to Hepatitis A in Healthy Adults
in Various Countries

Country	Approximate % Antibody Positive
Switzerland	30
USA	45
Senegal	75
Belgium	80
Taiwan	90
Israel	95
Yugoslavia	95

In vitro culture of HAV has only recently been successful when it was propagated in primary explant cell cultures of marmoset liver and fetal rhesus kidney cells.

Biochemical characterization of HAV is incomplete, but it appears to be a picornavirus containing single-stranded RNA. The antigen has been localized to the cytoplasm of hepatocytes in infected marmosets. Antigenic detection of HAV is currently performed only in experimental laboratories.

Serologic studies of the antibody response in man and primates show that as the concentration of HAV in stool falls, there is a rise in IgM antibody to HAV (anti-HAV IgM). This antibody is usually detectable shortly before or at the onset of clinical hepatitis and is found in the sera of all acutely infected persons (Figure 72.1). Total IgM is also increased during this stage of the illness and C3 is

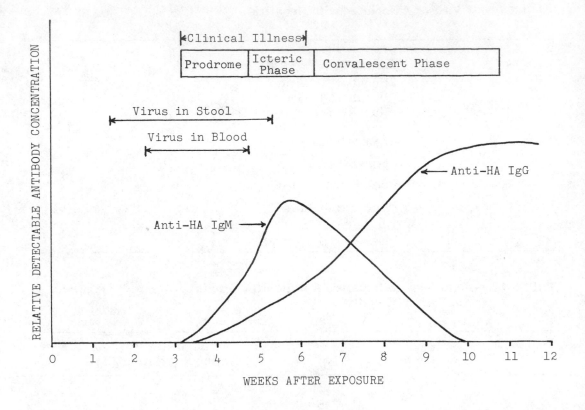

FIGURE 72.1   Hepatitis A: Serum antibody response in relation to the clinical course in a "typical case" of HAV infection.

decreased. These findings suggest that circulating immune complexes comprised of anti-HAV IgM and HAV could be playing a role in the pathogenesis of disease.

Following the onset of clinical illness, there is a gradual rise in IgG antibody to HAV (anti-HAV IgG) in the serum. This antibody persists for years, possibly life-long. There is a gradual decrease in the anti-HAV IgM over several weeks follow-ing clinical illness. Thus, the serodiagnosis of acute HAV infection depends upon either the demonstration of an elevated anti-HAV IgM on a single acute serum sample or the demonstration of a fourfold rise in anti-HAV IgG titer on paired acute and convalescent sera. A single positive anti-HAV IgG sample would only confirm a past infection with HAV. No demonstrable change in anti-HAV IgG from acute to convalescent sera would suggest the hepatitis was not due to HAV.

Infection with HAV is usually spread from person to person by the fecal-oral route, and cases may be sporadic or associated with epidemics or outbreaks that have an identifiable point source. Once infected, an individual may begin excret-ing virus in the stool as early as 9 days. Viral excretion continues intermittently in the stools for a variable period, usually reaching a maximum concentration 5-15 days before peak SGPT levels, and excretion may continue as long as 14 days after peak SGPT levels. Usually peak virus excretion occurs a few days before and at the onset of clinical symptoms. The preclinical incubation period is 15-45 days.

Epidemiologic evidence suggests that anicteric patients are as infectious as icteric patients. Infants and children are frequently asymptomatic.

Viremia also occurs in HAV infection and studies in human volunteers suggest
that the infectious agent is in blood as early as 2.5 weeks before and as late as 2
weeks after the onset of symptoms. Infection by transfusion occurs rarely. No
viremic carrier state has been described in hepatitis A.

Hepatitis B Virus (Table 72.3)

Hepatitis B virus is believed to be a DNA virus in a unique class. The infectious
virion appears on electron microscopy to be a double-shelled, spherical particle
which is 42 nm in diameter with a central core (Figure 72.2). This has been named

TABLE 72.3   Antibody to Hepatitis B Surface Antigen in Various Countries

Country	Approximate % Antibody Positive
Switzerland	3
Belgium	5
USA	10
Israel	15
Yugoslavia	35
Senegal	60
Taiwan	80

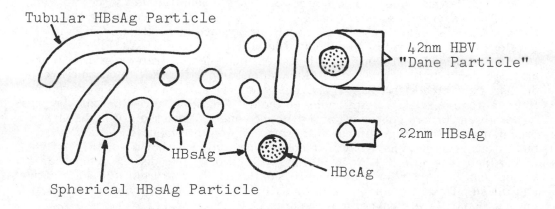

FIGURE 72.2 Schematic representation of hepatitis B virus and its associated
antigens.

the Dane particle following its description by Dane et al. The core is about 27 nm in diameter and contains specific antigenic material known as the hepatitis B core antigen (HBcAg). The core antigen has been isolated from the nuclei of infected hepatocytes where it is presumably replicated. The core contains circular double-stranded DNA and DNA-dependent DNA polymerase of the virus. The outer envelope has the chemical composition of a lipoprotein and contains hepatitis B surface antigen (HBsAg). This material is antigenically identical to that of smaller (22 nm diameter) round and tubular particles which are produced in the cytoplasm of infected hepatocytes and found in high quantities in infected patients' blood. The discovery of this (HBsAg) antigen by Blumberg et al. (first called the Australia antigen) led to a tremendous flurry of investigation of hepatitis which is still in progress by investigators all over the world. Careful serologic analysis has shown that HBsAg particles share a common group-specific antigen *a* and generally at least two mutually exclusive subdeterminants, *d* or *y* and *w* or *r*. Thus, four principal phenotypes *adw, adr, ayw,* and *ayr* have been recognized. There is no known correlation between subtype and severity of illness, chronicity, or other outcome of infection. The *ad* subtype is the most common type in North America, Northern Europe, Asia, and the Pacific, while *ay* is the predominant type in Africa, the Middle East, and the Mediterranean area. Other subdeterminants have been identified but their importance is unknown.

Magnius and Espmark in 1972 identified still another antigen associated with HBsAg-positive serum which is now called the e antigen (HBeAg). This appears to be a soluble protein antigen which is distinct from HBsAg and HBcAg. It is smaller than HBsAg and is nonparticulate. The presence of HBeAg has been linked with infectivity, and it is found almost exclusively in HBsAg-positive blood. This link with infectivity suggests that the e antigen is associated with the intact HBV. Exactly where the e antigen resides in HBV is unclear; recent evidence suggests that HBeAg is a subcomponent or a breakdown product of the HBV core. Other investigators have suggested it may be an expression of the viral genome in the host. Several reports have shown that persistence of HBeAg is associated with chronic liver disease. Others have found that the e antigen status did not correlate closely with liver histology in chronic HBV carriers.

The development of antibody to e antigen (anti-HBe) occurs before anti-HBs appears. Serum containing anti-HBe is generally less infectious than serum containing HBeAg. Studies have shown that some sera containing anti-HBe may still have infectious HBV and such sera are infectious when inoculated into susceptible animals. Thus, as a general rule, HBsAg-positive sera should be considered potentially infectious regardless of the presence or absence of e antigen. Once anti-HBs develops there is much less likelihood of infectivity.

A new antigen, delta antigen (HBδAg) has been demonstrated by direct immunofluorescence to be in the liver cell nuclei of some patients with chronic liver disease associated with HBsAg. The delta and core antigen determinants appear to be mutually exclusive. Antibodies to the delta antigen (anti-HBδ) may be present or absent in sera containing anti-HBc, however. There seems to be a higher prevalence of this antigen in patients from the Mediterranean (e.g., Italy) area, but extensive surveys have not been done. One study has shown a significantly higher incidence of anti-HBδ in patients with chronic liver disease compared with asymptomatic carriers or acute hepatitis patients. The nature of the delta antigen and the significance of the association with delta antibody in some patients with chronic hepatitis are unknown at the present time.

Transmission of HBV is due to inoculation of infected blood or blood-contaminated products, or person-to-person contact (see Chapter 26). The incubation period of hepatitis B varies, usually averaging 60-90 days but ranging from 15 to 210 days. In general, the higher the inoculum, the shorter the incubation period.

Using sensitive techniques (e.g., RIA or ELISA), HBsAg can be detected in 80-90% of patients with acute HBV infection (Figure 72.3). HBsAg becomes detectable about 6 weeks after infection and persists for variable lengths of time, usually 10-12 weeks. During this period of antigenemia the HBeAg appears in the blood as does the antibody to the core antigen. Clinical symptoms are often insidious in onset. During acute symptomatic hepatitis B the diagnosis can usually be established by the presence of HBsAg in serum. Occasionally a sample of blood will be taken when neither HBsAg nor anti-HBs is detected but the anti-HBc is present (see Figure 72.3). In such cases the diagnosis is usually confirmed on a subsequent blood test when the anti-HBs becomes positive. This period of negative HBsAg and negative anti-HBs is probably due to immune-complex formation and small undetectable levels of the HBsAg and antibody. This is usually short-lived, but may last for weeks. Therefore, in patients with a negative HBsAg in serum, an anti-HBc should be done to try to rule in or out HBV as a cause of acute hepatitis.

Non-A, Non-B Hepatitis

The identification of specific markers for hepatitis A and hepatitis B made it possible to carefully examine sera from hepatitis patients. Screening blood for HBsAg

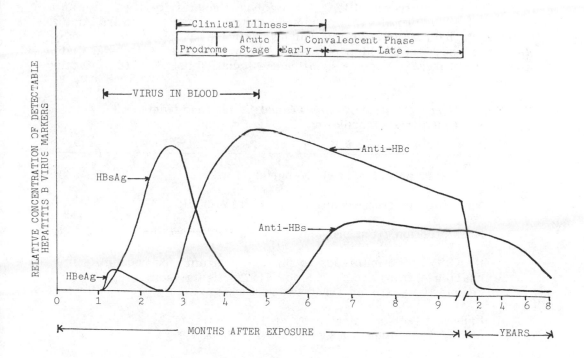

FIGURE 72.3 Hepatitis B: Serum antibody responses in relation to the clinical course in a "typical case" of HBV infection.

also decreased the incidence of posttransfusion hepatitis but only by about 30%. Most cases of posttransfusion hepatitis were (and still are) due to an agent (or agents) with an average incubation period somewhere between the incubation periods of hepatitis A and hepatitis B. Further evidence for additional hepatitis viruses came from the reports of multiple attacks of hepatitis in drug addicts, each episode with features of acute hepatitis. Much has been learned from transmission studies from patients to chimpanzees (Table 72.4). Until reliable serologic testing is available, diagnosis depends on ruling out HAV, HBV, Epstein-Barr virus, cytomegalovirus, and other causes of hepatitis, including other known viruses and infectious agents, toxic or drug-induced hepatitis, and other causes of a hepatitis-like syndrome.

Chronic Hepatitis and Hepatocellular Carcinoma

Some patients with acute hepatitis B or NANBH do not recover normally from their hepatitis. The persistence of hepatitis B surface antigen (HBsAg) in the blood for 6 months or longer is termed the "carrier" state and is usually associated with chronic hepatitis. Many of these patients had anicteric hepatitis with few, if any, symptoms. About two-thirds of HBsAg carriers have a mild, chronic, persistent hepatitis (CPH) and 1-5%/year will develop anti-HBs, often with resolution of the hepatitis. The course of chronic hepatitis is unpredictable and quite variable. Some individuals develop chronic active hepatitis (CAH), a more aggressive form of hepatitis. The prognosis of CAH is worse than CPH and is more likely to progress to cirrhosis. Persistent HBeAg, DNA polymerase activity, high-titer anti-HBc, and high elevations of liver chemistries indicate a poor prognosis. Factors influencing the natural history of chronic hepatitis are unknown.

In some areas of the world, particularly Africa, Asia, the Pacific and Mediterranean areas, there has been a significant association between HBV infection

TABLE 72.4   Characteristics of NANB Hepatitis Learned from Chimpanzee Inoculation

Incubation period $\sim$ 7 wk (range 2-22 wk)

No serologic cross-reactivity with HAV or HBV

No protection from previous HAV or HBV infection

NANBHV infection leads to protection against subsequent challenge from some, but not all, patients' sera, suggesting there are at least two viruses

Immune electron microscopy of liver extracts of infected animals suggests viral etiology

Prolonged viremic carrier state exists in some patients (similar to HBV)

and hepatocellular carcinoma. In these areas there is usually exposure to HBV at early age with up to 20% of the population identified as carriers of the virus. In these populations cirrhosis and hepatocellular carcinoma occur subsequent to HBV infection with alarming frequency. Also hepatoma has been associated with chronic persistent hepatitis without cirrhosis in about 25% of the cases. Recent prospective studies in Taiwan and Japan have demonstrated in those populations that chronic HBV infection is a significant risk factor for the development of hepatoma. It is possible that hepatocellular carcinoma is the cumulative result of several cofactors which may include genetic, immunologic, dietary, and others. At present there is no proof that HBV infection causes hepatocellular carcinoma, but in many areas of the world is highly significantly associated with it. The finding of a chronic viral hepatitis and associated hepatocellular carcinoma in woodchucks provides an experimental model to study the relationship and hopefully shed light on the human disease.

Recently, evidence suggests that NANBH leads to chronic hepatitis with a frequency equal to or greater than HBV. A chronic carrier state also has been described for NANBH. Since more than one virus is likely to cause NANBH, more investigation is necessary before the natural history of this form of chronic hepatitis is known. There is no convincing evidence at the present time that hepatitis A progresses to chronic hepatitis.

Selected Bibliography

Aach, R. D. and Kahn, R. A.: Post-transfusion hepatitis. Current perspectives. *Ann Intern Med* 92:539-546, 1980.

Bradley, D. W.: Hepatitis A virus infection. Pathogenesis and serodiagnosis of acute disease. *J Virol Meth* 2:31-45, 1980.

Bradley, D. W., Maynard, J. E., Cook, E. H., Ebert, J. W., Gravelle, C. R., Tsiquaye, K. N., Kessler, H., Zuckerman, A. J., Miller, M. F., Ling, C-M., and Overby, L. R.: Non-A/non-B hepatitis in experimentally infected chimpanzees: Cross-challenge and electron microscopic studies. *J Med Virol* 6:185-201, 1980.

Czaja, A. J. and Davis, G. L.: Hepatitis non-A, non-B. Manifestations and implications of acute and chronic disease. *Mayo Clin Proc* 57:639-652, 1982.

de Franchis, R., D'Arminio, A., Vecchi, M., Ronchi, G., Ninno, E. D., Parravicini, A., Ferroni, P., and Zanetti, A. R.: Chronic asymptomatic HBsAg carriers: Histologic abnormalities and diagnostic and prognostic value of serologic markers of the HBV. *Gastroenterology* 79:521-527, 1980.

Feinstone, S. M., Kapikian, A. Z., and Purcell, R. H.: Hepatitis A: Detection by immune electron microscopy of a viruslike antigen associated with acute illness. *Science* 182:1026-1028, 1973.

Gravelle, C. R., Hornbeck, C. L., Maynard, J. E., Schable, C. A., Cook, E. H., and Bradley, D. W.: Hepatitis A: Report of a common-source outbreak with recovery of a possible etiologic agent. II. Laboratory studies. *J Infect Dis* 131: 167-171, 1975.

Guyer, B., Bradley, D. W., Bryan, J. A., and Maynard, J. E.: Non-A, non-B hepatitis among participants in a plasmapheresis stimulation program. *J Infect Dis* 139:634-640, 1979.

Hoofnagle, J. H., Dusheiko, G. M., Seeff, L. B., Jones, E. A., Waggoner, J. G., and Bales, Z. B.: Seroconversion from hepatitis B e antigen to antibody in chronic type B hepatitis. *Ann Intern Med* 94:744-748, 1981.

Hoofnagle, J. H., Gerety, R. J., Ni, L. Y., and Barker, L. F.: Antibody to hepatitis B core antigen: A sensitive indicator of persistent viral replication. *N Engl J Med* 290:1336-1340, 1974.

Irwin, G. R., Allen, R. G., Segal, H. G., Allen, A. M., Putnak, J. R., Cannon, H. G., and Top, F. H., Jr.: Serodiagnosis of hepatitis B virus infection by antibody to core antigen. *J Infect Dis* 136:31-36, 1977.

Kabiri, M., Tabor, E., and Gerety, R. J.: Antigen-antibody system associated with non-A, non-B hepatitis detected by indirect immunofluorescence. *Lancet* 2:221-224, 1979.

Koff, R. S.: *Viral Hepatitis.* John Wiley & Sons, New York, 1978, p. 242.

Krugman, S., Giles, J. P., and Hammond, J.: Infectious hepatitis: Evidence for two distinctive clinical, epidemiological and immunological types of infection. *JAMA* 200:365-373, 1967.

Krugman, S. and Gocke, D. J.: *Viral Hepatitis.* W. B. Saunders Co., Philadelphia, 1978, p. 147.

Provost, P. J. and Hilleman, M. R.: Propagation of human hepatitis A virus in cell culture in vitro (40422). *Proc Soc Exp Biol Med* 160:213-221, 1979.

Realdi, G., Alberti, A., Rugge, M., Bortolotti, F., Rigoli, A. M., Tremolada, F., and Ruol, A.: Hepatitis B e antigen to anti-HBe in chronic hepatitis B virus infection. *Gastroenterology* 79:195-199, 1980.

Rizzetto, M., Canese, M. G., Gerin, J. L., London, W. T., Sly, D. L., and Purcell, R. H.: Transmission of the hepatitis B virus-associated delta antigen to chimpanzees. *J Infect Dis* 141:590-602, 1980.

Rizzetto, M., Shih, J. W. K., Gocke, D. J., Purcell, R. H., Verme, G., and Gerin, J. L.: Incidence and significance of antibodies to delta antigen in hepatitis B virus infection. *Lancet* 2:986-990, 1979.

Shirachi, R., Shiraishi, H., Tateda, A., Kikuchi, K., Ishida, N.: Hepatitis "C" antigen in non-A, non-B post-transfusion hepatitis. *Lancet* 2:853-856, 1978.

Tabor, E., Mitchell, F. D., Goudeau, A. M., and Gerety, R. J.: Detection of an antigen-antibody system in serum associated with human non-A, non-B hepatitis. *J Med Virol* 4:161-169, 1979.

Tabor, E., Seeff, L. B., and Gerety, R. J.: Chronic non-A, non-B hepatitis carrier state. Transmissible agent documented in one patient over a six-year period. *N Engl J Med* 303:140-143, 1980.

Takahashi, K., Akahane, Y., Gotanda, T., Mishiro, T., Imai, M., Miyakawa, Y., and Mayumi, M.: Demonstration of hepatitis B e antigen in the core of Dane particles. *J Immunol* 122:275-279, 1979.

Tong, M. J., Stevenson, D., and Gordon, I.: Correlation of e antigen, DNA polymerase activity, and Dane particles in chronic benign and chronic active type B hepatitis infections. *J Infect Dis* 135:980-984, 1977.

Vitvitski, L., Trepo, C., Prince, A. M., and Brotman, B.: Detection of virus-associated antigen in serum and liver of patients with non-A, non-B hepatitis. *Lancet* 2:1263-1267, 1979.

Zuckerman, A. J. and Howard, C. R.: *Hepatitis Viruses of Man.* Academic Press, New York, 1979, p. 269.

73

NORWALK AND HAWAII AGENTS
Ronica M. Kluge, M.D.

The Norwalk-like agents have been responsible for outbreaks of diarrheal illness in many parts of the world. The clinical aspects of disease caused by these agents are detailed in Chapter 23. Agents included in this group are listed in Table 73.1; Norwalk agent is considered the prototype.

Microbiology

There is strong evidence supporting the belief that the Norwalk agents are viruses. Efforts to cultivate the particle have been unsuccessful, however, and the nucleic acid content of the genome has not yet been determined. The agent resembles parvovirus (DNA) in size, density and stability, yet appears to contain a single 66,000 dalton protein which is more characteristic of calcivirus (RNA). The Norwalk agent is 27 nm in diameter, round, and unenveloped (Table 73.2).

Epidemiology

Norwalk-like agents appear to be responsible for one-third of epidemic nonbacterial gastroenteritis. Outbreaks have been reported in most age groups and do not have a seasonal predilection. The agents have been documented to cause outbreaks in the United States, Japan, England, and Australia, and no doubt are responsible for disease in other countries as well. Settings in which outbreaks have occurred include families, communities, schools, cruise ships, camp grounds, and nursing homes. Contaminated water and food have been incriminated. The agent is also transmitted by the fecal-oral route. Serologic studies indicate that Norwalk

654

TABLE 73.1   Norwalk-like Agents

Agent	Country
Norwalk	U.S.
Hawaii	U.S.
Ditchling	England
Cockle	England
Montgomery County	U.S.
W	England
Parramatta	Australia
Colorado	U.S.
SRV	Japan
Marin County	U.S.

TABLE 73.2   Biologic Properties of Norwalk-like Agents

Size	27 nm
Shape	Round
Density (CsCl)	$1.38-1.41$ g/cm^3
Stability	
Ether	20% for 24 hr
Acid	pH 2.7 for 3 hr
Heat	60° for 30 min

agent is worldwide and fairly ubiquitous. Antibody appears in early childhood in undeveloped countries, and by late adolescence in the United States. Two-thirds of adults in this country have detectable antibodies.

Pathogenesis

Because no good animal or organ culture models are available for Norwalk agent disease, the pathogenesis has been studied in volunteers with experimentally induced infections. The agent causes morphologic changes in the small-bowel mucosa, leaving the stomach and colon mucosae normal in appearance. The histologic changes include blunting of villus projections, mitochondrial swelling, distorted microvillae, crypt hypertrophy, and mild intracellular edema. Malabsorption of fat and xylose occurs during the acute illness, and decreased levels of brush-border enzymes are present. The histologic changes persist at least 4 days, but resolve by 2 weeks. More severe symptoms appear to be associated with more severe histologic changes, but even some asymptomatic volunteers have morphologic derangement of the intestinal mucosa. Symptoms in patients with gastroenteritis due to Norwalk virus are listed in Table 73.3.

Laboratory Diagnosis

Routine laboratory tests to detect Norwalk-like agents and their antibodies are not available. The agents can be detected by immune electron microscopy, and this technique has been adapted for use in estimating antibody levels to the agents. However, immune electron microscopy remains a research tool. Radioimmunoassays have been developed which allow identification of the Norwalk agent in stool and measurement of antibodies in serum. The reagents needed for the assay are available in short supply, making this test also one restricted to research laboratories. Inability to propagate the agent in cell or organ culture has hampered the development of simple, readily available diagnostic tests.

Immunology

Norwalk agent-induced disease is associated with a rise in serum antibodies and occurs in naturally acquired as well as induced illness. The serologic response appears to be short-lived (less than 2 years). When volunteers are rechallenged with Norwalk agent, those who were symptomatic on first challenge will become symptomatic again, and both episodes are accompanied by significant rises in antibody. Interestingly, volunteers who did not become ill on initial challenge will not develop illness on rechallenge. These individuals fail to show seroconversion. The latter data suggest that factors other than immune ones may play a role in protection. One hypothesis is based on genetic control of susceptibility: some individuals may lack a receptor required for entry of the Norwalk agent into mucosal

TABLE 73.3   Symptoms in Patients with Gastroenteritis Due to
Norwalk Virus

Symptom	Approximate %
Nausea	90
Vomiting	85
Diarrhea	85
Abdominal cramps	80
Headache	70
Fever	65
Sore throat	10

TABLE 73.4   Antigenic Relationships of Norwalk-like Agents

Distinct	Related
Norwalk	MC
Hawaii	
Ditchling	W
Paramatta	
SRV	

cells. Another hypothesis suggests that repeated exposures to the agent are required before a serologic response is detectable. This might explain the relative absence of antibody to Norwalk agent in children and its gradual appearance among adolescents and young adults.

There are at least three distinct serotypes of Norwalk-like agents (Table 73.4). Cross-challenge studies in volunteers have shown that disease caused by either Norwalk or Hawaii agent does not protect against heterologous challenge. Serologic studies show that the two agents do not share surface antigens. On the other hand, the Norwalk and Montgomery County agents share some surface antigens. Cross-challenge experiments with these two agents have shown significant immunity to the heterologous agent. Antigenic relatedness is being worked out for the entire group of Norwalk-like agents.

Vaccines to prevent Norwalk-like agent disease will not be possible until we have the technology to allow in vitro propagation of the agent. This is further impeded by lack of animal models of infection.

Selected Bibliography

Agus, S. G., Dolin, R., Wyatt, R. G., Tousimis, A. J., and Northrup, R. S.: Acute infectious nonbacterial gastroenteritis: Intestinal histopathology. *Ann Intern Med* 79:18-25, 1973.

Blacklow, N. R. and Cukor, G.: Viral gastroenteritis. *N Engl J Med* 304:397-406, 1981.

Christopher, P. G., Grohmann, G. S., Millsom, R. H., and Murphy, A. M.: Parvovirus gastroenteritis – a new entity for Australia. *Med J Aust* 1:121-124, 1978.

Dolin, R., Blacklow, N. R., DuPont, H., Buscho, R. F., Wyatt, R. G., Kasel, J. A., Hornick, R., and Chanock, R. M.: Biological properties of Norwalk agent of acute infectious nonbacterial gastroenteritis. *Proc Soc Exp Biol Med* 140: 578-583, 1972.

Dolin, R., Levy, A. G., Wyatt, R. G., Thornhill, T. S., and Gardner, J. D.: Viral gastroenteritis induced by the Hawaii agent. Jejunal histopathology and serologic response. *Am J Med* 59:761-768, 1975.

Greenberg, H. B., Valdesuso, J., Yolken, R. H., Gangarosa, E., Gary, W., Wyatt, R. G., Konno, T., Suzuki, H., Chanock, R. M., and Kapikian, A. Z.: Role of Norwalk virus in outbreaks of nonbacterial gastroenteritis. *J Infect Dis* 139: 564–568, 1979.

Greenberg, H. B., Wyatt, R. G., Valdesuso, J., Kalica, A. R., London, W. T., Chanock, R. M., and Kapikian, A. Z.: Solid-phase microtiter radioimmunoassay for detection of the Norwalk strain of acute nonbacterial, epidemic gastroenteritis virus and its antibodies. *J Med Virol* 2:97–108, 1978.

Holmes, I. H.: Viral gastroenteritis. *Prog Med Virol* 25:1–36, 1979.

Kapikian, A. Z., Gerin, J. L., Wyatt, R. G., Thornhill, T. S., and Chanock, R. M.: Density in cesium chloride of the 27 nm "8FIIa" particle associated with acute infectious nonbacterial gastroenteritis: Determination by ultracentrifugation and immune electron microscopy. *Proc Soc Exp Biol Med* 142:874–877, 1973.

Kapikian, A. Z., Wyatt, R. G., Dolin, R., Thornhill, T. S., Kalica, A. R., and Chanock, R. M.: Visualization by immune electron microscopy of a 27 nm particle associated with acute infectious nonbacterial gastroenteritis. *J Virol* 10:1075–1081, 1972.

Kogasaka, R., Sakuma, Y., Chiba, S., Akihara, M., Horino, K., and Nakao, T.: Small round virus-like particles associated with acute gastroenteritis in Japanese children. *J Med Virol* 5:151–160, 1980.

Murphy, A. M., Grohmann, G. S., Christopher, P. J., Lopor, W. A., Davey, G. R., and Millson, R. H.: An Australia-wide outbreak of gastroenteritis from oysters caused by Norwalk virus. *Med J Aust* 2:329–333, 1979.

Parrino, T. A., Schreiber, D. S., Trier, J. S., Kapikian, A. Z., and Blacklow, N. R.: Clinical immunity in acute gastroenteritis caused by Norwalk agent. *N Engl J Med* 297:86–89, 1977.

Schreiber, D. S., Blacklow, N. R., and Trier, J. S.: The mucosal lesion of the proximal small intestine in acute infectious nonbacterial gastroenteritis. *N Engl J Med* 288:1318–1323, 1973.

Schreiber, D. S., Trier, J. S., and Blacklow, N. R.: Recent advances in viral gastroenteritis. *Gastroenterology* 73:174–183, 1977.

Wyatt, R. G., Dolin, R., Blacklow, N. R., DuPont, H. L., Buscho, R. F.,. Thornhill, T. S., Kapikian, A. Z., and Chanock, R. M.: Comparison of three agents of acute infectious nonbacterial gastroenteritis by cross-challenge in volunteers. *J Infect Dis* 129:709–714, 1974.

74

ROSEOLA
Robert II. Waldman, M.D.

Roseola is an acute febrile illness mainly of infants and young children between the ages of 6 months and 3 years. It goes by a variety of names, including exanthema subitum and sixth disease. More than 95% of the cases are seen in children under 30 months of age, and 75% are seen in children between the ages of 6 and 18 months.

It is believed to be a viral illness, the best evidence being that the disease has been transmitted by injecting bacteria-free serum from children with the illness into susceptibles. Similar experiments have been done by injecting monkeys and producing illness. Other evidence that the disease is a viral infection is its similarities to other viral exanthems, and lifelong immunity follows the illness.

The disease is worldwide in distribution and is most often seen in late spring and midautumn. There are no epidemics, but the disease is only somewhat contagious, with the attack rate after exposure being low.

The incubation period is 10-15 days and the prodrome is absent or very mild, consisting of only a slight runny nose and scratchy throat. Then there is the sudden onset of fever, usually up to 40°C or higher, lasting for 3-5 days. Despite the high fever the child does not look particularly ill. Other signs and symptoms during this period are minor, with vomiting and constipation fairly common, and cervical and postauricular lymphadenopathy also occurring. Classically, as the fever falls a rash appears. The rash is rubelliform, i.e., maculopapular, 2-3 mm in diameter, which fades on pressure. It begins on the trunk or neck, then spreads to the arms and legs usually sparing the cheeks and region above the nose. The rash lasts for a few hours to a few days and does not result in desquamation. The diagnosis is made by the typical clinical picture of high fever with the rash appearing as the patient defervesces.

The differential diagnosis (Table 74.1) includes rubella (different because of the facial distribution, its rareness in infancy, and the occurrence of epidemics),

TABLE 74.1   Differential Diagnosis of Childhood Exanthems

Disease	Conjunctivitis	Pharyngitis	Rhinitis	Enanthem
Exanthema subitum	+/-	0	+/-	0
Measles	++	0	+	+
Rubella	+/-	+/-	+/-	+/-
Enterovirus infection	0	+/-	+/-	0
Scarlet fever	+/-	++	+/-	0
Infectious mononucleosis	0	+	0	0
Drug rash	0	0	0	0

measles (in roseola the rash is less elevated, less red, and does not show crescentic grouping, and in measles the fever persists during the rash, and there is prominent cough, runny nose, conjunctivitis, and Koplik's spots), and might also include erythema infectiosum, scarlet fever, enterovirus infection, infectious mononucleosis, meningococcemia, drug rash, and sunburn.

Laboratory abnormalities are minimal and spinal fluid is normal when it has been examined. Patients usually have a neutropenia which becomes a leukocytosis after a few days.

The prognosis is virtually 100% recovery, and the only complication is the occasional febrile convulsion.

Treatment is the use of antipyretics to keep the temperature below 39°C. Isolation of infected children is completely unnecessary.

Selected Bibliography

Kempe, C. H., Shaw, E. B., Jackson, J. R., et al.: Studies on the etiology of exanthema subitum (roseola infantum). *J Pediatr* 37:561, 1950.

Oski, F.: Roseola infantum. *Am J Dis Child* 101:376, 1961.

Shapiro, L.: The numbered diseases: First through sixth. *JAMA* 194:680, 1950.

75

ERYTHEMA INFECTIOSUM
Robert H. Waldman, M.D.

Erythema infectiosum, also called "fifth disease," is a benign exanthematous disease of children (Table 75.1). Although usually recognized in epidemics, it probably is also endemic. The latter is difficult to recognize because the disease is so mild and because it is so similar to other exanthems.

Although the disease is most common in children aged 5-14, it may be seen in infants and adults who have come in contact with cases. The disease is probably spread by inhaled droplets. It is more common in winter and spring and is worldwide in distribution.

Erythema infectiosum is presumed to have a viral etiology: the disease has many similarities to the other exanthems (Table 75.2), and is mildly contagious. The agent has not been isolated.

Clinical evaluation is the only way to diagnose erythema infectiosum. The incubation period is 4-14 days. The prodrome is mild, usually consisting of headache, malaise, low-grade fever, anorexia, and nausea.

The rash, if classic, is diagnostic. It appears 1-2 days after the onset of prodromal symptoms, beginning on the face. Children usually have circumoral pallor with a bright red, but not painful, confluent macular rash on the cheeks. This has been described as a "slapped cheek" appearance. The rash is faint on the rest of the body, with the arms and legs more commonly involved than the chest, back, and abdomen. The palms and soles are not usually involved. On the body, the rash is evanescent, lace-like, serpentine, and sometimes annular. Pruritus is common, but mild. Some children have urticaria-like edema. The rash is classically intensified by sunlight, exertion, or emotion. It usually lasts for up to 7 days, but may recur within the next week.

The disease is more severe in adults, with fever, adenopathy, and malaise persisting longer than the illness in children. The arthritis is usually seen only in adults, and is like that seen in rubella.

TABLE 75.1   Historic Classification of Exanthematous
              Childhood Infections

1. Measles

2. Scarlet fever

3. Rubella

4. Duke's disease (probably a subgroup of rubella - no
   longer in separate category)

5. Erythema infectiosum

6. Roseola

TABLE 75.2   Comparison of Some Characteristics of
              Exanthematous Diseases

	Incubation Period	Age	Season	Duration	Rash
Measles	10-14 days	Children (occasionally adults)	Winter, spring	7-10 days	Maculopapular, confluent, face and then down body
Rubella	12-23 days	Children (occasionally adults)	Spring	3-5 days	Maculopapular, faint, even non-existent
Roseola	10-15 days	Infants	Spring, fall	5-7 days	Maculopapular, appears as fever falls
Erythema infectiosum	4-14 days	Children and adults	Summer, early fall	2-5 days	Variable, maculopapular, vesicular, petechial, or absent

The differential diagnosis includes scarlet fever, rubeola, rubella, roseola, and enterovirus infection.

Treatment consists of lotions and antipruritic agents. Quarantine measures are unnecessary because they are probably ineffective and the disease is benign.

From epidemiologic studies, it appears that immunity persists for life and that the lifetime infection rate is about 90%. There is no evidence that the disease is teratogenic.

Selected Bibliography

Ager, E. A., Chin, T. D. Y., and Poland, J. D.: Epidemic erythema infectiosum. *N Engl J Med* 275:1326, 1966.

Balfour, H. H.: Fifth disease: Full fathom five. *Am J Dis Child* 130:239, 1976.

Balfour, H. H., May, D. B., Rotte, T. C., Phelps, W. R., and Schiff, G. M.: A study of erythema infectiosum: Recovery of rubella virus and echovirus 12. *Pediatrics* 50:285, 1972.

Balfour, H. H., Schiff, G. M., and Bloom, J. E.: Encephalitis associated with erythema infectiosum. *J Pediatr* 77:133, 1970.

Greenwald, P. and Bashe, W. J., Jr.: Epidemic of erythema infectiosum. *Am J Dis Child* 107:30, 1964.

Lauer, B. A., MacCormack, J. N., and Wilfer, C.: Erythema infectiosum. An elementary school outbreak. *Am J Dis Child* 130:252, 1976.

Wadlinton, W. B.: Erythema infectiosum. *JAMA* 192:58, 1965.

76

CAT-SCRATCH DISEASE
Robert H. Waldman, M.D.

Cat-scratch disease is a benign infection usually caused by the scratch of a cat and characterized by regional lymphadenitis. The etiologic agent is unknown, but generally thought to be a virus or possibly a chlamydia. The illness has occasionally followed skin injury with a splinter or thorn presumably contaminated with cat secretions.

Pathologically, the involved lymph nodes show granulomatous abscess formation with an intense polymorphonuclear leukocyte response, often with central necrosis and giant cells. If there is no suppuration of the node the histopathologic findings may be difficult to differentiate from Hodgkin's disease. Since the histologic findings are not pathognomonic, the diagnosis depends upon the clinical findings.

Clinically, since the skin injury may be trivial, a definite history of exposure to a cat is not always available. It is also surprising how infrequently one finds multiple cases among children in the same household exposed to the same infectious cat. An extremely helpful finding is the occasional development of an erythematous papule at the site of the scratch.

One week to several months after the exposure, the patient usually notices the development of painful enlargement of regional lymph nodes. This involves the axillary nodes most commonly, with cervical nodes being involved next in frequency. The nodes may become as large as 10 cm in diameter, are usually soft and fluctuant, and may drain spontaneously. If the nodes are not removed surgically, or do not drain spontaneously, the enlargement and other symptoms of the disease gradually subside over a period of several weeks to a few months.

Accompanying the lymphadenopathy there is usually, but not invariably, nonspecific constitutional symptoms such as fever and malaise. Rarely, patients develop an encephalitic picture. The lymphadenopathy subsides in several weeks to a few months.

As mentioned earlier, the diagnosis is essentially clinical. Involved lymph nodes are histopathologically nonspecific. A skin test preparation has been used, but is not commercially available. One can be prepared from material aspirated from an involved node, diluted 1:5 in saline, and heat inactivated for 1 hr at 56°C for 2 successive days. One-tenth milliliter is injected intracutaneously and read at 24-48 hr. The reaction is considered positive if there is an indurated papule of > 0.5 cm which is surrounded by erythema of > 1.5 cm.

It is important to differentiate cat-scratch fever from other causes of lymph-adenopathy, particularly those that are treatable with antimicrobial agents, the most important one probably being tuberculosis. Cat-scratch fever can usually be differentiated from tularemia, infectious mononucleosis, Hodgkin's disease, sar-coidosis, and lymphogranuloma venereum since patients have chronic, suppurative, solitary or regional lymphadenopathy.

The prognosis is prolonged but benign, and there have been no fatalities.

Treatment is "benign neglect" unless the lymph node becomes suppurative, in which case it should be removed. There is no evidence that antibiotic therapy is beneficial.

Selected Bibliography

Carithers, H. A., Carithers, C. M., and Edwards, R. O., Jr.: Cat scratch disease: Its natural history. *JAMA* 207:312, 1969.

Carithers, H. A., Carithers, C. M., and Edwards, R. O., Jr.: Cat scratch disease: The larger view. *Pediatrics* 43:629, 1969.

Johnson, W. C. and Helvig, E. B.: Cat scratch disease. Histopathic changes in the skin. *Arch Dermatol* 100:148, 1969.

Margileth, A. M.: Cat scratch disease: The larger view. *Pediatrics* 43:631, 1969.

Margileth, A. M.: Cat scratch disease: Non-bacterial regional lymphadenitis: The study of 145 patients and a review of the literature. *Pediatrics* 42:803, 1968.

Pollen, R. H.: Cat scratch encephalitis. *Neurology* 18:1031, 1968.

Rice, J. E. and Hyde, R. M.: Rapid diagnostic method for cat scratch disease. *J Lab Clin Med* 71:166, 1968.

Spaulding, W. B. and Hennessy, J. N.: Cat-scratch disease, a study of 83 cases. *Am J Med* 28:504, 1960.

Warwick, W. J.: The cat scratch syndrome; many diseases or one disease. *Prog Med Virol* 9:256, 1967.

Winship, P.: Pathologic changes in so-called cat scratch fever. Review of find-ings in lymph nodes of 29 patients and cutaneous lesions of two patients. *Am J Clin Pathol* 23:1012, 1953.

77

KAWASAKI SYNDROME
Robert H. Waldman, M.D.

Kawasaki syndrome, also known as mucocutaneous lymph node syndrome, is an acute febrile illness of unknown etiology, and thought to be an infectious disease by many. It is seen almost exclusively in children under 5 years of age, with half of the cases in children under 2 years. The disease affects boys slightly more frequently than girls, and 80% of the fatalities from this disease occur in boys. There have been a few case reports in older children and young adults. The disease is endemic in Japan and sporadic but increasing in incidence in the United States (Table 77.1). There has been no known person-to-person transmission of the disease nor have common exposures of patients been identified. Pathologically the disease appears very similar to infantile polyarteritis nodosa. Diagnostic considerations are listed in Tables 77.2-77.5.

The patients nearly always have fever, usually higher than 40°C, lasting 5 or more days. The conjunctival infection is more common on the bulbar conjunctiva than the palpebral. Usually a single cervical node is enlarged, but occasionally there are multiple nodes involved. The lymph node is usually minimally tender. The most serious involvement is cardiac, and coronary artery involvement is the cause of death in the small number of patients who do not recover. Thirty percent of patients have been shown to have coronary artery aneurysms. The most consistent laboratory findings are thrombocytosis and an elevated erythrocyte sedimentation rate.

The mortality is 1-2%, and patients who die are typically male, have a marked elevation of the erythrocyte sedimentation rate, are under 1 year of age, and have prolonged fever and rash. In those who survive but have coronary artery involvement demonstrated by arteriography, about one-half have permanent changes.

There is no known beneficial treatment, although aspirin has been reported in an uncontrolled trial to be beneficial. There is no evidence that corticosteroids lead to improvement.

TABLE 77.1   Racial Incidence of Mucocutaneous Lymph Node
Syndrome in U.S.

Race	Per 100,000, < 8 yr old
Oriental	2.74
Black	1.03
Caucasian	0.43

TABLE 77.2   Diagnosis of Mucocutaneous Lymph Node Syndrome

Must have five or all of the following:

≥ 5 days of fever

Bilateral conjunctival injection

One or more changes in lips or oral cavity

Dryness, redness, or fissuring of lips
Strawberry tongue
Erythema of oropharyngeal mucosa

Changes in extremities

Erythema of palms or soles
Indurative edema of hands or feet
Desquamation of fingertips

Erythema multiforme rash without vesicles or crusts

Cervical lymphadenopathy

TABLE 77.3   Incidence of Characteristic Findings in Kawasaki Disease

Characteristic	Approximate Incidence (%)
Fever	95
Conjunctival congestion	90
Dryness, redness, and/or fissuring of lips	90
Redness and dryness of oral and pharyngeal mucosa	90
Red palms and/or soles	90
Rash: morbilliform, erythema multiforme, or scarlatiniform	90
Strawberry tongue	75
Cervical adenopathy	75
Edema of hands and/or feet	75
Carditis	70
Desquamation of fingertips during convalescence	95

TABLE 77.4   Other Abnormalities Seen in Mucocutaneous Lymph Node Syndrome

Electrocardiographic	↑ PR interval ↑ ST interval ↓ R waves Flat T waves
Diarrhea	
Urinary	Proteinuria Sterile pyuria
Hematologic	Leukocytosis with shift to left Anemia ↑ Erythrocyte sedimentation rate Thrombocytosis
Arthralgias/arthritis	
Aseptic meningitis	
Mild jaundice	
Transverse nail furrow 1-2 mo postonset	

TABLE 77.5   Differential Diagnosis of Kawasaki Disease

Infectious mononucleosis	Rubella
Leptospirosis	Measles
Scarlet fever	Rocky Mountain spotted fever
Serum sickness	Scalded skin syndrome
Systemic lupus erythematosus	Juvenile rheumatoid arthritis

Selected Bibliography

Bell, D. M., Brink, E. W., Nitzkin, J. L., Hall, C. B., Wulff, H., Berkowitz, I.D., Feorino, P. M., Holman, R. C., Huntley, C. L., Meade, R. H., III, Anderson, L. J., Cheeseman, S. H., Fiumara, N. J., Gilfillan, R. F., Keim, D. E., and Modlin, J. F.: Kawasaki syndrome: Description of two outbreaks in the United States. *N Engl J Med* 304:1568, 1981.

Fujiwara, H. and Hamashima, Y.: Pathology of the heart and Kawasaki disease. *Pediatrics* 61:100, 1978.

Glanzer, J. M., Galbraith, W. B., and Jacobs, J. P.: Kawasaki disease in 28-year-old man. *JAMA* 244:1604, 1980.

Melish, M. E.: Kawasaki syndrome: A new infectious disease? *J Infect Dis* 143:317, 1981.

Morens, D. M., Anderson, L. J., and Hurwitz, E. S.: National surveillance of Kawasaki disease. *Pediatrics* 65:21, 1980.

Morens, D. M. and O'Brien, R. J.: Kawasaki disease in the United States. *J Infect Dis* 137:91, 1978.

Neches, W. H.: Mucocutaneous lymph node syndrome. Coronary artery disease and cross-sectional echocardiography. *Am J Dis Child* 133:1233, 1979.

Yanagihara, R. and Todd, J. K.: Acute febrile mucocutaneous lymph node syndrome. *Am J Dis Child* 134:603, 1980.

78

SLOW VIRUSES
Robert H. Waldman, M.D.

Slow virus infections are characterized by a very long incubation period, a protracted clinical course usually ending in death, and single organ involvement, i.e., the central nervous system. These presumed infections have a limited range of host susceptibility. Although slow virus is an accepted name for this group of diseases, it is not a particularly good one, since there is no evidence that the presumed viruses are slow in any way; it is just that the clinical manifestations develop slowly (Figure 78.1).

The best studied of these diseases are those of animals, i.e., scrapie and visna. The human slow virus infections can be conveniently divided into two categories: (1) those caused by common viruses but with uncommon manifestations, and (2) those caused by unique agents, presumed to be viruses (Tables 78.1-78.3).

Subacute Sclerosing Panencephalitis

This is a rare disease of children and young adults, with a mean age of onset of 10 years. The evidence is strong that the disease is caused by measles or a related virus, possibly an "incomplete" or "defective" form of the virus. It is clearly a different disease from postinfectious or postvaccination encephalitis which is seen within weeks of infection or immunization. Patients have a very high serum and cerebrospinal fluid antibody titer to measles, even higher than that seen shortly after naturally occurring measles infection. Viral antigen has been demonstrated in neurons and glial cells, and measles virus has been isolated when brain cells were co-cultivated with continuous tissue culture cell lines. Virus has also been isolated from lymph nodes of patients with the disease. Some minor differences between the virus isolated from patients with SSPE and measles virus have been detected. These differences are seen immunologically and by RNA

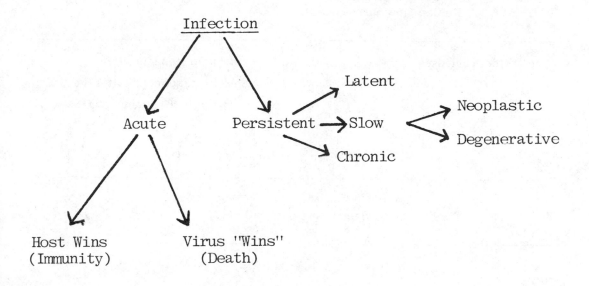

FIGURE 78.1   Patterns of virus infection.

TABLE 78.1   Various Types of Virus–Host Relationships

Virus	Infection	Characteristics	Examples
Eliminated	Acute	Short incubation period; results in death or complete recovery; if recovery, person usually immune	Smallpox
Persistent	Latent	Acute infection, periodic recurrences; virus not recoverable by usual methods during remissions; host's immune response apparently ineffective in eradicating infection	Herpes viruses
	Chronic	Virus persists and recoverable	Hepatitis B
	Slow	Long incubation, lethal	Kuru
	Intermediate	Characteristics of both "chronic" and "slow"	SSPE

TABLE 78.2   Human Slow Virus Diseases

Conventional viruses	Subacute sclerosing panencephalitis
	Progressive rubella panencephalitis
	Progressive multifocal leukoencephalopathy
Unconventional agents	Kuru
	Creutzfeldt-Jakob disease

TABLE 78.3   Possible Slow Virus Diseases

Multiple sclerosis
Amyotrophic lateral sclerosis
Parkinson's disease
Alzheimer's disease

hybridization. The SSPE virus contains approximately 10% more genetic information, suggesting that the SSPE virus is a recombinant of measles plus another virus. Others have hypothesized that SSPE virus is more closely related to canine distemper virus.

Children affected by the disease are more often rural than urban dwellers and usually have had measles infection at a relatively early age. The relationship between these various observations is unclear. An important question is why the rare patient gets SSPE when measles infection is so common. It has been hypothesized that there is an immunologic abnormality in the host. The evidence for this is that defective cell-mediated immunity to the nucleocapsid antigen of the measles virus and a hyperimmune antibody response to measles virus have been shown in SSPE patients.

Histopathologically, the brain of patients with SSPE shows perivascular cuffing with lymphocytes and plasma cells, diffuse mononuclear infiltration of the gray and white matter, demyelination, and eosinophilic Cowdry's type A inclusion bodies in the nucleus and cytoplasm of the cortical neurons. These inclusion bodies contain measles virus nucleocapsid.

The incidence of the disease is approximately one case per million children, with a male/female ratio of 3:1, and most cases in the United States are seen in the Southeast. However, the disease has been seen in nearly all parts of the world. The incidence seems to be decreasing, possibly secondary to measles vaccine use. As mentioned earlier, patients usually have a history of measles infection before the age of 2. The disease very rarely has been seen in children who have received the measles vaccine. The latent period between measles infection and the onset of SSPE averages 5-6 years.

The disease begins insidiously, first with behavioral and personality changes and decreased school performance (Table 78.4). The correct diagnosis rarely is made at this stage. Within weeks to months patients develop neurologic changes,

TABLE 78.4   Clinical Stages of SSPE

Stage 1	Subtle changes in intellectual skills, mood swings, inappropriate affect; drooling and changes in speech are less common
Stage 2	Myoclonic jerks, clumsiness, ataxia, choreoathetosis; ocular changes in ∿ 50%: cortical blindness, optic atrophy, etc.; unusual in this stage - grand mal seizures
Stage 3	Marked mental deterioration, coma, opisthotonus, decerebrate or decorticate posturing, autonomic nervous dysfunction; death often in this stage due to infection
Stage 4	Patient calmer, nearly total loss of cortical function; purposeless responses - eye movements, episodic laughing or crying; severe autonomic nervous dysfunction; death from vasomotor collapse or infection

usually in motor function, with myoclonic jerks, seizures, and choreoathetosis. Later, patients show signs of cerebral degeneration, coma, and hypothalamic dysfunction. Later still, patients become mute and develop cortical blindness.

The diagnosis is made on the basis of the clinical picture, along with spinal fluid, serologic, and electroencephalographic changes. There is a high serum and spinal fluid measles antibody titer. Other features of the cerebrospinal fluid are not particularly helpful. There is usually no abnormality in the cell count, and the markedly elevated protein content in the spinal fluid represents the marked elevation in antimeasles antibody. The EEG is characteristic showing the "suppression burst pattern."

The course is progressively downhill to death over a period of 1-8 years, with the average survival from diagnosis being 4 years. There have been rare reports of arrest in the progression of the disease, and even rarer reports of remission. The treatment is inosiplex (Isoprinosine) 100 mg/kg/day which may, if begun early in the course of the disease, lead to arrest of the disease and even significant recovery (Figure 78.2). Therefore, it is important to consider SSPE in the differential diagnosis of any child with a change in behavior and personality or decreased school performance.

There is considerable speculation, and some evidence, that multiple sclerosis is also a slow virus disease. As with SSPE, most of the evidence suggests that measles or a related virus is the etiology, but the evidence is far less firm than for SSPE, or for any of the other suspected slow virus diseases.

Progressive Multifocal Leukoencephalopathy

This is a rare demyelinating disease seen generally in patients with marked impairment of cell-mediated immunity. Most commonly these are patients with

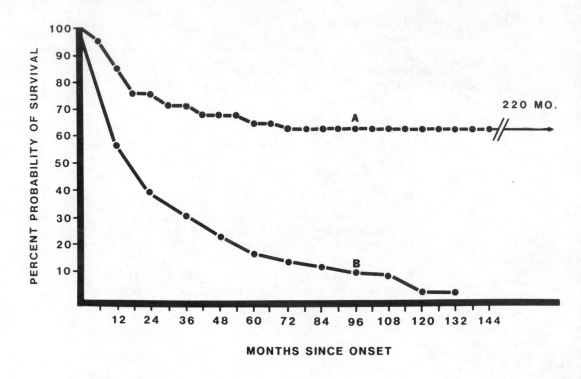

FIGURE 78.2   Survival from onset of SSPE of (A) cases treated with inosiplex (Isoprinosine), and (B) cases treated in a variety of other ways, excluding the use of Isoprinosine. (Courtesy of Newport Pharmaceuticals, Inc.)

lymphoproliferative malignancies, transplant patients, or patients with systemic lupus erythematosus receiving corticosteroids, but there have been a very few patients in whom no demonstrable immunologic defect has been discovered.

The etiology is a group of related viruses which are members of the papovavirus group. The most common species has been named the JC virus, after the initials of the patient from whom the virus was first isolated. Although the disease is rare, serologic studies show it to be a common infection, since antibody is found in 70-80% of adults. Primary infection appears to occur in infancy and early childhood, and is thought to be completely asymptomatic. The mode of transmission is unknown, although virus is found in urine of some normal people, and excretion has been noted to be increased during pregnancy. Antibody to the virus is found in people worldwide.

Pathologically patients have noninflammatory plaques in the white matter with demyelinization. Oligodendroglia cells in the periphery of the plaques contain intranuclear inclusion bodies. Brains of patients with the disease contain very large amounts of the virus.

Clinical findings are variable depending upon the location of most intense central nervous system involvement. Patients usually have paralysis, mental deterioration, blindness, ataxia, and sensory loss. Brain stem or spinal signs are less common. Spinal fluid is normal and the electroencephalogram is nonspecific. Papovavirus antibody titers are not helpful since, as mentioned before, most people have antibody. However, the diagnosis usually can be made on the basis of evidence for central nervous system involvement clinically in a patient with one of the predisposing diseases. Definite diagnosis can be made by obtaining a brain biopsy and showing virus by immunofluorescence. The prognosis is grim, with all patients dying, usually within a year. Treatment with antiviral agents has not been effective.

Progressive Rubella Panencephalitis

This is an extremely rare disease, with only a handful of cases having been reported. It is found primarily in older children who have had congenital rubella. Pathologically the brains show perivascular lymphocytes and plasma cells, gliosis, but no inclusion bodies. The disease begins with intellectual deterioration at about age 11-12, and the children develop seizures, myoclonus, cerebellar ataxia, and corticospinal tract signs. Patients have a high titer of spinal fluid rubella antibody. The course is progressively downhill with death occurring after several years.

Kuru

This is a disease found only in the eastern highlands of Papua New Guinea, among the Fore tribe. The disease is a result of cannibalism with consumption of the brain. With the outlawing of cannibalism, the disease is disappearing. It is seen much more commonly in women than men, and the explanation for this is that the men usually do not eat the brain. At the height of prevalence of the disease, nearly 90% of the Fore women developed it, and it was the most common cause of death in this tribe.

Pathologically the brain appears normal grossly, but microscopically there are marked neuronal loss and gliosis, most prominently in the cerebellum, brain stem, the thalamus, and basal ganglia.

Clinically patients demonstrate the insidious onset of cerebellar ataxia with little or no dementia. Spinal fluid is normal.

The course is one of relentless progression (Table 78.5) with death usually occurring within a year due to burns and sepsis.

TABLE 78.5   Clinical Stages of Kuru

Ambulant	Subjective unsteadiness, ataxic gait, convergent strabismus, shivering-like truncal tremor, dysarthria
Sedentary	Needs support for walking, rigidity of limbs, clonus, emotional lability with outbursts of pathologic laughter, no mental deterioration or sensory changes
Terminal	Unable to sit without support, urinary and fecal incontinence, bulbar signs, inanition, decubitus ulcers, and pneumonia

Creutzfeldt-Jakob

This is a rare disease, with an incidence of about 1:1 million population, worldwide in distribution, usually occurring in the 30- to 50-year-old age group. There is no evidence of person-to-person spread except iatrogenically. There have been interesting but tragic cases of transmission by corneal transplantation or by the use of brain probes. About 15-20% of cases are familial. The infectious and possibly viral etiology of this disease, like that of kuru, has been shown by transmission to chimpanzees, which develop a very similar clinical picture after a very prolonged incubation period.

Pathologically the brains of patients with Creutzfeldt-Jakob disease show intracellular vacuolization of neurons leading to spongiform degeneration, with reactive astrocytes, then development of plaques similar to the senile plaques of Alzheimer's disease. This has led to postulation that the latter, a much more common disease, is also a result of a slow virus infection.

Patients develop the insidious onset of dementia with a progressive downhill course leading to death, usually within a year, usually as a result of bronchopneumonia.

The cases of iatrogenic transmission of Creutzfeldt-Jakob disease have led to investigation into the methodology for sterilizing equipment that might transmit the viral agent. It has been found that the Creutzfeldt-Jakob and kuru agents are extremely difficult to inactivate, leading to speculation that they represent a type of microorganism which is different from viruses or other known infectious agents (Tables 78.6 and 78.7). Equipment may be sterilized using Chlorox, ether, iodine, or strong detergents.

TABLE 78.6   Are Kuru and Creutzfeldt-Jakob Disease Caused by Viruses?

For	Against
Filterable	Infection induces no inflammatory response
Self-replicating	Long incubation period
Enter an eclipse phase	Chronic progressive pathology
Host specificity	No remissions or recoveries
Appear to be strains of different virulence and pathogenicity	No antigenicity
	"Degenerative" histopathology
	Lack of interferon stimulation
	No inclusion bodies
	No virus particles seen by electron microscopy
	No detectable infectious nucleic acid
	Resistant to formaldehyde, proteases, nucleases, heat, ultraviolet light, ionizing radiation
	No decrease in cell-mediated immunity during the infection

TABLE 78.7   Comparison of Kuru and Creutzfeldt–Jakob Disease

Feature	Kuru	CJD
Age	> 4 yr	> 18
Insidious onset	+	+
Dementia	+/-	+
Sensory defects	+-/	+
Geographic distribution	Papua New Guinea	Worldwide

Selected Bibliography

Asher, D. M., Gibbs, C. J., Jr., and Gajdusek, D. C.: Pathogenesis of subacute spongiform encephalopathies. *Ann Clin Lab Sci* 6:84–103, 1976.

Brown, P., Tsai, T., and Gajdusek, D. C.: Seroepidemiology of human papovaviruses. *Am J Epidemiol* 102:331–340, 1975.

Chatigny, M. A. and Prusiner, S. B.: Biohazards of investigations on the transmissible spongiform encephalopathies. *Rev Infect Dis* 2:713–724, 1980.

Coleman, D. V., Wolfendale, M. R., Daniel, R. A., Dhanjal, N. K., Garder, S. D., Gibson, P. E., and Field, A. M.: A prospective study of human polyomavirus infection in pregnancy. *J Infect Dis* 142:1–8, 1980.

Detels, R., Brody, J., McNew, J., and Edgar, A.: Further epidemiological studies of subacute sclerosing panencephalitis. *Lancet* 2:11–14, 1973.

Duffy, P., Wolf, J., Collins, G., DeVoe, A. G., Streeten, B., and Cowen, D.: Possible person-to-person transmission of Creutzfeldt–Jakob disease. *N Engl J Med* 290:692–693, 1974.

Gajdusek, D. C.: Unconventional viruses and the origin and disappearance of kuru. *Science* 197:943–960, 1977.

Gajdusek, D. C. and Zigas, V.: Degenerative disease of the central nervous system in New Guinea. The endemic occurrence of "kuru" in the native population. *N Engl J Med* 257:974–978, 1957.

Hall, W. W., Kiessling, W. R., and ter Meulen, V.: Studies on the membrane protein of subacute sclerosing panencephalitis and measles viruses. *Nature* 272:460–462, 1977.

Huang, A. S.: Viral pathogenesis and molecular biology. *Bacteriol Rev* 41:811–821, 1977.

Kahana, E., Alter, M., Braham, J., and Sofer, D.: Creutzfeldt–Jakob disease: Focus among Libyan Jews in Israel. *Science* 183:90–91, 1974.

Mattson, R. H.: Subacute sclerosing panencephalitis recovery associated with isoprinosine therapy: Report of a case. *Neurology* 24:383, 1974.

Mehta, P. D., Kane, A., and Thorman, H.: Quantitation of measles virus–specific immunoglobulins in serum, CSF and brain extract from patients with subacute sclerosing panencephalitis. *J Immunol* 118:2254–2261, 1977.

Padgett, B. L. and Walker, D. L.: New human papovaviruses. *Prog Med Virol* 22: 1–35, 1976.

Padgett, B. L., Walker, D. L., Zultrein, G. M., Eckroade, R. J., and Dessel, B. H.: Cultivation of papova-like virus from human brain with progressive multifocal leucoencephalopathy. *Lancet* 1:1257–1260, 1971.

Rima, B. K. and Martin, S. J.: Persistent infection of tissue culture cells by RNA viruses. *Med Microbiol Immunol* 162:89–118, 1976.

Rockwell, D., Rubens, F. L., Winkelstein, A., and Mendelow, H.: Absence of immune deficiencies in a case of PML. *Am J Med* 61:433–436, 1976.

Sever, J. L., Krebs, H., Ley, A., Horta-Barbose, L., and Rubenstein, D.: Diagnosis of subacute sclerosing panencephalitis: The value of and availability of measles antibody determination. *JAMA* 228:604, 1974.

ter Meulen, V. and Hall, W. W.: Slow virus infections of the nervous system: Virological, immunological and pathogenetic considerations. *J Gen Virol* 41: 1–25, 1978.

Weiner, L. P., Herndon, R. M., Narayan, O., Johnson, R. T., Shah, K., Rubinstein, L. J., Preziosi, T. J., and Conley, F. K.: Isolation of virus related to SV_{40} from patients with progressive multifocal leukoencephalopathy. *N Engl J Med* 286:385–390, 1972.

79

CHLAMYDIA

Rama Ganguly, Ph.D. and
Robert H. Waldman, M.D.

The genus *Chlamydia,* previously called *Bedsonia,* consists of a group of obligate intracellular parasites that exhibit a unique developmental cycle. They are important human pathogens, as well as causing widespread infections in birds and mammals. As a result, these agents are responsible for significant economic losses.

Etiology

The chlamydiae are small, nonmotile, gram-negative organisms which reproduce only within host cells. They are not viruses (Table 79.1). The chlamydial elementary body (0.3 μm in diameter) is capable of extracellular existence and infection; when it comes in contact with the host cell membrane it is taken up by phagocytosis. The elementary body contained within a cytoplasmic vesicle then enlarges to form into the large, less dense, noninfectious reticulate body. The latter then undergoes binary fission during the next 24-48 hr and aggregates to form what is called an inclusion body (0.6-1.0 μm diameter). Subsequently the latter "reorganizes" to form numerous small, dense elementary bodies which upon release from the host cell can invade other cells. In chlamydial diseases the presence of inclusion bodies can be demonstrated.

Mice and guinea pigs can be infected with the chlamydiae, and these organisms can be grown in the yolk sac of chicken embryos, as well as in tissue cultures. Chlamydiae are divided into group A, *C. trachomatis* and group B, *C. psittaci* (Table 79.2).

TABLE 79.1   Characteristics Which Differentiate *Chlamydia* from Viruses

Gram-negative (cell wall similar to other gram-
negative bacteria)

Possess both RNA and DNA

Reproduce by binary fission

Possess ribosomes

Susceptible to antibiotics

Epidemiology

Chlamydiae can infect a wide range of host species. Group A organisms infect humans primarily via mucosal membranes of the eye and genitourinary tract. Transmission of infection is through direct contact. They cause murine pneumonitis. Group B organisms have a broader host range infecting birds and mammals, and can be transmitted to humans from birds having ornithosis. The organism is also transmitted from person to person by droplets. In birds and mammals the infection may be manifested in the forms of pneumonitis, polyarthritis, enteritis, or encephalitis.

The characteristics of the various types of chlamydial infections are outlined in Table 79.3. Trachoma is one of the most important human infectious diseases with approximately 400 million cases occurring each year. It is associated with lower socioeconomic conditions and lack of hygiene. A significant proportion (6-10 million) of these infections result in total blindness. Trachoma occurs only in humans.

The agent for trachoma inclusion conjunctivitis (TRIC) is found in the genital tract and is transmitted by sexual contact. The "inclusion" part of the name comes from the inclusion bodies, which are seen in cells scraped from the conjunctiva. Since the disease is rather mild clinically, most cases remain undetected. The infection is transmitted to newborns via the birth canal and usually becomes evident in the week after birth. In addition to transmission by sexual contact, the infection can be transmitted to adults from swimming pools (inadequately chlorinated) or by direct contacts with fingers and from contaminated towels.

Lymphogranuloma venereum (LGV) is a "minor" venereal disease with approximately 500 cases reported in the United States per year. Not much is known regarding the infectivity of LGV and its natural course. There is some evidence that the disease can persist for a very long period.

Ornithosis is transmitted to humans from birds by the inhalation of dried infected feces. As in birds, the disease in humans may be latent or active. During crowding and shipment this infection may become evident in apparently healthy birds. The incidence is higher in autumn. Approximately 50 cases of severe infection are reported in the United States each year, usually in bird-handlers.

TABLE 79.2   Differentiation of *Chlamydia* spp

	Inhibited by Neuraminidase	Pathogenic for		Sensitive to Sulfonamides	Principal Hosts
		Monkey Eyes	Mouse Brains		
C. trachomatis					
Serotypes A–K (trachoma, inclusion conjunctivitis, urethritis, etc.)	+	+	–	+	Humans
Serotype L (LGV)	–	–	+	+	Humans
C. psittaci	–	–	–	–	Birds and mammals

TABLE 79.3   Various *C. trachomatis* Syndromes

Disease	Transmission	Serotypes
Trachoma	Fomites, flies, close personal contact	A, B, Ba, C
Nongonococcal urethritis in men, epididymitis, proctitis	Sexual intercourse	D-K
Cervicitis, salpingitis, dysuria-pyuria syndrome in women	Sexual intercourse	D-K
Neonatal conjunctivitis (inclusion conjunctivitis), pneumonia	Passage through birth canal	D-K
Inclusion conjunctivitis in childhood	Swimming pool water	D-K
Lymphogranuloma venereum	Sexual intercourse	L1, L2, L3

May also be involved in etiology of Reiter's syndrome, endocarditis, and otitis media

Pathology

In trachoma, the disease begins with the sudden onset of inflammation of the conjunctiva. This leads to leukocyte migration, follicle formation under the conjunctiva, followed by vascularization as well as infiltration of the cornea. The resultant effect is scarring of the conjunctiva and blindness. This process is usually enhanced by simultaneous bacterial infections. A TRIC infection also involves the cervical epithelial and urethral lining often causing very mild or no clinical symptoms. However, in the newborns infected via the birth canal, acute purulent conjunctivitis may be evident as a transient manifestation without scars or pannus. In adults inclusion conjunctivitis with follicles may cause corneal opacities. Chlamydial neonatal infection often is followed by pneumonia and/or otitis media.

The primary painless lesions in LGV are vesicular and inconspicuous. However, the development of enlarged matted inguinal and femoral lymph nodes ensues; these are often painful and fluctuant. The lymph nodes contain granulomas and may completely obstruct the draining lymph channels causing tremendous enlargement of the genitalia (elephantiasis). Women also develop proctitis due to perirectal drainage of the vaginal lymphatics. Rectal stricture and perforation also develop as late complications of LGV. Vulvular carcinoma occurs at a higher rate in women who have had LGV.

Ornithosis may lead to fatal pneumonitis and may involve various organs in addition to the lungs. Thus, jaundice, acute thyroiditis, and meningitis may be manifested. Death may result from pulmonary insufficiency and toxemia.

Clinical Manifestation

Trachoma starts suddenly with conjunctival inflammation. Follicular hypertrophy occasionally followed by pannus and conjunctival scarring are typical clinical features (Table 79.4).

Conjunctivitis manifests as purulent inflammation, usually without pannus or conjunctival scarring. It starts with a sticky exudate, often unilateral. It is usually benign and self-limited but recent studies indicate that it may result in micropannus, conjunctival scars, and later relapse.

In the neonate, it has been recognized only recently that chlamydiae are a frequent cause of pneumonia. The infant, aged 1–3 months, exhibits paroxysmal cough, respiratory distress, and bilateral infiltrates, frequently preceded by conjunctivitis. Chlamydial pneumonia may account for as many as 30% of the pneumonias in infants under 6 months of age, and its prevalence may be as high as 20% of babies born to infected mothers.

Nongonococcal urethritis in men is characterized by a scanty mucoid urethral discharge, dysuria, and culture and Gram stain results negative for *Neisseria gonorrhoeae*. While only 0–7% of controls have *C. trachomatis* isolated from their urethras, 30–50% of patients with nongonococcal urethritis have been shown to have that organism. Similarly, postgonococcal urethritis in many, or most cases, is due to chlamydial infection and is explained by coincident infection with the gonococcus and *C. trachomatis*. Treatment with an antibiotic which is effective only against *N. gonorrhoeae* will result in the chlamydiae remaining and continuing to cause infection. Chlamydiae are also a cause, and possibly a major cause, of epididymitis.

TABLE 79.4   Clinical Characteristics of Trachoma

Diagnosis: two or more of the following:

Follicles on upper tarsal conjunctiva or limbus
Epithelial or subepithelial keratitis
Pannus formation
Scars causing impaired vision and distortion of eyelids

Staging:
I. Immature follicles
II. Well-developed follicles, papillary hyperplasia, pannus and infiltration
III. Follicular necrosis and beginning of scarring
IV. Follicles and infiltrates replaced by scar, with corneal opacification and distortion of eyelids

In women, chlamydiae cause cervicitis, salpingitis, urethritis, and also probably endometritis and premature birth. The relationship to cervicitis is not as definite as that to nongonococcal urethritis in men. Normal sexually active women have chlamydiae isolated in about 10% of the attempts, whereas about 20% of women with cervicitis have chlamydiae isolated. It is estimated that 35-60% of salpingitis cases are caused by chlamydiae. The salpingitis is characterized as being less acute than that caused by gonococcus, but with a high risk of leading to infertility.

Another problem in women that has been related to chlamydial infection is the acute urethral syndrome. This syndrome is characterized by the usual symptoms associated with cystitis, most prominently dysuria. Patients have pyuria but bacterial cultures are sterile. In a significant number of these patients, chlamydial infection has been documented.

Other diseases which have been related to chlamydial infection are proctitis and pneumonia in adults. With respect to the latter, the association was first documented in immunocompromised patients and more recently, in otherwise normal individuals.

Lymphogranuloma venereum has an incubation period of 1-4 weeks and starts with systemic symptoms of fever, headache, and myalgia. Primary genital lesions are inconspicuous and painless but are followed by painful, enlarged inguinal and femoral lymph nodes (buboes). The disease may progress to destroy the vulva and urethra. "Elephantiasis" of the genitalia may result from lymphatic obstruction.

Ornithosis may be manifested by pneumonic consolidation, fever, and chills. Frequently the disease may be asymptomatic with minor respiratory manifestations. The incubation period varies from 1 to 3 weeks.

Laboratory Diagnosis

Conjunctival scrapings may be used to inoculate cell cultures and yolk sacs of chick embryos. Fluorescent-labeled antibody may be used to identify the inclusion bodies. Lymphogranuloma venereum may be diagnosed by isolation of the agent from lymph node aspiration or biopsy. A rise in serum antibody can be measured using the complement-fixation test. The Frei skin test, which is not entirely specific, demonstrates delayed hypersensitivity reaction to the killed, injected organisms. Ornithosis is diagnosed by injecting blood or sputum of patients in the acute stage into cell cultures or embryonated eggs. The pathogen is then identified by using fluorescent antibody staining. Complement-fixing and infectivity-neutralizing antibodies can also be assayed.

Immunity

Chlamydial infections do not elicit enduring immunity. Diseases produced by the chlamydiae often assume chronic and relapsing patterns. Effective immunity for a few months has been shown to develop after experimental eye infections in animals. On the other hand, pneumonia and other forms of infections in birds do not result in complete protection. Infectivity-neutralizing antibodies prevent spread of infection in host cells but they are ineffective in influencing the intracellular existence of already established parasites. Local antibodies in secretions and cellular immunity may play protective roles but these have not been investigated in detail. Ocular trachoma in man often does not elicit circulating antibodies or delayed hypersensitivity reactions to Frei antigens, but may produce local secretory antibodies.

In neonatal pneumonitis a pronounced titer of specific antibody develops against the infecting strain. This can be detected by microimmunofluorescent tests. In the early phase of the disease, LGV patients often develop hypergammaglobulinemia. Positive reactivity for rheumatoid factor as well as for cryoglobulins is common. It is not yet certain if LGV infection induces effective immunity. Cell-mediated immunity develops and is usually retained lifelong indicating possible latency of the infection. The frequency of relapses of the disease also supports this contention.

Treatment, Control, and Prevention

Because the chlamydiae are intracellular parasites, it is required that antimicrobial agents be able to penetrate the host cells. Tetracycline and chloramphenicol are the drugs of choice to treat infections from *C. psittaci* and *C. trachomatis*. Rifampin also has been shown to be effective against these organisms.

Treatment of trachoma by both topical and systemic administration of drugs results in recovery from the overt, acute clinical disease, but often the disease assumes a latent form and relapses occur in spite of treatment. Vaccine field trials in humans have demonstrated that the immunity elicited can significantly reduce the clinical attack rates. Vaccinees who become infected with chlamydiae demonstrate restricted formation of inclusion bodies in conjunctival specimens. This could play a significant role in reducing the transmission rate and the magnitude of the epidemic. However, the immunity elicited with the vaccines, either in animal models or in human subjects, appears to be transient. Personal hygiene and sanitary measures are helpful in restricting the spread of infection.

Lymphogranuloma venereum is treated with either tetracycline or sulfonamides. There is no vaccine available against LGV.

Tetracycline, the drug of choice for ornithosis, can bring about a rapid cure. Vaccination against ornithosis has not been successful. Often tetracycline is included in poultry feed as prophylaxis.

Selected Bibliography

Beem, M. O. and Saxon, E. M.: Respiratory tract colonization and distinctive pneumonia syndrome in infants infected with *Chlamydia trachomatis*. *N Engl J Med* 296:306-310, 1977.

Bowie, W. R., Alexander, E. R., Floyd, J. F., Holmes, J., Miller, Y., and Holmes, K. K.: Differential response of chlamydial and ureaplasma-associated urethritis to sulfafurazole and aminocyclitol. *Lancet* 2:1276-1278, 1976.

Caldwell, H. D., Kuo, C. C., and Kenny, G. E.: Antigenic analysis of chlamydiae by two-dimensional immunoelectrophoresis. Parts I and II. *J Immunol* 115:969-975, 1975.

Dhir, S. P., Hakomori, S., Kenny, G. E., and Grayston, J. T.: Immunochemical studies on chlamydial group antigen. Presence of a 2-keto-3-deoxy carbohydrate as immunodominant group. *J Immunol* 109:116-122, 1972.

Evans, R. T. and Taylor-Robinson, D.: Detection of *Chlamydia trachomatis* in rapidly produced McCoy cell monolayers. *J Clin Pathol* 33:591-594, 1980.

Felman, Y. M. and Nikitas, J. A.: Nongonococcal urethritis. A clinical review. *JAMA* 245:381, 1981.

Fraser, C. E. O., McComb, D. E., Murray, E. S., and MacDonald, A. B.: Immunity to chlamydial infections of the eye. IV. Immunity in owl monkeys to reinfection with trachoma. *Arch Ophthalmol* 93:518-521, 1975.

Ghadirian, F. D., and Robson, H. G.: *Chlamydia trachomatis* genital infections. *Br J Vener Dis* 55:415-418, 1979.

Grayston, J. T. and Wang, S. P.: New knowledge of chlamydiae and the diseases they cause. *J Infect Dis* 132:87-105, 1975.

Gump, D. W., Dickstein, S., and Gibson, M.: Endometritis related to *Chlamydia trachomatis* infection. *Ann Intern Med* 96:61, 1981.

Hale, G. L. and Hinds, M. W.: Male urethritis in King County, Washington, 1974-75. I. Incidence. *Am J Public Health* 68:20-25, 1978.

Harrison, H. R., English, M. G., Lee, C. K., and Alexander, E. R.: *Chlamydia trachomatis* infant pneumonitis: Comparison with matched controls and other infant pneumonitis. *N Engl J Med* 298:702-708, 1978.

Holmes, K. K.: The *Chlamydia* epidemic. *JAMA* 245:1718, 1981.

Hoshiwara, I., Oster, B., Hanna, L., Cignetti, F., Coleman, V. R., and Jawet, Z. E.: Doxycycline treatment of chronic trachoma. *JAMA* 224:220-223, 1973.

Jones, B. R.: The prevention of blindness from trachoma. The Bowman Lecture 1976: President's Introduction. *Trans Ophthalmol Soc U K* 95:16-33, 1975.

Komaroff, A. L., Aronson, M. D., and Schachter, J.: *Chlamydia trachomatis* infection in adults with community-acquired pneumonia. *JAMA* 245:1319, 1981.

Lewis, V. J., Thacker, W. L., and Mitchell, S. H.: Demonstration of chlamydial endotoxin-like activity. *J Gen Microbiol* 114:215-216, 1979.

Moulder, J. W.: The relation of the psittacosis group (chlamydia) to bacteria and viruses. *Ann Rev Microbiol* 20:107-130, 1966.

Quinn, T. C., Goodell, S. E., Mkrtichian, E., Schuffler, M. D., Wang, S. P., Stamm, W. E., and Holmes, K. K.: *Chlamydia trachomatis* proctitis. *N Engl J Med* 305:195, 1981.

Richmond, S. J. and Sparling, P. F.: Genital chlamydial infections. *Am J Epidemiol* 103:428-435, 1976.

Schachter, J.: Chlamydial infections (Parts 1, 2, and 3). *N Engl J Med* 298:428, 490, 540, 1978.

Schachter, J., Sugg, N., and Sung, M.: Psittacosis: The reservoir persists. *J Infect Dis* 137:44-49, 1978.

Swanson, J., Eschenbach, D. A., Alexander, E. R., and Holmes, K. K.: Light and electron microscopic study of *Chlamydia trachomatis* infection of the uterine cervix. *J Infect Dis* 131:678–687, 1975.

Treharne, J. D., Darougar, S., and Jones, B. R.: Modification of the microimmunofluorescence test to provide a routine serodiagnostic test for chlamydial infection. *J Clin Pathol* 30:510, 1977.

Wang, S. P. and Grayston, J. T.: Immunological relationship between genital TRIC, lymphogranuloma venereum, and related organisms in a new microtiter indirect immunofluorescent test. *Am J Ophthalmol* 70:367–374, 1970.

80

MYCOPLASMA
Rashida A. Khakoo, M.D.

Mycoplasmas have been known pathogens of birds and mammals for many years. *Mycoplasma* as a cause of human disease has been documented relatively recently compared with the disease in animals. In 1943 the occurrence of cold agglutinins was demonstrated in a significant percentage of patients with primary atypical pneumonias. In 1944, Eaton and co-workers isolated a filtrable agent, initially thought to be a virus, from the sputa of patients with atypical pneumonias. Growth of the agent on agar was reported in 1962 and proof provided that the agent was a *Mycoplasma*. A definite role for *M. pneumoniae* in human disease was established by subsequent studies in volunteers. *Mycoplasma pneumoniae* is a common cause of pneumonia in young adults, particularly in closed populations. It occurs in endemic and epidemic forms. Although the pathogenesis is not entirely clear, attachment to specific receptors on the epithelial cell surface appears to be the initial event. Immunologic mechanisms may be responsible in part for pathogenesis.

Microbiology

Mycoplasmas are the smallest free-living organisms. They lack a cell wall and can reproduce in cell-free medium. On agar, they exhibit a characteristic colony morphology: the center of the colony is embedded in the agar giving it a "fried egg" appearance. Mycoplasmas have a triple-layered membrane and require sterols for growth. *Mycoplasma pneumoniae* is about 10 x 200 mm and is filamentous. It requires yeast extract and serum for growth.

Epidemiology

Infections with *M. pneumoniae* occur in many different areas of the world in endemic and epidemic form. Outbreaks occur in closed populations, e.g., military or college. The percentage of pneumonias caused by *M. pneumoniae* varies depending upon the population studied and the different periods of the study. Mycoplasmal infections occur throughout the year, but epidemics occur more commonly in summer and fall. Illness caused by *M. pneumoniae* occurs most frequently in schoolaged children and young adults, and occasionally, in younger children and the elderly. The usual incubation period is 2-3 weeks. Close contact is most likely required for spread. Families with a greater number of infections are more likely to have younger parents and more young children compared to those with smaller numbers of infection. The interval between cases in family studies is 3 weeks. Spread occurs slowly in families or other closed populations, but a high percentage of susceptible persons eventually become infected. Prolonged carriage of *M. pneumoniae,* even in the face of treatment with antimicrobials, may be important in epidemiology.

Pathogenesis and Pathology

Mycoplasma pneumoniae has a predilection for the respiratory tract. The exact mechanism by which *M. pneumoniae* induces cell injury is not known. The organism attaches to the cell surface by means of a specialized tip structure which may represent a high concentration of binding sites. It is the accepted view that mycoplasmas attach to sialic acid moieties on the host cell surface. The close association of adhering mycoplasmas and their host cells may lead to local concentration of toxic metabolites which may cause cell damage. In organ cultures, ciliostasis is the most pronounced early manifestation of injury. The cilia are later damaged and lost. This is followed by loss of superficial epithelial cells.

Pathogenesis of *M. pneumoniae* pneumonia may be immune-mediated, at least in part. Infections are usually asymptomatic or mild in young children but pneumonia is more likely to occur in older children and young adults. Systemic or local antigen-antibody or cell-mediated immune reactions may be responsible for damage. Circulating immune complexes have been demonstrated during acute illness and may play a role in local damage or systemic manifestations. The lack of radiologic findings in patients with immunodeficiency syndromes and *M. pneumoniae* infection also suggests that pulmonary infiltrates in immunocompetent individuals may result from an immunologic reaction. Despite lack of pulmonary infiltrates, these patients may have very serious symptoms. Therefore, immune mechanisms may be protective, yet damaging. Autoantibodies to different organs appear during mycoplasmal infections. The role that these play in the pathogenesis is not known.

Because illness caused by *M. pneumoniae* is usually self-limited there is little information on pathology. Interstitial pneumonia and acute bronchiolitis are the usual features. The pathology of *M. pneumoniae* has been well studied in animal models, particularly the hamster in which the characteristic lesion is peribronchial.

Mechanisms of recovery from *M. pneumoniae* infections are not entirely clear. Local accumulation of antibody, particularly IgA, seems to be important in host defenses. This antibody might be associated with inhibition of attachment of *M. pneumoniae* to respiratory epithelium. *Mycoplasma pneumoniae* can be lysed by complement. Phagocytosis and killing of opsonized mycoplasmas by polymorphonuclear leukocytes and macrophages also occur. The duration of immunity to mycoplasma is not known. Second episodes of infection and pneumonia can occur.

Diagnosis

Clinical

The patient may present with pharyngitis, tracheobronchitis, pneumonia, bullous myringitis, or otitis media (Table 80.1). Younger children are more likely to have mostly upper respiratory tract involvement. Pulmonary symptoms may be exacerbated in patients with chronic obstructive pulmonary disease.

The onset is usually insidious and most of the symptoms are nonspecific. Initially there is fever, headache, and malaise. This is followed by cough which is a very prominent symptom. Cough is usually nonproductive but can be productive of mucoid sputum. Purulent sputum and hemoptysis are rare. Patients may complain of sore throat, earache, or substernal chest pain. Physical examination usually reveals a patient who does not appear particularly ill. Patients with immunodeficiency syndrome and sickle cell anemia have more severe illness.

Myringitis, occasionally with bullae and hemorrhages, may occur. In a challenge study of volunteers, myringitis developed in 13 of 52 volunteers infected with *M. pneumoniae*. Hemorrhagic bullous myringitis occurred less frequently. In the setting of natural infection, myringitis is not as common; *M. pneumoniae* has been isolated from the middle ear fluid.

Physical examination of the chest may be unremarkable, but occasional rales or rhonchi may be heard. Rarely, signs of consolidation and pleural effusion may be present.

The occurrence of clinically significant hemolytic anemia is uncommon. It characteristically occurs 2-5 weeks after the onset of symptoms. By the end of the first week of infection, cold agglutinins occur in one-third to three-fourths

TABLE 80.1   Clinical Manifestations of *M. pneumoniae* Infection

Respiratory	Coryza
	Pharyngitis
	Bullous myringitis
	Tracheobronchitis
	Pneumonia
	Pleural effusion
Nonrespiratory	Hemolytic anemia
	Thrombocytopenia
	Migratory polyarthritis
	Hepatitis
	Myo- and/or pericarditis
	Erythema multiforme
	Meningoencephalitis
	Guillain-Barré syndrome

of patients with *M. pneumoniae* pneumonia. Cold agglutinins are IgM antibodies which react with the I antigen of erythrocytes. An altered antigen may stimulate the synthesis of antibody which cross-reacts with erythrocyte I antigen. Cold agglutinins attach to erythrocytes and fix complement at reduced temperatures in the extremities. The damaged erythrocytes have a shortened survival and are phagocytosed by the cells of the reticuloendothelial system. The severity of the clinical manifestations is determined by the degree of antibody-binding to erythrocytes, which in turn depends upon the thermal environment of the patient, the concentration of cold agglutinins, and the thermal maximum of the cold agglutinin molecules present. Patients usually present with anemia, jaundice, and indirect hyperbilirubinemia. Other hematologic manifestations include thrombocytopenia and disseminated intravascular coagulation.

Eleven to thirty-three percent of patients with *M. pneumoniae* infections are reported to have exanthems. The rashes described are erythematous, macular or papular, papulovesicular, urticarial, petechial, or morbiliform. Erythema multiforme major and minor are also reported and *M. pneumoniae* can be isolated from bullous lesions. The most common sites of the rashes are the extremities and trunk. The rash appears during the febrile period and usually persists for 2 weeks or longer. Two-thirds of the patients receive antimicrobial therapy before the appearance of the rash, so in some patients it may be secondary to antimicrobials or to a combination of *M. pneumoniae* infection and antimicrobials. A mechanism similar to that occurring in infectious mononucleosis might be responsible.

The neurologic syndromes in association with *M. pneumoniae* infections include meningitis, meningoencephalitis, transverse myelitis, seizures, Guillain-Barré syndrome, brain stem dysfunction, peripheral and cranial neuropathy, cerebellar ataxia, hemiplegia, coma, psychosis, and decerebration. Neurologic symptoms may occur during or several weeks following the respiratory symptoms. In some cases, patients with nervous system findings may not have had preceding respiratory complaints. Cerebrospinal fluids in patients with neurologic syndromes have shown increased or normal protein content, normal glucose levels, zero to several hundred leukocytes, with varying differentials. The pathogenesis of the central nervous system disorders is unclear although *M. pneumoniae* has been isolated from the brain. Recovery following neurologic involvement is usually slow but complete. Occasionally, residual deficits persist.

Pericarditis, myocarditis, and myopericarditis have been reported. In one retrospective series, pericarditis and myocarditis were present in 8.5% and 1.8%, respectively, of patients with *M. pneumoniae* diagnosed serologically. *Mycoplasma pneumoniae* has been isolated from pericardial fluid and left ventricular blood at autopsy.

Myalgia and arthralgia are common, and arthritis also occurs. The joint symptoms usually begin 3-8 days after the onset of respiratory symptoms. The larger joints are most frequently involved.

Nonspecific gastrointestinal symptoms such as anorexia, nausea, vomiting, and diarrhea may occur. Pancreatitis has been reported. Mild elevations of transaminases and alkaline phosphatase may occur.

Mycoplasmal infections should be suspected clinically in children and young adults who present with respiratory symptoms, particularly when symptoms are out of proportion to signs. The diagnosis should be considered also in patients presenting with respiratory complaints and one or more of the features mentioned previously, or in any patient with atypical pneumonia. The diagnosis is confirmed by laboratory tests.

Laboratory

The leukocyte count is usually normal although marked leukocytosis with left shift may occur. Leukopenia may occasionally occur.

Cold agglutinins usually appear during the second or third week after the onset of symptoms. The titers drop fairly rapidly after reaching the maximum, in most cases they are no longer demonstrated in significant titer by 4-6 weeks. The height of the cold agglutinin titer is related to the severity of symptoms, the extent of the pulmonary lesions , and the duration and the height of fever. Cold agglutinins are not specific for mycoplasmal infections since they may occur in other viral infections, nonmycoplasmal-induced hemolytic anemias, and lymphoproliferative disorders. However, the majority of cold agglutinin-positive pneumonias with cold agglutinin titers of $\geq$ 1:128 are caused by *M. pneumoniae*.

Other serologic tests for measuring antibodies to mycoplasmas are available. Of these, the complement-fixation test is most commonly used. A fourfold or greater rise in titer is significant.

Mycoplasma pneumoniae can be cultured from the sputum or a throat swab. It has also been isolated from other sites: middle ear fluid, bullous lesions or erythema multiforme major, cerebrospinal fluid, and the brain.

The findings on chest roentgenograms vary. The infiltrates are usually patchy, reticular, interstitial, or have mixed interstitial-acinar pattern. Lower lobe involvement is more common. Occasionally, other lobes may be involved. Lobar involvement is uncommon. Pleural effusions may be present but are usually small and have the characteristics of an exudate. Gram stain of the sputum shows a few polymorphonuclear leukocytes with no predominant organism.

The differential diagnosis of *M. pneumoniae* pneumonia includes viral infections, Legionnaires' disease, Q fever, psittacosis, tularemia, tuberculosis, and fungal infections. With Q fever, tularemia, and psittacosis, epidemiologic history is of help. These diagnoses can be confirmed by various serologic tests. For primary tuberculosis, history of contact, smears, and cultures of sputum would be helpful to differentiate from an infiltrate caused by *M. pneumoniae*. Hilar adenopathy is a feature of primary tuberculosis, whereas it is extremely unusual in *M. pneumoniae* pneumonia. Viral pneumonia may be difficult to distinguish clinically from *M. pneumoniae* pneumonia. Cold agglutinins can be positive in viral pneumonia but usually in low titer. Patients with Legionnaires' disease are generally older and have more severe disease than those with *M. pneumoniae* pneumonia. Also, patients with Legionnaires' disease are more likely to present with unexplained encephalopathy, hematuria, and elevation of serum glutamic oxaloacetic transaminase. In the absence of extrapulmonary symptoms and signs, it may be difficult to distinguish clinically between *M. pneumoniae* pneumonia and Legionnaires' disease.

Treatment and Prognosis

Erythromycin or tetracycline is used for the treatment of *M. pneumoniae* pneumonia. Both have been associated with clinical improvement and have been shown to reduce the length of illness. Erythromycin is about 50 times more active in vitro than tetracycline. In vivo, both seem to be of about equal efficacy. The choice of one antimicrobial over the other may be dictated by factors other than just the presence of *M. pneumoniae* pneumonia, e.g., treatment of a child, pregnant patient, or a patient in whom Legionnaires' disease appears to be the major differential diagnosis. In all these situations erythromycin would be indicated. In patients in whom psittacosis or Q fever are major differentials, tetracycline would be indicated. The usual adult dosage of erythromycin or tetracycline is 250–500 mg every 6 hr, given for 7–10 days. Longer courses of 2–3 weeks are proposed by some authorities since incomplete relief of cough and occasional clinical relapses have been observed after the shorter course. It has been shown that *M. pneumoniae* is not eradicated from the respiratory tract for several weeks in the presence of antimicrobial therapy. Persistence of organisms cannot be explained by insufficient antimicrobial concentrations or development of resistance.

The mortality is very low. Morbidity however can be significant in terms of symptoms and days lost from school or work.

Prevention

Several experimental vaccines have been, and are being evaluated. Inactivated *M. pneumoniae* vaccines relieve the illness rate by about one-half.

Selected Bibliography

Brunner, H., Greenber, H. B., James, W. D., Horsewood, R. L., Couch, R. B., and Chanock, R. B.: Antibody to mycoplasma in nasal secretions and sputa of experimentally infected human volunteers. *Infect Immun* 8:612–620, 1973.

Chanock, R. M.: Mycoplasma infections of man. *N Engl J Med* 273:1199–1205, 1257–1264, 1965.

Chanock, R. M., Fox, H. H., James, W. D., Gutekunst, R. R., White, R. J., and Senterfit, L. B.: Epidemiology of *M. pneumoniae* infection in military recruits. *Ann N Y Acad Sci* 143:484–496, 1967.

Chanock, R. M., Hayflick, L., and Barile, M. F.: Growth on artificial medium of an agent associated with atypical pneumonia and its identification as PPLO. *Proc Nat Acad Sci* 48:41–49, 1962.

Cherry, J. D., Hurwitz, E. S., and Welliver, R. C.: *Mycoplasma pneumoniae* infections and exanthems. *J Pediatr* 87:369–373, 1975.

Denny, F. W., Clyde, W. A., and Glezen, W. P.: *Mycoplasma pneumoniae* disease: Clinical spectrum, pathophysiology, epidemiology and control. *J Infect Dis* 123:74–92, 1971.

Finland, M., Peterson, O. L., Allen, H. E., Samper, B. A., and Barnes, M. W.: Cold agglutinins. II. Cold isohemagglutinins in primary atypical pneumonia of unknown etiology with a note on the occurrence of hemolytic anemia in these cases. *J Clin Invest* 24:458–473, 1945.

Foy, H. M., Grayston, J. T., Kenny, G. E., Alexander, E. R., and McMahan, R.: Epidemiology of *Mycoplasma pneumoniae* infections in families. *JAMA* 197:859–866, 1966.

Foy, H. M., Kenny, G. E., McMahan, R., Mansey, A. M., and Grayston, J. T.: *Mycoplasma pneumoniae* pneumonia in an urban area. Five years of surveillance. *JAMA* 214:1666–1672, 1970.

Foy, H. M., Ochs, H., Davis, S. D., Kenny, G. E., and Luce, R. R.: *Mycoplasma pneumoniae* infections in patients with immunodeficiency syndromes. Report of four cases. *J Infect Dis* 127:388-393, 1973.

Greenburg, H., Helms, C. M., Brunner, H., and Chanock, R. M.: Asymptomatic infection of adult volunteers with a temperature sensitive mutant of *Mycoplasma pneumoniae*. *Proc Nat Acad Sci* 71:4015-4019, 1974.

Griffin, J. P. and Crawford, Y. E.: Association of *Mycoplasma pneumoniae* infection with primary atypical pneumonia. *Am Rev Respir Dis* 100:206-212, 1969.

Helms, C. M., Viner, J. P., Sturm, R. H., Renner, E. D., and Johnson, W.: Comparative features of pneumococcal, mycoplasmal and Legionnaires' disease pneumonias. *Ann Intern Med* 90:543-547, 1979.

Hernandez, L. A., Urquhart, G. E. D., and Dick, W. C.: *Mycoplasma pneumoniae* infection and arthritis in man. *Br Med J* 2:14-16, 1977.

Jacobson, L. B., Longstreth, G. F., and Edginston, T. S.: Clinical and immunologic features of transient cold agglutinin hemolytic anemia. *Am J Med* 54:514-521, 1973.

Mufson, M. A., Chang, V., Gill, V., Wood, S. C., Romansky, M. J., and Chanock, R. M.: The role of viruses, mycoplasmas and bacteria in acute pneumonia in civilian adults. *Am J Epidemiol* 86:526-544, 1967.

Murray, H. W., Masur, H., Senterfit, L. B., and Roberts, R. B.: The protean manifestations of *Mycoplasma pneumoniae* infection in adults. *Am J Med* 58:229-262, 1975.

Peterson, O. L., Ham, T. H., and Finland, M.: Cold agglutinins (autohemagglutinins) in primary atypical pneumonias. *Science* 97:167, 1943.

Razin, S.: The mycoplasmas. *Microbiol Rev* 42:414-470, 1978.

Rifkind, D., Chanock, R., Krawetz, H., Johnson, K., and Knight, W.: Ear involvement (myringitis) and primary atypical pneumonia following inoculation of volunteers with Eaton agent. *Am Rev Respir Dis* 85:479-489, 1962.

Sands, M., Satz, J. E., Turner, W. A., and Soloff, L. A.: Pericarditis and perimyocarditis associated with active *Mycoplasma pneumoniae* infection. *Ann Intern Med* 86:544-548, 1977.

Shames, J. M., George, R. B., Holliday, W. B., Rasch, J. R., and Mogabgab, W. J.: Comparison of antibiotics in the treatment of mycoplasmal pneumonia. *Arch Intern Med* 125:680-684, 1970.

Shulman, S. T., Bartlett, J., Clyde, W. A. Jr., and Ayoub, E. M.: The unusual severity of mycoplasmal pneumonia in children with sickle-cell disease. *N Engl J Med* 287:164-167, 1972.

Stanbridge, E. J.: A reevaluation of the role of mycoplasmas in human disease. *Ann Rev Microbiol* 30:169–187, 1976.

Vitullo, B. B., O'Regan, S., deChadarevian, J., and Kaplan, B.: *Mycoplasma pneumoniae* associated with acute glomerulonephritis. *Nephron* 21:284–288, 1978.

81

RICKETTSIA
Larry G. Reimer, M.D.

The rickettsiae are small, obligate, intracellular bacteria transmitted from a specific arthropod host to specific vertebrate hosts including humans. Except for *Coxiella burnetii* which may survive for many years in dust or soil, the rickettsiae must be transmitted directly from arthropod to vertebrate animal and back again, or from arthropod to arthropod to survive. Infection in humans is only incidental to this rickettsial life cycle, except for epidemic typhus, because the major reservoirs for rickettsiae are lower vertebrate species.

Human rickettsial infections may be asymptomatic or life threatening, sporadic or epidemic. Epidemic typhus, scrub typhus, trench fever, and Q fever all have had a major impact on the outcome of past military conflicts. For example, 1 million soldiers were said to have been incapacitated during World War I by trench fever. On the other hand, asymptomatic seroconversion after exposure to rickettsiae is well documented as is isolated, sporadic infection.

Rickettsiae cause specific disease entities such as spotted fever, typhus, scrub typhus, or Q fever, with specific manifestations and epidemiology for each (Table 81.1). In general, however, all rickettsial diseases are characterized by acute onset, headache, high fever with true rigors, myalgias, and arthralgias (Table 81.2).

Since these bacteria require special techniques for laboratory cultivation and present significant risk for laboratory workers, rickettsiae are not routinely cultured from patients clinically. Instead diagnosis depends upon serologic testing in appropriate clinical settings.

Treatment of rickettsial diseases should reflect the overall severity of the diseases produced (Table 81.3). A disease without risk of death like rickettsialpox should not be treated with chloramphenicol which itself may have life-threatening toxicity. The use of vaccines has similar considerations (Table 81.4).

Manifestations of individual rickettsial diseases will follow.

TABLE 81.1   Major Rickettsial Diseases

Disease Group	Rickettsial Species	Arthropod Vector	Vertebrate Host	Geographic Distribution	Unique Features
Spotted Fevers					
Rocky Mountain spotted fever	*R. rickettsii*	Tick	Rodents, dogs	Western Hemisphere	Centripedal rash
Rickettsialpox	*R. akari*	Mites	Mice, rats	U.S., Russia, Africa, Mediterranean	Vesicular rash
Boutonneuse fever	*R. conorii*	Tick	Rodents, dogs	Africa, Asia	Primary lesion
Siberian tick typhus	*R. sibirica*	Tick	Rodents	Russia	Primary lesion
Queensland tick typhus	*R. australis*	Tick	Marsupials	Australia	Primary lesion
Typhus					
Epidemic typhus	*R. prowazekii*	Louse	Man, squirrels	Universal	Epidemic disease, late recurrence, CNS symptoms
Endemic typhus	*R. typhi*	Flea	Rats, mice	Universal	Mild disease
Scrub Typhus	*R. tsutsugamushi*	Trombiculid mites	Rodents	Asia, Western Pacific	Primary lesion, adenopathy
Trench Fever	*Rochalimaea quintana*	Louse	Man	Europe, Russia, Africa, South and Central America	Primary lesion, extracellular growth
Q Fever	*C. burnetii*	Tick (unnecessary)	Sheep, cattle, goats	Universal	Respiratory pathogen, infection from vertebrate carrier

TABLE 81.2   Common Presentations of Rickettsial Diseases

Acute onset	Headache
Fever $\geq$ 102°C	Arthralgias
True rigors	Myalgias
Rash*	Conjunctivitis

*Except Q fever

TABLE 81.3   Treatment of Rickettsial Diseases

Disease	Tetracycline	Chloramphenicol
Rocky Mountain spotted fever	Yes	Yes
Rickettsialpox	Yes	No
Epidemic typhus	Yes	Yes
Endemic typhus	Yes	Yes
Scrub typhus	Yes	Yes
Trench fever	Yes	No
Q fever	Yes	No

Microbiology

In the past, rickettsiae were not thought to be bacteria because they only grew intracellularly, were directly transmitted from one host to another, and were smaller than other bacteria. Neither were they thought to be viruses because they were too large and could be treated with antibiotics. We know now that these microorganisms are true bacteria by their method of reproduction, genetic composition with both RNA and DNA, cell-wall composition, and overall composition of protein, carbohydrates, and lipids.

The family Rickettsiaceae includes three genera that are pathogenic to man (Table 81.1). The organisms are coccoid to bacillary and may occur singly, in pairs of cocci, or in pairs of rods. Rickettsiae have cell walls with gram-negative characteristics, but they are not well visualized by this method. They are visualized much better by using alternative stains such as Machiavello, Gimenez, and Giemsa.

Rocky Mountain Spotted Fever

Rocky Mountain spotted fever (RMSF) is an acute illness of variable severity characterized by high fever, headache, myalgias, and rash. This is the most common rickettsial disease in the United States and has been increasing in occurrence since about 1960. Although the disease was originally described in American

TABLE 81.4   Immunity and Vaccination in Rickettsial Diseases

Disease	Natural Immunity	Vaccine Available	Vaccine Use
Rocky Mountain spotted fever	Incomplete	Yes	Yearly booster, exposed persons
Rickettsialpox	Complete	No	
Epidemic typhus	Incomplete[1]	Yes[2]	Epidemics
Endemic typhus	Complete[3]	Yes[2]	Not recommended
Scrub typhus	Incomplete[4]	No	
Trench fever	Incomplete	No	
Q fever	Complete	Yes	Laboratory workers, animal processors

[1]Protection against reinfection complete, but recrudescent illness in some individuals common

[2]Not manufactured in the United States

[3]Protection against both endemic and epidemic typhus

[4]Protection complete for strain of organism, but second infection with another strain occurs

Indians in western Montana and was initially reported only in the Rocky Mountain region, RMSF is now diagnosed much more frequently in the eastern United States, especially along the Appalachian mountain range.

Rickettsia rickettsii causes the disease which is transmitted to man by several tick species. Dermacentor andersoni, a wood tick in the western United States, and D. variabilis, a dog tick in the eastern United States, are the most common vectors while Amblyomma americanum, D. occidentalis, Haemaphysalis leporispalustris, and A. cajennense also carry the organism. There is some evidence, however, that the rickettsial organisms carried by these other tick species do not infect humans. Rickettsia rickettsii does not harm its tick host and is passed transovarially to the offspring. Humans are infected by transfer of the organism from the tick mouth parts into a bite wound or from tick feces rubbed into the wound. Similar transfer results in infection of multiple other mammalian species which provide a constant reservoir for perpetuating carriage in tick vectors.

Pathogenesis

After entering the body through skin bites, the organism enters the bloodstream and invades the endothelial cells of capillaries and arterioles. The endothelial cells swell and proliferate. Mononuclear and plasma cells invade the surrounding smooth muscle and the adventia creating a vasculitis. The vascular effects occur throughout the body and result in thrombosis, microinfarction, and leakage of plasma into perivascular tissue with resultant edema and intravascular hypovolemia.

In addition to diffuse vasculitis, patients may demonstrate thrombocytopenia and disseminated intravascular coagulation. The mechanism is unknown.

Clinical Manifestations

Patients generally present with the sudden onset of high fever, chills, severe headache, and myalgias, often with anorexia, nausea, abdominal pain, and photophobia, 2-12 days after exposure to ticks. Shorter incubation periods correlate with higher inocula of organisms and more severe disease. The rash, found in over 95% of the patients, usually begins 3-5 days after onset of illness, but it may be seen as early as the first day. This rash begins as a red, blanching, macular eruption on the wrists, ankles, palms, and soles. Over 3-5 days the rash spreads centripedally to involve all skin areas and transforms through maculopapular, petechial, and purpuric stages resembling those seen in meningococcemia. Variation in the rash has been noted, e.g., onset may be delayed for several days, and it may begin on the trunk rather than the extremities, although it eventually tends to become most prominent on the extremities in all patients.

Other manifestations of the disease may include nonpitting edema of the face and lower extremities; neurologic changes including delirium, coma, and grand mal seizures; thrombocytopenia; disseminated intravascular coagulation; pneumonitis with or without radiologic changes; acute renal impairment with multifocal perivascular interstitial nephritis; splenomegaly and hepatomegaly; and when most severe, vascular collapse and death.

Diagnosis

Initial management of patients must rely upon clinical suspicion when patients present with a compatible illness and history of exposure since definitive diagnosis will take many days to weeks. Nonspecific laboratory findings include leukopenia ($2000-4000/mm^3$) during the first week of illness followed by leukocytosis in the second week. Mild anemia, thrombocytopenia, prolonged prothrombin and partial thromboplastin times, mild elevations of liver transaminases and bilirubin levels, and increased creatinine levels may be seen. These usually occur in more severe cases. Diffuse or localized infiltrates may be seen on chest roentgenograph.

The organism is not cultured routinely in clinical settings, and diagnosis is dependent upon serologic methods. The most widely available and easiest test is the Weil-Felix reaction. Human antibodies to various rickettsial organisms are known to agglutinate surface antigens of *Proteus vulgaris* types OX-2, OX-19, and OX-K. Such agglutination may be demonstrated by day 5 of illness and usually by day 12. The Weil-Felix test is positive in other rickettsial illnesses with some selectivity by the *Proteus* OX type (Table 81.5), although cross-reactions are common. The Weil-Felix test is often negative in RMSF, and conversely patients with recent infections with *Proteus vulgaris* or other rickettsiae may have positive titers. Specific serologic testing by complement-fixation (CF) is now preferred. A rise in CF titer is not seen until the second or third week of illness, or later when patients receive early therapy. As with other serologies, a single high titer by Weil-Felix or CF will suggest rickettsial disease, but a fourfold or greater rise in titer from acute to convalescent stages is needed for definitive diagnosis. A promising new technique for early diagnosis by demonstration of immunofluorescent antibody on skin biopsy has been described.

TABLE 81.5   Weil-Felix Reactions in Rickettsial Diseases*

Disease	Proteus OX-2	Proteus OX-19	Proteus OX-K
Rocky Mountain spotted fever	Yes	Yes	No
Rickettsialpox	No	No	No
Epidemic typhus	No	Yes	No
Endemic typhus	No	Yes	No
Scrub typhus	No	No	Yes
Trench fever	No	No	No
Q fever	No	No	No

*Specificity not absolute. Many false-positive and false-negative reactions oc-
cur. Complement-fixation preferred for all diseases

Treatment

Early recognition and institution of specific antimicrobial therapy are important.
Rickettsiae are sensitive to tetracyclines and chloramphenicol. Most patients
should be treated with tetracycline because of its lower toxicity, but chloramphenicol may be used in patients who are profoundly ill, pregnant, under 8 years of
age, or when differentiation from meningococcal disease is not quickly discernible.
In addition to specific antimicrobial therapy, general supportive measures
such as appropriate fluid replacement and general nursing care are important.
Although the major pathologic change is a vasculitis, antiinflammatory agents
including steroids have not been shown to alter the course of illness.

Prognosis

Before the introduction of antibiotics 20-40% of patients with RMSF died. The
mortality now is from 3 to 10% with many deaths occurring in patients who are diagnosed too late. Complications during illness include pneumonia with secondary
bacterial pathogens, acute renal failure, distal gangrene, and internal hemorrhage.
Recovery may be prolonged, lasting several weeks to months. Early therapy does
not always shorten the duration of illness and may result in relapse. Early therapy
also delays antibody response so that serologic testing may not show titer rises
for several weeks.

Immunity and Prevention

Natural infection provides some protection against reinfection, although second
episodes have occurred. A vaccine containing inactivated rickettsiae has been
used but provides only limited protection and is only recommended for people with

recurrent exposure to ticks in high-risk areas. Immunity essentially lasts through one summer season, and patients needing protection must be revaccinated yearly.

Limiting exposure to tick vectors is much more important than vaccination. People should avoid tick-infested areas when possible and check themselves frequently for ticks when in such areas. Ticks require several hours to attach firmly and feed thus removal within 3-4 hr will effectively prevent disease. When ticks are found they should be removed by gentle traction to avoid crushing or leaving mouth parts. Tick repellants may be helpful. Widespread use of insecticides to reduce tick populations has not reduced disease incidence, but application of insecticides to limited, populated areas such as walking paths may help reduce exposure.

Rickettsialpox

Rickettsialpox occurs primarily in crowded urban centers and is caused by *R. akari*. An outbreak in New York City in 1979 suggested that rickettsialpox may be an important unrecognized cause of illness in the United States.

The disease is transmitted to humans by bites from mites which commonly parasitize mice and rats. Humans are incidental hosts in the mice/rat-mite cycle. Most reports of illness have come from large cities in the United States, but the disease has been recognized in Russia and parts of Africa.

Little is known about the disease since pathologic investigation has been limited to examination of skin biopsy material. Epidermal infiltration with mononuclear cells and vacuolization of the basal layer of the dermis are seen. Subdermal capillary changes with endothelial cell proliferation and perivascular inflammatory cells suggest a vasculitis.

Within a few days of exposure a primary papular lesion develops at the site of the bite wound. Over several days the papule progresses to a small vesicle which eventually dries, forming an indurated eschar from 0.5 to 3.0 cm in diameter. Regional adenopathy is usually present. The primary lesion persists for 3-4 weeks and then heals.

Shortly after appearance of the primary lesion, within 9-14 days of exposure, patients present with fever, shaking chills, headache, myalgias, and arthralgias, and often cough, sore throat, and abdominal complaints. One to four days after onset of these systemic symptoms a generalized papular rash develops that vesiculates, then crusts, similar to lesions of chickenpox. The rash may involve mucous membranes, but tends to spare the palms and soles. There may be as few as five or six lesions or as many as 100. Vesiculation does not always occur. Lesions remain hyperpigmented after healing but do not form scars. The total illness lasts 2-3 weeks.

This disease is probably underreported simply because it is not considered. An outbreak of illness similar to chickenpox that includes adults in crowded conditions should suggest this disease.

Routine laboratory tests usually show leukopenia in the first week followed by normal to elevated white blood cell counts later. Other tests are generally unremarkable.

Serologic conversion by CF or indirect fluorescent antibody tests are helpful but cross-react with other rickettsiae of the spotted fever group. In situations where differentiation cannot be made on clinical grounds, other spotted fever group antigens can be absorbed first, followed by indirect immunofluorescence which still should be positive for *R. akari*.

Treatment with tetracycline is effective and can be used to shorten the course of the illness. Given the relatively benign nature of the disease, chloramphenicol should not be employed. Therapy may prolong the time necessary for a specific antibody response to occur.

The disease is mild with no major complications or sequelae. Relapse or recurrent disease has not been reported.

Infection probably results in lifelong immunity to rickettsialpox, but not to other spotted fevers. No vaccine has been developed. Control of rats and mice is most important in disease prevention.

Other Spotted Fevers

Other forms of spotted fever can be differentiated from RMSF primarily by geographic distribution, species of rickettsiae, and species of tick vector. These other spotted fevers differ clinically from RMSF only in that an ulcerated lesion at the site of tick bite is more likely. Rocky Mountain spotted fever and rickettsialpox are the only spotted fever infections known to occur in the United States.

Epidemic Typhus

Similar to RMSF, epidemic or louse borne typhus may be a dramatic illness with significant morbidity and mortality. Personal hygiene has essentially eliminated the risk of epidemic typhus in the United States, but in other parts of the world with close living conditions, infrequent bathing, and infestation with body lice, the disease remains common and occasionally epidemic.

The disease is caused by *R. prowazekii*. Until recently it was believed that humans were the single vertebrate host capable of transmitting the organism from one body louse to another. The intermediate stage is necessary since this organism is not transmitted directly or transovarially between arthropod vectors. *Rickettsia prowazekii* has now been identified in flying squirrels in the eastern United States, and eight patients with serologic evidence of recent infection were reported by the Centers for Disease Control in 1980. How much risk people have of developing louse-borne typhus by exposure to flying squirrels is not clear.

People generally become infected when feces from lice carrying the organism are deposited on abraded skin areas. Airborne transmission has been suggested to occur with shaking of clothes harboring louse feces.

Pathogenesis

The pathology in epidemic typhus is quite similar to that in RMSF. Once inside the skin, the organism invades the bloodstream, causes a widespread vasculitis with thrombosis, hemorrhage, and perivascular fluid leakage, resulting in edema and focal areas of necrosis. Patients may develop interstitial pneumonitis, myocarditis, or panencephalitis. Fluid losses into the extravascular compartment may result in vascular collapse and death.

Clinical Manifestations

The incubation period for epidemic typhus is 5-23 days after which patients suddenly develop high fever, chills, malaise, severe headache, and myalgia. Conjunctivitis, photophobia, and painful eye movements often are present. After 3-9 days a macular rash appears first on the trunk and abdomen, in contrast to the rash of RMSF, and then spreads over the rest of the body usually sparing the face, palms, and soles. The rash changes from macular, to maculopapular, and then to purpural over several days before desquamating during convalescence. Meningoencephalitis often becomes the major manifestation of illness after the first week, with any combination of meningeal signs, psychosis, fluctuating mental status, or cranial nerve deficits. In severe cases with disease progression, patients may develop pneumonitis with diffuse interstitial infiltrates, myocarditis with tachycardia and hypotension, and renal failure. Untreated patients who recover begin to convalesce after the second week of illness, but recovery takes 3-4 weeks.

Diagnosis

In the usual setting in outbreaks of the disease the diagnosis is possible on clinical grounds. More sporadic cases, as might now be seen in this country, require serologic methods because, as with RMSF, cultures of the organism are not recommended. The Weil-Felix test can again be used with *Proteus* OX-19 antigen demonstrable after 7-8 days. However, cross-reactions with other rickettsiae and proteus infections do occur, and only about half the patients with disease develop positive titers. Specific testing of acute and convalescent serum to antigens of *R. prowazekii* is preferred and is most widely done by CF. General laboratory studies are similar to those in RMSF.

Treatment

Tetracycline and chloramphenicol are both effective and should be used with the same considerations as in RMSF. General supportive care is again important.

Prognosis

Without treatment the mortality is about 20%. Early recognition and antibiotic treatment will eliminate deaths. Complications during illness include bacterial pneumonia, otitis, parotitis, and peripheral gangrene. Despite extensive involvement of major organ systems during the acute illness, survivors usually recover completely. Possible chronic deficits in mental function, seizures, cranial nerve palsies, or personality changes do occur.

Late recurrence of the disease, up to 50 years after the original illness, is possible from surviving reservoirs of the organism in lymphoid tissue. This late recrudescence is known as Brill-Zinsser disease. Except for a milder illness of shorter duration, the clinical picture is identical to original attacks of epidemic typhus. All recent cases of apparent typhus in the United States, except those related to flying squirrels, have been Brill-Zinsser disease. The diagnosis is based on a rise in CF titer. The Weil-Felix reaction is generally not positive in recurrent disease.

Immunity and Prevention

Both killed and attenuated, live vaccines have been used to interrupt transmission of the disease in epidemic situations with some success, but the duration and completeness of protection from individual vaccines are unclear. Vaccine is not available in the United States.

The best approach to disease prevention is to destroy lice with insecticides. This can be done on a small or large scale depending upon the population at risk. In this country limitation of exposure to flying squirrels in rural areas may help prevent disease.

Endemic Typhus

Endemic or murine typhus is a mild disease occasionally affecting man after contact with rat fleas carrying the causative organism, R. typhi (mooseri).

Endemic typhus occurs throughout the world including occasional cases in the southern United States. Humans are infected incidentally when a rat flea deposits feces containing R. typhi on broken skin, by inhalation, or by invasion through the conjunctiva. Rickettsia typhi has been found in human fleas, human lice, ticks, and mites in some parts of the world. The role these other arthropods and their usual vertebrate hosts play in human infection is unknown.

The pathogenesis of endemic typhus is identical to that for epidemic typhus except that the disease is much milder. The explanation for the benign nature of this disease is unclear since R. typhi is very close antigenically to R. prowazekii.

Again, symptoms generally are acute onset of fever, chills, headache, myalgias, and arthralgias. Rash occurs after several days of illness in about 50% of the patients generally beginning on the trunk and later spreading to the extremities. The rash is variable in occurrence and distribution, and does not progress to petechial or purpuric lesions. Involvement of kidneys, liver, heart, and brain is absent or mild. Illness generally lasts 2 weeks or less with few complications.

The disease should be considered in patients with compatible illness and exposure to rats. Since the disease is mild it will often be confused with a nonspecific viral illness until the rash appears. Routine laboratory tests are generally normal. Definite diagnosis can be suggested by a positive Weil-Felix reaction to Proteus OX-19, but, again, this test may be negative. Specific serology to R. typhi by CF is available. Cross-reactions with R. prowazekii occur, but differentiation between these two illnesses can usually be made on clinical grounds.

Treatment should be limited to tetracycline since the disease is mild. Chloramphenicol is effective and could be used in unusually severe infections. Mortality and morbidity in untreated patients are unusual, and long-term sequelae are rare. Recrudescent disease, as occurs in epidemic typhus, has not been seen.

A single episode of illness provides lasting immunity not only to endemic typhus, but to epidemic typhus as well. Given the mild nature of the disease, vaccine development would not seem to be necessary. Reduction in populations of rats and their fleas is a helpful method of disease prevention.

Scrub Typhus

Scrub typhus or tsutsugamushi disease is a disease of variable severity limited to Asia and the western Pacific countries. The disease, caused by R. tsutsugamushi, is similar to other typhus-like illnesses but can be distinguished to some extent by a prominent lesion at the site of entry and by regional adenopathy. Rickettsia tsutsugamushi has more antigenic variability than other rickettsial species making the disease variable, serologic diagnosis more difficult, and immunity incomplete following infection. The disease is transmitted to man from bites of trombiculid mites or chiggers. Mite vectors can incidentally transmit the disease to other vertebrates in addition to man.

Pathologic lesions in scrub typhus have not been studied to the same extent as in RMSF or epidemic typhus. However, the lesions seen are predominantly vasculitic. Interstitial pneumonitis, meningitis, myocarditis, and nephritis may occur.

Presenting symptoms are as described previously for other typhus-like diseases with the addition of an easily recognized lesion at the site of entry. This lesion begins as a small papule that enlarges, ulcerates, and later forms an eschar. A rash similar to that seen in endemic typhus is usually present. Regional and

generalized adenopathy may be seen. Patients commonly have bronchitis or interstitial pneumonitis. Less common are myocarditis, nephritis, and meningitis.
Mild cases are a common cause of fever of unknown origin in endemic areas.

The diagnosis depends mainly on consideration of the disease, as with other
rickettsiae. Routine laboratory tests generally show a leukopenia during the first
week followed by leukocytosis in the second to third week. Anemia is uncommon,
but thrombocytopenia and clotting abnormalities consistent with disseminated intravascular coagulation may be seen. Elevated liver function tests and azotemia
occur occasionally. The Weil-Felix test to *Proteus* OX-K has been considered
helpful but is positive in as few as 25% of patients and may be positive in patients
with past illness. Specific CF and indirect immunofluorescent methods provide
more reliable results, but vary depending upon geographic location.

Rickettsia tsutsugamushi infection also should be treated with tetracycline or
chloramphenicol plus general supportive measures as needed. Recurrent disease
is common in those patients treated early and a second single dose of chloramphenicol 1 week after completing initial therapy is often employed. Reported
mortality from this disease has varied widely from < 1% to as high as 60% perhaps reflecting differences in particular strains of the organism. Complications
may occur as in epidemic typhus or RMSF.

Direct control of mites with insecticides, and insect repellants applied to the
skin in endemic areas help prevent the disease.

Trench Fever

Trench fever was first recognized during World War I when an estimated 1 million
soldiers in Europe were stricken. The disease was not observed again until recognized as a major cause of illness in soldiers on the Russian front during World
War II.

As with epidemic typhus, trench fever is prevalent only under crowded, unsanitary conditions since infection is transmitted to humans by body lice. The organism gains entry through broken skin or the conjunctiva. Trench fever is caused
by *Rochalimaea quintana,* formerly *Rickettsia quintana*. The bacterium is unique
among the rickettsiae in that it can grow extracellularly, and multiplies freely
within the louse gut. Humans are the only known vertebrate reservoir for infection. *Rochalimaea quintana* is now thought to exist in central and eastern Europe,
Russia, and in limited areas of Central America, South America, and Africa.

The disease has rarely resulted in death and pathologic material has not been
well studied. Biopsy specimens suggest that trench fever is also primarily a vasculitis of small vessels.

The disease has variable characteristics, from asymptomatic seroconversion
to a chronic, relapsing illness. The illness begins in most patients with an influenza-like illness with acute onset of fever, chills, headache, severe myalgias, conjunctivitis, and retro-orbital pain. Then about an equal number of patients have
either a single illness lasting 1-2 weeks or multiple relapsing illnesses spanning
weeks to as long as 10 years. During World War II soldiers were frequently unable
to perform for a period of 9-10 weeks. Most patients develop a rash consistent
with typhus, although its onset may occur any time during the course of the disease. Splenomegaly is often present, but major organ involvement is not found
either by symptoms or laboratory tests. Even though the disease is mild, a dramatic component of trench fever is the continuous bacteremia throughout periods
of relapse and remission. This latent bacteremia serves as a mechanism for long-
term continuation of endemicity in areas infested with lice.

Routine laboratory testing is generally normal. The Weil-Felix reactions are all negative in trench fever. Specific serologic conversion by CF, hemagglutination, or enzymatic immunoassay is necessary to confirm the diagnosis. The disease must be considered in places where a combination of lice infestation and crowding exists.

Rochalimaea quintana is susceptible in vitro to multiple antibiotics including tetracycline. There is little clinical experience with antimicrobial therapy, and although treatment with tetracycline appears effective its effect on the relapse rate and chronic carriage is unclear. Except for multiple recurrences trench fever is a benign illness. Chronic sequelae and directly related mortality are rare.

It is doubtful that patients become immune given the long duration of illness and persistent bacteremia. No vaccine is available. Control of louse vectors is essential for limiting disease. Human-to-human transmission is possible via blood transfusion from bacteremic donors. An appropriate epidemiologic history in blood donors from endemic areas is important.

Q Fever

Q fever is unique among the rickettsial diseases in that transmission to humans is generally by inhalation of dust contaminated with the causal agent, *Coxiella burnetii*. Humans may also be infected by ingesting contaminated milk or meat. While *C. burnetii* parasitizes certain species of ticks, humans are infected directly from vertebrate hosts, predominantly sheep, cattle, and goats. The organism requires an intracellular environment for growth, but can survive in a dormant state for years in contaminated soil. Recent work suggests that the long term stability of the organism is possible because of a sporogenic phase in *C. burnetii*'s life cycle. Infection may occur miles downwind from areas where contaminated material initially enters the environment.

The organism is particularly hazardous for laboratory workers. Most of the cases in the United States in recent years, including some large epidemics, have been related to laboratory work either directly with the organism or with research animals, especially pregnant ewes, harboring the organism. Exposure, limited to walking once past a room housing infected sheep, has resulted in infection. Laboratory outbreaks have actually been most hazardous to uninvolved employees exposed to contaminated air rather than to involved investigators who are usually already immune.

Coxiella burnetii is worldwide in distribution. The greatest concentration of organisms is in the placenta, and most infections occur in the spring during birthing season. Despite the extreme contagiousness of *C. burnetii* from soil and animals, human-to-human transmission rarely occurs.

Pathogenesis

Pathologic lesions are usually limited to the lungs where interstitial pneumonitis with a peribronchiolar and perivascular inflammatory reaction is seen. In patients with elevated liver function tests, liver biopsies have shown granulomatous hepatitis. In chronic infection endocarditis with typical valvular lesions is described.

Diagnosis

The disease is variable, extending from inapparent infection to a chronic disease ending in fatal endocarditis. The usual patient presents 10-20 days after exposure with acute onset of high fever, shaking chills, severe headache, and myalgias.

After 4-5 days the patients develop dry cough and pleuritic chest pain with interstitial infiltrates on a chest radiograph. For inapparent reasons infection in laboratory workers seldom includes respiratory symptoms or radiologic changes. Unlike other rickettsial diseases, rash has not been described for Q fever. In uncomplicated illness symptoms last from 4-5 days to as long as 3-4 weeks. Relapses over a period of several months may occur.

Acute illness may be accompanied by hepatosplenomegaly, abdominal pain, and elevated liver function tests, with granulomatous hepatitis. Abdominal complaints in association with unexplained fever have led to unnecessary laparotomies in a few patients. The hepatitis is self-limited without resulting in chronic liver disease.

There are rare patients who do not clear the infection who may develop clinical endocarditis 6 months to 20 years after the initial infection. The aortic valve is involved 80% of the time. Most infections involve valves with prior damage, and Q fever endocarditis has been reported on prosthetic valves. Diagnosis is difficult since routine blood cultures will be negative, and disease develops so long after the initial exposure that an epidemiologic history may not be helpful. Until recently all cases of Q fever endocarditis resulted in death.

Q fever must be considered in patients with typical acute illnesses who are exposed to livestock. Illness is similar to acute viral syndromes but should be suggested by higher fever, true rigors, and debilitating headache. The diagnosis should be considered also in patients with undiagnosed interstitial pneumonitis, hepatitis, or culture-negative endocarditis. Routine laboratory tests are similar to those in other rickettsial diseases. Most patients have mildly elevated liver transaminases whether or not they have documented granulomatous hepatitis.

Specific diagnosis is made by CF. Surface antigens of *C. burnetii* change depending upon whether the organism is outside an animal host (phase II) or active within a host (phase I). Initial infection in humans is usually with phase II forms which may convert to phase I in ongoing chronic infection. Serologic response can be specifically measured for either of these two phases. The acute form, or phase II antibody, is present within 12-15 days of infection, rises to a peak within 2-3 weeks, and then slowly declines over months to years. In mild illness phase I antibody rises only minimally or not at all, but in patients with chronic disease or endocarditis, phase I antibody rises after the first month and remains at high levels. Persistent phase I antibody levels greater than 1:256 by CF are diagnostic of chronic Q fever disease and highly suggestive of endocarditis. A good response to therapy in such cases is best demonstrated by a falling phase I antibody level.

Treatment

The disease is generally self-limited, but the duration of constitutional symptoms may be shortened with tetracycline therapy. Early treatment delays the onset of measurable serum antibodies, but probably does not cause relapse.

Patients with pneumonitis or hepatitis should be treated for several days beyond the duration of clinical illness.

Treatment of endocarditis has been difficult because effective antimicrobial drugs are not bactericidal to the organism. Recent reports suggest long-term therapy with oral tetracycline for up to 40 months or until phase I antibody is below 1:200. Indications for valve replacement are the same as with other forms of endocarditis but include failure to respond serologically.

Prognosis

The disease is generally benign with only rare complications. Chronic recurrent disease occurs in 1-5% of patients as does endocarditis which now has about a 25% mortality risk.

Immunity and Prevention

A single episode of illness provides lasting immunity to Q fever but not to other rickettsial diseases. Multiple vaccines with either phase I or phase II antigen, alive or killed, have been tested, but none is entirely satisfactory. All are immunogenic but also produce significant local or systemic ill effects in 25-50% of vaccinees. Such reactions are related to preexisting immunity which may be demonstrated by skin test response. Vaccination is safe and should only be necessary in those with no skin test reaction. Vaccination is now recommended for nonimmune laboratory workers handling *C. burnetii* and possibly new employees in animal-processing facilities.

Prevention of natural disease is difficult because carriage is common in domestic animals. Rigid control of research facilities where the organism or pregnant domestic animals are used is mandatory to prevent laboratory outbreaks.

Selected Bibliography

Brettman, L. R., Lewin, S., Holzman, R. S., Goldman, W. D., Marr, J. S., Kechijian, P., and Schinella, R.: Rickettsialpox: Report of an outbreak and a contemporary review. *Medicine* 60:363-372, 1981.

Burgdorfer, W.: A review of Rocky Mountain spotted fever (tick-borne typhus), its agent, and its tick vectors in the United States. *J Med Entomol* 12:269-278, 1975.

Donohue, J. F.: Lower respiratory tract involvement in Rocky Mountain spotted fever. *Arch Intern Med* 140:223-227, 1980.

Dupont, H. L., Hornick, R. B., Levin, H. S., Rapoport, M. I., and Woodward, T. E.: Q fever hepatitis. *Ann Intern Med* 74:198-206, 1971.

Hattwick, M. A. W., O'Brien, R. J., and Hanson, B. F.: Rocky Mountain spotted fever: Epidemiology of an increasing problem. *Ann Intern Med* 84:732-739, 1976.

Kimbrough, R. C., III, Ormsbee, R. A., Peacock, M., Rogers, W. R., Bennetts, R. W., Raaf, J., Krause, A., and Gardner, C.: Q fever endocarditis in the United States. *Ann Intern Med* 91:400-402, 1979.

Kishimoto, R. A., Stockman, R. W., and Redmond, C. L.: Q fever: Diagnosis, therapy, and immunoprophylaxis. *Mil Med* 144:183-187, 1979.

McCaul, T. F. and Williams, J. C.: Developmental cycle of *Coxiella burnetii*: Structure and morphogenesis of vegetative and sporogenic differentiations. *J Bacteriol* 147:1063-1076, 1981.

McDade, J. E., Shepard, C. C., Redus, M. A., Newhouse, V. F., and Smith, J. D.: Evidence of *Rickettsia prowazekii* infections in the United States. *Am J Trop Med Hyg* 29:277-284, 1980.

Meiklejohn, G., Reimer, L. G., Graves, P. S., and Helmick, C.: Cryptic epidemic of Q fever in a medical school. *J Infect Dis* 144:107-113, 1981.

Moe, J. B. and Pederson, C. E.: The impact of rickettsial diseases on military operations. *Mil Med* 145:780-785, 1980.

Riley, H. D., Jr.: Rickettsial diseases and Rocky Mountain spotted fever - Part I. *Curr Prob Pediatr* 11(5):1-46, 1981.

Riley, H. D., Jr.: Rickettsial diseases and Rocky Mountain spotted fever - Part II. *Curr Prob Pediatr* 11(6):1-38, 1981.

Varma, M. P. S., Adgey, A. A. J., and Connolly, J. H.: Chronic Q fever endocarditis. *Br Heart J* 43:695-699, 1980.

Walker, D. H. and Mattern, W. D.: Rickettsial vasculitis. *Am Heart J* 100:896-906, 1980.

Walker, D. H. and Mattern, W. D.: Acute renal failure in Rocky Mountain spotted fever. *Arch Intern Med* 139:443-448, 1979.

Wilson, H. G., Neilson, G. H., Galea, E. G., Stafford, G., and O'Brien, M.F.: Q fever endocarditis in Queensland. *Circulation* 53:680-684, 1976.

Woodward, T. E., Pedersen, C. E., Jr., Oster, C. N., Bagley, L. R., Romberger, J., and Snyder, M. J.: Prompt confirmation of Rocky Mountain spotted fever: Identification of rickettsiae in skin tissues. *J Infect Dis* 134:297-301, 1976.

82

STAPHYLOCOCCUS
Roger G. Finch, M.B.

Definition

The staphylococcus was first recognized in pus by Koch, cultured in liquid medium by Pasteur and shown to consist of two species, S. aureus and S. epidermidis, by Rosenbach. The name was coined by Ogston from the Greek word staphyle meaning " a cluster of grapes." It belongs to the family Micrococcaceae which includes one other genus, Micrococcus.

The two species of staphylococci are widely distributed in the normal flora of the skin and to a lesser extent on mucous membranes. Staphylococcus epidermidis is almost universally present on the skin, whereas colonization with S. aureus is found in 20-60% of persons. The anterior nares and perineum are the most heavily colonized areas. Among hospital employees colonization rates are frequently higher than in the general population. Colonization tends to fluctuate from time to time as does the particular colonizing strain.

Staphylococcal infections range from the trivial to the life threatening. Minor skin sepsis in the form of pustules is an almost universal experience. However, impaired host defenses, particularly a loss of the normal integrity of the skin and mucous membranes, permit more deep-seated infection. This may disseminate via the blood and lymphatics and establish metastatic foci of infection or may produce a fulminating septicemic state.

The opportunistic character of S. aureus is frequently seen in hospitals where it remains one of the leading causes of nosocomial infection. Infection may be sporadic in these institutions, and reflects the many opportunities for person-to-person transmission. Newborn nurseries and intensive care units are particularly vulnerable to epidemics of S. aureus infection.

Microbiology

The staphylococcus is a nonmotile, non-spore-forming, and rarely encapsulated organism ranging from 0.7 to 12 μm in diameter. In stained smears of pus it appears as grape-like clusters of gram-positive cocci, although some pairs and single organisms also can be seen.

The staphylococci are able to grow on a wide variety of unenriched laboratory media and are not difficult to isolate. They will grow in both aerobic and anaerobic conditions, since they are facultative organisms, but occasional strains require carbon dioxide for growth. They will grow at temperatures ranging from 10 to 45°C, and can survive at 60°C for 30 min and for several months at 4°C.

The colonies on nutrient agar or sheep blood agar are domed, circular, and 1-3 mm in diameter. On sheep blood agar S. aureus frequently produces a small zone of clear hemolysis whereas S. epidermidis rarely does so. In addition, the color of the colonies ranges from white, cream, orange, to yellow. Although S. epidermidis tends to form white colonies, and hence its former name S. albus, color is not a reliable method for differentiating between the two species.

Both species can survive in a 10% salt medium. Staphylococcus aureus usually ferments mannitol whereas S. epidermidis does not. These two features are utilized by incorporating salt and mannitol into agar and using it as a selective medium.

Several enzymes are produced by both species of Staphylococcus (Table 82.1). Catalase acts on hydrogen peroxide to release oxygen, and its presence is used to differentiate staphylococci from streptococci. Coagulase has a thrombokinase-like action and coagulates human plasma. It exists in two antigenically distinct forms, bound and free. The bound form is readily demonstrable on a glass microscope slide by emulsifying a colony of S. aureus with a drop of plasma, producing immediate clumping of bacteria within a fibrin web as a result of the conversion of fibrinogen to fibrin. The free coagulase, which is present extracellularly, is demonstrated by the incubation of S. aureus in human plasma. A coagulum will form in 1-4 hr. The presence of coagulase differentiates S. aureus from S. epidermidis. There is little evidence to suggest that it acts as a virulence factor, but it is simply a marker which helps differentiate the more virulent S. aureus from the less virulent S. epidermidis.

Staphylococcus aureus elaborates several other enzymes, including lipase, lysozyme, lactic acid dehydrogenase, protease, hyaluronidase, fibrinolysin, acid phosphatase, desoxyribonuclease, and penicillinase (β-lactamase). With the exception of penicillinase, the importance of the other enzymes in the pathogenesis of staphylococcal disease is unclear. However, lipase-positive strains have the ability to form boils, whereas lipase-negative strains appear to produce increased quantities of hyaluronidase and are associated with a greater tendency to disseminate locally and produce bacteremia.

Several toxins are produced by S. aureus (see Table 82.1) with varying properties. There are four hemolysins, α, β, γ, and ∂ which have several properties in addition to their in vitro ability to hemolyze erythrocytes. α-Toxin has cytotoxic leukocidal, and dermonecrotic properties, and it is antigenic. It also produces platelet aggregation and spasm of smooth muscle. ∂-Toxin has similar properties but is nonantigenic. Both α- and ∂-toxins act nonenzymatically on cell membranes to increase cell permeability. β-Toxin is a sphingomyelinase and is responsible for the hemolysis of erythrocytes at 37°C following overnight refrigeration.

Leukocidin consists of two antigenic proteins, S and F, which act synergistically on polymorphonuclear leukocyte cell membrane phospholipid and result in cell permeability without lysis but with eventual death of the cell.

TABLE 82.1   Enzymatic, Toxigenic, and Antigenic Characteristics of
               S. aureus

Enzymes

Coagulase	Protease
Catalase	Hyaluronidase
Lipase	Fibrinolysin
Lysozyme	Deoxyribonuclease
Lactic acid dehydrogenase	Penicillinase
Acid phosphatase	

Toxins

Hemolysins	Enterotoxins
Leukocidin	Exfoliatin

Antigens

Teichoic acid	Protein A

Another clinically important group of toxins are the enterotoxins produced by approximately 50% of strains of *S. aureus*. There are five antigenically distinct enterotoxins, A–E, detectable by gel-diffusion precipitin formation. These enterotoxins are important causes of staphylococcal food poisoning. *Staphylococcus aureus* multiplies in the contaminated foods, usually cooked meats, cream-filled pastries, custards, and milk products, as a consequence of inadequate refrigeration. The toxin is therefore present at the time of ingestion, is rapidly absorbed from the gut mucosa, and acts on the central nervous system to produce vomiting. It is in fact a neurotoxin. Another toxin thought to be important in staphylococcal food poisoning is the ∂-toxin described previously. This inhibits water reabsorption and hence is responsible for the diarrhea. Because the toxins are preformed, symptoms develop quickly, i.e., within 6 hr. The toxins can withstand heat at 100°C for several minutes. This temperature will kill the staphylococci but the toxins remain active and can be demonstrated in affected foods.

Another agent, exfoliatin, can produce severe cutaneous exfoliation, particularly in infancy where the condition is known as Ritter's disease. In older children and adults the same condition is called toxic epidermal necrolysis or more descriptively, the staphylococcal scalded skin syndrome. The toxin has a molecular weight (MW) of about 20,000, has an affinity for the stratum granulosum of the epidermis, and produces splitting of the desmosomal bridges. Most strains producing the disease belong to phage group II of which phage 71 is the most frequently isolated.

Teichoic acid is found in the cell wall of both *S. aureus* and *S. epidermidis*. In the former it is linked to ribitol to form ribitolteichoic acid, of which there are two antigenically distinct forms, α and β. In *S. epidermidis* it is linked to glycerol. Teichoic acid antibodies have been found in high titer in patients with endovascular staphylococcal infection, such as endocarditis, and in patients with deep-seated staphylococcal infection such as osteomyelitis and empyema. This is in contrast to patients with uncomplicated staphylococcal infections. The detection of these antibodies may prove useful in indicating the type and severity of infection and/or the response to antimicrobial therapy. However, infections caused by *S. epidermidis* and occasional streptococcal infections have also induced a high titer of teichoic acid antibodies.

Protein A is a cell-wall antigen found in most *S. aureus* in varying concentrations. It has a MW of 13,000 and has the unique property of binding specifically to the Fc fragment of the immunoglobulin molecules IgG_1, IgG_2, and IgG_4 from several animal species, including man.

This interaction of protein A with IgG can fix complement and also produce a hypersensitivity reaction when injected into guinea pigs and rabbits. The interaction has also proved useful for detecting microbial antigens by the attachment of the homologous antibody to protein-A-rich *S. aureus*. Interaction of the microbial antigen with the Fab fraction of the IgG produces visible agglutination of the tagged staphylococci.

A few strains of *S. aureus* produce capsules. The colonial appearance on enriched medium is mucoid, and a capsule swelling, or quellung reaction, can be demonstrated with appropriate antisera. The capsule has a similar function to that of the pneumococcus, i.e., it is antiphagocytic.

Epidemiology

Most persons have experienced a staphylococcal infection at some time or other. Staphylococcal infections may be endogenous or exogenous depending upon whether the source of the organism is from the host's normal flora or is acquired from other persons or the environment. Endogenous infections usually account for the sporadic wound infections seen in hospitals. However, staphylococcal infections also can be epidemic and endemic within the hospital environment and this reflects the ubiquitous presence of this organism. Epidemics of *S. aureus* were fairly common events in newborn nurseries in the late 1950s and 1960s, and these organisms were the cause of serious neonatal skin sepsis as well as maternal infection. The recognition that the majority of hospital personnel are asymptomatic carriers of *S. aureus* has led to an understanding of the transmission and spread of *S. aureus* and to methods aimed at its control.

The nose and perineum are the main sites of carriage. Nasal carriers shed few organisms during normal breathing and speech. However, the skin of these persons is usually colonized, and when squames are shed they act as a vehicle for airborne contamination of the environment. The degree of desquamation varies. Approximately 10% of healthy young men and only 1% of young women are profuse "dispersers" of *S. aureus*. The risks are considerably increased should the individual be suffering from a desquamative dermatosis. On the other hand, direct contact is quantitatively more important in the transmission of *S. aureus*. Sweat droplets contain many thousands of bacteria and a punctured surgical glove is more hazardous than airborne transmission. Smaller numbers of organisms may be transmitted from contact with objects such as towels, bedding, and basins which have been contaminated by an infected patient or an asymptomatic carrier. The risks are magnified in the presence of frank suppurative states, such as the presence of a boil or paronychia, where environmental contamination is great despite the wearing of an occlusive dressing. Health care personnel with such infected lesions should not have patient contact until the lesions have healed.

The high prevalence of staphylococcal carriage within the hospital makes it difficult to know the source of an infective strain, particularly since most strains will be penicillin-resistant and indistinguishable from nonvirulent strains on the basis of antimicrobial sensitivities. The susceptibility of *S. aureus* to a wide range of bacteriophages has proved useful in epidemiologic studies. The test strain is inoculated onto nutrient agar and then a set of phages is dropped onto the plate. The pattern of lysis is recorded and represents the phage type of that particular strain of *S. aureus*. The phage patterns can then be compared and may indicate the source of a pathogenic strain. There are three main phage groups. Group I contains many of the hospital epidemic strains such as type 52A/79. Group II encompasses many of the strains producing skin sepsis in infancy, while group III includes many of the antibiotic-resistant and enterotoxin-producing strains.

Diagnostic Features

Clinical

Staphylococcal skin infection is extremely common and usually of minor importance. The varieties of infection range from folliculitis, furunculosis, and carbuncle formation, which are localized necrotizing lesions that heal with scar formation, to impetigo, cellulitis, and toxic epidermal necrolysis, which have the ability to spread locally. It is often clinically difficult to differentiate staphylococcal cellulitis and impetigo from disease caused by *Streptococcus pyogenes*.

Staphylococcal infections of the skin frequently localize by virtue of the intense inflammatory response which proves an effective barrier against spread. However, hematogenous and lymphatic spread can occur and result in metastatic infection in one or multiple sites. Osteomyelitis, arthritis, perinephric abscess, endocarditis, and central nervous system infections are the result of hematogenous seeding. In hospitals, intravenous infusion devices are an important source of staphylococcal bacteremia and septic thrombophlebitis.

Staphylococcal pneumonia is fortunately uncommon but can follow viral infections of the upper respiratory tract, most notably influenza A and measles. Consolidation, abscess formation, pneumatoceles, and a high mortality characterize this virulent form of pneumonia. In addition, *S. aureus* is frequently present in the sputum of patients suffering from cystic fibrosis and is thought to be related to the higher salt concentration of mucosal secretions in these patients.

Wounds, either accidentally or surgically induced, are frequently contaminated with *S. aureus,* which usually originate from the patients' own normal flora, but on occasion, it may be acquired from the environment or hands of attendants. The risks of infection are increased considerably if a foreign body is present in the wound. Suture material can act in a similar fashion, and experimentally as few as 100 organisms have established a skin abscess.

Urinary tract infections are rarely caused by *S. aureus* although *S. epidermidis* is responsible for a few infections, especially in sexually active women.

Staphylococcal infections of the gastrointestinal tract include staphylococcal food poisoning, previously described, and enterocolitis, in which there is invasion of the mucosa with systemic as well as local features and a significant mortality. It usually occurs in debilitated hospitalized patients, most commonly following major surgery for which broad-spectrum antibiotics such as tetracycline or chloramphenicol have been prescribed. The effect of the antibiotic is to suppress the normal bowel flora with overgrowth of drug-resistant *S. aureus.* It was also well described before the use of antibiotics indicating that they are not absolutely essential for its development.

Toxic shock syndrome is an acute febrile illness with multisystem involvement. The syndrome typically begins with fever, vomiting and profuse, watery diarrhea, sometimes accompanied by sore throat, headache, and myalgias, and usually progressing to hypotension and shock within 48 hr. The disease occurs primarily in young women, usually during or immediately following the menstrual period.

Treatment

The tendency for S. aureus to form abscesses reinforces the need for judicious surgical drainage of such material. For the management of systemic staphylococcal infections there are many classes of antibiotics from which to choose and these are summarized in Chapter 6. However, the safest and most effective agent is still penicillin. Unfortunately, more than half the isolates from community-acquired staphylococcal infections, and approximately 90% of hospital-acquired infections elaborate the enzyme penicillinase, which hydrolyzes the β-lactam ring of penicillin and renders the organism insusceptible. Penicillinase is plasmid coded and transmitted by transduction from one S. aureus to another. It was present in nature at a low frequency before the introduction and widespread use of penicillin, and it has been suggested that naturally occurring penicillin molds are responsible for its presence.

Penicillin should be used to treat S. aureus infection only if susceptibility can be shown by laboratory testing. Penicillinase-producing strains will also be resistant to ampicillin, amoxicillin, carbenicillin, and ticarcillin. The penicillinase-resistant penicillins are recommended for the treatment of S. aureus infections. These include oxacillin, dicloxacillin, nafcillin, and methicillin. The latter drug is the prototype agent and can only be given by the parenteral route. There is little difference in efficacy between the agents although factors such as protein-binding, peak serum levels, gastrointestinal absorption, and toxicity vary (see Chapter 6 for a more detailed assessment).

Occasional strains of S. aureus are resistant to methicillin and therefore to this class of penicillins. Methicillin resistance may be most sensitively detected in the laboratory at temperatures of 30-35°C. These strains appear to be less virulent, but in the hospital environment where host resistance may be low and antibiotic use is high, serious disease can result.

Another problem associated with this class of penicillins is the phenomenon of tolerance. A few pathogenic strains have been shown to be inhibited by methicillin at the usual concentrations, but instead of being killed by similar concentrations, these strains are able to tolerate four- to sixteenfold higher concentration of drug before they are killed. This phenomenon may prove clinically important where host defenses are inadequate to kill inhibited pathogens, such as with staphylococcal endocarditis.

The cephalosporins also have excellent antistaphylococcal activity and are widely used for treatment of staphylococcal infections. It should be noted that methicillin-resistant strains are usually resistant to the cephalosporins as well.

Other antistaphylococcal agents include clindamycin, erythromycin, and vancomycin. However, clindamycin is less widely used for the treatment of staphylococcal disease because of the associated complication of pseudomembranous colitis. Staphylococcus aureus may become resistant to erythromycin during therapy and may also show cross-resistance to clindamycin. The aminoglycosides are not primarily antistaphylococcal agents, although serum levels may be adequate for treatment of uncomplicated infections. Furthermore, plasmid-coded resistance for the aminoglycosides by the enzyme acetyltransferase has been recognized recently among selected strains of S. aureus and may reflect the widespread use of these agents.

Vancomycin is a potent antistaphylococcal antibiotic which has proved valuable for the management of serious staphylococcal infections, most notably endocarditis and enterocolitis in penicillin hypersensitive patients and in the treatment of infections caused by methicillin-resistant staphylococci. Thrombophlebitis and ototoxicity are the main toxic effects. The latter occurs more frequently in patients with renal insufficiency, so careful dosage adjustment is essential in such patients.

Staphylococcus epidermidis is less predictable in its susceptibility to antibiotics. It is frequently resistant to penicillin and also commonly resistant to the penicillinase-resistant group of drugs. Most strains are susceptible to the cephalosporins. In the rare situations where *S. epidermidis* is truly pathogenic there is a strong need for guidance from the bacteriology laboratory in the choice of antibiotic.

Selected Bibliography

Fekety, F. R.: The epidemiology and prevention of staphylococcal infection. *Medicine* 43:593-613, 1964.

Forsgren, A.: Immunological aspects of Protein A. In: *Microbiology 1977.* American Society for Microbiology, Washington, DC, 1977, pp. 353-355.

Iannini, P. B. and Crossby, K.: Therapy of *Staphylococcus aureus* bacteremia associated with a removable focus of infection. *Ann Intern Med* 84:558-560, 1976.

Lacey, R. W.: Antibiotic resistance plasmids of *Staphylococcus aureus* and their clinical importance. *Bacteriol Rev* 39:1-32, 1975.

Rasmussen, J. E.: Toxic epidermal necrolysis: A review of 75 cases in children. *Arch Dermatol* 111:1135-1139, 1975.

Tuazon, C. U., Sheagren, J. N., Choa, M. S., Marcus, D., and Curtin, J. A.: *Staphylococcus aureus* bacteremia: Relationship between formation of antibodies to teichoic acid and development of metastatic abscesses. *J Infect Dis* 137: 57-62, 1978.

83

STREPTOCOCCUS
Roger G. Finch, M.B.

Definition

Streptococci are widely distributed throughout the animal kingdom. In man they form part of the normal flora of the mouth, skin, upper respiratory, gastrointestinal, and female genital tracts. It is therefore not surprising that streptococcal infections occur in several of these sites. Historically, most emphasis has been placed on the group A streptococcus (*S. pyogenes*) because of its ready identification in association with suppurative infections of the pharynx, skin, and female genital tract and the important nonsuppurative complications of acute glomerulonephritis, rheumatic fever and erythema nodosum. However, other streptococci have assumed increasing importance in infections of man. Of these, group B streptococci, enterococci, and anaerobic streptococci have attracted most attention. *Streptococcus pneumoniae* remains an important pathogen and is described in Chapter 84.

Microbiology

The streptococci belong to the family Lactobacillaceae. They are gram-positive cocci which appear spherical but can occasionally be ovoid or elongated. They occur in chains which vary in length according to factors such as temperature, culture medium, and previous exposure to antibiotics. In general, longer chains are formed in liquid cultures. In pus, pairs and single organisms may also be present. Streptococci grow well at 35-37°C on media such as brain heart infusion or trypticase soy, particularly if it is enriched with blood or serum. Streptococci vary from being facultative anaerobes, to strict anaerobes, or microaerophilic in their requirements. Their energy is acquired primarily from the fermentation of

718

sugars. All streptococci, with the exception of anaerobic ones, produce lactic acid from glucose. This accumulates in the medium and finally inhibits growth. They do not produce catalase, which differentiates them from staphylococci. The further identification of streptococci is based on a number of characteristics:

Hemolysis

Many streptococci produce hemolysins which vary in concentration and ability to lyse erythrocytes from a wide variety of animal sources, such as sheep, rabbit, horse, and human (Table 83.1). When incubated under anaerobic conditions on 5% blood agar three main varieties of hemolysis are recognized.

1. β-Hemolysis: total hemolysis of erythrocytes extending radially from the colony, recognized as a completely clear zone around the colony.
2. α-Hemolysis: a smaller inner zone of nonhemolyzed cells and an outer zone of completely hemolyzed cells which can only be appreciated by microscopic examination. The agar appears greenish owing to discoloration by a reductant of hemoglobin.
3. γ-Hemolysis: erythrocytes remain unaltered and there is therefore no change in the appearance of the medium.

Most strains of group A streptococci are β hemolytic, whereas most strains of enterococcus are nonhemolytic on sheep blood agar. The oral streptococci, of which there are many species, frequently produce α-hemolysis on blood agar and are traditionally lumped together and called *Streptococcus viridans* in recognition of this green hemolysis. The limitation of classifying streptococci according to their hemolytic characteristics is that it is not species-specific and is only a guide to the identification of the particular streptococcus. For example, streptococci belonging to groups A, C, and G frequently look alike on blood agar and produce a similar zone of β-hemolysis.

Group Antigen

Lancefield first identified the presence of the cell-wall, C, or carbohydrate antigen that gives the streptococcus its group designation. This antigen may be extracted by the treatment of an overnight broth culture with hot dilute hydrochloric acid and reaction of the extract with homologous rabbit antiserum to form a precipitin. The C antigen is determined by the terminal sugar residue on the oligosaccharide side chain, which for group A streptococci is N-acetylglucosamine, and for group C streptococci is N-acetylgalactosamine. There are in excess of 20 group antigens identifiable by letters A through U (excluding I). Very few groups contain streptococci regularly pathogenic to man. Groups A, B, and D are well recognized and groups C, F, and G occasionally produce human disease. The viridans streptococci belong to a variety of groups, but *S. salivarius,* which is associated with endocarditis, often belongs to group K. The remaining groups of streptococci are rarely pathogenic to man, but are important as pathogens in animals. The limitations of this antigen classification of streptococci include the inability to detect group antigens in all streptococci and the rather poor correlation between the presence of a particular group antigen and speciation. There are a few groups that contain but a single species, such as group A *(S. pyogenes)* and group B *(S. agalactiae).* Many groups, such as group D, contain several streptococcal species.

The biologic properties are more specific but more exacting to determine. They include a wide range of biochemical properties, identification of extracellular

TABLE 83.1   Classification of Streptococci

Species	Group	Hemolysis	Disease(s)	Normal Habitat	Other
S. pyogenes	A	β (rarely γ)	Pharyngitis, skin infections, pneumonia rarely, also non-infectious sequelae (rheumatic fever, poststreptococcal glomerulonephritis)	Nasopharynx, skin, rectum	Bacitracin-sensitive
S. agalactiae	B	β (α, γ)	Neonatal sepsis and meningitis, puerperal infections, urinary tract infections and endocarditis rarely	Nasopharynx, genital tract	May be bacitracin-sensitive
S. equi	C	β (α, γ)	Rare: skin and wound infections, endocarditis	Nasopharynx, skin	
S. canis	G	β (α, γ)	Rare: skin and wound infections, endocarditis	Nasopharynx, skin	
S. fecalis (enterococci)	D	β *or* γ (rarely α)	Endocarditis, rarely peritonitis, urinary tract infections	Gastrointestinal and genital tracts	Penicillin-resistant
S. bovis	D	β *or* γ (rarely α)	Endocarditis, urinary tract infections	Gastrointestinal and genital tracts	Penicillin-sensitive

Viridans streptococci		α	Endocarditis, sinusitis	Oropharynx
S. sanquis	H			
S. salivarius	K			
S. mutans and others	None			
Anaerobic streptococci	None	γ	Sinusitis, lung abscess, empyema, pneumonia, brain abscess	Oropharynx, gastrointestinal and genital tracts
S. pneumoniae (pneumococcus)	None	α, γ	Pneumonia, otitis media, sinusitis, meningitis	Oropharynx

products and other cellular antigens that vary from species to species. These will be discussed below, as they relate to individual species.

Streptococcus pyogenes

Numerically, *S. pyogenes* is responsible for the majority of streptococcal disease in humans. The pyogenic infections are preponderantly epithelial and involve the upper respiratory tract, skin, and in the past, the postpartum endometrium. Many of these infections are minor and even asymptomatic, but they can be responsible for significant morbidity. Furthermore, the nonsuppurative complications of *S. pyogenes* infections, namely rheumatic fever and acute glomerulonephritis, are extremely important.

Streptococcus pyogenes possesses the group A cell-wall polysaccharide antigen and the majority of strains are β-hemolytic on blood agar prepared from either sheep, horse, or rabbit blood. In addition, 95% of group A streptococci are inhibited by low concentrations of the antibiotic bacitracin, which is useful as a presumptive test for the identification of *S. pyogenes*. Care to use a heavy pure inoculum of the streptococcus, low-potency discs (0.04 U), careful quality control testing, and the recognition that any zone of inhibition should be considered a positive test, will avoid difficulties in interpretation of the bacitracin test.

Cellular Products

M antigens are present on cell surface fimbriae of about 50% of clinical isolates of group A streptococcus. There are more than 60 type M antigens recognizable and the number continues to increase. The M antigen is a virulence factor, destroyed by trypsin and antiphagocytic in nature. Type-specific antibodies are protective, although early antibiotic treatment can inhibit the rate and strength of their formation. M-negative (M-) strains are relatively avirulent but can revert to (M+) by infecting mice and reisolating the organism.

Capsule

Most group A streptococci possess a capsule of varying thickness composed of hyaluronic acid. It is present in young cultures and readily diffuses into the medium. It is responsible for the surface appearance of the colony on blood agar. Mucoid colonies have an abundance of hyaluronic acid, whereas glossy colonies are made up of cells deficient in this acid. Hyaluronic acid is not immunogenic but is an important virulence factor owing to its antiphagocytic action. *T antigens* are protein antigens which resist proteolysis but are heat- and acid-labile. They are not virulence factors and their distribution is unrelated to the presence of M antigen. Their identification is of value in typing *S. pyogenes* for epidemiologic purposes. With the M and T typing systems about 90% of strains can be identified (Table 83.2).

Extracellular Products

Streptococci elaborate many extracellular proteins which are immunogenic, thus measurement of the antibody response provides a marker for streptococcal infection. They are also important in explaining some of the in vivo and in vitro effects of these organisms. *Streptolysin O* and *streptolysin S* are two hemolysins elaborated by most strains of *S. pyogenes*. They are responsible for the hemolysis of

TABLE 83.2   Products of *S. pyogenes*

Cellular

    M antigen

    Capsule

    T antigen

Extracellular

    Hemolysins

    Streptokinase

    Streptodornase

    Hyaluronidase

    NADase

    Proteinase

    Amylase

    Esterases

    Erythrogenic toxin

erythrocytes in laboratory media and are differentiated by the fact that streptolysin S is oxygen-stable, cell-bound, and leukotoxic but not antigenic, unlike streptolysin O which is reversibly inactivated by oxygen and is antigenic, hence the detection of circulating antistreptolysin O antibodies is helpful in indicating streptococcal infection. *Streptokinase* catalyzes the conversion of plasminogen to plasmin and is fibrinolytic. It is assumed that it aids the spread of streptococci in the tissues by breaking down fibrin. *Streptodornase* is a deoxyribonuclease which depolymerizes the DNA that accumulates in tissues from killed polymorphonuclear cells and tissue debris. Both streptokinase and streptodornase have the ability to liquefy pus and this effect has been used clinically. The two are also useful markers of immunologic competence and hence are frequently used in skin tests of patients since most adults will react to these products as a result of previous exposure to these antigens. *Hyaluronidase* is a potent enzyme which acts on the matrix of connective tissue; the ability of *S. pyogenes* to spread in the tissues is frequently attributed to this enzyme. Other enzymes include nicotinamide adenine dinucleotidase (NADase), proteinase, amylase, and esterases. *Erythrogenic toxin* is responsible for the rash of scarlet fever. The ability to elaborate erythrogenic toxin, of which there are three antigenic types, is dependent upon the presence of a bacteriophage. Such streptococci are described as lysogenized. The quantity of erythrogenic toxin elaborated is variable and is reflected by the varying severity of the rash. The intradermal injection of erythrogenic toxin in a nonimmune individual produces erythema and edema; such a reaction is called a positive Dick test after its originator. Occasional strains of *Staphylococcus aureus* and group C and G streptococci may also elaborate erythrogenic toxin (see Table 83.2).

Streptococcus pyogenes Infections

Pharyngitis

Streptococcus pyogenes is the most common bacterial cause of pharyngitis. It is particularly common between the ages of 5 and 15 years and has a peak incidence in the winter and spring. It is more often seen in temperate climates and is transmitted from person to person by direct contact, with droplet transmission playing a minor role. Sporadic cases are usual but epidemics occur among the military and among schoolchildren.

Clinically the symptoms range from mild to severe. Classically, there is sudden onset of fever, headache, and pharyngitis, followed by an exudative tonsillitis or pharyngitis with cervical adenitis, all resolving in 3-4 days. There is extreme variability in these findings and nonexudative streptococcal pharyngitis certainly occurs. The symptoms are in no way diagnostic and can mimic viral pharyngitis. Hence, a throat culture is essential to confirm the diagnosis. The peripheral white cell count may show an increased number of polymorphonuclear neutrophils.

Suppurative complications are unusual but include peritonsillar abscess (called quinsy), sinusitis, otitis media, mastoiditis, and lymphadenitis. Scarlet fever may develop if the *S. pyogenes* produces erythrogenic toxin. A fine generalized erythematous rash develops which is more intense on the trunk and inner aspects of the limbs. Petechiae may develop, particularly over pressure areas. The throat will show changes similar to the uncomplicated pharyngitis, although the tongue may be bright red with prominent papillae (raspberry tongue) and changing to a coated tongue with projecting papillae (strawberry tongue). There may also be circumoral pallor. The rash fades over the course of 3-6 days and eventually desquamates from the head downward. This desquamation is quite characteristic and may be the first evidence to indicate the nature of the rash.

In epidemics of streptococcal pharyngitis patients with all grades of severity are seen and many will be asymptomatic yet have positive throat cultures. In addition to treating the overt cases it is also important to treat the asymptomatic carrier who can act as a reservoir for the continuation of an epidemic.

Streptococcal Skin Sepsis

Erysipelas usually affects the face or head and occurs at the extremes of life. There is spreading erythema with an elevated, well-demarcated edge to the rash, tightness of the skin, and considerable tenderness, together with systemic features of chills, fever, and even rigors. It frequently spreads over the bridge of the nose and results in marked periorbital swelling. *Pyoderma* covers a variety of lesions including impetigo, cellulitis, and secondary infections of wounds, burns, and dermatoses. *Impetigo* is a superficial vesicular rash on an erythematous base which rapidly progresses to crust formation and eventual healing without scarring. There may be itching or burning and the lesions may be exudative. It is highly infectious and is most frequently seen in young children, particularly in summer and autumn in tropical climates where uncovered skin and possibly minor trauma and insect bites are factors in the epidemiology. *Streptococcus pyogenes* can be isolated from the lesions, particularly if the vesicles or crusts are first cleansed and elevated before taking a swab culture. The infection can be indolent but responds to topical and systemic antibiotics. The latter are preferred for their more predictable effect and to eradicate nasopharyngeal streptococci that are usually of the same M type as the cutaneous strains and frequently present simultaneously.

Streptococcal cellulitis and wound infections can be dramatic in their presentation with high fever, leukocytosis, and a rapidly and diffusely spreading cellulitis, which is usually extremely tender. Postoperative wound infections and burn infections may originate from the patient or from one of his medical attendants who may harbor S. pyogenes in the nose, throat, or even the rectum. Lymphangitic spread with regional adenitis is a fairly common accompaniment of streptococcal pyoderma. Furthermore, bacteremic spread is more frequently associated with cutaneous streptococcal disease than with nasopharyngeal infections, thus osteomyelitis, meningitis, and suppurative thrombophlebitis may complicate streptococcal pyoderma.

Puerperal fever from S. pyogenes infection of the denuded endometrial surface fortunately is rarely seen today. Endometritis is more commonly caused by anaerobic streptococci.

Nonsuppurative Complications of S. pyogenes Infection

The nonsuppurative complications of S. pyogenes infection include rheumatic fever, acute glomerulonephritis, and erythema nodosum. Much of the evidence for this is based on epidemiologic observations while pathophysiologic evidence still remains inconclusive.

Rheumatic fever (RF) differs from acute poststreptococcal glomerulonephritis (GN) in that there does not appear to be any specific rheumatogenic strain of S. pyogenes. Furthermore, rheumatic fever follows only streptococcal pharyngitis, whereas GN may complicate either streptococcal pharyngitis or pyoderma. Repeated attacks of RF are not uncommon and usually can be attributed to repeated streptococcal infections as indicated by culture results and serologic testing, and here the efficacy of chemoprophylaxis with penicillin is undisputed.

The pathogenesis of RF is not understood although there is good evidence to support an immunologic basis for the disease. Persistent circulating antibodies to the group C polysaccharide antigen have been found in patients with rheumatic heart disease and have been shown to cross-react with the glycoprotein component of heart valves. Other streptococcal antigens, such as a fraction of the M protein, have been identified and cross-react with the sarcolemma or sarcoplasm of the heart and smooth muscle of vessel walls.

Rheumatic fever can occur at any age, but has a peak frequency in those 5-14 years old. It tends to occur 2-4 weeks following an episode of streptococcal pharyngitis. Patients will have clinical signs and symptoms related to inflammation of the joints, the cardiovascular, or the central nervous systems. See Table 83.3 for accepted diagnostic criteria for RF.

In contrast to RF the epidemiologic relationship between nephritogenic strains of S. pyogenes from the skin or pharynx is better defined, although the pathophysiology is still far from certain. The nephritogenic pharyngeal strains of streptococci are many but are preponderantly M types 1, 4, 6, and 12, of which the latter is the most common. The M types associated with streptococcal pyoderma include 2, 49, 52, 55, 57, 60, of which M49 predominates and is the classic Red Lake strain associated with epidemic GN on an Indian reservation. In addition to the variation in M types, the latent period from infection to the onset of GN differs and occurs about 10 days following a throat infection or approximately 21 days following skin sepsis. Pyoderma appears to be a more frequent antecedent to GN in tropical countries. This separation of streptococci into rheumatogenic and nephritogenic strains is not absolute, but the rarity of RF and GN occurring simultaneously in an individual stresses the fact that there must be important differences either in the strain or host response to infection.

Pathologically the findings in the kidney in GN are those of an immune-complex nephritis with "lumps and bumps" of fibrin, complement, and IgG, deposited along the glomerular basement membrane. A similar picture has been produced experimentally in rabbits with nephritogenic strains.

TABLE 83.3   Revised Jones' Criteria for Diagnosis of Rheumatic Fever*

Major

　　Carditis
　　Polyarthritis
　　Chorea
　　Erythema marginatum
　　Subcutaneous nodules

Minor

　　Previous rheumatic fever or rheumatic heart disease
　　Arthralgia
　　Fever
　　Acute phase reactants
　　Prolonged PR interval

Evidence of streptococcal infection

　　Increased titer of streptococcal antibodies
　　Positive throat culture for group A streptococcus
　　Recent scarlet fever

*Presence of two major, or of one major and two minor criteria, indicates high
probability that patient has rheumatic fever. Evidence of preceding streptococcal infection strengthens diagnostic possibility

The clinical picture is associated with the abrupt onset of malaise, headache,
edema, hypertension, oliguria, and dark urine caused by the presence of hematuria, proteinuria, and casts. Throat or skin cultures may be positive for S. pyogenes,
and the serology of paired sera confirms recent streptococcal infection. The antistreptolysin O titer is elevated more frequently with pharyngeal infections,
whereas anti-NADase and antihyaluronidase titers are frequently higher in streptococcal pyoderma.
　　Recurrent attacks of GN are rare and long-term chemoprophylaxis to the index case is not indicated. However, in epidemic situations, prophylactic penicillin
given early enough may prevent attacks of GN, by preventing or aborting streptococcal infections. Antibiotic prophylaxis may also prevent secondary spread of
infection within the community by eradicating the carrier state.
　　Erythema nodosum is a hypersensitivity vasculitis developing after a variety
of microbial or drug stimuli of which streptococcal pharyngitis is one. It is characterized by hot, red, tender subcutaneous nodules over the skin along the extensor surfaces of the extremities. The lesions are 2-5 cm in diameter and vary in
number according to the severity of the attack. Lesions heal completely within
1-2 weeks without scar formation. Recurrent attacks occur in a small percentage
of persons. Severe attacks may have accompanying systemic features of malaise,
fever, chills, arthralgia, adenitis, and albuminuria, in addition to the local features of streptococcal pharyngitis. Treatment of the streptococcal infection is

indicated as well as symptomatic management with salicylates and occasionally corticosteroids if symptoms are severe.

Treatment

Penicillin remains the drug of choice for the treatment and prevention of *S. pyogenes* infections. Despite its widespread use resistance to penicillin has not occurred, in contrast to the experience with tetracycline, erythromycin, and clindamycin, where resistant strains have emerged. Both streptococcal pharyngitis and pyoderma respond satisfactorily to a single injection of a long acting penicillin such as benzathine penicillin 1.2 million U, or phenoxymethyl penicillin 250 mg (400,000 U) q.i.d., p.o. for 10 days (Table 83.4). Ten-days treatment is necessary to eradicate pharyngeal colonization and prevent relapse or transmission to another individual although symptomatic improvement (usually with or without treatment) is generally noted after 3-4 days. As implied from the previous statement, the purpose of treatment is not symptomatic or immediate benefit, but the prevention of the nonsuppurative complications. Topical preparations such as bacitracin, are rapidly effective in impetigo but poststreptococcal nephritis has occurred in association with topical therapy and probably results from simultaneous nasopharyngeal colonization which will not be eradicated. Chemoprophylaxis for the prevention of recurrent attacks of rheumatic fever is effective. The risks of cardiac involvement increase significantly with each recurrence and hence the importance of preventive therapy. Recurrences are unusual 5 years after an initial attack and rare beyond the age of 21 years, hence some authorities feel that chemoprophylaxis can be discontinued at this age, while others feel it should be continued indefinitely owing to the exposure of young adults to children with streptococcal disease. Either benzathine penicillin G 1.2 million U once monthly, or penicillin V 250 mg daily by mouth are effective, while sulfadiazine 1.0 g daily is an effective alternative in the penicillin hypersensitive patient (Table 83.5).

TABLE 83.4   Eradication of Streptococci in Patients with Pharyngitis

Penicillin	Treatment Failure (Approximate %)
7-day course	31
10-day course	18

TABLE 83.5   Prophylaxis of Rheumatic Fever

Antibiotic Regimen	Recurrence Rate*
Parenteral benzathine penicillin	0.4
Oral penicillin	5.5
Oral sulfadiazine	2.8

*Rate/100 patient years

Group B Streptococcus

The group B streptococcus S. agalactiae has assumed increasing importance as a cause of a wide variety of infections, in particular neonatal sepsis. Historically it was and remains a cause of bovine mastitis. Human infections were sporadic until the late 1960s when perinatal infections increased alarmingly; the organism is now the leading cause of perinatal sepsis in some centers. In addition to neonatal infections, S. agalactiae has been recognized as a cause of serious infection in patients with cirrhosis, diabetes mellitus, and those who are immunocompromised by their treatment or their disease. Septicemia, cellulitis, osteomyelitis, peritonitis, and urinary tract infections all have been described. Epidemiologic studies have indicated that S. agalactiae may be found in the vagina, rectum, and throat of pregnant women. Approximately 25–35% of pregnant women have positive vaginal cultures at the time of delivery. Furthermore, approximately 75% of infants born to these women will have the organism present on the skin or mucous membranes within 48 hr of delivery. There is also evidence for the venereal transmission of S. agalactiae since the same serotypes have been found in the male urethra of sexual partners.

Microbiology

Streptococcus agalactiae is indistinguishable from S. pyogenes by Gram stain. However, the colonies on 5% sheep blood agar are quite distinctive; S. agalactiae forms gray, mucoid colonies 1–2 mm in diameter usually with a small zone of β-hemolysis, although a few strains are nonhemolytic. Orange pigment production occurs under anaerobic conditions provided the medium contains sufficient starch. Streptococcus agalactiae is usually bacitracin-resistant, will hydrolyze esculin and hippuric acid, but will not ferment mannitol. It also produces a positive cAMP reaction of synergistic hemolysis with a β-hemolytic strain of S. aureus. Antigenically, the group B streptococci possess a group polysaccharide antigen, and are of a variety of polysaccharide type-specific antigens, namely Ia, Ib, II, and III.

Type III strains are the most important cause of neonatal meningitis and appear to occur more frequently in infants born to mothers deficient in type III antibodies. These are IgG and can therefore cross the placenta. In addition to type-specific opsonic antibody, complement is also necessary for the efficient phagocytosis of these bacteria. The majority of newborn group B streptococcal infections can be divided into either an early-onset, acute illness developing within 5 days of birth, or a later-onset one at about 4 weeks. The early-onset disease is associated with obstetric complications such as prolonged rupture of membranes or premature onset of labor. Sepsis is overwhelming with respiratory distress, apnea, and both clinical and radiographic features that make differentiation from the respiratory distress syndrome difficult. Blood cultures are usually positive and cerebrospinal fluid cultures are positive in about 30%. Other sites, such as the ear, oropharynx, umbilicus, and gastric contents may also yield S. agalactiae on culture. These isolates are usually the same serotype as those obtained from the maternal vagina or rectum. The incidence of this early-onset infection lies between 3.4 and 4.2/1000 live births and has a mortality of about 50%. The later-onset infections occur around 4 weeks of age, although they may be seen from 10 days to 4 months and take the form of a pyogenic meningitis. In some centers it has eclipsed Escherichia coli as the most important cause of neonatal meningitis. Mortality is lower, at 20%, but approximately 50% of the survivors have neurologic sequelae. The mode of transmission of the group B streptococcus is less clear-cut in the late-onset than in the early-onset disease and reflects the great-er opportunities that occur for colonization following delivery. Serotype II pre-dominates and may reflect specific neurotropism on the part of this serotype.

Streptococcus agalactiae remains uniformly sensitive to penicillin although it appears to be killed more slowly and requires higher concentrations of the drug than does *S. pyogenes*. Neonatal group B streptococcal sepsis should be treated with dosages of penicillin G ranging from 150,000 to 250,000 U/kg/day intravenously in four divided doses. Prevention of group B streptococcal neonatal sepsis is ob-viously desirable and vaccination of pregnant women to produce opsonic antibody is under investigation. Chemoprophylaxis of either the mother or infant is an al-ternative approach, but the ubiquitous nature of the organism makes selection of high-risk infants difficult.

Enterococcus

The enterococci include several species of streptococci found in the alimentary tract such as *S. faecalis* and *S. faecium*. They differ from other streptococci in their ability to survive at pH 9.6 in a 6.5% salt medium, ferment mannitol, hy-drolyze bile esculin, and survive heating for 30 min at 60°C. Their colonies are usually nonhemolytic on sheep blood agar although occasional strains are β-hemo-lytic. They also possess teichoic acid as the group-specific antigen which is syn-onymous with the Lancefield group D antigen.

Clinically they are responsible for a small percentage of urinary tract infec-tions which may be a source of bacteremia following instrumentation of the lower urinary tract. In patients with prosthetic or damaged heart valves there is a risk of infective endocarditis which can be difficult to eradicate unless a two-drug regimen is employed. Enterococci tend to be more resistant than other strepto-cocci to the effect of penicillin but exhibit synergistic susceptibility to an amino-glycoside, such as gentamicin or streptomycin, in combination with penicillin or ampicillin. This combination is also indicated for the chemoprophylaxis of entero-coccal endocarditis and is discussed in Chapter 19.

Streptococcus bovis is not an enterococcus but shares the group D antigen with the enterococci. It differs from these organisms by its inability to ferment mannitol, or to survive a high salt concentration or pH of 9.6. Furthermore, it is far more sensitive to penicillin than the enterococcus and serious infections, in-cluding endocarditis, usually respond to penicillin therapy alone. Bacteremia caused by *S. bovis* has been associated with gastrointestinal pathology, most not-ably colon cancer, and hence *S. bovis* bacteremia should include a careful evalu-ation of the patient for underlying disease.

Anaerobic Streptococci

The anaerobic streptococci, or peptostreptococci, are important members of the normal flora of the upper respiratory tract, female genital tract, and to a lesser degree the gut. They are probably the second most frequent genus of anaerobic bacteria to be isolated from clinical infections and are of major importance in fe-male genital tract sepsis.

Peptostreptococcus anaerobius and *P. intermedius* are the species most com-monly isolated. They grow well on both solid and broth media. The former is a strict anaerobe, whereas the latter is frequently microaerophilic. Several species are, in fact, microaerophilic on subculture and require an increased carbon diox-ide content for their growth.

Several factors predispose to the development of infection with these micro-organisms. There is usually antecedent tissue damage. This may be either surgi-cally induced, associated with postpartum denuding of the endometrium, or ma-lignancy. Common sites of infections include the endometrium, infected follow-ing delivery or abortion or as part of acute or chronic pelvic inflammatory disease, and vaginal cuff infections following vaginal hysterectomy. These pelvic infec-tions may spread locally or via the lymphatics and blood stream to produce para-metritis, pelvic cellulitis, abscess, and septic thrombophlebitis with blood stream dissemination and infected emboli to the lungs.

Most of these infections are anaerobic and polymicrobic. Occasionally a syn-ergistic infection occurs which may produce a myositis, fasciitis, or anterior ab-dominal-wall gangrene. Anaerobic streptococci are frequently isolated in associ-ation with other anaerobic bacteria or facultative bacteria such as *S. aureus*.

Selected Bibliography

Anthony, B. F. and Okada, D. M.: The emergence of group B streptococci in in-fections of the newborn infant. *Am Rev Med* 28:355-369, 1977.

Duma, R. J., Weinbert, R. T., Medrek, T. F., and Kunz, L. J.: Streptococcal in-fections. *Medicine* 48:87-127, 1969.

Gorbach, S. L. and Bartlett, J. G.: Anaerobic infections. *N Engl J Med* 290:1177-1184, 1237-1245, 1289-1294, 1974.

Kaplan, E. L., Bascam, F. A., Chapman, S. S., and Wannamaker, L. W.: Epidemic acute glomerulonephritis associated with type 49 streptococcal pyoderma. I. Clinical and laboratory findings. *Am J Med* 48:9-27, 1970.

Moellering, R. C., Watson, B. K., and Kunz, L. J.: Endocarditis due to group D streptococci. Comparison of disease caused by *Streptococcus bovis* with that produced by enterococci. *Am J Med* 57:239-250, 1974.

Wannamaker, L. W.: Differences between streptococcal infections of the throat and of the skin. *N Engl J Med* 282:23-30, 78-85, 1970.

84

STREPTOCOCCUS PNEUMONIAE
Roger G. Finch, M.B.

Definition

Streptococcus pneumoniae was first recognized in sputum in 1881 by Pasteur in France and Sternberg in the United States. It belongs to the group of cocci known as the pyogenic cocci which includes *Staphylococcus aureus, Streptococcus pyogenes,* and the *Neisseria* spp, *N. gonorrhoeae* and *N. meningitidis.* It remains the most common cause of acute bacterial pneumonia and a leading cause of meningitis in adults. Until recently *S. pneumoniae* has been fully susceptible to penicillin. However, strains causing disease and resistant to penicillin have recently been reported from both South Africa and the United States.

Microbiology

Streptococcus pneumoniae is a gram-positive, nonmotile, encapsulated coccus. In pathologic specimens it occurs in pairs with the cocci appearing lancet-shaped with their short axis in parallel. Single organisms as well as short chains also occur. The tendency to appear in pairs in clinical specimens justified the now obsolete name *Diplococcus pneumoniae.*

The organisms are relatively fastidious, surviving drying and exposure to physiologic saline poorly. They have complex nutritional requirements which are generally satisfied by enriched media such as brain heart infusion, tryptic soy, and thioglycollate, if supplemented with 5 10% whole or defibrinated blood obtained from sheep, horse, rabbit, or man. Although most strains are facultative anaerobes, rare strains are strict anaerobes. Approximately 5-10% of strains grow only in an atmosphere of increased carbon dioxide.

Following 18-24 hr incubation on sheep blood agar the colonies are about 1 mm in diameter, round, and domed. Certain serotypes, such as types 3 and 37, produce large mucoid colonies. The colonies are surrounded by a zone of α-hemolysis which makes differentiation from α-hemolytic streptococci difficult. However, with prolonged incubation, autolysis results in the sinking of the central portion of the colonies to create the appearance of either a nailhead or a checker. If incubated anaerobically β-hemolysis is seen. In liquid media growth tends to be diffuse although sedimentation occurs with prolonged incubation.

Glucose is essential for growth. However, the consequent production of lactic acid causes a fall in pH which is then inhibitory to growth. This can be prevented by the addition of buffering agents. The optimum pH for growth is pH 7.6. Pneumococci survive poorly outside the pH range 7-7.8.

Although *S. pneumoniae* grows aerobically it is related to anaerobic bacteria by its lack of a cytochrome system. It utilizes oxygen through a flavoprotein enzyme system with hydrogen peroxide being an end product. This is inhibitory to growth because *S. pneumoniae,* in keeping with other streptococci, lacks the catalase necessary for the degradation of hydrogen peroxide. This explains the need for the addition of blood to growth media; the erythrocytes provide a source of catalase.

Inulin fermentation differentiates *S. pneumoniae* from most α-hemolytic streptococci. Furthermore, the surface action of bile, bile salts, or sodium dodecyl sulfate brings about the rapid dissolution of the organisms and is the basis for the *bile solubility* test which is almost specific for *S. pneumoniae.* It can be carried out either with a broth suspension, or by dropping the liquid solution directly onto a colony of the organism. Bile salts activate the enzyme, L-alanine-muramyl-amidase, which brings about this phenomenon.

Cellular Products

Capsule

The pneumococcal capsule is the major antigenic determinant and virulence factor. There are at least 84 recognizable capsular serotypes of *S. pneumoniae.* The difference among serotypes is due to the antigenic differences in the composition of the capsular polysaccharide. The antigenic structure has been established for only a few serotypes. For example, serotype 3 is composed of repeating units of cellobiuronic acid. Cellobiuronic acid is also found in serotypes 1 and 8 which probably explains the occasional cross-reactions seen between these serotypes. Occasional cross-reactions are seen with other bacteria, such as *Klebsiella, Salmonella,* α-hemolytic and nonhemolytic streptococci.

The capsule is antiphagocytic and virulence is approximately proportional to the size of the capsule. Serotype 3 is a particularly virulent strain and possesses a large capsule and also produces large mucoid colonies on blood agar. Occasional serotypes are unencapsulated and hence avirulent. Their colonies appear granular (rough) as opposed to the usual mucoid (smooth) appearance. The transition from smooth (S) to rough (R) can be brought about by repeated subculturing or growing in the presence of anticapsular antibody.

The capsule is not readily visible in clinical specimens. However, it can be demonstrated by mixing with type-specific antiserum which renders the capsule more refractile and also causes it to increase in thickness. This is the basis of the *capsule swelling* or quellung test.

The antigenic variation of the capsule is responsible for the numerical serotype accorded to a particular strain. Unfortunately there are two numerical systems extant, an American and a Danish system. Although most strains are readily identified by both a Danish and American notation, one or two serotypes are not interchangeably accommodated.

C Substance

A cell-wall carbohydrate or C substance is made up of galactosamine-6-phosphate in combination with phosphorylcholine and some fractions of cell-wall mucopeptides. It is antigenic and forms part of the Forssman antigen of the pneumococcus which is precipitated by a β-globulin in the presence of Ca^{2+}. This β-globulin is also known as the *C-reactive protein* which is found nonspecifically in several acute infectious conditions as well as some noninfectious diseases.

M Protein

The M protein is similar to that of group A streptococcus but is not antiphagocytic and does not give rise to protective antibodies.

Extracellular Products

Pneumolysin O

Pneumolysin O is a hemolysin which is oxygen-labile. It is antigenic and has both dermonecrotic and lethal properties in experimental animals as well as producing hemolysis of erythrocytes.

Neuraminidase

Neuraminidase is produced by fresh isolates. It cleaves N-acetylneuraminic acid from sugars on both glycolipids and glycoproteins.

Epidemiology

Streptococcus pneumoniae forms part of the normal flora of the upper respiratory tract of man and other mammals. It can be isolated from the pharynx in 5-70% of the population (Table 84.1), with the higher isolation rates in the winter and

TABLE 84.1   Pharyngeal Carriage Rate of Pneumococcus

Age (yr)	%
0-5	38
6-11	28
12-16	9
Adults (with children)	19
Adults (without children)	6

early spring. It is responsible for more than 75% of acute bacterial pneumonias in the community and for the majority in hospitalized patients. There are an estimated half million or more cases of pneumococcal pneumonia annually in the United States. Table 84.2 summarizes the case-fatality rate from pneumococcal infections. Males are more susceptible than females in a ratio of 3:2. Blacks are also more susceptible than whites. The disease tends to be sporadic, although epidemics have occurred in the military. Disease is more common in the elderly (Table 84.3) and in patients with chronic lung disease, congestive heart failure, diabetes mellitus, bronchogenic carcinoma, alcoholism, sickle cell disease, and patients with granulocytopenia, multiple myeloma, or hypogammaglobulinemia. Secondary pneumonia complicating influenza is often caused by *S. pneumoniae.* South African novice goldminers have a high rate of pneumococcal pneumonia, as do the natives of Papua New Guinea.

Bacteremia is detected in 20-30% of patients with pneumococcal pneumonia. Surveys of pneumococcal bacteremia in adults have shown that 12 capsular types, 1-8, 12, 14, 18, and 19, account for 84% of bacteremic infections and 77% of deaths associated with bacteremia. In children eight serotypes, 1, 3, 6, 7, 14, 18, 19, and 23, account for 70% of infections.

TABLE 84.2   Case-Fatality Rate From Pneumococcal Infection

Age (yr)	Bacteremic Pneumococcal Pneumonia (%)	Extrapulmonary Pneumococcal Infection, With or Without Pneumonia (%)
14-29	3	20
30-49	15	35
50-69	40	50
70+	55	75
Overall	25	45

TABLE 84.3   Pneumococcal Pneumonia Fatality Rates (%) Related to Age of Patient and Type of Therapy

Age (Yr)	None	Antiserum	Sulfonamides	Penicillin
20	∿ 10	5	3	1
50	45	35	25	8
≥ 70	70	70	40	15

Other pneumococcal infections of major importance are pneumococcal meningitis, of which there are an estimated 4800 infections annually, and otitis media,
which afflicts approximately 20% of children under 2 years of age.

The organism is spread by means of droplets or direct oral contact, with indirect spread from freshly soiled respiratory articles occurring less commonly. Person-to-person spread leads to colonization, and colonization is a prerequisite for
infection, but the two events are not closely related. Therefore, person-to-person
spread only rarely leads to acquisition of the disease. Thus illness is unusual among
contacts, and isolation precautions are not recommended. However, recent experience in South Africa with strains resistant to several antibiotics, including penicillin, has shown a high rate of spread among patients and medical attendants; this
may stimulate a reappraisal of the need for isolation should penicillin-resistant
strains become more widespread.

Pathogenesis and Pathology

Both natural as well as humoral and cellular host defenses are important in protecting against pneumococcal infection. This is well illustrated by considering
factors which lead to the development of pneumococcal pneumonia. The various
anatomic defenses include the epiglottis, which protects the trachea from aspiration; the mucociliary escalator and cough reflex, which maintain the tracheobronchial toilet; and the lung lymphatics and alveolar macrophages, which rid the lungs
of particulate matter including bacteria.

Preexisting disease (e.g., viral infections and chronic bronchitis), as well as
impairment of consciousness and protective reflexes from any cause, congestive
heart failure, and alcoholism, all provide circumstances in which the pneumococcus can overcome the natural host defenses and multiply in the lung parenchyma.
The organism's capsule is antiphagocytic and enables rapid multiplication to occur.
Other virulence factors such as toxins have not been detected and the mechanisms
by which pneumococci produce disease still remain unclear. The sequence of congestion, cellular infiltration, and resolution typical of lobar pneumonia is discussed in Chapter 16.

In the absence of antibacterial therapy, resolution is dependent upon the production of type-specific opsonic antibody which fixes complement and renders the
bacteria vulnerable to phagocytosis. This occurs from day 6 to day 12 following
the start of infection, at which time resolution is often dramatic, with lysis of the
fever by "crisis" and rapid recovery. Mortality under these circumstances was
30%; it has been reduced to approximately 5% by the early use of penicillin.

Other pneumococcal infections are frequently the result of bacteremic spread.
These include septic arthritis, endocarditis, and meningitis. However, pneumococcal meningitis may complicate structural defects which permit communication
between the nasopharynx and paracranial spaces and the subarachnoid space. These
defects are usually traumatic in origin, although they may occasionally be due to
congenital abnormalities. Recurrent attacks of pneumococcal meningitis should
lead to a search for such defects.

Contiguous spread accounts for otitis media, mastoiditis, and sinusitis from
upper respiratory tract infections; and pericarditis, pleuritis, and empyema from
lower respiratory tract infections.

Primary pneumococcal peritonitis is seen in association with ascites and cirrhosis, and less commonly in children with the nephrotic syndrome.

Anatomic or functional asplenia is well recognized as predisposing to pneumococcal bacteremia, which may be fulminant and complicated by disseminated

intravascular coagulation and even the Waterhouse-Friderichsen syndrome. This syndrome is associated with a high fatality rate, and is most often seen in patients with fulminant meningococcemia.

Following splenectomy there is impaired clearance of bacteria such as pneumococci, with lowered concentrations of circulating antibody, IgM, and frequently tuftsin, a naturally occurring tetrapeptide probably manufactured by the spleen, which stimulates phagocytosis. The risk of pneumococcal sepsis appears greatest in children who have undergone splenectomy, either for trauma or for the management of Hodgkin's disease. The situation in the adult is less clear-cut. Even patients who have undergone splenectomy for the staging of lymphoma have not consistently shown a higher risk of sepsis unless there is an additional complicating factor, such as granulocytopenia.

In diseases such as hypogammaglobulinemia and particularly multiple myeloma, deficient opsonic antibody formation increases the risk of sepsis from encapsulated bacteria, including S. pneumoniae.

Pneumococcal polysaccharide antigen is detectable in several body fluids including blood, cerebrospinal fluid, and urine in association with infection. With meningitis, the persistence and titer of polysaccharide antigen correlate with the severity of the illness and its prognosis. Prolonged high levels forebode complications, including death.

Diagnostic Features

Clinical

Pneumonia is the most common infection produced by S. pneumoniae. The pneumonia is lobar and most commonly affects the right lower, right middle, or left lower lobe, since bronchial secretions tend to gravitate most readily to these lobes in the recumbent patient. There may be an antecedent upper respiratory viral infection. The onset is often abrupt and heralded by a shaking chill in most patients and associated with a rapid rise in temperature and pulse rate.

Severe pleuritic pain and cough, productive of purulent and often "rusty" sputum, follow and are associated with rapid shallow respirations and even mild cyanosis. The illness persists with fever, cough, and pleuritic pain for 7-10 days when resolution occurs by crisis with defervescence, diaphoresis, and dramatic clinical improvement. The early use of antibiotics aborts the illness so that resolution by crisis is uncommon.

Physical examination confirms the presence of consolidation, usually confined to a single lobe. Evidence of a pleural friction rub or coexistent pleural effusion is common. Circulatory collapse and congestive heart failure may develop, while ileus and herpes labialis are also frequently seen.

Other infections such as meningitis are often primary but may complicate pneumonia. The clinical features are not sufficiently remarkable to permit differentiation from other pyogenic meningitides. The same applies to septic arthritis, endocarditis, and the upper respiratory infections, or to otitis media, mastoiditis, and sinusitis.

Laboratory

Examination of clinical samples is essential for the diagnosis of pneumococcal infection. Sputum should be freshly expectorated and smears made for gram stain. The presence of pus cells and large numbers of gram-positive diplococci is very suggestive of pneumococcal infection, particularly if a capsule is discernible.

Culture on blood agar in 5% CO_2 will yield α-hemolytic colonies that may have the characteristic appearance of *S. pneumoniae* or appear mucoid. Confirmatory tests include bile solubility and more frequently, susceptibility to 5 µg optochin (ethyl hydrocuprein HCl), determined by placing a 6-mm optochin disc on a heavy inoculum of *S. pneumoniae* on blood agar and incubating aerobically overnight. A zone diameter greater than 18 mm indicates susceptibility. This test is extremely reliable in differentiating *S. pneumoniae* from other α-hemolytic streptococci.

Serotyping is not normally carried out. However, for epidemiologic studies the *quellung* reaction is satisfactory. Antimicrobial susceptibility testing of *S. pneumoniae* to penicillin has not been a usual practice. However, the recent description of penicillin-resistant strains may alter this. Apart from penicillin, approximately 10% of the strains are resistant to tetracycline and a smaller percentage resistant to erythromycin, clindamycin, and chloramphenicol.

Bacteremia is present in 20-30% of persons with pneumococcal pneumonia. It is therefore of value to draw blood cultures if the patient has not had antibiotic therapy. Antibiotic therapy rapidly clears pneumococcal bacteremia rendering blood cultures unrewarding.

Previous antibiotic therapy also adversely affects the value of sputum culture, since pneumococci are rapidly cleared from the sputum, or they may take up the stain poorly and appear gram-negative. In addition there may be overgrowth of gram-negative bacilli, which may render the results of sputum culture misleading. In fact, only approximately 50% of the patients with bacteremic pneumococcal pneumonia have sputum cultures positive for *S. pneumonia*. Rejection of inadequate sputum samples by the diagnostic laboratory by screening for the presence of more than 10 squamous epithelial cells per low-power field (x 100), thereby suggesting oropharyngeal contamination, has been proposed as a means of improving the reliability of sputum cultures.

Mouse inoculation studies are not routine practice. However, the white mouse is extremely susceptible to encapsulated pneumococci. One colony-forming unit injected intraperitoneally (IP) can cause death. Homogenized sputum samples injected IP result in the phagocytosis of the normal flora but multiplication of the pneumococcus, which can often be isolated in pure culture from the peritoneum and heart blood.

Other body fluids such as cerebrospinal fluid, and empyema, joint, and pericardial fluid should be examined by Gram stain, after centrifugation if necessary, to detect low concentrations of organisms and then cultured on blood agar.

With pneumococcal meningitis there is usually a marked CSF polymorphonuclear predominance, with a cell count higher than $500/mm^3$, protein elevation (50-1500 mg/100 ml), and depressed CSF glucose (0-45 mg/100 ml).

Pneumococcal polysaccharide antigen can be detected in body fluids by counterimmunoelectrophoresis. This test has achieved popularity as a rapid (1-hr) method for diagnosing pneumococcal meningitis. High-potency antiserum is required. Antigen has also been detected in serum, urine, joint, pleural, and pericardial fluid.

Differential Diagnosis (Table 84.4)

Pneumonia

The majority of bacterial pneumonias other than that caused by *S. pneumoniae* are commonly bronchopneumonic and necrotizing, to greater or lesser degrees. The lung architecture in pneumococcal pneumonia is usually preserved, thus resolution is complete. This is in sharp contrast to infections caused by *S. aureus*,

TABLE 84.4   Conditions Commonly Misdiagnosed as Pneumonia

Pulmonary infarction

Acute bronchitis

Pulmonary tuberculosis

Congestive heart failure

Lung abscess

hemolytic streptococci, *K. pneumoniae, Pseudomonas aeruginosa,* and other gram-negative bacilli. Widespread disease is usual and lung abscess relatively frequent with these pathogens.

Mycoplasma pneumoniae pneumonia affects predominantly children and young adults and is usually more insidious in onset and is associated with myringitis, pharyngitis, circulating cold agglutinins in approximately 50% of patients, and complement-fixing antibodies.

Viral pneumonias may be difficult to distinguish but often have definite prodromata of an upper respiratory tract viral infection. Agents to be considered include influenza, adenovirus, rhinovirus, coxsackievirus, echovirus, respiratory syncytial virus, measles, and varicella.

Pneumococcal meningitis must be differentiated from meningococcal infection in the adult and *Haemophilus influenzae* and meningococcal meningitis in the child. In the neonatal period, group B streptococcus and *E. coli* predominate. Although recognition of the gram-positive diplococci on smear is helpful, caution must be exerted if the patient has had antibiotics before admission which may render the organisms gram-variable or scanty.

Treatment

Penicillin remains the drug of choice for the treatment of all pneumococcal infections. The organism is exquisitely sensitive although rare strains from South Africa and Minnesota have been relatively resistant. For treatment of pneumococcal pneumonia 600,000 U of aqueous crystalline penicillin G every 12 hr is adequate. In contrast, pneumococcal meningitis in adults should be treated with 12-20 million U penicillin G intravenously daily. In penicillin-hypersensitive patients, erythromycin, clindamycin, or a cephalosporin are appropriate choices. The use of tetracycline to treat pneumococcal pneumonia is controversial. Although there have been some reports of what was feared to be increasing tetracycline resistance, recent studies suggest that clinical isolates are only rarely resistant.

The recognition of empyema, pericarditis, and metastatic septic arthritis is an indication for surgical aspiration and drainage.

Immunology and Prevention

The pneumococcal polysaccharide capsule is antiphagocytic. Immunity is type-specific and relies upon the development of opsonic anticapsular antibodies. Before penicillin became available, serotherapy was successfully used for the treatment of pneumococcal infection. Pneumococci may activate the terminal complement components, C3 to C9, by either the classic or alternative complement pathways. Activation of either pathway produces cleavage of C3 and the fixation of opsonically active C3b to the bacterial surface. C3-dependent opsonization via the classic pathway is more important in acquired immunity. Activation of the classic pathway is initiated through immune complexes composed of capsular polysaccharide and type-specific anticapsular antibody, while the alternative pathway appears to be activated by the cell-wall C polysaccharide.

Asplenia increases the risks of pneumococcal infection particularly in childhood. Splenectomy appears to decrease the efficiency of bloodstream clearance of pneumococci and increases mortality in intravenously infected mice. Similarly in splenectomized rats and man the antibody response to intravenously injected microbial and cytologic antigens is depressed.

Purified capsular polysaccharide injected subcutaneously or intramuscularly produces protective type-specific immunity and has been effective in preventing pneumococcal pneumonia and bacteremia. A polyvalent pneumococcal vaccine is commercially available (Pneumovax) and contains 50 µg each of 14 polysaccharide antigens to *S. pneumoniae* types 1-4, 6, 8, 9, 12, 14, 19, 23, 25, 51, 56 (United States nomenclature). These serotypes currently account for approximately 80% of pneumococcal disease in the United States and Europe. The vaccine is currently approved for use in persons 2 years of age or older in whom there is an increased risk of morbidity and mortality from pneumococcal pneumonia. The risk factors include: (1) persons with chronic heart disease, chronic bronchopulmonary disease, chronic renal failure, diabetes mellitus, or other chronic metabolic disorders; (2) persons in chronic care facilities; (3) persons convalescing from severe disease; and (4) persons 50 years of age or older (although data are not convincing that healthy individuals aged 50-70 are at increased risk). Antibodies appear to persist for at least 5 years, although the duration of effectiveness is uncertain. In children under 2 years of age, the antibody response is unreliable.

The vaccine also appears effective in preventing pneumococcal bacteremia in persons over 2 years of age with sickle cell disease and in persons who have undergone splenectomy or who have impaired splenic function. In persons with multiple myeloma, nephrotic syndrome, or lymphoproliferative diseases, the antibody response is either poor or variable.

The vaccine is well tolerated, producing minor local erythema and soreness at the injection site, while fever is unusual, short-lived, and almost never more than 38°C. The question of whether or not the vaccine will result in a shift of serotypes causing disease remains to be determined.

Complications

Mortality from pneumococcal pneumonia increases with age and the presence of underlying disease. The overall mortality before the use of antibiotics was 30%; it is now about 5%. Leukopenia, bacteremia, multilobar involvement, an extrapulmonary focus, circulatory collapse, disseminated intravascular coagulation, or infection before age 1 year or after 55 are all bad prognostic indicators.

Infections with serotype 3 tends to be more virulent and the rare occurrence of lung abscess with *S. pneumoniae* appears to be associated with this serotype.

Contiguous spread to involve the pleural and pericardial cavities has been discussed, as has metastatic infection to the meninges, joints, or endocardium.

Between 50 and 70% of patients with pneumococcal meningitis recover. Sequelae are unusual but include deafness, seizures, hydrocephalus, subdural effusions, and hemiparesis.

Postpneumococcal glomerulonephritis is rare, but reduced C3 levels and electron microscopic evidence of a mesangial proliferative glomerulonephritis have been reported.

Selected Bibliography

Austrian, R.: Random gleanings from a life with the pneumococcus. *J Infect Dis* 131:474-484, 1975.

Austrian, R.: Prevention of pneumococcal infection by immunization with capsular polysaccharides of *Streptococcus pneumoniae:* Current status of polyvalent vaccines. *J Infect Dis* 136:S38-S42, 1977.

Editorial: Resistant pneumococci. *Lancet* 2:803-804, 1977.

Murray, P. R. and Washington, J. A., II: Microscopic and bacteriologic analysis of expectorated sputum. *Mayo Clin Proc* 50:339-344, 1975.

Smit, P., Oberholzer, D., Hayden-Smith, S., Koornhof, H. J., and Hilleman, M. R.: Protective efficacy of pneumococcal polysaccharide vaccines. *JAMA* 238:2613-2616, 1977.

Winkelstein, J. A. and Tomasz, A.: Activation of the alternative pathway by pneumococcal cell walls. *J Immunol* 118:451-454, 1977.

85

CORYNEBACTERIA
Robert H. Waldman, M.D.

By far the most important species of corynebacteria is *Corynebacterium diphtheriae*. Diphtheria is an extremely important disease historically because it represents one of the finest accomplishments of twentieth century biomedical scientific advance (Table 85.1). This advance is represented most importantly by the remarkable decrease in mortality from this illness and also by the complete understanding of the pathogenesis of this disease. With respect to the latter, diphtheria may well be the best understood major infectious disease.

The disease has intrigued investigators not only because it is the result of exotoxin production by the organism, but also because only those organisms infected with a bacteriophage that carries the genetic information for toxin production cause it. Thus the disease is the result of an infection that could be thought of as being caused by a bacterium which is itself infected with a virus, i.e., analogous to a Shakespearean play within a play.

Microbiology

Corynebacterium diphtheriae is an aerobic, pleomorphic, unencapsulated, nonmotile, gram-positive, coccobacillus, often with terminal polar masses. An important characteristic is its formation of black pigment on tellurite medium; however, it is not the only organism that does this, an important example being the staphylococci. Another important characteristic is that on Gram stain, organisms tend to arrange themselves at varying angles which overlap, resulting in what is called "Chinese figures."

These organisms have been divided into types on the basis of the degree of blackness of the colonies as seen on tellurite medium (Table 85.2). This typing is

TABLE 85.1   Historical Summary of Diphtheria

Loeffler	1884	Bacterial etiology, postulated exotoxin production
Roux and Yersin	1888	Demonstrated presence of toxin
Behring and Kitasato	1890	Development of antiserum
Ramon	1924	Immunization with toxoid

TABLE 85.2   *C. diphtheria* Types

| Type | Properties | |
	Bacillus	Colony
Gravis	Short, uniformly staining	Low, circular
Intermedius	Long, pleomorphic, clubbed	Small
Mitis	Long, pleomorphic, prominent granules	"Poached egg"

commonly misconstrued as an indication of the virulence of the organism. Although organisms of the mitis type often do cause less severe disease, typing is of almost no practical importance in the individual patient.

As indicated earlier, organisms are pathogenic when they are parasitized by a bacteriophage carrying the *tox*⁺ gene. Toxigenicity can be ascertained by immunoprecipitation testing using organisms grown on agar and antiserum placed in a trough or filter paper strip near the suspect colony.

There are many similar saprophytic organisms found in the upper respiratory tract of most individuals as part of their normal flora. These diphtheroids can be differentiated by carbohydrate fermentation. Diphtheroids occasionally cause disease in compromised individuals, e.g., causing sepsis and endocarditis in heroin addicts and in patients who have undergone cardiovascular surgery.

Corynebacterium minutissimum causes erythrasma, which will be briefly discussed at the end of this chapter. *Propionebacterium acnes* is associated with comedones and was formerly classified as *C. acnes*. *Gardnerella vaginalis* has, in the past, also been classified as a *Corynebacterium* sp.

Epidemiology

Historically, diphtheria was a disease primarily of children, but more recently has been seen in older age groups, thus today approximately one-third of the cases are adults. The explanation of this is that very young children are usually protected by passive immunity of maternal origin, but as this immunity wanes with age, the child becomes more susceptible in the absence of artificial immunization or immunizing subclinical infection. The disease is more common during the winter months and in more crowded living situations because person-to-person transmission from infected respiratory secretions or skin exudate is the method of contagion. Asymptomatic nasopharyngeal carriage is relatively common and important in the transmission of the organism. As would be expected the incidence is higher in poor, crowded, and unimmunized populations.

Humans are the only host for this organism and the distribution is worldwide. The disease usually occurs in epidemic form. There are about 200 cases each year in the United States, and the occurrence has been decreasing fairly steadily since the early years of this century (Table 85.3). The explanation for this decrease, from one of the leading causes of death in this country to a rare disease, is not completely understood. The advent of antibiotics occurred well after the disease was declining. Immunization undoubtedly has played some role, but whether this is a major or a minor role is speculative. It is probable that a major cause of the decline of the disease has been the general improvement in public health and hygiene, e.g., a decrease in crowded living conditions. It has also been speculated that the decrease is a part of some natural periodicity of the disease.

The severity of the disease is greater in patients under the age of 14. The incubation period is 2-6 days.

TABLE 85.3   Incidence of Diphtheria in the United States

Year	Cases/100,000 Population
1920	1500
1930	500
1940	150
1950	40
1960	0.50
1970	0.05
Aged 1 yr	0.03
10	0.03
15-20	0.01
25-30	0.05
30-50	0.12
> 50	0.06

Pathogenesis and Pathology

The exotoxin is not as potent as botulinum toxin, but certainly is quite potent, the lethal dose being about 130 ng/kg body weight. A great deal is known about the biochemistry of the adverse effects of the toxin on cell function, but this is beyond the scope of this chapter. Suffice it to say that the toxin disrupts protein synthesis. The toxin is absorbed from the mucosa of the upper respiratory tract and from the skin, leading to myocarditis and neuritis. In the heart fatty degeneration of myocardial cells is seen, and if the patient survives complete healing results. In the nervous system, fatty degeneration of the white matter, specifically the myelin sheaths, is seen.

Diagnosis

The diagnosis is clinical and should be made on the basis of the proper epidemiologic setting: i.e., a poor, unimmunized person living in crowded conditions; the history of sore throat and fever; and the typical findings on physical examination. It should be realized, however, that the severity of the disease ranges widely, from asymptomatic infection to a rapidly fatal illness. The fever and sore throat are usually mild to moderate, but the patient looks toxic and has fairly marked cervical lymphadenopathy.

The anatomic site and extent of the infection determine the symptoms and the severity. The mildest form is usually seen in patients with anterior nasal involvement. These patients usually have a thick mucopurulent, bloodstained discharge. More severe is faucial (or tonsillar) involvement. Patients have a grayish-green membrane which is difficult to dislodge with a swab, leaving bleeding points with removal of a portion of the membrane. Patients have dysphagia, moderate-sized and tender cervical lymph nodes, and soft-tissue swelling. An important differential diagnostic finding is the extratonsillar spread of the membrane that is seen in diphtheria but not in other causes of tonsillitis. In pharyngeal disease one finds spread to the soft palate and uvula. In this form of disease the whole anterior neck may become edematous and mildly tender, leading to the description of such patients as having a "bull neck." The patient is usually extremely toxic, weak, and limp. The most severe form is laryngeal and bronchial, and such patients have hoarseness, stridor, and cyanosis. The membrane must be removed to avoid suffocation. Other more unusual mucosal lesions are conjunctival involvement and otitis media. As with other forms of pharyngitis, e.g., infectious mononucleosis, patients with diphtheria may have a coexistent streptococcal pharyngitis.

Diphtherial skin involvement is much more common in tropical and subtropical areas, in native Americans, and also in alcoholics living in very crowded and unsanitary living conditions. The skin lesions are very nonspecific, and may present as ulcers or boils. Diphtheria may also be a secondary phenomenon in patients with preexisting skin disease.

Myocarditis is seen in about two-thirds of patients with diphtheria, usually coming on 5-7 days after the onset of respiratory symptoms, but it may actually develop after patients have recovered from the respiratory disease. The myocarditis is manifested by conduction system disturbances and circulatory failure, usually proportional to the extent of the upper respiratory involvement. First-degree heart block is seen in about 15-20% of diphtheria patients.

Neurologic involvement comes on even later than the myocarditis. One form of the disease is bulbar, with palatine paralysis resulting in dysphagia and/or nasal regurgitation of liquids. Peripheral neuropathy, usually mainly motor involvement, occurs in 5-15% of diphtheria patients (Table 85.4). A very late form of neuro-logic disease, occurring up to 3 months after the onset of the infection, is a pic-ture similar to Guillain-Barré syndrome.

Other manifestations of diphtheria, all very uncommon, are thrombocytopenia, infective endocarditis, and renal failure due to tubular disease.

The differential diagnosis includes infectious mononucleosis, which can usu-ally be differentiated on the basis that the membrane or exudate is whitish and confined to the tonsils; streptococcal pharyngitis, a white exudate, red throat, and more severe pain; Vincent's angina, which has gum involvement and a distinctive Gram stain of the exudate; peritonsillar abscess (quinsy); candidal pharyngitis; and poliomyelitis.

The laboratory is of only minor importance in the diagnosis and management of patients with diphtheria. The Gram, methylene blue, or toluidine blue stain of throat swab material is positive in about half of the patients. Culture on Loeff-ler's medium, or blood agar, is positive in about 70% of the patients. However, culture is not very helpful because institution of proper therapy should not be withheld pending culture results. As mentioned earlier, group A streptococci also are commonly found, being isolated in about one-third of the patients.

Because of the neuropathy, spinal fluid has been examined in many patients and may show an increase in cells, or an increased protein content, or both.

Treatment

The keystone of treatment is antitoxin, and the critical point in the use of anti-toxin is that the sooner it is used, the better the outcome (Table 85.5). Antitoxin is probably of no benefit if it is given more than 48 hr after the onset of the dis-ease. Since the antitoxin is horse serum, intradermal or conjunctival testing for hypersensitivity should be done before it is administered. If the testing for hyper-sensitivity is positive, then the patient must be desensitized. In any case, whether the testing is positive or negative, epinephrine should be present at the bedside because reactions are frequent. The dose and route of administration of the anti-toxin depend upon the severity of the disease; the patient should receive 20,000-100,000 U either intramuscularly or intravenously.

If the patient has symptoms or signs of myocarditis, he should be admitted to a cardiac care unit for careful fluid and electrolyte management, and given digi-talis preparations and antiarrhythmic agents as needed. A temporary pacemaker may be needed.

TABLE 85.4   Complications of Diphtheria

Complication	Incidence (% of Cases)	Mortality (%)
Myocarditis	10	50
Bronchopneumonia	8	70
Bulbar paralysis	4	20
Peripheral nerve palsies	2	15

TABLE 85.5   Dosage of Antitoxin in Treatment of Diphtheria

Clinical Situation (Location and Severity)	U/Kg Body Weight
Nasal or mild pharyngeal	500-1000
Moderately severe pharyngeal	1500
Severe pharyngeal	2000
Laryngobronchial	2500

Other supportive measures are physical therapy to prevent permanent complications of the neuropathy, tracheostomy, and bronchoscopy. Corticosteroids are unproved but usually are used in patients who are in danger of developing laryngeal obstruction.

Antibiotics are of less importance but should be used. Procaine penicillin, 600,000 U intramuscularly b.i.d. for 14 days, or erythromycin, 30-40 mg/kg/day for 14 days should be used. There have been no reports of organisms resistant to penicillin or erythromycin. Cephalosporins and penicillinase-resistant penicillins should not be used. One week after cessation of antibiotic therapy cultures should be taken to determine whether or not the patient has become a carrier. If the culture is positive then the patient should be treated with erythromycin.

Prognosis

The overall mortality has not changed in the past 50 years, and is about 5-15%. The prognosis depends upon the immune status of the patient, the toxigenicity of the organism, the anatomic location of the infection (Table 85.6), the age of the patient (Table 85.7), and coexisting illness. Myocardial involvement causes about half of the mortality and about 30% of patients with electrocardiographic changes will die. Atrioventricular or left bundle-branch blocks are particularly bad prognostic signs and are associated with a mortality of $\geq$ 60%.

The neuropathy is usually completely reversible in a matter of several weeks, but a few patients may be left with some residua.

TABLE 85.6   Area of Involvement and Mortality in Diphtheria

Region	% Total Cases	Mortality (%)
Tonsils-pharynx	60	2
Larynx	8	7
Nose	8	9
Bronchi	< 5	90

TABLE 85.7   Fatality Rate by Age

Age (yr)	Approximate Fatality Rate (%)
< 5	15
5-19	8
≥ 20	5

Immunity and Prevention

The protective antitoxin level is generally considered to be ≥ 0.01 U/ml serum, although some experts say even less than that level is sufficient. It is interesting that immunized individuals with negligible antitoxin levels still have less severe disease if they become infected. Very young children are usually protected by passive maternal antibody. Studies have shown that in the United States few adults over the age of 40 possess protective levels of antitoxin. In the past, when the disease was more common, adults were usually immune because they received natural boosting of their antibody titers.

The vaccine for diphtheria is formalin-detoxified toxin. It is quite effective but protection is *not* lifelong, and the duration of immunity is probably shorter than that following tetanus toxoid, the immunizing agent with which diphtheria toxoid is usually combined (Table 85.8). A common error is to not give the combined diphtheria-tetanus toxoids to adults but after a certain age, to give tetanus toxoid alone. A general rule is to always give the combination of tetanus and diphtheria toxoids. Although the ideal periodicity of diphtheria toxoid and tetanus toxoid boosting is different, this is probably neither immunologically nor clinically of any practical significance. Immunization does not prevent nasopharyngeal or skin carriage of the organism.

Recovery from the disease usually leaves the patient solidly immune, but because of exceptions to this, immunization of recovered patients should be carried out. It would appear that about 10% of survivors are at least partially susceptible.

The Schick test has been used to determine susceptibility (Table 85.9). A minute amount of toxin is injected intradermally. A local reaction, reaching maximum intensity in 4-7 days, is by convention called a positive test, but it means that the patient is not immune. No reaction means that the recipient has ≥ 0.0005 antitoxin U/ml of serum but probably ≥ 0.02 U. Some individuals develop a pseudopositive reaction which is caused by contaminants in the injected material and can be detected by a similar reaction to heat-inactivated toxin. Although there has been some controversy with respect to the meaning of a negative Schick test, for all intents and purposes over the years it has held up as an indication of immune status.

Epidemics can be controlled by immunization plus identification and antibiotic treatment of carriers. Quarantine has been shown to be ineffective.

TABLE 85.8   Immunization Against Diphtheria

Recommended for neonates	6 wk: DPT[1] 0.5 ml
	10 wk: DPT 0.5 ml
	14 wk: DPT 0.5 ml
	6-12 mo: DPT 0.5 ml
	5 yr: DT[2]
	At least every 10 yr: dT
If no previous immunization	
< 12 yr	Now: DT 0.5 ml
	In 6 wk: DT 0.5 ml
	In 6-12 mo: DT 0.5 ml
	At least every 10 yr: dT
> 12 yr	Now: dT[3] 0.5 ml
	In 6 wk: dT 0.5 ml
	In 6-12 mo: dT 0.5 ml
	At least every 10 yr: dT
Exposure to suspect case	
If no previous immunization	As above
Full course of primary immunization	
And booster in previous 10 yr	None
No booster in past 10 yr	0.5 ml dT

[1]DPT: diphtheria-pertussis-tetanus vaccine
[2]DT: pediatric diphtheria-tetanus vaccine
[3]dT: adult-type diphtheria-tetanus vaccine

TABLE 85.9   Schick Test

Antigen Injected				Reaction	Interpretation
Toxin		Toxoid			
36 hr	120 hr	36 hr	120 hr		
-	+	-	-	Positive	Not immune
-	-	-	-	Negative	Immune
+	-	+	-	Pseudo	Immune and allergic

Erythrasma

Erythrasma is a superficial skin infection characterized by slowly spreading, pruritic, reddish-brown macular patches which are finely scaled, wrinkled, and typically found in the genitocrural area, and caused by *C. minutissiumin*. The diagnosis can be made by seeing the organism on Gram stain of material obtained by placing a glass slide against a skin lesion, or by a coral-red fluorescence using a Wood's lamp. The lesions may be asymptomatic or cause fairly severe pruritus. Untreated, the disease may be chronic, with remissions and exacerbations. The differential diagnosis includes tinea versicolor and tinea cruris, candidiasis, contact dermatitis, intertrigo, and seborrheic dermatitis. Severe erythrasma may resemble psoriasis or discoid lupus. Patients should be treated with erythromycin, 1 g/day for 5-7 days. Treatment should not be continued until the lesions have completely cleared because this may take several weeks.

The disease is more common in tropical areas and in patients with diabetes or other debilitating illnesses.

Selected Bibliography

Boquet, P. and Pappenheimer, A. M., Jr.: Interaction of diphtheria toxin with mammalian cell membranes. *J Biol Chem* 251:5770-5778, 1976.

Brooks, G. F., Bennett, J. V., and Feldman, R. A.: Diphtheria in the United States, 1959-1970. *J Infect Dis* 129:172-178, 1974.

Carpenter, J. L. and Blom, J.: *Corynebacterium equi* pneumonia in a patient with Hodgkin's disease. *Am Rev Respir Dis* 114:235-239, 1976.

Collier, R. J.: Diphtheria toxin: Mode of action and structure. *Bacteriol Rev* 39:54-85, 1975.

Crossley, K., Irvine, P., Warren, J. B., Lee, B. K., and Mead, K.: Tetanus and diphtheria immunity in urban Minnesota adults. *JAMA* 242:2298-2300, 1979.

Edsall, G.: Passive immunity to diphtheria and tetanus in the newborn. *J Infect Dis* 134:314-315, 1976.

Gerry, J. L. and Greenough, W. B., III: Diphtheroid endocarditis: Report of nine cases and review of the literature. *Johns Hopkins Med J* 139:61-68, 1976.

Johnson, W. D. and Kaye, D.: Serious infections caused by diphtheroids. *Ann N Y Acad Sci* 174:568-576, 1970.

Koopman, J. S. and Campbell, J.: The role of cutaneous diphtheria infections in a diphtheria epidemic. *J Infect Dis* 131:239-244, 1975.

McCloskey, R. V., Eller, J. J., Green, M., Mauney, C. U., and Richards, S. E. M.: The 1970 epidemic of diphtheria in San Antonio. *Ann Intern Med* 75:495-503, 1971.

McCloskey, R. V., Green, M. J., Eller, J., and Smilack, J.: Treatment of diphtheria carriers: Benzathine penicillin, erythromycin, and clindamycin. *Ann Intern Med* 81:788-791, 1974.

Munford, R. S., Ory, H. W., Brooks, G. F., and Feldman, R. A.: Diphtheria deaths in the United States, 1959-1970. *JAMA* 229:1890-1893, 1974.

Nathenson, G. and Zakzewski, B.: Current status of passive immunity to diphtheria and tetanus in the newborn. *J Infect Dis* 133:199-201, 1976.

Nelson, L. A., Peri, B. A., Rieger, C. H. L., Newcomb, R. W., and Ruthberg, R. M.: Immunity to diphtheria in an urban population. *Pediatrics* 61:703-710, 1978.

Pappenheimer, A. M., Jr.: Diphtheria toxin. *Ann Rev Biochem* 46:69-94, 1977.

Pappenheimer, A. M., Jr. and Gill, D. M.: Diphtheria. Recent studies have clarified the molecular mechanisms involved in its pathogenesis. *Science* 182:353-358, 1973.

Pheifer, T. A., Forsyth, P. S., Durfee, M. A., Pollock, H. M., and Holmes, K. K.: Nonspecific vaginitis. Role of *Haemophilus vaginalis* and treatment with metronidazole. *N Engl J Med* 298:1429-1434, 1978.

Porschen, R. K., Goodman, Z., and Rafai, B.: Isolation of *Corynebacterium xerosis* from clinical specimens. *Am J Clin Pathol* 68:290-293, 1977.

Sarkany, I., Taplin, D., and Blank, H.: Incidence and bacteriology of erythrasma. *Arch Dermatol* 85:578-582, 1962.

Sarkany, I., Taplin, D., and Blank, H.: Organisms causing erythrasma. *Lancet* 2:304-305, 1962.

Sarkany, I., Taplin, D., and Blank, H.: The etiology and treatment of erythrasma. *J Invest Dermatol* 37:283-290, 1961.

Simmons, L. E., Abbott, J. D., Macaulay, M. E., Jones, A. E., Ironside, A. G., Mandal, B. K., Stanbridge, T. N., and Maximescu, P.: Diphtheria carriers in Manchester: Simultaneous infection with toxigenic and nontoxigenic mitis strains. *Lancet* 1:304-305, 1980.

Thompson, N. L. and Ellner, P. D.: Rapid determination of *Corynebacterium diphtheriae* toxigenicity by counterimmunoelectrophoresis. *J Clin Microbiol* 7:493-494, 1978.

Van Scoy, R. E., Cohen, S. N., Geraci, J. E., and Washington, J. A.: Coryneform bacterial endocarditis. Difficulties in diagnosis and treatment, presentation of three cases, and review of literature. *Mayo Clin Proc* 52:216-219, 1977.

Weiner, M. and Werthamer, S.: *Corynebacterium aquaticum* septicemia. *Am J Clin Pathol* 64:378-381, 1975.

Zalma, V. M., Older, J. J., and Brooks, G. F.: The Austin, Texas, diphtheria outbreak. Clinical and epidemiological aspects. *JAMA* 211:2125-2129, 1970.

86

LISTERIA
Robert H. Waldman, M.D.

The only species of *Listeria* that is pathogenic for humans is *L. monocytogenes*, so named because it caused a monocytic response in rabbits when they were experimentally infected. Interestingly, and a cause of some confusion, *L. monocytogenes* usually does not cause a monocytic peripheral leukocyte response in infected humans. *Listeria monocytogenes* is the prototype of the facultative, intracellular, opportunistic pathogen. It is generally of low virulence, infection being dependent upon the organism's ability to survive and replicate in host macrophages. Usually only people who have defective macrophage-killing capacity (discussed in more detail later) become infected with this organism.

Microbiology

Listeria monocytogenes is a gram-positive rod. This fact is important because it is the only organism with these characteristics that causes meningitis. It is weakly hemolytic and aerobic or microaerophilic. It is flagellated and optimally motile at 25°C or lower, an important distinguishing characteristic for identification in the microbiology laboratory.

A characteristic which has great clinical importance is that *Listeria* is commonly confused with diphtheroids which are frequent contaminants of bacterial cultures of various specimens. Therefore, the clinician must beware when the clinical laboratory informs him that a "contaminant" is thought to be a "diphtheroid." *Listeria* may be differentiated from diphtheroids in that the latter are club-shaped and form "Chinese figures." *Listeria* may also mimic diplococci in Gram stains of clinical specimens.

Listeria grows on blood agar as a translucent or gray colony, 1-2 mm in diameter and often surrounded by a small zone of β-hemolysis. There are several serotypes of *L. monocytogenes*.

Epidemiology

The organism is ubiquitous, widespread in the animal kingdom, and commonly isolated from poultry, livestock, pets, fish, as well as animal feeds and sewage. Despite this association with common animals, the infection is probably not a zoonosis, i.e., animal-to-human transmission rarely if ever occurs and in addition, most cases occur in urban residents.

Listeria monocytogenes is part of the normal intestinal flora in 0.5-5% of people. In the past, there has been some question as to whether or not the intestinal flora organisms are pathogenic, but they almost certainly are, and this is probably the source of infection in immunosuppressed patients. The organism is found in about one-fourth of healthy household contacts of patients with listeriosis.

The disease occurs sporadically, except for rare perinatal epidemics. Listeriosis is increasing in frequency, undoubtedly related to the general increase in infections caused by opportunistic organisms in immunosuppressed patients.

Pathology and Pathogenesis

The diseases caused by L. monocytogenes can be divided conveniently into two types. The first is perinatal, in which the infection is acquired in utero or during delivery. Infection commonly leads to stillbirth, with the babies showing the pathologic syndrome of granulomatous septicemia (disseminated miliary necrotizing granulomas, most intense in the liver). Newborns who acquire the organism during delivery may develop septicemia and/or meningitis. About one-fourth of all reported cases of listeriosis occur in newborns under 4 weeks of age (Table 86.1).

The second type of disease occurs in adults. In the past it has been stated that approximately one-half of these adult patients are immunologically normal, at least as far as the sensitivity of our immunologic measurements can determine. The proportion of normals who contract listeriosis is undoubtedly falling. Any patient who is immunosuppressed, either as a result of an underlying disease state, or secondary to a therapy which causes an impairment in host defenses, may develop listeriosis. However, the best correlation seems to be with patients who are receiving corticosteroids, most especially renal transplant patients. The most common manifestation is meningitis or other central nervous system infection such as cerebritis. Other manifestations of listeriosis are conjunctivitis, endocarditis, pneumonia, pyoderma, septicemia without meningitis, urethritis, and rectal abscess.

TABLE 86.1   Fatal Neonatal Listeriosis

% of Births	% of Perinatal Deaths
0.1-0.3	1.0-7.0

Diagnosis

Clinical

The most frequent symptoms are fever and various central nervous system disturbances. Most commonly, patients with listerial meningitis have an abrupt onset of their symptoms and rapid progression to coma. Usually the illness is similar to that caused by the pyogenic organisms, e.g., meningococcal meningitis, but the illness also may be more chronic.

Next to meningitis, the most common clinical syndrome is bacteremia without signs of central nervous system involvement. Other clinical presentations of listerial infection are endocarditis, peritonitis, polyserositis, and cutaneous infections.

Helpful clinical findings in newborns with granulomatous septicemia are whitish granulomas on mucous membranes and skin papules.

Laboratory

Spinal fluid findings are highly variable. The spinal fluid virtually always has an abnormal increase in cell count, but this may be predominantly polymorphonuclear or monocytic. The protein content of the spinal fluid is nearly always elevated, most commonly in the 100-300 mg/100 ml range. Identifying these organisms on a Gram stain is difficult, because the organisms are not easily seen, especially if one is not specifically looking for them. Most of the organisms are found intracellularly.

Culture of the organism from spinal fluid is also difficult because listeria is a fairly fastidious organism and also because, as mentioned earlier, the laboratory may discard it as a "diphtheroid contaminant."

The inflammatory response in humans, as manifested by a peripheral white count elevation, or cells in an infected area, is predominantly polymorphonuclear, but for reasons which are not understood, patients may show a lymphocytic response similar to that seen in infectious mononucleosis. Patients with listerial infection may also have a false-positive heterophil test, which has led in the past, to the erroneous conclusion that *L. monocytogenes* was the cause of infectious mononucleosis.

Treatment

The organism is sensitive in vitro to many antibiotics, including penicillin, ampicillin, erythromycin, cephalosporins, aminoglycosides, chloramphenicol, and tetracycline. Despite this sensitivity to cephalosporins, there is an interesting case report of a patient who developed the disease while taking cephalothin. Occasional strains have been isolated which appear to be resistant to one or more of the antibiotics. In vitro synergy has been shown between the penicillins and aminoglycosides. This has led to the suggestion that the combination therapy be used in the treatment of *L. monocytogenes* infection. Unfortunately, this, as well as other questions regarding the most efficacious therapy, has not been studied in controlled situations. The best we have are clinical impressions, usually based on a fairly small number of patients. Realizing these limitations, my recommendation is to use ampicillin, 400 mg/kg/day, for 2-4 weeks. In immunosuppressed patients, the longer course of therapy is recommended. In patients who are extremely ill, or who do not seem to be responding to ampicillin, an aminoglycoside should be added to the regimen. In patients who are allergic to penicillin, tetra-cycline, or erythromycin should be used.

A particularly difficult question is whether or not immunosuppressive therapy should be continued in a patient infected with *L. monocytogenes*. This question commonly arises in a patient who has received a renal transplant. Since there certainly have been "cures" of patients continuing to receive their immunosup-pressive therapy, if the patient is not extremely ill an attempt should be made to treat the patient while continuing the immunosuppressive therapy.

Prognosis and Complications

Untreated, nearly 100% of the patients die of the infection. With antibiotic treatment, the mortality has been reduced to 20-33%. A poor prognosis corre-lates with lower spinal fluid glucose levels. A 100% survival can be expected in patients who have an initial spinal fluid glucose concentration of greater than 40 mg/100 ml. Survivors rarely have permanent sequelae.

Recently reported complications of *L. monocytogenes* meningitis include re-lapse or cerebritis in renal transplant patients. Cerebritis is the earliest clinical stage of inflammation of the brain, before the accumulation of macroscopic pus. Patients develop fever, focal neurologic signs, positive technetium scintiscans (frontal and/or parietal lobes), but usually have a negative computerized axial tomography scan. The spinal fluid may be normal, but blood cultures are usually positive. About one-third of transplant patients who are treated less than 3 weeks for their original *L. monocytogenes* meningitis will relapse. These observations are the basis for the recommendation of prolonged therapy for *L. monocytogenes* meningitis in transplant patients.

Immunology and Prevention

Infection with *L. monocytogenes* in animal models is the prototype for study of cell-mediated immunity and the function of the activated macrophage. The ac-tivated macrophage possesses enhanced ability to phagocytize and destroy intra-cellular pathogens. This appears to apply to the human situation as well, since listeriosis occurs in patients with diseases, or receiving therapy, that interfere with T-lymphocyte and/or macrophage function.

Selected Bibliography

Etheredge, E. E., Light, J. A., Perloff, L. J., et al.: *Listeria monocytogenes* men-ingitis in a transplant recipient. *JAMA* 234:78-79, 1975.

Gantz, N. M., Myerowiitz, R. C., Medeiros, A. A., et al.: Listeriosis in immuno-suppressed patients: A cluster of 8 cases. *Am J Med* 58:637-643, 1975.

Isiadinso, O.: *Listeria* sepsis and meningitis: A complication of renal transplanta-tion. *JAMA* 234:842-843, 1975.

Lavertter, A., Leedom, J. M., Mathies, A. W., Ivler, D., and Wehrle, P. F.: Men-ingitis due to *Listeria monocytogenes:* A review of 25 cases. *N Engl J Med* 285:598-603, 1971.

Macnair, D. R., White, J. E., and Graham, J. M.: Ampicillin in the treatment of *Listeria monocytogenes* meningitis. *Lancet* 1:16–17, 1968.

Mangi, R. J., Kundargi, R. S., Quintiliani, R., and Andriole, V. T.: Development of meningitis during cephalothin therapy. *Ann Intern Med* 78:347, 1973.

Medoff, G., Kunz, L. J., and Weinberg, A. N.: Listeriosis in humans: An evaluation. *J Infect Dis* 123:247–250, 1971.

Schroter, G. P. J.: *Listeria monocytogenes* and encephalitis. *Arch Intern Med* 138:198–199, 1978.

Watson, G. W., Fuller, T. J., Elms, J., and Kluge, R.M.: *Listeria* cerebritis. *Arch Intern Med* 138:83–87, 1978.

87

CLOSTRIDIA
Roger G. Finch, M.B.

Definition

Clostridia are ubiquitous, spore-forming, anaerobic bacteria. Although frequently present in the gut and on mucosal surfaces of man and animals they are predominantly involved in the putrefaction of plant and animal matter in nature. There are 63 recognized species of which about 30 have been associated with human infections. Clostridia have anaerobic or microaerophilic growth requirements, are proteolytic and saccharolytic, and produce several toxins and enzymes, which include some of the most lethal substances known.

Tetanus, botulism, and gas gangrene are among the most feared of clostridial diseases, although clostridial gastrointestinal intoxications are much more common. Tetanus, gas gangrene, and the rarer wound botulism are true infections which contrast with food-associated botulism and *Clostridium perfringens* food poisoning which are intoxications.

Microbiology

Clostridia are large, gram-positive, anaerobic or microaerophilic bacilli that form endospores. All strains pathogenic to man are motile with the exception of *C. perfringens,* and all strains, except *C. perfringens* and *C. butyricum,* are unencapsulated.

Growth requirements vary considerably. *Clostridium tetani* is a strict anaerobe, while *C. perfringens* is less fastidious, and *C. histolyticum* will grow poorly in air (microaerophilic). The absence of cytochromes and the inability to produce catalases or peroxidases reflect their anaerobic metabolism. Both spores and vegetative bacilli require a reduced environment for multiplication thus explaining their natural habitat and the circumstances under which they produce human disease.

The spores are refractile, larger than the parent bacillus, and fail to stain by the Gram method. Terminal spores are typical of *C. tetani,* but in other species they are central or subterminal in position. Spores resist drying, heat, and some common disinfectants. The spores of *C. tetani* have been known to survive for 10 years and still germinate.

A wide variety of enzymes and toxins are produced by the clostridia. These are frequently described both by their action and by a letter of the Greek alphabet. Table 87.1 illustrates several of the enzymes and exotoxins produced by *C. perfringens,* which is the most commonly isolated member of the genus. Of these enzymes and exotoxins, *C. perfringens* α-toxin (lecithinase) is responsible for much of the cytotoxicity associated with gas gangrene. Two other toxins, *tetanospasmin* and *botulinum toxin,* are the cause of tetanus and botulism, respectively, and will be discussed later.

Isolation of clostridia on fresh blood agar can be achieved at 37°C in an oxygen-free atmosphere. Thioglycolate and cooked meat broth are suitable broth media. The colonial appearance of many clostridia is irregular with a tendency to spread over the surface of solid media. On the other hand, *C. perfringens* shows characteristic smooth, convex colonies, 2-4 mm in diameter, with a double zone of hemolysis on blood agar. *Clostridium tetani,* although difficult to isolate, produces a fine film over the surface of solid media.

Speciation is dependent upon the ability of the organism to denature proteins such as milk (proteolysis), or carbohydrates such as glucose, maltose, lactose, and sucrose (saccharolysis). Further information can be gained from the ability to hydrolyze gelatin and from gas chromatographic studies.

It is useful to demonstrate toxin production for strains of *C. perfringens, C. tetani,* and *C. botulinum.* Lecithinase production (α-toxin) can be recognized in vitro using lecithin agar. Antitoxin added to the agar surface of one-half of the plate inhibits the action of the toxin on lecithin (Nagler reaction). *Botulinum toxin* and *tetanospasmin* are lethal to mice and can be demonstrated in unprotected animals using antitoxin-protected animals and heat-inactivated toxin as controls.

Epidemiology

Clostridium tetani

The spores of *C. tetani* are present in the soil, house and hospital dust, and feces of animals, but rarely of humans. To produce disease the spores must gain entry into the tissues and germinate. This requires a reduction in tissue oxygen brought about by tissue enzymes, ischemia, or the presence of other bacteria. These circumstances are met by surgical or accidental trauma, such as lacerations, burns, compound fractures, gunshot wounds, criminal abortions, and ethnic practices associated with smearing animal dung over the severed umbilical cord of newborns. In recent years, shared contaminated narcotic drugs, needles, and syringes have been associated with tetanus among addicts. However, many patients develop tetanus in the absence of known trauma. There may be only minor evidence of past injury, such as a penetrating injury from a thorn.

In the United States the majority of the population is immunized and this is reflected in the declining incidence of tetanus to less than 200 cases each year. The majority of these occur during the spring and summer months. The overall

TABLE 87.1   Selected C. *perfringens* Toxins Indicating Their Effect or Enzymatic Action and Their Distribution Among Strains

Action or Enzyme	Toxin								
	Alpha	Beta	Delta	Epsilon	Theta	Iota	Kappa	Mu	Nu
Capillary permeability	+					+			
Collagenase							+		
Deoxyribonuclease									+
Gut permeability			+	+					
Hemolytic	+		+		+				
Hyaluronidase								+	
Lecithinase	+								
Necrotizing	+	+		+	+	+			
Neurotoxic		±							
Produced by C. *perfringens* types	ABCDE	BC	BC	BD	ABCDE	E	ABCDE	ABCDE	ABCDE

incidence of neonatal tetanus is about 2/1 million live births with the highest incidence among blacks. The mortality is extremely high both in neonatal tetanus and in patients over 50 years of age who develop tetanus.

Clostridium botulinum

Spores of *C. botulinum* are widely distributed in soil, inland lakes and sea beds, on vegetation, and in the intestinal tract of birds, fish, and mammals. Botulism is most commonly associated with home-preserved foods such as meat, fish, fruit, and vegetables. Commercial products are rarer sources, but canned tuna fish, peppers, and mushrooms have all produced outbreaks of botulism. Inadequate sterilization or a leaking container are responsible for the presence of spores which on germination and lysis intoxicate the food. The food may or may not show evidence of spoilage dependent upon the particular type of *C. botulinum*.

From 1899 to 1977, 766 outbreaks of botulism have been reported in the United States involving 1961 persons of whom 999 died. A mortality of 60% was common in the past although improved medical management has reduced this to 15.7% for the period 1970-1977. Type A, B, E, and F toxins are associated with human disease (Table 87.2) Type A predominates and is seen most frequently in outbreaks from the western United States. Type E is seen more frequently in Canada, Japan, and Scandinavia, whereas type B accounts for most European outbreaks. Types C and D botulism produce disease in cattle and fowl. Rarely botulism may follow contamination of a wound or laceration.

Histotoxic Clostridial Infections

Histotoxic clostridial infections include *gas gangrene* (myonecrosis) and *clostridial cellulitis*. The histotoxic infections are differentiated from the more common clostridial food poisoning.

Gas gangrene follows the introduction of clostridial spores into ischemic and devitalized tissues. These spores are widely distributed but are particularly plentiful in fertile soil. They are also occasionally present in the gastrointestinal and female genital tract.

Gas gangrene is usually traumatic in origin and classically is associated with war wounds such as penetrating injuries, bullet and shrapnel wounds, and compound fractures. An estimated 10% of wounds in World War I and 1% in World War II developed gas gangrene. In peacetime gas gangrene fortunately occurs in less than 0.1% of traumatic or postoperative wounds. Gas gangrene of the uterus is uncommon now that criminal abortions are less frequent.

TABLE 87.2   Human Botulism

Toxin Type	Geographical Site of Outbreak
A	USA, USSR
B	USA, Northern Europe, USSR
E	Northern Europe, Canada, USA, Japan, USSR
F	Denmark, USA

Clostridial cellulitis follows infection of tissues rendered ischemic and devitalized by accidental or surgical trauma. The infection is not uncommonly polymicrobial with anaerobic streptococci or facultative gram-negative bacteria also present. Although fascial planes are invaded and gas is produced, myonecrosis is absent and toxin production is minimal.

Simple contamination of wounds by pathogenic clostridia is fairly common yet most will heal without significant sequelae. From time to time clostridial bacteremia is recognized in association with such varying states as septic abortion, pneumonia in alcoholics, and gastroenteritis. It is noteworthy for the absence of significant constitutional symptoms and probably represents colonization of the mucosal surfaces from which the clostridia gain access to the blood.

Food Poisoning

In contrast to the histotoxic clostridial infections which are relatively uncommon, clostridia are second only to staphylococci as a bacterial cause of food poisoning. Illness develops within 12-24 hr and is the result of ingestion of contaminated food. Toxin is produced from lysis of the remnants of vegetative bacilli that have undergone sporulation in the gut lumen. The spores are heat-resistant and survive the cooking process. Gravies, meats, and stews that have been allowed to stand at room temperature for several hours are the foods most commonly associated with illness. Most outbreaks of *C. perfringens* food poisoning are caused by type A strains.

Enteritis necroticans is caused by toxin-producing type C strains of *C. perfringens*. The disease was prevalent in Germany following World War II but is now mainly confined to Papua New Guinea where it is called *pig-bel*. Illness follows the ingestion of infected pork during ritual native feasts. The disease is severe, producing abdominal pain, bloody diarrhea, dehydration, and the small bowel may become gangrenous, resulting in toxemia, shock, and death.

Pathogenesis and Pathology

Tetanus

Tetanus is caused by the neurotoxin, *tetanospasmin,* which is released from the vegetative bacilli of *C. tetani* when they lyse. To produce vegetative forms the spores must germinate in an environment of low oxygen tension. Lacerations, abrasions, compound fractures, and burns which have been inadequately debrided and contain foreign bodies and devitalized tissues provide an ideal environment for germination. Tetanus may complicate the most trivial of wounds, and spores can remain dormant in tissues for several years. Infection with *C. tetani* remains localized with minimal effects, no suppuration, and no progression to gangrene. Once released, *tetanospasmin* travels centrally up the peripheral nerves by a process of retrograde intraaxonal transport. Lymphatic and blood-borne spread probably plays only a minor role. In experimental trials the rate of transportation has been shown to be 0.5-3.0 mm/hr. Once the central nervous system is reached *tetanospasmin* becomes fixed to gangliosides and acts on the presynaptic junctions thereby impairing the release of inhibitory neurotransmitters, such as γ-aminobutyric acid and acetylcholine. This leads to hyperactivity of the motor neurons of the spinal cord and brain stem with subsequent local and generalized hyperreflexia and muscle spasm.

Botulism

Botulism is caused by any one of six antigenically distinct toxins (A–F) which are relatively heat-labile requiring about 10 min at 100°C for inactivation. Human disease has not been reported with types C or D. The toxin is absorbed from mucosal surfaces or wounds and is not inactivated by gastric acid or gastrointestinal enzymes. Once absorbed the toxin is transported via the blood and lymphatics to the nervous system, where it becomes fixed to the presynaptic terminals of cholinergic nerve fibers, thereby blocking the release of acetylcholine and interfering with motor nerve function, although nerve conduction remains intact. The brain stem nuclei are affected to a greater degree than those of spinal origin. There is considerable interspecies variation in the lethality of botulinum toxin. Part of this difference is related to differences in affinity of the toxins for nervous tissue.

The development of type-specific antitoxin plays no role in the clinical recovery from botulism since the dose of toxin required to produce an antibody response is lethal. Hence the administration of polyvalent antitoxin plays a vital role in the management of botulism.

Wound botulism differs from food-associated disease by the necessity for germination and multiplication of C. botulinum in the tissues. It is a true infection.

Histotoxic Clostridial Infection

Clostridial spores will not germinate in tissues with a normal oxygen concentration. If the reduction-oxidation potential is lowered germination occurs. Such conditions are found in ischemia following either traumatic interruption or compression of the blood supply by hematoma, edema, foreign body, or the ischemia of small-vessel disease as occurs in diabetes mellitus. The histotoxic exoenzymes and toxins allow rapid spread along fascial planes with gas formation and myonecrosis, which is the hallmark of gas gangrene. Lecithinase (α-toxin) is the most virulent of the toxins produced by C. perfringens (see Table 87.1) and acts on cell membranes to produce myonecrosis and hemolysis. Proteolysis, fermentation, and gas production further disrupt tissues causing necrosis, compression of blood vessels, and an extension of the hypoxic environment. Bacteremia and toxemia progress rapidly to shock, renal failure, and if not reversed, death. Macroscopically the muscles involved are swollen, ischemic, and gray to purple. The exudate contains numerous gram-positive bacilli but few pus cells, reflecting the destructive action of toxins on these cells.

Clostridial Food Poisoning

C. perfringens type A toxin is heat-labile, although the spores are relatively heat-stable, and is responsible for food-associated clostridial disease. Illness follows ingestion of food such as meat dishes and gravies which have been contaminated either before or after cooking. Slow cooling at room temperature provides suitable anaerobic conditions for C. perfringens to multiply. Once swallowed further multiplication and then sporulation occur in the small bowel. As sporulation occurs the toxin is produced and released into the lumen of the gut as the remnants of the vegetative bacilli lyse. Symptoms occur from 8 to 24 hr after ingestion. Type A toxin causes fluid accumulation in the gut lumen and diarrhea.

Food poisoning by C. perfringens differs from that caused by Staphylococcus aureus since the enterotoxin is not preformed and requires bacterial multiplication to take place in the bowel following ingestion.

Diagnostic Features

Tetanus

Clinical

Tetanus is a clinical diagnosis and takes the form of (1) *generalized* tetanus or (2) the much rarer *local* tetanus. In *generalized tetanus* there is initially restlessness, irritability, mild fever, and headache. The patient remains alert unless the level of consciousness is impaired by complications or treatment. *Generalized tetanus* is often first manifested by muscular spasm producing trismus or "lockjaw," while in the neonate lethargy, difficulty sucking, weakness, poor cry, loss of hand control, weak gag reflex, and ophthalmoplegia are most prominent. Progressive muscle spasms involve much of the voluntary musculature and produce characteristic spasms of the facial musculature (*risus sardonicus)*, arching of the trunk (*opisthotonus)*, neck stiffness, and board-like abdominal rigidity. Spasms increase in frequency and duration from a few seconds to several minutes and become progressively more painful and exhausting. They are triggered by a variety of internal and external stimuli such as coughing, movement, distension of bowel or bladder, noise, light, or drafts. The severity of the disease is inversely proportional to the length of incubation. The most severe cases develop symptoms within 3 days and the milder cases more than 14 days following the initial injury.

Local tetanus produces muscle spasm in the area adjacent to the wound. Muscle spasms are frequently mild but can persist for several weeks before subsiding. Only rarely do symptoms become generalized.

Another rare variety of local tetanus is *cephalic tetanus* where craniofacial injury produces tetanic involvement of the cranial nerves. The facial nerve is most frequently involved with resulting trismus. The incubation period is short, and mortality is high.

Autonomic nervous system dysfunction often accompanies severe forms of tetanus and, in recent years, has been a feature of tetanus seen among drug addicts. Labile blood pressure, sweating, vasoconstriction, tachycardia, cardiac dysrhythmias, and cardiac arrest are all recognized. Hyperpyrexia may complicate the hypermetabolic state that is the consequence of both muscular overactivity and increased sympathetic activity.

Laboratory

Clostridium tetani is a strict anaerobe and is isolated from only about one-third of patients with tetanus. Wounds positive by culture for *C. tetani* do not automatically progress to tetanus, which essentially remains a clinical diagnosis.

The cerebrospinal fluid is usually normal and the EEG and EMG are diagnostically unhelpful. There is often a mild to moderate leukocytosis.

Botulism

Clinical

Symptoms and signs develop 12-36 hr after food ingestion, although the incubation period ranges from a few hours to about a week according to the amount of toxin consumed. The essential features of botulism are those of a rapidly progressive symmetric impairment of cranial nerve function producing diplopia, dysphagia, and dysarthria, with descending motor weakness or paralysis. The pupils are fixed and dilated, and nystagmus is common. There are no sensory changes and the sensorium remains clear. Gastrointestinal symptoms of nausea, vomiting, dry mouth, abdominal cramps, and distension are frequent, particularly with type E toxin. Retention of urine is common. The pulse is normal or slow unless hypotension develops, and the temperature is not elevated in the absence of infective complications. This constellation of features occurring in more than a single individual points to a common source and should readily suggest the diagnosis. However, there is considerable variability in the rate of onset and severity of symptoms dependent upon the amount of toxin swallowed.

Laboratory

Routine hematologic and biochemical tests are normal unless complications develop. The ECG may show nonspecific ST and T wave changes. The identification of botulinum toxin in the serum or the contaminated food is the only definitive means of laboratory confirmation. A portion of the food should be kept refrigerated until tested using unprotected and antitoxin-protected mice in which serum or an aqueous extract of the food is injected intraperitoneally. Heat-inactivated samples are used as controls. Pretreatment of the test samples with trypsin enhances the virulence of toxins, particularly type E. Paralysis and death of the mice occur from a few hours to 5 days following injection. Contaminated food can also be subcultured anaerobically. Prior heat treatment of a sample may increase the chance of isolation by eliminating contaminating bacteria. All isolates should be tested for toxin production.

Histotoxic Clostridial Infections

Clinical

    Gas Gangrene

The clinical features of gas gangrene reflect the systemic toxemia and local effects of gas-producing myonecrosis of a surgically or traumatically contaminated wound. Symptoms develop rapidly within a few hours to a few days. Anxiety, restlessness, fever, and tachycardia may be rapidly followed by hypotension, oliguric renal failure, and death. Hemolysis and hemoglobinuria can be profound. The wound becomes characteristically painful, tense, and swollen, with bronze discoloration of the skin, and later bleb formation containing purplish fluid and accompanied by crepitus. The underlying muscle becomes pale, necrotic, and gangrenous.

    Uterine gas gangrene is frequently the result of criminal abortions although it may complicate prolonged labor or premature rupture of the membranes. There is a watery foul smelling vaginal discharge in addition to the features of systemic toxemia.

    Clostridial Cellulitis

In contrast to gas gangrene clostridial cellulitis is of gradual onset with less local pain and swelling and little toxemia. Gas may be detected in the subcutaneous tissues as infection tracts along fascial planes. The muscles are not involved.

    Simple Clostridial Wound Contamination

Surgical or traumatic wounds may yield a variety of clostridial species on culture yet there are no features to suggest histotoxicity. A positive culture finding does not indicate that treatment is required although the wound should be carefully inspected and debrided if necessary.

Laboratory

Gas Gangrene

A Gram stain of the exudate will show the presence of numerous typical gram-positive bacilli with few polymorphonuclear leukocytes. Most cases of gas gangrene are caused by *C. perfringens* which grows readily on blood agar under anaerobic conditions. Blood cultures also may be positive.

Gas in the tissues can be demonstrated roentgenographically. Intravascular hemolysis and hemoglobinuria may be detected. A peripheral leukocytosis is common.

Clostridial Cellulitis

The Gram stain and culture of the exudate will reveal the presence of a *Clostridium* sp. Blood cultures may also be positive as are the soft-tissue x-rays for gas.

Differential Diagnosis

Tetanus

Strychnine poisoning is the only condition that might be confused with tetanus. Trismus may complicate a variety of orodental infections such as a dental abscess and Ludwig's angina. Neck stiffness may suggest a pyogenic meningitis which can be excluded by examination of the cerebrospinal fluid. Rabies generally produces difficulties with swallowing and respiration and a history of an animal bite may be forthcoming. The immune history of the patient is helpful since tetanus is uncommon in a fully immunized patient.

Tetany and hysteria may mimic tetanus initially, while phenothiazines may produce trismus.

Botulism

Isolated attacks of botulism can be confused with the Guillain-Barré syndrome, encephalitis, or stroke. However the bilateral symmetry and absent sensory changes should help differentiate botulism from these conditions. Acute myasthenia gravis will be accompanied by muscle fatigue and respond to edrophonium, chloride. Several chemical intoxications should be considered, including methyl alcohol, organic phosphorus compounds, and atropine overdose which produces a dry mouth and dilated pupils. The dry mouth may result in a sore throat which may suggest diphtheria. Severe forms of paralytic fish and shellfish poisoning produce ataxia, bulbar and respiratory paralysis, and marked paresthesias, which differentiate them from botulism.

When the abdominal symptoms are severe acute gastrointestinal infections, intoxications, and acute abdominal surgical conditions require consideration.

Histotoxic Clostridial Infections (Table 87.3)

The profound toxemia and rapid progression of the disease are the main features that differentiate clostridial gas gangrene from streptococcal myonecrosis. A Gram stain of the exudate is also helpful in differentiating the two conditions.

TABLE 87.3   Causes of Gas in Soft Tissues

Clostridium spp

E. coli

Klebsiella spp

Peptostreptococcus spp

Bacteroides spp

Fusobacterium spp

S. pyogenes

Mixed bacteria: facultative and anaerobic species

Noninfectious: e.g., trapped air following trauma or surgery

Meleney's synergistic gangrene is a rare complication of trauma or surgery. The gangrenous process is superficial, slowly progressive, and without systemic symptoms, although severe local pain is characteristic. Bacteriologically there is a mixture of anaerobic cocci with facultative anaerobes such as *S. aureus, Streptococcus pyogenes* and coliforms.

Clostridial cellulitis must be differentiated from *necrotizing fasciitis* and a condition similar to Meleney's synergistic gangrene, *synergistic necrotizing cellulitis*. These conditions are more acute than Meleney's infection with marked systemic symptoms and higher mortality. Both are complicated by gas formation and on culture yield a mixture of anaerobic cocci, *Bacteroides,* and Enterobacteriaceae.

Finally *nonclostridial crepitant cellulitis* may result from any gas-forming organism and is seen in association with *Escherichia coli, Klebsiella, Bacteroides* and peptostreptococci, often in mixed culture. This form of cellulitis is often seen in patients with diabetes mellitus.

Treatment

Tetanus

Treatment is directed toward removal of the source of *tetanospasmin* by wound debridement, neutralization of unfixed circulating toxin, and supportive care during the period required for fixed toxin to be metabolized.

The initiating wound, which may be trivial or inconspicuous, should be surgically debrided of all devitalized tissue and foreign material, followed by irrigation of the open wound with hydrogen peroxide. Antibiotic therapy plays a minor role but penicillin G by intravenous injection is usually prescribed. Tetracycline is an alternative drug in patients allergic to penicillin.

Human tetanus immune globulin (TIG) should be given as soon as the diagnosis is made: 3000-10,000 U are given intramuscularly in divided sites as a single dose.

Supportive measures require both intensive medical and nursing care. Muscle spasms can be minimized by reducing external stimulation from light, noise, cold, and pain, but if frequent and severe may necessitate control with diazepam or curare and intermittent positive pressure ventilation. Intubation has the added advantage of protecting the airway which may be threatened by trismus, laryngeal spasm, and aspiration secondary to dysphagia. Tracheostomy may be necessary.

Attention to fluid balance and the nutritional state is essential. Autonomic disturbances demand careful monitoring with close attention paid to the blood pressure, cardiac rate and rhythm, and body temperature.

Botulism

The treatment of botulism is directed toward (1) elimination of any nonabsorbed toxin, (2) neutralization of unfixed toxin, (3) maintaining body functions during the period necessary for the metabolism of fixed toxin.

Symptoms generally develop within 12-36 hr following the ingestion of contaminated food. The shorter the incubation period the worse the illness and higher the mortality. It is therefore appropriate to attempt gastric lavage and purgation, in an attempt to eliminate any residual unabsorbed toxin.

Specific antitoxin is of proven efficacy, particularly with type E botulism. Two preparations are available, a trivalent antitoxin (ABE) and a polyvalent antitoxin (ABCDEF). Both are available from the Centers for Disease Control, Atlanta. They are of equine origin, and hence test doses and precautions against serum sickness should be used. When treating botulism one vial (8 ml) of trivalent antitoxin is injected intravenously and another vial intramuscularly. This dose is often repeated after 2-4 hr. Each vial contains 7500 U type A, 5500 U type B, and 8500 U of type E antitoxins.

Bulbar involvement leading to respiratory failure is the immediate life-threatening problem and demands constant monitoring of cardiorespiratory function with early tracheostomy and artificial ventilation. Penicillin is occasionally recommended to eliminate C. botulinum that was ingested with the food. Another drug that is occasionally used is guanidine, which increases acetylcholine release; its use has been associated with some clinical and electromyographic evidence for improvement.

Histotoxic Clostridial Infections

Early and thorough debridement of all infected, ischemic, or necrotic tissue, and the removal of all foreign material, is the mainstay of the management of gas gangrene. Such debridement may demand amputation of a limb or hysterectomy as a lifesaving maneuver.

High-dose, parenteral benzylpenicillin (10-20 million U/day) is administered to eliminate residual clostridial multiplication. Polyvalent equine antitoxin is of unproven value but may be given early in the disease: 40,000 U of either trivalent or pentavalent antitoxin is given intravenously and repeated at 4- to 6-hr intervals with due precautions against hypersensitivity reactions. Hyperbaric oxygen at 3 atms has been used at selected centers to limit the degree of tissue requiring debridement. Clinical improvement can be dramatic, although the need for debridement frequently remains and should not be delayed if clinical deterioration persists. In addition to these specific forms of management general supportive measures directed at maintaining blood pressure and renal function should not be ignored.

Clostridial cellulitis also requires adequate surgical debridement which is frequently less extensive than that needed in gas gangrene. Penicillin should be given to eliminate vegetative clostridia.

Immunology and Prevention

Tetanus

An attack of tetanus does not provide immunity against future infection. Tetanus toxoid is formalin-inactivated toxin and can be used untreated, precipitated, or adsorbed with alum, aluminum phosphate, or aluminum hydroxide. Adsorbed toxoid is a more effective immunizing agent. Routine immunization of infants is begun at 1-3 months of age when tetanus toxoid is given in combination with diphtheria and pertussis vaccine (DPT). Three doses at intervals of 4-6 weeks with booster doses 1 and 4 years later are recommended. Booster doses at 10-year intervals will maintain effective immunity throughout life. Serum levels of antitoxin in excess of 0.01 U/ml are considered protective and are detectable within 1 month following immunization and persist for 10 years.

Adverse reactions to tetanus toxoid are infrequent but include local reactions, urticaria (with or without angioneurotic edema), and rarely serum sickness and peripheral neuropathy. Reactions are uncommon in childhood but increase with age. They are more common in women and in those individuals who are overimmunized. Although plain toxoid is less reactogenic, it is also less immunogenic than the aluminum-adsorbed preparation. Reactions are less frequent if the vaccine is given by intramuscular injection.

One of the main factors in the prevention of tetanus is the prompt treatment of contaminated or potentially contaminated wounds and the assessment of the immune status of the injured person (Table 87.4). All wounds should receive prompt surgical toilet. Provided the wound is clean and minor and tissue damage

TABLE 87.4   Tetanus Immunoprophylaxis

Immunization History (Number of Doses)	Clean, Minor Wounds		All Other Wounds	
	Toxoid	TIG[1]	Toxoid	TIG
Uncertain	+	−	+	+
0-1	+	−	+	+
2	+	−	+	±[2]
3 or more	±[3]	−	±[4]	−

[1]TIG = tetanus immune globulin of human origin

[2]Only if wound is more than 24 hr old

[3]Only if more than 10 yr since last dose

[4]Only if more than 5 yr since last dose

is negligible, immunoprophylaxis should be restricted to a complete course of tetanus toxoid in the nonimmune, one or more doses to complete a course, or a single booster dose in those whose last dose was more than 10 years earlier. Tetanus immune globulin is not necessary. For all other wounds, in particular those that are contaminated, frankly infected, or have devitalized tissue or foreign material present, immunoprophylaxis should include both tetanus toxoid and passive protection with human tetanus immunoglobulin 250 U intramuscularly for the nonimmune, those with uncertain immune status, those with only a previous single dose of toxoid, and those whose wounds are older than 24 hr and have received only two previous doses of tetanus toxoid.

Human tetanus immunoglobulin has a half-life of about 25 days and provides protective levels of antitoxin (> 0.01 U/ml) for 4 weeks.

Patients who have suffered an attack of tetanus should be actively immunized. This can be effectively started during hospitalization since the therapeutic use of human tetanus immunoglobulin does not appear to interfere with the immune response to tetanus toxoid.

Botulism

Once botulism has been diagnosed early notification is essential to identify the source of the disease. Commercially prepared food requires batch identification and recall and a thorough investigation into the processing and canning procedures. Botulism associated with domestic bottling or canning of foodstuffs can only be prevented by constant education and awareness of the hazards of inadequate or faulty sterilization.

Wound botulism, although rare, emphasizes the need for thorough cleansing and debridement of all potentially infected wounds.

Great care should be observed in the laboratory-handling of all materials suspected of containing *C. botulinum* toxin. Ingestion, inhalation, or absorption through the eye or a break in the skin may prove fatal. Polyvalent botulinal toxoid is available from the Centers for Disease Control, Atlanta, for the active immunization of laboratory staff handling intoxicated material.

Histotoxic Clostridial Infection

Gas gangrene can only be effectively prevented by the thorough cleansing and removal of devitalized and foreign material from a contaminated wound. Antibiotics or antitoxin used prophylactically have no role to play.

Gas gangrene may complicate elective surgical procedures, most notably lower limb amputation for ischemic disease such as occurs in association with diabetes mellitus. Disease appears to result from fecal contamination of the skin infecting relatively ischemic stumps. In addition to sporicidal skin preparations, prophylactic penicillin G is recommended by some authorities to cover the perioperative and immediate postoperative period in these patients.

Clostridial Food Poisoning

The prevention of food poisoning is dependent upon a high standard of hygiene in individuals concerned with the preparation of food. Adequate cooking and sufficient refrigeration space should be available to permit storage of foods if they are to be kept for more than a few hours. Storage of meats, stews, and sauces at room temperature provides circumstances for the germination of microbes including *C. perfringens* and should be avoided.

Complications and Prognosis

Tetanus

The overall mortality exceeds 50%, although in specialist centers it is less than 10%. Neonates and persons over 50 years have the worst prognosis. The clinical course and severity also permit the prognostic division of tetanus into *mild, moderate,* and *severe* categories. (1) *Mild* attacks have an incubation period of more than 14 days and a slow onset of symptoms. Trismus is present but dysphagia is absent and generalized spasms if present are mild and short-lived. (2) *Moderate* attacks have an incubation period ranging from 10 to 14 days, although symptoms develop over 3-6 days. Trismus is marked, dysphagia is usually present and reflex spasms are more frequent and severe. (3) *Severe* attacks have an incubation period of less than 10 days and symptoms develop rapidly in less than 3 days. Dysphagia is severe, muscle spasms are frequent and violent, and cyanosis often occurs. Death results from asphyxiation, secondary atelectasis, aspiration pneumonia, bronchopneumonia or pulmonary embolus. Other complications include fecal impaction, urinary retention, acute gastric ulcers, and decubiti, in addition to the problems attendant upon prolonged intensive care and ventilatory support. Muscle spasms may be sufficiently violent to produce rupture of muscles.

Botulism

The case-fatality rate has fallen steadily over the years. For the period 1970-1979 it was 15.7%. This decline reflects improved medical care with ventilatory support and the prompt use of antitoxin. In general the severity of the illness reflects the quantity of toxin ingested. Mortality is high in infant botulism, in the elderly, and in those with type E botulism. The main complications are the result of the progressive bulbar paralysis producing respiratory failure and dysphagia. Aspiration pneumonia, bronchopneumonia and atelectasis, and cardiac arrhythmias may complicate the illness. Prolonged ventilatory support may be required; periods up to 88 days resulting in a successful outcome have been recorded.

Histotoxic Clostridial Infection

The major factor determining the outcome in gas gangrene is the time from onset to diagnosis and from diagnosis to adequate debridement. The fulminant nature of gas gangrene must be appreciated if survival is to be improved. In addition to the local effects of gas gangrene, severe toxemia can precipitate hypotension, shock, and acute renal failure (secondary to acute tubular necrosis or to bilateral cortical necrosis). Intravascular hemolysis, hemoglobinemia, and hemoglobinuria may be profound. Mortality due primarily to overwhelming infections is less than 10%, although overall mortality from gas gangrene and its complications is still about 30%.

Clostridial cellulitis carries a much better prognosis provided it is recognized and treated before progressing to gas gangrene.

Clostridial Food Poisoning

Death from clostridial food poisoning is uncommon, although gastrointestinal symptoms may be severe, particularly in the elderly and very young. Fluid and electrolyte losses from diarrhea can be severe and require replacement, sometimes intravenously.

Selected Bibliography

Anonymous: *Botulism in the United States, 1899-1977*. U.S. Department of Health, Education and Welfare, Public Health Service, Centers for Disease Control, 1979.

Arnon, S. S., Midusa, T. F., Clay, S. A., Wood, R. M., and Chin, J.: Infant botulism: Epidemiological, clinical and laboratory aspects. *JAMA* 237:1946-1951, 1977.

Darke, S. G., King, A. M., and Slack, W. K.: Gas gangrene and related infection, classification, clinical features and aetiology, management and mortality. A report of 88 cases. *Br J Surg* 64:104-112, 1977.

Edmondson, R. S. and Flowers, M. W.: Intensive care in tetanus: Management, complications and mortality in 100 cases. *Br Med J* 1:1401-1404, 1979.

Fraser, D. W.: Preventing tetanus in patients with wounds. *Ann Intern Med* 84: 95-97, 1976.

Gorbach, S. L. and Thadepalli, H.: Isolation of *Clostridium* in human infections: Evaluation of 114 cases. *J Infect Dis* 131(suppl):S81-S85, 1975.

Parker, M.T.: Postoperative clostridial infections in Britain. *Br Med J* 3:671-676, 1969.

Sanders, R. K. M., Martyn, B., Joseph, R., and Peacock, M. L.: Intrathecal anti-tetanus serum (horse) in the treatment of tetanus. *Lancet* 1:974-977, 1977.

Thomas, M., Noah, N. D., Male, G. E., Stinger, M. F., Kendall, M., Gilbert, R. J., Jones, P. H., and Phillips, K. D.: Hospital outbreak of *Clostridium perfringens* food-poisoning. *Lancet* 1:1046-1048, 1977.

Weinstein, L. and Barza, M. A.: Gas gangrene. *N Engl J Med* 289:1129-1131, 1973.

88

ANTHRAX
Roger G. Finch, M.B.

Anthrax is a zoonosis sporadically transmitted to man following occupational exposure to infected animals or their products, such as fur, wool, or skin. It is a disease which has been recognized from antiquity. The term anthrax is derived from the Greek "anthrakos" which means coal, and graphically describes the black eschar so characteristic of this skin infection. Cutaneous anthrax is the most common form of disease although pulmonary, gastrointestinal, and occasionally meningeal infections occur.

Microbiology

Anthrax is caused by the aerobic, spore-forming organism, *Bacillus anthracis,* a large nonmotile gram-positive bacillus with squared ends. The organism varies in size from 1-1.3 by 3-10 μm and has spores which are either central or paracentral.

Bacillus anthracis will grow on most laboratory media over a wide temperature range. Blood agar plates incubated aerobically at 35°C overnight are satisfactory for most purposes. The colonies are nonhemolytic, flat, off-white and with an irregular margin, often with comma-shaped outgrowths. The growth is quite tenacious and forms spicules when picked up.

A capsule is demonstrable if the organism is grown on sodium bicarbonate agar incubated in 5% CO_2. Virulent strains appear mucoid under these circumstances. The capsule is a virulence factor and has antiphagocytic properties. Another confirmatory test is lysis by a γ phage which can be read from 6 to 18 hr after phage inoculation. Biochemical testing further assists in the differentiation from other *Bacillus* spp most notably *B. cereus.* Animal inoculation studies using mice, rabbits, or guinea pigs provide confirmatory tests of pathogenicity; death usually occurs from 2 to 5 days after inoculation, and the organism is demonstrable on culturing animal heart blood, spleen, or liver.

The spores of the *B. anthracis* are killed by boiling for 10 min, although in nature they can survive for many years on animal hides and in the soil. Persistence in the soil is dependent upon the ambient temperature and degree of humidity. Sporulation occurs most readily at temperatures above 89°F, whereas below 68°F sporulation is slow and the vegetative forms of the organism have difficulty surviving.

Epidemiology

Most animal species are susceptible to anthrax although the disease is more frequent among herbivores. Infection in animals usually follows ingestion of infected food. Such infections tend to be rapidly fatal. Large concentrations of bacteria are present in body fluids including blood, urine, saliva, and feces. When the animal dies, widespread contamination of the surrounding area occurs which can persist for years as a result of sporulation. Another source of infection for animals is infected imported bone and fish meal, barley, and maize.

Humans are incidentally infected as a result of contact with infected animals or their products, most notably hair, fur, and hide. Cutaneous anthrax usually results, although inhalation produces a rapidly progressive pneumonia with septicemia. The infection is often occupational. Pulmonary anthrax used to be common among workers in the wool industry and was known as wool-sorters' disease.

Cutaneous anthrax may also result from contact with infected bone and fish meal. In addition, infected bristles in shaving brushes were once a source of cutaneous anthrax before such material was sterilized. Occasionally anthrax is acquired accidentally from gardening or horticultural exposure. Table 88.1 summarizes the epidemiology of anthrax in the United States from 1916 to 1975.

Pathogenesis and Pathology

Cutaneous anthrax follows inoculation which results in a sore known as a "malignant pustule." This consists of a central area of necrosis with an eschar, surrounded

TABLE 88.1   Number of Cases and Deaths from Anthrax in the United States

	Cases	Deaths
	Approximate Number/Year	
1916–1925	150	30
1926–1935	90	12
1936–1945	60	10
1946–1955	25	3
1956–1965	15	1
1966–1975	5	0

by vesicles which contain blood or serous material. The surrounding soft tissues are inflamed, with edema which is often extensive and may impinge on vital structures. Involvement of the regional lymph nodes is usual.

Pulmonary anthrax is a rapidly progressive disease usually accompanied by features of septicemia with cardiovascular collapse and death, often in association with renal failure and pulmonary edema. Laryngeal edema and hemorrhagic mediastinitis often accompany the pneumonia which is characterized by extensive edema, hemorrhage, patchy consolidation, and pleural effusion which is often blood-stained. The mediastinal lymph nodes show necrosis and hemorrhage and contain organisms.

Gastrointestinal anthrax is rare. The bowel is inflamed and edematous with the formation of a semipurulent, brownish exudate together with mesenteric lymph node enlargement. Gastrointestinal hemorrhage may complicate necrosis at the site of primary infection, often in the small bowel, where a "malignant carbuncle" may be present.

Diagnostic Features

Clinical

Cutaneous Anthrax

Following an incubation period of 2-3 days cutaneous anthrax starts as a small papule. Within a day, vesicles appear around the papule. These increase in size and become blue, black, or hemorrhagic. The central area ulcerates and dries to form a dark eschar which is slightly depressed. This becomes black over the course of the next day or so and enlarges to form the malignant pustule, which is usually 2-3 cm in diameter. The surrounding area of edema is often extensive. Pruritus is common but pain is absent or mild. The regional lymph nodes are usually tender and enlarged.

Systemic symptoms of fever, chills, malaise, nausea, and anorexia occur but are usually mild and sometimes absent. Rigors are uncommon. The temperature may be moderately elevated.

Pulmonary Anthrax

The onset is rapid with fever, malaise, cough, vomiting, and frequently hemoptysis, coming on within the course of a few hours. The temperature is raised, the pulse rapid, and the patient is usually sweating. Shortness of breath and cyanosis may develop. The chest generally shows widespread crepitations. The disease progresses rapidly over the course of a day or so and is usually fatal with death occurring from septicemia, shock, renal failure, and progressive pneumonia with hypoxia.

Gastrointestinal Anthrax

Gastrointestinal anthrax is rare and usually occurs in tropical or subtropical areas. The evolution is rapid with diffuse abdominal pain and symptoms and signs suggestive of peritonitis in addition to features of generalized septicemia. Gastrointestinal bleeding may occur together with complications of shock, renal failure, and progressive peritonitis. The disease is often fatal, although prompt treatment has proved successful.

Laboratory Features

The diagnosis of cutaneous anthrax is confirmed by isolation of *B. anthracis*. Swabs of vesicular fluid or material from beneath the margins of the eschar should be taken. The diagnosis may be suggested by the Gram-stained appearance and fluorescent antibody staining where this is available. Other forms of anthrax require a very high index of suspicion and taking sputum and blood for culture, and in the case of gastrointestinal disease, swabs of the peritoneal exudate if laparotomy has been performed. Other investigations are nonspecific but include the demonstration of a polymorphonuclear leukocytosis in the severe forms of the disease. The chest radiograph in pulmonary anthrax may show diffuse infiltrations and consolidation together with pleural effusion.

The laboratory should handle all samples from suspected cases of anthrax with care, although normal safety precautions should be adequate to prevent the staff from becoming infected.

Differential Diagnosis

Cutaneous Anthrax

In its early stages it may be difficult to differentiate cutaneous anthrax from other skin papules, although the evolution of the lesion should enable a diagnosis to be made. Boils contain pus unlike the lesion of anthrax. The history of occupational exposure is helpful.

Pulmonary Anthrax

It is extremely difficult to differentiate this from other overwhelming forms of pneumonia unless there is a history of an occupational exposure. The obvious acute infective nature of the illness should assist in the differentiation of the accompanying features of acute pulmonary edema and hemoptysis from other causes.

Gastrointestinal Anthrax

The diagnosis is usually made microbiologically, often at autopsy, although laparotomy may suggest the diagnosis if a malignant carbuncle is evident. Otherwise it is not possible to separate its presentation from the many causes of an acute abdomen associated with a rapidly progressive infective illness.

Treatment

Cutaneous Anthrax

The disease varies in severity yet responds promptly to antibiotic treatment. *Bacillus anthracis* is sensitive to penicillin, tetracycline, erythromycin, chloramphenicol, and streptomycin. Penicillin is the drug of choice and 2–4 million U/day should be administered parenterally. The response is rapid, and oral treatment can be continued following the initial parenteral therapy. Once the local lesion is sterilized, complete resolution will take about a week. Local treatment is unnecessary, apart from keeping it clean.

Pulmonary and Gastrointestinal Anthrax

Penicillin, although the drug of choice, is rarely selected initially. However, broad-spectrum therapy if it includes penicillin or ampicillin may prove effective. Chloramphenicol, if given for intraabdominal sepsis, would also be appropriate treatment. Supportive treatment is essential and is directed to the correction of hypoxemia, electrolyte imbalance, renal failure, and disseminated intravascular coagulation where these exist.

Immunology and Prevention

The disease is uncommon, and hence evidence for protection following a primary infection is difficult to establish although indirect hemagglutinating antibodies can be detected. However, second attacks of cutaneous anthrax have been reported.

The prevention of anthrax in man is directed toward its control in animals and toward reducing the risk of exposure to infected animal products. The carcasses of animals dying from anthrax should be cremated promptly or buried, and the surrounding ground disinfected with chlorinated lime. Infected bedding, straw, and manure also should be incinerated to reduce environmental contamination by bacilli or spores.

The control of anthrax in imported animal products such as hides, wool, and bones is difficult and expensive. However, autoclaving or treatment with sodium hypochlorite is effective in disinfecting these materials. Education of employees and the use of protective clothing should help reduce the hazards or allow early recognition.

A vaccine is available for workers at special risk and requires three injections. However, immunity is short-lived, and antibodies tend to wane by 6 months.

Complications and Prognosis

Cutaneous Anthrax

This generally resolves without complications, although extensive skin involvement with edema may cause pressure on vital structures such as the trachea or larynx, while involvement of the face may threaten the eye. Secondary infection may also occur; however mortality is less than 1%.

In contrast, pulmonary or gastrointestinal anthrax is usually rapidly fatal although treatment successes have been reported.

Selected Bibliography

Gold, H.: Anthrax: Report of 117 cases. *Arch Intern Med* 96:387-396, 1955.

LaForce, F. M., Bumford, F. H., Feeley, J. C., Stokes, S. L., and Snow, D. B.: Epidemiologic study of a fatal case of inhalation anthrax. *Arch Environ Health* 18:798-805, 1969.

Lamb, R.: Anthrax. *Br Med J* 1:157-159, 1973.

Nalin, D. R., Sultana, B., Sahunja, R., Islam, A. K., Rahim, M. A., Islam, M., Costa, B. S., Mawla, N., and Greenough, W. B.: Survival of a patient with intestinal anthrax. *Am J Med* 62:130-132, 1977.

89

ERYSIPELOTHRIX INSIDIOSA
Roger G. Finch, M.B.

Erysipeloid, a rare condition caused by *Erysipelothrix insidiosa,* primarily involves the skin and uncommonly produces systemic infection. Many infections are occupational in origin and secondary to contact with pigs and other wild or domestic animals in whom the organism causes a variety of diseases.

Microbiology

Erysipelothrix insidiosa, previously named *E. rhusiopathia,* is a slender, pleomorphic, gram-positive bacillus, 0.5-2.5 μm long by 0.2-0.4 μm wide. It is nonencapsulated, nonsporing, nonmotile, and microaerophilic in its growth requirements, producing either small groups, or chains, or long filamentous forms. It can be isolated on ordinary nonselective media, producing smooth, round, and transparent colonies 0.5-1 mm in diameter. It should be differentiated from *Listeria monocytogenes, Corynebacterium* spp, and *Bacillus* spp, by the absence of catalase, of motility, and of hemolysis on blood agar, as well as its failure to produce spores.

Epidemiology

Infection with *E. insidiosa* is widespread among both wild and domestic animals, most notably pigs, cattle, and sheep, as well as birds and fish. Human infection is essentially an occupational hazard among abattoir workers, farmers, fish handlers, butchers, and those who handle animal skins and furs and thus come into contact with infected material. There is a male preponderance of cases as well as a greater frequency in the summer and early fall.

Pathogenesis and Pathology

Inoculation of the skin through an abrasion or laceration is the usual mechanism of acquiring the organism. The hands are the most common sites for infection although more proximal infections are seen. The disease is generally self-limiting and characterized by a lesion which is raised with an erythematous edge that spreads peripherally while the central area fades. It is accompanied by a marked inflammatory response which includes mast cells and lymphocytes as well as some tissue necrosis. The organisms tend to be deep within the lesion, thus skin biopsy is frequently necessary for microbial isolation, although sampling the advancing edge of the lesion may also prove successful.

Bloodstream infection is uncommon but can result in endocarditis and septic arthritis.

Diagnostic Features

Clinical

Following inoculation through the skin there is a short incubation period of 1-4 days, rarely longer. The local lesion known as *erysipeloid* (or erysipeloid of Rosenbach after its original describer) then develops over the course of a few days. This consists of a raised lesion which is violaceous, painful, and accompanied by localized itching, burning, or throbbing which spreads peripherally over the course of a few days. Constitutional symptoms of fever and malaise are uncommon, although lymphangitis and lymphadenitis may occur. As the lesion spreads its center becomes pale but remains violaceous at its periphery. Suppuration is not a feature of this condition. The lesion tends to regress spontaneously after 1-3 weeks with complete resolution.

Laboratory

Bacterial isolation is best achieved from biopsy material of the spreading edge of the lesion. The bacillus grows facultatively on common laboratory media including blood agar.

Should blood stream invasion occur then routine blood culture media are satisfactory for bacterial isolation.

Differential Diagnosis

The migratory violaceous appearance of erysipeloid is unique and its localization to the distal upper limbs characteristic. Secondary infection with *Staphylococcus aureus* or *Streptococcus pyogenes* may cause diagnostic problems on occasion.

Treatment

Erysipeloid is usually self-limited, subsiding spontaneously over a few days to 3 weeks. It is accompanied by brownish discoloration of the skin but rarely desquamates.

Erysipelothrix insidiosa is susceptible in vitro to penicillin, erythromycin, and the cephalosporins. The local disease may be abbreviated by the use of a single injection of benzathine penicillin G or by more prolonged oral therapy, while systemic infection will require high-dose parenteral therapy.

Immunology and Prevention

Infection does not produce lasting immunity, although specific agglutinins can be detected in convalescent serum.

The disease is primarily an occupational hazard. There are no specific preventive measures available.

Complications and Prognosis

The local disease is essentially benign and self-limited, although relapses may occur. Metastatic infection involving the heart valves carries a significant mortality as well as running the risk of complications such as embolic phenomena.

Selected Bibliography

Grieco, M. and Sheldon, C.: *Erysipelothrix rhusiopathiae. Ann N Y Acad Sci* 174: 523, 1970.

Klander, V., Kramer, D., and Nicholas, L.: *Erysipelothrix rhusiopathiae* septicemia diagnosis and treatment. *JAMA* 122:938, 1943.

Nelson, E.: Five hundred cases of erysipeloid. *Rocky Mount Med J* 52:40, 1955.

Price, J. E. L. and Bennett, W. E. J.: The erysipeloid of Rosenbach. *Br Med J* 2: 1060-1066, 1951.

Simerkoff, M. S. and Rahal, J. J.: Acute and subacute endocarditis due to *Erysipelothrix rhusiopathiae. Am J Med Sci* 266:53-57, 1973.

90

LACTOBACILLUS
Roger G. Finch, M.B.

Lactobacilli are normally present in the mouth, gastrointestinal and female genital tracts and characteristically produce lactic acid from glucose fermentation, hence their name. In man they are uncommonly overtly pathogenic although recognized to be associated with dental caries. Nonetheless, they have been responsible for occasional reports of endocarditis, arthritis, endometritis, dental abscess, and bacteremia.

Microbiology

Lactobacilli are gram-positive, nonsporing, nonmotile, catalase- and oxidase-negative bacilli. They are either anaerobic or facultatively anaerobic and attack glucose and other sugars fermentatively, resulting in lactic acid production either alone (homofermentative) or with other metabolic products (heterofermentative). They are able to tolerate relatively acid conditions even as low as pH 3-4. The genus contains several species, including *L. acidophilus, L. plantarum, L. leichmanii,* and *L. casei* which have been pathogenic to man on occasion.

Epidemiology

In general lactobacilli are quite harmless to man and found in large numbers in the gut and vagina. In the latter site they constitute the predominant member of the normal flora during the reproductive years where they play a role in maintaining the vaginal pH around 4.5 through their action on vaginal glycogen and glucose. The maintenance of such a low pH is probably protective against infection with less acid-tolerant pathogens. Döderleins bacillus, present in the vagina, is now known not to represent a single species but reflects a number of *Lactobacillus* spp of which *L. acidophilus* predominates.

Pathogenesis and Pathology

The rare occasions when lactobacilli produce disease are usually secondary to a breech in those mucosal surfaces which harbor these organisms as part of their normal flora. Infections have complicated pregnancy, producing postpartum endometritis and periomphalitis in the neonate, and have followed bowel perforation to produce intraperitoneal abscess and bacteremia. Endocarditis on damaged or prosthetic heart valves is also a recognized complication of bacteremia. Localized suppuration of the oropharynx also may occur and be complicated by bacteremia.

Lactobacilli are also found in association with dental caries, although oral streptococci, most notably *Streptococcus mutans,* are likely to be the major microbial pathogen in this disease.   Acid production by lactobacilli can attack the mineral component of dentine and enamel.

Diagnostic Features

There are no pathognomonic features of localized or systemic infection with lactobacilli. The comparative rarity of such infections and knowledge that they are common members of the normal flora may result in their being dismissed as "contaminants." This is less likely to occur when they are isolated from blood, particularly if done so repeatedly.

Lactobacilli are not fastidious in their growth requirements and can be isolated from blood with standard blood culture media. Isolation from abscess cavities is achieved on routine media if incubated in an anaerobic atmosphere, and identification is confirmed by colonial appearance, Gram stain, fermentation, and catalase reactions.

Treatment

Several antibiotics are inhibitory to lactobacilli including penicillin, ampicillin, clindamycin, cephalothin, and vancomycin, although there is some variability in susceptibility between the species. Penicillin and ampicillin are the most active and therefore the drugs of choice. However, despite satisfactory inhibition of growth there is sometimes a striking difference in the amount of drug necessary to kill the organisms. For example, there are reports of relapse in lactobacillus endocarditis despite daily dosage of penicillin in excess of 20 million U intravenously, followed by subsequent cure with dosages up to 48 million U daily.

There is in vitro evidence for synergistic inhibition of growth by combinations of penicillins or ampicillin with either gentamicin or streptomycin, although clinical confirmation of the efficacy of such combinations is needed. It is thus apparent that deep-seated infections with lactobacilli require careful laboratory monitoring and sensitivity testing to determine the optimum antibiotic regimen.

In addition to antibiotic therapy, surgical drainage of purulent material remains an essential part of the management of such infections.

Immunology and Prevention

No definitive deficiencies in either humoral or cellular immune mechanisms have been described. Heroin addiction and poor dental hygiene are among the potentially preventable predisposing causes.

Complications and Prognosis

The prognosis for most forms of lactobacillus infection is good once a diagnosis is made and treatment and antibiotic therapy begun with or without surgical drainage, as appropriate.

In contrast lactobacillus endocarditis carries a much worse prognosis. It is generally subacute in its presentation, frequently involves either the mitral or aortic valves, and appears to be complicated by a relatively high frequency of systemic arterial embolization, most notably to the aortofemoral and intracerebral vessels.

Selected Bibliography

Axelrod, J., Keusch, G. T., Bottone, E., Cohen, S. M., and Hirschman, S. Z.: Endocarditis caused by *Lactobacillus plantarum*. *Ann Intern Med* 78:33-37, 1973.

Bayer, A. S., Chow, A. W., Betts, D., and Guze, L. B.: Lactobacillemia report of nine cases. *Am J Med* 64:808-813, 1978.

Bayer, A. S., Chow, A. W., Concepcion, N., and Guze, L. B.: Susceptibility of 40 lactobacilli to six antimicrobial agents with broad gram-positive anaerobic spectra. *Antimicrob Agents Chemother* 14:720-722, 1978.

Sharpe, M. E., Hill, L. R., and LaPage, S. P.: Pathogenic lactobacilli. *J Med Microbiol* 6:281-286, 1973.

Tennebaum, M. J. and Warner, J. F.: *Lactobacillus casei* endocarditis. *Ann Intern Med* 82:539, 1975.

91

NEISSERIA AND VEILLONELLA
Larry G. Reimer, M.D.

Neisseria gonorrhoeae and *Neisseria meningitidis* are the only common organisms pathogenic to man which appear as gram-negative cocci on smear (Table 91.1). Other nonpathogenic but morphologically similar members of the family Neisseriaceae including other *Neisseria* spp *(N. lactamicus, N. sicca, N. subflava, N. flavescens,* and *N. mucosa)*, *Branhamella catarrhalis,* and *Moraxella* spp are usually present in the upper respiratory tract of humans and rarely cause bacteremia, endocarditis, pulmonary infection, and meningitis. *Acinetobacter* is also a member of this family of organisms although it usually appears as short gram-negative rods and causes opportunistic infections in compromised patients.

 Veillonella parvula is the only anaerobic gram-negative coccus in man and is part of the normal flora of the oropharynx, gastrointestinal tract, and genitourinary tract. While it does not possess significant pathogenic properties, it will occasionally be part of mixed anaerobic infections adjacent to these locations.

Microbiology

The Neisseriae are nonmotile organisms usually appearing in pairs although clusters and tetrads also may be seen. *Neisseria gonorrhoeae* and *N. meningitidis* may be differentiated from the other nonpathogenic Neisseriae by failure to grow at 22°C and by characteristic patterns of carbohydrate degradation (Table 91.2). An important property of Neisseriae is their ability to oxidize dimethyl- or tetramethyl-p-phenylenediamine which is used as a laboratory test to differentiate these organisms from most other inhabitants of the upper respiratory and genitourinary tracts.

 On solid media *N. gonorrhoeae* grows as one of five colony types distinguishable by size, morphology, color, presence of surface pili, and several other characteristics. Types 1 and 2 alone are associated with human infection. Strains

TABLE 91.1   Gram-Negative Cocci in Humans

Neisseria spp

    N. *gonorrhoeae*

    N. *meningitidis*

    N. *lactamicus*

    N. *sicca*

    N. *subflava*

    N. *flavescens*

    N. *mucosa*

Branhamella catarrhalis

Moraxella spp

    M. *lacunata*

    M. *nonliquefaciens*

    M. *osloensis*

    M. *phenylpyruvica*

    M. *atlantae*

    M. *urethralis*

TABLE 91.2   Carbohydrate Degradation Patterns of Neisseriae

Specie	Glucose	Maltose	Lactose	Sucrose
N. *gonorrhoeae*	+	0	0	0
N. *meningitidis*	+	+	0	0
N. *lactamicus*	+	+	+	0
N. *sicca*	+	+	0	+
N. *subflava*	+	+	0	±
N. *flavescens*	0	0	0	0
N. *mucosa*	+	+	0	+

also differ in requirements for basic substances such as amino acids, a characteristic used to divide strains into different auxotypes. One auxotype in particular,
that requiring arginine, hypoxanthine, and uracil (the AHU- auxotype), is the most
frequent cause of disseminated gonococcal infection (DGI). Gonococci are usually encapsulated and may or may not be covered with pili which are composed
primarily of protein. All strains have another surface protein which can be used
to serotype different isolates. Gonococci are also coated with a lipopolysaccharide
which differs for each colony type.

Neisseria meningitidis has a polysaccharide capsule which is the basis for
grouping strains into one of eight serogroups: A, B, C, X, Y, 29E, and W-135. A
surface protein is also present which can further separate groups into serotypes.
Certain serogroups and serotypes are more virulent than others, and typing is
helpful in studying pathogenic mechanisms. However, typing is of little practical
importance in sporadic cases for predicting disease outcome.

Veillonella parvula, being the only common anaerobic gram-negative coccus
in man, is usually identified by Gram stain alone. The organism does reduce nitrate and has a characteristic pattern on gas-liquid chromatography if confirmatory studies are needed.

Pathogenesis and Pathology

The pathogenic mechanisms for N. gonorrhoeae and N. meningitidis are not entirely understood (Table 91.3). While some people develop fulminant disease, others either become asymptomatic carriers or are not colonized at all. Some of the
difference can be accounted for by strain variation, but human factors are also
important.

Meningococcemia and DGI are much more likely to occur in patients deficient
in complement components C5, C6, C7, or C8. Acquired natural immunity is also
important in that while most people have serum antibodies that are bactericidal
to Neisseriae, patients who develop systemic illness may either lack antibody or
have blocking antibodies that permit infection to occur. Sex hormones may also
be important since women, who are much more likely to develop DGI, usually have
onset of symptoms during menses or pregnancy.

Factors associated with virulence of N. gonorrhoeae are presence of pili,
smooth lipopolysaccharide, certain capsular types, secretion of IgA protease, and
possibly the presence of leukocyte association (LA) factor. Pili are important in
promoting attachment of the organism to mucosal epithelial cells for initiation
of infection, and possibly in resisting phagocytosis. The surface capsule and LA
factor are also postulated as important in resistance to phagocytosis and to destruction by polymorphonuclear leukocytes. Lipopolysaccharide has been shown
experimentally to destroy the cilia on human fallopian tube epithelial cells. Immunoglobulin A protease specifically cleaves IgA molecules, inactivating secretory antibody defenses against the organism.

Strains associated with DGI are unusual: they are less likely to cause local
infection despite colonization, yet more likely to cause dramatic systemic illness.
The mechanism for dissemination of these strains is unclear, although an important factor appears to be resistance to human serum killing activity.

Pathologic lesions in DGI reflect direct infection and tissue destruction at
involved sites. Immunologic mechanisms including immune complexes also may
play a role.

The meningococcus is also covered by a polysaccharide capsule that limits
phagocytosis. Pili present on the surface may be important for attachment to
epithelial cells. The major virulence factor for meningococcus, however, is its

TABLE 91.3   Presumed Mechanisms in Neisserial Infection

Host

   C5, C6, C7, C8 complement deficiency
   Sex hormones (menstrual cycle)
   Absent serum bactericidal activity

Bacterial

   Gonococcus

      Colony type 1 or 2
      Pili
      Lipopolysaccharide
      Capsule
      ? LA factor
      IgA protease
      AHU- auxotype

   Meningococcus

      Pili
      Capsule
      Lipopolysaccharide (endotoxin)

---

production of lipopolysaccharide, an endotoxin that can reproduce the major manifestations of fulminant meningococcal infection in experimental animals.

Fulminant meningococcemia with the Waterhouse-Friderichsen syndrome is characterized pathologically by diffuse vascular injury with thrombosis and infarction of multiple organs, renal cortical necrosis, and shock lung. Myocarditis is commonly present with evidence of congestive failure. Disseminated intravascular coagulopathy usually follows and, in association with fluid loss from vascular injury, results in hypovolemia, shock, and death.

Clinical Manifestations

Typical gonorrhea was discussed in Chapter 36 and meningococcal meningitis in Chapter 42.

Disseminated gonococcal infection usually occurs in the setting of asymptomatic carriage of *N. gonorrhoeae* with a variable clinical presentation usually falling into one of two major categories (Table 91.4). At some point, often during a menstrual period or pregnancy, the organism enters the blood stream. Patients most often present during this bacteremic phase with the acute onset of fever, chills, sterile polyarthritis of wrists, hands, ankles, and knees, tenosynovitis in one or more of these locations, and one to ten skin lesions, usually on the extremities, which typically progress from papules to hemorrhagic pustules over 2-3 days.

Meningococcemia may have a much more profound impact but is also variable (Table 91.5). About 50% of patients have associated meningitis. Five to fifteen

TABLE 91.4   Manifestations of Disseminated Gonococcal Infection

Dermatitis-polyarthritis syndrome

Fever
Sterile polyarthritis
Tenosynovitis
Pustular rash
Bacteremia

Monoarticular syndrome

Fever
Suppurative monoarticular arthritis

Intermediate forms

TABLE 91.5   Manifestations of Meningococcemia

Acute bacteremia with or without meningitis

Waterhouse-Friderichsen syndrome

Transient bacteremia

Chronic intermittent bacteremia

percent present with Waterhouse-Friderichsen syndrome, a disease with acute onset, high fever, nausea, vomiting, delirium, rapidly progressing purpural or hemorrhagic rash of skin and mucous membranes, renal failure, respiratory insufficiency, shock, and death. Most patients have a less severe form characterized by fever, chills, headache, myalgias, arthralgias, and a rash occurring in crops on any part of the body, progressing from petechial to purpuric. Rare patients may develop benign, transient meningococcemia with fever alone which resolves without therapy, or they may have chronic intermittent meningococcemia with periods of fever associated with maculopapular rash and arthralgias. Symptomatic periods are brief, and the whole syndrome may last for weeks to months. Nonbacteremic illness caused by meningococcus includes pneumonia, endocarditis, pericarditis, and urethritis.

Veillonella parvula is isolated occasionally from mixed cultures in patients who present with orofacial, pulmonary, intraabdominal or genitourinary abscesses and tissue infections. The organism may be isolated rarely in blood cultures from patients after dental procedures or during the course of one of the above infections. The clinical course of such patients is typical for anaerobic infections in general.

Diagnosis

Disseminated gonococcal infection and meningococcemia are best recognized by their clinical manifestations since cultures, especially for *N. gonorrhoeae,* may be negative. Arthralgia or arthritis with pustular rash in sexually active, healthy, young adults should always suggest DGI, and a rapidly progressive purpuric rash with systemic toxicity is most likely meningococcemia. In suspected DGI, cultures of the pharynx, urethra, and rectum in addition to blood and joint fluid are essential because cultures from any one site may be negative, and systemic infection generally occurs in association with asymptomatic colonization at some mucosal site. Rapid transport of specimens to the laboratory or placement of material into adequate transport media, such as Stuart or Amies broths, is essential to assure viability of these organisms. Strains of gonococci associated with DGI are often sensitive to vancomycin which is incorporated into gonococcal selective media. When DGI is suspected laboratories should always inoculate plain chocolate agar in addition to modified Thayer-Martin, Martin-Lewis, or New York City agar. Patients with suspected meningococcemia should routinely have blood and CSF cultures. The disease may also be diagnosed rapidly by specific counter-immunoelectrophoresis.

Patients with DGI and meningococcemia usually present with elevated white blood counts and often have elevated liver function tests with other laboratory studies generally normal. When Waterhouse-Friderichsen syndrome is present, patients have leukopenia, thrombocytopenia, prolonged prothrombin and partial thromboplastin times, and laboratory tests confirming acute renal failure and respiratory insufficiency.

Veillonella will grow in usual anaerobic culture media employed in clinical laboratories and can be diagnosed by its isolation in such cultures or by the presence of gram-negative cocci seen on smears of infected material.

Treatment

Disseminated gonococcal infection is best treated with parenteral penicillin G, although ampicillin, tetracycline, and erythromycin can also be used. Strains of gonococci associated with DGI are usually very sensitive to penicillin and generally respond rapidly. Penicillinase-producing *N. gonorrhoeae* have not been associated with DGI acquired in the United States, although imported cases have been reported. With the increasing number of penicillinase-positive strains recognized in this country, failure to respond to therapy should suggest the possibility of penicillin resistance and the need for susceptibility testing and penicillinase assays. Suppurative arthritis can generally be managed by closed aspiration of the involved joint, as needed, in addition to the systemic antibiotic.

Meningococcemia is best treated with high-dose parenteral penicillin G. Penicillin-allergic patients may be treated with chloramphenicol. In fulminant disease general supportive care with appropriate fluid management, use of pressor agents, and respiratory support may improve the outcome.

Veillonella is sensitive to penicillins, cephalosporins, clindamycin, and chloramphenicol. It can be treated with any of these agents appropriate for control of other organisms present or the site involved.

Prognosis and Complications

Disseminated gonococcal infection is usually a self-limited disease, although rare patients may develop endocarditis, meningitis, or myopericarditis with outcomes typical for those diseases.

Meningococcemia has a 5-10% overall mortality, and patients with fulminant disease rarely survive. Less dramatic illness is often complicated by an immune-complex disease which manifests as sterile oligoarticular or monoarticular joint effusion.

Immunity and Prevention

Single episodes of gonorrhea do not prevent subsequent recurrence. Since attempts to control gonorrhea by public health measures have had little impact on this epidemic disease, attempts are in progress to develop vaccines using lipopolysaccharide or pilus protein. Pilus protein appears particularly promising in that a specific antibody response can be demonstrated after vaccination, and gonococci are unable to attach to epithelial cells and initiate infection in vaccinated individuals.

Natural immunity to meningococcal infection certainly occurs since disease is unusual beyond the pediatric age group. Colonization with meningococci of one serogroup provides variable cross-protection to other serogroups or serotypes in addition to the colonizing strain. Patients with complement or immunoglobulin deficiency states are not protected and may suffer multiple recurrences of systemic disease with similar strains. Vaccines to groups A and C meningococci have been developed and were discussed in Chapter 42. Antibiotic prophylaxis of close personal contacts with rifampin or minocycline is recommended.

Selected Bibliography

Carlson, B. L., Fiumara, N. J., Kelly, J. R., and McCormick, W. M.: Isolation of *Neisseria meningitidis* from anogenital specimens from homosexual men. *Sex Trans Dis* 7:71-73, 1980.

Davis, C. E. and Arnold, K.: Role of meningococcal endotoxin in meningococcal purpura. *J Exp Med* 140:159-171, 1974.

Eisenstein, B. I. and Masi, A. T.: Disseminated gonococcal infection (DGI) and gonococcal arthritis (GCA): I. Bacteriology, epidemiology, host factors, pathogen factors, and pathology. *Sem Arthritis Rheum* 10:155-172, 1981.

Goldschneider, I., Gotschlich, E. C., and Artenstein, M. S.: Human immunity to the meningococcus. I. The role of humoral antibodies. *J Exp Med* 129:1307-1326, 1969.

Handsfield, H.H.: Disseminated gonococcal infection. *Clin Obst Gynecol* 18:131-142, 1975.

Handsfield, H.H., Knapp, J. S., Diehr, P. K., and Holmes, K. K.: Correlation of auxotype and penicillin susceptibility of *Neisseria gonorrhoeae* with sexual preference and clinical manifestations of gonorrhea. *Sex Trans Dis* 7:1-5, 1980.

Holmes, K. K., Counts, G. W., and Beaty, H. N.: Disseminated gonococcal infection. *Ann Intern Med* 74:979-993, 1971.

Masi, A. T. and Eisenstein, B. I.: Disseminated gonococcal infection (DGI) and gonococcal arthritis (GCA): II. Clinical manifestations, diagnosis, complications, treatment, and prevention. *Sem Arthritis Rheum* 10:173-197, 1981.

Medical Staff Conference: Meningococcus. *West J Med* 127:314-324, 1977.

Melly, M. A., Gregg, C. R., and McGee, Z. A.: Studies of toxicity of *Neisseria gonorrhoeae* for human fallopian tube mucosa. *J Infect Dis* 143:423-431, 1981.

Mirrett, S., Reller, L. B., and Knapp, J. S.: *Neisseria gonorrhoeae* strains inhibited by vancomycin in selective media and correlation with auxotype. *J Clin Microbiol* 14:94-99, 1981.

Morello, J. A. and Bohnhoff, M.: *Neisseria* and *Branhamella,* In: E. H. Lennette, A. Balows, W. J. Hausler, Jr., and J. P. Truant (eds.): *Manual of Clinical Microbiology,* 3rd ed. American Society for Microbiology, Washington, D.C., 1980, pp. 111-130.

Morse, S. A.: The biology of the gonococcus. *Crit Rev Microbiol* 7:93-189, 1979.

Rice, P. A. and Goldenberg, D. L.: Clinical manifestations of disseminated infection caused by *Neisseria gonorrhoeae* are linked to differences in bactericidal reactivity of infecting strains. *Ann Intern Med* 95:175-178, 1981.

Schaad, U. B.: Arthritis in disease due to *Neisseria meningitidis.* *Rev Infect Dis* 2:880-888, 1980.

Sippel, J. E.: Meningococci. *Crit Rev Microbiol* 8:267-302, 1981.

Tramont, E. C., Sadoff, J. C., Boslego, J. W., Ciak, J., McChesney, D., Brinton, C. C., Wood, S., and Tukafuji, E.: Gonoccoccal pilus vaccine. Studies of antigenicity and inhibition of attachment. *J Clin Invest* 68:881-888, 1981.

92

ENTEROBACTERIACEAE
Ronica M. Kluge, M.D.

The Enterobacteriaceae comprise a large number of gram-negative bacilli, widely distributed in nature and frequently pathogenic for humans. Normal inhabitants of the large bowel of animals and humans, the organisms tend to cause disease when mechanical barriers are breached (trauma, surgery, perforation, instrumentation), particularly in the host with an altered immune status. Enterobacteriaceae are a leading cause of hospital-acquired infections in this country.

Microbiology and Pathogenesis

Microbiologic characteristics and members of the family Enterobacteriaceae are listed in Tables 92.1 and 92.2. Because of technologic advances such as DNA homology determinations, the taxonomy of these organisms is in a state of flux.

Enterobacteriaceae may be motile or nonmotile, the motile ones possessing peritrichous flagella in contrast to pseudomonads and vibrios which have polar flagella. The H antigens are located on the flagella and may play a role in pathogenesis of disease, although this has not been proved conclusively.

Enterobacteriaceae may have a well-defined capsule (e.g., *Klebsiella*), a loose covering (e.g., *Escherichia coli*), or no capsule at all. Some capsular antigens are listed in Table 92.3. These antigens appear to be important in the pathogenesis of certain diseases such as typhoid fever, meningitis, pyelonephritis, and diarrhea caused by *E. coli*.

The bacterial cell wall contains the somatic or O antigen. This antigen is composed of repeating polysaccharide units and, within certain genera, allows for serologic subgrouping. Attached to the O antigen is endotoxin, made up of the core lipopolysaccharide (common to a particular genus) and the lipid A moiety (common to all gram-negative bacilli). The core antigen must play a role in

TABLE 92.1   Characteristics of Enterobacteriaceae

Gram-negative bacilli, nonsporeforming
Aerobic (facultatively anaerobic)
Reduce nitrates to nitrites
Ferment glucose, forming acid alone, or acid and gas
Oxidase-negative

TABLE 92.2   Members of the Enterobacteriaccae Family

Escherichia	Klebsiella
Shigella	Enterobacter
Edwardsiella	Serratia
Salmonella	Proteus
Arizona	Morganella
Citrobacter	Providencia
Yersinia	Erwinia
Hafnia	

TABLE 92.3   Capsular Antigens

Antigen	Organism
K	E. coli
Vi	S. typhi, Citrobacter
M	Salmonella, Arizona, E. coli
Capsular	Klebsiella

pathogenesis of disease since the presence and level of antibody to core antigen are correlated with protection against shock and death in patients with gram-negative bacteremia. A great deal of evidence suggests that the lipid A moiety is responsible for the clinical signs and symptoms of gram-negative septicemia (see Chapter 47).

Some of the Enterobacteriaceae produce enterotoxins that act directly on the gastrointestinal tract to cause symptoms. *Shigella*, certain *E. coli* and *Salmonella* are prototypes for toxin production. Other virulence factors include the ability to penetrate epithelial lining of the gut (*Salmonella, Shigella*), adherence to mucosal cells (*E. coli*), and the presence of large antiphagocytic capsules (*Klebsiella*). A number of hemolysins and a variety of enzymes are produced by Enterobacteriaceae, but the role of these products in pathogenesis is only speculative. Table 92.4 lists the more common diseases caused by the Enterobacteriaceae.

Escherichia

Escherichia coli is the preponderant organism of the large bowel. It is usually motile, ferments lactose, and produces gas from glucose fermentation. *Escherichia coli* is a frequent cause of urinary tract infection (UTI), bacteremia, and meningitis among newborns. It is especially important as a cause of nosocomial infections. Up to 90% of UTI are caused by *E. coli.* The strains responsible for UTI belong to a handful of O serotypes. Whether these serotypes are more virulent in some fashion, or merely more frequent colonizers of the gut is not known. *Escherichia coli* causes most of the gram-negative bacteremias. These organisms usually gain entry to the blood stream from a focus in the urinary tract, skin, respiratory tract, or from an intravenous device site. Newborns are particularly susceptible to *E. coli* meningitis. Seventy-five percent of the strains causing neonatal *E. coli* meningitis are of a single capsular antigen, K1. Why these strains seem so virulent for newborns is not known. Certain *E. coli* strains are responsible for diarrhea in infants and among travellers of all ages. The diarrhea results from either toxin production or epithelial invasion by the organism. Two types of toxin, heat-labile and heat-stable, are produced. The labile toxin resembles cholera toxin in its action: stimulates cAMP production and results in loss of fluid and electrolytes into the gut lumen. The mechanism of action of the stable toxin is related to the activation of cGMP with similar clinical results. Other less common infections caused by *E. coli* include pneumonia, arthritis, skin and soft tissue, endophthalmitis, peritonitis, intraabdominal abscess, brain abscess, osteomyelitis, sinusitis, and endocarditis.

Shigella

Shigella spp (*S. dysenteriae, S. flexneri, S. boydii* and *S. sonnei*) (Table 92.5) are nonmotile, nonencapsulated, do not produce hydrogen sulfide, and except for some *S. flexneri,* do not produce gas from carbohydrate fermentation. Most shigellae do not ferment lactose, although some *S. sonnei* will do so very slowly. *Shigella* spp cause diarrheal illness which ranges in severity from mild to severe (dysentery). It is a particular problem among infants and young children in day-care centers, among institutionalized persons, and in developing countries. *Shigella* strains capable of producing diarrheal illness have invasive properties although they rarely penetrate beyond the mucosa. The invasiveness is thought to be the primary pathogenic mechanism. An additional virulence factor is the production of an enterotoxin which causes fluid accumulation in ligated rabbit ileal loops. The enterotoxin also has cytotoxic effects on the intestinal mucosa. Rarely, shigellae invade the blood stream and cause pneumonia, arthritis, or keratoconjunctivitis. Shigellae are also reported to cause hemolytic-uremic syndrome.

TABLE 92.4   Most Common Diseases Caused by Enterobacteriaceae

Organism	Disease
E. coli	UTI
	Bacteremia
	Neonatal meningitis
	Diarrhea
	Nosocomial infections
Shigella	Diarrhea
	Bacteremia
E. tarda	Diarrhea
Salmonella	Enteric fever (typhoid, paratyphoid)
	Bacteremia
	Diarrhea
A. hinshawii	Bacteremia
	Diarrhea
Citrobacter	UTI
	Bacteremia
	Wound infection
Yersinia	Plague
	Enterocolitis
	Mesenteric adenitis
Klebsiella	UTI
	Bacteremia
	Pneumonia
	Nosocomial infections
Enterobacter	UTI
	Nosocomial infections
Serratia	Nosocomial infections
Proteus	UTI
Morganella morgagnii	Nosocomial infections
Providencia	Nosocomial infections
Erwinia	Nosocomial infections
H. alvei	Nosocomial infections

TABLE 92.5   *Shigella* Serotype Isolates

Serotype	Approximate % of Total
S. sonnei	65
S. flexneri	30
S. boydii	4
S. dysenteriae	1

Edwardsiella

Edwardsiella tarda produces hydrogen sulfide as well as lysine and ornithine de-carboxylases, but does not ferment lactose. In the laboratory it may be distin-guished from a salmonella by its ability to produce indole. The pathogenetic mechanisms are not well defined for this organism. The usual clinical illness pro-duced is a gastroenteritis. Less common infections include meningitis, soft-tissue infections, liver abscess, and bacteremia.

Salmonella

With rare exception, *Salmonella* spp are motile, but do not ferment lactose. Most produce hydrogen sulfide and produce acid and gas from glucose fermentation. *Salmonella typhi* does not produce gas from fermentation of glucose and its pro-duction of hydrogen sulfide may be minimal. Taxonomists differ in their schemes for classifying *Salmonella,* with one camp listing only three species (*S. typhi,* *S. cholerae-suis,* and *S. enteritidis),* and one giving each antigenic type the status of a species (e.g., *S. dublin, S. derby, S. heidleberg*). In all, over 1700 serotypes have been described. From an epidemiologic standpoint, it is useful to categorize the *Salmonella* by host preference and adaptation (Table 92.6). For example, man is the only natural reservoir for *S. typhi,* and swine are the major reservoir for

TABLE 92.6   **Examples of Host Preference of *Salmonella* Serotypes**

Host	Serotype
Man	S. typhi
	S. paratyphi group
	S. sendai
Fowl	S. gallinarum-pullorum
Cattle	S. dublin
Swine	S. cholerae-suis

S. cholerae-suis. In man, salmonellae cause primarily enteric fever, diarrheal illness, or bacteremia. Virulent salmonellae, such as Vi-containing *S. typhi,* can
penetrate the epithelial lining of the small intestine and pass into the subepithe-
lium (lamina propria) where the organisms are ingested by macrophages. Salmonellae thereby gain access to lymphoid tissue, the blood stream, and distant organs. Early investigators believed the clinical manifestations of typhoid fever
were all due to circulating endotoxin. However, there is evidence to support the
additional role of synthesis and release of endogenous pyrogen from *S. typhi* inflammatory lesions in pathogenesis. The salmonellae which cause gastroenteritis
probably do so through the combined mechanisms of tissue invasion and enterotoxin production. Bacteremia from salmonellae is more common in infants, the
elderly, and those with underlying diseases such as lymphoproliferative disorders,
hemoglobinopathies, and schistosomiasis. Other salmonella infections include endocarditis, arthritis, osteomyelitis, meningitis, pneumonia, and focal abscesses of
kidney, liver, spleen, or aneurysms. Biliary tract infection may result in chronic
asymptomatic intestinal carriage.

Arizona

Arizona hinshawii, serologically related to the *Salmonella,* produces hydrogen sulfide, liquefies gelatin, and ferments lactose and malonate. Its natural reservoirs
are reptiles and poultry. The organism causes bacteremia and diarrhea in these
species as well as in humans. The pathogenesis of *A. hinshawii* infections in man
has not been elucidated. Localized infections (lung, liver, bone, joint, middle ear)
due to *A. hinshawii* have been reported but they are rare.

Citrobacter

This genus is also related to the *Salmonella,* but unlike *Salmonella* they will grow
in the presence of potassium cyanide. There are two major species: *C. freundii*
which is indole-negative and hydrogen sulfide-positive, and *C. diversus* which is
indole-positive and hydrogen sulfide-negative. Both ferment malonate to some
extent. Little is known about the mechanisms by which the organisms cause disease. However, citrobacter are implicated in urinary tract and wound infections,
bacteremia, neonatal meningitis, and other nosocomial infections. Rare cases of
endocarditis, pneumonia, and brain abscess have been reported.

Yersinia (Table 92.7)

Three species are included in this genus: *Y. pestis, Y. enterocolitica,* and *Y. pseudotuberculosis.* Primarily pathogens of animals, yersinia can also produce disease
in humans. Yersinia share the major characteristics of Enterobacteriaceae (see
Table 92.1). They manifest bipolar staining and do not ferment lactose. *Yersinia
pestis* is nonmotile, whereas the other two species are motile (peritrichous

TABLE 92.7 *Yersinia* spp

Yersinia:	pestis
	enterocolitica
	pseudotuberculosis

flagella) at room temperature. There are three biotypes of *Y. pestis.* The organism produces endotoxin, exotoxins, and an antiphagocytic substance (fraction 1) which are involved in pathogenesis. *Yersinia pestis* reaches humans via infected fleas from animal reservoirs to cause either pneumonic or bacteremic illness (plague). The presenting manifestations in plague are listed in Table 92.8. *Yersinia enterocolitica* and *Y. pseudotuberculosis* are urease-positive which helps distinguish them from *Y. pestis.* There are 34 serotypes of *Y. enterocolitica.* There is experimental evidence supporting the role of tissue invasion and enterotoxin production in pathogenesis of illness due to *Y. enterocolitica* (enterocolitis, mesenteric adenitis). Bacteremia and a reactive polyarthritis have been reported as well. Abscess of liver and spleen, osteomyelitis, and meningitis are caused rarely by *Y. enterocolitica.* There are at least five serotypes of *Y. pseudotuberculosis* that are thought to cause disease in humans by mechanisms similar to *Y. enterocolitica.* Mesenteric adenitis is the most frequent illness due to *Y. pseudotuberculosis;* bacteremia and reactive polyarthritis are rare.

Klebsiella (Table 92.9)

Klebsiella have the human large bowel as their natural habitat. They are nonmotile, encapsulated lactose fermenters which do not produce hydrogen sulfide. Most strains will grow in potassium cyanide and can use citrate as a sole carbon source. *K. oxytoca* is indole-positive, the other species are indole-negative. Klebsiella have prominent polysaccharide capsules which probably play a role in their virulence (antiphagocytic). More than 70 capsular types have been identified. A frequent cause of UTI and bacteremia, particularly of nosocomial origin, klebsiella also cause primary pneumonia in debilitated individuals such as alcoholics. *Klebsiella ozaenae* causes a chronic atrophic rhinitis and *K. rhinoscleromatis* produces a granulomatous, destructive process in the upper respiratory tract called scleroma.

TABLE 92.8   Presenting Manifestations in Plague

	Approximate %
Prostration	75
Headache	55
Chills	40
Vomiting	35
Confusion	30
Cough	25
Abdominal pain	20
Chest pain	15

TABLE 92.9   *Klebsiella-Enterobacter-Serratia* spp

Klebsiella:	*pneumoniae*
	ozaenae
	rhinoscleromatis
	oxytoca
Enterobacter:	*aerogenes*
	cloacae
	agglomerans
Serratia:	*marcescens*
	liquefaciens
	rubidaea

Enterobacter (see Table 92.9)

Enterobacter spp are related to *Klebsiella*. Like klebsiella, enterobacter do not produce hydrogen sulfide, are indole-negative lactose fermenters, grow in the presence of potassium cyanide, and can utilize citrate as a sole carbon source. *Enterobacter* differs from *Klebsiella* in being motile. The mechanisms of pathogenesis for humans have not been clarified. Enterobacter rarely cause primary infections, but are incriminated in hospital-acquired infections, for example UTI and bacteremia.

Serratia (see Table 92.9)

Serratia is also related to *Klebsiella*. These organisms are motile and do not produce hydrogen sulfide; they ferment lactose slowly, if at all. Many produce pink or red pigment. Serratia are unique among the Enterobacteriaceae in their production of extracellular DNAse. Strains of *Serratia* virulent for humans (i.e., blood isolates) are resistant to the complement-dependent bactericidal activity of normal serum. Serratia rarely cause primary infections but have been responsible for a number of nosocomial epidemics. Pneumonia, UTI, and bacteremia are frequent. Less common infections include endocarditis, arthritis, meningitis, and osteomyelitis.

Proteus (Table 92.10)

Proteus strains have the ability to deaminate phenylalanine. These organisms are motile and generally do not ferment lactose. *Proteus mirabilis* is indole-negative, whereas *P. vulgaris* is indole-positive; both produce hydrogen sulfide. Proteus produce urease which may account for their prominence as urinary tract pathogens. Other virulence factors include their flagella (motility) and pili (adherence). Besides the genitourinary tract, proteus cause infections of the lung, blood stream, and wounds, which are generally acquired in the hospital.

TABLE 92.10   *Proteus-Morganella-Providencia* spp

Proteus:	*mirabilis*
	vulgaris
Morganella:	*morgagnii*
Providencia:	*stuartii*
	alcalifaciens
	rettgeri

Morganella (see Table 92.10)

Morganella morgagnii, previously called *Proteus morgagnii,* was reclassified on the basis of DNA homology studies and anomalous biochemical reactions. *Morganella morgagnii* shares certain characteristics of the *Proteus* group: phenylalanine deaminase, motility, and urease production. It is indole-positive but does not produce hydrogen sulfide. In contrast to *Proteus, M. morgagnii* swarming can be inhibited by 2% agar. This organism causes nosocomial infections of the urinary and respiratory tracts.

Providencia (see Table 92.10)

Similar to *Proteus* and *Morganella, Providencia* spp produce phenylalanine deaminase. However, providencia generally do not produce urease or hydrogen sulfide and do not possess decarboxylases. Although a producer of urease, *Proteus rettgeri* has been reassigned to the *Providencia* group on the basis of DNA homology determinations. The *Providencia* organisms often cause hospital-acquired infections. Bacteremia, UTI, wound infection, and pneumonia have been reported.

Erwinia

Erwinia isolates may be lactose-positive or lactose-negative and often produce a yellow pigment. They do not produce hydrogen sulfide and are negative for decarboxylases and for alanine dihydrolase. Primarily plant pathogens, these organisms have been recovered from human sources, particularly in nosocomial infections and/or debilitated hosts. The mechanism by which they produce disease in humans has not been elucidated.

Hafnia

Hafnia alvei is related to the *Klebsiella-Enterobacter-Serratia* group. The organism is lactose-negative and nonmotile. Pathogenic mechanisms are not known. These organisms have been implicated in nosocomial infections.

Selected Bibliography

Cohen, M. L. and Gangarosa, E. J.: Nontyphoid salmonellosis. *South Med J* 71: 1540, 1978.

Donta, S. T., Sack, D. A., and Wallace, R. B., et al.: Tissue-culture assay of antibodies to heat-labile *Escherichia coli* enterotoxins. *N Engl J Med* 291:117, 1974.

Elin, R. J. and Wolff, S. M.: Biology of endotoxin. *Ann Rev Med* 27:127, 1976.

Evans, D. J., Jr. and Evans, D. G.: Three characteristics associated with enterotoxigenic *Escherichia coli* isolated from man. *Infect Immun* 8:322, 1973.

Giannella, R. A., Rout, W. R., and Formal, S. B.: Effect of indomethacin on intestinal water transport in salmonella-infected Rhesus monkeys. *Infect Immun* 17:136, 1977.

Hornick, R. B. and Greisman, S. E.: On the pathogenesis of typhoid fever. *Arch Intern Med* 138:357, 1978.

Hornick, R. B., Greisman, S. E., Woodward, T. E., et al.: Typhoid fever: Pathogenesis and immunologic control. *N Engl J Med* 283:686, 739, 1970.

Johnson, R. H., Lutwick, L. I., Huntley, G. A., and Vosti, K. L.: *Arizona hinshawii* infections. *Ann Intern Med* 85:587, 1976.

Kaijser, B.: Immunity of *Escherichia coli*: K-antigen and its relation to urinary tract infection. *J Infect Dis* 127:670, 1973.

Kantor, H. S., Tao, P., and Wisdom, C.: Action of *Escherichia coli* enterotoxin: Adenylate cyclase behavior of intestinal epithelial cell in culture. *Infect Immun* 9:1003, 1974.

Leino, R. and Kalliomaki, J. L.: Yersiniosis as an internal disease. *Ann Intern Med* 81:458, 1974.

Levine, M. M., Dupont, H. L., Formal, S. B., et al.: Pathogenesis of *Shigella dysenteriae* 1 (Shiga) dysentery. *J Infect Dis* 127:261, 1973.

McCabe, W. R.: Immunoprophylaxis of gram-negative bacillary infections. *Ann Rev Med* 27:335, 1976.

McCabe, W. R., Bruins, S. C., Craven, D. E., et al.: Cross-reactive antigens: Their potential for immunization-induced immunity to gram-negative bacteria. *J Infect Dis* 136(suppl):S161, 1977.

McCabe, W. R., Carling, P. C., Bruins, S., et al.: The relation of K-antigen to virulence of *Escherichia coli*. *J Infect Dis* 131:6, 1975.

McCabe, W. R., Kreger, B. E., and Johns, M.: Type specific and cross-reactive antibodies in gram-negative bacteremia. *N Engl J Med* 287:261, 1972.

Meyers, B. R., Bottone, E., Hirschman, S. Z., et al.: Infections caused by micro-organisms of the genus *Erwinia. Ann Intern Med* 76:9, 1972.

Orskov, F., Orskov, I., Jann, B., et al.: Serology, chemistry and genetics of O and K antigens of *E. coli. Bacteriol Rev* 41:667, 1977.

Pazin, G. J. and Braude, A. I.: Immobilizing antibodies in urine. 2. Prevention of ascending spread of *Proteus mirabilis. Invest Urol* 12:129, 1979.

Robbins, J. B., McCracken, G. H., Gotschich, E. C., et al.: *Escherichia coli* K1 capsular polysaccharide associated with neonatal meningitis. *N Engl J Med* 290:1216, 1974.

Ryder, R. W., Wachsmuth, I. K., Buxton, A. E., et al.: Infantile diarrhea produced by heat-stable enterotoxigenic *Escherichia coli. N Engl J Med* 295:849, 1976.

Silverblatt, F. J.: Host-parasite interaction in the rat renal pelvis. A possible role for pili in the pathogenesis of pyelonephritis. *J Exp Med* 140:1696, 1974.

Simberkoff, M. S., Ricupero, I., and Rahal, J. J., Jr.: Host resistance to *Serratia marcescens* infection: Serum bactericidal activity and phagocytosis by normal blood leukocytes. *J Lab Clin Med* 87:206, 1976.

Ulshen, M. H. and Rollo, J. L.: Pathogenesis of *Escherichia coli* gastroenteritis in man – another mechanism. *N Engl J Med* 302:99, 1980.

Une, T.: Studies on the pathogenecity of *Yersinia enterocolitica*. 1. Experimental infection in rabbits. *Microbiol Immunol* 21:349, 1977.

vonReyn, C. F., Weber, N. S., Tempest, B., et al.: Epidemiologic and clinical features of an outbreak of bubonic plague in New Mexico. *J Infect Dis* 136:489, 1977.

Yu, V. L.: *Serratia marcescens.* Historical perspective and clinical review. *N Engl J Med* 300:887, 1979.

93

PSEUDOMONADACEAE
Ronica M. Kluge, M.D.

Pseudomonas spp include a large variety of aerobic, gram-negative bacilli which do not ferment carbohydrates. They are found widely dispersed in soil and water. Some species are plant pathogens, others cause disease primarily in animals. Pseudomonads are also opportunistic invaders of humans (e.g., cystic fibrosis, neutropenia, burns, immunosuppression).

Microbiology and Pathogenesis

The microbiologic characteristics of *Pseudomonadaceae* are listed in Table 93.1. Species of the family are listed in Table 93.2.

    Pseudomonadaceae have cell walls which are similar to those of the *Enterobacteriaceae* and made up of approximately 60% lipid and polysaccharide, 30% protein and 10% peptidoglycan. Somatic, or O, antigens have been utilized for serogrouping, but the system is at best cumbersome. Most *P. aeruginosa* produce pyocyanines which permit typing; other *Pseudomonas* strains do not have this characteristic. The importance of endotoxin in the pathogenesis of disease caused by *P. aeruginosa* is controversial. Endotoxin produced by this organism is much less potent than endotoxin from *Enterobacteriaceae*.

    P. aeruginosa also produces a slime layer loosely attached to the cell surface, consisting of polysaccharide, nucleic acid, lipid and protein. Slime is considered a virulence factor, as it impedes phagocytosis. Purified slime preparations injected into a mouse model reproduce the toxic manifestations of infections by live organisms. Type-specific antislime antibodies afford protection in an animal model.

    Pseudomonadaceae usually have pili which may also be virulence factors. Pili are believed to be involved in attachment of the organism to biological surfaces and in resistance to phagocytosis.

TABLE 93.1   Characteristics of *Pseudomonadaceae*

Gram-negative bacilli, nonsporeforming

Aerobic (facultatively anaerobic)

Nonfermentative

Oxidize carbohydrates to acid but not gas

Catalase-positive

Polar monotrichous or tuft of flagella

TABLE 93.2   Members of the *Pseudomonadaceae* Family

P. aeruginosa	*P. alcaligenes*
P. fluorescens	*P. pseudoalcaligenes*
P. putida	*P. diminuta*
P. pseudomallei	*P. vesiculare*
P. mallei	*P. stutzeri*
P. cepacia	*P. maltophilia*
P. acidovorans	*P. putrefaciens*
P. testosteroni	*P. paucimobilis*

The cellular products of *Pseudomonadaceae* are best characterized for *P. aeruginosa* strains and include a variety of exotoxins and enzymes (Table 93.3). Exotoxin A, a single polypeptide chain weighing 71,500 daltons, is the most potent toxin on a weight basis. It is heat labile and becomes active when cleaved by proteases. Exotoxin A has been detected in the serum of patients with *P. aeruginosa* bacteremia. High-titer antibodies to exotoxin A appear to offer some protection against mortality from *P. aeruginosa* bacteremia. Exotoxins B and C cause shock and death in mice, dogs, and monkeys, but their role in human disease is less well defined.

P. aeruginosa produces several proteolytic enzymes, including protease, elastase and collagenase. These products may play a role in pathogenesis of localized infection. Specifically, an elastase is thought to be important in the development of necrotizing vasculitis, which is often present within *P. aeruginosa* infected tissue.

The role of the hemolytic factors produced by *P. aeruginosa* is not clear and that of leukocidin is only speculative for human disease.

TABLE 93.3   Proven and Potential Virulence Factors of *P. aeruginosa*

Proven:	slime
	pili
	exotoxin A
Potential:	endotoxin
	exotoxin B, C
	protease
	elastase
	collagenase
	hemolytic factors
	leukocidin

Epidemiology

Host factors (Table 93.4) assume great importance in diseases caused by *Pseudomonadaceae* (Table 93.5). Patients who are granulocytopenic due to underlying disease, or therapy for same, are at greater risk to develop *P. aeruginosa* colonization and subsequent infection. The presence or absence of opsonophagocytic antibodies appears to relate directly to outcome in patients with *P. aeruginosa* bacteremia. Patients with cystic fibrosis are particularly prone to colonization by mucoid strains of *P. aeruginosa*; in fact, such isolates are recovered rarely from other than cystic fibrosis patients. Patients with extensive burns also appear to be at risk to develop *P. aeruginosa* infections. Many other *Pseudomonas* strains (e.g., *P. cepacia, P. fluorescens, P. stutzeri*) are primarily acquired as in-hospital infections and may be considered opportunists. *P. pseudomallei* is a common soil inhabitant in Southeast Asia but not in the United States.

P. aeruginosa

This organism is responsible for 10-20% of all gram-negative bacteremias, but responsible for 30-50% of gram-negative bacteremias in the immunocompromised

TABLE 93.4   Host Factors in Infections Caused by *Pseudomonadaceae*

Granulocytopenia

Opsonophagocytic antibodies

Local immunity (e.g., cystic fibrosis)

Depressed/defective cellular immunity

TABLE 93.5   Most Common Diseases Caused by *Pseudomonadaceae*

Organism	Disease
P. aeruginosa	Bacteremia
	Endocarditis
	Pneumonia
	UTI
	Malignant otitis externa
P. pseudomallei	Melioidosis
P. mallei	Glanders
Others	Nosocomial infections

host.   *P. aeruginosa* bacteremia has a 70% mortality. Ecthyma gangrenosum occurs in 5-10% of patients with *P. aeruginosa* bacteremia; biopsy shows necrotizing vasculitis with vessel invasion by the organism. Endocarditis due to *P. aeruginosa* occurs primarily in drug addicts or in those with prosthetic cardiac valves. Pneumonia due to this organism is most likely to occur in the elderly or otherwise debilitated patient. The pneumonic process is usually necrotizing and may be accompanied by bacteremia or empyema. *P. aeruginosa* urinary tract infections occur following instrumentation, obstruction or multiple courses of antimicrobials. Osteomyelitis due to this organism is seen in drug addicts, following puncture wounds of the foot in children, and in diabetics. Central nervous system infection is rare and usually nosocomially acquired in patients with head trauma and/or cranial surgery. *P. aeruginosa* causes external otitis, and in selected patients (diabetics, immunosuppressed) the process can become a fulminant, destructive one involving cartilage and bone. Sixty-five to eighty-five percent of patients with cystic fibrosis are colonized with *P. aeruginosa* strains, usually of the mucoid variety. Interestingly, these patients rarely become bacteremic.

P. pseudomallei

This organism has marked variations in uptake of stains and often appears bipolar, or like a safety pin. As mentioned previously, it is found primarily in Southeast Asia, where it can be isolated from soil, water and produce. The greatest number of melioidosis cases occurs in Vietnam, Cambodia, Laos, Thailand, Malaysia and Burma. The organism gains entrance to the body by inhalation or through skin abrasions. Clinically, the disease takes several forms (Table 93.6), and there is evidence supporting the occurrence of a large number of subclinical infections for every symptomatic one. Most common is the acute pulmonary infection which varies in onset (gradual to abrupt) and severity (mild to overwhelming). Tachypnea may occur out of proportion to fever or findings in physical/roentgenographic examinations. The upper lobes are usually involved, and cavitation occurs frequently, leading to its confusion with pulmonary tuberculosis. In the septicemic form, the patient is extremely toxic, with high temperatures and cyanosis. In addition to chest findings, muscle tenderness and hepatosplenomegaly may be present. The course is often so rapidly fatal that therapy cannot be instituted.

TABLE 93.6   Clinical Forms of Melioidosis

Acute localized, suppurative

Acute pulmonary

Acute septicemic

Chronic suppurative

P. mallei

This organism causes disease primarily in equine animals, but it is occasionally transmitted to humans. Glanders is almost nonexistent in horses in the United States today, hence human cases are extremely rare in this country. Sporadic glanders in humans occurs in South/Central America, Asia, and Africa. The organism resembles *P. pseudomallei* morphologically. Clinical presentations vary, depending upon portal of entry, but in general resemble the four forms of melioidosis (see Table 93.6). Skin inoculation usually results in a nodule and associated lymphangitis. Inoculation of mucous membranes results in purulent discharge and development of ulcerating granulomatous lesions. The septicemic form is fulminant and frequently fatal; it is accompanied by a diffuse papular eruption. Inhalation infection results in lobar or bronchopneumonia with systemic toxicity. The chronic, suppurative form of the disease presents with multiple skin and muscle abscesses, and lymphadenopathy.

Others

The other *Pseudomonas* strains listed in Table 93.1 are recovered variously in plant, soil, and water samples and not infrequently in the hospital environment. Generally considered contaminants, each has been documented to cause infection in the occasional patient. Such infections are often nosocomially acquired, and they tend to occur in selected patients (elderly, debilitated, immunosuppressed, following surgery or other instrumentation, those on long-term, broad spectrum antibiotics, and patients on ventilatory equipment).

Selected Bibliography

Baltch, A. L., Griffin, P. E., and Hammer, M.: *Pseudomonas aeruginosa* bacteremia: Relationship of bacterial enzyme production and pyocine types with clinical prognosis in 100 patients. *J Lab Clin Med* 93:600, 1979.

Berkelman, R. L., Lewin, S., Allen, J. R., et al.: Pseudobacteremia attributed to contamination of povidone - iodine with *Pseudomonas cepacia. Ann Intern Med* 95:32, 1981.

Clayton, A. J.,Lisella, R. S., and Martin, D. G.: Melioidosis: A serological survey in military personnel. *Mil Med* 138:24, 1973.

Crane, L. R., Tagle, L. C., and Palutke, W. A.: Outbreak of *Pseudomonas paucimobilis* in an intensive care facility. *JAMA* 246:985, 1981.

Everett, E. D. and Nelson, R.A.: Pulmonary melioidosis: Observations in thirty-nine cases. *Am Rev Respir Dis* 112:331, 1975.

Gilardi, G. L.: Infrequently encountered *Pseudomonas* species causing infection in humans. *Ann Intern Med* 77:211, 1972.

Jones, L. F., Zakanycz, J. P., Thomas, E. T., et al.: Pyocin typing of *Pseudomonas aeruginosa:* A simplified method. *Appl Microbiol* 27:400, 1974.

Liu, P. V.: Extracellular toxins of *Pseudomonas aeruginosa. J Infect Dis* 130:594, 1974.

Liu, P. V., Abe, Y., and Bates, J. L.: The role of various fractions of *Pseudomonas aeruginosa* in its pathogenesis. *J Infect Dis* 108:218, 1961.

Nonoyama, S., Kojo, H., Mine, Y., et al.: Inhibitory effect of *Pseudomonas aeruginosa* on the phagocytic and killing activities of rabbit polymorphonuclear leukocytes: Purification and characterization of an inhibitor of polymorphonuclear leukocyte function. *Infect Immun* 24:394, 1979.

Pavlovskis, O. R., Voelker, F. A., and Shackelford, A. H.: *Pseudomonas aeruginosa* exotoxin in mice: Histopathology and serum enzyme changes. *J Infect Dis* 133:253, 1976.

Pollack, M., Callahan, L. T., and Taylor, N. S.: Neutralizing antibody to *Pseudomonas aeruginosa* exotoxin in human sera: Evidence for in vivo toxin production during infections. *Infect Immun* 14:942, 1976.

Pollack, M. and Young, L. S.: Protective activity of antibodies to exotoxin A and lipopolysaccharide at the onset of *Pseudomonas aeruginosa* bacteremia in man. *J Clin Invest* 63:276, 1979.

Sensakovic, J. W. and Bartell, P. R.: The slime of *Pseudomonas aeruginosa:* Biological characterization and possible role in experimental infection. *J Infect Dis* 129:101, 1974.

Soave, R., Murray, H. W., and Litrenta, M. M.: Bacterial invasion of pulmonary vessels: *Pseudomonas* bacteremia mimicking pulmonary thromboembolism with infection. *Am J Med* 65:864, 1978.

94

BRUCELLA: BRUCELLOSIS

Rama Ganguly, Ph.D.

The genus *Brucella* consists of a group of organisms that cause diseases in domestic animals. Humans may become an accidental host as an occupational hazard or by contact with contaminated animal products. Human-to-human transmission of the disease has not been reported.

Etiology

Brucella are gram-negative nonmotile, nonsporeforming coccobacilli. They consist of three major species: *B. melitensis* (infects goats and sheep), *B. abortus* (infects cattle), and *B. suis* (infects pigs). This is not an absolute division in that both humans and domestic animals are susceptible to all three species. Another specie, *B. canis*, is known to have caused several outbreaks in dogs. These species may be characterized on the basis of their need for CO_2 for growth, hydrogen sulfide produced during growth, sensitivity to dye (basic fuchsin and thionin), urease activity, and agglutination by monospecific antisera. These organisms grow optimally at 37°C under aerobic conditions. Animal serum, glucose, vitamins, salts, and protein digest in media enhance their growth. It usually takes several days before the growth is detected on agar plates. The colonies are usually smooth, moist, transparent, glistening, and about 1 mm in diameter. They may undergo mutation to rough or mucoid types of colonies in laboratory media resulting in the loss of virulence. Loss of somatic antigen (O) may also render them nonagglutinable by homologous sera. *Brucella* have two cell-wall carbohydrate antigenic determinants (A and M) present on the lipopolysaccharide protein complex. The amounts of these antigens vary in the three species. Immunologic cross-reactivity occurs between *Brucella, Yersinia, Francisella,* and *Vibrio.* Toxins other than endotoxin have not been described.

Epidemiology

Brucella organisms are ubiquitous and are related to animal diseases. Goats, cattle, swine, sheep, and dogs carry these organisms under natural conditions. They may be infected via skin and mucous membrane surfaces such as the gastrointestinal and genitourinary tracts, and conjunctivae. They cause abortion in animals and may be shed in secretions, urine, and milk of infected animals for prolonged periods. The disease may be spread to other animals by contact with contaminated milk, tissues, and placenta. Because of the prophylactic vaccination measures against brucellosis, the incidence of cattle abortion has declined, but the infection is still spread in cattle in an endemic form.

Unpasteurized milk and milk products may be major sources of human infection. In the United States, at present, most cases occur from contact with infected materials, e.g., in abattoir workers, veterinarians, laboratory workers, and dairy farming employees. Inhalation of infected aerosols in a slaughter house may be another source of the spread of the disease. *Brucella suis* causes most of the diseases in man. Erythritol which is present in animal uteri enhances multiplication of the organisms. This entity is not present in human tissues and therefore does not contribute to colonization of the pathogen. *Brucella* may survive for long periods in damp soil, water, and refrigerated carcasses of infected animals but may be destroyed in 2-4 hr in direct sunlight. The disease in animal herds left untreated may cause significant economic loss. In 1977, 37 states, Puerto Rico, and Guam reported 233 cases of human brucellosis to the Centers for Disease Control.

Pathogenesis

The pathogens entering the host via skin abrasion or mucous membrane surfaces are phagocytized and transported to the regional lymph nodes. They multiply within the phagocytes which lyse, leading to bacteremia. Intracellular growth of the organisms in macrophages enables the pathogens to establish long-term infection despite the presence of antibody. They preferentially grow in placental tissue. *Brucella* also grow well in the mammary glands of lactating animals and are shed in milk. The animal fetus may be infected or aborted. Brucellar infection in dairy cattle is detected by the screening milk ring test (MRT) which measures the brucellar agglutinin. In humans, granuloma formation, abscess formation, and even caseation may occur in a variety of organs, including liver, placenta, lymph nodes, subcutaneous tissues, testis, ovary, kidney, and brain. Chronic, latent, and relapsing infections are frequent. Formation of activated macrophages is important for eradicating this intracellular parasite. Classic undulant fever may be observed and is thought to be caused by endotoxin release from the organisms. Organisms surviving in various tissues may lead to the Jarisch-Herxheimer reaction upon antibiotic treatment. In the chronic state of the disease granulomas are formed consisting of epithelioid cells, giant cells, and lymphocytes.

Clinical Manifestations

Brucellosis in humans may assume any one of the following forms: carrier (or asymptomatic) brucellosis, acute brucellosis, relapsing brucellosis, brucellosis localized in various organs, and vaccine-acquired (strain 19) brucellosis. The incubation period may be 3 days to several months or years. Weakness, fatigue, chills, sweats, anorexia, headache, malaise, weight loss, arthralgia, anxiety, or even mental depression may be seen. The fever tends to be intermittent with diurnal variation. Splenomegaly or lymphadenopathy may occur. The disease is usually self-limited, but chronic forms of the disease may linger for 1-20 years with relapses. Complications of the disease result from the granulomatous lesions formed in various tissues and organs and include infective endocarditis, meningitis and meningoencephalitis, osteomyelitis, acute suppurative arthritis, bursitis, and renal brucellosis. Because of the various types of nonspecific manifestations observed in brucellosis, differential diagnosis includes influenza, malaria, typhoid fever, typhus, tularemia, miliary tuberculosis, and some noninfectious diseases. Analysis of the source of contact may be useful for diagnostic purposes.

Laboratory Diagnosis

Repeated blood cultures should be done in the acute febrile stage. Also spleen, liver, and bone marrow biopsies may be used for bacteriologic isolation. Cerebrospinal fluid testing is warranted in the presence of CNS symptoms. Serologic diagnosis involves the standard tube agglutination test which is very sensitive and reproducible. The test utilizes selected and standardized antigens of the three major species. Cross-reactivity with other organisms usually gives a lower titer than with the homologous antigen. The recently developed card agglutination test is a very rapid method of diagnosis/screening and it correlates in 90% of the cases with the tube agglutination test. In the initial stage of the disease, IgM agglutinating antibodies are present. Depending upon age, sex, and geographic location relatively high titers of brucellar antibodies are found in normal people. A titer of > 1:160 using the standard agglutination test may be considered as presumptive evidence of active infection. A four-fold or greater rise in antibody, whatever the titer, is definitive evidence of active disease. The antibody titer falls fairly rapidly with successful treatment, although the titer may chronically remain fairly high.

Immunity

Patients develop cell-mediated immunity to antigens from the organism, and this can be tested using the preparation Brucellergen. This cell-mediated immunity and the consequent activation of macrophages correlate with control of the infection and eradication of the intracellular pathogen. This immunity is not long lasting and second infection and/or reactivation occurs.

Treatment

Tetracycline (2 g/day p.o.) is the drug of choice.   Streptomycin and tetracycline in combination have been found to be highly effective in severe cases as well as in preventing relapses (Table 94.1). Treatment is usually continued for at least 3 weeks. In experimental animals rifampin has been highly effective, which may be related to its ability to penetrate cells.

Prevention

Control of the disease in man is related to the control of infections in animals. In recent years pasteurization of milk and various eradication programs have helped in reducing the incidence of the disease. However, during the last 5 years, for yet

TABLE 94.1   Treatment of Brucellosis

Regimen	Total Dose	Relapse Rate (Approximate %)
Tetracycline + streptomycin	40 g 30 g	1-10
Tetracycline alone	$\geq$ 40 g	5-10
Trimethoprim-sulfamethoxazole	120-160 tablets	10-20
Sulfonamide + streptomycin	60 g 30 g	30-35
Chloramphenicol alone Streptomycin alone Sulfonamide alone	24 g 30 g 60 g	> 40

undetermined reasons, there has been an upswing in human cases in the United States mostly from contact with infected cattle. There is an attenuated vaccine that has been developed (*B. abortus* strain 19) for cattle. This has reduced the rate of abortion and bacterial shedding in milk. No vaccines are available for human use.

Selected Bibliography

Alausa, O. K.: Brucellosis: Socioeconomic problems and control in various countries. *Trop Geogr Med* 32:5-11, 1980.

Eckman, M. R.: Brucellosis linked to Mexican cheese. *JAMA* 232:636-637, 1975.

Elberg, S. S.: Immunity to brucella infection. *Medicine* 52:339-356, 1973.

Fox, M. D. and Kaufman, A. F.: Brucellosis in the United States, 1965-1974. *J Infect Dis* 136:312-316, 1977.

Heck, F. C., Williams, J. D., and Pruett, J.: Interpretation of spectrophotometric absorbance values to define results of enzyme-linked immunosorbent assays. *J Clin Microbiol* 11:398-401, 1980.

Kaneene, J. M., Nicoletti, P., Anderson, R. K., Muscoplat, C. C., and Johnson, D. W.: Cell-mediated immune responses in cattle adult-vaccinated with *Brucella abortus* strain 19 and in cattle infected with *Brucella abortus* field strain. *Am J Vet Res* 40:1503-1509, 1979.

Meyer, M. E.: Evolution and taxonomy in the genus *Brucella:* Concepts on the origins of the contemporary species. *Am J Vet Res* 37:199-202, 1976.

Munford, R. S., Weaver, R. E., Patton, C., Feeley, J. C., and Feldman, R. A.: Human disease caused by *Brucella canis:* A clinical and epidemiological study of two cases. *JAMA* 231:1267-1269, 1979.

Philippon, A. M., Plommet, M. G., Kazmierczak, A., Marly, J. L., and Nevot, P.A.: Rifampin in the treatment of experimental brucellosis in mice and guinea pigs. *J Infect Dis* 136:482-488, 1977.

Spink, W. W.: The significance of bacterial hypersensitivity in human brucellosis: Studies on infection due to strain 19 *Brucella abortus. Ann Intern Med* 47: 861-874, 1957.

Tabatabai, L. B., DeYoe, B. L., and Ritchie, A. E.: Isolation and characterization of toxic fractions from *Brucella abortus. Infect Immun* 26:668-679, 1979.

95

BORDETELLA
Robert H. Waldman, M.D.

There are three species of *Bordetella* that are of clinical significance to humans. One, *B. bronchiseptica,* is an animal pathogen rarely transmitted to humans, and therefore is of very minimal importance; the second, *B. parapertussis,* is relatively unimportant and causes a milder version of the illness caused by the *Bordetella* organism that is of major importance, *B. pertussis.* Before 1900, pertussis was a significant cause of infant morbidity and mortality, but the incidence has fallen greatly as a result of immunization and also social and nutritional improvements (Tables 95.1 and 95.2).

Microbiology

Bordetella pertussis was first isolated from a case of whooping cough by Bordet and Gengou. The organism is a minute, gram-negative coccobacillus. It has a capsule and pili and is best isolated on the medium developed by Bordet and Gengou consisting of blood, glycerin, and potato extract. Upon repeated passage on artificial medium the organism undergoes changes analogous to the smooth-to-rough change which many gram-negative organisms undergo, and which for *B. pertussis* has been denoted as changing from phase I, virulent, through phase IV, nonpathogenic.

Epidemiology

The disease is spread by inhaling droplets, and patients are most infectious before the onset of the classic whooping cough symptoms during the nonspecific catarrhal phase. The disease is worldwide in distribution and affects children, newborns

TABLE 95.1 Infant Mortality from Pertussis

	Deaths/1000 Infants
In the past	
1900	4.4
1920	2.3
1935	1.3
Today	
Guatemala	5.2
Ecuador	3.0
Honduras	2.7
Peru	1.9
England and Wales	0.01
U.S.	0.003

TABLE 95.2 Factors Other than Immunization that May Have Played a Role in Decrease in Pertussis Incidence

General improvement in socioeconomic status

Better hygiene and nutrition

Improvements in supportive therapy

Decreased virulence of *B. pertussis*

Decreased % of population in high-risk group (< 5 years)

in particular. Two-thirds of the deaths from pertussis occur in infants under 1 year of age. As opposed to most infectious diseases, there is probably no completely asymptomatic carrier state. The reported number of cases has remained stable for the past 10 years, i.e., about 2300 cases and about 10 fatalities per year. Although the latter is a fairly accurate number, it is undoubtedly an underestimate.

Bordetella parapertussis is of very minor importance in the United States, but is relatively more common in certain countries where it has been searched for, e.g., Denmark, Czechoslovakia, and the USSR.

Pathogenesis

Bordetella pertussis is not invasive, but apparently causes disease by attaching to the ciliated epithelium of the respiratory tract and producing a toxic substance. Histopathologically, masses of organisms are seen on the luminal surface, beneath which the bronchial epithelium is damaged with infiltration of polymorphonuclear leukocytes. There is also a peribronchial inflammatory response and interstitial pneumonia. Further pulmonary pathology is a result of bronchial obstruction by mucous plugs and/or secondary bacterial infection leading to bronchopneumonia. Pathologically, the two main sequelae of whooping cough are bronchiectasis and microscopic hemorrhages in the brain.

Diagnosis

Whooping cough always should be a clinical diagnosis. There is some question as to whether or not the clinical syndrome can be caused by certain viruses, e.g., adenoviruses. It is generally thought that the isolation of viruses from patients with pertussis probably represents coincidental infection or viral reactivation secondary to the stress of the illness.

The incubation period is about 7 days. The illness begins with the "catarrhal" stage, which is very difficult to differentiate from the myriad other causes of viral upper respiratory syndromes, i.e., there is nothing that would make one suspect pertussis, except epidemiology. The symptoms are coryza, sneezing, lacrimation, cough, and low-grade fever. The child is usually listless and irritable. This is followed by the classic paroxysmal stage of the disease. The cough which was present in the catarrhal stage gradually takes on the characteristic whooping nature. The cough, instead of improving as one would expect in the course of the usual viral respiratory infection, becomes more severe. It comes on in characteristic spasms, i.e., episodic bouts of coughing, followed by seemingly lifesaving inhalation, the "whoop." The whoop is usually accompanied, preceded, or followed by vomiting. The spasms of coughing occur three to four times a day in the milder cases, to as often as every few minutes. The spasms are accompanied by cyanosis and in the worst cases by convulsions. The paroxysmal stage lasts from 1 to 3 weeks. Next is the convalescent stage, which is a period of variable length, during which the child slowly regains strength, but continues to have some coughing which is not of the whooping type, but is more of a nagging nature, even appearing to be a habit. The convalescent stage may last up to 2 months.

In older children and adults pertussis is much milder, does not usually cause serious spasms of coughing, and is identical to any other cause of bronchitis or a rather severe upper respiratory infection.

The laboratory diagnosis is made by culturing the organism; however, cultures are most often positive during the catarrhal phase of the disease when one least expects the diagnosis clinically. During the paroxysmal stage, culture is usually negative. The organism grows optimally on Bordet-Gengou or blood charcoal media. The identity of the organism isolated on one of these media is confirmed by growth characteristics and agglutination. The diagnosis can also be made by immunofluorescence on nasal pharyngeal swab material.

The differential diagnosis includes the etiologies of any other type of severe bronchitis, but with other etiologies, the cough is not spasmodic, and that caused by a foreign body should not have been preceded by a catarrhal stage.

Immunology and Prevention

Infection probably confers immunity lasting about 15-20 years. The protective antigen is not known, but is thought to be part of the cell wall, and antibody to it may confer immunity. Serum agglutination titers correlate fairly well with protection. On the other hand, passive administration of immune serum globulin is of no value, and there is apparent lack of transfer of immunity from mother to fetus. These observations could be explained by the fact that the protective antibody is of the IgM or secretory IgA classes, but this has not been examined carefully.

Pertussis immunization is an extremely controversial subject. Although it is at least somewhat effective, it is also associated with unwanted side effects. The degree of its protective efficacy is unclear. The vaccine is a suspension of inactivated bacteria, containing a large number of antigens, both protective and possibly toxic. Fatal reactions are estimated to occur in about 1-2:10 million doses. Permanent sequelae occur in about 1:300,000 doses. On the other hand, this is far less than the fatalities or permanent sequelae associated with the disease itself. Some authorities have suggested that with a decreasing disease occurrence there is more harm associated with the vaccine than benefit, and that routine pertussis immunization should be discontinued. On the other hand, others have suggested that the current practice of not recommending the vaccine for children over the age of 7, or adults, be changed because the lowered occurrence of the disease has lessened natural immunity leading to a large susceptible population. Table 95.3 gives the suggested immunization schedule for pertussis.

The most common vaccine side effects are fever and local pain, erythema, and the development of a nodule (Table 95.4). These occur in about half of vaccinees and are treated symptomatically. The fever usually comes on within several hours of the injection and is generally mild to moderate. Much more worrisome are the "screaming" and "shock" reactions (Table 95.5). The screaming

TABLE 95.3   Immunization Schedule for Pertussis [1]

Dose	Age
1	6 wk or as soon thereafter as possible
2	4-8 wk after 1st dose[2]
3	4-8 wk after 2nd dose
4	About 1 yr after 3rd dose
5	Before entering kindergarten or elementary school (not necessary if 4th dose received after age 4)

[1]Given as DTP (along with diphtheria and tetanus toxoids) intramuscularly

[2]Interruption or delay in recommended schedule does *not* require restarting, regardless of time elapsed between doses

TABLE 95.4   Mild to Moderate Reactions to Pertussis Immunization

Reaction	Approximate %
Local	
Swelling	40
Redness	35
Pain	30
Fever	
$\geq$ 38°C	25
$\geq$ 39°C	5
$\geq$ 40°C	1
Irritability	35
Anorexia	15
Drowsiness	15

TABLE 95.5   Severe Side Effects of Pertussis Immunization

Side Effect	Estimated Occurrence*
Persistent screaming	70-2000
Collapse or shock	60-300
Convulsion(s) (with or without fever)	40-700
Encephalopathy	1-30

*Per million doses given

reaction occurs within a few hours of the injection and is characterized by a high-pitched, "encephalitic" cry, different from any other the child has ever had, and the parents usually observe that the vaccinee cannot be comforted nor can the crying be controlled. After several hours of screaming, the child falls asleep and awakens apparently completely normal. The shock reaction is characterized by decreased activity, lethargy, unresponsiveness, pallor, and hypotension, which occur within 12 hr of injections, but are very rarely fatal. The shock and screaming reactions have no sequelae. The most severe reaction to the vaccine is encephalopathy (Table 95.6) which comes on within 48 hr of immunization, is fatal in 2-15%, and leads to serious sequelae, i.e., persistent convulsions, hemiplegia, or psychomotor retardation, in about 50%. It occurs in approximately 1:100,000 vaccinees, and follows infection as well as immunization. It is this side effect of

TABLE 95.6 Characteristics of Postpertussis Encephalopathy

Males predominate

Not related to age of immunization,
  size of dose, or whether first or
  subsequent dose

Manifestations: changes in consciousness,
                 convulsions,
                 paresis

Mortality ∿ 15%

Permanent sequelae ∿ 30%

TABLE 95.7 Contraindications to Further Pertussis Immunization

Occurrence of any of following after previous
  pertussis immunization:

      Collapse or shock
      Persistent screaming episode
      Temperature ≥ 40.5°C
      Convulsion
      Alteration in consciousness
      Neurologic abnormality
      Systemic allergic reaction
      Thrombocytopenia
      Hemolytic anemia

Neurologic disease

immunization which has led some investigators to reevaluate the standard use of pertussis vaccine and to various approaches that are intended to minimize its occurrence. The most reasonable approach is to be sure that a parent is questioned when the child returns for subsequent doses of the vaccine, and if any serious side effect occurred with a preceding dose (Table 95.7) further immunization is contraindicated. The pathogenic mechanisms of the postpertussis immunization encephalopathy are unknown. It has been postulated that impurities from the media in which the organism is grown are responsible. The organism contains many biologically active substances; perhaps one of these is responsible for the encephalopathy. Some of these substances are agglutinogens, a hemagglutinin, endotoxin, a heat-labile toxin, lymphocyte-promoting factor, and insulin-stimulating activity.

Antibiotics are useful in preventing the spread of the infection. The drug of choice is erythromycin, which should be given to the patient and to close contacts who are under 1 year of age and to unimmunized contacts under 7 years old. Other

818   Organisms

TABLE 95.8   Complications of Whooping Cough

Pressure effects

Inguinal or umbilical hernia
Rectal prolapse
Mucosal hemorrhage
Petechiae
Rare: pneumothorax, subcutaneous
emphysema, subdural hematoma

Neurologic (temporary or permanent)

Convulsions
Paralysis
Deafness
Blindness
Aphasia
Mental retardation

Respiratory

Bronchopneumonia
Atelectasis
? Bronchiectasis

---

antibiotics which are efficacious are chloramphenicol and tetracycline. In addition to receiving antibiotics, close contacts should be immunized if they are under 7 years old, and if they have not completed the complete four-dose schedule, or if they have not received a booster immunization within the past 3 years.

Treatment

Antibiotics have no effect on the course of the disease, except for being useful in the treatment of secondary pneumonia. Hyperimmune serum has been used but there is no evidence that it is beneficial.   General supportive measures including oxygen and good hydration are essential.
Table 95.8 lists the complications that may result from whooping cough.

Selected Bibliography

Altemeier, W. A., III and Ayoub, E. M.: Erythromycin prophylaxis for pertussis. *Pediatrics* 59:623, 1977.

Balagtas, R. C., Nelson, K. E., Levin, S., and Gotoff, S. P.: Treatment of pertussis with pertussis immune globulin. *J Pediatr* 79:203, 1971.

Baraff, L. J., Wilkins, J., and Wehrle, P. F.: The role of antibiotics, immunizations, and adenoviruses in pertussis. *Pediatrics* 61:224, 1978.

Barkin, R. M. and Pichichero, M. E.: Diphtheria-pertussis-tetanus vaccine: Re-actogenecity of commercial products. *Pediatrics* 63:256, 1979.

Bemis, D. A., Greisen, H. A., and Appel, M. J. G.: Pathogenesis of canine borde-tellosis. *J Infect Dis* 135:753, 1977.

Bradstreet, C. M. P., Tannahit, A. J., and Edwards, J. M.B.: Detection of *Borde-tella pertussis* antibodies in human sera by complement-fixation and immu-nofluorescence. *J Hyg* 70:75, 1972.

Church, M. A.: Evidence of whooping-cough-vaccine efficacy from the 1978 whooping-cough epidemic in Hertfordshire. *Lancet* 2:188, 1979.

Edsall, G.: Present status of pertussis vaccination. *Practitioner* 215:310, 1975.

Griffith, A. H.: Pertussis vaccine and convulsive disorders of childhood. *Proc R Soc Med* 67:16, 1974.

Griffith, A. H.: Reactions after pertussis vaccines: A manufacturer's experience and difficulties since 1964. *Br Med J* 1:809, 1978.

Katz, S. L. and Wilfert, C. M.: New thoughts on pertussis. *Pediatrics* 63:941, 1979.

Kendrick, P. L.: Can whooping cough be eradicated? *J Infect Dis* 132:707, 1975.

Koplan, J. P., Schoenbaum, S. C., Weinstein, M. C., and Fraser, D. W.: Pertussis vaccine - an analysis of benefits, risks and costs. *N Engl J Med* 301:906, 1979.

Kulenkampff, M., Schwartzman, J. S., and Wilson, J.: Neurological complications of pertussis inoculation. *Arch Dis Child* 49:46, 1974.

Lautrop, H.: Epidemics of parapertussis: 20 years' observation in Denmark. *Lancet* 1:1195, 1971.

Lewis, F. A., Gust, I. D., and Bennet, N. M.: On the aetiology of whooping cough. *J Hyg* 71:139, 1973.

Linneman, C. C.: *Bordetella parapertussis:* Recent experience and review of lit-erature. *Am J Dis Child* 131:560, 1977.

Linneman, C. C., Jr. and Nasenberry, J.: Pertussis in the adult. *Ann Rev Med* 28:179, 1977.

Linneman, C. C., Ramundo, N., Perlstein, P. H., Minton, S. D., Englender, G. S., McCormick, J. B., and Hayes, P. S.: Use of pertussis vaccine in an epidemic involving hospital staff. *Lancet* 2:540, 1975.

Miller, C. L. and Fletcher, W. B.: Severity of notified whooping cough. *Br Med J* 1:117, 1976.

Morse, J. H., Kong, A. S., Lindenbaum, J., and Morse, S. I.: The mitogenic effect of the lymphocytosis promoting factor from *Bordetella pertussis* on human lymphocytes. *J Clin Invest* 60:683, 1977.

Morse, S. I. and Morse, J. H.: Isolation and properties of the leucocytosis- and lymphocytosis-promoting factor of *Bordetella pertussis*. *J Exp Med* 143:1483, 1976.

Nelson, J. D.: The changing epidemiology of pertussis in young infants: The role of adults as reservoirs of infection. *Am J Dis Child* 132:371, 1978.

Pereira, M. S. and Candeias, J. A. N.: The association of viruses with clinical pertussis. *J Hyg* 69:399, 1971.

Pittman, M.: Pertussis toxin: The cause of harmful effects and prolonged immunity of whooping cough. A hypothesis. *Rev Infect Dis* 1:401, 1979.

Pollard, R.: Relation between vaccination and notification rates for whooping cough in England and Wales. *Lancet* 1:1180, 1980.

OTHER GRAM-NEGATIVE BACILLI
Ronica M. Kluge, M.D.

The microbiologic features of *Haemophilus*, *Francisella*, *Pasteurella* (other than *P. pestis*), and miscellaneous gram-negative bacilli will be considered in this chapter. *Campylobacter* is discussed in Chapter 24 and *Yersinia* in Chapter 92 in regard to microbiology and pathogenesis.

Haemophilus

Members of the genus *Haemophilus* and their general laboratory characteristics are listed in Tables 96.1 and 96.2. These organisms are strict parasites, requiring accessory erythrocyte factors for in vitro growth (X and/or V). Factor X can be replaced by hematin, factor V by NAD (coenzyme I), NADP (coenzyme II), or nicotinamide nucleoside. The members of the genus vary in their production of polysaccharide capsules, their need for increased carbon dioxide, and their ability to produce hemolysis (Table 96.3).

Haemophilus influenzae is separable into six antigenically distinct types (a–f) on the basis of the composition of the polysaccharide capsule. Type b contains pentose sugars (ribose and ribitol), whereas the other types contain either a hexose or hexosamine moiety in the capsule. Types a, b, and c share certain antigenic determinants with pneumococci; type b cross-reacts with a number of other organisms, including certain enteric bacilli. Most *H. influenzae* that are documented to cause disease are encapsulated and almost all of these are type b. The organism's cell wall contains lipopolysaccharide similar to that found in other gram-negative bacilli.

Haemophilus influenzae resides exclusively in humans, particularly in their upper respiratory tracts and is spread by inhalation of infected droplets. The organism is distributed worldwide and generally causes endemic disease (Table 96.4).

TABLE 96.1   Members of the Genus *Haemophilus*

Pathogenic for humans	*H. influenzae*
	H. parainfluenzae
	II. aphrophilus
	H. paraphrophilus
	H. aegyptius
	H. ducreyi
Rarely pathogenic for humans	*H. haemolyticus*
	H. parahaemolyticus

TABLE 96.2   General Characteristics of *Haemophilus*

Minute, gram-negative coccobacilli
Nonmotile, nonsporeforming
Aerobic (facultatively anaerobic)
Pleomorphic, often bipolar staining
Require factors X and/or V
Polysaccharide capsules in many strains

TABLE 96.3   Differential Characteristics of *Haemophilus*

	Requirement For			
	X	V	CO_2	Cause Hemolysis
H. influenzae	+	+	−	−
H. parainfluenzae	−	+	−	−
H. aphrophilus	+	−	+	−
H. paraphrophilus	−	+	+	−
H. aegyptius	+	+	−	−
H. ducreyi	+	−	+	Slight
H. haemolyticus	+	+	−	+
H. parahaemolyticus	−	+	−	+

TABLE 96.4   The Most Common Diseases Caused by *Haemophilus*

Organism	Disease
H. influenzae type b	Meningitis
	Pneumonia
	Epiglottitis
	Bacteremia
	Cellulitis
	Otitis
H. influenzae, untypable	Bronchitis
	Pneumonia
H. parainfluenzae	Epiglottitis
	Meningitis
	Endocarditis
H. aphrophilus and *H. paraphrophilus*	Sinusitis
	Endocarditis
H. aegyptius	Purulent conjunctivitis
H. ducreyi	Chancroid

Outbreaks occur in certain closed populations (e.g., day-care centers); predisposing factors are listed in Table 96.5. Age is particularly important: newborns are rarely infected (protected by maternal antibody); whereas most *H. influenzae* infections occur among those aged 3 months to 3 years. The secondary attack rate for contacts of primary cases of *H. influenzae* meningitis and epiglottitis is similar to that in contacts of patients with meningococcal meningitis. Antibody to the ribose-ribitol phosphate polymer of the type b capsule (PRP) promotes complement-mediated phagocytosis and bacteriolysis in vitro, enhances bacterial clearance in vivo, and provides protection against disease in animal models and humans. Unfortunately, those in greatest need of protection, i.e., children aged 2-15 months, respond poorly, if at all, to PRP immunization.

Type b *H. influenzae* is a common cause of meningitis, pneumonia, epiglottitis, cellulitis, and bacteremia without a focus in young children. It also can be responsible for otitis, sinusitis, pericarditis, and septic arthritis in this age group. In adults, *H. influenzae* type b usually causes bacteremia, meningitis, pneumonia, or arthritis. Unencapsulated strains are frequently incriminated in pneumonia and

TABLE 96.5   Factors Predisposing to Haemophilus Infections

Age

Sickle cell disease

Splenectomy

Agammaglobulinemia

Treated Hodgkin's disease

Alcoholism

---

exacerbations of bronchitis in adults. Clinical manifestations are discussed in the specific disease-related chapters (meningitis, pneumonia, etc.).

Haemophilus parainfluenzae is responsible for most of the infections caused by other Haemophilus spp. It frequently causes epiglottitis, meningitis, and endocarditis and has been reported to produce otitis, pneumonia, septicemia, arthritis, and conjunctivitis. Haemophilus aphrophilus causes sinusitis, endocarditis, otitis, and pneumonia, as well as some cases of osteomyelitis, wound infections, and brain abscess. Haemophilus paraphrophilus has been reported as the causative agent in some patients with epiglottitis, endocarditis, brain abscess, and osteomyelitis. Haemophilus aegyptius, considered by some authorities to be indistinguishable from the biotype III H. influenzae, causes purulent conjunctivitis in young children.

Haemophilus ducreyi has a unique appearance on smears from clinical material: the organisms tend to aggregate in chains, and the chains between mucous strands give a picture resembling railroad tracks or a darting school of fish. This organism, found throughout the world, causes chancroid, a sexually transmitted infection. The incubation period ranges between 2 and 5 days. The lesion appears as a tender papule, becomes pustular, and then breaks down leaving a painful, shallow ulcer with ragged, undermined edges. Generally confined to the genital and perineal areas, the lesions are associated with regional lymphadenopathy in 30-50% of the patients. Chancroid is discussed more completely in Chapter 36.

Haemophilus haemolyticus and H. parahaemolyticus are not believed to be pathogenic for humans.

Francisella

Francisella tularensis, the sole human pathogen in this genus, has been known previously as Bacterium, Bacillus, Pasteurella, and Brucella tularensis. Although similar in many respects to the plague bacillus (Yersinia pestis), authorities believe its special growth requirements warrant a separate classification for F. tularensis (Table 96.6). It is a small (0.2 by 0.5 μm), poorly staining, gram-negative bacillus that is frequently pleomorphic. This organism is a strict aerobe, catalase-negative, that ferments glucose, maltose, and mannose, producing acid without gas. It will not grow on ordinary culture media, because it requires cysteine or other sulfhydral-containing compounds. Those strains of F. tularensis virulent for man metabolize citrulline and ferment glycerol; they are associated most often with tick-borne tularemia in rabbits. Less virulent strains do not metabolize citrulline and seldom ferment glycerol; they are associated with waterborne disease

TABLE 96.6   Characteristics of *Francisella*

Small, gram-negative coccobacillus

Nonmotile, nonencapsulated

Bipolar, though takes stain poorly

Obligate aerobe

Requires cysteine

TABLE 96.7   Sources of Human Infection With *F. Tularensis*

Mammals	Birds
Rabbits	
Hares	
Squirrels	Amphibians
Moles	
Muskrats	
Beavers	Fish
Deer	
Woodchucks	
Sheep	Invertebrates
Cattle	Ticks
Cats	Deerflies
	Mosquitoes

of rodents. *Francisella tularensis* contains a number of antigens: (1) a protein which cross-reacts with *Brucella,* (2) a polysaccharide, and (3) cell-wall and envelope components that are responsible for endotoxin-like activity.

The organism is found throughout the Northern Hemisphere and is recovered from a wide variety of mammals, birds, and invertebrates (Table 96.7). Rabbits, hares, and ticks are the primary reservoir in the United States. The portal of entry is through broken skin, mucous membranes, or rarely the respiratory tracts. The usual incubation period is 3-5 days, after which the patient has the abrupt onset of fever, chills, and malaise, and develops one of the clinical syndromes listed on Table 96.8. All forms are associated with painful, regional lymphadenopathy except the typhoidal disease. Diagnosis is frequently dependent upon a serologic titer rise (fourfold or more), although the organism can be recovered from clinical specimens when an appropriate medium is used. Streptomycin is considered the drug of choice and should be administered for 7-10 days. Mortality is less than 1%; immunity following infection is usually lifelong.

The only other member of the genus, *F. novicida,* is not believed to be pathogenic for man.

TABLE 96.8   Clinical Forms of Tularemia

Type	%	Fever	Adenopathy	Ulceration	Other
Ulceroglandular	75–85	+	+	+	–
Glandular	5–10	+	+	–	–
Typhoidal	5–15	+	–	–	Prostration, weight loss
Oculoglandular	1–2	+	+	–	Purulent conjunctivitis
Oropharyngeal	< 1	+	+	–	Exudative pharyngitis

TABLE 96.9   Members of the Genus *Pasteurella*

Pathogenic for humans	*P. multocida*
Rarely pathogenic for humans	*P. haemolytica*
	P. pneumotropica
	P. ureae

TABLE 96.10   Characteristics of *Pasteurella*

Small, ovoid, gram-negative bacilli
Bipolar staining
Aerobic (facultatively anaerobic)
Nonmotile, nonsporeforming

Pasteurella

The genus *Pasteurella* comprises a heterogenous group of organisms that are primarily animal pathogens (Table 96.9). Their general microbiologic features are outlined in Table 96.10. The *Pasteurella* spp are oxidase- and catalase-positive. They have a fermentative metabolism, producing acid from glucose, mannitol, and sucrose. Their indole and urease reactions are variable, as is their ability to produce hemolysis. *Pasteurella ureae* has no known animal reservoir and is of questionable significance in humans; *P. multocida* is the only one of this group that causes human infections with any regularity (Table 96.11).

Virulent *P. multocida* strains are encapsulated; the capsule is made up of polysaccharides and is type-specific. The cell wall contains endotoxin-like activity. *Pasteurella multocida* is part of the normal oral, pharyngeal, and gastrointestinal flora in a variety of domestic and wild animals and is sometimes responsible for disease in these hosts. Humans usually become infected by cat or dog bites. The patient typically presents with a soft-tissue infection of the hand, arm, or leg, associated with prominent regional adenopathy. Fever, if present, is low grade. If the bite penetrates deeply, osteomyelitis may develop. Although septicemia has been reported rarely in otherwise normal individuals, it may be more likely to occur in a patient with a compromised reticuloendothelial system (e.g., cirrhosis). Septicemia can produce metastatic foci of infection such as meningitis or brain abscess. Patients with chronic respiratory tract diseases (upper or lower) may develop infections due to *P. multocida*. The organism is sensitive to a number of antimicrobial agents, but penicillin is the drug of choice.

TABLE 96.11   Most Common Diseases Caused by *Pasteurella*

Organism	Disease	
P. multocida	Wound infections following dog or cat bites	
	Septicemia	
	Pulmonary infections	
P. haemolytica	Pneumonia in cattle and sheep	
	Septicemia in lambs	
	Fowl cholera	
P. pneumotropica	Pneumonia	
	Septicemia	In laboratory rats, mice, and guinea pigs, and in cats and dogs
	Peritonitis	
	Conjunctivitis	
	Abscess	

Others (Table 96.12)

Acinetobacter calcoaceticus exists as two variants, *A. anitratum* and *A. lwoffi*. *Acinetobacter* are very plump coccoid or coccobacillary organisms that frequently appear gram-variable on stain. They are aerobic, nonmotile, and can be highly pleomorphic. *Acinetobacter* are oxidase-negative, catalase-positive, and generally nitrate-negative. The organisms tend to be fimbriated. *Acinetobacter* are common isolates from soil and water and are recovered from skin, mucous membranes and gastrointestinal tracts of some normal individuals. It is frequently necessary to distinguish between colonization and true infections when *Acinetobacter* spp are recovered from clinical specimens. The organism is a documented cause of hospital-acquired infections in particular situations (Table 96.13), but it has also been reported to cause community-acquired pneumonia. These latter infections tend to occur in those elderly who have chronic diseases such as alcoholism, hematologic malignancies, and renal failure. *Acinetobacter* may be highly resistant to multiple antimicrobial agents.

    Actinobacillus actinomycetemcomitans is a small gram-negative organism that is coccoid or coccobacillary, nonmotile, and very slow growing. It may take up to a week for the colonies to become visible under laboratory conditions, although growth is enhanced in the presence of increased carbon dioxide. *Actinobacillus* is distinguished from *Cardiobacterium hominis* and *Eikenella corrodens* on

TABLE 96.12   Diseases Caused by Miscellaneous Gram-Negative Bacilli

Organism	Disease
Acinetobacter calcoaceticus	Nosocomial UTI, sepsis, pneumonia Community pneumonia
Actinobacillus actinomycetemcomitans	Endocarditis, endarteritis Cerebral abscess Skin and soft-tissue infections
Aeromonas hydrophilia	Gastroenteritis Skin and soft-tissue infections Necrotizing myositis Bacteremia
Alcaligenes faecalis	Bacteremia Nosocomial UTI
Cardiobacterium hominis	Endocarditis
Chromobacterium violaceum	Skin abscess Bacteremia
Eikenella corrodens	Deep abscesses
Flavobacterium meningosepticum	Meningitis in neonates Nosocomial infections

TABLE 96.13   Predisposing Factors and *Acinetobacter* Infections

---

Tracheostomy

Ventilator therapy

Broad-spectrum antibiotic therapy

Multiple indwelling catheters

Old age

Underlying chronic disease

---

the basis of producing catalase, reducing nitrate, and being oxidase-negative. Most strains ferment glucose, levulose, and maltose. First recognized in mixed cultures from patients with *Actinomyces* infection, *Actinobacillus* has been documented as a sole organism causing endocarditis, endarteritis, and brain abscess, as well as skin and soft-tissue infections. It is often sensitive to penicillin.

Aeromonas spp are gram-negative bacilli that are nonsporeforming, motile, and facultatively anaerobic. They produce beta-hemolysis and ferment carbohydrates to form acid and gas. *Aeromonas* are oxidase positive which distinguishes them from Enterobacteriaceae. *Aeromonas hydrophilia* is the most important member of the genus in terms of infecting humans. Other species of the genus are primarily pathogenic for poikilotherms (fish, frogs, snakes, lizards). *Aeromonas hydrophilia* is a common inhabitant of water and soil. It has been implicated in cholera-like disease in India, skin and soft-tissue infections, necrotizing myositis, and bacteremia. Rarely, meningitis and endocarditis due to *A. hydrophilia* have been reported. The bacteremia is likely to occur in the immunocompromised individual. Most *A. hydrophilia* isolates are sensitive to chloramphenicol and the aminoglycosides.

Alcaligenes spp are gram-negative bacilli with peritrichous flagella; they are oxidase- and catalase-positive, nonsaccharolytic, and urease-negative. The genus includes a number of organisms without species status as well as four identified species. *Alcaligenes faecalis* is the specie most often incriminated in human infections. It is part of the gastrointestinal flora in some normal individuals. This specie is reported to cause bacteremia and urinary tract infections, almost exclusively in the hospital setting. The organism is usually sensitive to colistin.

Cardiobacterium hominis is a slow-growing, nonmotile, gram-negative bacillus which is pleomorphic with bulbous ends and irregular staining when grown on agar without yeast. With yeast added to the medium, the organisms are uniform rods 0.5 by 2 μm. Supplemental carbon dioxide and increased humidity enhance growth. *Cardiobacterium hominis* is oxidase-positive and catalase-negative; it does not reduce nitrates, but is indole-positive. The organism ferments dextrose, sucrose, and maltose to form acids. *Cardiobacterium hominis* is part of the normal mouth and upper respiratory tract flora, recoverable from two-thirds of throat cultures. It has been linked to bacteremias and endocarditis of natural and prosthetic valves. The endocarditis presents with an indolent course, patients being ill up to 18 months before the diagnosis is confirmed. Isolates of *C. hominis* are usually highly sensitive to penicillin.

Chromobacterium violaceum is a gram-negative bacillus which produces a characteristic violet to dark purple pigment on overnight incubation. It is a common inhabitant of soil and water. This organism is best known for causing fatal infections in animals (pigs, water buffalo, gibbons) but is a rare cause of disease in humans. The typical case occurs in the southeastern United States or is imported from Southeast Asia. A relatively minor skin lesion with regional adenopathy progresses rapidly to septicemia and necrotizing metastatic abscesses (skin, liver). Most cases reported have been fatal. *Chromobacterium violaceum* is generally sensitive to the aminoglycosides and chloramphenicol.

Eikenella corrodens is a slow-growing, facultatively anaerobic, pleomorphic bacillus. It is nonmotile, nonsporeforming, and does not produce a capsule. Its initial growth is in the form of a depression rather than a raised colony, and subsequent growth is spreading in concentric circles. The colonies are often pale yellow and have the characteristic odor of bleach. The organism is oxidase-positive, catalase-negative, and reduces nitrates. *Eikenella corrodens* is part of the normal mouth and upper respiratory tract flora. Frequently recovered as part of a mixed microbial infection, *E. corrodens* has been incriminated as the sole pathogen in deep abscesses (abdominal, brain), endocarditis, meningitis, and arthritis. Predisposing factors to *E. corrodens* infection include old age, ruptured viscus, carcinoma, and intravenous drug abuse (methylphenidate). The organism is sensitive to penicillin, chloramphenicol, and the broad-spectrum penicillins (carbenicillin, ticarcillin).

The *Flavobacterium* group are long, thin, nonmotile gram-negative bacteria with slightly bulbous ends. They are oxidase- and catalase-positive and produce a pale-yellow pigment. *Flavobacterium* are indole-positive and capable of liquifying gelatin. They produce a distinctive lavender-green discoloration on blood agar. The most important species for humans is *F. meningosepticum* which is recovered commonly from soil, water, and moist environments within the hospital. *Flavobacterium meningosepticum* causes disease primarily in newborns, particularly premature infants. Meningitis, with or without septicemia, is the most common infection. Adults are much less commonly affected. *Flavobacterium* spp are highly resistant to many antibiotics; appropriate therapy must be based on specific susceptibilities.

Selected Bibliography

Blazevic, D. J.: Current taxonomy and identification of nonfermentative gram-negative bacilli. *Human Pathol* 7:265-275, 1976.

Brooks, G. F., O'Donoghue, J. M., Rissing, J. P., et al.: *Eikenella corrodens,* a recently recognized pathogen. *Medicine* 53:325-342, 1974.

Burke, D. S.: Immunization against tularemia: Analysis of the effectiveness of live *Francisella tularensis* vaccine in prevention of laboratory-acquired tularemia. *J Infect Dis* 135:55-60, 1977.

Chunn, C. J., Jones, S. R., McCutchan, J. A., et al.: *Haemophilus parainfluenzae* infective endocarditis. *Medicine* 56:99-113, 1977.

Crawford, S. A., Evans, J. A., and Crawford, G. E.: Necrotizing fasciitis associated with *Haemophilus aphrophilus. Arch Intern Med* 138:1714-1715, 1978.

Davis, W. A., II, Kane, J. G., and Garagusi, V. F.: Human Aeromonas infections: A review of the literature and a case report of endocarditis. *Medicine* 57:267-277, 1978.

Elster, S. K., Mattes, L. M., Meyers, B. R., et al.: *Hemophilus aphrophilus* endocarditis: Review of 23 cases. *Am J Cardiol* 35:72-79, 1975.

Gaisin, A. and Heaton, C. L.: Chancroid: Alias the soft chancre. *Int J Dermatol* 14:188-197, 1975.

Geraci, J. E., Greipp, P. R., Wilkowske, C. J., et al.: *Cardiobacterium hominis* endocarditis. Four cases with clinical and laboratory observations. *Mayo Clin Proc* 53:49-53, 1978.

Glew, R. H., Moellering, R. C., Jr., and Kunz, L. J.: Infections with *Acinetobacter calcoaceticus (Herellea vaginicola):* Clinical and laboratory studies. *Medicine* 56:79-97, 1977.

Granoff, D. M., Congeni, B., Baker, R., Jr., et al.: Countercurrent immunoelectrophoresis in the diagnosis of *Haemophilus influenzae* type b infection. *Am J Dis Child* 131:1357-1362, 1977.

Handsfield, H. H., Totten, P. A., Fennel, C. L., et al.: Molecular epidemiology of *Haemophilus ducreyi* infections. *Ann Intern Med* 95:315-318, 1981.

Henriksen, S. D.: *Moraxella, Neisseria, Branhamella,* and *Acinetobacter. Ann Rev Microbiol* 30:63-83, 1976.

Hubbert, W. T. and Rosen, M. N.: II. *Pasteurella multocida* infection in man unrelated to animal bite. *Am J Publ Health* 60:1109-1117, 1970.

Kilian, M.: A taxonomic study of the genus *Haemophilus* with the proposal of a new species. *J Gen Microbiol* 93:9-62, 1976.

Lucas, G. L. and Bartlett, D. H.: *Pasteurella multocida* infection in the hand. *Plastic Reconst Surg* 67:49-53, 1981.

Lynn, D. J., Kane, J. G., and Parker, R. H.: *Haemophilus parainfluenzae* and influenzae endocarditis: A review of forty cases. *Medicine* 56:115-128, 1977.

Miller, L. G.: Further studies on tularemia in Alaska: Virulence and biochemical characteristics of indigenous strains. *Can J Microbiol* 20:1585-1590, 1974.

Pulverer, G. and Ko, H. L.: *Actinobacillus actinomycetemcomitans:* Fermentative capabilities of 140 strains. *Appl Microbiol* 20:693-695, 1970.

Rudin, M. L., Michael, J. R., and Huxley, E. J.: Community-acquired acinetobacter pneumonia. *Am J Med* 67:39-43, 1979.

Schneerson, R. and Robbins, J. B.: Induction of serum *Haemophilus influenzae* type b capsular antibodies in adult volunteers fed cross-reacting *Escherichia coli* 075:K100:H5. *N Engl J Med* 292:1093-1096, 1975.

Teres, D.: ICU-acquired pneumonia due to *Flavobacterium meningosepticum. JAMA* 228:732, 1974.

Teutsch, S. M., Martone, W. J., Brink, E. W., et al.: Pneumonic tularemia on Martha's Vineyard. *N Engl J Med* 301:826-828, 1979.

Victoria, B., Baer, H., and Ayoub, E. M.: Successful treatment of systemic *Chromobacterium violaceum* infection. *JAMA* 230:578-580, 1974.

Wallace, R. J., Jr., Musher, D. M., and Martin, R. R.: *Hemophilus influenzae* pneumonia in adults. *Am J Med* 64:87-93, 1978.

Ward, J. I., Fraser, D. W., Baraff, L, J., et al.: *Haemophilus influenzae* meningitis. A national study of secondary spread in household contacts. *N Engl J Med* 301:122-126, 1979.

97

CURVED RODS - VIBRIOS
Rama Ganguly, Ph.D.

Taxonomy

The vibrios are gram-negative, motile rods, usually curved (the comma bacillus) with a single polar flagellum. They are placed in the family Spirilaceae and are nonsporing as well as noncapsulated. They are facultative anaerobes, ferment glucose without gas, and are hydrogen sulfide-negative. *Vibrio cholerae* (the classic and the El Tor biotype) is the causative agent for choleraic diarrhea. Robert Koch discovered the cholera vibrio in 1884. *Vibrio parahaemolyticus* is the causal agent for a form of acute food poisoning in Japan, the United States, and Southeast Asia. *Vibrio fetus* infects domestic animals and is the causative agent for abortion in cattle and sheep. All vibrios have O and H antigens. *Vibrio cholerae* strains are distinguished from other vibrios on the basis of their somatic antigen (O subgroup 1). Species other than *V. cholerae* are often referred to as noncholera vibrios or nonagglutinating vibrios (NAG). Such vibrios are agglutinable, however, by their own antisera and may produce cholera-like or mild diarrhea. Many nonpathogenic vibrios are found in nature, mostly in water and fish.

Vibrio cholerae

Bacteriology

There are two serotypes of *V. cholerae,* called Inaba and Ogawa, based on the presence of a subsidiary O antigen. An intermediate serotype, Hikojima, is also known to exist. The biotype El Tor vibrios, which were initially distinguished from the classic *V. cholerae* on the basis of their hemolytic properties, were thought to be nonpathogenic. Subsequently Gotschich, in 1906, isolated hemolytic *V. cholerae* strains from the dead bodies of pilgrims seen at the El Tor quarantine station in Egypt. El Tor vibrios were also found to be the causative agents for endemic cholera in Celebes, Indonesia, in 1939. Subsequently, this El Tor vibrio became the causative agent for the seventh pandemic of cholera.

Epidemiology

Cholera has been endemic in the Indian subcontinent since the beginning of recorded history. A series of six pandemics of cholera have ravaged the world between 1817 and 1923 spreading over most of the globe along the trade routes. As indicated previously, the seventh pandemic started from a focus in Indonesia in 1961. Between 1963 and 1966, it spread to Korea, China, Philippines, West Pakistan, Afghanistan, Iran, southern USSR, and Iraq. During this pandemic, cholera was introduced repeatedly into countries such as Japan, the United Kingdom, and Australia but was eliminated promptly due to improved sanitation and health measures. Cases of cholera, Inaba serotype, have been reported from Louisiana, United States, probably related to eating crab meat from the coastal areas of the Gulf of Mexico. Strains of *V. cholerae,* Inaba and El Tor, also have been isolated from the sewage system of Louisiana, but the source of infection remains unknown at this time. El Tor vibrio appears to be hardier than the classic *V. cholerae* and therefore more easily isolated from night soil and water. The infection/case ratio of El Tor is higher (25:1-100:1) compared with the classic type (5:1-10:1). This indicates that almost all infections remain asymptomatic or occur as mild atypical diarrhea and go unrecognized. Thus the occurrence of cases represents the tip of the iceberg.

Man is the only known natural reservoir of this disease. Cholera is transmitted in a cyclic manner by the fecal-oral route in which environment, especially water, plays a most important part. Table 97.1 shows the viability of *V. cholerae* in food, water, and fomites. An abundant supply of pure water and improved sanitation can break this cycle and eliminate the disease. Following naturally acquired cholera, a relatively short period of immunity develops and therefore, reinfection frequently develops. Because the reinfection and asymptomatic carrier states are so frequent, quarantine and isolation measures are not useful.

Laboratory

The technique for laboratory diagnosis of *V. cholerae* in clinical cases is relatively simple since a large number of vibrios, 10^7-10^9/ml of stool, are usually present. Using dark-field microscopy, or fluorescent antibody techniques, diagnosis may be achieved within a few minutes with 80-90% accuracy. Cholera stool may be streaked on nutrient agar plates and colonies may be detected with a stereoscope within 4-5 hr. The organisms are then confirmed by slide agglutination with O group serum and typed using Ogawa and Inaba antisera. Various transport and enrichment media have been used for cholera stool, especially for use in the later stage of the disease or to detect carriers, e.g., trypticase taurocholate tellurite broth or alkaline peptone water at a high pH (8-9.2). Various selective and nonselective agar media are available for isolation of vibrios: nutrient agar, bile salt agar, vibrio agar, TCBS (Difco, BBL, Oxoid). Biotype El Tors are distinguished from classic *V. cholerae* strains by their infra-subspecific characteristics.

TABLE 97.1   Viability of *V. cholerae* (El Tor) in Food and Water*

	Period of Survival (Days)	
Articles	Room Temperature (30–32°C)	Refrigeration (5–10°C)
Cooked food	2–5	3–5
Fresh vegetables	1–7	7–10
Fish and shellfish	2–5	7–14
Fruits	1–3	3–5
Beverages (beer, cola drinks, and carbonated water)	1	1
Milk and milk products	7–14	14 or more
Grains	1–3	3–5
Sea water	10–13	60
Tank or well water	7–13	18

*Modified from Barua, D.: Survival of cholera vibrios in food, water and fomites, *In: Principles and practice of cholera control.* Public Health Papers No. 40. World Health Organization, Geneva, 1970, pp. 29–30

Pathogenesis and Pathophysiology

The pathogenesis of cholera is relatively simple. After the organism gains entrance by the oral route, it multiplies in the small intestine, producing a potent enterotoxin. The latter acts on the mucosal cells of the small bowel causing them to secrete large amounts of isotonic fluid faster than the colon can absorb it. The result is a watery isotonic diarrhea (rice-water stool). The rapid gastrointestinal loss of isotonic fluid is responsible for all of the clinical signs and symptoms of cholera. Since *V. cholerae* poorly survives at low pH, the stomach acidity acts as the first line of host defense. Approximately 10^6 organisms introduced orally after neutralization of stomach acidity can produce disease in 50% of the human volunteers. The degree of production of the enterotoxin by the infecting *Vibrio* strain directly correlates with the severity of the clinical disease. Cholera enterotoxin acts locally on the gut tissue and stimulates the activity of the enzyme adenylcyclase. The latter in turn converts ATP to cAMP and results in secretion of chloride and inhibition of sodium absorption. Large amounts of potassium bicarbonate are also lost in cholera stool. Thus electrolyte imbalance in addition to severe fluid loss occurs. The enterotoxin (a protein of 82,000 mol wt) is composed of A and B subunits connected with noncovalent bonds. The B subunit mediates binding of the enterotoxin to membrane ganglioside (GM_1) receptors and the subunit A is responsible for activation of adenylcyclase. Other enteropathogens *(Escherichia coli* and *Salmonella typhimurium)* produce toxins that immunologically cross-react with vibrio enterotoxin. The laboratory abnormalities in cholera include severe metabolic acidosis, hemoconcentration, and marked elevation of the plasma proteins. Delay in treatment results in renal failure and problems associated with hypokalemia.

Treatment

The intravenous replacement of the water and electrolytes lost in the stool is the basis of treatment of cholera. By adequate replacement of lost fluid all the clinical signs and symptoms can be reversed and mortality reduced to less than 1%. After admission, replacement of the fluid lost is undertaken as quickly as possible until an easily palpable radial pulse is restored. With severe dehydration and cardiovascular collapse, the fluid deficit is about 10% of the patient's body weight (i.e., 5 L for a 50-kg patient). The second phase of fluid replacement therapy is maintenance therapy which is adjusted to subsequent fluid loss due to continued diarrhea after admission. A useful adjunct to cholera therapy is antibiotic administration, e.g., tetracycline 500 mg by mouth every 6 hr for 48 hr. Antibiotic treatment reduces the duration of diarrhea and the time of vibrio excretion, but cannot substitute for fluid replacement therapy.

Immunity

As indicated earlier, immunity developing from clinical cholera is of short duration. Because the enterotoxin acts locally in the small bowel, local mucosal immunity is of great importance. However, various cholera vaccines administered parenterally induce 30-80% protection for 3-6 months as indicated from several field trials. Research is underway to develop an attenuated cholera strain to be employed as a live oral vaccine. Combined whole cell-toxoid vaccines are also being developed to induce both antibacterial and antitoxic immunities against the disease.

Vibrio parahaemolyticus

Vibrio parahaemolyticus is ubiquitous in temperate and subtropical coastal waters. The isolation of the organism also varies with the seasons. Eating raw fish is the major cause of acute food poisoning due to *V. parahaemolyticus* in Japan. More than 10^5 viable organisms are required to induce illness. Production of hemolysin on special media (Wagatsuma's agar) by the organism is referred to as the Kanagawa phenomenon and is probably related to greater disease-producing capability. Existence of enterotoxin(s) has been suggested but more work is needed in this area. Some reports indicate that this pathogen might possess some degree of invasiveness. The best means of prevention is to avoid inadequately cooked seafoods.

Selected Bibliography

Berry, L. J.: Bacterial toxins. *Crit Rev Toxicol* 5:239–318, 1977.

Blake, P. A., Allegra, D. T., Snyder, J. D., Barrett, T. J., McFarland, L., Casaway, C. T., Feeley, J. C., Craig, J. P., Lee, J. V., Puhr, N. D., and Feldman, R. A.: Cholera – a possible endemic focus in the United States. *N Engl J Med* 302: 305–309, 1980.

Burrows, W. and Havens, I.: Studies on immunity to Asiatic cholera. V. The absorption of immune globulin from the bowel and its excretion in the urine and feces of experimental animals and human volunteers. *J Infect Dis* 82:231– 250, 1948.

Finkelstein, R. A. and Lospalluto, J. J.: Crystalline cholera toxin and toxoid. *Science* 175:529–530, 1972.

Fujino, T., Sakaguchi, G., Sakazani, R., and Takeda, Y. (eds.): *International symposium on* Vibrio parahaemolyticus. Sept. 17–18, 1973, Tokyo, Japan. Saidon Pub. Co. Lts, Tokyo, 1–261, 1974.

Ganguly, R., Clem, L. W., Bencie, Z., Sinha, R., Sakazake, R., and Waldman, R. II.: Cholera immunology. III. Antibody response in the intestinal secretions of volunteers immunized with various cholera vaccines. *Bull WHO* 52: 323–330, 1975.

Levine, M. M., Nalin, D. R., Craig, J. P., Hoover, D., Berquist, E. J., Waterman, D., Holley, H. P., Hornick, R. B., Pierce, N. P., and Libonati, J. P.: Immunity of cholera in man: Relative role of antibacterial versus antitoxic immunity. *Trans R Soc Trop Med Hyg* 73:3–9, 1979.

MacKan, D. M.: Cholera: The present world situation. *Trans R Soc Trop Med Hyg* 73:1–2, 1979.

Mekalanos, J. J., Collier, J. R., and Romig, W. R.: Enzymatic activity of cholera toxin: Relationships to proteolytic processing, disulfide bond reduction and subunit composition. *J Biol Chem* 254:5855–5861, 1979.

Mhalu, F. S., Mmari, P. W., and Ijumba, J.: Rapid emergence of El Tor *Vibrio cholerae* resistant to antimicrobial agents during first six months of fourth cholera epidemic in Tanzania. *Lancet* 1:345–347, 1979.

Pollitzer, R.: *Cholera.* Geneva World Health Organization: Monograph Series, No. 43, 11–1019, 1959.

Principles and Practice of Cholera Control. Geneva World Health Organization, Public Health Papers No. 40, 9–139, 1970.

Richards, R. L., Moss, J., Alving, C. R., Fishman, P. H., and Brady, R. O.: Choleragen (cholera toxin) a bacterial lectin. *Proc Natl Acad Sci* 76:1673–1676, 1979.

Spiers, J., Stavrie, S., Konawalchur, J.: Assay of *Escherichia coli* heat-labile enterotoxin with Vero cells. *Infect Immun* 16:617–622, 1977.

Van Heyningen, S. V.: Cholera toxin. *Biol Rev* 52:509-549, 1977.

Yancey, R. J., Willis, D. L., and Berry, L. J.: Role of motility in experimental cholera in adult rabbits. *Infect Immun* 22:387-392, 1978.

98

BACTEROIDACEAE
Ronica M. Kluge, M.D.

The Bacteroidaceae comprise the most common anaerobic gram-negative bacilli pathogenic for humans. They are normal inhabitants of the oropharynx, large intestine, and female genital tract but cause disease under certain circumstances.

Microbiology and Pathogenesis

The bacteroides are nonsporeforming obligate anaerobes, pleomorphic (filamentous, rounded ends), and they take Gram stain poorly. They may be divided conveniently into three groups (Tables 98.1 and 98.2): *B. fragilis, B. melaninogenicus,* and *B. oralis.*

 Bacteroides fragilis originally was thought to consist of five subspecies, but DNA homology and serologic information have led microbiologists to declare them five distinct species. In addition, *B. fragilis* has a polysaccharide capsule that distinguishes it from the other four organisms. *Bacteroides fragilis* can ferment a number of carbohydrates to form acids. They also grow in the presence of 20% bile. This organism produces a number of enzymes including fumarate reductase, alkaline phosphatase, and bile-salt-deconjugating enzymes. Most clinical isolates of *B. fragilis* produce superoxide dismutase and catalase.

 The presence of endotoxin in *B. fragilis* is in dispute. Some investigators believe endotoxin is present, although in a greatly decreased amount and a reduced potency when compared with the endotoxin from Enterobacteriaceae. Others find that the *B. fragilis* outer-membrane complex lacks some of the classic components of endotoxin and that the material neither kills chick embryos nor induces a local Shwartzman reaction in rabbits.

 All clinical isolates of *B. fragilis* possess a polysaccharide capsule which is highly antigenic and is believed to be a major virulence factor. Only these

TABLE 98.1   Members of the *Bacteroides* spp and Their Usual
Human Habitat

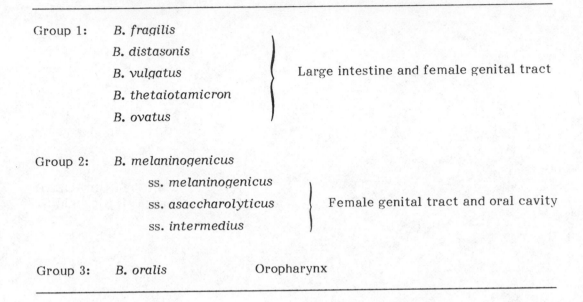

Group 1:   *B. fragilis*
            B. distasonis
            B. vulgatus   } Large intestine and female genital tract
            B. thetaiotamicron
            B. ovatus

Group 2:   *B. melaninogenicus*
                ss. *melaninogenicus*
                ss. *asaccharolyticus*   } Female genital tract and oral cavity
                ss. *intermedius*

Group 3:   *B. oralis*   Oropharynx

TABLE 98.2   Distinguishing Characteristics of *Bacteroides* spp

	Inhibited By Bile	Catalase	Black Pigment	Capsule
B. fragilis	–	+	–	+
B. melaninogenicus	+	–	+	+
B. oralis	+	–	–	–

encapsulated strains are capable of causing abscesses in animal models in the absence of other microbes. The capsular material also seems to impede phagocytosis. Other *Bacteroides* spp in this group, such as *B. distasonis* and *B. thetaiotamicron,* do not have this capsule and rarely cause human infection.

The *B. melaninogenicus* group contains three subspecies (see Table 98.1). This group is distinguished by its production of brown/black pigment when grown on blood agar. *B. melaninogenicus,* in contrast to *B. fragilis,* is inhibited by bile and lacks catalase (see Table 98.2). Members of this group fluoresce red under ultraviolet light, and they produce a number of enzymes, such as collagenase, which may play a role in pathogenesis. As with *B. fragilis, B. melaninogenicus* does not have the classic endotoxin but does produce a polysaccharide capsule.

Bacteroides oralis is a single species and resembles *B. melaninogenicus* bacteriologically except for absence of brown/black pigment production. Almost nothing is known about its mechanism(s) of causing disease.

Epidemiology

There is a high concentration of *B. fragilis* in the normal human colon, and it is a frequent commensal in the normal female genital tract. It is not surprising, therefore, that this organism is a frequent cause of both infection localized to, and bacteremia from, these sites. Such infections usually follow abdominal or pelvic trauma, surgical procedures, or ruptured viscus (Table 98.3).

Bacteroides melaninogenicus is part of the normal flora in the adult oropharynx, female genital tract, and gastrointestinal tract. This organism is acquired later in life than other *Bacteroides* spp (e.g., it is not found in the oral cavity until after puberty), and this may explain why it so infrequently causes infections in children. *Bacteroides melaninogenicus* rarely acts alone to cause infection but is present with other anaerobes.

Bacteroides oralis is present in the oropharynx, principally as part of the gingival crevice and plaque flora.

Clinical Disease (Table 98.4)

Bacteroides fragilis causes or contributes to about two-thirds of the intraabdominal infections. These infections usually occur as a result of fecal contamination and often result in abscess formation. This specie is frequently the causal organism in necrotizing fasciitis originating from the genital tract, in postabortion septicemia, and in infections following hysterectomy. Bacteroidaceae cause 5–10% of all bacteremias, and *B. fragilis* is responsible for 80% of these. As expected, the source of the bacteremia is the gastrointestinal or genitourinary tracts in most instances. *Bacteroides fragilis* is isolated in 15% of pleuropulmonary infections, almost always as part of a complex flora. Its role in the pathogenesis of pulmonary infections is not well understood. Other infections in which *B. fragilis* has been implicated include skin and soft-tissue (e.g., decubitus ulcers, diabetic ulcers) and osteomyelitis.

Bacteroides melaninogenicus is an important pathogen in anaerobic pleuropulmonary infections. It is recovered in 30–35% of aspiration and necrotizing pneumonias, lung abscesses, and empyema. This organism is responsible for a large number of oral cavity infections, especially periodontal disease and dental-space infections. Contiguous spread can lead to involvement of neck, jaw, and

TABLE 98.3   Predisposing Factors to Bacteroidaceae Infections

Trauma or surgery

Alcoholic liver disease

Diabetes mellitus

Malignancy (solid tumors)

Atherosclerosis

Prematurity

End-stage renal disease

TABLE 98.4   Most Common Diseases Caused by Bacteroidaceae

Organism	Disease
B. fragilis group	Intraabdominal abscess Female pelvic infections Bacteremia Pleuropulmonary infections
B. melaninogenicus group	Pleuropulmonary infections Orodental infections
B. oralis	Orodental infections

retropharyngeal spaces. *Bacteroides melaninogenicus* is reportedly found as part of the flora in 15% of intraabdominal and in 10% of female genital tract infections. It can cause necrotizing skin and soft-tissue infections, and it occasionally results in bacteremia.

Bacteroides oralis appears to be an important cause of orodental infections, often mixed with other anaerobes. It also is found as part of the flora in some anaerobic pulmonary infections. Rarely, *B. oralis* has been reported as the causal agent in infective endocarditis.

Selected Bibliography

Bartlett, J. G.: Anaerobic bacterial pneumonitis. *Am Rev Respir Dis* 119:19, 1979.

Bartlett, J. G., Moon, N. E., Goldstein, P. R., et al.: Cervical and vaginal bacterial flora: Ecologic niches in the female lower genital tract. *Am J Obstet Gynecol* 130:658, 1978.

Bjornson, A. B. and Bjornson, H.S.: Participation of immunoglobulin and the alternative complement pathway in opsonization of *Bacteroides fragilis* and *Bacteroides thetaiotamicron*. *Rev Infect Dis* 1:347, 1979.

Brook, I., Controni, G., Rodriguez, W. J., et al.: Anaerobic bacteremia in children. *Am J Dis Child* 134:1052, 1980.

Chow, A. W. and Guze, L. B.: Bacteroidaceae bacteremia: Clinical experience with 112 patients. *Medicine* 53:93, 1974.

Finegold, S. M., Bartlett, J. G., Chow, A. W., et al.: Management of anaerobic infections. *Ann Intern Med* 83:375, 1975.

Galgiani, J. N., Busch, D. F., Brass, C., et al.: *Bacteroides fragilis* endocarditis, bacteremia and other infections treated with oral or intravenous metronidazole. *Am J Med* 65:284, 1978.

Grohn, M.: Endotoxins of gram-negative anaerobic bacteria. *Infection* 8(suppl 2): S138–S139, 1980.

Hansen, S. L.: Variation in susceptibility patterns of species within the *Bacteroides fragilis* group. *Antimicrob Agents Chemother* 17:686, 1980.

Hofstad, T. and Sveen, K.: The chemotactic effect of *Bacteroides fragilis* lipopolysaccharide. *Rev Infect Dis* 1:342, 1979.

Kaspar, D. L.: Chemical and biological characterization of the lipopolysaccharide of *Bacteroides fragilis* subspecies *fragilis*. *J Infect Dis* 134:59, 1976.

Kaspar, D. L., Hayes, M. E., Reinap, B. G., et al.: Isolation and identification of encapsulated strains of *Bacteroides fragilis*. *J Infect Dis* 136: 75, 1977.

Kaspar, D. L., Onderdonk, A. B., Polk, B. F., et al.: Surface antigens as virulence factors in infection with *Bacteroides fragilis*. *Rev Infect Dis* 1:278, 1979.

Kaspar, D. L. and Seiler, M. W.: Immunochemical characterization of the outer membrane complex of *Bacteroides fragilis* subspecies *fragilis*. *J Infect Dis* 132:440, 1975.

Polk, B. F. and Kaspar, D. L.: *Bacteroides fragilis* subspecies in clinical isolates. *Ann Intern Med* 86:569, 1971.

Rotimi, V. O., Faulkner, J., and Duerden, B. I.: Rapid methods for identification of clinical isolates of gram-negative anaerobic bacilli. *Med Lab Sci* 37:331, 1980.

Simon, G. L., Klempner, M. S., Kaspar, D. L., and Gorbach, S. L.: Alterations in opsonophagocytic killing by neutrophils of *Bacteroides fragilis* associated with animal and laboratory passage: Effect of capsular polysaccharide. *J Infect Dis* 145:72, 1982.

Thompson, S. E., III, Hager, W. D., Wong, K-H, et al.: The microbiology and therapy of acute pelvic inflammatory disease in hospitalized patients. *Am J Obstet Gynecol* 136:179, 1980.

99

LEGIONNAIRES' DISEASE
Roger G. Finch, M.B.

Legionnaires' disease (LD) is an acute febrile illness usually associated with pneumonia. Asymptomatic infection and acute febrile illness without lung involvement also occur. It has been estimated that LD is responsible for 0.5-1.5% of all pneumonias in the United States. The disease occurs in both epidemic and sporadic forms and is the result of infection with a bacillus originally associated with the outbreak of disease among persons attending the Legionnaires' Convention in Philadelphia in 1976.

Microbiology

The bacillus of LD has been named *Legionella pneumophila*. It possesses unique characteristics which justify the formation of a new genus. It was originally isolated from lung tissue obtained at autopsy and cultured in the peritoneal cavity of guinea pigs and in the yolk sac of embryonated hens' eggs. Subsequently it has been isolated on a variety of enriched solid media such as charcoal yeast extract agar supplemented with ferric pyrophosphate and L-cysteine, or on Mueller-Hinton agar supplemented with 1% hemoglobin and 2% Isovitalex. It will grow aerobically at 35°C, preferably in an atmosphere of 2.5% CO_2. The colonies are pinpoint after 3 days incubation but increase in size when incubation is prolonged to 7 days. They then appear circular, convex, gray, and glistening. Occasionally 2 weeks incubation may be necessary. Brown pigment occurs in areas of confluent growth and the colonies may also fluoresce yellow under ultraviolet light.

Legionella pneumophila appears gram-negative with conventional staining but takes up safranin poorly. Fortunately, it stains well with spirochetal stains, such as the Dieterle silver stain, which renders the bacillus dark brown to black.

This stain readily demonstrates the bacillus in tissue sections. The organism is a pleomorphic bacillus varying in size from 0.4 to 0.8 µm wide and 2.0 to 4.0 µm long, although occasional bacilli reach 20 µm in length.

Serologic tests have defined six antigenically distinct serogroups. The serologic method of choice is a direct or indirect fluorescent antibody technique which is highly sensitive and produces very few cross-reactions with bacteria of other genera.

Epidemiology

Legionnaires' disease occurs in both epidemic and sporadic forms. The incubation period ranges from 2 to 10 days. It is more prevalent in the summer and fall.

The epidemic form of the disease was intensively studied following an outbreak of acute febrile pneumonia in July 1976, in Philadelphia among persons attending an American Legion convention. One hundred eighty-two people became ill and 29 died (16%). A further 39 cases with five deaths were recognized among other persons who had been in the vicinity. The age range of infected persons in the Philadelphia outbreak was 3-82 years (mean 54.7 years) and occurred preponderantly in men (M/F, 3.5:1). The estimated attack rate was 1.6%. Underlying disease was associated with a higher risk of infection and increased mortality. The most common preexisting illnesses were hypertension, arteriosclerotic cardiovascular disease, chronic lung disease, peptic ulcer disease, and malignancy. No definite source for the bacterium was established, although the airborne route was strongly suspected.

Serologic testing of stored sera from previously undiagnosed outbreaks of acute respiratory illness in Washington and Philadelphia has shown that these were also due to LD. Epidemics subsequent to July 1976 have also been recognized. Some of these have involved hospitalized patients who have had renal transplants, chronic renal failure, or malignant disease. In fact, those at greatest risk of contracting LD appear to be males of middle age or older who smoke, or persons receiving adrenocorticosteroids or other immunosuppressing agents, or those who have serious underlying disease.

Sporadic cases of LD have been recognized throughout the United States, as well as Canada, Australia, Great Britain, the Netherlands, Sweden, and Israel.

In contrast to the epidemics of pneumonia, an epidemic in Pontiac, Michigan, produced a self-limited illness of fever, headache, malaise, and myalgia, without pneumonia or fatalities.

The source of the bacillus is unknown although environmental sources have been suspected. Several outbreaks have been temporally related to nearby soil excavations while the bacillus has also been isolated from water in an air-conditioning system, cooling towers, evaporative condensers, as well as a creek.

Pathogenesis and Pathology

The lungs are the organs most consistently involved in LD. The macroscopic appearance is of a lobar or multilobar pneumonia with frequent evidence of a fibrinous pleurisy. Pleural effusions are uncommon and when present are small.

Microscopically there is a patchy yet extensive inflammatory exudate which predominates within the alveoli. The exudate is rich in polymorphonuclear neutrophils, macrophages, and fibrin. Terminal bronchioles also show inflammatory involvement when in direct continuity with consolidated lobules, although the larger bronchioles, bronchi, and trachea are usually spared. Interstitial edema and infiltration of the alveolar septae occur in relation to the affected air spaces, although there appears to be little destruction of the alveolar septal framework. However, in severe cases the alveolar epithelium may desquamate. Bacteria may be demonstrated within the inflammatory exudate by direct fluorescence or the silver Dieterle stain. They are most abundant within the alveoli with relatively few seen in the larger airways. Many bacilli appear within macrophages and also have been demonstrated in pleural exudate. These histopathologic changes are not specific for LD. However, the demonstration of appropriately stained bacilli in conjunction with the clinical illness is certainly considered to be diagnostic.

Diagnostic Features

Clinical

The earliest symptoms of LD are malaise, myalgia, and headache (Table 99.1). Within a day or so shaking chills and fever occur. The temperature rises rapidly, frequently exceeds 38.9°C, and remains elevated and unremittent. Patients usually have a cough which is unproductive or productive of only small amounts of mucoid sputum. Pleuritic chest pain occurs in about one-third of the patients but hemoptysis is unusual. The respiratory symptoms predominate, with progressive dyspnea, tachypnea, and cyanosis which may require mechanical ventilation. Abdominal discomfort, vomiting and diarrhea may also be present (Table 99.2).

Examination will confirm a lobar or multilobar pneumonia with scattered rales, occasionally signs of consolidation and a pleural friction rub. Fever is almost universally present and may exceed 40°C. A relative bradycardia is frequently recognized. Disorientation, confusion, and obtundation may be present at the height of the illness.

TABLE 99.1   *Legionella pneumophila* – Clinical Manifestations

Malaise	Cough
Myalgias	Pleuritic pain
Headache	Tachypnea
Fever	Rales
Shaking chills	Tachycardia

TABLE 99.2   *Legionella pneumophila* – Extrapulmonary Manifestations

Watery diarrhea

Abdominal distention

Abdominal pain

Vomiting

Relative bradycardia

Laboratory (Table 99.3)

Abnormalities of the chest radiograph are the rule. Patchy lobar interstitial infiltrates frequently progress to involve multiple lobes with frank consolidation. Bilateral involvement is seen in about half the patients with a predilection for the lower lobes. Effusions are uncommon and of mild degree. Cavitation is rare. Radiographic resolution lags behind clinical resolution and may take up to 8 weeks.

Sputum examination is frequently unremarkable. Macroscopically it appears mucoid and microscopically shows few inflammatory cells and scanty organisms which yield a normal flora on culture. Secondary bacterial invasion with gram-negative bacilli may occur in patients with chronic lung disease. *Legionella pneumophila* is rarely isolated from sputum, even on specifically enriched media, although occasional reports demonstrating the bacillus in sputum have been published. Pleural exudates, tracheal aspirates, and bronchial brushings, all have yielded the organism on subculture. Direct fluorescent antibody examination and silver Dieterle staining of lung biopsy material may also demonstrate the bacillus.

Leukocytosis is present in four-fifths of the patients. A shift to the left and the presence of band forms are frequent. Thrombocytopenia may be present. The erythrocyte sedimentation rate is increased. Hyponatremia is not uncommon, and in some patients suggests the syndrome of inappropriate antidiuretic hormone secretion. An absolute hypophosphatemia also has been observed.

Disturbances of liver function producing an elevated SGOT, alkaline phosphatase, total bilirubin, and particularly LDH, are frequent. Renal function is generally normal although urinalysis may show moderate proteinuria and microscopic hematuria. Occasional patients develop acute tubular necrosis usually as a terminal phenomenon secondary to hypotension.

Arterial blood gas analysis shows hypoxemia and hypocarbia relative to the degree of lung involvement.

Serologic testing is the most reliable means of confirming the diagnosis owing to the difficulties associated with culture of the bacillus. Indirect fluorescent antibody testing of serum drawn at the time of onset of the illness and 3 weeks later will usually show seroconversion with a fourfold rise in titer to $\geq$ 1:64. Occasionally the antibody response occurs later. A single titer of > 1:128 is considered to indicate seropositivity. The test appears to be specific with few cross-reactions reported. Titers peak at about 5 weeks and remain elevated for several months.

TABLE 99.3 *Legionella pneumophila* - Laboratory

Chest roentgenogram: patchy infiltrates to frank consolidation

Proteinuria, hematuria

Abnormal liver function tests

Hyponatremia (syndrome of inappropriate ADH secretion)

Sputum smear: mononuclear cells

No organisms

Special cultures: charcoal yeast extract agar

Direct immunofluorescent staining of respiratory secretions

Serum antibody rise

Differential Diagnosis

Several viral and bacterial pneumonias must be considered in the differential diagnosis (Table 99.4). The initial symptoms of LD resemble influenza. However, the early and frequently extensive degree of lung involvement is unusual for influenza. Influenza epidemics are more frequent in the winter and LD is more commonly seen during the summer and fall. Sporadic cases may prove difficult to differentiate without confirmatory serologic testing. Adenovirus and respiratory syncytial virus pneumonias may closely mimic LD and are considered in Chapters 71 and 52 respectively.

Among bacterial pneumonias, psittacosis and Q fever should be considered. Here an exposure history is usually helpful but the definitive diagnosis is again serologic. *Mycoplasma pneumoniae* pneumonia is probably the illness most likely to be confused with LD. The clinical features are very similar; however, *M. pneumoniae* pneumonia occurs uncommonly over the age of 35, unlike LD which is a disease of middle and later life. Circulating cold agglutinins are found in about half the patients with *M. pneumoniae* infection and only rarely in LD. The definite diagnosis is again serologic. For both *M. pneumoniae* and LD, erythromycin is the antibiotic of choice.

Treatment

Several antibiotics show good activity against *L. pneumophila* in vitro, but clinical experience with erythromycin has shown it to be the most effective agent. Case-fatality rates among patients in the 1976 Philadelphia epidemic were lowest for those treated with erythromycin. Guinea pigs challenged with a lethal dose of organisms are protected by prior treatment with erythromycin.

Rifampin shows the greatest in vitro activity against the bacillus. However, the possibility of developing drug resistance to rifampin warrants caution in its use as a single agent. Early experimental information in animals suggests that erythromycin and rifampin in combination may prove more effective. Erythromycin, 0.5-1.0 g every 6 hr, is recommended in adults and 15 mg/kg every 6 hr for children other than neonates.

Prevention

Until the source of *L. pneumophila* is known with certainty primary prevention remains difficult. Person-to-person spread appears uncommon, if it exists, and respiratory isolation of a patient with LD does not appear justified. However, the high frequency of LD among patients with renal homograft transplants, or among those patients who are on immunosuppressive therapy may justify alternative hospital facilities should LD be prevalent in one institution.

The possibility of immunization against LD should be considered now that the bacillus has been isolated. The justifications for a vaccine include the estimated incidence of 0.5-1.5% of all pneumonias in the United States and the fatality rate of 15-20%. Information concerning the degree of protection afforded by naturally acquired infection, and whether or not this is modified by the use of antibiotics is lacking.

TABLE 99.4 Comparison of Various Features of the Atypical Pneumonias

	Legionnaires' Disease	Mycoplasmal Pneumonia	Psittacosis	Q Fever	Influenza, Parainfluenza or Adenovirus	Histoplasmosis	Coccidioidomycosis
Incubation period (days)	2–10	12–21	7–14	14–35	1–3	3–21	7–28
Age	Middle to elderly	Children and young adults	Adult	Adult	All	All	All
Person-to-person transmission	0	+	Rare	0	+	0	0
Underlying disease, smoking, alcohol	+	0	0	0	Some	Some	0
Upper respiratory symptoms	0	+	+/–	0	+	+/–	+/–
Pleural effusion	20–30% (small)	10–25% (small)	Rare	Rare	Rare	Rare	Common
Treatment	Erythromycin	Erythromycin or tetracycline	Tetracycline	Tetracycline	None	Amphotericin B (under certain circumstances)	Amphotericin B

TABLE 99.5   Legionellaceae

L. pneumophila

Serogroups 1-6, group 1 most important

L. bozemanii

Includes WIGA

L. micdadei

Does not produce β-lactamase
Includes TATLOCK and HEBA
Pittsburgh pneumonia

L. dumoffii

Includes TEX-KL

L. gormanii

L. longbeachae

Complications and Prognosis

Asymptomatic infections occur and short-lived, self-limiting infections without lung involvement are well recognized. The major complication of LD is progressive respiratory failure with cyanosis, tachypnea, hypoxemia, and the requirement for oxygen and ventilatory support. Progressive and overwhelming toxemia with high fever, obtundation, and subsequent hypotension and irreversible shock are also seen. Hemorrhage secondary to thrombocytopenia or consumptive coagulopathy is another serious and sometimes fatal complication. Acute oliguric renal failure is usually, but not always, secondary to a period of hypotension and may require dialysis.

Neurologic complications include a toxic confusional state, amnesia, altered personality, abnormalities of gait and muscle tone, and encephalopathy. Most will disappear with recovery, although symptoms and signs related to encephalomyelitis may persist for several months before improvement.

Complications and mortality tend to be more frequent in those patients with preexisting disease, most notably chronic lung disease, malignancy, chronic renal failure, diabetes mellitus, and those receiving immunosuppressive agents. Mortality varies from 14 to 19% of infected persons.

Other Legionellae

There have been other cases of pneumonia which clinically resemble Legionnaires' disease and from which previously unrecognized organisms have been isolated. These gram-negative bacilli have characteristics which are similar to *L. pneumophila,* such as ability to grow on charcoal yeast extract agar but not on the more commonly used media. Pittsburgh pneumonia was identified as a nosocomial infection in immunocompromised patients. The nomenclature for these various organisms is complicated by their very recent identification. A recent classification, obviously subject to change, is listed in Table 99.5.

Selected Bibliography

Bock, B. V., Kirby, B., Edelstein, P. H., George, W. L., Snyder, K., Owens, M. L., Hatayama, C., Haley, C. E., Lewis, R. P., Meyer, R. D., and Finegold, S. M.: Legionnaires' disease in renal transplant recipients. *Lancet* 1:410-413, 1978.

Brenner, D. J., Steigerwalt, A. G., and McDade, J. E.: Classification of the Legionnaires' disease bacterium: *Legionella pneumophila,* genus novum, species nova, of the family Legionellaceae, family nova. *Ann Intern Med* 90:656, 1979.

Broome, C. V., Goings, S. A. G., Thacker, S. B., Vogt, R. L., Beaty, H. N., Fraser, D. W., and the Field Investigation Team: The Vermont epidemic of Legionnaires' disease. *Ann Intern Med* 90:573, 1979.

Cordes, L. G., Wilkenson, H. W., Gorman, G. W., Fikes, B. J., and Fraser, D. W.: Atypical *Legionella*-like organisms: Fastidious water-associated bacteria pathogenic for man. *Lancet* 2:927, 1979.

Foy, H. M., Broome, C. V., Hayes, P. S., Allan, I., Cooney, M. K., and Tobe, R.: Legionnaires' disease in a prepaid medical-care group in Seattle 1963-1975. *Lancet* 1:767, 1979.

Fraser, D. W., Tsao, T. R., Orenstein, W., Parkin, W. E., Beecham, H. J., Sharrar, R. G., Harris, J., Mallison, G. F., Martin, S. M., McDade, J. E., Shepard, C. C., Brachman, P. S., and the Field Investigation Team: Legionnaires' disease, description of an epidemic of pneumonia. *N Engl J Med* 297:1189-1197, 1977.

Fraser, D. W., Wachsmuth, I. K., Bopp, C., Feeley, J. C., and Tsai, T. F.: Antibiotic treatment of guinea pigs infected with agents of Legionnaires' disease. *Lancet* 1:175-178, 1978.

Gump, D. W., Frank, R. O., Winn, W. C., Jr., Foster, R. S., Jr., Broome, C. V., and Cherry, W. B.: Legionnaires' disease in patients with associated serious disease. *Ann Intern Med* 90:538, 1979.

Hebert, G. A., Thomason, B. M., Harris, P. P., Hicklin, M. D., and McKinney, R. M.: "Pittsburgh Pneumonia Agent": A bacterium phenotypically similar to *Legionella pneumophila* and identical to the TATLOCK bacterium. *Ann Intern Med* 92:53, 1980.

Kirby, B. C., Snyder, K. M., Meyer, R. D., and Finegold, S. M.: Legionnaires' disease: Clinical features of 24 cases. *Ann Intern Med* 89:297-309, 1978.

Lattimer, G. L., Rhodes, L. V., III, Slaventi, J. S., Galgon, J. P., Stonebreaker, V., Boley, S., and Haas, G.: The Philadelphia epidemic of Legionnaires' disease: Clinical, pulmonary, and serologic findings 2 years later. *Ann Intern Med* 90: 522, 1979.

McDade, J. E., Shepard, C. C., Fraser, D. W., Tsai, T. R., Redus, M. A., Dowdle, W. R. and the Laboratory Investigation Team: Legionnaires' disease. Isolation of a bacterium and demonstration of its role in other respiratory disease. *N Engl J Med* 297:1197-1203, 1977.

Sanford, J. P.: Legionnaires' disease - the first thousand days. *N Engl J Med* 300: 654-655, 1979.

Thornsberry, C., Baker, C. N., and Kirven, L. A.: In vitro activity of antimicrobial agents in Legionnaires' disease bacterium. *Antimicrob Agents Chemother* 13: 78-80, 1978.

Tsai, T. F., Finn, D. R., Plikaytis, B. D., McCauley, W., Martin, S. M., and Fraser, D. W.: Legionnaires' disease: Clinical features of the epidemic in Philadelphia. *Ann Intern Med* 90:509, 1979.

Wong, K. H., Schalla, W. O., Arko, R. J., Bullard, J. C., and Feeley, J. C.: Immunochemical, serologic, and immunologic properties of major antigens isolated from the Legionnaires' disease bacterium. Observations bearing on the feasibility of a vaccine. *Ann Intern Med* 90:634, 1979.

100

SYPHILIS

Rama Ganguly, Ph.D. and
Robert H. Waldman, M.D.

Syphilis is an infectious disease affecting only humans, usually transmitted by sexual contact, and caused by the spirochete *Treponema pallidum*. Beginning late in the fifteenth century the disease was rampant for several decades in Western Europe and was given the name syphilis after a mythical shepherd by the early epidemiologist Fracastorius (1530). Schaudinn and Hoffman first discovered the causal agent in 1905.

Etiology

Treponema pallidum is a thin, delicate organism with tapering ends, 5-15 μm in length, with a transverse diameter of 0.25 μm. It divides by binary fission and is extremely sensitive to various physical and chemical agents, including heat. It survives poorly outside the human body and has never been cultured in vitro. It is wrapped around by 6-14 corkscrew axial filaments or flagella, which give the organism its characteristic motility. The spirochetes possess endotoxins and their cell walls contain muramic acid. The organism can be grown in certain animal models, the one most commonly used being the rabbit.

Epidemiology

Syphilis is endemic throughout the world. The organism enters the body through minute abrasions in the epithelium during direct contact. The infectious dose is very low, and nonvenereal transmission is uncommon, except in the case of congenital, or prenatal, syphilis. Most new cases of syphilis occur during the most sexually active period, i.e., 15-40 years. There has been a rapid increase in the number of cases in homosexuals. For the most recent year from which data are available, the reported number of cases in the United States was about 22,000 for primary and secondary syphilis, and about 400-500 for congenital syphilis. It is estimated that only about 12% of the cases are reported. It is also estimated that an even greater number of people have asymptomatic and undetected infection and therefore serve as a large reservoir of the infection.

Pathogenesis and Pathology

After penetration of a small break in the epithelium, the bacteria multiplies at the site, followed by migration to regional lymph nodes within a few hours or days. In 10-90 days, with an average of 21 days, a firm, usually nontender, solitary cutaneous ulcer, the chancre, develops, accompanied by painless enlargement of the regional lymph nodes. The chancre is the classic lesion of *primary syphilis* (Table 100.1). Multiple genital lesions also may occur, and the chancre may be extragenital in about 10% of cases. The chancre results from an intense cellular infiltration consisting mainly of mononuclear and plasma cells. There are a large number of organisms present in the lesion and in the extracellular fluid exuding from it. The chancre heals spontaneously.

Secondary syphilis (Table 100.2) begins 2 weeks to several months following the primary manifestation. The classic manifestation is a generalized symmetric skin rash, involving the mucous membranes and the palms and soles of the feet. The lesions of secondary syphilis also may involve the eyes, bones, joints, central nervous system, liver, and kidney. Patients commonly have malaise and fever. The secondary lesions contain very large numbers of organisms, and the inflammatory infiltrate consists of mononuclear and plasma cells. There is swelling of the capillary endothelium, but necrosis is minimal or absent, and lesions heal slowly but without scarring.

The primary and secondary stages of syphilis may go completely unrecognized, or recognized and treated inadequately, and then are followed by *latent syphilis* (Table 100.3). Latent syphilis is characterized by no signs or symptoms, but a positive serology (antibody response to the infection, see later discussion). The latent stage may continue for many years, not uncommonly for the life-time of the patient.

TABLE 100.1   Characteristics of Primary Syphilis

History of sexual contact often of doubtful reliability

Painless ulcer on genitalia, perianal area, pharynx, tongue, lip: 2-6 wk after exposure

Nontender regional adenopathy

Fluid from lesion: spirochetes by immunofluorescence or dark-field microscopy

Serology may or may not be positive

TABLE 100.2   Characteristics of Secondary Syphilis

Generalized maculopapular rash

Mucous membrane lesions: patches and ulcers

Weeping papules (condylomas) in moist skin areas

Generalized nontender lymphadenopathy

Fever

Lesion scrapings have myriads of spirochetes

Serology always positive

Less common manifestations: meningitis, hepatitis, osteitis, arthritis, iritis

TABLE 100.3   Characteristics of Latent Syphilis

No physical signs

History of syphilis inadequately treated

Specific serologic test positive

In about half of the untreated patients with syphilis, 2–40 years after the latent stage begins, *late (tertiary) syphilis* develops (Table 100.4). There are many different manifestations of late syphilis. One of the characteristic manifestations is the development of the gumma, a large granuloma characterized by extensive caseation and necrosis. They may be found in the skin, mucous membranes, bones, or viscera, and histopathologically are composed of epithelioid giant cells surrounded by macrophages, lymphocytes, and plasma cells.

Other manifestations of late syphilis result from obliterative endarteritis of the terminal arterioles and small arteries, involving the central nervous system (Table 100.5), the aorta, and the musculoskeletal system.

Very few organisms are present in the lesions of late syphilis, and it is thought that the tissue damage results from the host's immune response to treponemal antigens persisting in the tissues.

Lesions of congenital (prenatal) syphilis (Table 100.6) in general resemble those of acquired syphilis of comparable duration. Fetuses who have been massively infected in utero may be stillborn or die shortly after birth. Those who survive may develop lesions early (less than 2 years) or later in life, up to 40 years of age.

TABLE 100.4   Late (Tertiary) Syphilis

Neurosyphilis

Asymptomatic
Meningovascular
Tabes dorsalis
General paresis

Cardiovascular: aortitis, AI, aneurysms

Gumma

TABLE 100.5   Neurosyphilis

Meningovascular

Seizures (generalized or focal)
Stroke

Parenchymatous

General paresis

Changes in personality, affect, sensorium,
    intellect, insight, judgment
Hyperactive reflexes
Argyll Robertson pupil
Optic atrophy

Tabes dorsalis

Ataxia
Impotence
Bladder disturbances
Peripheral neuropathy
Romberg's sign
Cranial nerves II-VII involvement

Diagnosis

The diagnosis and staging of syphilis are important for purposes of treatment and
for public health preventive measures, and require integration of the history,
physical findings, and laboratory testing (Tables 100.7 and 100.8). Early primary
syphilis can be diagnosed only by demonstration of organisms seen on examination
of material from a chancre. Two methods are used to identify the organism, either dark-field examination or fluorescent antibody staining. Examining a wet
preparation under the dark-field microscope, *T. pallidum* is seen as a rotating,
twisting, and undulating microorganism. For fluorescent antibody staining, a

TABLE 100.6   Characteristics of Congenital Syphilis

Early:	Osteochondritis	Jaundice
	Snuffles	Neurologic signs
	Rash	Lymphadenopathy
	Anemia	Mucous patches
	Hepatosplenomegaly	
Late:	Frontal bosses	Hutchinson's incisors
	Short maxillas	Mulberry molars
	Saddle-nose	Sternoclavicular thickening
	Protruding mandible	Clutton's joints
	Interstitial keratitis	Saber-shins
	Nerve deafness	Flaring scapulas
	High palatal arch	

fixed specimen is reacted with fluorescein-tagged antibody to *T. pallidum*. In addition to examining exudate from a chancre, either of these methods can be used to identify the pathogen from a skin or mucous membrane lesion of secondary syphilis, including the secondary stage of congenital syphilis. One warning with respect to interpretation of the dark-field examination is the occasional contamination of the specimen with commensal spirochetes which may be found in normal genital secretions.

The important diagnostic approach to syphilis is serologic (Table 100.9). The important specimens for serologic examination are blood, serum, and cerebrospinal fluid. Very little is known about the nature of the antigens that elicit the antibody responses in a patient with syphilis. Both specific antitreponemal and nonspecific antibody responses occur. The nonspecific (Wasserman) reaction tests for antibody to cardiolipin or, more exactly, diphosphatidylglycerol. This antibody is a very sensitive screening test for the early stages of syphilis, and there are many different techniques used, e.g., the Venereal Disease Research Laboratory (VDRL) tests, the rapid plasma reagin (RPR) test, and the automated reagin (ART) tests. These nonspecific tests are positive in a variety of diseases other than syphilis, e.g., malaria, leprosy, infectious mononucleosis, and systemic lupus erythematosus (Table 100.10).

There are also several different tests for the measurement of specific treponemal antibodies: the fluorescent antibody test (FTA-ABS), the most commonly used specific antibody test; the hemagglutination reaction; and the *Treponema pallidum* immobilization (TPI) test, which requires the use of live organisms. Nonspecific, e.g., VDRL, antibodies decline with the passage of time and/or with treatment, whereas specific treponemal antibodies nearly always persist for the life-time of the patient. In some patients with a very high titer of antibody, the nonspecific test may give a false-negative result using undiluted serum, whereas when diluted considerably a positive result is obtained. This is called the prozone phenomenon and is caused by the complete coating of antigen by antibody molecules, thereby not allowing the agglutination or flocculation of the particles.

TABLE 100.7   Laboratory Tests for Antibody Detection in Syphilis

---

Nonspecific antibody test

> VDRL or RPR: The Venereal Disease Research Laboratory test or rapid plasma reagin test for nontreponemal (reagin) antibody which has as an endpoint flocculation of a cholesterolized cardiolipin-lecithin antigen.

Specific antibody test

> FTA: The fluorescent treponemal antibody test for treponemal antibody: Detected by incubating serum (or CSF) with whole nonviable *T. pallidum* (Nichols strain) antigen fixed to a glass slide and made fluorescent (visible) by the addition of fluorescein-conjugated antihuman globulin.

> FTA-ABS: The fluorescent treponemal antibody absorption test: Performed as in FTA above but with the additional step of first diluting the serum (or CSF) in a "sorbent" prepared from Reiter strain treponema to absorb out cross-reacting group antibody induced by saprophytic nonpathogenic treponemes.

> FTA-ABS-IgM: The fluorescent treponemal antibody absorption test for IgM: Treponemal antibody performed as in FTA-ABS above except a specific anti-IgM fluoresceinated conjugate is used.

> MHA-TP: The microhemagglutination assay for *T. pallidum:* Performed by absorbing serum (or CSF) with sorbent and then incubating with erythrocytes sensitized with cellular components of Nichols strain of *T. pallidum.* In the presence of treponemal antibody agglutination of erythrocytes occurs.

> TPI: The *Treponema pallidum* immobilization test: Performed by incubating live motile *T. pallidum* with serum and complement. Immobilization of the treponemata occurs in the presence of treponemal antibody.

> Reiter: Reiter protein (extract of treponeme) complement fixation.

Treatment

Early treatment is of utmost importance to prevent the destructive features of late (tertiary) and congenital (prenatal) syphilis. *Treponema pallidum* is killed, albeit slowly, by extremely low concentrations of penicillin, the drug of choice (Table 100.11).

Immunity and Prevention

Immune mechanisms in syphilis are very poorly understood. As is clear from the earlier discussion, antibodies develop during the course of the disease, but apparently do not stop its progression in the absence of treatment. Patients with latent

TABLE 100.8   Recommendations for the Laboratory Diagnosis of Syphilis

Neonatal congenital

> Rising VDRL titer diagnostic
>
> Positive FTA-ABS-IgM suggestive but not diagnostic (10% false-positive)
> Negative FTA-ABS-IgM does not exclude diagnosis (35% false-negative)

Primary

> Dark-field examination of primary lesion *
>
> FTA-ABS more likely to be positive (85%) than either MHA-TP (65%) or
> VDRL (70%); a rising VDRL titer in the presence of a positive FTA-ABS
> is diagnostic

Secondary

> Dark-field examination of mucosal or cutaneous lesion *
>
> Positive VDRL in the presence of a positive FTA-ABS or MHA-TP

Late

> Latent, late benign, and cardiovascular: positive FTA-ABS or MHA-TP
> on serum and a normal CSF examination
>
> Neurosyphilis: Positive FTA-ABS or MHA-TP on serum with CSF demon-
> strating any one or all of the following:
>
> > ≥ 5 white cells/mm^3
> > > 40 mg% protein
> > Positive VDRL (the FTA or FTA-ABS on CSF is of uncertain signifi-
> > cance and therefore not recommended)

*Care must be taken to avoid contamination by commensal spirochetes from
 genitalia

TABLE 100.9   Comparative Results of Serologic Tests for Syphilis in Various Stages of Disease and in Nonsyphilitics

| Test | Neonatal/Congenital | Stages of Disease | | | | | | Nonsyphilitics |
		Primary	Secondary	Early Latent	Late Latent	Late (Benign, Cardiovascular, Neurosyphilis)	Neurosyphilis (Cerebrospinal Fluid Serology)	False-Positive Serum[1]
VDRL	Must be differentiated from maternal VDRL. Only a rising titer diagnostic	70%	99%	95%	72%	70%	22–61%	Frequent occurrence, but usually in low titer
FTA-ABS	Must be differentiated from maternal FTA-ABS[2]	85	99	99	96	97	Variable[3]	0.5–1%; patients with hyperglobulinemia and/or antinuclear factor
MHA-TP	Insufficient data	65	96	~95	~95	~95	Insufficient data	Less than 1.5%, although some studies reported a higher rate of false-positivity (9%), particularly with sera demonstrating false-positive VDRL
TPI	Insufficient data	50–60	95	94	89	93	Insufficient data	Rare

[1] False-positive treponemal and reagin antibody tests will occur regularly in nonsyphilitic treponemal disease such as yaws and pinta.

[2] The FTA-ABS-IgM has been used to distinguish fetal from maternal treponemal antibody. However, the technique is not well standardized; 10% false-positives (in part may be due to nontreponemal fetal IgM directed against maternal IgG) and 35% false-negatives reported, particularly in cases acquired late in pregnancy.

[3] The specificity and sensitivity are not well established. The FTA appears to be more sensitive than the FTA-ABS which in turn is more sensitive than the FTA-IgM test.

Modified from Bracero, et al. *Mt Sinai J Med* 45:289–292, 1979.

TABLE 100.10   False-Positive Serologic Tests

Infectious Diseases	Noninfectious
Leprosy	SLE
Pneumococcal pneumonia	Drug addiction
SBE	Rheumatoid arthritis
Chancroid	Transfusions
Scarlet fever	Pregnancy
Leptospirosis	Aging
Relapsing fever	
Rat-bite fever	
Rickettsial disease	
Trypanosomiasis	
Vaccinia	
Mycoplasmal	

TABLE 100.11   Treatment

Primary, secondary, and early latent

    Benzathine penicillin 2.4 x 10^6 U IM, or
    Procaine penicillin 600,000 U IM daily x 8, or
    Tetracycline or erythromycin 500 mg p.o. q.i.d. x
      15 days

Late latent or tertiary

    Benzathine penicillin 2.4 x 10^6 U IM weekly x 3, or
    Procaine penicillin 600,000 U IM daily x 15, or
    Tetracycline or erythromycin 500 mg p.o. q.i.d. x 30 days

Neurosyphilis

    Aqueous crystalline penicillin G 12-24 x 10^6 U daily
      IV x 8

Congenital (prenatal)

    Normal CSF: benzathine penicillin 50,000 U/kg IM
    Abnormal CSF: aqueous 50,000 U/kg IM or IV x 10 days

TABLE 100.12   Nonvenereal Treponematoses

Yaws

Pinta

Endemic syphilis (bejel, skerljevo)

---

or late syphilis are resistant to reinfection and will not develop a chancre when exposed. On the other hand, patients treated in the early stages of the disease are susceptible to reinfection. Passive immunization using serum with high antibody titers delays development of syphilis upon exposure. There is evidence that patients develop cell-mediated immune (CMI) reactions to the organism in the later stages of the disease, but the role of CMI is unclear. The mucoid envelope of the pathogen renders it highly resistant to phagocytosis. Experimental vaccines are being studied, and animal studies have been promising. The only effective method of control currently available, or in the immediate future, is prompt reporting, identification, and treatment of infected persons and contacts.

Table 100.12 lists the nonvenereal treponematoses, which will be discussed in Chapter 101.

Selected Bibliography

Becker, G. D.: Late syphilitic hearing loss: A diagnostic and therapeutic dilemma. *Laryngoscope* 89:1273-1288, 1979.

Bracero, L., Wormser, G. P., and Bottone, E.: Serologic tests for syphilis: A guide to interpretation in various stages of disease. *Mt Sinai J Med* 45:289-292, 1979.

Brown, W. J.: Status and control of syphilis in the United States. *J Infect Dis* 124:428, 1971.

Campisi, D. and Whitcombe, C.: Liver disease in early syphilis. *Arch Intern Med* 139:365-366, 1979.

Clark, E. G. and Danbolt, N.: The Oslo study of the natural course of untreated syphilis. *Med Clin N Am* 48:613, 1964.

Drusui, L. M., Topf-Olstein, B., and Levy-Zombek, E.: Epidemiology of infectious syphilis at a tertiary hospital. *Arch Intern Med* 139:901-904, 1979.

Duncan, W. C., Knox, J. M., and Wende, R. D.: The FTA-ABS test in darkfield-positive primary syphilis. *JAMA* 228:859-860, 1974.

Dunlop, E. M., Al-Eqaily, S. S., and Houang, E. T.: Penicillin levels in blood and CSF achieved by treatment of syphilis. *JAMA* 241:2538-2540, 1979.

Fitzgerald, T. J. and Johnson, R. C.: Surface mucopolysaccharides of *Treponema pallidum*. *Infect Immun* 24:244-251, 1979.

Fitzgerald, T. J., Johnson, R. C., and Ritzi, D. M.: Relationship of *Treponema pallidum* to acidic mucopolysaccharides. *Infect Immun* 24:252-260, 1979.

Gnoda, Y.: Therapeutic effect of oral doxycycline on syphilis. *Br J Vener Dis* 55:110-115, 1979.

Hunter, E. F., McKinney, R. M., Maddison, S. E., and Cruce, D. D.: Double-staining procedure for the fluorescent treponemal antibody absorption (FTA-ABS) test. *Br J Vener Dis* 55:105-108, 1979.

Jaffee, H. W.: The laboratory diagnosis of syphilis. *Ann Intern Med* 83:846, 1975.

Jongensen, D.: Epidemiology of gonorrhea and syphilis in South Australia (1966-1977). *Br J Vener Dis* 55:131-137, 1979.

Magnuson, H. J., Thomas, E. W., Olansky, S., et al.: Inoculation syphilis in human volunteers. *Medicine* 35:33, 1956.

Metzger, M.: Role of humoral versus cellular mechanisms of resistance in the pathogenesis of syphilis. *Br J Vener Dis* 55:94-98, 1979.

Musher, D. M. and Schell, R. F.: The immunology of syphilis. *Hosp Pract* 10:45-50, 1975.

Peter, C. R., Thompson, M. A., and Wilson, D. L.: False positive reaction in the rapid plasma reagin-card, fluorescent treponemal antibody-absorbed and hemagglutination treponemal syphilis serology tests. *J Clin Microbiol* 9:369-372, 1979.

Platts, W. M.: Epidemiology of gonorrhea and syphilis in New Zealand. *Br J Vener Dis* 55:138-141, 1979.

Rockwell, D. H., Yobs, A. R., and Moore, M. B.: The Tuskeegee study of untreated syphilis; the 30th year of observation. *Arch Intern Med* 114:792, 1964.

Rudolph, A. H.: Serologic diagnosis of syphilis: An update. *South Med J* 69:1196, 1976.

Sparling, R. F.: Diagnosis and treatment of syphilis. *N Engl J Med* 284:642, 1971.

Speer, M. E., Taber, L. H., Clark, D. B., et al.: Cerebrospinal fluid levels of benzathine penicillin G in the neonate. *J Pediatr* 91:996, 1977.

Tramont, E. C.: Persistence of *Treponema pallidum* following penicillin G therapy. *JAMA* 236:2206, 1976.

Wade, T. R. and Huntley, A.: Multiple penile chancres: An atypical manifestation of primary syphilis. *Arch Dermatol* 115:227, 1979.

Zoller, M., Wilson, W. R., and Nadol, J. B.: Treatment of syphilitic hearing loss: Combined penicillin and steroid therapy in 29 patients. *Ann Otol Rhinol Laryngol* 88:160-165, 1979.

101

TREPONEMAL DISEASES OTHER THAN SYPHILIS
Robert H. Waldman, M.D.

Although syphilis is by far the most important treponemal disease in the United States and throughout the world, there are nonsyphilitic diseases caused by organisms with many similarities to *Treponema pallidum*. These diseases have several common characteristics, including those that are different from syphilis, as well as those that are held in common with syphilis (Table 101.1). Infection with one of these treponemata, including *T. pallidum,* seems to render the host immune to infection with another organism from this genus.

Yaws

Yaws is found in remote populations of the Caribbean, Central and South America, Africa, Sri Lanka, and India. The disease is rapidly decreasing in frequency in the Americas, at least partially as a result of case-finding, and the treatment of patients and contacts with penicillin. Thirty years ago there were nearly 50,000 new cases each year, whereas there were 400 or fewer cases last year. However, the prevalence may be increasing in some areas of Africa. There is no animal reservoir and the disease is transmitted from person-to-person mainly by direct contact, and possibly to a lesser extent by flies. The disease, usually acquired as a child, is caused by the organism *T. pertenue*.

The pathology of the disease is granulomatous lesions of the skin, mucous membranes, and bone, but without perivascular cuffing, as is seen in syphilis. Chronic infection leads to disfigurement and disability.

The primary lesion is a single painless papule which develops 3–4 weeks after exposure, usually on the legs or hands. The papule degenerates into an ulcer which gradually enlarges, and may reach 7 cm in diameter. Regional lymphadenopathy also develops. Secondary lesions develop 6–12 weeks later and persist for months

TABLE 101.1   Comparison of Nonsyphilis Treponemal Infections and Syphilis

	Syphilis	Nonsyphilis Treponemes
Differences	Worldwide	Tropical
	Venereal	Nonvenereal
	Visceral involvement	Visceral involvement
	Severe and fairly frequent	Rare
Similarities	Organisms seen by dark-field or immuno-fluorescence	
	Has not been possible to culture on artificial media	
	Serologic tests for syphilis are positive	
	Disease can be divided into stages, i.e., primary, secondary and, in some, tertiary	
	Penicillin-, erythromycin-, and tetracycline-sensitive	

to years. These lesions are similar to the primary lesion. They heal, leaving a depigmented spot, which is anesthetic. Lesions on the feet evolve into nodules. The tertiary lesions are gummatous, with bony changes which are disfiguring. Involvement of the digits and facial bones leads to shortening of the digits and leonine facies and facial horns.

The diagnosis is made on clinical, epidemiologic, serologic, and bacteriologic evidence. The serologic response is the same as in syphilis, and the bacteriologic proof, when available, is the demonstration of organisms by dark-field examination. The treatment is a single injection of long-acting penicillin.

Pinta

Pinta is a disease with many similarities to yaws, except that bony involvement is extremely rare, and the disease is almost entirely limited to skin changes. Pinta, which means spotted, is caused by *T. carateum*. It is found only in rural areas of South and Central America, especially in Mexico and Colombia, in coastal regions, and along river banks.

The primary lesion is a nonulcerative, erythematous, pruritic papule, usually in young children, which evolves into a dark plaque. Secondary lesions are similar. They occur within a year of the primary, mainly on the extremities. As the lesions age they become scaly, atrophic, and depigmented. Rarely, tertiary lesions are found in the central nervous system and/or aorta.

TABLE 101.2   Comparison of Yaws, Pinta, and Endemic Syphilis

	Yaws	Pinta	Endemic Syphilis
Organism	*T. pertenue*	*T. carateum*	*T. pallidum*
Geographic distribution	Rural, tropical	Central and South America - rural, tropical	Africa, Southeast Asia, Arabian Peninsula - rural, temperate
Age distribution of acquisition of infection	2-3 yr	Adolescents	6-16 yr
Primary lesion	Large papillomatous	Scaly, erythematous papules	Not usually seen
Secondary	Papulosquamous	Pintids	Mucous patches
Tertiary	Gummas of skin, bones and joints	Depigmentation	Gummas of skin and bones

Endemic Syphilis

Endemic syphilis, which goes by many regional names, the most well known probably being bejel and skerljevo, is caused by an organism indistinguishable from *T. pallidum;* but it is not a venereal disease. It is transmitted by body contact and fomites. It is found in dry areas of the eastern Mediterranean and Southeast Asia.

The primary lesion is a moist ulcer of the skin or mucous membrane, usually appearing during childhood. Secondary lesions are similar to those of venereal syphilis and appear long after the healing of the primary lesion. Tertiary lesions are similar to those of venereal syphilis.

Table 101.2 summarizes the comparative features of yaws, pinta, and endemic syphilis.

Selected Bibliography

Garner, M. F., Backhouse, J. L., Cook, C. A., and Roeder, P. J.: Fluorescent treponemal antibody absorption (FTA-ABS) test in yaws. *Br J Vener Dis* 46: 284-286, 1970.

Hopkins, D. R.: After smallpox eradication: Yaws? *Am J Trop Med Hyg* 25:860-865, 1976.

Hopkins, D. R.: Yaws in the Americas, 1950-1975. *J Infect Dis* 136:548-554, 1977.

Hudson, E. H.: Endemic syphilis - heir of the syphiloids. *Arch Intern Med* 108: 1-4, 1961.

Kuhn, U. S. G., III, Varela, G., Chandler, F. W., Jr., and Osuna, G. G.: Experimental pinta in the chimpanzee. *JAMA* 206:829, 1968.

Lees, R. E. M.: A selective approach to yaws control. *Can J Public Health* 64: 52-56, 1973.

102

LEPTOSPIROSIS
Robert H. Waldman, M.D.

Leptospirosis is a zoonosis caused by *Leptospira interrogans*. It is a difficult disease to understand from the medical literature because of confusion regarding the taxonomy of *Leptospira*, and the various clinical syndromes which have been described. Human disease is caused by one species, *L. interrogans*, made up of 16 serogroups (Tables 102.1 and 102.2) and 130 serotypes. Any of these serotypes may cause any of the various manifestations of the disease, including mild to severe syndromes, but there is a tendency for certain serotypes to cause more severe disease. The disease has many manifestations, and these various manifestations historically have been given different names, e.g., Weil's disease or Fort Bragg fever. This phenomenon is not unheard of in medicine; however, it is possibly more complicated with leptospirosis as a result of the difficulty in growing and identifying the organism, and the extremely nonspecific nature of the signs and symptoms in many patients.

Microbiology

Leptospira are tightly coiled spirochetes which do not stain with the usual laboratory bacterial stains. They are aerobic, and grow on artificial media, such as Fletcher's semisolid or Stuart's liquid media. They grow slowly, appearing in 6-14 days, but occasionally as long as 5 weeks are required.

Epidemiology (Table 102.3)

The organism is found throughout the world and is mainly an infection of wild and domestic animals (Table 102.4). Humans are an incidental host. Infected animals

TABLE 102.1   Serogroups of *L. interrogans*

Icterohaemorrhagiae
Javanica
Celledoni
Canicola
Ballum
Pyrogenes
Cynopteri
Autumnalis
Australis
Pomona
Grippotyphosa
Hebdomadis
Bataviae
Tarassovi
Panama
Shermani

TABLE 102.2   Serogroup Etiology of Leptospirosis

Serogroup	Approximate % of Total
Icterohaemorrhagiae	30
Canicola	25
Autumnalis	15
Pomona	10

have prolonged asymptomatic infection with leptospiruria persisting for several months and occasionally, up to a few years. The organism is transmitted to humans most commonly by contact with contaminated water or soil. The conditions which optimize survival of the organism in water or soil are warm temperatures, alkaline pH, and the absence of chemical pollutants. The disease is most commonly seen in humans in summer and early autumn. At greatest risk are people who are exposed because of occupational or recreational activities, i.e., veterinarians, dairy workers, abattoir workers, miners, farmers, fish and poultry workers, hunters, fishermen, and people who swim in natural fresh water. Dogs and rats are the most common source of infection in the United States (Table 102.5).

The organism enters through abraded skin (it is unknown whether or not it can penetrate intact skin) or mucous membranes. The organism is acquired by direct contact with urine or tissues, or indirect contact with contaminated water, soil, or vegetation. There is no person-to-person transmission. The incubation period is 1-2 weeks.

TABLE 102.3   Epidemiologic Features of Leptospirosis

Survival of organism in nature	Enhanced by alkaline pH of animal urine, ground water, and soil
	Optimum conditions: days to weeks
Geographic distribution	General
	Concentration in southern U.S.
Seasonality	Concentrated in summer and early autumn
Age of patients	Most during childhood through middle age (because of increased hazards resulting from recreational and occupational activities)
Occupational exposure	Construction
	Farm
	Veterinary
	Abattoir
Recreational	Swimming in contaminated waters
	Hunting
Exposure to infected pets or rodents	
Incubation period	Usually 7-14 days

TABLE 102.4   Animal Hosts of *Leptospira*

Most Common Sources of Human Infection	Others
Rodents	Horses
Dogs	Skunks
Cattle	Raccoons
Swine	Foxes
	Opossums
	Armadillos

TABLE 102.5   Animal Source of Leptospirosis

Animal	Approximate % of Total
Dogs	30
Cattle/swine	10
Rodents	8
Wildlife	5
Unknown	45

Diagnosis

Clinical (Table 102.6)

The disease is biphasic, and during the first stage organisms are present in the blood and spinal fluid. This is followed by the immune phase which correlates with the appearance of IgM antibodies. Renal disease is a result of acute tubular necrosis and interstitial nephritis.

The first phase usually lasts 4-9 days and is characterized by the abrupt onset of high spiking fevers, chills, frontal headaches, prostration, and severe myalgias. The latter most commonly involve the thighs, low back, and calves; muscle tenderness and rigidity are common. Patients also may have abdominal and/or chest pains, nonproductive cough, conjunctival suffusion, relative bradycardia, and pharyngeal erythema. In more severe cases patients may have bleeding, jaundice, and nephritis. Various types of rashes are common, with the most frequent being macular or maculopapular. In Fort Bragg fever the characteristic finding is patchy erythema over the pretibial area, hence the other name for this syndrome, pretibial fever. In leptospirosis, splenomegaly and lymphadenopathy are unusual.

After the leptospiremic phase, patients are usually afebrile and feel relatively well for 1-5 days. The immune phase is much more variable than the leptospiremic one. Patients have many or most of the same symptoms as in the first phase, plus the common finding of meningeal inflammation. In the immune phase less common findings are iridocyclitis, optic neuritis, peripheral neuropathy, rash, and endocarditis. The immune phase is usually short, with fever lasting only 1-3 days.

Laboratory

The organism may be demonstrated in blood, urine, or spinal fluid by dark-field examination. The organism is seen in the blood and spinal fluid during the first 10 days of illness, but may be found in urine for up to 6 weeks following the onset of disease. Liver function abnormalities and an elevated bilirubin level are commonly found, as is an elevation in the blood urea nitrogen or creatinine concentrations. Spinal fluid findings are consistent with aseptic meningitis. Agglutinin titers rise at about day 7, persist for many years, and may be helpful in making the diagnosis.

TABLE 102.6   Major Clinical Findings in Patients with Leptospirosis

Finding	% of Patients
Fever	75
Headache	65
Stiff neck	40
Myalgias	40
Spinal fluid pleocytosis	35
Jaundice	35
↑ CSF protein	30
Nausea and/or vomiting	30
Hematuria	25
Proteinuria	20
Oliguria	15
Rash	15
Chills	10
Conjunctivitis	9

TABLE 102.7   Initial Diagnosis in Patients with Leptospirosis

Initial Clinical Impression	Approximate % of Cases
Meningitis	30
Hepatitis	15
Encephalitis	10
Fever of unknown origin	9
Pneumonia	2
Influenza	2
Leptospirosis	25

The most serious form of the disease is called Weil's syndrome. It is caused classically by the serogroup Icterohaemorrhagiae. In this form of the disease jaundice and renal failure are pronounced.

Differential Diagnosis

The differential diagnosis of leptospirosis is immense because of the nonspecific and varied nature of the signs and symptoms. Of particular significance in the differential diagnosis are hepatitis, yellow fever, and relapsing fever (Table 102.7).

Therapy

Antibiotics are of doubtful value in the treatment of leptospirosis, particularly if begun after the first few days of the leptospiremic phase. Penicillin, streptomycin, tetracycline, and erythromycin all are effective in vitro.

Prognosis and Complications

Fatal cases are almost always jaundiced, and patients with jaundice have approximately a 15% mortality. Complications are endocarditis, massive hemorrhage, and iridocyclitis. The disease can be prevented only by controlling the animal reservoir and avoiding contact.

Selected Bibliography

Adler, B. and Faine, S.: Host immunological mechanisms in the resistance of mice to leptospiral infections. *Infect Immun* 17:67, 1977.

Adler, B. and Faine, S.: The antibodies involved in the human immune response to leptospiral infection. *J Med Microbiol* 11:387, 1978.

Berman, S. J., Tsai, C. C., Holmes, K. K., et al.: Sporadic anicteric leptospirosis in South Vietnam. A study in 150 patients. *Ann Intern Med* 79:167, 1973.

Bey, R. F. and Johnson, R. C.: Protein-free and low-protein media for the cultivation of leptospirae. *Infect Immun* 19:562, 1978.

Buckler, J. M. H.: Leptospirosis presenting as erythema nodosum. *Arch Dis Child* 52:418, 1977.

Burke, B. J., Searle, J. F., and Mattingly, D.: Leptospirosis presenting with profuse haemoptysis. *Br Med J* 2:982, 1976.

Durham, R. J. L., Owens, G. G., and Weddridge, M. A. W.: Leptospirosis as a cause of erythema nodosum. *Br Med J* 2:403, 1976.

Edwards, G. A., and Dorum, B. M.: Human leptospirosis. *Medicine* 39:117, 1960.

Feigin, R. D., Lebes, L. A., Jr., Anderson, D., et al.: Human leptospirosis from immunized dogs. *Ann Intern Med* 79:777, 1973.

Fraser, D. W., Glosser, J. W., Francis, D. P., et al.: Leptospirosis caused by sero-type Fort-Bragg. *Ann Intern Med* 79:786, 1973.

Hall, H. E., Hightower, J. A., Rivera, R. D., Byrne, R. J., Sandel, J. E., and Woodward, T. E.: Evaluation of antibiotic therapy in human leptospirosis. *Ann Intern Med* 35:981, 1951.

McCrumb, F. R., Jr., Skockard, J. L., Robinson, C. R., Turner, L. H., Lewis, D. A., Maisey, C. W., Kelleher, M. F., Gleischer, C. A., and Smadel, J. E.: Leptospirosis in Malaya. I. Sporadic cases among military and civilian personnel. *Am J Trop Med Hyg* 6:238, 1957.

Ooi, B. S., Chen, B. T. M., Tan, K. K., and Khoo, O. T.: Human renal leptospirosis. *Am J Trop Med Hyg* 21:336, 1972.

Tatlock, H.: Studies on virus from a patient with Fort Bragg (pretibial) fever. *J Clin Invest* 26:287, 1977.

Thierman, A. B.: Incidence of leptospirosis in the Detroit rat population. *Am J Trop Med Hyg* 26:970, 1977.

Thorsteinsson, S. B., Sharp, P., Musher, D. M., and Martin, R. R.: Leptospirosis: An underdiagnosed cause of acute febrile illness. *South Med J* 68:217, 1975.

Tong, M. J., Rosenberg, E. B., Vetteri, B. A., and Tsai, C. B.: Immunological response in leptospirosis. Report of three cases. *Am J Trop Med Hyg* 20:625, 1971.

Turner, L. H.: Leptospirosis. *Br Med J* 1:321, 1969.

Wong, M. L., Kaplan, S., Dunkle, L. M., et al.: Leptospirosis: A childhood disease. *J Pediatr* 90:532, 1977.

103

RELAPSING FEVER AND RAT–BITE FEVER
Robert H. Waldman, M.D.

Relapsing Fever

Relapsing fever is caused by the spirochete genus, *Borrelia*. The disease is an acute bacterial infection characterized by recurrent febrile attacks separated by afebrile intervals. There are two types of relapsing fever, the louse-borne and the tick-borne varieties. The former is seen in epidemics in Asia, Africa, and Europe. The latter is usually endemic, but occasionally does occur in epidemics and is found in America, as well as the areas where the louse-borne variety is found.

Unlike other spirochetes, i.e., *Treponema* and *Leptospira*, *Borrelia* stain easily with the usual laboratory dyes. *Borrelia recurrentis* causes louse-borne relapsing fever. The tick-borne variety is caused by several species. Each is carried by a particular species of tick which transmits the disease (Table 103.1).

In the United States only the tick-borne variety of relapsing fever is found, and the disease usually occurs in late spring and summer, but it has been seen in winter months among campers. It is most common in the western states. The rodent population is the animal reservoir for the disease. Relapsing fever is transmitted by saliva or excreta of the tick during the feeding process. The disease is transmitted by soft ticks which do not cause pain while biting, and thus there is often no history of a tick bite. The tick remains infective for several years and the organism can be passed congenitally by the female tick to its offspring.

Louse-borne relapsing fever is seen under crowded, unsanitary, and cold conditions, such as during wars, large migrations of population, or destitution. There is no animal reservoir of the disease. Transmission occurs through abraded skin or mucous membranes from crushed lice, e.g., following scratching. Lice are infective for life, which is about 1 month. There has not been a case diagnosed in the United States during the twentieth century.

TABLE 103.1   Tick and *Borrelia* Species Responsible for Relapsing
Fever in U.S.

Tick Species	*Borrelia* spp
Ornithodoros hermsi	*B. hermsii*
O. turicatae	*B. turicatae*
O. parkeri	*B. parkeri*

Organisms are eliminated by the humoral immune response; however, a clone of the bacteria will show antigenic change. This clone reproduces during the afebrile period, leading to recurrence which is characteristic of the disease. Why *Borrelia* alone among the bacteria seem to have this capability and characteristic is not known.

Following an incubation period of about 7 days patients have the very abrupt onset of fever, rigors, headache, arthralgias, myalgias, fever up to 41°C, and prostration. Other less common clinical findings are vomiting and diarrhea, cough, chest pain, sore throat, and delirium. A macular rash is fairly commonly found on the trunk and/or extremities. Other findings in severe cases are mucosal hemorrhages and bleeding into the skin, lymphadenopathy, muscle tenderness, jaundice, and hepatosplenomegaly. The latter, if it occurs, is usually found late in the course of the disease. Splenomegaly is found in 40% of patients with tick-borne disease, and 75% of those with louse-borne relapsing fever (Table 103.2). Jaundice is uncommon in tick-borne, but is found in one-third of those with louse-borne relapsing fever. Signs of meningeal irritation are commonly seen in severe disease.

An attack ends with the rapid fall in temperature, drenching sweat, weakness, and lethargy. The duration of the primary attack averages 3 days for tick-borne, and 5.5 days for louse-borne relapsing fevers.

After a period of 1-2 weeks recurrence develops, identical to the primary attack, except that it is likely to be shorter and milder. There is usually only one recurrence in patients with louse-borne relapsing fever, but there may be several in patients with tick-borne disease.

The organism may be identified in blood smears taken during acute attacks. Thick or thin smears should be stained with Wright's or Giemsa stains. In severe disease the organism may be found in urine or spinal fluid as well. A more sensitive method of isolating the organism is by inoculation of young laboratory mice and then performing daily smears from tail blood beginning 24 hr after inoculation. There are no other characteristic laboratory findings (Table 103.3). Patients may have changes resembling acute bacterial meningitis in spinal fluid.

Other diseases which should be considered in the differential diagnosis of relapsing fever are given in Table 103.4.

The treatment of choice is tetracycline, with chloramphenicol, erythromycin, and penicillin as alternatives. Patients occasionally develop the classic Herxheimer reaction with antibiotic treatment. This usually can be treated symptomatically but may require intravenous fluids and/or corticosteroids.

Patients usually recover with the rare fatalities occurring in the old, the debilitated, or the very young. Possibly because the epidemic disease is more likely to occur in these groups, the fatality rate is higher in louse-borne relapsing fever.

TABLE 103.2   Comparison of Clinical Characteristics of Relapsing Fever

Characteristic	Louse–Borne	Tick–Borne
Age	∿ one-fourth are children	Most young adults and older children
Sex	Females > males	Males > females
Fatalities	40% untreated, ∿ 5% treated	< 5%
Duration of primary attack	5.5 days	3.5 days
Duration of afebrile interval	9.2 days	6.8 days
Number of relapses	1	3
Splenomegaly	75%	40%
Hepatomegaly	65%	15%
Jaundice	35%	7%
Respiratory symptoms	35%	15%
Rash	9%	25%
CNS involvement	30%	9%

Despite the low fatality rate, there is a substantial amount of morbidity associated with relapsing fever. Patients may suffer prolonged depression, headache, back pains, and lethargy. More serious are the neurologic and ophthalmologic complications. Anterior uveitis occurs in about 15% of patients and may result in residual visual impairment. The anterior uveitis is usually bilateral and occurs during the second or third febrile attack. Neurologic complications are cranial nerve palsies or various types of limb paralyses. These usually resolve completely.

The disease results in immunity to repeated attack, but the duration of this immunity is unknown. The disease can be prevented partially by the use of lousicides and tick repellents. In endemic areas, the body should be examined frequently for the presence of ticks.

TABLE 103.3   Laboratory Findings in Relapsing Fever

Finding	Approximate % or Mean
Serologic test for syphilis	
Blood	5
CSF	Rare
Proteus OX-K agglutinins	
Louse-borne ≥ 1:40	90
≥ 1:1000	30
Tick-borne ≥ 1:40	30
Complement-fixation test for *Borrelia*	50
Positive blood smear	70
Positive animal inoculation	85
CSF (lumbar puncture done in patients with symptoms or signs)	
Cells	$950/mm^3$
Protein	95 mg/dl
Glucose	75 mg/dl
Organism	10%

TABLE 103.4   Differential Diagnosis of Relapsing Fever

Disease	Difference
Malaria and dengue	Febrile episodes shorter
Leptospirosis	Conjunctival suffusion
Rat-bite fever	Bite history, inflammatory reaction at site of bite
Rocky Mountain spotted fever	Rash typically different (first on limbs, involves palms and soles)

Rat-Bite Fever

There are actually two rat-bite fevers, a streptobacillary form caused by *Streptobacillus moniliformis,* and the spirillary form, caused by *Spirillum minus* (Table 103.5). The latter is also known by its Japanese name, sodoku. The two diseases are similar clinically, but not identical, with both producing chills, rash, and intermittent or relapsing fever, as well as a skin lesion at the bite site, and regional lymphadenopathy. One of the major differences is that only the streptobacillary form is commonly accompanied by migratory polyarthritis.

TABLE 103.5   Differentiation of Rat-Bite Fever Caused by *Spirillum minus* and *Streptobacillus moniliformis (Streptothrix muris)*

	S. minus	*S. moniliformis* *(S. muris)*
Bacteriology	Gram-negative, spiral	Microaerophilic, gram-negative, pleomorphic
Incubation period	> 10 days	< 10 days
Local skin reaction at site of bite	+	−
Regional lymphadenopathy	+	Rare
Chills	+	Rare
Arthritis	Rare	+
Leukocytosis	Rare	+
Complications	Very rare	Uncommon but severe
Mortality	∿ 6%	∿ 13%
Isolation of organism	Animal inoculation	Artificial medium
Specific serology	−	+
False-positive serologic test for syphilis	> 50%	< 25%

Streptobacillus moniliformis is an aerobic, pleomorphic bacillus, which is gram-negative, nonencapsulated, nonmotile, and sensitive to penicillin, erythromycin, tetracycline, and chloramphenicol in vitro. *Spirillum minus* is a short, thick, spiral, gram-negative organism with flagella, and is sensitive to penicillin and tetracycline in vitro.

Rat-bite fever occurs throughout the world but with increased frequency in urban areas because of poor sanitation and an increased rat population. The spirillary form occurs mainly in Japan and the Far East. The streptobacillary form is the main cause of rat-bite fever in the United States. More than half of all cases occur in children under 12 years of age.

About half of all rats carry *S. moniliformis* as part of their normal flora. Thus the disease is an occupational hazard of laboratory workers and occurs following about 10% of rat bites. The reservoirs for the organisms are rats and mice. In addition to being transmitted by rat bites, occasionally another animal bite such as that of the mouse, cat, or squirrel will transmit the disease. There is no direct person-to-person transmission of the disease. In the case of the streptobacillary form, milk contaminated by rat secretions caused an outbreak several years ago. Because of the location of this outbreak, whenever disease is transmitted other than by a bite, it is known as Haverhill fever.

The incubation period for the streptobacillary form is less than 10 days, for the spirillary form it is 7-21 days.

Clinically, patients have the abrupt onset of fever, chills, headache, rash, myalgias, and lymphangitis. As mentioned previously, migratory polyarthritis is seen in the streptobacillary form, occurring in about 50% of patients. The rash in the streptobacillary form is either morbilliform or petechial and may involve the palms and soles. Hepatosplenomegaly is uncommon.

Characteristically in the spirillary form, the bite site which had healed becomes inflamed. The febrile attack lasts 3-4 days, then subsides only to flare up again after a few days. Relapses have been described as occurring for years after the primary bite. Arthritis is very uncommon in the spirillary form.

Streptobacillus is isolated most readily using trypticase soy agar and broth enriched with 20% horse or rabbit serum incubated in 8% CO_2. The organism may be isolated from blood, joint fluid, or pus. Serologic testing may be helpful, using the agglutination test. The serologic test for syphilis is positive in about 25% of patients.

The organism in the spirillary form cannot be cultured in vitro, so mouse inoculation is necessary. The organism may be seen on the smear from the patient's blood or pus from an infected site. Patients may have a biologically false-positive test for syphilis.

The differential diagnosis of rat-bite fever includes viral and rickettsial infections but usually can be differentiated on the basis of recurrences, rash, and arthralgias (Table 103.6).

Penicillin is the accepted therapy, given in a dosage of 1.2 million U/day for 7 days. Erythromycin is the alternative choice in patients who are allergic to penicillin. The streptobacillus is also sensitive to tetracycline and streptomycin, and the spirillary form is sensitive to streptomycin.

The complications of the streptobacillary form are endocarditis, bronchitis and pneumonia, arthritis, and brain abscess. Patients with the spirillary form have complications less often, but these include epididymitis, myocarditis, meningitis, and pleurisy. Infants and young children frequently develop anemia, weight loss, and severe diarrhea.

Untreated, the streptobacillary form lasts 1-2 months with about a 10% fatality rate. The spirillary form will last for years untreated but with a lower mortality.

TABLE 103.6   Differential Diagnosis of Rat-Bite Fever

Acute viral exanthems

Rickettsial infections

Drug reactions

Septic arthritis

Leptospirosis

Collagen-vascular diseases

Secondary syphilis

Neisserial infections

Influenza

Infective endocarditis

Acute rheumatic fever

Malaria

Relapsing fever

Lymphoma/leukemia

Prevention is accomplished by rat control and care in dealing with laboratory animals. It is suggested (although not proved) that penicillin is effective in preventing development of the disease following a rat bite. Pasteurization of milk prevents Haverhill fever.

Selected Bibliography

Beeson, P. B.: Problem of etiology of rat bite fever: Report of two cases due to *Spirillum minus. JAMA* 123:332, 1943.

Boyer, K. M., Munford, R. S., Maupin, G. O., et al.: Tick-borne relapsing fever: An interstate outbreak originating at Grand Canyon National Park. *Am J Epidemiol* 105:469, 1977.

Brown, T. M. and Neuemaker, J. C.: Rat bite fever: Review of American cases with reevaluation of its etiology and report of cases. *Bull John Hopkins Hosp* 70:201, 1942.

Bryceson, A. D. M., Parry, E. H. O., Perine, P. L., et al.: Louse-borne relapsing fever. A clinical and laboratory study of 62 cases in Ethiopia and a reconsideration of the literature. *Quart J Med* 39:129, 1970.

Burke, W. A., Kwong, O., and Halpern, R.: Rat bite fever due to *Streptobacillus moniliformis:* Report of two cases. *Calif Med* 91:356, 1959.

Butler, T., Jones, P. K., and Wallace, C. K.: *Borrelia recurrentis* infection: Single-dose antibiotic regimens and management of Jarisch–Herxheimer reaction. *J Infect Dis* 137:573, 1978.

Cole, J. S., Stoll, R. W., and Bulger, R. J.: Rat-bite fever: Report of three cases. *Ann Intern Med* 71:979, 1969.

Edell, T. A., et al.: Tick-borne relapsing fever in Colorado. *JAMA* 241:2279, 1979.

Gallaway, R. E., Leven, J., Butler, T., et al.: Activation of mediators of inflammation and evidence of endotoxemia in *Borrelia recurrentis* infection. *Am J Med* 63:933, 1977.

Gilbert, G. L., Cassidy, J. F., and Bennett, N. M. K.: Rat bite fever. *Med J Aus* 58:1131, 1971.

Holmgren, E. B. and Tunevall, G.: Rat bite fever. *Scand J Infect Dis* 2:71, 1970.

Lambe, D. W.: Haverhill fever and rat-bite fever. *Am J Clin Pathol* 62:444, 1974.

Portnoy, B. L., Satterwhite, T. K., and Dyckman, J. D.: Rat-bite fever misdiagnosed as Rocky Mountain spotted fever. *South Med J* 72:607, 1979.

Robertson, A.: Causal organism of rat bite fever in man. *Ann Trop Med* 18:157, 1924.

Roughgarden, J. W.: Antimicrobial therapy of rat bite fever. *Arch Intern Med* 116:39, 1965.

Southern, P. M. and Sanford, J. P.: Relapsing fever. A clinical and microbiological review. *Medicine* 48:129, 1969.

Thompson, R. S., Burgdorfer, W., Russell, R., and Francis, B. J.: Outbreak of tick-borne relapsing fever in Spokane County, Washington. *JAMA* 210:1045, 1969.

Watkins, C. G.: Rat bite fever. *J Pediatr* 28:429, 1946.

104

TUBERCULOSIS
Andrew P. Matragrano, M.D.

Throughout recorded history tuberculosis has been one of the most serious public health problems facing mankind. In the developed countries of the world, because of the availability of effective chemotherapy and vigorous public health measures, the prevalence of tuberculosis has decreased markedly, and deaths due to tuberculosis have been drastically reduced (Table 104.1). Even with this triumph many problems remain – changing patterns of disease, persistent rates of extrapulmonary tuberculosis, emergence of drug-resistant organisms, infection in immunosuppressed hosts. In the underdeveloped nations tuberculosis remains one of the most prevalent infectious diseases and one of the leading causes of death.

Microbiology

The causative agent, *Mycobacterium tuberculosis,* is a straight or slightly curved rod, which does not produce pigment and does not grow at room temperature (20-25°C). It is virulent for laboratory animals such as guinea pigs. *Mycobacterium tuberculosis* has the ability to accumulate niacin, whereas the other mycobacteria possess an enzyme which converts free niacin to niacin ribonucleotide. Tubercle bacilli are obligate aerobes and require in addition, carbon dioxide, carbon from glycerol and glucose, nitrogen from asparagine and ammonium, hydrogen, oxygen, phosphorus, potassium, magnesium, and iron. The organisms can be cultured on an appropriate medium, such as Lowenstein-Jensen agar at 37°C, in an atmosphere at 3-10% CO_2, in 6-8 weeks. Guinea pig inoculation is also an effective method of detecting tubercle bacillus but because of the cost, is reserved for special situations, e.g., specimens that are positive on microscopy but yield negative cultures. The organism can be demonstrated on stained specimens

TABLE 104.1   Tuberculosis Mortality (per 100,000 Population)

	White		Black	
	Male	Female	Male	Female
1900	150	130	490	400
1930	60	50	200	200
1947 (before streptomycin introduced)	40	26	100	70
1952 (before INH)	20	7	50	30
1960	8	3	20	9
1970	3	1	9	4

of fluid and tissue. The two methods in common use are carbolfuchsin stains (Ziehl-Neelsen or Kinyoun) and fluorochrome dyes (auramine, rhodamine).

Pathogenesis (Figure 104.1)

Tuberculous infection results from inhalation of airborne tubercle bacilli in droplet nuclei smaller than 10 μm in diameter. These travel down to the terminal alveoli without impaction on ciliated epithelium, thus avoiding removal. Other modes of transmission (e.g., ingestion of dairy products from tuberculous cattle, leading to infection of intestinal mucosa and subsequent mesenteric lymphatic spread) rarely occur in the United States, but they continue to be important mechanisms in developing countries.

In the alveolus of the nonimmune host the tubercle bacillus incites an inflammatory reaction, first mediated by polymorphonuclear leukocytes followed by macrophages, which phagocytize the bacilli but permit intracellular multiplication. With time, macrophages tend to coalesce and fuse to form a granuloma with lymphocytes at the periphery. During this time the dissemination to hilar nodes occurs along lymphatic channels to the thoracic duct, followed by hematogenous spread to multiple sites in all organs, with the same basic pathologic process occurring at each site. Two to ten weeks after the initial infection, the central portion of each lesion undergoes necrosis, resulting in a yellow, cheesy, or caseous material, containing organisms and cellular debris. At this time, there is development of cell-mediated immunity (delayed hypersensitivity). The acquired immune response inhibits the multiplication of the tubercle bacillus but does not destroy all the organisms. Hence bacilli within foci of infection may remain viable for long periods, capable of multiplying and dividing if local immunity is lowered. At the periphery of these multiple scattered sites fibrocytes grow and deposit collagen, encasing the area of caseous necrosis. Eventually, these lesions undergo

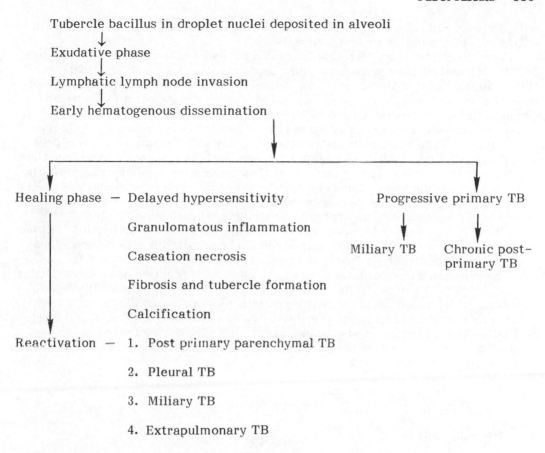

Tubercle bacillus in droplet nuclei deposited in alveoli

↓

Exudative phase

↓

Lymphatic lymph node invasion

↓

Early hematogenous dissemination

Healing phase — Delayed hypersensitivity   Progressive primary TB

Granulomatous inflammation

Caseation necrosis   Miliary TB   Chronic post-
                                               primary TB

Fibrosis and tubercle formation

Calcification

Reactivation — 1. Post primary parenchymal TB

2. Pleural TB

3. Miliary TB

4. Extrapulmonary TB

FIGURE 104.1   Schematic summary of the pathologic course of tuberculosis infection.

complete fibrosis and calcification. Should any of these lesions reactivate at a later time due to the waning of cell-mediated immunity (CMI), the primary process will be caseation necrosis in the parenchyma of an organ such as lung or kidney, or else an intense exudative, inflammatory reaction on a serous membrane, such as pleura or peritoneum.

Diagnosis

Tuberculin Skin Test

The tuberculin skin test continues to be an important diagnostic tool. The Mantoux method is the most reliable and will be the only form discussed here. In this technique purified protein derivative, stabilized with Tween 80 (polysorbate) and standardized to 5 tuberculin U/0.1 ml is injected intradermally (0.1 ml) on the volar surface of the forearm. This is read in 48-72 hr by measuring the area of induration. Ten millimeters or more of induration constitutes a positive test; 5-9 mm of induration can reflect infection by *M. tuberculosis* or an atypical mycobacterium and is considered a positive test in patients who have been in close contact with a confirmed case, or who have clinical or x-ray evidence of disease. A skin test with 4 mm of induration or less is negative.

A positive tuberculin test signifies that a patient has developed CMI to a protein component of the tubercle bacillus. Since atypical mycobacteria share certain proteins found in *M. tuberculosis,* induration of less than 10 mm may reflect infection with atypical organisms. A positive tuberculin skin test may also be found in those vaccinated with BCG. The size of a positive reaction does not strongly correlate with active disease; 10% of patients with pulmonary tuberculosis have negative tuberculin tests, although many will become tuberculin-positive during therapy. Those with large reactions, i.e., 20 mm, are two to four times more likely to develop active tuberculosis than those with smaller reactions. The phenomenon of skin anergy has been described in many clinical circumstances. To evaluate anergy as a cause of a negative tuberculin skin test, several other common antigens, such as mumps, trichophytin, or candida, should be implanted at the same time. If this procedure does not resolve the question of anergy, and if clinical circumstances justify it, the patient should be sensitized with dinitrochlorobenzene and repeat skin testing performed with this substance.

The common causes of a false-negative tuberculin reaction are summarized in Table 104.2. A more difficult source of error is the occurrence of false-positive tests which result from the booster effect. In most cases this is due to infection by atypical mycobacteria, and the size of the reaction is increased by repeated doses of antigen. It also occurs in patients who were infected in the past with *M. tuberculosis,* whose delayed hypersensitivity waned, only to be stimulated by repeated doses of antigen.

Clinical Manifestations

Primary Tuberculosis

Primary tuberculosis is that form which occurs following the introduction of tubercle bacillus into the alveoli of a previously uninfected host. Most infected patients will go through the entire process outlined earlier up to the healing phase without clinical illness, the only evidence of infection being a positive PPD and possibly a Ghon's focus or Ranke's complex on a roentgenogram. Other patients, especially children, may manifest a fever, occasionally with erythema nodosum. In a small percentage of patients, however, more serious clinical illness may be produced due to either a heavy inoculum of very virulent organisms or a delay in the development of CMI, both of which permit very rapid multiplication of organisms at the primary site, producing tuberculous pneumonia. The tuberculous pneumonia can spread through the bronchi, as well as to the hilar nodes, causing compression on the bronchi. Rarely, there is massive hematogenous dissemination.

Progressive primary tuberculosis is usually a disease of infants and young children whose CMI may not be fully developed, or who may have prolonged contact with an active case of tuberculosis, e.g., parents or grandparents. The symptoms of progressive primary tuberculosis are usually mild – anorexia, weight loss, night sweats, lethargy, cough, chest pain, and dyspnea. With more extensive disease, however, the symptoms may be markedly increased. Occasionally, patients may present with altered mental status, including frank coma or seizures, due to meningeal involvement. On physical examination the patient may be febrile and tachypneic. Examination of the chest may reveal signs of consolidation or localized wheezing and diminished breath sounds due to the bronchial compression by enlarged nodes. In cases of massive dissemination, choroidal tubercles, peripheral adenopathy, or hepatosplenomegaly may be found. In cases of meningeal

TABLE 104.2   Reasons for a Negative Tuberculin Reaction

"True" negative

    Patient related

        Patient never infected with *M. tuberculosis*
        INH prophylaxis begun within 3 months of
            skin test conversion

"False" negative

    Patient related

        Suppressed delayed hypersensitivity

            Viral infection; live virus vaccine
            Leukemia, lymphoma
            Sarcoidosis
            Amyloidosis
            Overwhelming *M. tuberculosis* infection
            Uremia
            Immunosuppressive therapy

        Too early in course of infection
        Atypical mycobacterial organisms
        Elderly

    Tuberculin related

        Incorrect dilution
        Incorrect diluent
        Inactivated by sunlight
        Adsorbed to container
        Bacterial contamination

    Administration related

        Incorrect route

    Interpretation related

        Improper reading

infection, altered mental status, convulsions, or focal neurologic deficits suggestive of basilar involvement may be found.

The roentgenographic picture of progressive primary tuberculosis includes airspace consolidation, due to filling up of alveoli with exudative products of reaction to the organisms, located usually in the lower lobes. Cavitation rarely occurs, but endobronchial spread to other areas of the lung is common. Lymph node enlargement, at times massive, occurs in nearly all cases. Atelectasis commonly occurs in the anterior segment of the right upper lobe and medial segment of the right middle lobe due to the compressive effects of the nodes on the airway. Pleural effusion occurs rarely in children but is a more common

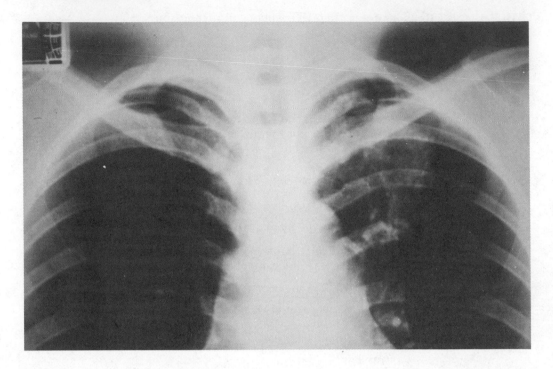

FIGURE 104.2 Typical apical infiltrates of tuberculosis.

manifestation of primary tuberculosis in adults. In cases of massive hematogeneous dissemination, a miliary pattern may be seen in the lung fields.

The diagnosis of primary tuberculosis is made by a positive tuberculin skin test (in certain cases the conversion can actually be documented), the characteristic roentgenographic pattern, as well as bacteriologic confirmation from smear and culture of sputum, body fluid, or biopsy material. In young children it is often necessary to isolate acid-fast organisms from morning gastric washings. Because of the propensity of children to develop tuberculous meningitis, a spinal tap should be performed and fluid cultured.

Progressive primary tuberculosis in young children may be rapidly fatal. Before the advent of chemotherapy, most deaths occurred within 1 year of diagnosis. The mortality was highest when the disease occurred in a child under 4 years of age and when the primary lesion was large. Death was usually due to meningitis, in most cases associated with miliary dissemination, protracted hematogenous tuberculosis, and extensive progressive pulmonary disease. With chemotherapy, most patients have an excellent response with clearing of infiltrates and decrease in the size of enlarged lymph nodes; the frequency of reactivation later in life is also greatly reduced. Residual distortion of the bronchial tree with resultant bronchiectasis, as well as permanent collapse of the involved lobe, may occur. Calcification of the peripheral pulmonary lesion produces the well-known Ghon's focus, often accompanied by calcified hilar nodes (Ranke's complex).

Reactivation

Postprimary, or reactivation, tuberculosis results from the recrudescence of previous foci of infection due to a breakdown in cellular immunity permitting dormant

organisms to multiply. The most common site of reactivation is the Simon's focus, established during the initial primary hematogenous dissemination in the upper
portion of the lung. This is a preferred site for the organism because of the higher
O_2 tension in the apex of the lung. Pulmonary tuberculosis is the most common
clinical form of tuberculosis in the adult population.

The precise reason for reactivation is unclear. In some cases depressed cellular immunity has been attributed to old age, malnutrition, alcoholism, diabetes,
uremia, silicosis, malignancy (Hodgkin's disease, other lymphoreticular neoplasms,
and solid tumors), and immunosuppressed states including the use of steroids. In
other cases, e.g., chronic obstructive pulmonary disease, the defect in cellular immunity or other host defense mechanisms is unknown. The risk of reactivation is
highest in the first year after initial infection, and declines thereafter.

The primary process is caseation necrosis with macrophages, epithelial cells
and giant cells, dead and viable bacilli, and lymphocytes, forming tubercles at the
periphery of the central area of necrosis. The caseous contents are emptied out
via the airways, and then fibroblasts invade the areas of caseation and lay down
collagen. Healing thus occurs by fibrosis, contraction, and closure of cavities left
by caseation necrosis. Because CMI is effective in adjacent tissues and within the
lymphatic system, spread by way of lymphatics to hilar nodes and then to other
organs does not occur. Lymph node enlargement rarely occurs in reactivation pulmonary tuberculosis; however, since organisms multiply in the center of the necrotic area, the lesion may progress. It may erode blood vessels or break into a
bronchus, spreading the contents to other areas of the lung.

A patient with reactivation tuberculosis may be asymptomatic even with advanced disease. The onset more commonly is insidious with gradual development
of constitutional symptoms, i.e., malaise, fatigue, anorexia, weight loss, myalgias,
night sweats, amenorrhea. Pulmonary symptoms usually follow – cough with mucopurulent sputum and occasional hemoptysis, chest pain due to inflammation of
the tracheobronchial tree, and dyspnea. Rarely, this disease may resemble an
acute bacterial pneumonia, with high fever, chills, rapid pulse, productive cough,
or an upper respiratory infection with nasal congestion, rhinorrhea, cough, and
sputum production. The physical examination may be entirely normal or have
findings disproportionate to the extent of disease as seen on x-ray. There may be
evidence of volume loss, i.e., elevated diaphragm, decreased movement of the
chest, deviated trachea, and breath sounds suggestive of consolidation and cavitation. Emaciation is common. A thorough search for other foci of tuberculosis
should be made on physical examination.

Reactivation tuberculosis is usually localized to the apical and posterior segments of the upper lobes and occasionally to the superior segment of the lower lobe
because of the higher pO_2 in these areas (Figure 104.2). The x-ray picture may consist of an airspace consolidation in the exudative phase; later in the course, irregular, angular, and fibrotic shadows appear, often with evidence of volume loss.
Cavities, usually with thick walls in the active phase of the disease, may appear.
In certain cases of advanced disease patchy consolidation may appear in sites distant from the primary lesion owing to endobronchial spread of caseous material.

Occasionally reactivation tuberculosis may develop in the lower lobes, usually
on the right side, secondary to transbronchial perforation of a hilar lymph node.
Almost all of these patients are over 40 years of age, and several conditions are
thought to predispose – diabetes mellitus, pregnancy, silicosis, kyphoscoliosis. The
x-ray picture more often resembles bacterial or viral pneumonia with dense consolidation. Important clues to the diagnosis include the presence of hemoptysis,
a normal white count, prolonged but usually mild symptoms, and the presence of
cavitation, pleural effusion, and other residua of primary tuberculosis.

The diagnosis is usually established on the basis of a characteristic x-ray picture and positive acid-fast smears, usually easily obtainable in patients with exudative or cavitary lesions. In certain cases, sputum induction using aerosols or bronchoscopy may be required to obtain adequate specimens. When repeated smears are negative and the patient is clinically stable, it is legitimate to await culture confirmation of the diagnosis since the activity of the disease cannot be accurately assessed by x-ray alone.

Tuberculous Meningitis

Tuberculous meningitis is the most common central nervous system manifestation of tuberculosis. Similar to other manifestations of extrapulmonary tuberculosis, it results from rupture of a granuloma established during a previous hematogenous phase, in this instance, directly into the subarachnoid space. With the introduction of bacilli into the subarachnoid space, there is a violent inflammatory reaction with outpouring of a thick exudate of cells and proteinacious fluid, which tends to accumulate at the base of the brain. This causes compression of cranial nerves, as well as obstruction of cerebrospinal fluid drainage, resulting in hydrocephalus, especially in children. Because the propensity for development of acute tuberculous meningitis is highest within 3 months of infection, the highest prevalence of the disease formerly occurred in children. Since the primary infection rate has declined, however, more cases are now seen among older people who were infected earlier in life.

The duration of symptoms varies from 2 to 6 weeks before clinical presentation. Headaches, neck stiffness, visual disturbances, abnormal behavior, progressive deterioration in consciousness, and seizures are the most common symptoms. On physical examination the patient usually has an altered state of consciousness, ranging from drowsiness to frank coma. Fever is common. Neurologic abnormalities include signs of meningeal irritation, papilledema, and cranial nerve palsies. In certain cases, evidence of miliary disease, such as adenopathy, choroidal tubercles, hepatosplenomegaly, and basilar rales, is found. According to several studies the mental status upon admission is the most important prognostic factor, with those presenting in coma having the worst prognosis. The cerebrospinal fluid classically shows a lymphocytic pleocytosis (100-500 white blood cells with more than 50% lymphocytes), increased protein, low glucose, and low chloride levels; early in the course the cerebrospinal fluid may show a normal glucose level and polymorphonuclear predominance (Table 104.3). The importance of serial lumbar punctures in the early phase of the disease, especially when therapy is started on a presumptive diagnosis, cannot be overemphasized. The chest roentgenogram often manifests changes suggestive of tuberculosis, e.g., residua of primary disease, apical lesions, or in certain cases a miliary pattern. Since the parameningeal focus may originate in the spinal column, x-ray evaluation of the spine is indicated.

TABLE 104.3   Cerebrospinal Fluid Findings in Tuberculous Meningitis

	Approximate % in Various Series
Cell count $\geq$ 100/mm^3	60-85
Protein $\geq$ 100 mg/dl	70-80
Glucose $\leq$ 45 mg/dl	70-85

The tuberculin skin test is positive in almost all cases. Smears of the pellicle formed by centrifuging specimens of cerebrospinal fluid are positive in 10-22% of cases; cultures are positive in 38-88% of cases. Smears of sputum as well as examination of biopsies of liver, enlarged lymph nodes, and bone marrow may be helpful in cases of meningitis due to miliary dissemination. Since direct confirmation of the diagnosis on smear is rarely available and prognosis depends heavily on early therapy, treatment must be started on the weight of clinical evidence and suggestive laboratory data.

Pleural Tuberculosis

Pleural tuberculosis occurs most frequently in those under 25 years old, with the highest occurrence approximately 3-4 months after the initial infection. A pleural effusion develops due to the rupture of a subpleural caseous focus into the pleural space, or else the rupture of mediastinal nodes with spread of infected material into the mediastinal pleura. The presence of CMI is important in the development of the inflammatory reaction and the outpouring of cells and fluid into the pleural space. The onset can be insidious or abrupt, with cough, pleuritic chest pain, night sweats, dyspnea, weakness, and weight loss. On physical examination the temperature is usually elevated but may be normal, and there are physical findings consistent with a pleural effusion. On the roentgenogram there is usually a moderate pleural effusion, occasionally with enlarged lymph nodes or lesions suggestive of parenchymal pulmonary tuberculosis. Most patients will have a positive intermediate-strength tuberculin skin test. If tuberculosis is strongly suspected and the intermediate-strength tuberculin skin test is negative, a second-strength tuberculin (250 TU) is recommended. In certain cases, the tuberculin reaction may be negative initially and positive following thoracentesis, theoretically because of large amounts of antigen in the pleural fluid "tying up" most of the T lymphocytes, preempting their reacting to the intradermal antigen. The pleural fluid is characteristically a lymphocytic exudate, and the glucose concentration is usually normal or occasionally low. The diagnosis can occasionally be established by culture of the pleural fluid, but far more rewarding is the pleural biopsy, which provides material for histologic examination as well as culture. The diagnostic yield of the procedure in pleural tuberculosis is more than 90%. Pleural effusions secondary to tuberculosis usually resolve spontaneously even without therapy. Because 65% of these patients will develop active pulmonary tuberculosis without treatment, a course of chemotherapy is mandatory.

Genitourinary Tuberculosis

The genitourinary tract is a common site of extrapulmonary tuberculosis. Hematogenous seeding of the kidney occurs during the bacillemic phase following the primary infection, resulting in multiple bilateral granulomatous lesions of the glomeruli, most of which heal. These lesions, however, may progress or, at a later time, reactivate and rupture into a tubule; tubercle bacilli are then shed into the urine and form cavities in the kidney medulla as organisms lodge in the loop of Henle. The multiple lesions that result coalesce into cavities which may destroy the renal parenchyma and pelvis. In addition, organisms in the urine produce multiple lesions of the ureter and bladder. Clinically, renal tuberculosis can be entirely asymptomatic, the diagnosis being first suspected on the basis of an abnormal urine sediment. Symptoms are present for as short as 1 month or as long as 20 years before the diagnosis is made. The common symptoms include flank pain, hematuria, pyuria, and dysuria; in the absence of active infection elsewhere, constitutional symptoms, i.e., fever, weight loss, are unusual. In spite of extensive renal destruction, hypertension is infrequent. The physical examination is usually not helpful. An abnormal urine sediment with pyuria, hematuria, or both, not attributed to another cause, is found in almost all cases. Urine culture is the most important diagnostic test for renal tuberculosis. Optimum yield is obtained by culture of three early morning specimens; this method is superior and less costly than 24-hr collections. A positive culture is obtained in more than 80% of the patients. The tuberculin skin test is extremely useful, being positive in 90% of the patients. The chest x-ray may be entirely normal but, in a large number of patients, shows abnormalities suggestive of tuberculosis. The intravenous pyelogram is extremely useful diagnostically. Although many of the common abnormalities are nonspecific (i.e., calyceal dilatation, cortical scarring and filling defects, papillary cavities, renal calcification, or multiple strictures of the ureters), the presence of multiple abnormalities in the upper and lower urinary tract is strongly suggestive of the diagnosis.

Tuberculosis can invade the prostate, seminal vesicles, and epididymis. In many cases male genital tuberculosis results from direct infection of the urine, but hematogenous infection also occurs. A common presentation is that of a painful scrotal mass, the etiology of which is discovered on biopsy and culture. Because of the mechanism of infection, involvement of the upper urinary tract should be ruled out by IVP and urine cultures. Biopsy specimens should be submitted for fungal stains and cultures.

Tuberculosis of the female genital tract usually results from hematogenous seeding to the fallopian tubes. From the tubes the infection can spread upward to cause a pelvic peritonitis or perioopheritis, or downward to produce endometritis, cervicitis, or vaginitis. A large number of patients are in the childbearing years and present with a chief complaint of infertility. Other common manifestations are pelvic pain, usually low-grade and chronic, and abnormal vaginal bleeding or discharge. Physical examination often reveals a palpable adnexal mass, with cervical erosion seen less commonly. The diagnosis can be established by culture of the menstrual blood, or by cervical biopsy when erosion is present. A more reliable source for culture is endometrial tissue obtained by curettage performed at the end of the menstrual cycle, so that granulomas have the maximal time to develop. A negative culture on curettage does not rule out female genital tuberculosis if salpingitis is present without endometritis. In these cases direct visualization and biopsy via culdoscopy, laparoscopy, and possibly laparotomy are indicated.

Tuberculosis at Other Sites

Skeletal tuberculosis is one of the more common forms of extrapulmonary disease. Formerly seen most often in children within the first year after the primary infection, it is now more commonly seen in older adults. Joint infection usually involves the breakdown of a focus, established during the bacillemic phase in the epiphyseal portion of the bone which erodes into the joint space; here the inflammatory reaction results in formation of granulation tissue which destroys the joint space. In the spinal column, infection spreads to bone via the blood stream or from another focus of tuberculosis in the lung or pleura via lymphatic drainage. The infection begins in the vertebral body, with necrosis of the bony trabeculae and resultant vertebral collapse and angulation of the spine; abscess formation occurs along the anterior portion of the spinal column. The clinical presentation is usually one of pain, limitation of motion, and joint swelling, chiefly of weight-bearing joints. In more severe cases a "cold abscess" (an abscess with little evidence of inflammatory reaction) and draining sinus are present. In tuberculous spondylitis, back pain, as well as symptoms and signs of spinal cord compression, is seen.   The roentgenographic changes, while nonspecific for tuberculosis, are essential in documenting the extent of the disease and in following the progress during chemotherapy.   The tuberculin test is positive in almost all patients and is an important diagnostic clue.   Aspiration of a tuberculous joint yields fluid suggestive of chronic inflammation, with a high white cell count (more than 1000, usually with a polymorphonuclear predominance), high protein concentration (more than 3.5 g/100 ml), and low glucose content (usually 40 mg/100 ml less than the blood glucose).   Since the yield is poor on acid-fast stain of fluid aspirated from a joint or abscess, the more definitive procedure is biopsy of the synovium or vertebral body, with histologic examination and culture of that material.

Tuberculosis continues to be an important cause of pericarditis, accounting for 10% of all cases.   Tuberculous involvement of the pericardium can occur by hematogenous dissemination during the initial bacillemic phase or a later miliary stage, direct extension from adjacent tuberculous nodes, or, more rarely, from a tuberculous osteomyelitis of a rib or vertebra.   The clinical onset is usually insidious, and prominent symptoms include: a cough which is usually nonproductive and intractable, chest pain similar to that seen in pericarditis of other etiologies, night sweats, fever, weight loss, dyspnea, orthopnea, and ankle edema.   The prominent physical findings include fever, tachycardia, cardiomegaly, as well as more specific signs of pericardial effusion, e.g., distant sounds, friction rub, paradoxic pulse, hepatomegaly, distended neck veins, Kussmaul's sign, and peripheral edema. A pleural effusion is often present.   In addition to the characteristic globular heart a tuberculous etiology may be suggested by the presence of a Ranke's complex, enlarged nodes in the mediastinum, and evidence of parenchymal disease elsewhere on chest x-ray.

The rapid diagnosis of tuberculous pericarditis is important in improving the prognosis, since delay in diagnosis permits pericardial inflammation to affect the mechanical function of the myocardium and the development of constrictive pericarditis.   The tuberculin test is positive in almost all cases in most series, but a small percentage (5-10%) will be tuberculin-negative.   The presence of acid-fast bacilli on the sputum smear, or consistent findings in the pleural fluid and biopsy, may support the diagnosis.   An open pericardial biopsy is the procedure of choice because it provides therapeutic drainage through a pericardial window, as well as fluid and tissue for examination and culture.   The fluid is an exudate with a lymphocyte predominance, but cultures are positive in only approximately 40%. In most cases the tissue sections will provide an immediate diagnosis, whereupon therapy can be instituted.

Tuberculosis can involve any portion of the alimentary tract.   Inflammation and, at times, ulceration of the mucosa due to ingestion of tubercle bacilli, either from a tuberculous pulmonary source or from contaminated milk, are thought to be the primary mechanism.   These patients commonly present with abdominal pain of varying severity and location, weight loss, and other symptoms which may localize the lesion to a specific portion of the gastrointestinal tract.   Occasionally patients present with intestinal obstruction.   The radiographic findings in the gastrointestinal tract are nonspecific, but the combination of intestinal abnormality, such as obstruction, and a chest x-ray consistent with pulmonary tuberculosis may suggest the diagnosis.   Histologic examination and culture of the biopsy specimen obtained at laparotomy usually establish the diagnosis.

Tuberculous peritonitis results from breakdown of a focus in the peritoneum or mesenteric lymph node and occasionally from spillage of infected material from the fallopian tubes.   The usual symptoms are abdominal pain and/or swelling, fever, abdominal distention, and tenderness.   A significant percentage of patients will have evidence of another focus of tuberculosis outside the peritoneum.   The tuberculin skin test is positive in most cases at some time in the course, and repeat testing is advocated in those who are initially negative. The results of examination of the peritoneal fluid are variable, the most consistent finding being a protein content higher than 2.5 g. The diagnosis is most rapidly made by biopsy of the peritoneum either with a Cope needle or at laparoscopy, with confirmation usually obtained by culture of the biopsy specimen or peritoneal fluid. With prompt diagnosis and therapy, there is an excellent clinical response. Unfortunately, the diagnosis is often overlooked in alcoholics whose ascites is attributed to liver disease alone. Paracentesis and a tuberculin skin test should be performed in patients with ascites, especially if fever, abdominal pain, and tenderness are present.

Miliary Tuberculosis

Miliary tuberculosis is caused by massive hematogenous dissemination of tubercle bacilli which embolize to capillary beds, forming lesions which progress to caseation necrosis. In children this usually results from extensive lymph node invasion following the primary infection; in adults hematogenous dissemination occurs from breakdown of a tubercle in a lymph node adherent to a blood vessel, with outpouring of tubercle bacilli into the blood stream.

Clinically, symptoms including anorexia, weakness, fatigue, weight loss, cough, and progressive dyspnea can be present for several weeks before presentation. Occasionally, patients will appear acutely ill, in coma, or in frank respiratory failure. Hepatosplenomegaly, generalized lymphadenopathy, choroidal tubercles, and skin lesions are found, as well as evidence of pleural and pericardial effusion. Nuchal rigidity, altered mental status, and cranial nerve signs are often seen with meningeal involvement.

The radiographic appearance of miliary tuberculosis begins as pinpoint lesions scattered throughout the lung, which expand in size to form the classic 2-mm nodules, with areas of confluence especially at the bases. In more severe cases there may be dense alveolar shadows consistent with adult respiratory distress syndrome. X-ray changes may lag as long as 15 days behind the hematogenous dissemination. Therefore, if this diagnosis is strongly suspected, especially in patients with fever of unknown origin, serial x-rays may be extremely helpful.

The tuberculin skin test is an important diagnostic tool. Although anergy is seen, the tuberculin skin test is positive in more than 70% of the patients. Sputum smears are positive in approximately 30%, and cultures in approximately 60%. In certain patients where the diagnosis is uncertain and clinical circumstances justify it, direct evidence can be obtained by lung biopsy. This usually requires thoracotomy, although several studies report success with transbronchoscopic or needle biopsy. Biopsies of the liver, bone marrow, pathologic lymph nodes, and skin lesions are all important sources of diagnostic material for smear and culture. Since the presence of granulomas in the liver is nonspecific, this finding is diagnostic only if the organism is demonstrable by smear or culture. Since meningeal involvement is frequent in miliary tuberculosis, a lumbar puncture should form part of the routine evaluation of these patients.

Miliary tuberculosis is a serious illness with a significant mortality, especially since it often occurs in a medically compromised population. Early drug therapy is mandatory. Proper supportive care, especially in cases of coma or respiratory failure, improves the prognosis.

Prevention of Active Disease

The prevention of active disease in those at greatest risk is of extreme importance in the community control of tuberculosis. Isoniazid, 300 mg/day for adults, and 10 mg/kg/day (not to exceed 300 mg/day) in children, administered for 1 year is effective in preventing the development of active tuberculosis, presumably by decreasing the bacterial population in foci established during the initial bacillemic phase. Situations in which chemoprophylaxis should be considered are:

1. Contacts of an active case: Before administration a contact should be questioned about previous tuberculous disease, tuberculin skin test status, BCG vaccination, prior antituberculosis therapy, and any adverse reactions. A tuberculin skin test and chest x-ray should be performed. If the skin test is positive, i.e., > 5 mm, and there is no evidence of active disease on chest x-ray, then isoniazid should be administered for 1 year. If the skin test and chest x-ray are negative, isoniazid should be prescribed for 3 months in the following situations:
   a. A high probability of infection, i.e., household contact
   b. A high incidence of infection, i.e., positive skin test or active case among those with a similar degree of exposure
   c. A substantial risk should active disease develop, i.e., infants, children under 6, and those with suppressed immunity

After 3 months, therapy may be discontinued if a repeat tuberculin skin test is negative.

2. Newly infected persons: Patients who have had a conversion of the tuberculin skin test, i.e., tuberculin skin test reaction has increased by at least 6 mm from < 10 mm to > 10 mm within 2 years
3. Persons with a positive tuberculin skin test with an abnormal chest x-ray
4. Persons under age 35 with a positive tuberculin reaction
5. Special clinical categories: Patients with a positive tuberculin skin test should receive isoniazid prophylaxis in clinical situations where there is a high risk of developing active disease
   a. Prolonged steroid therapy
   b. Immunosuppressive therapy
   c. Diabetes
   d. Silicosis
   e. Hematologic and reticuloendothelial neoplasms
   f. Postgastrectomy

Before isoniazid therapy is started, one should rule out active pulmonary disease in those with abnormal chest x-ray. Patients should be evaluated for contraindications to isoniazid prophylaxis, such as (1) previous isoniazid-associated hepatic disease, (2) severe adverse reaction to isoniazid, or (3) acute liver disease of any etiology. Although isoniazid has been used during pregnancy for active tuberculosis without harmful effects to the fetus, it is generally recommended that prophylactic therapy be postponed until after delivery. Because in some individuals isoniazid may decrease excretion of diphenylhydantoin or enhance its effect, the dosage of diphenylhydantoin may have to be reduced to avoid toxicity.

Treatment

Currently, available chemotherapy has revolutionized the treatment of tuberculosis. The proper use of these drugs requires understanding of principles, such as the use of multiple drugs and prolonged therapy. It is well established that in a population of M. tuberculosis organisms, a certain number of mutants resistant to particular drugs will arise spontaneously (Table 104.4). The chance of resistance developing to any particular drug regimen increases in proportion to the number of organisms present. Situations with very large numbers are open cavitary pulmonary tuberculosis, cavitary renal tuberculosis, and miliary tuberculosis. If one drug were used, the number of resistant organisms might be sufficient to multiply and repopulate the entire lesion in a short time. With the use of multiple drugs, the number of mutant organisms resistant to both drugs is much reduced, making the growth of a drug-resistant population unlikely. For the same reason, should retreatment be necessary because of drug resistance, it is standard practice to introduce two new drugs to which the organisms are sensitive.

Antituberculosis therapy must be continued for a long period. Most of the drugs affect RNA, DNA, or protein synthesis; thus they are able to kill only metabolically active organisms. Because the metabolic rate of the tubercle bacillus is much slower than other bacteria, the bactericidal action of these drugs requires a longer time. In addition, the tubercle bacillus is capable of developing a dormant state after the metabolically active phase, and in this condition the antituberculosis drugs are only bacteriostatic, but they suppress the growth of organisms permitting the usual healing process to overcome residual infection. Recently, shorter regimens have been studied in which emphasis is placed on initial intensive chemotherapy during the active metabolic phase. Drugs such as isoniazid, pyrazinamide, and rifampin are effective in drastically reducing the number of organisms in a very short time. As a result, the total length of treatment can be reduced with minimal danger of reactivation.

The drugs commonly used in therapy of tuberculosis are listed in Table 104.5 along with potential toxicities. Routine drug sensitivity studies are usually not necessary for initial therapy; however, in cases where primary drug resistance is suspected, such as patients from an area where drug resistance is frequent, and certainly in all retreatment cases, such studies are warranted. The current recommendations for initial treatment of pulmonary tuberculosis are in a state of

TABLE 104.4   Prevalence of Spontaneous Antibiotic Resistant Mutants

Drug	Prevalence
Isoniazid (INH)	$1:10^6$ organisms
Rifampin	$1:10^8$
Streptomycin	$1:10^5$
INH *and* rifampin	$1:10^{14}$
INH *and* streptomycin	$1:10^{11}$

TABLE 104.5 Antituberculous Drugs

Drug	Dose Adult Daily	Twice Weekly	Side Effects
Isoniazid	300 mg	15 mg/kg	Peripheral neuritis; hepatitis
Rifampin	600 mg	600 mg	Hepatitis; accelerates metabolism of several other drugs; stains secretions orange
Ethambutol	15-25 mg/kg	50 mg/kg	Optic neuritis (very rare if dose ≤ 15 mg/kg)
Streptomycin	0.75-1 g	25-30 mg/kg	Eighth nerve damage; nephrotoxicity
Pyrazinamide	20-35 mg/kg	-*	Hepatotoxicity; hyperuricemia
Para-amino-salicylic acid	15-25 g	-	GI upset extremely common; hepatotoxicity
Capreomycin	1 g	1 g	Eighth nerve and renal toxicity
Kanamycin	0.5-1 g	-	Eighth nerve and renal toxicity
Cycloserine	750 mg	-	CNS - psychosis and seizures
Ethionamide	0.75-1 g	-	GI upset; hepatotoxicity

*Not recommended

flux. A satisfactory regimen for many years has been isoniazid (300 mg p.o., q.d.) and ethambutol (15 mg/kg q.d.) for 18 months in cases of disease with minimal infiltrates and thin cavities. Isoniazid (300 mg p.o., q.d.), ethambutol (15 mg/kg q.d.), and streptomycin (1 g IM, q.d.) should be administered until sputum "conversion" (becomes negative for organisms) in cases of extensive disease with large, thick-walled cavities, at which time the streptomycin can be discontinued and isoniazid and ethambutol continued for 18-24 months. More recent regimens have stressed the use of isoniazid and rifampin as an extremely effective bactericidal combination in the early treatment of pulmonary tuberculosis. In 1980, the Center for Disease Control recommended the following regimen for pulmonary tuberculosis where drug resistance was judged to be unlikely: INH 300 mg/day and rifampin 600 mg/day for 9 months with at least 6 months of negative sputum documented.

Miliary tuberculosis requires optimal initial therapy consisting of isoniazid, ethambutol, and streptomycin, or isoniazid and rifampin. Adjustment to a less toxic regimen can be made once the infection is clinically controlled. Pleural tuberculosis is adequately treated with only isoniazid and ethambutol.

Clinical management of patients should focus on detection of toxicity due to medication and assessment of efficacy of therapy. The probability of hepatitis secondary to isoniazid is increased in patients aged over 35, in those on isoniazid and rifampin, and in those with preexisting liver disease. Isoniazid-induced hepatitis is most often seen in the first few weeks after initiating therapy. All patients on this drug and other hepatotoxic agents should be followed at least monthly for symptoms suggestive of hepatitis, i.e., anorexia, malaise, nausea, weight loss, change in urine color, as well as fever, rash, pruritus, arthralgias, and myalgias. Liver function tests should be obtained at the start of therapy, but they should not be monitored at regular intervals unless symptoms develop. Patients on ethambutol should have baseline evaluation of visual acuity and color vision, with periodic determinations during therapy. Those on streptomycin should have a clinical assessment of vestibular function, measurement of serum creatinine concentration, and audiometry at the start of therapy and at monthly intervals.

Clinical variables such as weight gain and decrease in pulmonary and systemic symptoms should be followed as sensitive indicators of improvement. Sputum specimens are usually obtained on a monthly basis, but the most important specimens are those obtained 5-6 months into therapy; persistence of positive smears and cultures beyond this time is a strong indication of treatment failure. Chest x-rays obtained on a monthly basis were the usual routine in the past; however, it has been recognized that the radiographic appearance of cavities alone may be misleading and cannot be used to assess the activity of the disease without knowledge of the patient's bacteriologic status. In addition, radiographic improvement occurs too slowly to justify monthly x-ray evaluation. Therefore x-rays should be obtained only when there is a strong clinical indication.

The need for retreatment commonly occurs in the management of pulmonary tuberculosis. Some patients will relapse following conversion of sputum smears and cultures, usually because drugs were stopped too soon; fortunately, in these cases, the disease will respond to a resumption of the same drug. On the other hand, a patient with persistently positive sputum smears and cultures after 4-6 months of documented chemotherapy probably has resistant organisms, except in cases of silicosis or far-advanced cavitary disease, where decreasing numbers of organisms are noted on smear and culture and clinical improvement is noted. Resistance should also be suspected in patients who have had several relapses and irregular drug therapy. In such patients chemotherapy should be based on culture and drug sensitivity studies. If therapy must be started before cultures are available, two new drugs should be added that have never been used before. Many would recommend a three-drug regimen in retreatment cases where drug resistance has developed. When drug sensitivities are available, drugs to which the organism is resistant can be discontinued. Some authorities recommend the continuation of isoniazid despite demonstrated resistance.

Experimentally, corticosteroids are known to reduce the host reaction to mycobacteria and minimize exudation, fibrous deposition, and proliferation of granulation tissue. In tuberculous pericarditis, use of steroids (prednisone, 80 mg/day) has been beneficial in reducing inflammatory exudate and damage to the myocardium, as well as enhancing the reabsorption of fluid. Prednisone is recommended. In tuberculous meningitis prednisone is advocated in cases complicated by altered consciousness, increased intracranial pressure, or block in cerebrospinal fluid drainage. Obviously, such therapy should be used in conjunction with adequate chemotherapy and only in cases where the diagnosis is reasonably well established. Although no well-controlled study exists, many series show a definite advantage in the use of steroids, with more rapid reversal of cerebrospinal fluid abnormalities and improvement in mental status.

Modern chemotherapy has relegated surgery to an adjunctive role in the therapy of tuberculosis. In pulmonary tuberculosis resectional surgery may be lifesaving in cases of severe hemoptysis. Surgery is also occasionally performed to remove a cavity harboring large numbers of resistant organisms in retreatment cases which have failed on multiple drugs; reduction in the population of organisms may permit successful treatment of residual infection by remaining drugs. In tuberculous pericarditis, as noted previously, surgery is often employed to establish the diagnosis and promote drainage. Some authorities advocate a more extensive pericardiectomy to prevent recurrent tamponade and residual inflammatory damage to the myocardium. In gastrointestinal and peritoneal tuberculosis, surgery is often required to treat complications such as intestinal obstruction. With early diagnosis and therapy the number of such complications is reduced. In renal tuberculosis, surgery is indicated for complications, such as ureteral stricture, or for advanced unilateral renal tuberculosis complicated by bacterial infection and sepsis, hemorrhage, pain, newly developed severe hypertension, suspected malignancy, or inability to sterilize the urine with drugs alone. Female genital tuberculosis may require surgery to remove large pelvic masses and treat fistulas. In tuberculous arthritis, early chemotherapy produces satisfactory healing in most cases; surgery is indicated, however, for the correction of deformities and improvement of function. Most cases of tuberculous spondylitis are treated with chemotherapy before extensive damage occurs. Surgical intervention is indicated when there is extensive destruction and the possibility of vertebral collapse with resultant paraplegia exists.

Selected Bibliography

Addington, W. W.: The side effects and interactions of antituberculosis drugs. *Chest* 76:782, 1976.

Agner, R. C. and Gallis, H. A. : Pericarditis. Differential diagnostic considerations. *Arch Intern Med* 139:407, 1979.

Auerback, O.: Tuberculosis of the female genital organs. *Surg Gynecol Obstet* 95:712, 1942.

Berger, H. W. and Mejia, E.: Tuberculous pleurisy. *Chest* 63:88, 1973.

Berney, S., Goldstein, M., and Bishko, F.: Clinical and diagnostic features of tuberculous arthritis. *Am J Med* 53:36, 1972.

Bondurant, R. E. and Reid, D.: Ileocecal tuberculosis. *Am J Gastroenterol* 63:58, 1975.

Borhanmanesh, F., Hekmat, K., Vaezzadek, K., et al.: Tuberculous peritonitis. Prospective study of 32 cases in Iran. *Ann Intern Med* 76:567, 1972.

Buechner, H. A.: Short course chemotherapy for tuberculosis. A story of flawed studies. *Am Rev Respir Dis* 124:655, 1981.

Cantrell, R. W., Jensen, J. H., and Reid, D.: Diagnosis and management of tuberculous cervical adenitis. *Arch Otolaryngol* 101:53, 1975.

Carr, D. T., Karlson, A. G., and Stilwell, G. G.: A comparison of cultures of in-
    duced sputum and gastric washings in the diagnosis of tuberculosis. *Mayo
    Clin Proc* 42:23, 1967.

Christensen, W. I.: Genitourinary tuberculosis: Review of 102 cases. *Medicine*
    53:377, 1974.

Comstock, G. W. and Wolpert, S. F.: Tuberculin conversions: True or false?
    Am Rev Respir Dis 118:215, 1978.

Damergis, J. A., Lefterich, E. I., Cartin, J. A., et al.: Tuberculoma of the brain.
    JAMA 239:413, 1978.

Davidson, P. T. and Harowitz, I.: Skeletal tuberculosis. A review with patient
    presentations and discussion. *Am J Med* 48:77, 1970.

Ehrenkranz, N. J. and Kicklighter, J. L.: Tuberculosis outbreak in a general hos-
    pital: Evidence of airborne spread of infection. *Ann Intern Med* 77:377, 1972.

Escobar, J. A., Belsey, M. A., Duenas, A., et al.: Mortality from tuberculous men-
    ingitis reduced by steroid therapy. *Pediatrics* 56:1050, 1975.

Gammill, S. L. and Nice, C. M.: Tuberculous mesenteric lymphadenitis. *Am J
    Roentgenol Radium Ther Nucl Med* 117:346, 1973.

Gelb, A. F., Liffler, C., Brewin, A., et al.: Miliary tuberculosis. *Am Rev Respir
    Dis* 108:1329, 1973.

Glassroth, J., Robins, A. G., and Snider, D. E., Jr.: Tuberculosis in the 1980's.
    N Engl J Med 302:1441, 1980.

Greico, M. H. and Chmel, H.: Acute disseminated tuberculosis as a diagnostic
    problem. *Amer Rev Respir Dis* 109:554, 1974.

Haas, E. J., Madhaven, T., Quinn, E. L., et al.: Tuberculous meningitis in an urban
    general hospital. *Arch Intern Med* 137:1518, 1977.

Hageman, J. H., D'Esopo, N. D., and Glenn, W. W. L.: Tuberculosis of the peri-
    cardium. A long-term analysis of forty-four proven cases. *N Engl J Med*
    270:327, 1964.

Jones, F. L.: The relative efficacy of spontaneous sputa, aerosol-induced sputa
    and gastric aspirates in the bacteriologic diagnosis of pulmonary tuberculo-
    sis. *Dis Chest* 50:403, 1966.

Kennedy, D. H. and Fallon, R. J.: Tuberculous meningitis. *JAMA* 241:264, 1979.

Kent, D. C. and Schwartz, R.: Active pulmonary tuberculosis with negative tu-
    berculin skin reactions. *Am Rev Respir Dis* 95:411, 1967.

Khan, M. A.: Clinical and radiographic spectrum of pulmonary tuberculosis in the
    adult. *Am J Med* 62:1, 1977.

Kocen, R. S. and Parsons, M.: Neurological complications of tuberculosis: Some unusual manifestations. *Quart J Med* 29:17, 1970.

Long, M. W., Snider, D. E., and Farer, L.: U. S. Public Health Service Cooperative Trial of three rifampin-isoniazid regimens in the treatment of pulmonary tuberculosis. *Am Rev Respir Dis* 119:879, 1979.

Mayers, M. M., Kaufman, D. M., and Miller, M. H.: Recent cases of intracranial tuberculomas. *Neurology* 6:256, 1978.

Ortbals, D. M. and Avioli, L. V.: Tuberculous pericarditis. *Arch Intern Med* 139: 231, 1979.

Rosenberg, S. A., Seipp, C. and Sears, H. F.: Clinical and immunologic studies of disseminated BCG infection. *Cancer* 41:1771, 1978.

Sweany, H. C.: The pathology of primary tuberculous infection in the adult. *Am Rev Respir Dis* 39:236, 1939.

Tabrisky, J., Lindstrom, R. R. , and Peters, R.: Tuberculous enteritis. Review of a protean disease. *Am J Gastroenterol* 63:49, 1975.

Thompson, N. J., Glassroth, J. L., Snider, D. E., Jr., and Farer, L. S.: The booster phenomenon in serial tuberculin testing. *Am Rev Respir Dis* 119:587, 1979.

Vorherr, H., Massy, S., Fallet, R., et al.: Antidiuretic principle in tuberculous lung tissue of a patient with pulmonary tuberculosis and hyponatremia. *Ann Intern Med* 72:383, 1970.

Weaver, R. A.: Tuberculosis of the tongue. *JAMA* 235:2418, 1976.

Wolfe, J. H. N., Behn, A. R., and Jackson, B. T.: Tuberculous peritonitis and role of diagnostic laparoscopy. *Lancet* 1:852, 1979.

Wolfowitz, B. L.: Tuberculous mastoiditis. *Arch Otolaryngol* 95:109, 1972.

105

NONTUBERCULOUS MYCOBACTERIAL INFECTIONS
Rashida A. Khakoo, M.D.

Definition

Shortly after Robert Koch's discovery of the human tubercle bacillus, reports of isolations of other acid-fast bacteria from nonhuman sources began to appear, and soon isolations from human sources were also reported. In 1935 these organisms were first termed "atypical mycobacteria." Later such eponyms as anonymous, unclassified, nontuberculous, opportunistic, tuberculoid, and mycobacteria other than tubercle bacilli have been proposed. According to Wolinsky, the term nontuberculous mycobacteria seems most appropriate. Initially there was a lot of resistance in acceptance of these mycobacteria as agents causing disease because they were nonpathogenic for guinea pigs.

Microbiology

Several classification schemes for nontuberculous mycobacteria have been proposed. The classification by Runyon based on pigment production, rate of growth, and colony morphology, has been widely used (Table 105.1). With better techniques available for species identification of nontuberculous mycobacteria, the Runyon classification is of less significance. "Saprophytic" mycobacteria are commonly found in the environment and do not cause disease, except under very unusual circumstances. They may, however, be found in cultured material from humans, and therefore it is important to separate them from the strains just discussed. These usually "nonpathogenic" strains are listed in Table 105.2.

In the microbiology laboratory, the identification of different species is carried out by several different tests. Some of these include optimal temperature for growth, niacin production, nitrate reduction, arylsulfatase test, catalase test,

TABLE 105.1   Classification of Nontuberculous Mycobacteria

Species and Runyon Group	Clinical Significance	Growth Rate	Niacin Test	Nitrate Reduction	Tween Hydrolysis	Catalase 68°C	Arylsulfatase 3 Days	Urease	Serotyping Available
Group I									
Photochromogens (pigment in presence of light)									
M. kansasii	2	S	-	+	+	+	-	+	+
M. marinum	2	S	*	-	+	+	-		+
Group II									
Scotochromogens (pigment in dark)									
M. scrofulaceum	3-2	S	-	-	-	+			+
M. szulgai †	1	S	-	+	*	+	*	+	+
Group III									
Nonchromogens (no pigment)									
M. avium-intracellulare	2	S	-	-	-	+	-	-	+
M. xenopi	3	S	-	-	-	+	*	-	+
Group IV									
M. fortuitum	4-3	R	-	+	*	+	+	+	+
M. chelonei	4-3	R	*	-	-	+	+	+	+

*Some strains are positive, (1) only as pathogens; (2) usually as pathogens; (3) commonly as nonpathogens; (4) usually as nonpathogens; S slow, R rapid

†M. szulgai is scotochromogenic at 37°C and photochromogenic at 25°C

TABLE 105.2   Usually Nonpathogenic Strains

M. smegmatis

M. vaccae

M. parafortuitum

M. gordonae

M. gastri

M. terrae

M. flavescens

M. triviale

M. phlei

Tween hydrolysis, tellurite reduction, iron uptake, growth on MacConkey's agar, urea hydrolysis, and antimicrobial susceptibility patterns. Serologic classification and lipid analysis also have been used.

Epidemiology

No documented human-to-human transmission of disease due to nontuberculous mycobacteria has been reported. *Mycobacterium kansasii* has not been found in soil or dust but has occasionally been isolated from water samples in different areas of the world. *Mycobacterium marinum* may be found in fresh or salt water as a result of contamination from infected fish and other marine life. *Mycobacterium simiae* was recovered from monkeys imported from India. *Mycobacterium scrofulaceum* has been identified in raw milk and other dairy products, soil, water, and oysters, while *M. szulgai* has almost always been isolated from humans. *Mycobacterium avium* and *M. intracellulare* have been found in soil and raw milk. Strains of *M. fortuitum* have been found in water, soil, and dust.

Two species of nontuberculous mycobacteria have an unexplained geographic distribution: *M. intracellulare* disease is mostly found in the southeastern United States, western Australia, and Japan; disease due to *M. kansasii* has been reported most commonly from Chicago, Kansas City, England, and Wales. In some areas in the United States and in Germany both species are equally important as agents of pulmonary disease. Despite the geographic distribution, because of increased movement of people and chronicity of illness, a patient may present in a place far removed from where the disease was actually acquired. Detailed prevalence figures for all diseases caused by nontuberculous mycobacteria are not available for the following reasons: incomplete reporting; reports from large referral centers (therefore biased); lack of speciation of all isolates; and lack of documentation that the isolates are indeed responsible for disease. Estimates of the prevalence of nontuberculous mycobacterial disease, expressed as a percentage of total mycobacterial disease, have varied from 0.5 to 30%.

Pathogenesis and Pathology

From skin test data, it appears that large segments of the population are infected, but few develop disease, a situation somewhat similar to that for histoplasmosis. It is not clear whether the pulmonary disease is due to reactivation or to primary infection.

The route of infection is not entirely known. Since pulmonary disease occurs, airborne spread of infection via the respiratory route seems likely. For skin and subcutaneous infections caused by *M. marinum, M. ulcerans,* and *M. chelonei,* entry into skin by direct inoculation seems most likely. For cervical lymphadenopathy caused by nontuberculous mycobacteria, entry through a breach in the mucosa of the mouth or pharynx has been postulated. Nontuberculous mycobacteria have been cultured from the tonsils. The pathology of the affected tissues is very similar to that caused by *M. tuberculosis* with granulomas, giant cells, and presence of acid-fast organisms. A few differential points have been mentioned but none are discriminatory. In some patients with disseminated infections the granulomas may not be well formed or may be absent and the tissue may show just extensive necrosis.

Diagnostic Features

Clinical

Generally, pulmonary disease caused by nontuberculous mycobacteria is more indolent compared with that caused by *M. tuberculosis.* Most species of nontuberculous mycobacteria have been reported to cause pulmonary disease, but *M. kansasii* and *M. intracellulare* are the most common, and the disease is most often seen in white males 50 years of age or older. Most patients with disease due to *M. intracellulare,* and about half of those with disease due to *M. kansasii,* have an underlying lung disease such as chronic obstructive pulmonary disease, silicosis, pulmonary fibrosis, or bronchiectasis. Malignant disease is reported to be another risk factor. Approximately two-thirds of the patients with *M. kansasii* pulmonary disease are symptomatic, usually presenting with cough. A paucity of symptoms in the face of cavitary disease as shown by roentgenograms has been reported. Most patients have pulmonary infiltrates, cavitation, or both. Bilateral involvement is common when disease is caused by *M. kansasii* as compared with tuberculosis, and granulomatous nodules are fewer, pleural effusion seldom occurs, and cavitation occurs more frequently. The cavity walls are usually thin, and soft exudative infiltration is rarely seen. However, none of this is diagnostic in a particular patient. Pulmonary disease caused by *M. intracellulare* is indistinguishable from tuberculosis, except for the indolent course. Fifty percent of patients have far-advanced disease on initial presentation. Pulmonary disease caused by *M. scrofulaceum* is very rare, although the organism is a fairly frequent isolate from the sputum. All reported patients have been males with a duration of illness from 1.5 to 8 years. Industrial exposure to silica, arc welding fumes, or dust is common. Very few patients with pulmonary disease caused by *M. szulgai* have been reported and their clinical presentation is not much different from that produced by other nontuberculous mycobacteria. Approximately 50 patients with pulmonary disease due to *M. xenopi* have been reported. Megaesophagus is a predisposing factor to pulmonary disease caused by *M. fortuitum* or *M. chelonei.* It is more frequent in women and is often bilateral. The exact reason for the association of megaesophagus with pulmonary disease caused by nontuberculous mycobacteria is not clear. It is

postulated that as a result of the delayed transit and the rapid growth characteristics of these mycobacteria, a high inoculum may be produced which is then aspirated.

Lymphadenitis caused by nontuberculous mycobacteria usually occurs in children. The most common age group is 1.5-5 years. The nodes most commonly involved are those that drain the buccal mucous membranes, the submaxillary and
submandibular groups. Occasionally axillary, preauricular, epitrochlear, and inguinal nodes are involved, and the adenitis is most commonly unilateral. Axillary
adenitis has been associated occasionally with lesions on the palms, preauricular
adenitis with conjunctivitis, and inguinal adenitis with a lesion on the leg. Nodes
tend to suppurate readily with formation of sinuses and with prolonged drainage.
Most of the children feel well and there is no evidence of constitutional symptoms.
Chest roentgenograms are usually normal and there is usually no family history of
tuberculosis. Three species of nontuberculous mycobacteria, *M. scrofulaceum,*
M. avium-intracellulare, and *M. kansasii,* have been reported with lymphadenitis.

Mycobacterium marinum is associated with "swimming pool" or "fish tank
granuloma." Patients are usually children or young adults. Fingers, knees, or elbows are common sites of lesions. Most patients report antecedent trauma or an
abrasion of the area. The lesions are usually papuloverrucous with subsequent
progression to shallow ulceration. The lesions occasionally resemble the lymphocutaneous form of sporotrichosis. The duration of illness may be prolonged, but
the patients usually feel well and have no constitutional symptoms. Cutaneous
disease due to *M. marinum* usually remains localized to the skin; rarely involvement of synovium, bursa, tendons, and bone has been noted.

Chronic necrotizing skin ulcers caused by *M. ulcerans* were first reported from
Australia in 1948. Subsequently, patients with similar ulcers have been reported
from Africa and other parts of the world. The subcutaneous nodule has been recognized as the preulcerative stage. This is usually painless and may occur at any
site. Children aged 5-14 years are most commonly affected. Histology of the
nodule shows extensive necrosis of subcutaneous tissue with minimal inflammatory
response at the edges. Many acid-fast bacilli can be demonstrated in the necrotic
connective tissue. The ulcers are usually extensive with undermined edges.

Abscesses at the sites of trauma, surgery, and other infections have been reported with *M. fortuitum-chelonei.* Outbreaks of cutaneous abscesses due to *M.
chelonei* have been reported in patients undergoing venous stripping. The initial
lesions are hard nodules surrounded by an area of inflammation overlying the surgical incision. The nodules may become fluctuant and drain, and they are very indolent. The source of contamination may be certain skin disinfectants. Recently,
infections caused by *M. fortuitum* have been reported in patients who have undergone insertion of silicone prostheses for augmentation mammoplasty. The onset
of infection has been from 1 to 2 weeks to over a year following surgery. Clinically
the patients present with a painful swollen breast with little or no erythema or
drainage and no fever. The source of contamination remains unclear.

Disseminated infections have been reported with *M. kansasii, M. avium-
intracellulare, M. scrofulaceum,* and *M. fortuitum-chelonei.* Many of these patients have underlying hematologic diseases such as leukemia or are immunosuppressed by disease, drugs, or a combination of both. In some patients, the hematologic abnormalities (particularly pancytopenia) associated with *M. kansasii* may
be secondary to the disease. Disseminated *M. kansasii* infections have been reported more often in adults, whereas disseminated *M. avium-intracellulare* infections have been reported more frequently in children. Most patients with disseminated *M. kansasii* infections have underlying diseases, whereas those infected
with *M. intracellulare* and *M. scrofulaceum* usually do not. Many patients with
disseminated infections due to *M. fortuitum-chelonei* have either endocarditis or

are renal transplant recipients. Osteomyelitis, arthritis, synovitis, bursitis, and carpal tunnel syndrome have been reported due to nontuberculous mycobacteria. Arthritis has been reported involving the wrist and knee joints. Recently, osteo- myelitis of the sternum caused by *M. fortuitum-chelonei* has been reported follow- ing cardiac surgery. Contaminated bone cement has been suspected, but not docu- mented, as the source of infection. In children lytic lesions in different bones, in- cluding the ribs, sternum, skull, metacarpals, and metatarsals, have been reported. These commonly result in draining sinuses, and *M. scrofulaceum* or *M. intracellu- lare* have been isolated from bone biopsies or draining sinuses. Most of the non- disseminated bone and joint infections caused by nontuberculous mycobacteria are indolent, resembling disease caused by *M. tuberculosis.*

Although urine cultures frequently demonstrate nontuberculous mycobacteria, genitourinary tract disease is rare. Meningitis has been rarely documented as hav- ing been caused by nontuberculous mycobacteria. The role of these mycobacteria when cultured from cerebrospinal fluid at the same time as other organisms (e.g., *M. tuberculosis* or cryptococci) remains unclear. Keratitis and corneal ulcers with *M. fortuitum-chelonei* following trauma (foreign body) have been reported.

Recently porcine valves have been reported to be contaminated with *M. chel- onei*. Pericarditis and aortic root abscess have been reported to result from this. The source of contamination is unknown.

Laboratory

Since nontuberculous mycobacteria are found in the environment and in clinical specimens from patients without disease, and since criteria for disease are not firmly established, interpretation of cultures should take into account the known pathogenic potential of the specific isolate. Repeated isolation of the same spe- cies in sputum in large numbers (more than 100 colonies per culture) from patients who have clinical and/or radiologic evidence of disease is probably significant. However, sputum cultures may be intermittently, or even persistently, positive for *M. fortuitum-chelonei* or *M. gordonae* as a result of long-term colonization in patients with other underlying lung diseases. Isolation of nontuberculous myco- bacteria from a closed space (in the absence of environmental contamination of the specimen) or from tissue with consistent histopathologic changes is diagnostic.

The usefulness of differential skin tests for diagnosis of nontuberculous myco- bacterial infections is limited, although they may be helpful in epidemiologic stud- ies. Since many surface antigens are shared, cross-reactions occur. Also, stand- ardized skin test antigens are not generally available.

Differential Diagnosis (Table 105.3)

Treatment and Prognosis

The response to treatment of pulmonary disease caused by nontuberculous myco- bacteria depends mainly upon the susceptibility of the isolate to antituberculous agents. Recently, a much better response to chemotherapy of pulmonary disease caused by *M. kansasii* has been reported. Previously, culture negativity has been reported in 70% of patients with underlying lung disease and cavity closure in 35%. Relapse occurred in 10% and progression of disease in 20%. Recently, 92% of pa- tients on antituberculous treatment have demonstrated sputum conversion. Reg- imens containing rifampin are very effective in both initial and retreatment cases because most strains of *M. kansasii* are inhibited by 0.25-1 µg of rifampin. A

TABLE 105.3   Differential Diagnosis of Nontuberculous Mycobacterial Infections

Type of Infection	Differential Diagnosis	Comments
Pulmonary	Tuberculosis	Pulmonary nontuberculous mycobacterial infections (especially caused by *M. kansasii* and *M. intracellulare*) have more indolent course, more common in older white males with underlying disease. Culture is the only definitive way of differentiating
	Fungal Infection	
	Blastomycosis	Skin lesions often present with blastomycosis
	Histoplasmosis	Culture and serology helpful in diagnosis of fungal infections
	Coccidioidomycosis	History of residence or travel to endemic areas helpful
	Lung abscess	Location and predisposing factors different. Cavity usually thick-walled in abscess with air-fluid level
	Cavitating bronchogenic carcinoma	History, cytology, and biopsy of tissue usually helpful in diagnosis
Lymphadenitis	Tuberculosis	Nodes in tuberculosis are usually in supraclavicular area or posterior cervical triangle, more commonly bilateral. Pulmonary tuberculosis may be present. Constitutional symptoms are prominent
	Bacterial infections	Fever is usually present. Nodes may be warm and tender. Pharyngitis may be present
	Cat-scratch disease	Usually unilateral and suppurates - similar to nontuberculous mycobacterial infection. History of cat scratch would be important. Skin tests may help

TABLE 105.3 (Cont'd)

Type of Infection	Differential Diagnosis	Comments
	Infectious mono-nucleosis	Blood picture and heterophil antibody test and specific tests for Epstein-Barr virus would help
	Lymphoma	Involvement of other sites may be present. Biopsy is helpful
	Leukemia	Blood picture and bone marrow examination should help
Cutaneous		
M. marinum	Blastomycosis	Pulmonary lesions commonly present. Biopsy and culture helpful
	Chromoblasto-mycosis	Biopsy and culture necessary for diagnosis
	Foreign-body granuloma	History of trauma may be available. Absence of acid-fast bacteria on stain and culture
	Inoculation tuberculosis	Rare. Occupational history important. Biopsy and culture of lesion necessary
M. marinum "sporotricho-sis" type of infection	Sporotrichosis	History of work or hobby important. Biopsy and culture helpful
	Nocardial infection	Acid-fast stain and culture helpful
M. ulcerans infections (preulcera-tive stage nodule)	Nodular fasciitis; injection abscess; panniculitis	Biopsy with special stains is helpful to separate the nodule caused by M. ulcerans
M. fortuitum M. chelonei abscesses	Abscesses caused by other organisms particularly bacteria	Smears and cultures helpful

TABLE 105.3   (Cont'd)

Type of Infection	Differential Diagnosis	Comments
Disseminated infection	Disseminated tuberculosis	Stains and cultures of material from one or more sites
Disseminated infections with hematologic abnormalities	Lymphoma Leukemia	Blood smear, bone marrow examination helpful. However nontuberculous mycobacterial infection may be superimposed on underlying hematologic abnormality
Bone and joint infection	Bone infections caused by *M. tuberculosis*	Bone or synovial biopsy with culture helpful
	Fungal infection	Serology, stain, and culture may help
	Partly treated bacterial infection	History of previous antimicrobial therapy which resulted in some response
Genitourinary infections	Renal tuberculosis caused by *M. tuberculosis*	Urine culture
	Fungal infection	Blood, urine, stain, and culture

three-drug regimen consisting of rifampin, INH, and ethambutol for 2 years is recommended. Since 90% of sputum conversions in successful regimens occur within 4-6 months of beginning therapy, patients whose cultures remain positive at this time should be considered for alternative regimens, depending upon sensitivities. Very few patients require surgery. Slow progression, or rarely spontaneous remission, has been described in patients with untreated *M. kansasii* pulmonary disease. The mortality due to *M. kansasii* pulmonary disease is low.

Pulmonary disease caused by *M. avium-intracellulare* responds less well to drug treatment. A combined medical/surgical treatment is usually recommended. If a patient is a surgical candidate, his chances of achieving inactive status are about 75%. On medical treatment alone, the chance of attaining inactive status is 25-30%. It is likely that those who are selected to receive medical treatment alone have more extensive disease. The isolates are usually resistant to INH and other antituberculous agents. Four- to six-drug regimens have been recommended, including streptomycin, with appropriate alterations made according to sensitivity data. The combination therapy should be continued for at least 2 years or until it is obvious that the treatment is not beneficial. At the sixth or eighth month, appropriate resectional surgery should be considered.

The experience in treatment of pulmonary disease caused by *M. szulgai* and *M. xenopi* is limited. They are both relatively sensitive to antituberculous agents. Use of a combination of rifampin, ethambutol, and either ethionamide or streptomycin is recommended for *M. szulgai* and INH, rifampin, and streptomycin for *M. xenopi*.

Very few patients with pulmonary disease caused by *M. scrofulaceum* have been reported. The isolates are usually resistant to most antituberculous agents. Intensive multiple-drug regimens may be tried and surgery may be required.

Treatment of pulmonary infections caused by *M. fortuitum-chelonei* is difficult because of the resistance of these isolates to antituberculous therapy. In the patients with bilateral disease, surgical resection is not feasible. Recently *M. fortuitum* isolates have been reported to be sensitive to amikacin and to doxycycline; either of these drugs can be tried. However, studies are needed to document the usefulness of these agents in vivo.

The treatment of choice in lymphadenitis is total excision of the nodes, if possible. There are controversies regarding the use of antituberculous therapy. *Mycobacterium scrofulaceum* and *M. intracellulare* are quite resistant to antituberculous therapy, and children do well after node excision alone, therefore this is thought by many to be the treatment of choice.

The spectrum of cutaneous involvement with *M. marinum* is wide. Spontaneous healing of some lesions occurs. With very localized lesions, surgical excision, curettage, or electrodesiccation has been carried out. With more extensive lesions, chemotherapy is used. *Mycobacterium marinum* strains are usually resistant to INH but sensitive to rifampin and ethambutol. The use of tetracycline or trimethoprim sulfamethoxazole (TMP-SMX) has been reported. Since patients may undergo spontaneous remission, it is difficult to judge the efficacy of some therapeutic regimens. In patients who are judged to require chemotherapy, TMP-SMX or tetracycline can be tried. If there is no response, then a trial of a combination of rifampin and ethambutol for 6 weeks is suggested. Local heat treatment has also been reported to be beneficial. The prognosis of *M. marinum* infections is good. Surgery, usually with skin grafts, has been required for ulcers caused by *M. ulcerans*. There are conflicting reports on the use of chemotherapy. Streptomycin, rifampin, and local heat treatment have been used. Treatment of the preulcerative stage (nodule) is by excision and the patients seem to do fairly well. For abscesses caused by *M. fortuitum-chelonei,* incision and drainage are usually carried out.

The treatment of disseminated infections depends upon the species of nontuberculous mycobacteria involved. Combination chemotherapy is always used. Other supportive therapy may be required. Many of these patients have hematologic abnormalities and thus are subject to develop other infections. The mortality is high, mainly reflecting the underlying diseases.

The major treatment of bone and joint infections consists of surgical drainage and removal of infected synovium and bone. The role of antituberculous therapy is difficult to evaluate, except in those infected with *M. kansasii,* where it seems to be beneficial.

Combination chemotherapy, depending upon the sensitivities of infecting species, will be required for genitourinary tract disease. Since only a few patients have been reported, it is difficult to make judgments on response.

Very few patients with meningitis caused by these organisms have been reported. The treatment will depend upon the susceptibility of the infecting species.

The course of *M. fortuitum* keratitis has been reported to be chronic with spontaneous remissions and relapses. Hypopyon has been reported to occur. It is difficult to evaluate the effect of chemotherapy.

Selected Bibliography

Adams, R. M., Remington, J. S., Steinberg, J., and Seibert, J. S.: Tropical fish aquarium – a source of *Mycobacterium marinum* infections resembling sporotrichosis. *JAMA* 211:457–461, 1970.

Black, B. G. and Chapman, J. S.: Cervical adenitis in children due to human and unclassified mycobacteria. *Pediatrics* 33:887–893, 1964.

Burke, D. S. and Ullian, R. B.: Megaesophagus and pneumonia associated with *Mycobacterium chelonei*. A case report and a literature review. *Am Rev Respir Dis* 116:1101, 1977.

Chapman, J. S.: Atypical mycobacterial infections – pathogenesis, clinical manifestations and treatment. *Med Clin N Am* 51:503–517, 1967.

Fogan, L.: Atypical mycobacteria – their clinical, laboratory and epidemiologic significance. *Medicine* 49:243–255, 1970.

Foz, A., Roy, C., Jurado, J., Arteaga, E., Ruiz, J. M., and Moragas, A.: *Mycobacterium chelonei* iatrogenic infections. *J Clin Microbiol* 7:319–321, 1978.

Harris, G. D., Johanson, W. G., and Nicholson, D. P.: Response to chemotherapy of pulmonary infection due to *Mycobacterium kansasii*. *Am Rev Respir Dis* 112:31–36, 1975.

Johanson, W. G. and Nicholson, D. P.: Pulmonary disease due to *Mycobacterium kansasii,* an analysis of some factors affecting prognosis. *Am Rev Respir Dis* 99:73–85, 1969.

Jolly, H. W. and Seabury, J. H.: Infections with *Mycobacterium marinum*.   *Arch Dermatol* 106:32–36, 1972.

Lakowski, L. F., Marr, J. J., Spernoga, J. F., Frank, N. J., Barner, H. B., Kaiser, G., and Tyras, D. M.: Fastidious mycobacteria grown from porcine prosthetic heart valve catheters. *N Engl J Med* 297:101–102, 1977.

Lincoln, E. M. and Gilbert, L. A.: Disease in children due to mycobacteria other than *Mycobacterium tuberculosis*. *Am Rev Respir Dis* 105:683–714, 1972.

Molavi, A. and Weinstein, L.: In vitro susceptibility of atypical mycobacteria to rifampin. *Appl Microbiol* 22:23–25, 1971.

Mycobacterial infections associated with augmentation mammoplasty – Florida, North Carolina, Texas. *MMWR* 27(51):513, 1978.

Owens, D. W.: General medical aspects of atypical mycobacteria.   *South Med J* 67:39–43, 1974.

Philpott, J. A., Woodburne, A. R., Philpott, O. S., Schaefer, W. B., and Mollohan, C. S.: Swimming pool granuloma - a study of 290 cases. *Arch Dermatol* 88: 158-162, 1963.

Rauscher, C. R., Kerby, G., and Ruth, W. E.: A ten-year clinical experience with *M. kansasii*. *Chest* 66:17-19, 1974.

Schaefer, W. B., Wolinsky, E., Jenkins, P. A., and Marks, J.: *Mycobacterium szulgai* - a new pathogen, serologic identification and report of five new patients. *Am Rev Respir Dis* 108:1320-1326, 1973.

Shaad, U. B., Votteler, T. P., McCracken, G. M., and Nelson, J. D.: Management of atypical mycobacterial lymphadenitis in childhood. A review based on 380 cases. *J Pediatr* 95:356-360, 1979.

Uganda Buruli Group: Report II, Clinical features and treatment of preulcerative Buruli lesions (*Mycobacterium ulcerans* infection). *Br Med J* 2:390-393, 1970.

Wolinsky, E.: Nontuberculous mycobacteria and associated disease - state of the art. *Am Rev Respir Dis* 119:107-159, 1979.

Yeager, H. and Raleigh, J. W.: Pulmonary disease due to *Mycobacterium intracellulare*. *Am Rev Respir Dis* 108:547-552, 1973.

106

LEPROSY
Rashida A. Khakoo, M.D.

Leprosy is a chronic infectious disease mainly affecting skin, nasal mucosa, and nerves. The causative organism *Mycobacterium leprae* was first described by Hansen in Norway in 1874. It is estimated that there are at least 12 million cases of leprosy in the world. In the United States there has been an increase in the number of cases, with 244 seen in 1981 owing to immigrants from highly endemic areas. Some of these patients could present to physicians who have had little or no experience in the diagnosis and treatment of leprosy. Table 106.1 lists other diseases that may be considered in the differential diagnosis of this disease.

Etiology

Mycobacterium leprae is an acid-fast, slightly curved rod. The organism may be pleomorphic and may stain irregularly, giving a beaded appearance. It has not been cultivated in vitro, but it has been grown in foot pads of mice where the generation time is 12-1/2 days, far longer than any other bacterium. This model is usually used for drug screening and testing sensitivities of isolates from patients. In 1971, growth of *M. leprae* in the nine-banded armadillo was reported. The armadillo was chosen since its body temperature is 2-5°C lower than most mammals. Subsequently, natural infection of armadillos with leprosy-like disease has been seen. More recently, naturally acquired leprosy has been observed in mangabey monkeys imported from Africa.

TABLE 106.1   Differential Diagnosis of Leprosy

Manifestation	Other Diseases
Skin lesions	Fungal infections
	Yaws
	Vitiligo
	Leishmaniasis
	Mycosis fungoides
Positive ANA	Lupus
Positive syphilis serology	Syphilis
	Lupus
Acid-fast organisms	Disseminated tuberculosis

Epidemiology

Leprosy is generally thought to be transmitted from person to person by direct contact. The nasal discharge of patients with lepromatous leprosy contains large numbers of *M. leprae.* Infectivity is not high; the attack rate in household contacts of patients with multibacillary disease (large number of organisms) is only 5-10%. The incubation period is estimated to be 3-10 years or longer.

Leprosy occurs worldwide. Endemic areas are mainly in Asia (approximately one-fourth of all cases worldwide occur in India), Africa, and South America. In endemic areas, the prevalence rate is about 1%. The usual areas in the United States from which leprosy is reported are Louisiana, Texas, California, Florida, Hawaii, and recently from New York. Slightly more males than females are affected.

The percentage of cases of different types of leprosy varies in different parts of the world. In the United States, a significant percentage of patients have lepromatous or borderline leprosy (probably reflecting the rates in their countries of origin). In Africa, most cases are of the tuberculoid type (further described later).

It is postulated that genetic factors may play a role in differing susceptibility, but the data are inconclusive. Concordance rates in monozygotic twins are not as high as one would expect if genetic factors played a major role.

Pathogenesis, Pathology, and Immunology

Leprosy presents in a spectrum from mild to extensive, and the different clinical types are related to the degree of cell-mediated immune response. In 1966 Ridley and Jopling standardized the nomenclature of the various clinical forms of leprosy, advancing the concept of the two polar forms with a spectrum of forms between them. At one end of the spectrum is tuberculoid leprosy (TT), and at the other is lepromatous (LL). Between these are borderline-tuberculoid (BT), borderline (BB), and borderline-lepromatous (BL) forms. Subsequently, subpolar lepromatous (LLs) was added between BL and LL. The earliest lesion of leprosy may not show either clinically or histologically features of the various polar forms and is referred to as indeterminate.

Suppression of cell-mediated immunity has been demonstrated in patients with lepromatous leprosy. This suppression is specific for *M. leprae* and shows no improvement even after treatment. Nonspecific suppression of cell-mediated immune response also has been demonstrated in lepromatous leprosy and may be secondary to a number of factors, e.g., malnutrition or advanced disease. This improves once the patient's overall health improves and when the bacillary load decreases with therapy. Whether anergy for *M. leprae* precedes or follows the development of leprosy is not clear, nor is the mechanism for this specific immune nonresponsiveness. Patients with tuberculoid leprosy possess cell-mediated immunity and delayed-type hypersensitivity against *M. leprae.*

The distribution of T-cell subpopulations in the peripheral blood of lepromatous leprosy patients is normal. Most of the T cells in skin lesions of patients with lepromatous leprosy are suppressor T cells and there are no helper T cells. In contrast, in lesions of tuberculoid leprosy, in addition to epitheloid cells and giant-cell granulomas, the predominant T cells are of the helper type. It is postulated that these different T-cell subsets influence microbicidal activity of macrophages.

Serum immunoglobulins are normal or increased. Antibody responses to various vaccines are normal. A number of autoantibodies are also produced, and patients may have a false-positive VDRL, positive rheumatoid factor, or antinuclear antibodies (ANA).

Histopathologically, the skin lesions in tuberculoid leprosy contain well-formed granulomas composed of epitheloid cells, Langhan-type giant cells and lymphocytes, and few or no acid-fast bacilli. Dermal nerves are infiltrated with inflammatory cells or may appear completely destroyed. In contrast, skin lesions of lepromatous leprosy demonstrate numerous acid-fast bacilli within macrophages, referred to as foamy macrophages. Granulomas and Langhan-type giant cells are absent. Few lymphocytes are found in the lesions. As the lesions progress, eventually the whole dermis is replaced by macrophages containing the organisms. Typically, the macrophages are separated from the basal layer of the epidermis by a thin band of stroma called the clear zone. Acid-fast bacilli are demonstrated within Schwann cells and perineural cells. The destruction of axons is not as marked as in tuberculoid leprosy. Granulomas with macrophages laden with bacilli may occur in multiple sites, including the liver, lymph nodes, and bone marrow. In severe cases, bacillemia can be demonstrated by buffy-coat staining of blood.

Histopathologic findings of the other forms of leprosy vary depending upon the nearness to one or the other polar form. In the BT and BB forms, epithelioid cells are found but Langhans-type giant cells are usually not seen. Lymphocytic infiltration is greatest in the TT form, compared with the BT and BB forms. The bacilli are usually not found in the lesions of TT leprosy. More bacilli are found in the lesions of BT and BB forms. Nerve destruction is greatest in the TT form. In BL leprosy, there are fewer bacilli compared with the LL form and the number of lymphocytes is slightly greater.

In indeterminate lesions, there is infiltration of skin with mononuclear cells. Acid-fast bacilli may be seen in nerves.

Diagnosis

Clinical

The illness is usually insidious in onset. The indeterminate type may present with an erythematous or hypopigmented macule, which may heal or progress to one of the well-established forms. The classic lesion of tuberculoid leprosy is flat and well demarcated, hypopigmented with a raised border. Usually there is a single lesion, but occasionally more than one may be found. The distribution is asymmetric. The lesions may be found anywhere but classically are absent from warmer intertriginous areas. Usually, the lesions are hypesthetic or anesthetic. The loss of temperature sensation occurs before the loss of other sensory modalities. Enlargement of ulnar, greater auricular, and peroneal nerves is characteristic. Other nerves also may be involved. With progression, clawhand, wristdrop, or footdrop may occur, as well as loss of sensation in the areas supplied by the respective nerves. In BB leprosy, the number of lesions is greater. The lesions are less well defined and erythematous. Anesthesia is less marked and nerve infiltration is less intense.

In lepromatous leprosy, multiple erythematous macules are seen. These are distributed symmetrically and later evolve into papules and nodules. Thickening of the ear lobes sometimes occurs early. With increasing infiltrations, leonine furrowing of the face develops. Loss of eyebrows and eyelashes eventually occurs. The lesions are small and red, ultimately darken in the center and ulcerate. Obliterative, necrotizing vasculitis is seen (Lucio's phenomenon). Ocular involvement occurs mainly in the LL and BL types. Lesions that can potentially lead to blindness occur in about one-third of the patients. The eye lesions include lid infiltration, keratitis, lagophthalmos, choroidal involvement, and leprous pannus. Involvement of the throat may cause hoarseness and laryngeal obstruction. Destruction of peripheral nerves initially leads to glove-and-stocking distribution of sensory loss. With progression, other areas are involved. Eventually, superimposed trauma, infection, and worsening neuropathy lead to shortening and loss of digits.

Laboratory

In LL and BL forms, slit-skin smears will demonstrate the presence of acid-fast organisms. Nasal discharge or scraping of the nasal mucosa is also a good source for demonstrating bacilli. In addition to the usual stains, fluorescent microscopy has been used.

In tuberculoid leprosy, the diagnosis usually is based on the typical clinical appearance and skin biopsy. A biopsy is taken from the edge of the lesion and the deeper part of the dermis should be included. Acid-fast bacilli may be demonstrated in the BT and BB types and very rarely in the tuberculoid type using the Fite-Faraco stain.

The available skin test material is a crude preparation from lesions of patients with lepromatous leprosy. Positive reactions occur in two phases, the first at 24–48 hr with transient erythema and induration (Fernandez reaction). At 4 weeks, a nodule forms, and this is considered positive if the diameter is 5 mm or more. Histologic examination demonstrates granulomas. The lepromin test is not diagnostic for leprosy since many normal people will have a positive reaction. It is a useful test for grading the disease, usually being negative in LL and BL leprosy, markedly positive in tuberculoid leprosy, and slightly positive in the BT form.

Glomerulonephritis is seen in various forms of leprosy, with or without the presence of erythema nodosum leprosum (ENL). The deposition of immune complexes in the glomeruli seems to be the most likely explanation. Mesangial cell proliferation and endothelial cell swelling are seen. Immunofluorescent staining reveals deposits of IgG and C3.

Treatment

The treatment of leprosy involves a number of modalities: medical, physical therapy, surgery as required for complications, psychologic, and social rehabilitation. Patients do not need to be institutionalized; most patients can be treated as outpatients. Hospitalization is necessary only for acute complications. Because treatment of leprosy in many cases is prolonged, education of the patient and family regarding the disease and its complications is most important.

Until recently dapsone was the mainstay for the treatment of leprosy. An increasing incidence of secondary dapsone resistance has been reported, and more recently, cases of primary dapsone resistance have occurred. Another problem is bacterial persistence following monotherapy. These problems have led the study group of the World Health Organization (WHO) to recommend combination chemotherapy. The most effective regimens and their durations are not known. At present a study group has made the recommendations given in Table 106.2.

TABLE 106.2   Recommendations of WHO Study Group for Treatment of Leprosy

Types of Leprosy	Drugs and Dosages	Duration
Multibacillary leprosy (LL, BL, BB)	Dapsone 100 mg once daily (self-administered)	At least 2 years and until negative for organisms[1]
	Rifampin 600 mg once monthly (supervised)	
	Clofazimine 300 mg once monthly (supervised) and 50 mg daily (self-administered)	
Paucibacillary leprosy (TT, BT)	Dapsone 100 mg once daily (self-administered)	6 months[2]
	Rifampin 600 mg once a month (supervised)	

[1]Exact duration is not known. The objective is to reduce the bacillary population to an extent that resistant mutants are no longer present

[2]Follow closely for relapse. Restart regimen if relapse occurs

The study group recommends that the combined drug treatment for multibacillary patients should be offered to all newly diagnosed patients and to patients who have responded incompletely, have not responded, or have relapsed while on dapsone monotherapy.   Short-course chemotherapy of paucibacillary leprosy should be offered to all newly diagnosed patients, those who have relapsed, and those who are receiving dapsone monotherapy and have not yet completed 2 years of treatment.

For LL and BL leprosy caused by dapsone-resistant strains, a combination of clofazimine with rifampin or ethionamide for at least 2 years, followed by clofazimine monotherapy for life, or a combination of rifampin with ethionamide, indefinitely, has been recommended. Table 106.3 lists the side effects of these drugs.

In the United States, all drugs for leprosy except dapsone are considered investigational. Questions regarding therapy should be addressed to the National Hansen's Disease Center, Carville, Louisiana.

Complications and Prognosis

Complications usually follow the initiation of therapy, within the first year, but may be seen before drugs are administered. Erythema nodosum leprosum (ENL) is usually seen in LL and BL patients, and is an Arthus-type reaction mediated by

TABLE 106.3   Side Effects of Drugs Used in the Treatment of Leprosy

Drug	Side Effect
Dapsone	Hemolytic anemia, agranulocytosis, methemoglobinemia (usually with high dosages), skin rashes, exfoliative dermatitis, peripheral neuropathy, gastrointestinal complaints, cholestatic jaundice, infectious mononucleosis-like syndrome
Clofazimine	Skin pigmentation (may clear slowly when the drug is discontinued); gastrointestinal complaints (crystals deposited in the walls of the small bowel and mesenteric lymph nodes); intestinal obstruction may occasionally develop (dose-related effect); also decreased sweating and tearing
Rifampin	Hepatotoxicity, thrombocytopenia
Ethionamide	Hepatotoxicity and gastrointestinal complaints

immune complexes. Patients usually present with painful, tender nodules, arthritis, high fever, leukemoid reactions, lymphadenopathy, worsening neuritis, and iridocyclitis. The symptoms may last for months. The treatment of choice is thalidomide which, because of its teratogenic properties, should not be administered to women of childbearing age. In the United States, thalidomide is available only from the National Hansen's Disease Center at Carville, Louisiana. The usual dosage is 100 mg four times daily. The symptoms usually subside in 48-72 hr and the dosage can then be tapered over 1-2 weeks to a maintenance dosage of 100 mg daily. Antileprosy treatment should be continued. Prednisone is also effective in controlling symptoms and is recommended if neuritis is present or if thalidomide cannot be used. The usual initial dosage is 60 mg/day. This then can be tapered to an every-other-day schedule. Clofazimine is also fairly effective for ENL. For iridocyclitis, an ophthalmologist should be consulted. Local steroids are generally used.

Reversal reactions are thought to be caused by an increase in the patient's cell-mediated immune response to *M. leprae*. The existing skin lesions may become worse, become more erythematous and edematous, and may ulcerate. Fever and leukocytosis may occur. One of the most worrisome problems is impending loss of nerve function, most probably from increased inflammatory cell infiltration. Prednisone is generally recommended at a usual dosage of 50 mg/day. Several days after the symptoms are controlled, the dosage can be tapered.

Apart from reversal reactions and ENL, major complications of leprosy include the disabling deformities with subsequent loss of function. The stigma associated with leprosy unfortunately still persists in many cultures resulting in social and psychologic problems. With better education this should improve. An uncommon complication is amyloidosis. Overall mortality in leprosy is quite low.

Prevention

Examination of household contacts of patients is important. Follow-up at regular intervals for a few years is generally necessary. Family members should be educated regarding early signs of leprosy. Those contacts of multibacillary cases who are less than 25 years old, may be given dapsone for 3 years, although this is not a universally accepted recommendation. The results of BCG trials have yielded varying results from very good to very little protection.

Currently, there is a tremendous interest in a vaccine for leprosy. Use of *M. leprae,* grown in armadillos and then heat killed, is planned, but the demonstration of effectiveness of the vaccine will require several years. Another approach is combining *M. leprae* vaccine and BCG. This combined approach restores cell-mediated immunity in patients with lepromatous leprosy and promotes clearance of bacilli.

Selected Bibliography

Albert, D. A., Weisman, M. H., and Kaplan, R.: The rheumatic manifestations of leprosy (Hansen disease). *Medicine* 59:442-448, 1980.

Bach, M. A., Chatenoud, L., Wallach, D., Tuy, F. P. D., and Cottenot, F.: Studies on T cell subsets and functions in leprosy. *Clin Exp Immunol* 44:491-500, 1981.

Binford, C. H., Meyers, W. M., and Walsh, G. P.: Leprosy. *JAMA* 247:2283-2292, 1982.

Bullock, W. E., Fields, J. P., Brandriss, M. W.: An evaluation of transfer factor as immunotherapy for patients with lepromatous leprosy. *N Engl J Med* 287: 1053-1059, 1972.

Enna, C. D.: Rehabilitation of leprous deformity. *Ann Rev Med* 33:41-45, 1982.

Godal, T.: Immunological aspects of leprosy - present status. *Prog Allergy* 25: 211-242, 1978.

Grove, D. I., Warren, K. S., Mahmoud, A. A. F.: Algorithms in the diagnosis and management of exotic diseases. XV. Leprosy. *J Infect Dis* 134:205-210, 1976.

Jacobson, R. R.: The treatment of leprosy (Hansen's disease). *Hosp Formul* 17: 1076-1091, 1982.

Jariwala, H. J. and Kelkar, S. S.: Fluorescence microscopy for detection of *M. leprae* in tissue sections. *Int J Lepr* 47:33-36, 1979.

Levis, W. R., Schuman, J. S., Friedman, S. M., and Newfield, S. A.: An epidemiologic evaluation of leprosy in New York City. *JAMA* 247:3221-3226, 1982.

Maugh, T. II.: Leprosy vaccine trials to begin soon. *Science* 215:1083-1086, 1982.

Ng, W. L., Scollard, D. M., Hua, A.: Glomerulonephritis in leprosy. *Am J Clin Pathol* 76:321-329, 1981.

Opromolla, D. V. A., Tonello, C. J. S., McDougall, A. C., and Yawalkar, S. J.: A controlled trial to compare the therapeutic effects of dapsone in combination with daily or once-monthly rifampin in patients with lepromatous leprosy. *Int J Lepr* 49:393-397, 1981.

Ridley, D. S.: Reactions in leprosy. *Lepr Rev* 40:77-81, 1969.

Ridley, D. S. and Jopling, W. H.: Classification of leprosy according to immunity. A five-group system. *Int J Lepr* 34:255-273, 1964.

Saha, K. and Agarwal, S. K.: Immune deficit in patients with lepromatous leprosy: Its nature and relation to genetic factors, spectrum, and duration of the illness. *Int J Lepr* 47:1-6, 1979.

Sehgal, S. and Kumar, B.: Circulating and tissue immune complexes in leprosy. *Int J Lepr* 49:294-301, 1981.

Van Voorhis, W. C., Kaplan, G., Sarno, E. N., Horwitz, M. A., Steinman, R. M., Levis, W. R., Nogueira, N., Hair, L. S., Gattass, C. R., Arrick, B. A., and Cohn, Z. A.: The cutaneous infiltrates of leprosy: Cellular characteristics and the predominant T-cell phenotypes. *N Engl J Med* 307:1593-1597, 1982.

Weissman, J. B. and Neu, H. C.: Lepromatous leprosy masquerading as disseminated tuberculosis. *Am J Med* 67:113-116, 1979.

WHO Study Group: Chemotherapy of leprosy for control programmes. *WHO, Tech Rep Ser* 675:1-33, 1982.

107

ACTINOMYCETES

Robert H. Waldman, M.D. and
Melanie A. Fisher, M.D.

The actinomycetes are the fungus-like bacteria which derived their name from *aktino* (Greek for ray). This refers to the radial arrangement of the club-shaped elements formed in tissue by the major human pathogen in this group. The suffix *mykes* is the Greek for mushroom or fungus. The actinomycetes, along with the family which contains the mycobacteria, make up the order Actinomycetales.

They have long been considered to be fungi for the following reasons: their filamentous growth which leads to mycelial colonies; they cause chronic subcutaneous granulomatous abscesses; and some of these species grow on media which traditionally are used to grow fungi, such as Sabouraud's media.

The evidence that they are bacteria, however, is summarized in Table 107.1. Their taxonomy is summarized in Table 107.2.

Actinomyces

There are two species of the genus *Actinomyces* that are of medical importance: *A. bovis* and *A. israelii*. The characteristics of these organisms are outlined in Table 107.3. In tissue the organism grows into what is known as a sulfur granule, caused by mycelial clumps 1-2 mm in diameter, in a matrix of calcium phosphate; the sulfur granule is yellow white. When the organism is grown in culture, filaments are formed. However, in older cultures or in vivo, there is increased septation, leading to fragmentation into bacillary, or even coccoid forms, of irregular size, and appearing much like diphtheroids.

TABLE 107.1   Evidence That Actinomycetes Are Bacteria

Prokaryotic (i.e., lack a nuclear membrane)

Diameter of filaments: < 1 μm, much narrower than hyphae

Content of cell wall

    Contains muramic and diaminopinelic acids, characteristic of bacteria

    PAS-negative and contains no chitin or glucans, characteristic of fungi

Sensitivity to antimicrobial agents

    Growth inhibited by common antibacterial agents, all of which are innocuous for fungi

    Insensitive to polyenes, since cell membranes contain no sterols

Motile forms possess simple flagella of the bacterial type

There are anaerobic forms

They are parasitized by bacteriophages

TABLE 107.2   Taxonomy of Actinomycetes

Class: Schizomycetes

Order: Eubacteriales
Chlamydobacteriales
Pseudomonadales
Actinomycetales

Family: Mycobacteriaceae
Family: Actinomycetaceae
    Genus: *Nocardia*
    Genus: *Actinomyces*

Family: Streptomycetaceae
Family: Micromonosporaceae

TABLE 107.3   Characteristics of *Actinomyces*

Gram-positive pleomorphic, rod-shaped

Branching filaments 0.5-2 μm in diameter

Not acid-fast

No spore formation

Anaerobic or microaerophilic, growing better when CO_2 is added to medium

Grow on agar as white, spherical, or lobulated colonies

Require rich media, e.g., blood or brain-heart infusion

Poor growth below $37^\circ C$

Epidemiology

Actinomyces is not found in the soil or in vegetation, but it is easily isolated from the mouth. It can be cultured from most tonsils and nearly always from scrapings from around the teeth and gums. Although the organism is ubiquitous, the disease occurs mainly in rural areas. There is a male/female ratio of about 2:1. Actinomycosis is found in a worldwide distribution, but has been decreasing in frequency over recent years for reasons that are not readily apparent. Putting all of these somewhat unrelated facts together, it seems most reasonable that the disease is related to the presence of severely carious teeth, although this does not completely explain all of the observations.

What definitely has been established is that the disease in cattle is of no epidemiologic relationship to the human disease. There has been no animal-to-human transmission. Laboratory animals are generally not susceptible to the organism.

Pathogenesis

Actinomycosis is an opportunistic infection. It becomes invasive with severe caries and a great deal of necrotic tissue, secondary to trauma or aspiration, and rarely as a result of human bites, the latter being the only example of person-to-person transmission. The infection is almost always a mixed one, with primarily anaerobic bacteria being co-infecting organisms. Occasionally, one sees hematogenous dissemination leading to brain abscess and infective endocarditis.

Pathologically one sees abscess formation, the abscesses containing granules surrounded by polymorphonuclear leukocytes, with later a minimal amount of chronic granulomatous reaction with giant cells. Abscesses expand and eventually form burrowing, tortuous sinuses to the skin surfaces, ultimately leading to discharge of purulent material. Penetration onto mucosal surfaces is less common than onto skin surfaces. Bone invasion is uncommon, in contradistinction to the disease in cattle, in which involvement of the bones of the face leads to the disease lumpy jaw.

Clinical Manifestations

The classic picture of actinomycosis is cervical-facial involvement, which occurs in 30-40% of the cases. The subcutaneous tissue at the angle of the jaw and the adjacent areas of the neck is indurated (the so-called woody edema). The skin over this area is red, with one or more draining sinus tracts. Despite the appearance, pain is minimal. Chest involvement occurs in about 20% of the patients. Cough and fever are minimal at first, and there is pulmonary consolidation, pleurisy, and eventually, draining sinuses. Later the patient has weight loss, night sweats, and high fever. Abdominal involvement occurs in about half of the patients; the origin usually being the cecum and the appendix. An abdominal mass is present, and there are sinus tracts to the inguinal area. The disease may also spread retroperitoneally.

Diagnosis

Pus should be examined for sulfur granules. These range from being barely visible to several millimeters in diameter. The culture will almost always be positive for other organisms, even if washed sulfur granules are cultured. The organisms that one most commonly isolates are fusiform bacilli, anaerobic streptococci, and *Actinobacillus actinomycetemcomitans* (species incertae sedis). From the name of the latter, it is obvious that this organism has been found mainly in association with actinomycosis.

Serologic testing may be of occasional benefit. The agar double-diffusion test is positive in about 90% of the patients with disseminated disease. It is negative in patients with localized infection. One of the more interesting aspects of this test is that there are false-positive reactions in patients with tuberculosis, pointing out the similarities between these two organisms. Fluorescent antibody to the organism has been somewhat useful in identifying the bacteria in smears of tissue or exudates. There is no skin test that is of value in diagnosing actinomycosis.

Therapy

Untreated, the lesion spreads slowly but inexorably, and the prognosis is poor. Penicillin is the most effective antibiotic, and combined with drainage and debridement, one should expect a cure in most cases. The cervical-facial disease has a better prognosis (90% cure) than the thoracic or abdominal disease. Alternative antibiotics are tetracycline, chloramphenicol, and streptomycin.

Nocardia

There are three species of *Nocardia* that are of clinical importance: *N. asteroides, N. brasiliensis,* and *N. caviae.* The characteristics of the organisms are shown in Table 107.4. The velvety nature of the colonies is due to the aerial mycelia, but when they are smeared and stained the filaments break up into the bacillary or coccoid bodies. The sugar content of the pathogenic species is important in differentiating the organisms from the nonpathogenic species, of which there are nearly 40. The relatively slow growth of the organisms on culture may lead to difficulty in isolation, due to overgrowth with other bacteria.

TABLE 107.4   Characteristics of Nocardia

Optimum growth at 5-10% CO_2, 37°C

Not so fastidious, growing on simple media and at wide temperature range

Velvety colonies

On smear, appear bacillary or coccoid

Somewhat acid-fast

Pathogenic species contain arabinose plus galactose, or madurose

Somewhat slow growing, colonies not appearing until 48-72 hr

Nocardia are related to mycobacteria in several ways, with the similarities and differences shown in Table 107.5.

Epidemiology

Nocardia are saprophytes in soil, dust, plants, water; in essence, any decaying organic matter and many mammals are natural hosts. Nocard's original isolation was from cattle in Guadeloupe in 1888; however, the distribution is worldwide. The most common age group affected in man is between 20 and 50 years with a male/female ratio of about 3-4:1. This male preponderance is probably related to occupational exposure. There is probably no animal-to-human, or human-to-human transmission.

Pathogenesis

Humans are infected most commonly by inhaling organisms, but also may be infected by traumatic implantation through the skin, most commonly in the feet. The infection is much more common in patients with decreased host defenses, particularly those with lymphoreticular neoplasia or those receiving immunosuppressive agents, although more than half of the patients have no underlying disease.

The primary infection leads to a necrotizing pneumonia and abscess formation. There is very little inflammatory response, encapsulation, or granuloma formation. Sulfur granules are rare, and there is really very little that is distinctive pathologically. The infection may extend into the pleural cavity and then through the chest wall. Lymphohematogenous spread leads to metastatic infection in 20% of the patients, nearly all of whom have brain abscesses. A brain abscess may be seen in a patient with a relatively small pulmonary lesion. Occasionally, other organs are involved, with the pericardium, bone, kidneys, and eye being involved, in that order of frequency.

TABLE 107.5   Relationship of *Nocardia* and Mycobacteria

Similarities

Colonies resemble saprophytic mycobacteria

Somewhat acid-fast (younger cultures more than older), decolorized by acid alcohol

Serologically related

Some common bacteriophages

Differences

More rapid growth

Less acid-fast

Tendency to branch

Not resistant to 4% NaOH

Susceptibility to antituberculous drugs

Clinical Manifestations

Patients have a productive cough and fever. Sputum is not malodorous, but is thick, tenacious, purulent, and blood-tinged. There may be no leukocytosis and in general, the symptoms are fairly nonspecific. The patients may have various central nervous system symptoms, suggesting the presence of a brain abscess. Mycetomas, which contain granules, may cause bone destruction and sinus tracts.

Diagnosis

The diagnosis is made by isolating the organism. The lack of success in making the diagnosis is apparent from the fact that 40% of the diagnoses are made at autopsy. Biopsy material is an important source for culture. Histologic examination of biopsy material is less helpful, since the organisms are not easily seen (Figure 107.1). The best methods for staining the organism are the methenamine silver stain or the Brown and Brenn modification of the Gram stain. The laboratory must be warned of the possibility of infection with *Nocardia* spp, because of the slow growth of the organism.

Nocardia are occasional saprophytes of the upper respiratory tract, so a single isolate is of questionable significance.

No useful immunologic tests for the diagnosis of nocardiosis have been developed.

Treatment

Without treatment, most patients die in about 6 months. Even with treatment, patients with brain abscess have a high mortality, more than 80%. The treatment of choice is surgical drainage combined with antimicrobial agents. One of the

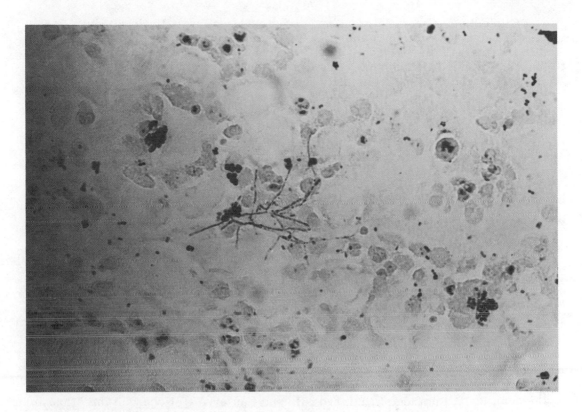

FIGURE 107.1   Gram stain of sputum showing *Nocardia* (in center of figure).

sulfonamides should be used alone or in combination with another drug. One needs to obtain a peak concentration of 12–15 mg% sulfonamide in the blood. Cycloserine has been used in combination with a sulfonamide. An alternative approach is to use the combination of trimethoprim and sulfamethoxazole (Septra; Bactrim). There are several reports of the effectiveness of dapsone. Many other antibiotics have been shown to be active in vitro but have not yet been proved in vivo. It is of interest that the antituberculous drugs are of no benefit in treating nocardial infections.

Mycetoma (Madura Foot)

Mycetomas may be caused by at least 20 different species of actinomycetes and fungi, most commonly *Nocardia* and *Streptomyces,* and the fungi *Madurella mycetomatis* and *Petriellidium boydii* (previously *Allescheria boydii*). The infection derives its name from the fact that it was first described in Madura, India, in 1712.

The disease is found worldwide but predominantly in tropical areas, with the Sudan the most common location. It is seen most frequently in adult males.

The infection occurs as a result of trauma resulting in granuloma formation with giant cells. Rarely, one sees lymphohematogenous spread.

Clinically one sees grotesque and disfiguring swelling with sinus tracts. Granules are common. Although the disease is most common in the feet, lesions may also be seen on the shoulders and buttocks of laborers, as well as on the back and hands. There is little pain or systemic symptoms or signs.

The diagnosis is made clinically and by the identification of granules. Culture is difficult because of the many different organisms that may cause the disease.

The therapy is appropriate antimicrobial agents with debridement, although the latter is not usually efficacious alone. Amputation may be needed.

Thermophilic Actinomycetes

While not an infectious disease, thermophilic actinomycetes do lead to illness, i.e., farmer's lung disease. This is a result of the immunologic reaction to inhaling these organisms. Two organisms which cause this disease are *Thermoactinomyces vulgaris* and *Micropolyspora faeni*.

Selected Bibliography

Adams, J. N. and McClung, D. M.: Comparison of the development cycles of some members of the genus *Nocardia.* *J Bacteriol* 84:206–216, 1962.

Aron, R. and Gordon, W.: Pulmonary nocardiosis. Case report and evaluation of current therapy. *S Afr Med J* 46:29–32, 1972.

Beaman, B. L., Burnside, J., Edwards, B., and Causey, W.: Nocardial infections in the United States, 1972–1974. *J Infect Dis* 134:286–289, 1976.

Butz, W. C. and Ajello, L.: Black grain mycetoma. *Arch Dermatol* 104:197–201, 1971.

Causey, W. A.: *Nocardia caviae:* A report of 13 new isolations with clinical correlation. *Appl Microbiol* 28:193–198, 1974.

Coleman, R. M. and George, L. K.: Comparative pathogenicity of *Actinomyces naeslundii* and *Actinomyces israelii.* *Appl Microbiol* 18:427–432, 1969.

Curry, W. A.: Human nocardiosis. A clinical review with selected case reports. *Arch Intern Med* 140:818–826, 1980.

Evans, R. A. and Benson, R. E.: Complicated nocardiosis treated with trimethoprim and sulfamethoxazole. *Med J Aust* 58:684–685, 1971.

Faias, N., Taplin, D., and Rebell, G.: Mycetoma. *Arch Dermatol* 99:215–225, 1969.

Filice, G. A., Beaman, B. L., Krick, J. A., and Remington, J. S.: Effect of human neutrophils and monocytes on *Nocardia asteroides:* Failure of killing despite occurrence of the oxidative metabolic burst. *J Infect Dis* 142:432, 1980.

Frazier, A. R., Rosenow, E. C., III, and Roberts, G. D.: Nocardiosis: A review of 25 cases occurring during 24 months. *Mayo Clin Proc* 50:657–663, 1975.

Geiseler, P. J., Check, F., Lamothe, F., and Anderson, B. R.: Failure of trimetho-prim/sulfamethoxazole in invasive *Nocardia asteroides* infection. *Arch Intern Med* 139:355–356, 1979.

Hoeprich, P. D., Brandt, D., and Parker, R. H.: Nocardial brain abscess cured with cycloserine and sulfonamides. *Am J Med Sci* 255:208–215, 1968.

Krick, J. A., Stinson, E. B., and Remington, J. S.: Nocardia infection in heart transplant patients. *Ann Intern Med* 82:18–26, 1975.

Laberge, D. E. and Stahmann, M. A.: Antigens from *Thermopolyspora polyspora* involved in farmer's lung. *Proc Soc Exp Biol Med* 121:463–468, 1966.

Lechevalier, M. P.: Identification of aerobic actinomycetes of clinical impor-tance. *J Lab Clin Med* 71:934–944, 1968.

Lechevalier, M. P., Horan, A. C., and Lechevalier, H. A.: Lipid composition in the classification of nocardial and mycobacteria. *J Bacteriol* 105:313–318, 1971.

Lerner, P. I.: Susceptibility of pathogenic actinomycetes to antimicrobial com-pounds. *Antimicrob Agents Chemother* 5:302, 1974.

Mohr, J. A. and Muchmore, H. G.: Maduromycosis due to *Allescheria boydii.* *JAMA* 204:335–336, 1968.

Orfanakis, M. G., Wilcox, H. G., and Smith, C. B.: In vitro studies of the com-bined effect of ampicillin and sulfonamides on *Nocardia asteroides* and results of therapy in four patients. *Antimicrob Agents Chemother* 1:215–220, 1972.

Yogev, R., Greenslade, T., Firbit, C. F., and Lewy, P.: Successful treatment of *Nocardia asteroides* infection with amikacin. *J Pediatr* 96:771–773, 1980.

E. Fungi

INTRODUCTION TO FUNGAL DISEASES
Robert H. Waldman, M.D.

Fungal infections are generally considered to be fairly rare and therefore do not receive as much emphasis as viral or bacterial diseases. However, they are more important than generally recognized, and are becoming ever more important as we have more patients who are immunosuppressed, either because of an underlying disease process or as a result of therapy.

It is of historic interest that a fungus was the very first microorganism proved to cause a human disease. Nearly 140 years ago *Microsporum audouinii* was shown to be the cause of tinea capitis. Even before the modern era of aggressive therapy of malignancies, more extensive surgical procedures, and transplantation, fungal infections were of great importance. Although thought to be relatively rare diseases, they were not. Histoplasmosis and coccidioidomycosis alone infect nearly half of the population of the United States. Obviously, almost all of these infections are mild or inapparent. Also, several major advances in treatment of fungal infections antedated this modern "immunosuppression" era.

As mentioned, since 1960, fungal infections have grown in importance because of the association with diseases which cause impaired host defenses. The best examples are patients with leukemia or lymphoma receiving treatment and transplant patients. Currently, serious fungal infections are found at autopsy in 2% of patients overall, 5-10% of patients with solid tumors, and in 20-50% of patients dying of leukemia. A large majority are not diagnosed or treated antemortem. Fifteen percent or more of renal transplant patients will have a fungal infection at some time in their course. Another important predisposing factor is large plastic intravenous catheters which are left in place for several days.

Classification

Fungi can be classified in several different ways, and different approaches are shown in Table I. From a practical clinical point of view, fungal infections are best divided into those which are superficial and those which are systemic. The superficial mycoses are described in detail in Chapter 108.

TABLE I   Classification of Fungi Commonly Pathogenic for Humans

Class	Representative Examples
Taxonomic	
Phycomycetes	*Rhizopus, Mucor*
Ascomycetes	*Aspergillus*
Deuteromycetes	Most human pathogens
Anatomic	
Superficial	*Trichophyton, Candida*
Subcutaneous	*Sporotrichum schenckii; Cladosporium* and *Fonsecaea* (chromoblastomycosis); and *Madurella* and others (maduromycosis)
Systemic	*Cryptococcus neoformans, Blastomyces dermatitidis,* etc.
Pathogenesis	
Opportunistic	*Candida, Aspergillus*
Sometimes opportunistic	*Cryptococcus neoformans*
Nonopportunistic	*Histoplasma capsulatum, Coccidioides immitis, Blastomyces dermatitidis*
Invasion	*Cryptococcus, Histoplasma*
Allergy	*Aspergillus*
Toxicosis	*Aspergillus flavus* food poisoning, mushroom poisoning

A helpful way to conceptualize the deep mycoses is to divide them into three major categories. The first category, at one end of the spectrum, is the opportunistic fungal infections. These fungi only rarely cause invasive or systemic disease in normal individuals. They are commonly part of the normal or indigenous flora of the respiratory, gastrointestinal, or female genital tract, and they may cause relatively mild, though troublesome, superficial infections. It is these fungi which have grown so important in recent years because they cause very severe infections in patients who have compromised host defenses. The best examples of this group are the *Candida* and *Aspergillus* spp.

The second category of deep mycoses can be thought of as true pathogens, since they appear to be pathogenic for nearly all people. They are not part of the normal flora, and when isolated must be thought of as a pathogen. However, there are "opportunistic" aspects of the fungal infections in this category, since some people are susceptible to severe types of illness caused by these fungi, while others have only mild or inapparent illness. There are racial and immunologic factors which have an effect on how one handles infection with the fungi in this group, somewhat analagous to tuberculosis. The best examples of fungi in this group are *Histoplasma capsulatum* and *Coccidioides immitis*.

The third group has only one member, and that is *Cryptococcus neoformans*. This organism behaves in an intermediate fashion, i.e., normal people, at least as far as can be determined by present day immunologic techniques, occasionally have serious infection with *C. neoformans,* developing cryptococcal meningitis. On the other hand, the disease is much more common in individuals with impaired host defenses, e.g., patients with Hodgkin's disease, or patients receiving corticosteroids for any reason. With the greater prevalence of patients who are immunosuppressed, normal people make up a smaller and smaller fraction of the total patient population with cryptococcal meningitis. It is not part of the normal flora and it does not cause trivial superficial mucosal or skin infections.

Treatment

While there are a great number of individual differences with respect to treatment of fungal infections, there are some common features which will be discussed here. A high index of suspicion, especially in patients with predisposing factors, is especially important in the management of invasive fungal infections because early institution of therapy is often a prerequisite for a successful outcome.

The mainstay of treatment of the deep mycotic infections is amphotericin B. This is a very effective, though fairly toxic, antifungal agent. Unfortunately, there is no other agent available that can reliably be used to treat most fungal infections, and there is none on the immediate horizon.

The approach to administering amphotericin B is outlined in Table II. Amphotericin B is given in 5% dextrose in water, at a concentration no higher than 10 mg/100 ml, and should be given over 2-6 hr. The preparation is complexed with desoxycholate as a colloidal suspension. Therefore, no electrolytes may be given in the same intravenous solution. There has been no noticeable decrease in effectiveness when amphotericin B is given every other day, rather than daily. In some situations, it has even been given every third day, thereby allowing patients who can stay outside of the hospital to live fairly normal lives. It has been recommended that the dose be adjusted depending upon the in vitro sensitivity of the organism, but this has not been shown to be of definite clinical value, and it certainly adds to the complexity of caring for the patient. For a sensitive organism, the usual inhibiting level of amphotericin B is 0.1-0.8 µg/ml. The dosage may be

TABLE II   Use of Amphotericin B

	Usual Patient	Emergency Situation, Patient Moribund or Rapidly Becoming So
Day 1	2 mg	5 mg "test" dose followed by 10 mg later same day
Day 2	5 mg	20 mg
Day 3	10 mg	30 mg
Subsequent days	Increase by 5 mg/day until patient stable or toxicity (usual renal) supervenes, then switch to q.o.d. dosage schedule, attempting to give 0.5-1.0 mg/kg, q.d.	Increase by 10 mg/day until patient stabilized or reach 1.0 mg/kg/day

adjusted to obtain a peak serum level of twice the minimal inhibiting concentration. The suspension is slightly light sensitive, but this is of no clinical significance, and therefore the intravenous solution does not have to be shaded from room light.

Excretion and plasma levels of amphotericin B are unaffected by renal or hepatic failure. Hemodialysis does not alter the blood levels.

Amphotericin B can be given intrathecally or intraventricularly, the usual dosage being 0.5 mg twice or thrice weekly.

As mentioned earlier, side effects of amphotericin B therapy are a major problem. Fever, malaise, chills, and vomiting are not dose-related, and can usually be mitigated by the concomitant administration of low-dose corticosteroids, such as 100 mg hydrocortisone in the intravenous bottle. The frequency of thrombophlebitis may be decreased by the use of 1000 U of heparin in the IV solution. Anemia and hypokalemia are dose-related toxicities but usually can be managed fairly easily. The most disturbing side effect is the nephrotoxicity of amphotericin B, which is dose-related and only partially reversible. The nephrotoxicity of the drug should not preclude its use when necessary. Many attempts have been made to try to prevent the nephrotoxicity of amphotericin B, but without uniform success. Such measures as administration of mannitol, and alkalinization of the urine have not been studied in a controlled fashion, but may be of some benefit.

Organisms do not usually become resistant to amphotericin B in the course of therapy. There have been some laboratory-derived resistant organisms, but these seem to be less virulent than the naturally occurring amphotericin-sensitive organisms.

Two similar antifungal agents are nystatin and natamycin. Nystatin is very similar to amphotericin B, but is too toxic for parenteral use. It is given topically or orally, which leads to negligible systemic absorption. Natamycin is a topical preparation which is used for the treatment of fungal keratitis, blepharitis, or conjunctivitis.

Miconazole represents a different class of antifungal agents. No serious renal or hepatic toxicity has been reported with the use of miconazole; however, side effects are fairly frequent, although probably not as severe as those following amphotericin B. About 30% of patients develop thrombophlebitis, a similar number develop hyponatremia, and a smaller number develop fever, chills, rash, or anemia. Miconazole may be of some use in the treatment of infections caused by *Candida, Coccidioides, Paracoccidioides, Cryptococcus,* and *Aspergillus.* It appears to be of limited usefulness in the treatment of meningitis or urinary tract infections. At this time, miconazole should be reserved for use in patients who have been treatment failures with other forms of antifungal therapy.

5-Fluorocytosine (flucytosine) is an agent which has the advantage of being absorbed following oral administration. It is relatively nontoxic except for bone marrow depression (seen primarily in face of renal dysfunction), but it has the significant disadvantage that organisms very quickly develop resistance in the course of therapy. It is ineffective in histoplasmosis, blastomycosis, and coccidioidomycosis. Its main value is that it is quite effective when used in combination with amphotericin B, and this has been especially well studied in the treatment of cryptococcal meningitis. 5-Fluorocytosine, as well as other agents, are receiving increasing attention in combinations as a way of treating fungal infections more effectively, with less toxicity, since it appears that lower doses of amphotericin B can be used. The mechanism of the synergistic activity is that amphotericin B increases the ability of a variety of agents to penetrate the fungal cytoplasmic membrane but avoids toxicity to human cells, since amphotericin B has very little similar effect on animal cell membranes. When used in combination, it is advisable to monitor blood levels of 5-fluorocytosine, to keep peak blood levels between 50 and 75 µg/ml.

Selected Bibliography

Bennett, J. E.: Chemotherapy of systemic mycoses. *N Engl J Med* 290:30–32, 320–323, 1974.

Bennett, J. E.: Flucytosine. *Ann Intern Med* 86:319–322, 1977.

Bindschadler, D. D. and Bennett, J. E.: A pharmacologic guide to the clinical use of amphotericin B. *J Infect Dis* 120:427–436, 1969.

Block, E. R., Jennings, A. E., and Bennett, J. E.: 5-Fluorocytosine resistance in *Cryptococcus neoformans. Antimicrob Agents Chemother* 3:649–656, 1973.

Butler, W. T., Bennett, J. E., Alling, D. W., Wertlake, P. T., Utz, J. P., and Hill, G. J., II: Nephrotoxicity of amphotericin B: Early and late effects in 81 patients. *Ann Intern Med* 61:175–187, 1964.

Cosgrove, R. F., Beezer, A. E., and Miles, R. J.: In vitro studies of amphotericin B in combination with the imidazole antifungal compounds clotrimazole and miconazole. *J Infect Dis* 138:681–685, 1978.

Curry, C. R. and Quie, P. G.: Fungal septicemia in patients receiving parenteral hyperalimentation. *N Engl J Med* 285:1221–1225, 1971.

Fass, R. J. and Perkins, R. L.: Five-fluorocytosine in the treatment of cryptococcal and candida mycoses. *Ann Intern Med* 74:535, 1971.

Kaufman, C. A., Carleton, J. A., and Frame, P. T.: Simple assay for 5-fluorocytosine in the presence of amphotericin B. *Antimicrob Agents Chemother* 9: 381-383, 1976.

Kauffman, C. A. and Frame, P. T.: Bone marrow toxicity associated with 5-fluorocytosine therapy. *Antimicrob Agents Chemother* 11:244, 1977.

Medoff, G. and Kobayashi, G. S.: Strategies in the treatment of systemic fungal infections. *N Engl J Med* 302:145-155, 1980.

Sarosi, G. A., Armstrong, D., Barbee, R. A., Bates, J. H., Campbell, G. D., George, R. B., Goldstein, R. S., Schaffner, W., and Stevens, D. A.: Treatment of fungal diseases. *Am Rev Respir Dis* 120:1393-1397, 1979.

Singer, C., Kaplan, M. H., and Armstrong, D.: Bacteremia and fungemia complicating neoplastic disease. A study of 364 cases. *Am J Med* 62:731, 1977.

Stevens, D. A., Levine, H. B., and Deresinski, S. C.: Miconazole in coccidioidomycosis. *Am J Med* 60:191, 1976.

108

SUPERFICIAL AND CUTANEOUS MYCOSES
Robert H. Waldman, M.D.

Dermatophytoses

Dermatophyte infections, also known as tinea or ringworm (Table 108.1), are caused by three genera of fungi which metabolize keratin. Therefore they are capable of growing on the superficial stratum corneum of the skin, the nails, or hair. There are many species of fungi which cause dermatophytoses, and a single specie may cause more than one type of clinical syndrome. Similarly, a single clinical syndrome, e.g., ringworm of the scalp, may be caused by several species. It is not usually possible, nor clinically important, to make a specific etiologic diagnosis in tinea infections.

The three genera of dermatophytes are *Epidermophyton,* which has only one specie, *E. floccosum,* which causes skin and nail infections but does not infect hair; *Microsporum,* which infects skin and hair, but not nails; and *Trichophyton,* which infects skin, hair, and nails (Tables 108.2 and 108.3).

The ecology of dermatophytes is varied (Table 108.4) with some being geophilic, i.e., found in soil, e.g., *M. gypseum.* Some are zoophilic, i.e., mainly pathogens of animals, and infecting humans by contact or as a result of fomites. An example is *M. canis,* which is transmitted to humans from puppies and kittens. (It is of interest that, like the human situation, *M. canis* does not usually cause infection of adult animals.) Several dermatophyte species are anthropophilic, i.e., are spread by either direct or indirect person-to-person contact. An example of an anthropophilic dermatophyte is *M. audouinii.*

Up to 90% of the population in temperate climates will have athlete's foot at some time in their lives, with *T. mentagrophytes* the most common causal agent.

Tinea capitis is related to socioeconomic factors. In Somalia, for example, the disease is found in more than one-third of boys 5-10 years of age.

TABLE 108.1   Clinical Types of Tinea Infections

Tinea capitis

Tinea favosa

Tinea barbae

Tinea corporis

Tinea imbricata

Tinea cruris

Tinea pedis

Tinea manuum

Tinea unguium

TABLE 108.2   Dermatophytes

Organism	Part of Dermis Involved	Clinical	
E. floccosum	Skin, nails	Tinea corporis, tinea pedis	
Microsporum spp	Skin, hair		Produces fluorescence with Wood's UV light
M. audouinii		Childhood epidemic tinea capitis	
M. canis		Tinea corporis	
M. fulvum		Sporadic tinea corporis, tinea capitis, and tinea barbae	
Trichophyton spp	Skin, hair, nails		
T. mentagrophytes		Tinea pedis and tinea unguium	
T. rubrum		Most common cause of tinea pedis and tinea unguium in U.S.	
T. soudanense		More inflammatory types of tinea capitis and tinea corporis	
T. tonsurans		Tinea capitis in all age groups	Common in slums

TABLE 108.3   Dermatophytes Most Commonly Associated with Clinical Syndromes

Tinea Syndrome	Site	Organisms
Capitis (epidemic)	Scalp	M. audouinii T. tonsurans
(nonepidemic)		M. canis T. verrucosum
Favosa	Scalp, torso	T. schoenleinii T. violaceum
Barbae	Beard	T. rubrum T. verrucosum
Corporis	Arms, legs, torso	T. rubrum T. mentagrophytes M. canis
Crurus	Genitocrural	T. rubrum T. mentagrophytes E. floccosum
Pedis and manus	Feet and hands	T. rubrum T. mentagrophytes
Unguium	Nails	T. rubrum T. mentagrophytes E. floccosum

TABLE 108.4   Ecology of Dermatophytes

Anthropophilic	Zoophilic	Geophilic
E. floccosum	M. canis (dogs, cats)	M. gypseum
M. audouinii	M. gallinae (birds	M. fulvum
T. mentagrophytes	T. mentagrophytes (rodents)	M. nanum
T. schoenleinii	T. verrucosum (cattle)	T. ajelloi
T. tonsurans	T. equinum (horses)	T. terrestre
T. violaceum	M. nanum (pigs)	
T. rubrum		

Moisture aids the growth of dermatophytes, with infections occurring most frequently at moist parts of the body surface. For example, athlete's foot only occurs where people wear shoes. There are other factors in pathogenesis, e.g., some of the organisms only grow in children before puberty. There is evidence that the skin acidity or other sebaceous gland changes which occur during adolescence turn a hospitable environment into a hostile one for the fungi.

Dermatophyte lesions are classically superficial, chronic, slow-spreading, and relatively asymptomatic. If symptoms are present, they usually are a result of secondary bacterial infection.

Tinea corporis, ringworm of the body, is usually pruritic, ringed, scaling, with central clearing, and with small vesicles at the periphery of the lesions. It is found on exposed parts of the body and is most commonly a result of a zoophilic dermatophyte.

Tinea pedis, athlete's foot, is the most common dermatophytic infection. It is seen in adults in the summer months, and presents as blisters on the instep of the foot, with interdigital scaling or, in severe cases, widespread fine scaling on the soles, with accentuation in the creases, leading to the term "moccasin foot."

Tinea capitis, ringworm of the scalp, is a persistent, contagious, often epidemic dermatophytic infection. It is usually asymptomatic, but patients may have some pruritus. The lesions are scaly, erythematous, and usually described as causing alopecia. However, the involved areas are not really bald, but the hairs are broken off at or near the surface of the skin. The infection occasionally involves the eyebrows. Most cases of tinea capitis are caused by *Microsporum* spp, which causes a brilliant green fluorescence when exposed to a Wood's lamp. Tinea capitis usually disappears at puberty.

Tinea barbae, ringworm of the beard, is pustular, or causes large, erythematous, edematous nodules with pustules on them, called kerions. Tinea cruris, jock-itch, is characterized by erythema of the groin and inner thighs, sharply margined with raised scaly borders. As indicated by its common name, it is very pruritic. Onchomycosis commonly accompanies superficial fungal infections elsewhere, and causes yellow discoloration of the nails.

The differential diagnosis of the various dermatophytoses includes psoriasis, erythema multiforme, and pityriasis rosea. Diagnosis is clinical, and as mentioned previously, identification of the exact etiologic agent is rarely necessary in terms of treatment of the individual patient. Diagnostic laboratory tests include microscopic examination of potassium hydroxide preparation of skin scrapings, fungal culture, and examination with a Wood's fluorescent light (Table 108.5).

TABLE 108.5   Laboratory Diagnosis of Superficial Fungal Infections

Direct demonstration: 15% KOH preparation of scrapings from lesion

Culture

Wood's (UV) light

Histopathologic sections of biopsy material stained with periodic acid-Schiff

Treatment involves topical and/or systemic agents, but it must be emphasized that since dermatophyte infections are rarely more than a nuisance causing very little morbidity and no mortality, a decision not to treat is valid, and if treatment is undertaken, it must be absolutely safe and also inexpensive. General measures that should be undertaken are keeping the skin dry and cool, and encouraging frequent clothing changes. Bacterial superinfection is a common problem, and should be treated appropriately. The topical agents of choice are 2% miconazole cream, or 1% clotrimazole cream or lotion.

Oral ketoconazole is quite effective, leading to a cure in about 80% of cases (Table 108.6). However, it is expensive and causes side effects. The recommended dosage is 4-8 mg/kg/day as a single oral dose, best taken on an empty stomach, with a maximum of 200 mg/day. The most common side effect is nausea which is often seen with the first few doses but usually rapidly disappears. Other side effects are dizziness, drowsiness, myalgias, pruritus, rash, gynecomastia, hepatitis, and "heartburn." Ketoconazole acts to cause defects in the fungal cell membrane by blocking biosynthesis of ergosterol.

Griseofulvin has been used much longer than ketoconazole but is also slightly more toxic. It is involved in many drug interactions, therefore a careful drug history should be obtained in any patient in whom griseofulvin is considered for use. It should not be given to pregnant or lactating women. It owes its effectiveness to its preferential accumulation in the stratum corneum of the skin. It should be used in 250 mg or 20 mg/kg doses orally one to four times per day (Table 108.7). The length of therapy depends upon the location of the infection, with tinea capitis usually requiring about 2 weeks for cure, and tinea unguium requiring 3-9 months.

TABLE 108.6   Comparison of Ketoconazole and Griseofulvin in Treatment of Dermatophyte Infections*

Drug	% Cured	P
Ketoconazole	83	
		0.005
Griseofulvin	32	

Mycology Observer 2 (3):4, 1982

TABLE 108.7   Treatment with Griseofulvin

Children	
< 1 yr	62.5 mg b.i.d.
1-5 yr	62.5 mg t.i.d.
6-12 yr	125 mg b.i.d. - t.i.d.
Adults	
≤ 60 kg	250 mg b.i.d.
> 60 kg	250 mg t.i.d.

Complications are unusual, but fungal invasion has been reported in immuno-suppressed patients. Scarring may result from the development of a kerion.

These infections are difficult to prevent, but certain steps are somewhat worthwhile. Children should not wear caps or hats which belong to schoolmates; cases of tinea capitis should be treated aggressively; and children should be checked to ensure that a cure has been effected. With respect to tinea pedis, the disease can be prevented by wearing open shoes or sandals.

Dermatophytid

This is a hypersensitivity reaction to dermatophyte infection elsewhere, usually tinea pedis, and the usual organism causing the dermatophytid is *T. mentagro-phytes.* The lesions occur as groups of vesicles usually on the hands, but they can be located elsewhere on the body. Most typically, they are on the sides and flexor aspects of the fingers and palms, or thenar and hypothenar surfaces. They are round, up to 15 mm in diameter, and intensely pruritic.

The trichophytin skin test is always positive in this condition, but this is of limited usefulness, except in a negative sense, i.e., to rule out the condition, since most people have a positive trichophytin skin test anyway. The lesions must be negative for presence of fungus.

The differential diagnosis includes contact dermatitis, dyshidrosis, and local-ized atopic dermatitis.

The treatment is to eradicate the infection on the feet or elsewhere. Topical corticosteroids may be used to control symptoms. Recurrences are common.

Mucocutaneous Candidiasis

Mucocutaneous candidiasis, or thrush, is seen as white patches on inflamed mu-cosa or skin (Table 108.8). The pathogenesis involves the warmth and moisture of body folds and mucous membranes. For other predisposing factors, see Chapter 116, *Candida,* but most prominent are diabetes, pregnancy, obesity with increased sweating, antibiotic therapy, oral contraceptives, anything which impairs cell-me-diated immunity, hypothyroidism, and iron deficiency. The most common sites are the mouth, tongue, pharynx, and vagina. Involvement of the esophagus leads to dysphagia, and anal involvement causes burning with defecation. The involved

TABLE 108.8   Mucocutaneous Candidiasis

Intertriginous

Thrush

Perleche (angles of lips)

Paronychia

skin is reddened with weeping lesions, usually involving intertriginous areas. Satellite vesicopustules are seen, and the lesions are severely pruritic. Other common areas for infection are the nails and paronychial skin.

Diagnosis is made by seeing mycelia and budding yeast microscopically using 15% KOH or by growing the fungus on Sabouraud's medium.

A more severe type of the disease is chronic mucocutaneous candidiasis which may be related to congenital absence of an ability to mount a cell-mediated immune reaction to the organism, which is covered in more detail in Chapter 116.

The differential diagnosis involves bacterial skin infections of intertriginous areas and paronychia by *Staphylococcus aureus* or gram-negative organisms, herpes simplex, pemphigus vulgaris, aphthous stomatitis, erythema multiforme, seborrheic dermatitis, tinea cruris, and erythrasma. Perleche must be differentiated from vitamin deficiency, secondary syphilis, and poorly fitting dentures.

Treatment involves eliminating the underlying predisposing factor if possible, keeping the involved areas of skin dry, and using topical nystatin, miconazole, or haloprogin. Chronic paronychia is treated with 3% thymol or chloroform. Chronic mucocutaneous candidiasis is treated with amphotericin B intravenously, ketoconazole, or experimentally, transfer factor.

Candidal infections of the skin and mucous membranes can be very difficult to eradicate, particularly in children.

Tinea Versicolor

Tinea versicolor is different from the other fungal infections of the skin in that it is even less invasive, more superficial, and virtually asymptomatic. Patients seek medical advice only for cosmetic reasons, except in rare cases. It is caused by *Pityrosporum orbiculare* (also known as *Malassezia furfur*).

It is a common but not particularly contagious infection, usually seen in young adults, particularly those who perspire a great deal. The yeast-like form of the organism is often present on normal skin and the disease results from its transformation to the mycelial phase. What causes this transformation is unknown.

Clinically, tinea versicolor is seen as small macules which do not tan. The macules themselves may be hypopigmented or may be darker than the surrounding skin in the wintertime. The lesions are scaly and velvety. They usually appear on the upper trunk, neck, shoulders, or face. The disease most often becomes evident in the summer because tanning makes the lesions noticeable. There may be very mild pruritus. The differential diagnosis is mainly with seborrheic dermatitis. The diagnosis is made by KOH preparation of scales, showing short, thick, tangled hyphae, with budding yeast cells. Under the Wood's lamp, there is yellow white to blue white fluorescence.

Treatment is with topical clotrimazole or miconazole, salicyclic acid lotions, or selenium sulfide lotions. The latter may cause irritation, especially at skin folds. Relapses are common and the skin may take several weeks to months to return to its normal appearance.

Selected Bibliography

Chretien, T. H., et al.: Efficacy of undecylenic acid-zinc undecylenic powder in culture-positive tinea pedis. *Int J Dermatol* 19:57, 1980.

De Villez, R. L. and Lewis, C. W.: Candidiasis seminar. *Cutis* 19:69, 1977.

Faergemann, J. and Fredricksoon, T.: An open trial of the effect of zinc pyrithione shampoo on tinea versicolor. *Cutis* 25:667, 1980.

Fuerst, J. F., et al.: Comparison between undecylenic acid and tolnaftate in the treatment of tinea pedis. *Cutis* 25:544, 1980.

Graybill, J. R. and Drutz, O. J.: Ketoconazole: A major innovation for treatment of fungal disease. *Ann Intern Med* 93:921, 1980.

Graybill, J. R., et al.: Ketoconazole treatment of chronic mucocutaneous candidiasis. *Arch Dermatol* 116:1137, 1980.

Joly, J., et al.: Favus. *Arch Dermatol* 114:1647, 1978.

Oskui, J.: Intermittent use of griseofulvin in tinea capitis. *Cutis* 21:689, 1978.

Quinones, C. A.: Tinea versicolor: New topical treatments. *Cutis* 25:386, 1980.

Shelley, W. B. and Wood, M. G.: New technic for instant visualization of fungi in hair. *J Am Acad Dermatol* 2:69, 1980.

Shelley, W. B. and Wood, M. G.: The stratum corneum biopsy for instant visualization of fungi. *J Am Acad Dermatol* 2:56, 1980.

Sorenson, G. W. and Jones, H. E.: Immediate and delayed hypersensitivity in chronic dermatophytosis. *Arch Dermatol* 112:40, 1976.

Vaffee, A. S.: Tinea nigra palmaris resembling malignant melanoma. *N Engl J Med* 283:1112, 1970.

Van Dersarl, J. V. and Sheppard, R. H.: Clotrimazole vs. haloprogin treatment of tinea cruris. *Arch Dermatol* 113:1233, 1977.

109

SPOROTRICHOSIS
H. Preston Holley, Jr., M.D.

Sporothrix schenckii is a dimorphic fungus; that is, it exists in the yeast form in tissue or at 37°C on enriched media, and in the mycelial form in nature or when cultured at room temperature. In nature, *S. schenckii* exists as a saprophyte and can be isolated from soil, plants, wood, straw, sphagnum moss, decaying vegetation, and other contaminated material. It has also been isolated from cats, dogs, and rodents.

Sporotrichosis poses an occupational hazard for farmers, florists, gardeners, forestry workers, horticulturists, and others who might come in contact with contaminated material. Wearing gloves and protective clothing can help prevent infection when handling potentially contaminated material. Masks have also been recommended during prolonged exposure to sphagnum moss, since sinus and pulmonary infections have resulted from aerosolization during the harvesting process.

Human infection usually occurs by accidental cutaneous inoculation from a contaminated source, such as thorns and splinters. The fungus rarely has been inoculated by bites of animals and insects. The resulting infection develops over 1-6 weeks at the site of subcutaneous implantation. The lesion may be a small ulcer or, more commonly, a subcutaneous nodule which becomes fixed to the skin. This nodule may ulcerate or remain intact. About 75% of patients develop subcutaneous nodules along the lymphatic drainage of the primary lesion. These eventually become fixed to the overlying skin and may ulcerate, discharging a thin pus. The connecting lymphatics become enlarged and indurated. This is the cutaneous lymphatic form of sporotrichosis. If the disease goes untreated, distant lymph nodes may become swollen without necrosis or drainage.

In some patients, the infection remains localized without lymphatic or other system involvement. This is known as the localized (fixed) cutaneous form (Table 109.1). It has been suggested that these patients have had previous exposure to the fungus and have developed immunity. Other investigators have isolated from

TABLE 109.1   Clinical Types of Sporotrichosis

Cutaneous	
Cutaneous lymphatic	Most common; firm subcutaneous nodules
Fixed cutaneous	No lymphatic involvement
Extracutaneous	
Localized extracutaneous	Skeletal most common; pulmonary can mimic tuberculosis
Disseminated	Rare; immunosuppressed patients

such patients strains of *S. schenckii* which grow at 35°C but not at 37°C. When these strains are injected intraperitoneally into mice, they do not produce infection. Whatever the reason, about 20% of patients present with lesions which remain localized to the skin.

Extracutaneous sporotrichosis is much less common than the cutaneous form (see Table 109.1). Localized extracutaneous foci may develop from contiguous spread from cutaneous lesions or accidental deep implantation. Occasionally such extracutaneous foci occur with no known source of infection. Examples of the localized form include infections of the bone, muscle, synovium, lungs, eyes, and genitourinary tract.

Disseminated sporotrichosis results from hematogenous dissemination from the primary lesion or from suppurating lymph nodes. Thus, the majority of patients with disseminated sporotrichosis will have skin or lymphatic involvement at the time of diagnosis. This is helpful in diagnosis, since biopsy and culture of these tissues are relatively simple. After skin, the most common site of involvement in disseminated sporotrichosis is bone and associated periosteum or synovium. However, any organ can be involved. When the skin or lymphatics are not actively involved at the time of presentation, diagnosis may be very difficult. Fever and an elevated erythrocyte sedimentation rate are usually present, but other signs and symptoms are usually related to the site of involvement. Articular involvement, for example, is associated with painful swelling of the involved joint. Most patients with disseminated sporotrichosis have some underlying immunological abnormality or are on immunosuppressive therapy. Disseminated sporotrichosis is usually fatal if untreated.

Pulmonary sporotrichosis may be a manifestation of either extracutaneous or disseminated disease. Lung infection can occur by inhalation of the fungus from an environmental source, or possibly by aspiration from oral contamination with the fungus. In primary infection, the upper lobes are usually involved. Pulmonary sporotrichosis often resembles tuberculosis with similar symptoms and a cavitary infiltrate on chest x-ray. In addition, several cases of coexisting sporotrichosis and tuberculosis have been reported. The lungs can also be involved following dissemination from cutaneous lymphatic disease. Primary infection of the lungs rarely leads to dissemination, however.

Diagnosis of sporotrichosis is made by culturing *S. schenckii* from the infected tissue. The fungus grows well when cultured on most of the common mycologic media (such as Sabouraud's dextrose agar with chloramphenicol and cycloheximide) incubated at 29-30°C. Aspiration of a nodule or biopsy of a draining ulcer bed is usually satisfactory for culture.

Direct microscopic examination of exudates has proven to be of little diagnostic value because of the small number of yeast cells in such specimens. Even in biopsy specimens of tissue, the cigarshaped yeast forms are not found easily. Special fungal stains increase the likelihood of finding the organism. Mycelial forms are not found in tissue. The direct fluorescent antibody stain has been useful for detecting *S. schenckii* in clinical specimens, but is of limited availability and is not used routinely. Cultures are often positive despite negative microscopic findings.

Serologic testing by tube agglutination or latex agglutination may be helpful diagnostically in culture-negative cases and is performed by the Centers for Disease Control in Atlanta, Georgia. The tube agglutination test is highly specific, and elevated serum titers correlate well with culturally proved infection. Sera from patients with various forms of sporotrichosis may show titers ranging from 1:4 to 1:128. A high or rising titer suggests active disease. Tube agglutination is positive in 95-100% of extracutaneous infections and in 75% of lymphocutaneous infections. Latex agglutination titers ≥ 1:4 are suggestive of active disease.

The typical histopathologic pattern in sporotrichosis is a combination of pyogenic and granulomatous reactions. The granulomas are typically small, and Langhan's giant cells can be seen occasionally. Asteroid bodies are sometimes seen in tissue, appearing as a central, nonstaining yeast cell with eosinophilic radiations and should alert one to the possibility of sporotrichosis. They are not specific, however, and can be seen in some other fungal infections as well. Another histologic pattern of pseudoepitheliomatous hyperplasia occurs in chronic sporotrichosis skin infection which may grossly be mistaken for cancer.

Host factors probably play a significant role in defense against *S. schenckii* infection. Experimental studies in athymic nude mice have shown that dissemination occurs readily and is more widespread than in normal mice, suggesting an important role for cellular immunity. Humoral immunity (opsonizing antibodies) is also probably important.

Therapy of lymphocutaneous, fixed cutaneous, and mucocutaneous sporotrichosis consists of saturated potassium iodide solution (1 g KI/ml distilled water). The dose is given orally in milk or juice, usually starting with 1/2 ml (5 drops) every 8 hr. This is increased by 1/2-1 ml/dose each day as tolerated until a dose of 3-4 ml every 8 hr is reached. If toxicity develops with salivary gland swelling, increased lacrimation, gastrointestinal irritation, or hyperkalemia, the drug can be stopped and restarted at a somewhat lower dosage. An acneiform rash may occur and usually does not warrant discontinuation of therapy unless it becomes severe. Treatment with the maximum dose tolerated is usually continued for at least 4 weeks after resolution of clinical disease. If treatment failure occurs with adequate doses, retreatment with potassium iodide has little chance for success.

A few patients with cutaneous sporotrichosis have responded to moist heat. These cases usually took 1-4 months to resolve. Thus, local heat can be combined with oral iodine therapy, but it is generally too inconvenient to be practical.

In cases of failure with potassium iodide, or in pulmonary or disseminated sporotrichosis, amphotericin B should be used. Amphotericin B is given at a dose of 0.5-0.8 mg/kg/day. Adequate therapy may require a total dose of 1.5-2.5 g. The side effects of amphotericin B therapy are outlined in the Introduction to Fungal Diseases (p. 935). Although resistance to amphotericin B has not been demonstrated, relapses have rarely been reported. A few patients have been successfully treated with dihydroxystilbamidine. The recommended dosage is 2 mg/kg dissolved in 5% glucose and given slowly intravenously. Therapy is continued for 10 days and then is stopped for 10 days. A total of three 10-day courses has been sufficient, but very few patients have been treated with this form of therapy. In general, relapses should be retreated with amphotericin B, and dihydroxystilbamidine used only if failure or severe allergy occurs.

A few patients with cutaneous sporotrichosis have been treated with ketoconazole, and in one report, two of three patients showed marked improvement. Until additional experience is reported, ketoconazole cannot be recommended as primary therapy, but may be an alternative in patients with localized disease who are allergic or do not respond to iodides.

The prognosis of both the cutaneous lymphatic and localized cutaneous forms of sporotrichosis is good and occasional spontaneous cures have been reported.

Selected Bibliography

Altner, P. C. and Turner, R. R.: Sporotrichosis of bones and joints. Review of the literature and report of six cases. *Clin Orthoped Rel Res* 68:138-148, 1970.

Blumer, S. O., Kaufman, L., Kaplan, W., McLaughlin, D. W., and Kraft, D. E.: Comparison evaluation of five serological methods for the diagnosis of sporotrichosis. *Appl Microbiol* 26:4-8, 1973.

Boehm, D., Lynch, J. M., Hodges, G. R., Abdou, N. I., Garrison, R. G., Lee, S. H., Bellome, J., and Barnes, W. G.: Disseminated sporotrichosis presenting as sarcoidosis: Electron microscopic and immunologic studies. *Am J Med Sci* 283:71-78, 1982.

Bulpitt, P. and Weedon, D.: Sporotrichosis: A review of 39 cases. *Pathology* 10: 249-256, 1978.

Crout, J. E., Brewer, N. S., and Tompkins, R. B.: Sporotrichosis arthritis. Clinical features in seven patients. *Ann Intern Med* 86:294-297, 1977.

Hachisuka, H. and Sasai, Y.: Development of experimental sporotrichosis in normal and modified animals. *Mycopathologica* 76:79-82, 1981.

Jung, J. Y., Almond, C. H., Campbell, D. C., Elkadi, A., and Tenorio, A.: Role of surgery in the management of pulmonary sporotrichosis. *J Thorac Cardiovasc Surg* 77:234-239, 1979.

Kown-Chung, K. J.: Comparison of isolates of *Sporothrix schenckii* obtained from fixed cutaneous lesions with isolates from other types of lesions. *J Infect Dis* 139:424-431, 1979.

Lynch, P. J., Vorhees, J. J., and Harrell, R. E.: Systemic sporotrichosis. *Ann Intern Med* 73:23-30, 1970.

Plouffe, J. F., Jr., Silva, J., Jr., Fekety, R., Reinhalter, E., and Browne, R.: Cell-mediated immune responses in sporotrichosis. *J Infect Dis* 139:152-157, 1979.

Rippon, J. and Adler, L.: Chronic pulmonary sporotrichosis. The importance of appropriate fungal serology. *Clin Microbiol Newsletter* 1:5-6, 1979.

Rohatgi, P. K.: Pulmonary sporotrichosis. *Southern Med J* 73:1611-1618, 1980.

Wilson, D. E., Mann, J. J., Bennett, J. E., and Utz, J. P.: Clinical features of extracutaneous sporotrichosis. *Medicine* 46:265-279, 1967.

Zvetina, J. R., Rippon, J. W., and Daum, V.: Chronic pulmonary sporotrichosis. *Mycopathologia* 64:53-57, 1978.

110

CHROMOMYCOSIS AND PHAEOHYPHOMYCOSIS
H. Preston Holley, Jr., M.D.

Chromomycosis (chromoblastomycosis) and phaeohyphomycosis are caused by de-matiaceous (darkly pigmented) fungi which most commonly produce localized skin and subcutaneous tissue infections. The tissue form of fungi causing chromomy-cosis is primarily a rounded, thick-walled, dark brown cell called a sclerotic body. These cells appear alone, in pairs, or in clusters and usually divide by septation rather than by budding. Phaeohyphomycosis, on the other hand, is caused by fungi which occur predominantly as dark-walled, septate hyphae in tissue. Table 110.1 lists some of the more common causes of these infections. Unfortunately, the taxonomy and nomenclature of many of these agents are still in dispute and there-fore many of these fungi have been reported under different names.

Chromomycosis (Chromoblastomycosis)

Chromomycosis has been reported from many areas of the world, most commonly from tropical and subtropical regions. Rural populations are preponderantly af-fected because the agents are saprophytic fungi found on grass, plants, and in soil. Males are more commonly infected owing to agricultural occupational exposure. The fungus enters through breaks in the skin associated frequently with minor trauma such as small cuts or puncture wounds. Most lesions occur on the distal portion of the legs, but infections of the arms, head, or trunk may be seen.

The initial lesion is usually a small papule which develops in a few days or weeks at the site of inoculation. Systemic symptoms are usually absent. The le-sion slowly grows into a verrucous, occasionally crusted, lesion at the average rate of about 1-cm diameter per year. If allowed to persist for several years, satellite lesions may develop and coalesce with the primary lesion. Trauma to the lesion may introduce secondary bacterial infection and ulceration. Older lesions

TABLE 110.1   More Common Fungi Causing Chromomycosis and
Phaeohyphomycosis

Chromomycosis	Phaeohyphomycosis
Cladosporium carrionii	*Alternaria alternata*
Fonsecaea compacta	*Cladosporium bantianum**
Fonsecaea pedorosoi	*Curvularia geniculata*
Phialophora verrucosa	*Drechslera hawaiiensis*
	Exophiala jeanselmei
	Wangiella dermatitidis

*Previously known as *Cladosporium trichoides*

may appear as large, cauliflower-like tumors. When the arms are involved, lesions are often dry, hyperkeratotic patches with no tumor formation.

Dissemination may occur through the superficial lymphatics and less commonly through the deep lymphatic channels. When lymphatic involvement occurs, a clinical picture resembling sporotrichosis develops. Fibrosis following repeated secondary infections may lead to elephantiasis in these patients.

Differential diagnosis includes blastomycosis, sporotrichosis, tuberculosis verrucosa cutis, tertiary syphilis, yaws, and verrucous leishmaniasis.

As mentioned, the typical sclerotic bodies can be found in biopsy specimens or on KOH preparations of scrapings. Occasionally hyphal elements may be seen in the horny layer of skin. Microabscesses with polymorphonuclear leukocytes can be seen. Langhans and foreign-body giant cells can also be found, usually in the dermis where there is extensive fibrous thickening.

The definitive diagnosis depends upon isolation of the etiologic agent from tissue. Because the agents causing chromomycosis cannot be distinguished in tissue, culture and identification are necessary. It is advisable to refer isolates to reference laboratories for identification since most laboratories do not have the expertise to identify and speciate them properly.

Treatment of localized lesions is surgical excision. The resection should be made well beyond the margin of the lesion and should extend down to the fascia. Attempts at electrocoagulation, topical freezing, and other local measures have met with failure in many cases. Inadequate removal may result in ulcers, recurrences in situ, and possibly dissemination.

Medical therapy has been successful in a few cases. Flucytosine (5-FC) has been the most successful agent in doses of 100-150 mg/kg of body weight per day divided into four equal doses. Certain of the fungi involved, such as *Cladosporium carrionii,* seem more susceptible to 5-FC than others. Vitamin D, intralesional amphotericin B, and thiabendazole have been reported to have some success in a few patients. The susceptibility of the fungi to various forms of therapy is quite variable, but they are often resistant in vitro to amphotericin B. Some authors have advocated combined amphotericin B/5-FC therapy. Experience with newer agents such as miconazole and ketoconazole is limited. Unfortunately, no overwhelmingly successful regimen for this disease is known.

Phaeohyphomycosis

As in chromomycosis, the lesions are primarily found on the skin of the lower extremities. The causative fungi (see Table 110.1) are found in soil, decaying organic material, and as plant saprophytes. Infection occurs by accidental inoculation or inhalation. Abscess formation and ulceration occur more commonly with phaeohyphomycosis than with chromomycosis. Early lesions may not be distinguishable clinically from those of chromomycosis, and biopsy and culture are necessary to make the diagnosis. The pathology is that of a granulomatous lesion with dark-walled hyphae present. Dissemination via lymphatics and presumably the bloodstream has been reported more commonly in phaeohyphomycosis. The brain seems to be particularly vulnerable and cerebral abscesses may be single or multiple. Many of the cases of disseminated disease have no apparent primary focus of infection. Disseminated cases are usually fatal. Phaeohyphomycosis may also present as an opportunistic infection in compromised patients.

Therapy is surgical excision where possible as in chromomycosis. The organisms are often resistant to standard antifungal agents. Amphotericin B has been successful in a few cases but may be only inhibitory in the concentrations achievable in serum.

Selected Bibliography

Ajello, L.: The gamut of human infections caused by dematiaceous fungi. *Jap J Med Mycol* 22:1-5, 1981.

Azulay, R. D. and Serruya, J.: Hematogenous dissemination in chromoblastomycosis. Report of a generalized case. *Arch Dermatol* 95:57, 1967.

Blank, H. and Rebell, G.: Thiabendazole activity against the fungi of dermatophytosis, mycetomas and chromomycosis. *J Invest Dermatol* 44:219-220, 1965.

Clark, R. F.: Chromoblastomycosis of the ear - successful intralesional therapy with amphotericin B. *Cutis* 24:326-328, 1979.

DiSalvo, A. F. and Chew, W. W.: *Phialophora gougerotii:* An opportunistic fungus in a patient treated with steroids. *Sabouraudia* 6:241-245, 1968.

Dixon, D. M. and Shadomy, H. J.: Taxonomy and morphology of dematiaceous fungi isolated from nature. *Mycopathologia* 70:139-144, 1980.

Fuste, F. J., Ajello, L., Threlkeld, R., and Henry, J. E.: *Drechslera hawaiiensis,* causative agent of a fatal fungal meningoencephalitis. *Sabouraudia* 11:59-63, 1973.

Hironaga, M. and Watanabe, S.: Cerebral phaeohyphomycosis caused by *Cladosporium bantianum:* A case in a female who had cutaneous alternariosis in her childhood. *Sabouraudia* 18:229-235, 1980.

Kaufman, S. M.: Curvularia endocarditis following cardiac surgery. *Am J Clin Pathol* 56:466-470, 1971.

Lopes, C. F., Resende, M. A., Alvarenga, R. J., Moreira, Y. K., and Ferreira, I.: 5-Fluorocytosine in the treatment of chromomycosis. *Curr Chemother* 1: 219-220, 1978.

Mauceri, A. A., Cullen, S. I., Vandevelde, A. G., and Johnson, J. E., III.: Flucytosine an effective oral treatment for chromomycosis. *Arch Dermatol* 109: 873-876, 1974.

Zaias, N.: Chromomycosis. *J Cutaneous Pathol* 5:155-164, 1978.

Zaias, N. and Rebell, G.: A simple and accurate diagnostic method in chromoblastomycosis. *Arch Dermatol* 108:545-546, 1973.

111

MYCETOMA
H. Preston Holley, Jr., M.D.

Mycetoma (maduromycosis, madura foot) is a chronic infection caused by a variety of filamentous eumycetes (true fungi) and actinomycetes. The infection usually begins on the foot and may progress to involve not only skin, but subcutaneous tissues, fascia, tendons, muscle, and bone.

Maduromycosis was originally described in India. Today, mycetoma is found worldwide between latitudes 15°S and 30°N, and is most commonly seen in northern Africa and southern Asia. The infection is also seen in the United States, Mexico, and Central and South America.

When the infection is caused by the eumycetes, it is known as eumycetoma (Table 111.1). Several species of actinomycetes, which are not true fungi, can cause similar infections known as actinomycetoma (see Table 111.1). The distinction between these two is important from the standpoint of therapy. In the United States, the most common causes of mycetoma are *Petriellidium boydii*, *Actinomyces israelii*, and *Nocardia* spp.

The organisms causing mycetoma are generally considered to be saprophytic soil inhabitants. Infection begins with the introduction of the organism into a minor abrasion, cut, or puncture of the skin. The foot is the most common site of infection, but other areas such as hands, arms, legs, chest, buttocks, and even the head may be involved. Mycetoma occurs most commonly in men between the ages of 20 and 40 years, presumably because of occupational exposure during cultivating or farming while not wearing shoes.

The disease often begins as a small papule or nodule which becomes indurated. Later, a vesicle may form. Abscess formation occurs as the lesion progresses and draining sinuses eventually result. The infection is destructive if allowed to progress and may involve all tissues from the skin to the bone. Usually this infection is not confused with bacterial osteomyelitis, but the x-ray appearance can be similar with osteolytic lesions and periosteal reactive changes. Systemic symptoms

TABLE 111.1   Agents of Mycetoma

Type of Mycetoma	Color of Grains	Species
Eumycetoma	White to yellowish	*Aspergillus nidulans* *Acremonium falciforme* *A. recifei* *Petriellidium boydii* *Zophia rosatii*
	Brown to black	*Exophiala jeanselmei* *Madurella mycetomatis*
	Black	*M. grisea* *Curvularia geniculata* *C. lunata* *Helminthosporium spiciferum* *Leptosphaeria senegalensis* *Pyrenochaeta romeroi*
Actinomycetoma	White to yellowish	*Actinomadura madurae* *Actinomyces israelii* *Nocardia asteroides* *N. brasiliensis* *N. caviae*
	Yellow to brownish	*Streptomyces somaliensis*
	Bright red	*Actinomadura pelletieri*
	Black	*Streptomyces paraguayensis*

are uncommon and fever suggests secondary bacterial infection. Pain is usually associated only with advanced lesions or concomitant bacterial infection.

Diagnosis is confirmed by finding the characteristic mycotic grains in draining material from the sinuses and abscesses. The grains are actual colonies of the infecting organism. Grains vary in color depending upon the etiologic agent (see Table 111.1). The grains are usually 0.2–3.0 mm in diameter and if seen should be cultured and examined histologically. Some of the agents produce grains which are characteristic, and presumptive diagnosis can be made on the basis of their morphology and staining character. The exact etiology can be ascertained only by culture and identification. Deep biopsy specimens are preferable for culture to avoid contamination by the bacteria and fungi present on the surface of the lesion. Sabouraud's dextrose agar is preferred for eumycetoma cultures. Actinomycetoma should also be cultured aerobically and anaerobically in brain-heart infusion agar at 35°C.

The differential diagnosis includes other fungal or bacterial osteomyelitis and botryomycosis, which is usually caused by *Staphylococcus aureus* and also is characterized by grains in a chronic, granulomatous, suppurative skin and soft-tissue infection. Botryomycosis can be differentiated on histologic section since bacteria are seen in Gram and methenamine silver stains, while periodic acid Schiff (PAS) and other fungal stains are negative.

Treatment of mycetoma depends upon the causative organism. Mycetoma is progressive and does not heal spontaneously. Hematogenous or lymphangitic spread fortunately occurs only rarely. There is no satisfactory medical treatment for most types of eumycetoma. Thorough removal of the involved area by excision or cautery has been successful in very early lesions. In more advanced cases amputation is often necessary. The recurrence rate is high if the amputation is made too close to the infected tissue margin. Amphotericin B has not proved useful. *Petriellidium boydii* is relatively susceptible to miconazole, and this agent might be useful.

Actinomycetoma often does respond to long-term medical treatment. *Actinomyces israelii* has been treated with large doses of penicillin G intravenously or phenoxymethyl potassium penicillin orally. Dapsone has also been reported to be effective. *Nocardia* spp are often sensitive to sulfonamides including sulfadiazine or sulfamethoxazole-trimethoprim. Streptomycin has been reported to be useful in combination with sulfamethoxazole-trimethoprim or dapsone for actinomycetoma and should be tried in stubborn cases. Therapy may take many weeks to months and should be longer with bone involvement. Treatment is generally continued for several months beyond clinical cure to reduce the chance of relapse.

In one report of eight cases of mycetoma treated with ketoconazole, there were no cures, but three had moderate regression of the lesions. Seven of these eight cases had actinomycetomas. Combination therapy with ketonazole has not been reported. Thus these early data are not particularly encouraging for this new oral antifungal agent, but further studies are needed.

Selected Bibliography

Barnetson, R. StC. and Milne, L. J. R.: Mycetoma. *Br J Dermatol* 99:227-231, 1978.

Butz, W. C. and Ajello, L.: Black grain mycetoma. A case due to *Madurella grisea*. *Arch Dermatol* 104:197-201, 1971.

Cuce, L. C., Wroclawski, E. L., and Sampaio, S. A. P.: Treatment of paracoccidioidomycosis, candidiasis, chromomycosis, lobomycosis, and mycetoma with ketoconazole. *Int J Dermatol* 19:405-408, 1980.

Kamalam, A., Subramaniyam, P., Augustine, S. M., and Thambiah, A. S.: Restoration of bones in mycetoma. *Arch Dermatol* 111:1178-1180, 1975.

Mahgoub, E. S.: Medical management of mycetoma. *Bull WHO* 54:303-310, 1976.

Mariat, F., Destombes, P., and Segretain, G.: The mycetomas: Clinical features, pathology, etiology and epidemiology. *Contrib Microbiol Immunol* 4:1-39, 1977.

Nitidandhaprabhas, P. and Sittapairochana, D.: Treatment of nocardial mycetoma with trimethoprim and sulfamethoxazole. *Arch Dermatol* 111:1345-1348, 1975.

Picou, K., Batres, E., and Jarratt, M.: Botryomycosis: A bacterial cause of mycetoma. *Arch Dermatol* 115:609-610, 1979.

Rogers, R. S., III and Muller, S. A.: Treatment of actinomycetoma with dapsone.
A report of infection with *Nocardia asteroides*. *Arch Dermatol* 109:529-534,
1974.

Saxena, P. S., Udawat, M. P., and Singh, H.: Unusual manifestations of mycetoma.
Trop Geogr Med 31:253-256, 1979.

Tight, R. R. and Bartlett, M. S.: Actinomycetoma in the United States. *Rev Infect Dis* 3:1139-1150, 1981.

Winslow, D. J. and Steen, F. J.: Considerations in the histologic diagnosis of
mycetoma. *Am J Clin Pathol* 42:164-169, 1964.

112

CRYPTOCOCCUS
Robert H. Waldman, M.D.

The most common clinical presentation of disease caused by infection with *Crypto-coccus* is subacute or chronic meningitis. Almost all of the disease is caused by the species *C. neoformans,* previously called *Torula histolytica.* Untreated, the disease is uniformly fatal and frequently occurs in patients who are immunosuppressed, but it can occur in apparently normal individuals.

Microbiology

Cryptococcus is an exception to the rule that pathogenic fungi are dimorphic, i.e., it is uniphasic and yeast-like with no mycelial form. It reproduces by budding, and the junction between the mother and daughter cells is narrow, in contradistinction to the broad junction seen with *Blastomyces.* The organism is 4-6 μm in diameter and is encapsulated, the capsule being 1-30 μm in diameter. The size of the capsule is probably not related to virulence, although totally unencapsulated organisms do show decreased virulence. The fungus grows well on Sabouraud's glucose agar at 20-37°C.

Epidemiology

The organism and disease have worldwide distribution, and the organism has been isolated from soil, foods, pigeon excreta, as well as the excreta of other animals. The organism does not infect pigeons and other birds but grows abundantly in avian intestines and feces. One-third to one-half of the patients with cryptococcosis have abnormalities in their immune systems. The most common diseases with which it is associated are Hodgkin's disease, non-Hodgkin's lymphoma, leukemia, sarcoidosis (even in the absence of corticosteroid treatment), and diabetes mellitus. Illness is seen more commonly in whites than blacks, and males have the disease three times more commonly than females.

Pathogenesis and Pathology

As mentioned, the organism is found in great numbers in the feces of pigeons and other birds. However, there is a large amount of evidence indicating that this is not the source of human disease. There is no history of exposure in most patients, clusters of infection are not seen, and although serotypes B and C cause most cases in southern California, this serotype has not been isolated in pigeon droppings or soil in this area. The portal of entry is probably the respiratory tract, but there has been no known person-to-person transmission of the disease. It is also unknown whether the most common manifestation of the disease, meningitis, is a result of immediate spread from the portal of entry, or a reactivation many years after the primary infection, in an analogous fashion to tuberculosis. Adding to the confusion about the pathogenesis of the disease is that laboratory workers have a high frequency of a positive skin test to cryptococcal antigens, but there are no reported cases of illness.

Pathologically there is usually not a granulomatous inflammatory response to the infection, but a plasma cell, lymphocytic, and macrophage response. Lesions are seen diffusely throughout the central nervous system, with the heaviest involvement usually in the basal ganglia of the brain. Therefore, the disease would be more accurately called a meningoencephalitis. Occasionally, large focal collections of involvement, which are cryptococcomas, are found in the brain.

Diagnosis

Meningitis caused by *C. neoformans* is usually chronic or subacute, although rarely it can cause an acute meningitis leading to death in 2-3 weeks. Headache of increasing severity is the most prominent symptom. Other common symptoms are vertigo, nausea, anorexia, visual disturbances, and mental deterioration (Tables 112.1 and 112.2). Signs of meningeal irritation are usually present. Signs consistent with a space-occupying lesion may also be found. In most patients the signs and symptoms come on insidiously over a period of weeks or months and are waxing and waning in intensity. In patients who are severely immunosuppressed, the disease may be very acute developing over 3-4 days.

Less common clinical findings include: painless skin abscesses seen in about 10% of patients; involvement of cranial nerves seen in about 20%; bone involvement, manifested as deep pain; and findings referable to the lungs. Skin lesions are acneiform, slowly enlarging, ulcerating, and may involve extensive areas (Table 112.3).

Patients with cryptococcal infection rarely have meningitis and pulmonary involvement at the same time. A patient with both is much more likely to have tuberculosis. Patients with pulmonary cryptococcosis usually have cough, scant sputum production which may be blood-streaked, and dull pain (Table 112.4). Chest x-ray reveals nodular infiltrates, usually in the lower lobes, and may show cavitation. Pulmonary cryptococcosis is much more common in patients with pre-existing pulmonary disease.

TABLE 112.1   Symptoms and Signs of Cryptococcal Meningitis

Headache	Intermittent, of increasing frequency and severity, usually frontal, temporal, or postorbital, may be accompanied by vomiting and vertigo
Disturbance of consciousness and orientation	Confusion, personality change, decreased memory, lethargy
Meningeal signs	Nuchal rigidity, positive Kernig's and Brudzinski's signs
Cranial nerve involvement	Hearing loss, diplopia, ophthalmoplegia, facial nerve palsy
Increased intracranial pressure	
Hyperreflexia, pathologic reflexes, ataxia, convulsions	
Fever	

TABLE 112.2   Clinical Findings Relative to Central Nervous System in Cryptococcal Meningitis

Progressive delirium and psychosis: 10%

Cranial nerve involvement: 20%

Meningeal signs: 50%

Common symptoms: headache, nausea, dizziness, irritability, somnolescence, clumsiness, impaired memory and judgment

TABLE 112.3   Cutaneous Cryptococcosis

Found in ∿ 10% of cases, usually in disseminated disease

Rarely is primary (no disease detectable elsewhere)

Patterns:

Cystic or firm subcutaneous swellings which ulcerate

Crusted granulomas

Plaques or nodules

Ulcers

Mucosal lesions in ∿ 3%

TABLE 112.4   Characteristics of Patients with Pulmonary Cryptococcosis

Feature	Approximate %
Presenting symptoms	
Fever	65
Chest pain	45
Weight loss	35
Dyspnea	25
Night sweats	25
Cough	15
Hemoptysis	7
Asymptomatic: discovered by routine x-ray	15
Diagnostic tests	
Positive sputum culture	35
Bronchoscopy	35
Open-lung biopsy	100

Next to meningitis is most common clinical manifestation of cryptococcal infection

Chest roentgenogram

Predilection for lower lung fields

Lesions range from solitary mass to diffuse infiltrates or scattered miliary nodules

Unusual: cavitation, calcification, hilar lymphadenopathy or pulmonary collapse

The most important diagnostic procedure is the lumbar puncture (Table 112.5). Examination by India ink is positive in about 30-60% of patients (Figure 112.1). The test is done by mixing a drop of sediment prepared from 3-5 ml of spinal fluid, with a drop of India ink. The test makes use of the fact that the capsule of the organism repels charcoal particles. One can also use the Wright's or PAS stains. One should also determine the presence of the polysaccharide antigen in the spinal fluid. This test is positive in about 90% of patients. Rabbit antibody to the polysaccharide antigen is coated on latex particles, and if a significant amount of antigen is present the particles agglutinate. False-positive results are found in patients with rheumatoid factor in their spinal fluid (rheumatoid factors being antiimmunoglobulin). The antigen should also be searched for in blood and urine. An alternative method for determining the presence of antigen is the complement-fixation test, but it is less sensitive and more difficult to perform. Antibody to cryptococcus should be measured in serum, and in spinal fluid, but it is of importance as a prognostic test, not a diagnostic one (see Table 112.11).

Spinal fluid should also be cultured and will yield the organism in 40-70%. However, to obtain a positive culture, repeated lumbar punctures may be necessary. In addition, because of the low number of organisms in the spinal fluid, large volumes of material should be cultured, larger than is usually sent for culture in patients suspected of having pyogenic meningitis. One may also filter the spinal fluid through a 0.45-μm filter and then culture the filter. Blood culture is positive in about 10% of the patients, and urine in about 30%. The organism usually grows in 3-7 days, but may take longer, and therefore the culture should be held for 1 month. The organism grows on a variety of culture media, including blood agar, but grows best on Sabouraud's. The cryptococcus will grow at room temperature or at 37°C. In addition to spinal fluid, blood, and urine, any skin lesion should be cultured. A positive result of the India ink, antigen-antibody detection, or culture is found in about 95% of the patients.

Other spinal fluid findings include an increased opening pressure, abnormal cell counts (usually mononuclear although polymorphonuclear leukocytes are commonly found), with the total count 40-400/mm^3, increased protein content (nearly always < 300 mg/dl), and in about 50% of patients, hypoglycorrhachia. The spinal fluid lactic acid level is increased as well but, as with the other spinal fluid findings just mentioned, this is not specific for cryptococcal meningitis.

TABLE 112.5   Diagnosis of Cryptococcal Meningitis

Test	Positive in % of Patients
India ink on spinal fluid	30-60
Culture	40-70
Antibody (serum)	About 40
Antigen (spinal fluid and/or serum)	80-90
One or more of above	95

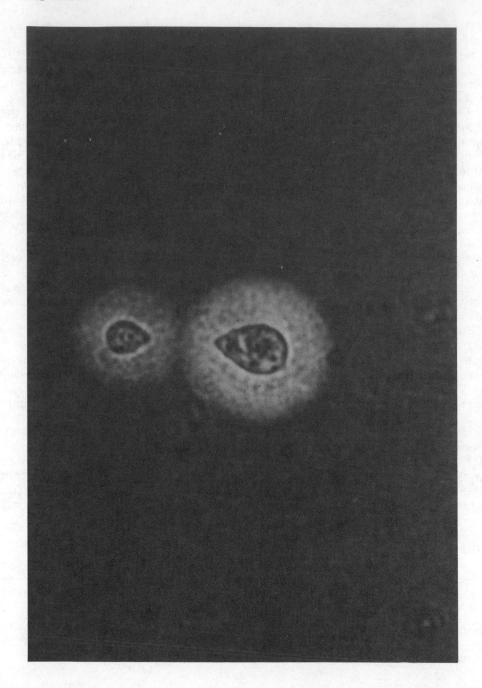

FIGURE 112.1   India ink of spinal fluid showing budding yeast and capsule typical of *Cryptococcus*.

The CAT scan is usually positive in cryptococcal meningitis, pointing out that cryptococcomas are present in nearly every patient. A bone scan is nearly always positive in patients with osseous involvement.

Treatment

The treatment of choice is combined therapy with amphotericin B and flucytosine (Tables 112.6 and 112.7). There are a variety of dosage schedules, all of which are of approximately equal efficacy. The one usually recommended is amphotericin, either 20 mg/day or 40 mg every other day, for 6 weeks (or 0.3 mg/kg/day or 0.6 mg/kg every other day) plus 150 mg/kg of flucytosine daily, in four divided doses. The advantage of the combination of amphotericin B and flucytosine is shorter hospitalization and reduced toxicity from the decreased total dosage of amphotericin B. The results are as good as, or slightly better than, amphotericin alone. The only disadvantage of the combined therapy is that nephrotoxicity caused by amphotericin B may lead to increased blood levels and serious toxicity from flucytosine (Table 112.8). Therefore, blood levels of the latter should be run and dosage decreased if blood levels are greater than 100 µg/ml. In addition, bone marrow depression should be watched for, with thrombocytopenia being the most common manifestation.

TABLE 112.6   Treatment

Amphotericin B only	
Duration	6–10 wk
Total dose	2–3 g
Shortcomings	
Treatment failures	About 25%
Relapse	About 25%
Nephrotoxicity	>80%
Amphotericin B + 5-FC	
6 wk of 20 mg amphotericin daily	
150 mg/kg 5-FC daily	
Advantages	
Shorter hospitalization	
Reduced toxicity	
Results at least as good	

TABLE 112.7   Amphotericin B (AmB) vs AmB + Flucytosine in Treatment of Cryptococcal Meningitis

	AmB	AmB + Flucytosine
Duration (wk)	10	6
AmB dosage (mg/kg/day)	0.4	0.3
Cured	30%	45%
Improved	15%	25%
Relapsed	15%	3%
Failed full course	20%	5%
Died during therapy	20%	25%

TABLE 112.8   Toxicity of Treatment

Amphotericin B

Nephrotoxicity - 80%, dose-dependent and largely reversible: decreased creatinine clearance, isosthenuria, decreased excretion of H^+, abnormal urine sediment, renal tubular acidosis, nephrocalcinosis

Immediate: chills, fever, nausea, vomiting, hypotension - 50 mg hydrocortisone added to infusion, plus antipyretics and/or antihistamines may be helpful

Thrombophlebitis: 1000 U heparin added to infusion may be helpful

Hypokalemia

Anemia (normocytic, normochromic)

Unusual: arrhythmias, hearing loss, anaphylaxis, hepatocellular

Minimized by alternate-day therapy

Flucytosine

Bone marrow: thrombocytopenia most commonly

Hepatic

Diarrhea

Miconazole has been used in the treatment of cryptococcal infections but has not been shown to be beneficial. It does not enter the spinal fluid in therapeutically significant concentrations but has been used intrathecally, in doses of 6-12 mg/day. The toxic side effects of miconazole are phlebitis, nausea and vomiting, skin rash and pruritus, anemia, hyponatremia, thrombocytosis, and hyperlipidemia. The drug may be antagonistic with amphotericin B, and therefore great care should be taken if a decision is reached to use the two drugs together. Similarly, ketoconazole has not been shown to be beneficial. Table 112.9 reviews other aspects of therapy.

The indications for treatment of pulmonary cryptococcosis are summarized in Table 112.10.

TABLE 112.9   Other Aspects of Therapy

Focal brain lesions

Should nearly always try medical therapy, since lesions often disappear (clinically and by CAT scan) with amphotericin B

Surgical excision: associated with high mortality

Intrathecal amphotericin B

Patients who relapse
Fail to respond
If nephrotoxicity precludes IV
Many complications of therapy

Investigational

Transfer factor
Aerosolized amphotericin B for pulmonary disease

TABLE 112.10   Indications for Treatment of Pulmonary Cryptococcosis

Progression of chest x-ray findings

Symptoms of increasing severity

Stable disease in patient who is susceptible to dissemination, e.g., malignancy, corticosteroid therapy

No treatment indicated in asymptomatic carriers, e.g., isolation of organism from sputum of patients with chronic bronchitis

Prognosis

Untreated, cryptococcal meningitis is uniformly fatal with 20% of the patients dead within the first year. The longest known survivor died after 16 years of the illness. With optimum treatment the mortality is still about 25%, and about 40% of the patients who are cured have significant neurologic sequelae.

The characteristics of the disease that are known to correlate with a poor prognosis are shown in Table 112.11. The only one of those factors which can be changed at the time of diagnosis is therapy with corticosteroids. However, lowering the steroid dosage significantly is often impossible or impractical because the underlying disease for which the steroids are being used may flare and adversely affect the outcome. Furthermore, decreasing the steroids may lead to exacerbation of cerebral edema.

Of more importance are the factors noted to be correlated with an increased chance of relapse after a course of therapy (Table 112.12). If these are present, some authorities recommend that therapy be prolonged, or that the total dose of amphotericin B be increased. However, it should be clearly stated that there are no controlled studies that prove more intensive therapy will decrease the chance of relapse.

TABLE 112.11   Poor Prognosis in Cryptococcal Meningitis

Markedly positive India ink test

Spinal fluid pressure > 300 mm

CSF glucose < 20 mg%

CSF leukocytes < 20 mm^3

Cryptococci isolated from other sites (e.g., blood, urine)

No detectable cryptococcal antibody

CSF antigen > 1:32

Patient with malignancy and/or receiving corticosteroids

Not poor prognostic factors

Advanced age

Persistently positive India ink test with negative culture

TABLE 12.12   Increased Chance of Relapse Following Therapy

No detectable antibody

Spinal fluid antigen > 1:8

Fall in CSF antigen during course of therapy
    < fourfold

Persistent malignancy and/or corticosteroid
    therapy

In follow-up of patients, spinal fluid examination occasionally reveals crypto-cocci by India ink examination, but cultures are negative. Such nonviable organisms are of no apparent significance, and their presence does not mean that the patient is in relapse. Experience has shown that if a patient is to relapse, he will do so within the first year of completion of therapy.

Hydrocephalus severe enough to require a shunt is a very poor prognostic sign, and these patients usually show progressive deterioration.

Immunity and Prevention

The protective mechanism against disease appears to be cell-mediated immunity via the activated macrophage. The best evidence for this is that the predisposing factors, e.g., corticosteroid therapy and Hodgkin's disease, have in common T-cell and macrophage defects. However, some patients who develop cryptococcal meningitis or other forms of disseminated disease, have no apparent defect in CMI. Some patients with no known predisposing disease have been shown to have T-cell abnormalities, but since these patients are fairly ill, it is unclear which is cause and which effect.

Interesting but incomplete work has been done with a humoral factor found in serum, but not in spinal fluid, which inhibits the growth of cryptococci. Further studies are necessary to elucidate whether or not this factor is deficient in patients who develop disseminated cryptococcal disease.

Selected Bibliography

Bennett, J. E.: Flucytosine. *Ann Intern Med* 86:319-322, 1977.

Bennett, J. E., Dismukes, W. E., Duma, R. J., Medoff, G., Sande, M. A., Gallis, H., Leonard, J., Fields, B. T., Bradshaw, M., Haywood, H., McGee, Z. A., Cate, T. R., Cobbs, C. G., Warner, J. F., and Alling, D. A.: A comparison of amphotericin B alone and combined with flucytosine in the treatment of cryptococcal meningitis. *N Engl J Med* 301:126-131, 1979.

Bindschadler, D. D. and Bennett, J. E.: Serology of human cryptococcosis. *Ann Intern Med* 69:45-52, 1968.

Diamond, R. D.: Effects of stimulation and suppression of cell-mediated immunity on experimental cryptococcosis. *Infect Immun* 17:187–194, 1977.

Diamond, R. D. and Allison, A. C.: Nature of the effector cells responsible for antibody-dependent cell mediated killing of *Cryptococcus neoformans. Infect Immun* 14:716–720, 1976.

Diamond, R. D. and Bennett, J. E.: Prognostic factors in cryptococcal meningitis. A study in 111 cases. *Ann Intern Med* 80:176–181, 1974.

Duperval, R., Hermans, P. E., Brewer, N. S., and Roberts, G. D.: Cryptococcosis, with emphasis on the significance of isolation of *Cryptococcus neoformans* from the respiratory tract. *Chest* 72:13–19, 1977.

Dykstra, M. A., Friedman, L., and Murphy, J. W.: Capsule size of *Cryptococcus neoformans:* Control and relationship to virulence. *Infect Immun* 16:129–135, 1977.

Einsenberg, R. S. and Oatway, W. H.: Nebulization of amphotericin B. *Am Rev Respir Dis* 103:289–292, 1971.

Ellner, J. J. and Bennett, J. E.: Chronic meningitis. *Medicine* 55:341–369, 1976.

Graybill, J. R. and Levine, H.B.: Successful treatment of cryptococcal meningitis with intraventricular miconazole. *Arch Intern Med* 138:814–816, 1978.

Gross, P. A., Patel, C., and Spitler, L. E.: Disseminated *Cryptococcus* treated with transfer factor. *JAMA* 240:2460–2462, 1978.

Kaplan, M. H., Rosen, P. P., and Armstrong, D.: Cryptococcosis in a cancer hospital. Clinical and pathological correlates in forty-six patients. *Cancer* 39: 2265–2274, 1977.

Lewis, J. L. and Rabinovich, S.: The wide spectrum of cryptococcal infections. *Am J Med* 53:315–322, 1972.

Macher, A. M., Bennett, J. E., Gadek, J. E., and Frank, M. D.: Complement depletion in cryptococcal sepsis. *J Immunol* 120:1686–1690, 1978.

Sapico, F. L.: Disappearance of focal cryptococcal brain lesion on chemotherapy alone. *Lancet* 1:560, 1979.

Schimpff, S. C. and Bennett, J. E.: Abnormalities in cell-mediated immunity in patients with *Cryptococcus neoformans* infections. *J Allergy Clin Immunol* 55:430–441, 1975.

Snow, R. M. and Dismukes, W. E.: Cryptococcal meningitis. Diagnostic value of cryptococcal antigen in cerebrospinal fluid. *Arch Intern Med* 135:1155–1157, 1975.

Sung, J. P., Campbell, G. D., and Crendahl, J. G.: Miconazole therapy for fungal meningitis. *Arch Neurol* 35:443–447, 1978.

113

NORTH AMERICAN BLASTOMYCOSIS
Robert M. D'Alessandri, M.D.

Introduction

The causative agent of North American blastomycosis was first identified by Gilchrist and Stokes in 1896. Until recently it was thought that the organism was found only in North America. However, several cases have been reported from Africa. Most cases have been reported from the Mississippi and Ohio River valleys and the southeastern United States.

Etiology

Blastomyces dermatitidis is a dimorphic fungus, growing in the yeast phase in vivo and at 37°C on enriched media. The mycelial form grows on Sabouraud's agar at room temperature. Generally, one to several weeks are required to produce mature colonies. The colonies are composed of mycelia with slender conidiophores bearing spherical to oval conidia (spores) which vary in size from 2 to 10 μm.

Epidemiology

Within the United States most cases of blastomycosis occur in Kentucky, Ohio, the Carolinas, Illinois, Michigan, Wisconsin, Iowa, Tennessee, Arkansas, Virginia, and West Virginia. A few cases are reported in Mexico and Canada. The source of the organism is generally thought to be the soil, although recovery from soil has been generally unsuccessful. The disease occurs ten times more frequently in men than women, affects all age groups, but is more common between the ages of 30 and 50. Primary cutaneous blastomycosis occurs rarely as a result of accidental percutaneous laboratory inoculation.

Pathogenesis

The usual portal of entry is the respiratory tract. The incubation period following inhalation of the fungus is quite variable and probably relates to the size of the inoculum. Hematogenous spread from lungs to skin may occur. Person-to-person or animal-to-human transmission is very unusual. However, spread by sexual intercourse has been reported. In lung tissue the reaction to B. dermatitidis generally consists of granuloma formation with giant cells and leukocytes in a central necrotic area. On occasion, granulomas without necrosis predominate and may be confused with sarcoidosis. On other occasions, polymorphonuclear leukocytes predominate with microabscess formation. Rarely, one may see very little tissue reaction with many organisms. In the skin the finding of pseudoepitheliomatous proliferation with an intraepithelial abscess is characteristic. However identification of organisms in tissue section remains essential for diagnosis.

Diagnosis

Clinical

Following inhalation of the fungus many patients remain asymptomatic demonstrating only skin test conversion. Others develop an influenza-like illness ranging from minimal to incapacitating symptomatology. A second form of the acute pulmonary disease consists of severe pleuritic pain of short duration. In the acute forms the findings on the chest roentgenogram are variable, ranging from small localized infiltrates to dense multilobe consolidation. Pleural effusion may develop. Perhaps the most characteristic radiographic finding is a perihilar mass mimicking carcinoma.

In general, cough, fever, malaise, sputum production, and chest pain are the most common symptoms of acute pulmonary disease. Physical findings are likewise nonspecific. Chronic pulmonary lesions may develop and include cavitation, fibrosis, and bronchiectasis. Following pulmonary infections, dissemination occurs. The interval is variable and 33 months or longer may intervene between pulmonary infection and presentation with disseminated disease. Cutaneous involvement is the most frequent site of dissemination and usually involves exposed areas such as the face and hands. Skin lesions tend to be chronic and resolve spontaneously. The lesions begin as small papules, gradually enlarge, and become verrucous and erythematous. These lesions may ulcerate and weep. The lesions enlarge eccentrically and appear serpigenous with pustules at the base. Healing begins centrally with a resultant atrophic nonpigmented scar. Regional lymphadenopathy is not usually associated with cutaneous blastomycosis. Most patients have a single lesion, although multiple lesions do occur.

The genitourinary tract is another common site of involvement, particularly the prostate, epididymus, and testes. Clinical findings include perineal and testicular pain and tenderness, hematuria, and pyuria. Dysuria rarely occurs. Osseous lesions develop in the vertebral column, long bones of the lower extremities, and flat bones. In children the skull is a frequent site of involvement. Extension into a joint space may occur. Pain at the infected site is common. Chronic osseous involvement may lead to sinus tract formation with persistent drainage. Psoas abscess may develop as a result of lumbar spine involvement and fistula formation. At autopsy granulomas are found in the spleen and liver in 40% of the cases. Central nervous system involvement occurs in about 10% of the cases, presenting as a mass lesion or as meningitis. The organism is cultured only rarely from the CSF. Involvement of the adrenals, pericardium, and endocardium has been reported.

Laboratory

The diagnosis of blastomycosis is missed frequently, not because the fungus is difficult to identify or isolate, but because blastomycosis is not considered in the differential. The diagnosis rests on isolation of the organism from appropriate cultures. Potassium hydroxide preparations of sputum or tissue exudates often reveal the thick-walled budding cells of *B. dermatitidis*. In tissue preparations, PAS, mucicarmine, and methenamine silver stains facilitate identification of the organism. Skin and serologic tests are unreliable and insensitive. Blastomycosis must be differentiated from other fungal infections such as coccidioidomycosis and histoplasmosis, tuberculosis, and lung cancer. Cutaneous blastomycosis may be confused with sporotrichosis.

Therapy

Amphotericin B is the mainstay of therapy for blastomycosis. Response to therapy is excellent and relapse is uncommon. All patients, even those with localized skin lesions, should receive a total of at least 1.5 g of amphotericin B. The use of 2-hydroxystilbamidine is primarily of historic interest since it appears to be less effective and at least as toxic as amphotericin B. Miconazole has been used successfully in patients unable to tolerate amphotericin B. Iodides have no place in the treatment of blastomycosis. Surgical drainage of abscesses is important adjunctive therapy. In vitro studies suggest that ketoconazole may be an effective oral agent in the treatment of infections caused by *B. dermatitidis*. Clinical studies are needed to determine efficacy.

Prognosis

With appropriate therapy, mortality has been reduced to less than 8% of all cases. If untreated, pulmonary disease slowly progresses with a fatal outcome. Occasionally spontaneous remissions occur with complete resolution of pulmonary lesions.

Selected Bibliography

Gonyea, E. F.: The spectrum of primary blastomycotic meningitis: A review of central nervous system blastomycosis. *Ann Neurol* 3:26-39, 1978.

Laskey, W. and Sarosi, G.: Endogenous activation in blastomycosis. *Ann Intern Med* 88:50-52, 1978.

Powell, D. A. and Schuit, K. E.: Acute pulmonary blastomycosis in children: Clinical course and follow-up. *Pediatrics* 63:736-740, 1979.

Sarosi, G. A., Hammerman, K. J., Tosh, F. E., and Kronenberg, R. S.: Clinical features of acute pulmonary blastomycosis. *N Engl J Med* 290:540-543, 1974.

Schwarz, J. and Salfelder, K.: Blastomycosis: A review of 152 cases. *Curr Top Pathol* 65:165-200, 1977.

114

HISTOPLASMOSIS
Charles E. Andrews, M.D.

Histoplasmosis is a disease caused by the dimorphic fungus *Histoplasma capsulatum*. Inhalation of the spores of this organism usually leads to a mild asymptomatic infection in man, but rarely a severe disseminated disease occurs. The classification developed by Goodwin et al., and listed in Table 114.1 is a useful categorization of the various clinical pictures. In endemic areas, most individuals become infected at some time during their lives. It has been estimated that over 30 million people have been infected. The frequency of occurrence of the various types of symptomatic infections is unknown, but they must be relatively rare. A case rate of between 1:100,000 and 1:500,000 for disseminated histoplasmosis is probably reasonable. The occasional symptomatic infection, rare complication, or opportunistic infection is of importance because appropriate treatment administered early may be lifesaving.

Microbiology

Histoplasma capsulatum is a dimorphic fungus and is identified by finding the characteristic large, round to pyriform tuberculate spores (7.5–15 μm in diameter) that develop when the organism is grown on Sabouraud's glucose agar at room temperature. In mammals *H. capsulatum* is primarily a parasite of the reticuloendothelial system and exists in the yeast phase in macrophages. It is rare to find the organism extracellularly. Specimens including sputum, gastric washings, heated aerosols, blood, bone marrow, or biopsies from open lesions from patients suspected of having histoplasmosis should be placed on brain-heart infusion glucose blood agar plates to which antibiotics have been added and incubated at 37°C. The organism is more likely to be isolated on this medium than Sabouraud's at room temperature. However, since any isolate must be transferred to this medium for identification, it is worthwhile to use it in initial isolation attempts.

974

TABLE 114.1   Classification of Histoplasmosis

Acute pulmonary histoplasmosis

Usual asymptomatic infection

Occasional symptomatic infection

Rare complications

Pericarditis

Mediastinal granuloma

Mediastinal fibrosis

Histoplasmoma

Opportunistic infections

Chronic pulmonary histoplasmosis
(structural defect)

Disseminated histoplasmosis (immune
defect)

Epidemiology

The development and use of the histoplasmin skin test, derived from the mycelial phase of the organism, have clarified the distribution of infection with this organism. Skin test reactivity to histoplasmin by state is shown in Figure 114.1 and illustrates that infection is most likely to occur in the central portion of the United States in the Ohio and Mississippi River valleys. The potentially airborne spores are most plentiful in moist fertile soil, especially if it has been enriched by avian or bat excreta. The factor or factors that facilitate growth of the organism in this environment are unknown. Thus human exposure to airborne spores in large numbers may be encountered in such activities as cleaning old chicken houses, spreading chicken manure, raking or bulldozing starling roosts, or spelunking. Most reported cases of acute infection have been associated with epidemics related to point sources involving those activities. The specific source of the organism is unknown in most patients since acute infections are usually undetected. The infection has never been transmitted from person to person.

Pathogenesis

The first event is the inhalation of the airborne spores. At the alveolar level the spores germinate to the yeast phase and are engulfed by macrophages. The fungus continues to divide and infected macrophages are found in the lymph channels and hilar lymph nodes. Hematogenous spread to secondary sites such as the liver and spleen occurs at this time. Specific cellular immunity develops about 2 weeks after the initial infection and the skin test becomes positive. In the lung, a small granulomatous reaction develops, and with larger infiltrates central necrosis may

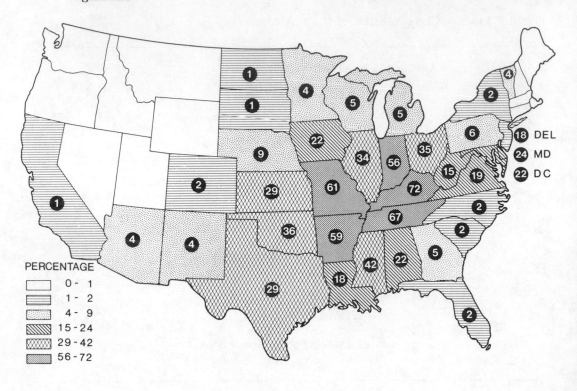

FIGURE 114.1   Geographic distribution of histoplasmin skin test positivity, indicative of endemicity of histoplasmosis.

occur. With healing, calcification frequently occurs in the center of the lesion both at the initial sites of infection and in secondary sites of involvement such as the lymph nodes, liver, and spleen. With heavy exposure to the organism, multiple areas of pulmonary infiltration may occur and the patient experiences a flu-like illness. These lesions usually heal with no specific treatment, but symptoms may persist for several weeks.

Macrophages infected with *Histoplasma* migrate to the mediastinal lymph nodes. Occasionally the nodes may produce a mass-like lesion and encroach on a bronchus or esophagus. The associated periadenitis may lead to pericarditis or pleuritis with effusion. Excessive fibrogenesis may occur with healing, and fibrous mediastinitis can result.

The caseous lesions in the lung usually heal with a thick fibrotic capsule. Occasionally capsule formation continues for years; such a lesion presents on the chest roentgenogram as an enlarging pulmonary nodule and may be confused with carcinoma if central calcification is not present.

Chronic pulmonary histoplasmosis occurs only in a lung that is already the site of chronic bronchitis or emphysema. The early lesion is a segmental interstitial pneumonitis with areas of focal necrosis. In lesions that persist, the pneumonitis involves bullous or emphysematous areas, the walls of which may become necrotic and then thickened by fibrous tissue. Necrotic material, which may or may not be infective, is aspirated into other parts of the lung. This material produces more fibrosis and scarring and destruction of the lung.

Rarely, the fungus may grow in secondary sites after hematogenous spread producing disseminated histoplasmosis. This occurs more frequently in infants and probably occurs only in individuals with cellular immune deficiencies. However, specific immune deficiencies have not been documented as yet in all patients. The reticuloendothelial system becomes crowded with organisms and fever, anemia, leukopenia, and hepatosplenomegaly develop. Gastrointestinal ulcerations, endocarditis, adrenal gland destruction, diffuse meningitis or central nervous system focal lesions, and ulcerative lesions of the skin and mucous membranes may occur.

Diagnosis

The diagnosis of histoplasmosis in the various forms of the disease is usually made by the clinical findings, including epidemiologic data, serologic studies, and appropriate cultures for the fungus.

A positive skin test with histoplasmin, a mycelial phase antigen, indicates previous infection with the fungus and should be used only for epidemiologic studies. In endemic areas, positive reactors occur so frequently that the test has little or no diagnostic value. Testing with histoplasmin also has the disadvantage of producing a booster effect on the complement-fixation test.

The complement-fixation test using either the whole yeast phase or histoplasmin as antigen is most useful in making the diagnosis of histoplasmosis. The antibody measured against either antigen is an IgG. A positive reaction in a serum dilution of 1:4 for the mycelial phase and 1:16 for the yeast antigen is usually considered significant. A fourfold difference in serial determinations is more significant than a single test. Precipitin and agglutination tests have been developed and technically are easier to perform but are less sensitive and specific when compared with the complement-fixation test.

Recovery of the organism from body fluids, bone marrow, or tissue is the most reliable way to make the diagnosis. These materials should be cultured on both glucose agar at room temperature and on cysteine blood agar at 37°C. The demonstration of tuberculate spores in mycelial growth is necessary for positive identification. Identification of the organism in tissues obtained by biopsy requires the use of the periodic acid-Schiff (PAS) procedure or the Gomori's methenamine silver stain.

The diagnosis of histoplasmosis in the usual asymptomatic infection is of course made only retrospectively. Calcified parenchymal lesions and hilar nodes by chest roentgenogram in an individual from the endemic area with a negative tuberculin test are generally accepted as evidence of previous infection.

Patients with the occasional symptomatic form of the disease usually present with a flu-like illness. Studies of epidemics indicate an incubation period of approximately 18 days. The complement-fixation test is usually positive a month after infection. Chest roentgenographic findings vary from normal to patchy nonsegmental opacities, usually in the lower lobes, with hilar node enlargement. Rarely a thin-walled cavity may be seen. The patches of infiltrate may clear in one area only to reappear in another. It is difficult to recover the organism from sputum in this form of the disease. The diagnosis is usually confirmed by demonstrating a fourfold rise in the complement-fixation titer.

Mediastinal involvement may lead to various clinical and roentgenologic manifestations depending upon the site and extent of the lesions. Pericarditis, superior vena caval syndrome, esophageal displacement or obstruction, and pulmonary arterial and venous obstruction may be produced by the enlarged mediastinal nodes and resultant fibrosis. A widened mediastinal shadow may be the only clue to the diagnosis, and special studies such as angiography may be necessary to delineate the lesions. By the time the fibrosis has progressed to the point of causing symptoms, it may be impossible to confirm the diagnosis of histoplasmosis. The organism can rarely be cultured from mediastinal nodes. Biopsy of the nodes and examination using PAS and silver stains may disclose the organisms, even when cultures are negative. Studies of the fibrous tissue are uniformly nonproductive. The complement-fixation test when positive is most useful in confirming the diagnosis.

Histoplasmoma is a common manifestation of histoplasmosis. It is usually a solitary lesion up to 3 cm in size and located in a lower lobe. Small satellite lesions may be present. Usually there is a central nidus or concentric rings of calcium present. The lesion may enlarge when new layers of fibrous tissue are laid down. Silver stains of surgically removed histoplasmomas usually reveal organisms, but cultures are sterile. Serologic tests for histoplasmosis are usually negative. The clinical problem is that of the management of a solitary pulmonary nodule. Surgical removal is indicated unless calcium is present or the lesion has remained stable by roentgenographic examination for 2-3 years.

Patients with chronic pulmonary histoplasmosis have symptoms similar to those of patients with tuberculosis: cough, low-grade fever, night sweats, and malaise (Table 114.2). This form of the disease was recognized as a significant

TABLE 114.2   Characteristics of Chronic Pulmonary Histoplasmosis

---

Males over 50 years old

Underlying chronic bronchitis and/or emphysema

20% asymptomatic; disease is discovered incidentally

Cough, malaise, easy fatigability, weight loss, low-grade fever

Chest pain, deep and aching, suggestive of carcinoma, found in 1/3

Hemoptysis, usually in cavitary disease, in ∿ 1/3

Dyspnea with progression

Chest radiograph mimics tuberculosis

Histoplasmin skin test of no diagnostic help

Complement-fixation test

    Negative in 25%
    Borderline in 40%
    Diagnostic in 35%
    Not helpful in determining prognosis or need for treatment

Definitive diagnosis: culturing *H. capsulatum* from sputum

Respiratory insufficiency is usual cause of death

---

entity among patients hospitalized in tuberculosis sanitoria. The radiograph of the chest mimics that seen in tuberculosis. Characteristically the apical and posterior segments are involved. The initial lesion is a patchy infiltrate, segmental in nature, and frequently located near the pleura. As the lesion progresses, some areas appear to clear while other areas become more dense, and the lobe appears to contract. With further progression, a cavity with thick walls may develop. The radiographic findings of emphysema are frequently present. The only way to make a definitive diagnosis is by demonstrating *H. capsulatum* in cultures of the sputum. At least six separate specimens should be submitted for culture. In patients with early pneumonic lesions and those with thin-walled cavities about one-third of the cultures will be positive. Patients with thick-walled cavities have positive cultures in 50–70% of the cases. These patients should be carefully studied for tuberculosis because of frequent coexistence of the two diseases.

It has been estimated that approximately 120 new cases of disseminated histoplasmosis occur in the United States each year. This form of the disease occurs in an immunocompromised host and is usually fatal if untreated (Table 114.3). Approximately one-third of the cases occur during the first year of life. Cough associated with the initial primary infection continues and malaise, anorexia, and weight loss develop. Fever may range from 100°F to 105°F (Table 114.4). Nausea, vomiting, and diarrhea are usually present. Hepatosplenomegaly is practically always present and most will have generalized lymphadenopathy. Anemia, leukopenia, and thrombocytopenia develop secondary to bone marrow involvement by the fungus (Table 114.5).

TABLE 114.3   Risk Factors for Fatal or Disseminated Histoplasmosis

Factor	Approximate % of Symptomatic Patients with Fatal or Disseminated Disease
Immunosuppression	
Present	75
Absent	6
Age	
< 55	10
> 55	25
Race	
Black	9
White	15
Chronic lung disease	
Present	15
Absent	10

TABLE 114.4   Presenting Symptoms in Disseminated Histoplasmosis

Symptom	% of Patients
Fever	70
Weight loss	65
Pulmonary (cough, dyspnea, etc.)	50
Oral lesions	25
Neurologic	20

TABLE 114.5   Hematologic Manifestations of Disseminated Histoplasmosis

Manifestation	% of Patients
Thrombocytopenia	50
Anemia	45
Splenomegaly	40
Leukopenia	25
Leukocytosis	10
Positive bone marrow culture	70

A few infants and adults have a more moderate form of the disease with many of the features present. With a less severe and more chronic course, focal lesions with destructive organ disease may occur. These patients may have endocarditis, meningitis, intestinal ulceration, or Addison's disease. Without treatment death occurs in 6-12 months.

Adults tend to have a milder more chronic disease. Unexplained weight loss, intermittent low-grade fever, and fatigue may be present for years. Eventually most of these patients will develop an oropharyngeal nodule or ulcer suggestive of malignancy. A biopsy of these lesions will lead to the correct diagnosis of histoplasmosis (Table 114.6).

The complement-fixation test is positive in about two-thirds of these patients. A Wright's stain smear and culture of the peripheral blood are usually positive for the fungus in the acute severe infant form of the disease (Table 114.7). Smears are less helpful in the adult forms of disseminated disease but cultures are still worthwhile. A bone marrow biopsy using methenamine silver stain is often helpful. Table 114.8 gives a summary of liver biopsy findings.

TABLE 114.6   Isolation of Organism in Disseminated Histoplasmosis

Specimen	% of Patients with Positive Culture
Oral lesion	90
Lymph node	70
Bone marrow	70
Sputum	60
Liver biopsy	55
Blood	55
Spinal fluid	45
Urine	45

TABLE 114.7   Culture Results in Disseminated Histoplasmosis

Correlation of blood and bone marrow culture: 1/3 with negative blood culture had + marrow; none with negative marrow had + blood

Urine culture relative to abnormal renal function: 40% of patients with positive culture had normal renal function

TABLE 114.8   Liver Biopsy Findings in Disseminated Histoplasmosis

Finding	% of Biopsies
Positive culture	55
Organisms seen microscopically	40
Granulomas	70

About one-half of the patients with disseminated histoplasmosis have adrenal insufficiency. Serum electrolyte and corticosteroid serum levels should be followed in these patients.

Treatment

Before the introduction of amphotericin B in 1956, there was no effective treatment for histoplasmosis. A few patients with the chronic pulmonary form had responded to surgery and bed rest, but the disseminated form was uniformly fatal. Subsequent experience has shown that the drug is an effective agent for the treatment of most cases but far from ideal. The drug has significant toxicity, must be given intravenously, and is not always effective. It is the standard, however, against which new drugs must be evaluated. Patients with the disseminated, chronic pulmonary, and rarely the acute symptomatic pulmonary forms of the disease should be treated. The outcome of therapy is dependent upon the stage of histoplasmosis when treatment is started, the presence or absence of other serious disease, and the patient's ability to tolerate the drug.

The diagnosis in patients with disseminated histoplasmosis should be confirmed by finding the organism in a peripheral blood or bone marrow smear, biopsy of a lesion, or culture of a body fluid before beginning amphotericin B therapy. The ideal is not known but a minimum of 35 mg/kg body weight total dose should be given. A 5-year survival rate of approximately 35% can be expected. The patient must be followed closely for evidence of clinical improvement after the drug is started. Conversion of a positive smear or culture of the organism to negative should be documented. If a relapse occurs, amphotericin B should be continued and therapy with ketoconazole considered.

Patients with chronic pulmonary histoplasmosis and a positive sputum culture should be treated with amphotericin B for a total dosage of at least 35 mg/kg body weight. The results of such treatment are listed in Table 114.9.

TABLE 114.9   Results of Therapy of Chronic Pulmonary Histoplasmosis

Sputum cultures usually become negative in 1-4 wk

Relapse

    15% of patients

    More common if unable to complete full course of treatment

    Usually within first 2 yr

    Should give second course of amphotericin B and a course of ketoconazole

Mortality

    Untreated: 55%

    Treated: 30%

TABLE 114.10   Criteria for Treatment of Patients with the Occasional Symptomatic Infection

---

A good history of exposure to the organism

An acutely ill patient with an illness of several weeks duration

A chest roentgenograph with diffuse involvement

A positive culture or fourfold or higher rise in the complement-fixation test

---

Amphotericin B has been used in patients with acute histoplasmosis to shorten the course of the illness and to prevent the rare occasion when the disease disseminates. The value of treatment in these circumstances is unknown. If this very toxic drug is to be used in a usually self-limiting disease, strict criteria should be used to select the patients (Table 114.10).

Selected Bibliography

Edwards, P. Q. and Palmer, C. E.: Nationwide histoplasmin sensitivity and histoplasmal infection. *Public Health Rep* 78:241-259, 1963.

Furcolow, M. L. and Brasher, C. A.: Chronic progressive (cavitary) histoplasmosis as a problem in tuberculosis sanitoriums. *Am Rev Tuberc Pulm Dis* 73:609, 1975.

Goodwin, R. A. and Des Prez, R. M.: Histoplasmosis. *Am Rev Respir Dis* 117: 929-956, 1978.

Goodwin, R. A., Loyd, J. E., and Des Prez, R. M.: Histoplasmosis in normal hosts. *Medicine* 60:231-266, 1981.

Goodwin, R. A., Owens, F. T., Snell, J. D., Hubbard, W. W., Buchanan, R. D., Terry, R. T., and Des Prez, R. M.: Chronic pulmonary histoplasmosis. *Medicine* 55:413-452, 1976.

Hawkins, S. S., Gregory, D. W., and Alford, R. H.: Progressive disseminated histoplasmosis: Favorable response to ketoconazole. *Ann Intern Med* 95:446-449, 1981.

Lehan, P. H. and Furcolow, M. L.: Epidemic histoplasmosis. *J Chron Dis* 5:489-503, 1957.

Naylor, B. A.: Low-dose amphotericin B therapy for acute pulmonary histoplasmosis. *Chest* 71:404-406, 1977.

Parker, J. D., Sarosi, G. A., Doto, I. L., Bailey, R. E., and Tosh, F. E.: Treatment of chronic pulmonary histoplasmosis: A National Communicable Disease Center Cooperative Mycoses Study. *N Engl J Med* 283:225–229, 1970.

Sarosi, G. A., Voth, D. W., Dahl, B. A., Doto, I. L., and Tosh, F. E.: Disseminated histoplasmosis: Results of long-term follow-up. A Center for Disease Control Cooperative Mycoses Study. *Ann Intern Med* 75:511–516, 1971.

Smith, J. W. and Utz, J. P.: Progressive disseminated histoplasmosis. A prospective study of 26 patients. *Ann Intern Med* 76:557, 1972.

Sutliff, W. D.: Histoplasmosis cooperative study. II. Chronic pulmonary histoplasmosis treated with and without amphotericin B. *Am Rev Respir Dis* 89: 641–650, 1964.

Zeidberg, L. D., Dillion, A., and Gass, R. S.: Some factors in the epidemiology of histoplasmin sensitivity in Williamson County, Tennessee. *Am J Public Health* 41:90, 1951.

115

COCCIDIOIDOMYCOSIS
Robert M. D'Alessandri, M.D.

Etiology

The causative agent of coccidioidomycosis is the diphasic fungus *Coccidioides immitis*. This saprophytic soil fungus was first discovered in Argentina, but most of the cases occur in the United States. In nature and on Sabouraud's agar *C. immitis* grows as a luxuriant mycelium, initially white, later turning tan or brown. The mycelium is composed of separate hyphae which mature to form arthrospores (arthroconidia) separated by empty cells. The arthrospores are barrel-shaped, 2-4 by 3-6 μm. Other fungi which produce arthrospores such as species of *Geotrichum* and *Arthroderma* may lead to misidentification. There is tremendous variation in the morphologic characteristics of *C. immitis*. As a result, inoculation of laboratory animals and the production of (1) the disease and (2) the spherule phase have traditionally been the only acceptable method of identification. As few as 10 arthrospores are able to produce pulmonary infection in primates. Microscopically in tissue, *C. immitis* appears as nonbudding, spherical, thick-walled structures of 10-80 μm in diameter, the spherule. Within the spherule numerous endospores may be identified. Reproduction of the fungus begins when the spherule ruptures and releases the endospores which in turn develop into spherules. This phase, unlike the arthrospore phase, is not infective.

    Coccidioides immitis requires no special media for growth and the arthrospores are hardy and resistant to drying. More than 200 cases of laboratory-acquired coccidioidomycosis have been reported. Therefore only laboratories skilled and equipped to handle this highly infectious agent should attempt transfer and identification of suspected cultures. Black, Filipino, and pregnant laboratory workers may be at particular risk.

Epidemiology

Nearly 200,000 cases of coccidioidomycosis are reported yearly in the United States. The disease appears to be restricted to the Western Hemisphere with the endemic zone extending from northern California to Argentina. The areas of greatest endemicity include the southwestern United States and northern Mexico. During the dry season, the fungus is absent from the desert surface but survives for months in the soil at depths of up to 20 cm in rodent burrows. Following the rainy season the desert surface becomes recolonized. The likelihood of infection is greatest whenever dry, windy conditions exist or whenever *C. immitis*-receptive soil is disturbed and arthrospores are aerosolized. Epidemics usually occur in the hot, dry months following the rainy season, often after the soil has been disturbed by agricultural operations, or archeological or housing excavations. As a result of several epidemics associated with archeological expeditions, the California State Department of Public Health recommends that those individuals who are skin test negative should not be allowed to participate in field work in endemic areas. Coccidioidomycosis is also recognized as an important occupational hazard, and partial control in excavating projects has been accomplished by local application of a fungicide. Coccidioidomycosis may be acquired by contact with infected fomites thousands of miles from an endemic zone.

In general, infection is acquired via the respiratory tract. On rare occasion, acquisition has occurred by cutaneous inoculation and is generally self-limited. A case of in utero transmission has been documented. Rodents, horses, cattle, sheep, cats, and dogs may be infected just as humans are. Animal-to-human or person-to-person transmission is unlikely.

Pathogenesis

The histopathologic response to the inhalation of arthrospores appears to be similar to that following infection with *Mycobacterium tuberculosis*. Classic granuloma formation occurs with giant cells and caseation. However, there appears to be a pathologic spectrum ranging from a suppurative, predominantly polymorphonuclear response, to one which is predominantly granulomatous. The suppurative response appears to be more predominant in disseminated disease and may indicate a relative lack of cell-mediated immunity. Following primary pulmonary infection, a pneumonitis develops with associated lymphatic spread of organisms frequently manifested by hilar adenopathy. Supraclavicular or scalene nodes may be involved by direct spread of organisms; this does not imply dissemination. Cavities or thin-walled cysts frequently develop and are usually transient; however, cavities may persist and may become secondarily infected. Solid granulomatous lesions often occur and may in later years require surgical removal because of the fear that they might represent a malignancy.

Dissemination is believed to occur via lymphatic and hematogeous spread and usually occurs within several weeks of primary infection. Any tissue of the body may be affected, but cancellous bones, such as ribs, skull, and limbs, are very commonly affected. Other organs commonly involved are the kidneys, spleen, and leptomeninges.

Diagnostic Features

Clinical

Most cases of coccidioidomycosis are asymptomatic. In approximately 40% of the patients, symptoms ranging from a mild flu-like illness to pneumonia develop. Generally the symptoms are mild, nonspecific, and not suggestive of coccidioidomycosis. In symptomatic disease the incubation period is from 1 to 4 weeks (average 10-16 days). The most frequent symptoms include dry cough, fever, headache, and chest pain (often marked) (Table 115.1). Chills, malaise, and rash occur in more than half of the patients. The chest pain is often pleuritic. Fever is accompanied by mild chills, and night sweats occur frequently. Headache is a frequent nonspecific symptom associated with febrile illnesses and not necessarily an indication of meningeal or CNS involvement. Lumbar puncture should be performed, as in most other febrile illnesses, whenever there is any question of meningeal involvement.

Early in the course of the illness a fine diffuse macular erythematous eruption develops over the extremities. Generally the rash disappears before the patient seeks medical attention. The rash may be confused with an allergic or contact dermatitis, the exanthem of measles, scarlet fever, heat rash, or urticaria. The etiology of the rash is unknown.

The complex of erythema nodosum or erythema multiforme, arthralgias, conjunctivitis, and pneumonitis make up the entity known as valley fever. Erythema nodosum (EN) and erythema multiforme may occur in otherwise asymptomatic individuals. Erythema nodosum occurs usually on the shins, is painful, asymmetric, occurs more commonly in women and Caucasians, and is generally regarded as a good prognostic indicator. It develops at approximately the same time the coccidioidin skin test becomes positive. Erythema multiforme tends to involve the upper torso, is often pruritic and may desquamate. Both eruptions usually subside within 2-6 weeks.

Radiographic abnormalities are common and variable and include lobar infiltration, scattered patchy infiltration, atelectasis, hilar adenopathy, and pleural effusion (Table 115.2).

TABLE 115.1   Symptoms of Primary Pulmonary Coccidioidomycosis

Symptom	% of Patients
Fever: usually low-grade	~ 80
Chest pain	~ 80
Cough: usually nonproductive	~ 70
Cutaneous lesions	~ 20
Arthralgias	~ 10
Nonspecific symptoms: malaise, chills, night sweats, headache, anorexia, pharyngitis (one or more)	~ 100

TABLE 115.2   Chest Roentgenogram Findings in Primary Pulmonary
Coccidioidomycosis

Finding	% of Patients
Pneumonitis	$\sim$ 70
Adenitis	$\sim$ 25
Cavitation	$\sim$ 8
Nodules	$\sim$ 5
Pleural effusion	$\sim$ 3
Normal chest	$\sim$ 3

Within 2-3 weeks symptoms of primary pulmonary coccidioidomycosis abate
(Table 115.3). If symptoms or radiographic abnormalities persist beyond 2 months,
then persistent coccidioidomycosis is said to have developed. This is manifested
by chronic progressive pulmonary involvement with resultant fibrosis and scarring (Table 115.4). Patients with persistent pneumonia are typically very ill with
fever, chest pain, cough, and often a fatal outcome.

Dissemination to extrapulmonary tissues appears to be dependent upon at least
five factors: race, sex, pregnancy, age, and immune status. Filipinos, blacks and
Mexicans are at significantly greater risk of dissemination and death. Coccidioidomycosis acquired late during pregnancy is associated with a higher maternal and
fetal mortality. In addition it would appear that the younger (under 5) and older
(50 or over) age groups are more susceptible to dissemination. The reason for this
association is unclear but may relate to waning cell-mediated immunity in the
elderly and an incompletely developed immune system in the young.

Immunosuppression, most commonly in the form of corticosteroid therapy,
may lead to reactivation and dissemination of coccidioidomycosis. Therefore, in
patients with a history of residence in endemic areas, skin and serologic testing
should be performed before steroid therapy. Dissemination tends to occur within
months of acquisition and usually involves the skin, bones, meninges, or genitourinary system (Table 115.5). The early clinical manifestations are subtle until
involvement of specific sites becomes manifest. The meninges are involved in
one-third to one-half of all cases of dissemination. Headache, stiff neck, and
confusion are early symptoms. Later manifestations reflect widespread meningeal
involvement with ventricular obstruction and the development of hydrocephalus.

Laboratory

The protean manifestations of coccidioidomycosis frequently complicate early
detection. In its classic form of fever, chest pain, pneumonic infiltrates, arthralgias, and erythema nodosum in an endemic area, the diagnosis presents little difficulty and requires only confirmatory laboratory studies. Unfortunately, the presentation is frequently not so clear and other diagnostic possibilities include viral
or bacterial pneumonia, tuberculosis, histoplasmosis, lymphoma, or other malignancies.

TABLE 115.3   Characteristics of Primary Coccidioidomycosis

Clinical	Pulmonary
	Cough
	Chest pain
	Skin
	Erythema nodosum
	Erythema multiforme
	Fever, chills, malaise
Chest x-ray	Infiltrate
	Pleural effusion
	Hilar adenopathy
Laboratory	Delayed hypersensitivity skin test:
	Becomes + 2-3 wk after onset of illness, remains + for life
	Antibody
	Precipitin test: + at 2 wk, does not persist
	Complement-fixation test: + at 2-4 wk, persists for many months
	Sputum
	Wet mount – spherules
	Culture may be +
Course	Usually self-limited
	Residual pulmonary changes in 5-10%
	Cavity
	Coin lesion
	Fibrosis

TABLE 115.4   Chronic Residual Thoracic Coccidioidal Lesions

Lung

  Fibrosis: most common
  Cavitation: about 5%, may be either
    thin- or thick-walled
  Coccidioidoma: caseous lesion with
    fibrous capsule
  Bronchiectasis

Pleura

  Empyema
  Pneumothorax and hydropneumothorax
    after cavity rupture

Pericardium

TABLE 115.5   Characteristics of Disseminated Coccidioidomycosis

Incidence	Rare: < 1% of total
	More common in nonwhites and
	  patients with impaired
	  immunity

Involved sites	Skin: most common
	Meninges: most serious, 40%
	  mortality
	Viscera: liver, spleen, pros-
	  tate, adrenals
	Bones and joints
	Lymph nodes
	Serous membranes: peritoneum,
	  pericardium

Ultimately the diagnosis of coccidioidomycosis may be confirmed by the identification in tissue sections of spherules. This requires special staining techniques.
In addition, cultures of clinical specimens may yield the diagnosis, but require
animal inoculation or special identification procedures since the morphologic appearance of mycelial growth is not characteristic. Because cultural identification
is difficult and hazardous and, in the case of CNS infection, frequently fails to
yield the organism, skin and serologic testing should be performed and often confirms the diagnosis (Table 115.6). However, it is important to note that patients

TABLE 115.6   Immunologic Tests in Primary Pulmonary Coccidioidomycosis

| Week of Illness | % Positive | | |
	Coccidioidin Skin Test	Precipitin	Complement-Fixation
1	∿90	∿50	∿10
2	∿95	∿85	∿20
3	∿99	∿90	∿30
8		∿45	∿80

with disseminated disease usually have a negative skin test and in some immuno-suppressed patients serologic tests are negative. At present there are two skin test antigens available: coccidioidin and spherulin. Coccidioidin is prepared from culture filtrates of the mycelial-arthrospore phase grown on synthetic media. The standard dilution is 1:100 and the test is positive if there is more than 5-mm induration at 24 or 48 hr. Patients with primary infection develop skin reactivity 3-21 days after the onset of illness, almost all within 1 week of the onset. Spherulin is the soluble fraction of the spherule-endospore phase produced in vitro. It possesses antigenic similarities to coccidioidin; however, there are some antigenic and physicochemical differences. Spherulin is more sensitive than coccidioidin and tends to be easier to standardize. More patients with disseminated disease react to spherulin, which has advantages and disadvantages. The advantage is with respect to its ability to help in the diagnosis of cases with negative coccidioidin reactions. The disadvantage is with respect to the prognostic value of a negative skin test in already diagnosed cases. Both skin test antigens must be diluted before administration to patients with erythema nodosum because of associated violent reactions. Neither skin test agent alters the complement-fixation titer for *Coccidioides,* but may elevate the serologic test for the yeast phase of *Histoplasma.*

In patients with disseminated disease or persistent infection, testing for IgG antibodies by complement-fixation should be performed. A low (< 1:16) or falling titer is a prognostically favorable sign. Conversely, rising or elevated titers generally indicate a poor response to infection and a poorer prognosis. This test is difficult and costly to perform and should be done in reference laboratories. Of greatest importance is the fact that more than 98% of patients with meningitis due to *C. immitis* will have detectable complement-fixing antibody in spinal fluid, and its presence in the CSF is diagnostic.

Treatment

In most patients with primary pulmonary coccidioidomycosis, symptomatic therapy only is required. However in patients with a high probability of dissemination and in patients with severe primary infection, antifungal therapy should be given.

In patients with persistent or progressive pulmonary infection antifungal treatment may reduce symptoms and limit the extent of the infection. Thin-walled cavities require no antifungal drug therapy. The clearest indication for aggressive antifungal therapy is in patients with disseminated disease, in whom the untreated mortality is 50% (Table 115.7).

Amphotericin B is the mainstay of therapy in coccidioidomycosis. Amphotericin B is fungistatic in vitro for *C. immitis,* and treatment failure is not related to fungal resistance. In severe infections the dose of amphotericin B should be 0.5-0.75 mg/kg/day intravenously (Table 115.8). With clinical improvement the dose may be lowered to 0.25-0.50 mg/kg/day. Alternate-day administration may also be effective but should be reserved for those patients improving clinically on daily therapy or for treatment of less severe infections. In patients with meningitis, intrathecal amphotericin B, in addition to intravenous drug, is recommended (0.5-1.0 mg four times weekly). However, prolonged intrathecal administration of amphotericin B results in arachnoiditis and occasionally a myelopathy. In addition, because of the mechanics of CSF flow, intrathecal administration often fails to deliver sufficient drug to infected sites. Cisternal injection avoids these problems. When repeated administration over a prolonged period appears to be necessary, an Ommaya intraventricular catheter-subcutaneous reservoir is the method of choice. Intraventricular amphotericin B should be continued at least until all CSF abnormalities and the CSF antibody titer return to normal.

TABLE 115.7   Indications for Intravenous Amphotericin B in Coccidioidomycosis

Severe primary infection with persistent fever, extending pulmonary disease, mediastinal adenopathy

Serologic evidence of persistent or extending disease, evidenced by rising titer of complement fixation (also titer > 1:64)

Evidence of spread to other organ systems from primary pulmonary focus

Negative skin test reaction to coccidioidin

Racial susceptibility, especially blacks and Filipinos

Perioperative coverage, beginning 2 weeks before surgical removal of coccidioidal lesion

Prophylaxis during pregnancy, in diabetics, during corticosteroid therapy being used for some other illness

TABLE 115.8   Treatment of Coccidioidomycosis

Primary (pulmonary)

Healthy adults and children	None
Infants	Amphotericin B, 0.1-0.5 g
Debilitated	Amphotericin B, 0.1-0.5 g (infants), 1-3 g (adults) + corticosteroids
Immunosuppressed, pregnant women, diabetics	Amphotericin B, 1-3 g
Progressive primary	Amphotericin B, 1-3 g
Residual pulmonary cavity	Surgery + amphotericin B, 1 g (+ intrapleural amphotericin B in patients with empyema)
Granuloma	Amphotericin B, 1-3 g

Disseminated

Meningitis	Amphotericin B, 1-3 g, + intracisternal or ventricular amphotericin B in certain cases, 0.25-0.5 mg/dose, also sometimes + corticosteroids
Skin, lymph nodes	Amphotericin B, 1-3 g IV, sometimes + local irrigation with 10% solution, or paste, and/or excision
Bones, viscera, GU tract, peritonitis	Amphotericin B, 1-4 g, sometimes + local irrigation and/or surgery

---

In addition to antifungal drug therapy, transfer factor has been used with varying success. Transfer factor frequently leads to conversion in skin test reactivity, lymphocyte transformation, and production of macrophage migration inhibitory factor. However whether or not there is any measurable clinical improvement has yet to be demonstrated.

Surgery is indicated to prevent rupture of an expanding pulmonary cavity, serious pulmonary hemorrhage, bronchopleural fistula, symptomatic mycetoma, or obstructive hydrocephalus. Surgery may be necessary to establish a diagnosis particularly in the patient with an isolated "coin" lesion or the immunosuppressed patient with pulmonary infiltrates.

Prevention

Since it is impossible to identify both the conditions under which infection occurs and the group that is at greatest risk, preventive measures may be possible to minimize the occurrence of severe coccidioidomycosis. Immunization of the population at risk would be a simple measure; unfortunately there is no effective vaccine available.

Selected Bibliography

Bayer, S. A., Guze, L. B., Yoshikawa, T. T., and Galpin, J. E.: Unusual syndromes of coccidioidomycosis. Diagnostic and therapeutic considerations. A report of 10 cases and review of the English literature. *Medicine* 55:131-152, 1976.

Catanzaro, A.: Pulmonary coccidioidomycosis. *Med Clin N Am* 64:461, 1980.

Caudill, R., Smith, C. E., and Reinarz, J.: Coccidioidal meningitis. A diagnostic challenge. *Am J Med* 49:360, 1970.

Deresinski, S. C., Lilly, R. B., Levine, H. B., Galgiani, J. N., and Stevens, D. A.: Treatment of fungal meningitis with miconazole. *Arch Intern Med* 137:1180-1185, 1977.

Deresinski, S. C. and Stevens, D. A.: Coccidioidomycosis in compromised hosts. *Medicine* 54:377-395, 1974.

Drutz, D. J. and Catanzaro, A.: Coccidioidomycosis, (Part I and II). *Am Rev Respir Dis* 117:559-585; 727-771, 1978.

Graybill, J. R., Lundberg, D., Donovan, W., Levine, H. B., Rodriquez, M. D., and Drutz, D. J.: Treatment of coccidioidomycosis with ketoconazole: Clinical and laboratory studies of 18 patients. *Rev Infect Dis* 2:661, 1980.

Heindl, I., Mickel, A., Pappagianis, D., and Werner, S. B.: An epidemic of coccidioidomycosis among archaeology students in northern California. *N Engl J Med* 286:507, 1972.

Pappagianis, D., Lindsay, S., Beall, S., and Williams, T.: Ethnic background and the clinical course of coccidioidomycosis. *Am Rev Respir Dis* 120:959, 1979.

Sarosi, G. A., Parker, J. D., Doto, I. L., and Tosh, F. E.: Chronic pulmonary coccidioidomycosis. *N Engl J Med* 283:325, 1970.

Sung, J. P.: Treatment of disseminated coccidioidomycosis with miconazole. *West J Med* 124:61-64, 1976.

116

CANDIDA

Robert H. Waldman, M.D. and
James C. Reynolds, M.D.

Candida is a yeast which commonly causes mild mucocutaneous infection, although it is capable of producing severe disease, especially in immunocompromised patients. It is a classic opportunistic organism, commonly found as part of the normal flora; severe disease with this organism was exceedingly rare up to the last 20–30 years. It is found in the oropharynx of approximately 30% of people, in intestines of about 65%, and in the vagina of 30–70% of women. The frequency of finding a *Candida* spp as part of the normal flora increases with debilitation. As implied from the previous sentences, the occurrence of systemic candidiasis has been increasing in recent years, and studies carried out in the last few years have shown that as many as 25% of leukemia patients have systemic candidal infection at autopsy.

Microbiology

Candida grows in yeast-like colonies and appears bacteria-like. The colonies are composed of single-cell, budding forms on the surface of the medium, plus hyphae which penetrate. Organisms from clinical specimens are gram-positive, and budding cells as well as pseudomycelia are seen.

There are many species of *Candida,* but the most important are *C. albicans,* which is responsible for about 75% of serious candidal infections; *C. tropicalis,* responsible for about 20% or more; and *C. parapsilosis,* the most common organism causing endocarditis.

The dimorphism of *Candida* is nutritionally governed. In the presence of fermentable carbohydrate, the organisms are found as budding yeast. In the absence of fermentable substrate, the cells elongate and form irregularly joined primitive hyphae, also called pseudohyphae. Blastospores are frequently produced at the nodes of the pseudohyphae, and in some species, chlamydiospores are produced at the end of the hyphae.

Epidemiology

Serious systemic infection with *Candida* is seen in a number of clinical situations, all of which have an adverse effect on one's host defenses. These are severe diabetes mellitus, cancer, cirrhosis, renal failure, blood dyscrasias, antibiotic therapy (by killing off the "good" normal flora), corticosteroids, cytotoxic drugs, radiation therapy, intravenous or urinary catheters, prosthesis, cachexia, and burns. For reasons which are not clear, oral contraceptive pills predispose women to candidal vaginitis. The gastrointestinal carriage rate of *Candida* spp goes up rapidly when patients are hospitalized, even in the absence of receiving antibiotics.

Candidal infections are especially common in patients with leukemia. In many patients, this infectious complication of a malignancy is diagnosed only at postmortem examination. Because of the nature of modern medical care, serious candidal infection is increasing in frequency, and in some hospitals, *Candida* organisms have become one of the more common isolates from blood cultures.

Pathogenesis

As with other opportunistic infectious diseases, the first step in candidal infection is colonization. This colonization is of the skin or, more commonly, of a mucosal surface. The mucosal surfaces usually involved are those of the gastrointestinal or female genital tracts, and less commonly the respiratory or urinary tracts. As mentioned previously, unless there is some breakdown in normal host defenses, there is no progression beyond this stage of colonization. Colonization proceeds to infection of the skin in moist areas occluded by tight, closely woven garments, in hot weather, and usually in overweight, diabetic patients. The chance of infection is further aided in patients who are receiving corticosteroids or antimicrobials.

Systemic infection is caused by a defect in granulocytes and/or cell-mediated immunity. The former seems to be much more important and may result from a quantitative deficit in granulocytes, or a functional defect. Patients with chronic mucocutaneous candidiasis (discussed later) appear to have normal granulocytes, both in numbers and in functional capability, but have a defect in T-cell activity. There is some evidence of genetic susceptibility to candidal infection linked to the HLA system.

Fungemia leads to secondary seeding of the kidneys, skin, and/or central nervous system. It is of interest that the lungs are relatively rarely involved, both as a site of initial infection, or as a site of involvement in fungemia, in contradistinction to the other most common opportunistic fungal infection, aspergillosis. Endocarditis with *Candida* almost always occurs on a previously damaged heart valve or on a prosthetic valve. In systemic candidal infection one finds diffuse microabscesses with both acute suppurative and chronic granulomatous inflammatory responses.

In patients with chronic mucocutaneous candidiasis one may find coexisting thymoma or one or another type of endocrinopathy.

Diagnosis

Clinical

The clinical manifestations of candidiasis can be conveniently divided into super-ficial localized disease and serious systemic disease. The former can further be divided into skin and mucosal involvement. As mentioned earlier, skin disease is located where skin integrity has been compromised, usually in moist areas, e.g., the axillary, inframammary, intergluteal fold, or groin areas, or external auditory canal. Patients who have their hands in water for prolonged periods during the day may develop chronic onychia caused by *Candida*.

Mucosae of any part of the body may be involved with *Candida*. Thrush is painful involvement of the buccal mucosa, tongue, and posterior pharynx, the involved areas being covered with a white to gray exudate with erythematous margins. Scraping the lesions leaves a bleeding surface. It is a fairly common disorder in newborns, but is also quite commonly seen today in asthmatics treated with corticosteroid inhalers, or patients receiving immunosuppressive therapy.

Perleche is angular stomatitis secondary to riboflavin deficiency with super-infection by *Candida*.

Bronchial involvement is an occupational disease of tea tasters, and is manifested by low-grade fever, cough, and patchy infiltrates.

Vulvovaginal and perianal involvement is usually secondary to the use of broad-spectrum antibiotics, with tetracycline being the most common offender, but it also occurs in patients using oral contraceptives, during pregnancy, or in diabetics. The symptoms usually begin shortly before the onset of menses. The most common manifestations are intense pruritus and a thick curd-like discharge. Men may be affected following sexual intercourse with women with candidal vaginitis. In addition to the itching, women may complain of dysuria, dyspareunia, and burning and itching after intercourse. In addition to the thick cheesy discharge, white patches adherent to the inflamed mucosa may be seen, but the examination may be quite benign.

Cystitis is almost always related to prolonged indwelling Foley catheter use and usually spontaneously resolves with correction of the underlying predisposing factors, most important being the removal of the catheter.

Esophagitis is usually associated with oral thrush. Patients complain of sub-sternal pain and dysphagia and may be fairly toxic, particularly infants. When examined by endoscopy, grey white patches are seen similar to those which patients with thrush have in their mouths. The diagnosis may also be made from characteristic changes seen on barium swallow.

A more recently described type of gastrointestinal involvement is erosive gastritis and/or duodenitis. Most cases have been reported in patients receiving cimetidine, and endoscopy is required to make the diagnosis.

Chronic mucocutaneous candidiasis is usually first detected in infancy or early childhood, but has been seen first in adolescence. The disease is character-ized by moderate to severe skin, nail, and mucosal involvement, quite refractory to therapy, with no other apparent underlying predisposing factor, and with coex-isting thymic or endocrinologic abnormalities (Table 116.1).

Systemic candidiasis may be divided into "benign fungemia" and serious, life-threatening disease (Table 116.2). The former is seen in patients with intravenous catheters who develop fungemia which resolves upon removal of the catheter. Differentiation of the benign from the more serious form of the disease is diffi-cult, since patients may have extensive disease without positive blood cultures, or a positive blood culture without significant disease. Invasive candidiasis is seldom

TABLE 116.1   Chronic Mucocutaneous Candidiasis

Characteristics	T-cell immunodeficiency Candidal infection of mucous membranes, skin, hair and nails Endocrinopathy in about 50% Familial in about 20%
Immune defect	Fairly specific: *Candida* and some antigenically close fungal genera; thus different from other known immunodeficiencies; since other host defenses are normal, systemic candidal infection is not a problem
Endocrinopathy	Usually several years after candidiasis Most common: hypoparathyroidism, Addison's disease Cause: autoantibodies
Other manifestations	Autoimmunity, e.g., pernicious anemia Alopecia, depigmentation Iron-deficiency anemia
Clinical variants	Early-onset chronic mucocutaneous candidiasis: most severe form, hypoparathyroidism and Addison's disease very rare Late-onset chronic mucocutaneous candidiasis: mild, in older individuals, no endocrinopathies Familial chronic mucocutaneous candidiasis: autosomal-recessive, mild to moderate, endocrinopathies uncommon Juvenile familial endocrinopathy with candidiasis: mild to moderate, hypoparathyroidism and/or Addison's disease usually present

diagnosed antemortem (in only 15-40% of patients) because the disease is manifested by completely nonspecific signs and symptoms and the lack of a reliable diagnostic laboratory test. The most common organs involved are the kidney, brain, myocardium, and eye. The most helpful signs are skin lesions, retinal involvement, and endocarditis. The "characteristic" skin lesion is a hemorrhagic macronodule, 0.5-1 cm in diameter, which is found in about one-sixth of patients with invasive candidiasis. Retinal lesions have been described as "the only pathognomonic clinical sign," and are focal, white, cottonball-like, chorioretinal lesions which rapidly progress to involve the vitreous.

Patients with endocarditis have very large vegetations, and emboli to large vessels are common. Patients are more likely to have splenomegaly and petechiae than are patients with endocarditis caused by other organisms.

TABLE 116.2 Differentiation Between Significant and Trivial Candidemia

Factor in Patients with Candidemia	% of Patients Who Were Shown to Have	
	Disseminated	Transient
Positive culture, three or more mucosal sites	50	20
Positive culture, any other site	90	90
Number of positive blood cultures		
Two or more	80	55
Five or more	15	0
Immunosuppressive therapy	85	30
Neutropenia	80	20

Although organisms are commonly found in the sputum, *Candida* rarely causes significant pulmonary disease. Other types of involvement are osteomyelitis, arthritis, myocarditis and meningitis. Peritonitis, associated with dialysis catheters, is increasing in frequency, and is most commonly caused by *C. tropicalis*.

Laboratory

The diagnosis of local lesions is fairly straightforward, since direct microscopic examination may be made of exudates or scrapings. However, cultures are less helpful since *Candida* organisms are such a common part of our indigenous flora. Material for direct examination should be mixed with potassium hydroxide. The presence of pseudohyphae or mycelia strongly suggests that the *Candida* is pathogenic and not merely an incidental saprophyte.

As mentioned earlier, the laboratory diagnosis of systemic candidiasis is more difficult. Blood cultures are positive in, at best, about half. Also, as previously mentioned, a positive culture may be simply a manifestation of transient fungemia. Therefore repeated blood cultures should be obtained after intravenous catheters and all possible foreign bodies have been removed.

The most helpful laboratory test is the identification of organisms, as well as their isolation by culture, from biopsy material. It is particularly important to take biopsy specimens of skin lesions, as well as ulcers of the gastrointestinal tract, which might be seen by endoscopy. Cultures should also be obtained of other material such as exudates and catheter tips.

Echocardiography has been extremely helpful in patients suspected of having endocarditis, since the vegetations are extremely large.

An area of very intense investigation in recent years is the immunologic diagnosis of invasive candidiasis. The immunologic approach presents an inherent problem in that nearly all patients with serious candidal infection are immunosuppressed and therefore do not respond well immunologically. In addition, since candidal colonization and skin and mucosal infection are common, normal people may already have received antigenic stimulation by the organisms. This is best exemplified by the delayed hypersensitivity skin test, which is of no value because it is positive in most normal people but negative in immunosuppressed patients. Various antibody tests have been tried, with only modest success. The precipitin test, measuring antibody against cytoplasmic antigens, becomes positive 10-14 days following the onset of systemic infection. It appears to be quite specific and may lack sensitivity; however, it could be useful as a screening test. Candidal-agglutinating antibody is not specific, but in combination with the precipitin test, may provide the specificity and sensitivity needed. Still another test is counter-immunoelectrophoresis; this test also gives mixed results and cannot be relied upon for definite diagnosis.

Another immunologic approach is the detection of antigen, analogous to the measurement of cryptococcal antigen, as a diagnostic procedure. The antigen that has been most thoroughly studied is mannan, a surface cell-wall polysaccharide. It has been detected in serum by counterimmunoelectrophoresis, hemagglutination-inhibition, and gas-liquid chromatography. Although there have been a few promising reports, the results so far have been inconsistent.

At the present time, a reasonable approach to diagnosing serious candidal infection in the absence of biopsy material for histopathologic examination and culture is to culture sputum, throat, stool, and blood. If any of these are positive, look for antigenemia or antibody if the tests are available. If one of these is positive institute therapy if the patient is immunosuppressed, particularly if neutropenic and febrile.

Prevention and Immunity

The most important aspect of prevention is to avoid predisposing factors, such as corticosteroid therapy, foreign bodies (particularly intravenous and urinary bladder catheters), and antibiotic therapy, particularly broad-spectrum. It appears that using steel needles rather than plastic, shorter length, and changing intravenous sites at least every 48 hr, lowers the chance of *Candida,* as well as other agents, causing infections complicating intravenous therapy. In leukemic patients, some recommend prophylactic oral nystatin or amphotericin B, but there is no evidence that this is effective. Similarly, there is no evidence that nystatin or amphotericin B in combination with antibiotics prevents a candidal superinfection, such as candidal vaginitis. Oropharyngeal candidiasis in asthmatics using inhaled corticosteroids can be partially prevented by gargling with water after each use.

Humans are normally protected from candidal infection by normal skin and mucosa, the T-cell system, and by polymorphonuclear leukocytes, possibly in combination with antibody and complement. Polymorphonuclear leukocytes damage hyphal elements, presumably by the release of lysosomal enzymes.

Treatment

The treatment for cutaneous candidiasis is topical nystatin, amphotericin B, clotrimazole, or miconazole (Table 116.3). There are no serious side effects of treatment with any of these agents, although local irritation may occur. Since the latter two agents are also effective against tinea, they are usually preferred because a patient may have mixed infection or the exact etiologic agent may be unknown. Treatment should be continued for 48 hr after the lesions have disappeared and the cultures are negative.

TABLE 116.3   Treatment of Candidal Infections

Manifestation	Treatment
Disseminated	Amphotericin B: intravenous, ∿ 0.7 mg/kg q.o.d., duration of 6-10 wk* 5-Fluorocytosine*: added (not alone) if organism is sensitive
Endocarditis	As above, plus removal of valve(s) and vegetations
Meningitis	Same as for disseminated
Peritonitis	Same, and/or continuous peritoneal dialysis with fluid containing 2-4 µg/ml amphotericin B
Urinary	Removal of foreign body, if possible, usually leads to spontaneous cure; may have to use amphotericin B irrigation: 50 mg/1000 ml
Oral	Nystatin or amphotericin B suspensions, tablets, or sucking on "vaginal" suppositories; cleansing of dentures and correction of poor fits, if present
Esophagitis	Oral nystatin, or low-dose (10-20 mg/day) intravenous amphotericin B given 5-14 days
Anogenital	Local therapy, plus, if persistent or severe, oral therapy to decrease intestinal *Candida* population
Chronic or severe mucocutaneous	Intravenous amphotericin B plus an immunostimulant such as transfer factor

*See Introduction to Fungal Diseases for details

For oral and esophageal candidiasis, one of the above agents should be used orally. They can be given as an oral suspension, or the patient can suck on a suppository. In troublesome esophageal infection, many clinicians use low-dose intravenous amphotericin B, i.e., 0.25-0.5 mg/kg for 5 days to 2 weeks.

In urinary tract infection, any predisposing factor should be removed, if possible. Amphotericin B bladder irrigation and/or oral flucytosine can be used. For bladder irrigation, 50 mg of amphotericin B is suspended in 1 L of 5% dextrose in water. Similar to esophageal candidiasis, with urinary tract disease, low-dose intravenous amphotericin B has been used.

Vaginal candidiasis can be treated with gentian violet, nystatin, or clotrimazole (or miconazole). Gentian violet, 1% in 10% alcohol, is effective, but its main drawback is that it stains clothing. It is still used in cases which are unresponsive to other agents. Nystatin vaginal tablets should be used for a minimum of 2 weeks. If the disease recurs, oral nystatin, in combination with the vaginal tablets, is recommended to eradicate a possible intestinal source of the organism. Nystatin vaginal tablets occasionally cause vaginal irritation making it difficult to clinically differentiate persistent disease from treatment. A culture should adequately differentiate the two.

Clotrimazole or miconazole are equal, or possibly more effective than nystatin, and the recommended treatment is for only 7 days. This class of drug has been shown to be effective in recurrent cases or in patients who have failed on nystatin. However, patients may have more side effects with clotrimazole or miconazole, including vaginal irritation and lower abdominal cramps. In patients who are pregnant, nystatin is recommended because there has been more experience with that drug.

The drug of choice for disseminated candidiasis is amphotericin B. Because this is an extremely serious infection, a large starting dose of 0.3 mg/kg is recommended, with rapid escalation to the full daily dosage of 1 mg/kg, if tolerated. Patients should be treated for about 6 weeks.

Flucytosine may be helpful in combination with amphotericin B. About half of the *Candida* strains are resistant to flucytosine before treatment is begun, and about two-thirds of the sensitive strains develop resistance during the course of therapy. Nonetheless, flucytosine is indicated if the organism is originally sensitive, since the patient may very well be cured before the organism has time to develop resistance. Although there are no controlled clinical trials comparing amphotericin B alone with amphotericin B plus flucytosine, in the mouse model the combination is more effective.

Miconazole given intravenously has been reported to be of some effect; however, there have been no direct comparisons with other forms of therapy, and the current recommendation is to use miconazole only in those patients who have failed on a regimen of amphotericin or amphotericin plus flucytosine.

A more recent drug from the clotrimazole-miconazole class is ketoconazole. It has been reported to be effective in both superficial and invasive candidiasis and has the advantage of being administered orally. It is given in a dosage of 200-400 mg/day, and reports suggest that it is particularly effective in chronic mucocutaneous candidiasis. It causes mild nausea and vomiting and should be taken with meals. There are some reports which suggest it may cause some liver toxicity. It should not be given to pregnant women.

Other therapeutic regimens which may prove to be effective with further clinical testing are the combinations of amphotericin B with rifampin or tetracycline (particularly minocycline); and immunotherapy (leukocyte transfusion, transfer factor, thymosin, and levamisole). In patients with candidal endocarditis the treatment is controversial. Most authorities recommend the combination of chemotherapy and surgical resection of the involved valve.

A final reminder that the most important aspect of therapy is the removal of predisposing factors, i.e., removal of a foreign body, stopping antibacterial agents, decreasing corticosteroid dosage, etc.

Prognosis and Complications

Only about 20-50% of patients show a beneficial response to treatment. The response rate is related to how quickly the diagnosis is made and therapy is started, to the severity of the underlying disease, and to whether or not immunosuppressive therapy can be discontinued. The fatality rate in candidal endocarditis is nearly 90%.

The complication rate of systemic candidal infection is high, including such things as blindness in patients with candidal eye involvement, and esophageal stricture following severe or prolonged esophagitis.

Selected Bibliography

Atkinson, A. J., Jr. and Bennett, J. E.: Amphotericin B pharmacokinetics in humans. *Antimicrob Agents Chemother* 13:271-276, 1978.

Bennett, J. E.: Flucytosine. *Ann Intern Med* 86:319-322, 1977.

Bodey, G. P. and Luna, M.: Skin lesions associated with disseminated candidiasis. *JAMA* 229:1466-1468, 1974.

Brandstetter, R. D. and Brause, B. D.: *Candida parapsilosis* endocarditis. Recovery of the causative organism from an addict's own syringes. *JAMA* 243:1073, 1980.

Edwards, J. E., Jr. (Moderator), Lehrer, R. I., Stiehm, E. R., Fischer, T.J., Young, L. S. (Discussants): Severe candidal infections. Clinical perspective, immune defense mechanisms, and current concepts of therapy. *Ann Intern Med* 89: 91-106, 1978.

Ezdinli, E. Z., O'Sullivan, D. D., Wasser, L. P., Kim, U., and Stutzman, L.: Oral amphotericin for candidiasis in patients with hematologic neoplasms. *JAMA* 242:258-260, 1979.

Filice, G., Yu, B., and Armstrong, D.: Immunodiffusion and agglutination tests for *Candida* in patients with neoplastic disease: Inconsistent correlation of results with invasive infections. *J Infect Dis* 135:349-357, 1977.

Fischer, T. J., Klein, R. B., Kershnar, A. G., Borut, T. C., and Stiehm, E. R.: Miconazole in the treatment of chronic mucocutaneous candidiasis: A preliminary report. *J Pediatr* 91:815-819, 1977.

Glew, R. H., Buckley, H. R.,Rosen, H. M., Moellering, R. C., Jr., and Fischer, J. E.: Serologic tests in the diagnosis of systemic candidiasis. Enhanced diagnostic accuracy with crossed immunoelectrophoreses. *Am J Med* 64:586-591, 1978.

Jarowski, C. I., Fialk, M. A., Murray, H. W., Gottlieb, G. J., Coleman, M., Steinberg, C. R., and Silver, R. T.: Fever, rash, and muscle tenderness: A distinctive clinical presentation of disseminated candidiasis. *Arch Intern Med* 138: 544-546, 1978.

Katz, M. E. and Cassileth, P. A.: Disseminated candidiasis in a patient with acute leukemia: Successful treatment with miconazole. *JAMA* 237:1124–1125, 1977.

Kirkpatrick, C. H. and Alling, D. W.: Treatment of chronic oral candidiasis with clotrimazole troches. A controlled clinical trial. *N Engl J Med* 299:1201–1203, 1978.

Kirkpatrick, C. H. and Windhorst, D. B.: Mucocutaneous candidiasis and thymoma. *Am J Med* 66:939–945, 1979.

Kressel, B., Szewczyk, C., and Tuazon, C. U.: Early clinical recognition of disseminated candidiasis by muscle and skin biopsy. *Arch Intern Med* 138:429–433, 1978.

Lew, M. A., Beckett, K. M., and Levin, M. J.: Antifungal activity of four tetracycline analogues against *Candida albicans* in vitro: Potentiation by amphotericin B. *J Infect Dis* 136:263–270, 1977.

Martin, E., Pancoast, S. J., and Neu, H. C.: *Candida parapsilosis* endocarditis: Medical and surgical cure. *Ann Intern Med* 91:870–871, 1979.

Masur, H., Rosen, P. P., and Armstrong, D.: Pulmonary disease caused by *Candida* species. *Am J Med* 63:914–925, 1977.

Meade, R. H., III.: Treatment of chronic mucocutaneous candidiasis. *Ann Intern Med* 86:314–315, 1977.

Medoff, G., Dismukes, W. E., Meade, R. H., III, and Moses, J. M.: A new therapeutic approach to *Candida* infections. *Arch Intern Med* 130:241–245, 1972.

Merz, W. G., Evans, G. L., Shadomy, S., Anderson, S., Kaufman, L., Kozinn, P. J., MacKenzie, D. W., Protzman, W. P., and Remington, J. S.: Laboratory evaluation of serological tests for systemic candidiasis: A cooperative study. *J Clin Microbiol* 5:596–603, 1977.

Miles, M. R., Olsen, L., and Rogers, A.: Recurrent vaginal candidiasis. *JAMA* 238:1836–1837, 1977.

Montgomerie, J. Z. and Edwards, J. E., Jr.: Association of infection due to *Candida albicans* with intravenous hyperalimentation. *J Infect Dis* 137:197–201, 1978.

Murray, H. W., Fialk, M. A., and Roberts, R. B.: *Candida* arthritis: A manifestation of disseminated candidiasis. *Am J Med* 60:587–595, 1976.

Myerowitz, R. L., Pazin, G. J., and Allen, C. M.: Disseminated candidiasis: Changes in incidence, underlying diseases, pathology. *Am J Clin Pathol* 68:29–38, 1977.

Oblack, D., Schwarz, J., and Holder, I. A.: Comparative evaluation of the candida agglutinin test, precipitin test, and germ tube dispersion test in the diagnosis of candidiasis. *J Clin Microbiol* 3:175–179, 1976.

Oriel, J. D. and Waterworth, P. M.: Effects of minocycline and tetracycline on the vaginal yeast flora. *J Clin Pathol* 28:403-406, 1975.

Rosner, F., Gabriel, F. D., Taschdjian, C. L., Cuesta, M. B., and Kozinn, P. J.: Serologic diagnosis of systemic candidiasis in patients with acute leukemia. *Am J Med* 51:54-62, 1971.

Rutgeerts, L. and Verhaegen, H.: Intravenous miconazole in the treatment of chronic esophageal candidiasis. *Gastroenterology* 72:316-318, 1977.

St. Hill, C. A., Finn, R., and Denye, V.: Depression of cellular immunity in pregnancy due to a serum factor. *Br Med J* 3:513-514, 1973.

Taschdjian, C. L., Kozinn, P. J., Cuesta, M. B., and Toni, E. F.: Serodiagnosis of candidal infections. *Am J Clin Pathol* 57:195-205, 1972.

Wingard, J. R., Merz, W. G., and Saral, R.: *Candida tropicalis:* A major pathogen in immunocompromised patients. *Ann Intern Med* 91:539-543, 1979.

Wise, G. J., Ray, B., and Kozinn, P. J.: The serodiagnosis of significant genito-urinary candidiasis. *J Urol* 107:1043-1046, 1972.

Young, R. C., Bennett, J. E., Geelhoed, G. L., and Levine, A. S.: Fungemia with compromised host resistance. *Ann Intern Med* 80:605, 1974.

117

ASPERGILLUS
Robert H. Waldman, M.D.

The fungus *Aspergillus* is interesting because of its "versatility" as a pathogen. It causes five different types of human disease, four of which involve very different pathogenic mechanisms. The diseases are (1) allergic bronchopulmonary aspergillosis, sometimes called hypersensitivity pneumonitis, the pathogenesis of which is an immune reaction to antigens from the organism; (2) mycetoma, which is caused by colonization of a preformed pulmonary cavity; (3) invasive pulmonary disease, a necrotizing bronchopneumonia; (4) disseminated infection; and (5) food poisoning, caused by a toxin produced by *Aspergillus flavus*.

After a brief description of the microbiology of *Aspergillus*, the various types of disease will be discussed separately, except for invasive pulmonary and disseminated infection, which will be discussed together. They are closely related, since the former usually is a precursor of the latter, and both occur virtually only in immunocompromised patients.

Microbiology

Aspergillus spp are part of the normal flora, particularly of the respiratory tract, but also occasionally in the gastrointestinal tract. Species also quite commonly colonize burn eschars and are found in the detritus in the external ear canal. The organism is found in the sputum and in tissue as dichotomously branched, septate hyphae. Spores may be formed in pulmonary cavities. *Aspergillus fumigatus* is most commonly associated with human disease, but occasionally, other species are also found (Figure 117.1).

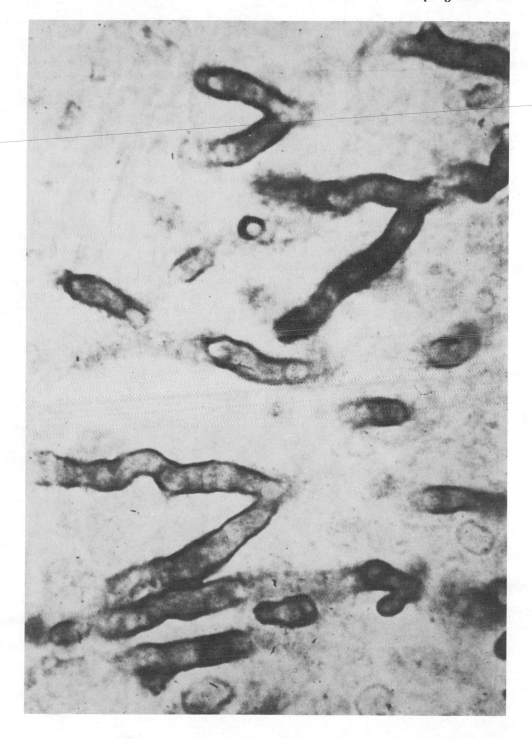

FIGURE 117.1   Sputum smears showing *A. fumigatus.* Note the characteristic conidial head.

Invasive and Disseminated Disease

Invasive and disseminated aspergillosis is the systemic mycosis which has the most rapidly increasing occurrence. This is because a greater number of immunosuppressed patients are surviving for a longer time, added to the fact that most other opportunistic infections are easier to diagnose and treat. Aspergillosis is now third in frequency, behind histoplasmosis and coccidioidomycosis. Unfortunately, this current trend of increasing prevalence of aspergillosis will probably continue. Aspergillosis is found at autopsy in over 10% of patients with acute leukemia. Of all patients with invasive aspergillosis, diagnosed either ante- or postmortem, 40% have acute lymphocytic leukemia, and 20% have acute myelogenous leukemia (Table 117.1). As another example of the type of patient who is prone to aspergillosis, it is one of the most common organisms infecting children with chronic granulomatous disease.

The organism can infect every organ system, but the most common organs involved are the lung (greater than 90% of patients), the gastrointestinal tract (about 20%), the central nervous system (about 15%), the liver (about 12%), and the urogenital tract (about 10%) (Table 117.2).

The organism causes disease by vascular invasion, growth in the lumen of the vessel, leading to infarction at that point, or following embolization. *Aspergillus* has a special propensity for patients who are neutropenic, receiving corticosteroid

TABLE 117.1   Preexisting Diseases in Patients with Invasive Aspergillosis

Disease	Approximate % of Patients
Acute lymphocytic leukemia	40
Acute myelogenous leukemia	20
Chronic myelogenous leukemia	10
Hodgkin's disease	5
Lymphoma	5
Other diseases of lymphoreticular system, including aplastic anemia, chronic lymphocytic leukemia, mycosis fungoides, multiple myeloma	10
"Autoimmune" disease, including systemic lupus erythematosus and polyarteritis nodosa	5

TABLE 117.2   Organ Involvement in Cases of Invasive Aspergillosis

Organ	Approximate % of Patients
Lung	95
Gastrointestinal tract	20
Brain	15
Liver	10
Kidney	10
Thyroid	10

therapy, and/or receiving broad-spectrum antibiotics. Aspergillosis is often ac-companied by, or accompanies *Pseudomonas* (in 15% of patients) or *Candida* (in about 13%) infection. It has also been reported following influenza virus infection.

The diagnosis is as challenging to the clinician and the clinical laboratory as any in medicine. There is nothing clinically characteristic, the laboratory is often not helpful, the patients are usually extremely ill, making invasive diagnostic pro-cedures dangerous, and the clinician is justifiably reluctant to begin therapy with-out good evidence, since the drug of choice, amphotericin B, is quite toxic and does not have a good record of success as far as eradication of the infection. Put-ting even more pressure on the clinician is that in this infection, early diagnosis is vitally important to eventual outcome.

The clinical picture is extremely variable, with pulmonary signs and symptoms common, but exhibiting no particular pattern. Empyema is rare but occasionally does occur. Hemorrhagic ulcerations may occur anywhere along the gastrointes-tinal tract, and if seen by the endoscopist, appropriate biopsy material for culture and histologic examination should be obtained. Necrotic cutaneous lesions, analo-gous to ecthyma gangrenosum, are occasionally seen. Ulcerations of the nasal mu-cosa also may be found, especially when the organism is *A. flavus*. The chest roentgenogram is normal in about 40% of patients, despite the fact that almost all of those are subsequently found to have pulmonary involvement. If the roent-genogram is abnormal, the whole gamut of abnormalities may be seen (Table 117.3).

The only way to make a definite diagnosis of invasive aspergillosis is to iso-late the organism from a specimen or site where it is not expected to be part of the normal flora, or to identify the organism in a histopathologic section. Fewer than 40% of patients have a positive culture before death. Blood cultures should be obtained, but are rarely positive. Sputum, throat, or nasal cultures are often positive in normal people, or people with other diseases, so a positive culture from the respiratory tract is very difficult to interpret. Studies have shown, however, if nose cultures are done serially in a susceptible population, the "conversion" from a negative to a positive culture is of definite predictive value. The best way to make the diagnosis is culture and histologic examination of biopsy material (Fig-ure 117.2). The procedures to obtain biopsy material usually have a high morbid-ity and mortality, and therefore it is recommended that they be carried out as early in the course of illness as possible, since the patient is more likely to be in better general condition and better able to tolerate the procedure.

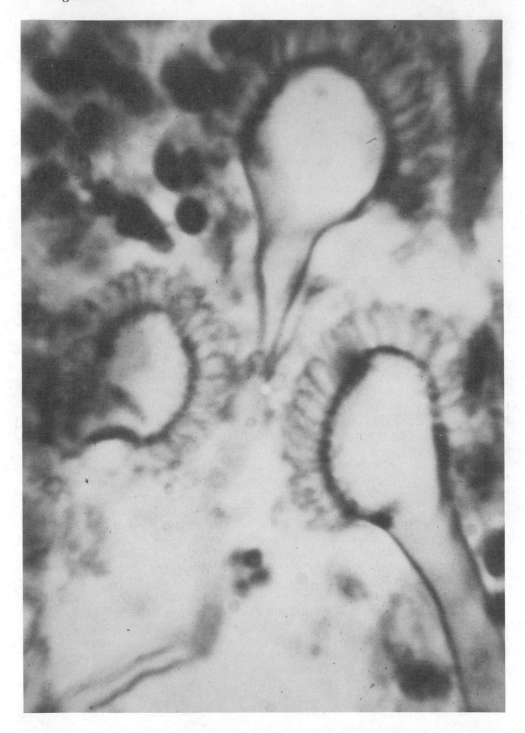

FIGURE 117.2   Stain from lung biopsy of patient with invasive pulmonary disease, showing characteristic segmented hyphae and acute angle of branch points.

TABLE 117.3   **Pulmonary Manifestations in Patients with Pulmonary Aspergillosis**

Manifestation	Approximate % of Patients
Necrotizing bronchopneumonia	35
Hemorrhagic infarction	30
Miliary microabscesses	10
Lobar pneumonia	10
Bronchitis	10
Focal abscesses	5
Solitary abscess	5

The inherent drawback to any type of test of immune reactivity in invasive aspergillosis is that patients are immunosuppressed and therefore unlikely to have a potent enough immune system to react reliably. Thus the aspergillus skin test may be helpful in some forms of disease associated with the organism, but is worthless to diagnose invasive aspergillosis. Serologic tests, such as the precipitin test, may convert from negative to positive in patients with invasive aspergillosis, but there are still too many false-negative and a few false-positive results, thereby limiting their usefulness.

Potentially of more usefulness is a test for antigen from the organism. This does not depend upon the host being able to mount an immune response, but uses one of a variety of immunologic tests with antibody made in an animal, to detect antigen in blood or another body fluid. A great deal of investigative work is currently going on in an attempt to develop a sensitive and specific test (Table 117.4).

In summary, because of the factors mentioned earlier concerning the importance of starting treatment early and the difficulty in making the diagnosis, it is generally felt that treatment should be started if the organism is found in the sputum of a febrile, neutropenic patient.

The drug of choice for treating invasive aspergillosis is amphotericin B, which is far from optimum, i.e., the organisms are usually somewhat resistant, results have been generally poor, and there is the relatively high toxicity. Another area of intensive investigation with respect to aspergillosis is the use of combinations of other agents with amphotericin B. 5-Fluorocytosine (flucytosine) exhibits in vitro synergy with amphotericin B against most clinical isolates. Rifampin also has been studied and appears to exhibit some synergy. A single agent which has been used in a few cases is clotrimazole. Other forms of therapy that have been used, with some success, are surgical resection in patients with localized pulmonary disease, and granulocyte transfusions.

The prognosis is extremely poor, and survival is related to early diagnosis, rapid and aggressive therapy, and remission of the underlying disease (e.g., leukemia or lymphoma).

TABLE 117.4   Immunologic Tests in Aspergillosis

Test	Normals	Colonization	Aspergilloma	ABPA	Invasive Disease
Skin test					
Immediate	Rarely	Rarely	25%	Nearly all	Rarely
Intermediate	Rarely	Rarely	Occasionally	Most	Rarely
Antibody					
IgE (RAST)	Rarely	Rarely	Occasionally	Nearly all	Rarely
IgG (Precipitin)	Rarely	Rarely	90%	60–75%	Occasionally
Antigen					
Radioimmunoassay	Rarely	Occasionally	Probably	Unknown	Usually

Allergic Bronchopulmonary Aspergillosis (Table 117.5)

This entity is not caused by the *Aspergillus* organism itself, but by the immune response to the organism. Nearly all patients have preexisting asthma. Typically, a patient, aged 15-35, has worsening of his asthmatic symptoms, with increased wheezing and sputum production, fever, and shortness of breath. Chest roentgenogram shows some consolidation or atelectasis, usually worse in the upper lobes. There is sputum and peripheral blood eosinophilia, unless the patient is receiving corticosteroids. The patient may cough up small yellow-brown mucous plugs, which, when stained, show hyphae, and aspergillus may be recovered on culture (in about 60% of patients). An important part of the syndrome is proximal, saccular bronchiectasis. This may not be present early in the course of the disease. Allergic bronchopulmonary aspergillosis (ABPA) may also accompany cystic fibrosis.

The immunopathogenic features are an immediate hypersensitivity reaction (type I, or wheal and flair) to intradermal *A. fumigatus* extract. In some patients, in addition to the immediate skin reaction, an Arthrus-like reaction (type III reaction) develops at 4-8 hr after the intradermal injection. Total serum IgE levels are elevated, and IgE antibody to *A. fumigatus* can be detected by the radioallergosorbent test (RAST). One can also usually detect serum IgG antibody by a precipitin test, which is most easily carried out by agar immunodiffusion. The prevailing opinion is that the pulmonary pathology results from a combined type I and type III reaction to aspergillus antigens, the reaction taking place in the submucosa of the bronchial tree. Patients may acquire the organism simply by colonization, since it is commonly part of the normal flora of the respiratory tract. Alternatively, spores may be inhaled from animals or decaying vegetation. Viscid mucus in the asthmatic or cystic fibrosis patients may favor colonization and replication of the organism.

TABLE 117.5   Allergic Bronchopulmonary Aspergillosis

Feature	Approximate Incidence (%)
Asthma	95
Sputum production	55
Hemoptysis (blood-tinged)	85
Pulmonary infiltrates	100
Precipitins	90
Positive skin test (types I and III)	95
Eosinophilia	100
A. fumigatus in sputum	60

The differential diagnosis presents some difficulties, since there are several other entities which can be confused with ABPA, e.g., asthma complicated by bacterial or viral pneumonia, mucous plugs leading to atelectasis in an asthmatic, bronchiectasis from some other cause, tuberculosis, eosinophilic pneumonia, various pulmonary vasculitides and granulomatoses and extrinsic allergic alveolitis (i.e., hypersensitivity pneumonitis) (Tables 117.6 and 117.7).

TABLE 117.6   Differential Diagnoses of Allergic Bronchopulmonary Aspergillosis

> Cystic fibrosis
>
> Tuberculosis
>
> Cancer
>
> Eosinophilic pneumonia
>
> Mucous plug
>
> Atelectasis
>
> Bronchiectasis

TABLE 117.7   Criteria for Diagnosis of Allergic Bronchopulmonary Aspergillosis

Suspect diagnosis	Asthma Eosinophilia Recurrent bouts of symptoms of acute bronchitis or pneumonia, with pulmonary infiltrates seen on chest roentgenograms
Probable diagnosis: 3 of 4 criteria	Positive immediate skin test Serum precipitins Elevated total serum IgE
Definite diagnosis: All 4	Positive sputum culture

or

Bronchograms demonstrating
  proximal saccular
  bronchiectasis

Note: Corticosteroid therapy may cause false-negative immunologic tests

The prognosis in ABPA is very good, the disease progressing to lung damage in a small minority of cases. This is important with respect to the choice of therapy, since the use of corticosteroids is somewhat controversial. The conservative approach is to eliminate the source of exposure, if known, and use bronchodilators, hydration, postural drainage, and bronchoscopy, if necessary, to remove plugs. A more aggressive approach is to add corticosteroids. There is no question that radiographic infiltrates clear and serum IgE levels decrease with the use of steroids. However, as mentioned above, most patients do quite well without steroids and their side effects can be significant. Pending further studies, it would seem prudent to reserve steroids for cases in which the disease is severe, or there is chronicity and deterioration as indicated by the history, chest roentgenograms, and/or pulmonary function tests (Table 117.8).

There is an additional immunologic disease caused by aspergillus. Malt workers may develop hypersensitivity pneumonitis (extrinsic allergic alveolitis) because of their exposure to barley dust heavily contaminated by *A. clavatus*.

TABLE 117.8   Protocol for Management of Allergic Bronchopulmonary Aspergillosis*

Prednisone 0.5 mg/kg daily for 2 wk or until complete clearing of chest roentgenogram

Prednisone 0.5 mg/kg q.o.d. for 3 mo

Repeat chest roentgenograms q. 4 mo x 6, then q. 6 mo x 4, then q. yr if no exacerbations

Serum IgE monthly for 2 yr, then q. 2 mo

Pulmonary function tests yearly

Therapy with prednisone resumed if there is significant worsening of symptoms, chest roentgenogram or pulmonary function tests, or significant increase in total serum IgE

---

*Recommended by Wang et al.

Aspergilloma

Aspergilloma (mycetoma or fungus ball) is a mass of fungal hyphae in preformed lung cavities (Figure 117.3). The fungus does not invade the cavity wall, but can cause irritation leading to bleeding. In addition to *Aspergillus,* other organisms can cause a mycetoma, including *Candida, Coccidioides,* phycomycetes, *Nocardia,* and *Sporotrichum.*

The diagnosis is made by chest roentgenogram, which shows a crescent-moon translucency beside a round density (Monod's sign). The mass usually moves when the patient assumes a lateral decubitus position. Mycetomas are almost always in the upper lobes.

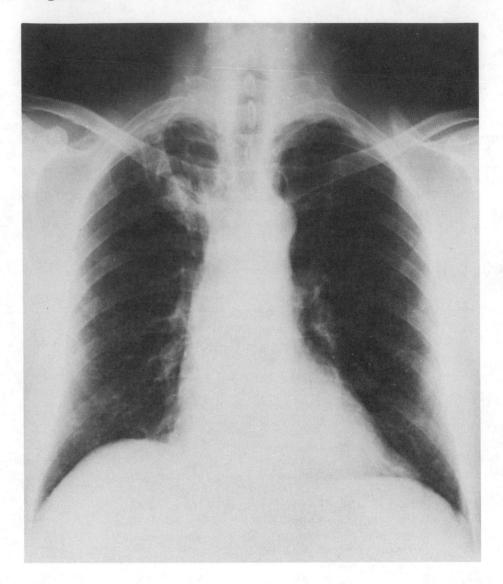

FIGURE 117.3   Chest x-ray from patient with aspergilloma ("fungus ball") in right upper lung field. X-ray courtesy of Dr. E. Morgan, Morgantown, WV.

    The immediate hypersensitivity skin test is positive in about 20% of these patients, and there are serum precipitins in over 90%.

    The only problem that patients may have with an aspergilloma is hemoptysis, which occurs in half to three-quarters of the patients. The hemoptysis is usually mild, but can become massive, even causing death. However, the prognosis in patients with a mycetoma is much more related to their underlying disease than to the fungus ball itself. Spontaneous lysis of the fungus ball occurs in 10-20% of patients. The risk of the aspergilloma becoming invasive or disseminated is negligible.

The main treatment is reassurance and benign neglect. Amphotericin B, either intravenously or by aerosol, is probably of no value. Surgery should be performed only if the hemoptysis is severe, frequent, or life-threatening.

Aflatoxicosis

Among the rarer causes of gastroenteritis is aflatoxicosis, which is caused by *A. flavus.* In hot climates the fungus grows on moldy grains, peanuts, and bread, producing large amounts of a toxin. Small amounts of the ingested toxin produce no symptoms; however, ingestion of large amounts causes nausea, vomiting, and diarrhea, and in rare cases, death. Chronic ingestion over many years leads to chronic liver disease.

Selected Bibliography

Aisner, J., Murillo, J., Schimpff, S. C., and Steere, A. C.: Invasive aspergillosis in acute leukemia: Correlation with nose cultures and antibiotic use. *Ann Intern Med* 90:4-9, 1979.

Aisner, J., Schimpff, S. C., and Wiernik, P. H.: Treatment of invasive aspergillosis: Relation of early diagnosis in treatment of response. *Ann Intern Med* 86: 539, 1977.

Codish, S. D. and Tobias, J. S.: Managing systemic mycoses in the compromised host. *JAMA* 235:2123-2134, 1976.

Codish, S. D., Tobias, J. S., and Hannigan, M.: Combined amphotericin B-flucytosine therapy in *Aspergillus* pneumonia. *JAMA* 241:2418-2419, 1979.

Fischer, J. J. and Walker, D. H.: Invasive pulmonary aspergillosis associated with influenza. *JAMA* 241:1493-1494, 1979.

Fraser, D. W., Ward, J. I., Ajello, L., and Plikaytis, B. D.: Aspergillosis and other systemic mycoses. The growing problem. *JAMA* 242:1631-1635, 1979.

Graves, T. S., Fink, J. N., Patterson, R., Kurup, V. P., and Scanlon, G. T.: A familial occurrence of allergic bronchopulmonary aspergillosis. *Ann Intern Med* 91:378-382, 1979.

Kitahara, M., Seth, V. K., Medoff, G., and Kobayashi, G. S.: Activity of amphotericin B, 5-fluorocytosine, and rifampin against 6 clinical isolates of *Aspergillus*. *Antimicrob Agents Chemother* 9:915-919, 1976.

Krammer, R. B. and Utz, J. P.: *Aspergillus* species endocarditis: The new face of a not so rare disease. *Am J Med* 56:506, 1974.

Nichols, D., Dopico, G., Braun, S., Imbeau, S., Peters, M. E., and Rankin, J.: Acute and chronic pulmonary function changes in allergic bronchopulmonary aspergillosis. *Am J Med* 67:631, 1979.

Pennington, J. E.: Aspergillus pneumonia in hematologic malignancy. *Arch Intern Med* 137:769-771, 1977.

Pennington, J. E.: Successful treatment of aspergillus pneumonia in hematologic neoplasia. *N Engl J Med* 295:426, 1976.

Rosenberg, M., Patterson, R., Mintzer, R., Cooper, B. J., Roberts, M., and Harris, K. E.: Clinical and immunologic criteria for the diagnosis of allergic bronchopulmonary aspergillosis. *Ann Intern Med* 86:405-414, 1977.

Rosenberg, M., Patterson, R., Roberts, M., and Wang, J.: The assessment of immunologic and clinical changes occurring during corticosteroid therapy for allergic bronchopulmonary aspergillosis. *Am J Med* 64:599-606, 1978.

Schaefer, J. C., Yu, B., and Armstrong, D.: An aspergillus immunodiffusion test in the early diagnosis of aspergillosis in adult leukemia patients. *Am Rev Respir Dis* 113:325, 1976.

Shaffer, P. J., Kobayashi, G. S., and Medoff, G.: Demonstration of antigenemia in patients with invasive aspergillosis by solid phase (protein A-rich *Staphylococcus aureus*) radioimmunoassay. *Am J Med* 67:627, 1979.

Varkey, B. and Rose, H. D.: Pulmonary aspergilloma. A rational approach to treatment. *Am J Med* 61:626-631, 1976.

Wang, J. L. F., Patterson, R., Roberts, M., and Ghory, A. C.: The management of allergic bronchopulmonary aspergillosis. *Am Rev Respir Dis* 120:87-92, 1979.

118

MUCORMYCOSIS

David A. Pitrolo, M.D. and
Robert H. Waldman, M.D.

Mucormycosis, or phycomycosis, is a disease produced by the fungi of the class Zygomycetes (Phycomycetes). The specific pathogens are included in the genera *Rhizopus, Mucor, Absidia,* and *Cunninghamella,* all bread molds. The organisms are characterized by nonseptate hyphae which are broad and branching.

Epidemiology

Mucormycosis is worldwide in distribution and the organism is ubiquitous. It usually exists on decaying vegetation and food products high in sugar content. It is found in the soil and air and has been recovered from hospital ventilation systems.

Pathogenesis and Pathology

Disease in the normal host is usually limited to minor infections such as paronychia, otitis externa, and dermatitis. In immunosuppressed patients, progressive, life-threatening illness may be produced. The majority of patients with significant mucormycosis are diabetics, especially those with acidosis. Also at risk are patients with hematologic malignancies, those with significant skin or mucosal injuries, and patients receiving cytotoxic or immunosuppressive therapy.

The fungal spore gains entry usually via inhalation but also via the gastrointestinal tract. The initial infection occurs most frequently in the mucosae of the nose, palate, or lower respiratory tract. The organism's pathogenicity is based on its ability to invade blood vessels, particularly arteries. Growth thus results in thrombus formation and necrosis of areas supplied by the vessel. The infection spreads by direct extension and also hematogenously.

Diagnosis

The rhino-ophthalmocerebral form of mucormycosis accounts for more than half of all reported cases. This form is most often associated with diabetes. While acidosis seems to exist as an important predisposing factor, diabetics under apparently good control remain susceptible. Although less common, acidosis associated with renal failure and dehydration also may predispose, as can the use of immunosuppressive agents in patients with leukemia and those who have reccived transplants. Presenting symptoms include headache, painful swelling of the face, epistaxis, and black nasal or ocular discharge. Patients may have fever, proptosis, tenderness of the sinuses, as well as a characteristic black eschar on the palantine or nasal mucosae. Physical findings are associated with abnormalities of cranial nerves II, III, IV, and VI, and impairment of VII and VIII occurring late in the disease. Fever and inflammation may not be present in severely immunocompromised patients, and the mucosa may appear only mildly ischemic. The disease may present initially as acute sinusitis. The diagnosis should be suspected in any diabetic with ketoacidosis whose mental status does not improve upon correction of the metabolic abnormalities.

The infection spreads to the central nervous system through the orbit or by penetrating the cribriform plate. The fungus may lead to cavernous sinus and internal carotid artery thrombosis. Brain infarcts then occur with a variety of clinical signs and symptoms. Blindness may develop secondary to interruption of retinal artery flow.

Since the nasal mucosa may be colonized with these organisms without causing disease, isolation of the organism from a nasal swab is not diagnostic. It is necessary to obtain a biopsy of the area, showing hyphal invasion of tissue and vessels. Sinus x-rays or tomograms often reveal mucosal thickening with clouding of the sinus cavity. More than one sinus is frequently involved. The presence of air-fluid levels is uncommon. Tomography or computerized axial tomography may demonstrate focal bony destruction, which is somewhat suggestive of mucormycosis.

When rhino- ophthalmocerebral disease is demonstrated, a lumbar puncture should be performed, although, even with CNS disease, the cerebral spinal fluid may be normal. The organism is rarely seen or cultured from spinal fluid. The spinal fluid findings are nonspecific, with an elevated pressure, slightly elevated protein, and a modest pleocytosis.

Pulmonary mucormycosis is usually associated with leukemia or lymphoma, especially in patients receiving chemotherapy. The fungus reaches the lung by inhalation or by hematogenous spread. Patients present with fever, pleuritic chest pain, dyspnea, and cough usually productive of only scant sputum. However, patients may present with life-threatening hemoptysis. Pulmonary mucormycosis may develop subsequent to a viral or bacterial infection, and exhibits no lobar propensity. The disease usually follows a rapid, progressive course, and the diagnosis is often made at postmortem examination. The chest roentgenogram shows patchy infiltrates which may progress to consolidation and then cavitation. Patients may have pleural effusions. The diagnosis must be established by biopsy, which demonstrates tissue invasion by the fungus. A positive sputum culture is very suggestive, but does not firmly establish the diagnosis. Perfusion scans of the lung show abnormalities secondary to vascular interruption by the fungus.

Cutaneous mucormycosis occurs over an area of previous injury, most often following a burn. The diagnosis should be suspected if a patient develops a fever and/or there is a change in appearance of the wound, especially if it begins to appear dark and necrotic. An early biopsy is the key to diagnosis. The use of Elastoplast has been associated with cases of cutaneous mucormycosis, and the organism has been cultured from unused stock of the material.

The stomach is the most frequently affected site for gastrointestinal mucormycosis, with the large bowel being the second most commonly involved area. Phycomycotic endocarditis has occurred on abnormal, as well as prosthetic valves. The vegetations produced are often large and quite likely to embolize. Myocardial infarction secondary to coronary artery involvement has been reported. Mucormycosis has also been implicated in cases of septic abortion and in osteomyelitis.

Disseminated mucormycosis may develop secondary to any of the primary infections described. Almost any organ may be affected and therefore the clinical presentation is variable. The disease usually is rapidly fatal.

A biopsy of the affected tissue is necessary for establishing the diagnosis of mucormycosis. Because an early diagnosis is crucial, it is necessary to perform fairly invasive procedures, often based on vague symptomatology in a susceptible patient. The tissue should be stained with Gomori's methenamine silver stain, and a piece of the tissue also should be crushed and suspended in KOH solution. The hyphae are nonseptate and demonstrate right-angle branching. The organism grows relatively rapidly and in a variety of media. There are no serodiagnostic techniques available.

Treatment and Prognosis

Successful treatment depends upon an early diagnosis, rapid initiation of therapy, aggressive surgical debridement, and correction of the underlying disease, if possible. Amphotericin B remains the only drug that has been efficacious. In vitro sensitivity testing correlates poorly with clinical results. Because of the severity of the disease, it is usually necessary to aggressively increase the dosage of amphotericin B to 0.7-1.0 mg/kg/day after the initial test dose is given. The total minimally effective dose is unknown, but it is usually recommended that patients receive 2.5-4 g.

Neutropenia is a poor prognostic sign; however, granulocyte transfusions have not been beneficial.

The prognosis is very poor; however, there are reports of survival of over 50% with early detection and aggressive treatment.

Selected Bibliography

Addlestone, R.: Rhinocerebral mucormycosis. *Radiology* 115:113-127, 1975.

Agger, W.: Mucormycosis, complication of critical case. *Arch Intern Med* 138: 925-927, 1978.

Brown, J.: Pulmonary and rhinocerebral mucormycosis. *Arch Intern Med* 137: 936-938, 1977.

Edwards, J. E., Howard, D. H., Lehrer, R., Segal, G. P., Sypherd, P. S., and Winston, D. J.: Mucormycosis. *Ann Intern Med* 93:93-108, 1980.

Marchensky, A.: The changing spectrum of disease, etiology and diagnosis of mucormycosis. *Human Pathol* 11:456-464, 1980.

Myers, B.: Rhinocerebral mucormycosis. *Arch Intern Med* 139:557-560, 1979.

Pillsbury, H.: Rhinocerebral mucormycosis. *Arch Otolaryngol* 103:600-604, 1977.

F. Protozoa

119

AMEBIASIS
Rashida A. Khakoo, M.D.

Gastrointestinal Amebiasis

Descriptions of dysentery were recorded by ancient cultures. However, only in
the nineteenth century did physicians become aware that there were different
types of dysentery and that there was occasionally liver involvement with dysentery. Ipecac bark (ipecacuanha) was used for treatment. Subsequent studies described the presence of amebae in the stool. The Russian physician Losch is cred-
ited with describing the first case of amebic dysentery. William Osler was the
first to describe a case of dysentery and liver abscess. Schaudinn differentiated
between the nonpathogenic and pathogenic amebae and he coined the term *Entamoeba histolytica* for the pathogenic variety because of its ability to destroy tissue.
     Amebiasis occurs worldwide, but with the prevalence varying tremendously.
In the United States, the disease occurs in immigrants, travelers who have returned from endemic areas, institutionalized patients, and homosexual males. The
disease is endemic in low socioeconomic areas. Recently, an epidemic occurred
following colonic irrigation at a chiropractic clinic. Lack of sterilization of the
irrigation machine most likely resulted in colonic inoculation of fecal material
from a previous patient.
     The spectrum of disease varies considerably from asymptomatic or mild to
severe or fulminating.

Etiology

Entamoeba histolytica belongs to the family Entamoebidae. The other specie
within the genus *Entamoeba* is *E. hartmanni,* a nonpathogen. *Entamoeba histolytica* exists in two forms – the trophozoite and the cyst. Two different types of

1022

trophozoite have been described: the smaller, 10-20 μm in diameter, referred to as noninvasive; and the larger, invasive, up to 50μm. The latter are hematophagous. The two forms are most likely the same organism. The factors required for change from a small noninvasive to the larger invasive form are not clear. Encystment occurs in the colon as the contents become more solid. The cysts measure 10-18 μm in diameter and when mature contain four nuclei. Young cysts contain chromatoid bodies. The cysts are passed in the feces. Following ingestion of the cyst, nuclear division occurs. The cyst wall is destroyed in the gastrointestinal tract and eight trophozoites are released.

Epidemiology

Humans are the usual reservoir for *E. histolytica*. Amebiasis is transmitted by the fecal-oral route from person to person. Outbreaks from contaminated food or water have been reported. Food handlers also may play a role in the transmission. The overall prevalence of amebiasis in the United States is estimated at 4%. Cysts of *E. histolytica* survive in soil for prolonged periods and are not affected by chlorine in the amount used in water purification procedures.

Pathogenesis and Pathology

The pathogenetic mechanisms in amebiasis are not clearly understood. It has been postulated that the virulence of amebae is related at least in part to their association with bacteria. Alteration of virulence has been postulated to result from the transfer of a factor from bacteria to amebae, but such a factor has not been isolated.

Cytolethal activity of *E. histolytica* has been demonstrated against a number of target cells including polymorphonuclear leukocytes. It has been demonstrated that the cytolethal effect occurs only following direct contact of amebae with target cells. Intact amebic microfilament function has been demonstrated to be important for the killing of target cells. Marked cytotoxic activity and no cytotoxic activity have been demonstrated from extracts of virulent and avirulent strains, respectively. It is thought that cytotoxic substances may be located intracellularly near the plasma membrane of the ameba and when there is contact with host cells, these substances may be released.

Following entry through the mucosa, extensive necrosis in the submucosa takes place; this results in the well-known "flask-shaped ulcer." The cecal and rectosigmoid areas are most frequently affected, but other parts of the colon and terminal ileum may be involved. Extensive ulceration may interfere with the blood supply resulting in more tissue necrosis. Microscopic examination demonstrates minimal inflammatory reaction and amebae at the edge of the lesions. The ulcer may extend to the serosa resulting in perforation and peritonitis. Amebae can enter the bloodstream during the invasive processes and be carried to distant parts of the body, most frequently the liver. Focal necrosis of hepatocytes occurs by means of direct cytotoxicity. Ischemia from amebic obstruction of the portal vein also occurs. Two different modes of presentation, acute and chronic, have been reported. In acute disease there is rapid expansion of the abscess, antigen excess, and formation of immune complexes. In chronic disease (preexisting antibody from a long residence in an endemic area) the growth of the abscess is limited. Amebae are found in the periphery of the abscesses and the center contains liquefied, brownish, necrotic liver tissue referred to as "anchovy sauce."

Immunologic mechanisms against *E. histolytica* are not completely understood. Why some patients remain asymptomatic and others develop severe or fulminating infection is not clear. Circulating antibodies are produced in 90-95% of the patients with invasive disease. A lower percentage of patients with asymptomatic amebiasis develop antibodies. From epidemiologic and clinical information, antibodies are not thought to be protective. Reinfection occurs in endemic areas despite the presence of antibodies. Although cultured amebae are lysed by serum, amebae from dysenteric stool are not. It is felt that serum factors may be important in limiting the extent of invasion, rather than in preventing attachment and colonization. Secretory IgA may play a role in protection. Coproantibodies have been found in a significant percentage of patients with intestinal amebiasis. The role of cell-mediated immunity in amebiasis also has been evaluated. During acute illness, suppression of cell-mediated immunity has been demonstrated. Lymphocytes from patients recovered from amebiasis demonstrate cytotoxic activity for amebae. Clinical observations of worsening of amebiasis following corticosteroid administration also suggest a possible role of cell-mediated immunity in recovery or reduction of invasion from amebae. Pregnant patients with amebiasis also have been reported to do poorly. Whether this is related to suppression of cell-mediated immunity, or to hormonal effects on the organism with altered virulence, or to other yet undefined factors is not clear.

Diagnosis

Clinical

Intestinal Amebiasis

There is a tremendous variation in the severity and the mode of presentation. The patient may be asymptomatic. In symptomatic patients, the onset is usually gradual with colicky, lower-abdominal pain, tenesmus, and frequent bowel movements. Right lower-quadrant tenderness may be present; constitutional signs are generally mild or absent. The stools usually contain blood and mucus. The symptoms may continue for several months. In more severe cases, the patient may appear quite ill with weight loss, prostration, frequent bloody stools, and marked abdominal tenderness. If perforation occurs leading to peritonitis, patients present with signs of acute abdomen. Occasionally a patient will present with a mass lesion in the colon (ameboma) which can mimic carcinoma.

Extraintestinal

The liver is the most frequent site of extraintestinal involvement (Tables 119.1 and 119.2). Only 30% of patients with hepatic amebiasis give a history of current or previous intestinal amebiasis. Hepatic amebic abscess may occur shortly after the onset of intestinal amebiasis, or much later. In acute cases, symptoms usually start abruptly. Patients with chronic illness are more likely to present with sweats and low-grade fever. Pain is usually felt in the right upper-quadrant and may be referred to the tip of the shoulder. Pain may be felt in the epigastrium or right lower chest. With long-standing illness, weight loss may occur. Physical examination demonstrates tenderness in the right upper-quadrant and usually a palpable liver. Point tenderness either over the liver or intercostal spaces may occur. An obvious bulge or fullness may be present in the right upper-quadrant or epigastrium. Dullness or rales in the right lower chest may be present.

TABLE 119.1   Presenting Complaints of Patients with Amebic Liver Abscess

Symptom	Approximate % of Patients
Fever	40
Right upper-quadrant abdominal pain	30
Diarrhea	15
Anorexia	5
Right shoulder pain	3

TABLE 119.2   Clinical Findings in Patients with Amebic Liver Abscess

Symptom	Approximate % of Patients
Anorexia	100
Fever	95
Night sweats	75
Nausea/vomiting	75
Chills	70
Diarrhea	65
(bloody)	50
Pain	
Right upper-quadrant abdominal	90
Right chest	50
Right shoulder	40
Back	30

The diagnosis of intestinal amebiasis should be suspected clinically in persons returning from endemic areas, in institutionalized patients, in male homosexuals with diarrhea or dysentery, or in patients presenting with unexplained bloody diarrhea. The diagnosis should be considered in patients presenting with features suggesting inflammatory bowel disease, particularly ulcerative colitis. The diagnosis of hepatic amebiasis should be suspected in patients in epidemiologic settings similar to those just given, who present with right upper-quadrant tenderness, hepatomegaly, and fever.

Laboratory

Immediate examination of a wet mount of a fresh stool specimen is extremely important in identifying motile trophozoites of *E. histolytica*-containing erythrocytes. A number of substances, e.g., antimicrobials, antiparasitic drugs, laxatives, antacids, barium sulfate, various types of enemas, bismuth, and kaolin, will cause the organisms to disappear from the stool or to be more difficult to identify. Repeated stool samples should be obtained. If the stool samples are negative, scraping from an ulcer during proctoscopy using a glass pipette or metal instrument, not cotton swabs, should be employed. Stools should be examined, if possible, by a reasonably experienced person. Initially a direct smear using saline can be carried out. Buffered methylene blue is useful for differentiating leukocytes from amebae. Although erythrophagocytosis by *E. histolytica* is considered a hallmark for the diagnosis of intestinal amebiasis, occasionally macrophages with ingested erythrocytes may be mistaken for amebae. Trichrome staining of both trophozoites and cysts is useful for better delineation of morphology. If cysts are not demonstrated on direct smear, a concentration technique should be employed. In studies carried out by the Centers for Disease Control, one of the most frequently encountered problems was mistaking leukocytes for *E. histolytica* resulting in false-positive results. There were also false-negative results occurring from failure to consider the diagnosis or from inappropriate handling of the specimens. In addition to examining stools immediately for trophozoites, polyvinyl alcohol should be used for preserving trophozoites so that the specimen will be available for restudy later or for sending the slide to the Centers for Disease Control. *Entamoeba histolytica* should be differentiated from the smaller nonpathogenic *E. hartmanni* using an ocular micrometer.

A number of serologic tests are available for diagnosis of amebiasis. The most commonly employed test is indirect hemagglutination, which is positive in 85-90% of the patients with amebic colitis. It is a very sensitive test but remains positive for many years (sometimes with high titer) following the acute illness. The agar gel diffusion precipitin test becomes negative in a significant percentage of patients within 6 months.

Hepatic Abscess

Leukocytosis with a shift to the left is usual (Table 119.3). Lower leukocyte counts are found in chronic disease along with mild anemia. The most common abnormal liver function test is elevation of alkaline phosphatase. It is much more likely to be elevated and to a greater degree in those with chronic disease. Elevated serum glutamic oxaloacetic transaminase (SGOT) correlates with the severity of the disease. Hyperbilirubinemia is very uncommon and is related to a poorer prognosis.

A chest roentgenogram may show elevated right hemidiaphragm and occasionally a pleural effusion. Radioisotope scanning, ultrasonography, or computerized tomography are utilized in demonstrating the hepatic abscess. The

TABLE 119.3   Laboratory Findings in Patients with Amebic Liver Abscess

Finding	Approximate % of Patients
Leukocytosis	90
Elevated prothrombin time	80
Anemia	70
Elevated alkaline phosphatase	60
Abnormal x-ray	
Elevated right hemidiaphragm	60
Right pleural effusion	35
Elevated SGOT	35
Stool positive for *E. histolytica*	25
Elevated bilirubin	20

abscess(es) is (are) usually in the right lobe. Single abscesses are more common in chronic disease and multiple abscesses in acute disease.

Serologic tests are helpful in making the diagnosis of hepatic amebiasis. Various tests for determination of antibody are always positive, except early in the illness. The titer of 1:128 is considered significant. Amebic antigen may be demonstrated in serum in approximately a quarter of the patients with hepatic abscess and much more frequently (92%) in pus aspirated from the hepatic abscess. *Entamoeba histolytica* is demonstrated very infrequently (15%) in the pus, probably because it is usually present at the border of the abscess.

Differential Diagnosis

In the differential diagnosis of intestinal amebiasis, other agents causing bloody diarrhea should be considered, e.g., *Shigella, Campylobacter,* and other causes of invasive bacterial diarrhea. Bacterial dysentery is abrupt in onset unlike amebiasis, which is usually insidious. Fecal leukocytes are much more likely to be present and in larger numbers in invasive bacterial diarrhea than in amebic dysentery. Ulcerative colitis and amebiasis may appear similar clinically. It is generally thought prudent to rule out amebiasis and other causes of invasive bacterial diarrhea before making a diagnosis of ulcerative colitis. Steroids have a detrimental effect in cases of amebiasis. Abnormal liver enzymes with right upper-quadrant tenderness may lead one to think of viral hepatitis or pyogenic liver abscess in addition to amebic liver abscess. In general, alkaline phosphatase is more likely to be elevated than SGOT in cases of infiltrative or "space-occupying" processes such as a hepatic abscess, whereas in viral hepatitis, elevations of SGOT and serum glutamic pyruvic transaminase, in addition to alkaline phosphatase, are more likely. Generally in viral hepatitis, unless complicated by an acute fulminating course or submassive necrosis, fever is unusual once liver function tests are abnormal, whereas with either amebic or pyogenic liver abscess fever may be present with abnormalities of liver function tests. A rash or arthralgias, which may occur with hepatitis B, are not present in cases of amebic hepatic abscess. Filling defects in the liver may be caused by a number of possibilities in addition to amebic liver abscesses, e.g., pyogenic liver abscess, cysts, and tumors.

Treatment

Drugs used for amebiasis differ in (1) their mode of action on different forms of ameba (trophozoite versus cysts), (2) toxicity, and (3) availability (routine versus from the Centers for Disease Control) (Table 119.4). The principles of therapy in symptomatic patients consist of eradicating the tissue and the intraluminal forms. Metronidazole is most effective against the tissue form and diiodohydroxyquin

TABLE 119.4   Treatment of Amebiasis

Problem	Drug	Usual Adult Dose
Asymptomatic patient	Diiodohydroxyquin	650 mg t.i.d. x 20 days
Stool examination demonstrating cysts	(Alternative diloxanide furoate*)	500 mg t.i.d. x 10 days
Symptomatic intestinal infection	Metronidazole plus	750 mg t.i.d. x 5 days
	diiodohydroxyquin	650 mg t.i.d. x 20 days
	(Alternative dehydroemetine* SC or IM plus	1 mg/kg/day (maximum dose 90 mg/day) x 5 days
	diiodohydroxyquin)	650 mg t.i.d. x 20 days
Extraintestinal	Metronidazole plus	750 mg t.i.d. x 5-10 days
	diiodohydroxyquin	650 mg t.i.d. x 20 days
	(Alternative dehydroemetine* SC or IM plus	1 mg/kg/day (maximum 90 mg/day) x 5 days
	chloroquine phosphate)	600 mg base daily x 2 days then, 300 mg base daily x 2-3 weeks

*Available from the Parasitic Diseases Branch, Centers for Disease Control

and diloxanide furoate are effective against the cysts. An alternative form of therapy for the tissue form is dehydroemetine. Because of its toxicity, particularly cardiac, it is not used as a first-line drug. Paromomycin also is occasionally used as an alternative agent in treatment of intestinal amebiasis.

Most amebic abscesses do not require drainage for therapy (Table 119.5). In cases of perforation known to be from amebiasis, resection is not advised. Drainage of the peritoneal cavity combined with appropriate antiamebic therapy is considered the best option.

Side effects of metronidazole include nausea, vomiting, diarrhea, metallic taste in the mouth, occasionally leukopenia, peripheral neuropathy, seizures, and mental confusion. Patients should be warned regarding Antabuse-like reactions. Since amebiasis may be a severe disease in pregnancy, the risk versus benefit of metronidazole should be weighed carefully. Metronidazole does cross the placenta and is secreted in breast milk. Animal studies have demonstrated its carcinogenic potential. For diiodohydroxyquin, the dosage and duration should not be exceeded because of the possibility of optic neuritis. Dehydroemetine is associated with cardiotoxicity, and therefore electrocardiographic monitoring should be carried out and the patient should be sedentary.

Complications and Prognosis

Rarely, perforation resulting in peritonitis will occur in the setting of intestinal amebiasis or hepatic abscess. Amebic liver abscess may rupture into the pleural cavity, lung, or pericardial cavity. Extension into the lung (giving rise to consolidation, abscess, or tracheobronchial fistula), or pleural cavity (empyema), usually occurs from the right lobe of the liver, and into the pericardial cavity from the left lobe. Extension is generally by contiguous spread. Hematogenous spread may rarely occur. With extension into the pleura or lung, patients usually complain of pleuritic chest pain, cough, dyspnea, and hemoptysis. The sputum may be reddish brown. Extension into the pericardium may be gradual or sudden. The patient usually will complain of chest pain and a pericardial rub may be present. Frank congestive heart failure also may occur. A brain abscess may rarely result from hematogenous spread. Cutaneous fistulae in the region of a hepatic abscess or in the perineum from intestinal amebiasis also may be seen.

The prognosis varies with the severity of the disease and the presence of complications. Pregnancy has been associated with the worst prognosis. The use of steroids is also associated with complications.

Prevention

Fecal contamination of food and water should be avoided. Boiling water for at least 10 min will result in killing of amebae. Since ordinary chlorination procedures are ineffective against *E. histolytica* cysts, water in endemic areas cannot

TABLE 119.5   **Indications for Aspiration of Amebic Hepatic Abscess**

Large size (> 10 cm)

Suspected impending rupture

Poor clinical response after 5 days of therapy

be regarded as "safe" with reference to amebiasis. Raw vegetables and fruits should be washed carefully before eating. Handwashing by infected persons should be emphasized. Enteric isolation should be instituted for affected hospitalized patients.

Primary Amebic Meningoencephalitis

Primary amebic meningoencephalitis caused by free-living amebae was first reported from Australia in 1965. Since then it has been reported from many parts of the world including Africa, Belgium, Britain, Czechoslovakia, and New Zealand. In the United States, most cases have been reported from Virginia, Florida, Texas, and Georgia. Of the primary amebic meningoencephalitides, the disease caused by *Naegleria fowleri* has been studied the most. It is a relatively rare disease and almost always fatal (only occasional survivors have been reported). Recently, cases of meningoencephalitis caused by *Acanthamoeba* have been reported. As compared with *Naegleria* meningitis, the course of meningitis caused by *Acanthamoeba* is subacute or chronic (Table 119.6).

The classification of free-living amebae is still controversial. The two genera that have been associated with human disease are *Naegleria* and *Acanthamoeba*. *Naegleria fowleri* trophozoites measure 10-20 μm. They contain a single nucleus, a large karyosome, distinct endoplasm and ectoplasm, food vacuoles, and a contractile vacuole. The cyst is 10 μm and has a single nucleus. The trophozoites of *Acanthamoeba* are larger than those of *Naegleria*. Cysts have a characteristic wrinkled double wall. With both genera, encystation occurs when the environmental conditions are less favorable.

TABLE 119.6   Differential Diagnosis of Amebic Meningoencephalitis

Naegleria	Bacterial meningitis (including partially treated)
	Viral meningitis (early)
Acanthamoeba	Partially treated bacterial meningitis
	Viral meningoencephalitis
	Tuberculous meningitis
	Fungal meningitis
	Parameningeal infectious focus
	Carcinomatous meningitis
	CNS vasculitis

Patients who develop primary amebic meningoencephalitis from *N. fowleri* are usually healthy children and young adults. *Naegleria* spp may be found in lakes contaminated with bacteria or other organic matter. A history of swimming or diving in fresh water lakes, heated indoor pools, or hot springs is usually obtained. Cases usually are seen during the summer. The incubation period is estimated to be 5-6 days. Since it is such an uncommon disease despite tremendous possibilities for exposure, host factors or factors related to the pathogen (e.g., the degree of contamination of the suspected water sources) may play a role. *Acanthamoeba* has been cultured from the nasopharynx of healthy individuals. Very few cases have been reported and the identification is usually morphologic. There is no increased incidence of recent swimming. Unlike patients with naeglerial meningoencephalitis, underlying diseases are usually present in patients with central nervous system involvement caused by *Acanthamoeba* spp.

On the basis of epidemiologic information, experimental infection, and pathologic findings in humans, it is postulated that *Naegleria* organisms enter the central nervous tissue following invasion of the olfactory epithelium and the cribriform plate. The mechanism that produces destruction of tissues is not clear. Central nervous system infection by *Acanthamoeba* has also been produced in experimental infections following intranasal instillation. Whether it is this route or other routes of infection that are involved in human infections is not clear.

Gross examination of the brain in cases of naeglerial meningitis demonstrates edema and the presence of purulent meningitis. The exudate is prominent over the sulci and the basal cisterns. Superficial hemorrhagic necrosis of the grey matter is also present. *Naegleria* organisms are usually found around the small blood vessels near the areas of necrosis. Examination of the brain in cases of acanthamoebic encephalitis shows widespread areas of necrosis. Both the cyst form and the trophozoites of *Acanthamoeba* may be identified in the affected areas.

Cases of keratitis caused by *Acanthamoeba* also have been reported. Direct entry rather than involvement by the systemic route seems most likely. Almost all patients have received steroids before the onset of disease. Exposure to water or contaminated material was reported in some cases.

The patient with *N. fowleri* meningoencephalitis usually presents with the sudden onset of headache and fever. Abnormalities in the senses of taste or smell have occasionally been reported. Rapid progression from neck stiffness and abnormalities of mental status to seizures and coma is usually observed. Death occurs around the fifth or sixth day of illness.

The presentation and the course of meningoencephalitis caused by *Acanthamoeba* are subacute to chronic. Fever, lethargy, altered mental status, and focal neurologic deficits may occur.

Patients with keratitis caused by *Acanthamoeba* present with eye pain and visual impairment. Examination demonstrates blepharospasm, hyperemia of the conjunctiva, and few keratic precipitates.

Cerebrospinal fluid from patients with *N. fowleri* meningoencephalitis demonstrates increased numbers of leukocytes ranging from several hundred to several thousand. The differential count shows a predominance of polymorphonuclear leukocytes. Erythrocytes may be present. Protein concentration usually is increased and glucose is decreased. *Naegleria* spp can be demonstrated by examination of a wet mount of the cerebrospinal fluid. Refrigeration or centrifugation of the cerebrospinal fluid should not be done before examination for *Naegleria* because the former may kill the organism, and the latter may result in decreased motility. *Naegleria* spp can be cultured on plain agar plates seeded with *Escherichia coli*. Both flagellation and the production of cysts can be observed in cultures.

The data on cerebrospinal fluid findings in patients with meningoencephalitis caused by *Acanthamoeba* are limited. Increased protein, low or normal glucose, and increased numbers of cells with a predominance of lymphocytes have been reported. The diagnosis usually has been made on the morphologic features of *Acanthamoeba* in the tissue rather than by culture.

The drug of choice for *N. fowleri* meningoencephalitis is amphotericin B. The agents used in the treatment of *E. histolytica* infections, metronidazole, chloroquine, emetine hydrochloride, and tetracycline, are not effective. Recently, combinations of amphotericin B with rifampin or tetracycline have been demonstrated to be synergistic in a mouse model of naeglerial meningoencephalitis. Successful treatment of a 9-year-old patient with intravenous and intrathecal amphotericin B, miconazole, and oral rifampin has been recently reported. More studies are needed to determine the efficacy of combined drug therapy.

The drug of choice for the treatment of meningoencephalitis caused by *Acanthamoeba* has not been determined. Use of a sulfonamide in the mouse model has resulted in decreased mortality. Topical amphotericin B and 5-fluorocytosine or pimaracin have been used for the treatment of keratitis in humans. Medical therapy usually is disappointing. Therapeutic keratoplasty is generally necessary.

The prognosis of *N. fowleri* meningitis is very poor; only occasional survivors have been reported. It is difficult to comment on the outcome of patients with meningoencephalitis caused by *Acanthamoeba* since very few cases have been reported, but it also seems to be poor. However, the course is subacute compared to naeglerial meningoencephalitis. Education of the public to avoid a known contaminated water source is important in prevention. Chlorination of water may not prevent the disease, but steam cleaning of water filters has been recommended.

Selected Bibliography

Adams, E. B. and MacLeod, I. N.: Invasive amebiasis. I. Amebic dysentery and its complications. *Medicine* 56:315-323, 1977.

Adams, E. B. and MacLeod, I. N.: Invasive amebiasis. II. Amebic liver abscess and its complications. *Medicine* 56:325-334, 1977.

Cleland, P. G., Lawande, R. V., Onyemelukwe, G., and Whittle, H. C.: Chronic amebic meningoencephalitis. *Arch Neurol* 39:56-57, 1982.

Duma, R. J. and Finley, R.: In vitro susceptibility of pathogenic *Naegleria* and *Acanthamoeba* species to a variety of therapeutic agents. *Antimicrob Agents Chemother* 10:370-376, 1976.

Duma, R. J., Helwig, W. B., and Martinez, A. J.: Meningoencephalitis and brain abscess due to a free-living amoeba. *Ann Intern Med* 88:468-473, 1978.

Ibarra-Pérez, C.: Thoracic complications of amebic abscess of the liver. Report of 501 cases. *Chest* 79:672-677, 1981.

Katzenstein, D., Rickerson, V., and Braude, A.: New concepts of amebic liver abscess derived from hepatic imaging, serodiagnosis, and hepatic enzymes in 67 consecutive cases in San Diego. *Medicine* 61:237-246, 1982.

Kean, B. H., Gilmore, H. R., and Van Stone, W. W.: Fatal amebiasis: Report of 148 fatal cases from the Armed Forces Institutes of Pathology. *Ann Intern Med* 44:831-843, 1956.

Key, S. N., III, Green, W. R., Willaert, E., Stevens, A. R., and Key, S. N., Jr.: Keratitis due to *Acanthamoeba castellani.* A clinicopathologic case report. *Arch Ophthomol* 98:475-479, 1980.

Krogstad, D. J., Spencer, H. C., and Healy, G. R.: Amebiasis. *N Engl J Med* 298:262-265, 1978.

Krogstad, D. J., Spencer, H. C., Healy, G. R., Gleason, N. N., Sexton, D. J., and Herron, C. A.: Amebiasis: Epidemiologic studies in the United States, 1971-1974. *Ann Intern Med* 88:89-97, 1978.

Mahajan, R. C. and Ganguly, N. K.: Amoebic antigen in immunodiagnosis and prognosis of amoebic liver abscess. *Trans R Soc Trop Med Hyg* 74:300-302, 1980.

Mahmoud, A. A. F. and Warren, K. S.: Algorithms in the diagnosis and management of exotic disease. XVII. Amebiasis. *J Infect Dis* 134:639-643, 1976.

Martinez, A. J., Duma, R. J., Nelson, E. C., and Moretta, F. L.: Experimental naegleria meningoencephalitis in mice. Penetration of the olfactory mucosal epithelium by *Naegleria* and pathologic changes produced: A light and electron microscope study. *Lab Invest* 29:121-133, 1973.

Patterson, M., Healy, G. R., and Shabot, J. M.: Serologic testing for amoebiasis. *Gastroenterology* 78:136-141, 1980.

Peters, R. S., Gitlin, N., and Libke, R. D.: Amebic liver abscess. *Ann Rev Med* 32:161-174, 1981.

Pomerantz, B. M., Marr, J. S., and Goldman, W. D.: Amebiasis in New York City 1958-1978: Identification of the male homosexual high risk population. *Bull NY Acad Med* 56:232-244, 1980.

Ravdin, J. I., Croft, B. Y., and Guerrant, R. L.: Cytopathogenic mechanisms of *Entamoeba histolytica. J Exp Med* 152:377-390, 1980.

Ravdin, J. I. and Guerrant, R. L.: A review of the parasite cellular mechanisms involved in the pathogenesis of amebiasis. *Rev Infect Dis* 4:1185-1207, 1982.

Robert, V. B. and Rorke, L. B.: Primary amebic encephalitis, probably from *Acanthamoeba. Ann Intern Med* 79:174-179, 1973.

Sheehan, D. J., Bottone, E. J., Pavletich, K., and Heath, M. C.: *Entamoeba histolytica:* Efficacy of microscopic, cultural, and serological techniques for laboratory diagnosis. *J Clin Microbiol* 10:128-133, 1979.

Thong, Y. H.: Clinical review - Primary amoebic meningoencephalitis: Fifteen years later. *Med J Aust* 1:352-354, 1980.

Thong, Y. H., Rowan-Kelly, B., and Ferrante, A.: Delayed treatment of experimental amoebic meningoencephalitis with amphotericin B and tetracycline. *Trans R Soc Trop Med Hyg* 73:336-337, 1979.

Thong, Y. H., Rowan-Kelly, B., and Ferrante, A.: Treatment of experimental naegleria meningoencephalitis with a combination of amphotericin B and rifamycin. *Scand J Infect Dis* 11:151-153, 1979.

Trissl, D.: Immunology of *Entamoeba histolytica* in human and animal hosts. *Rev Infect Dis* 4:1154-1184, 1982.

Yang, J. and Kennedy, M. T.: Evaluation of enzyme-linked immunosorbent assay for the serodiagnosis of amebiasis. *J Clin Microbiol* 10:778-785, 1979.

120

GIARDIASIS
Rashida A. Khakoo, M.D.

Definition

Giardia lamblia was previously thought to be nonpathogenic, but its role in causing disease has recently been better appreciated. It is the most commonly identified pathogenic intestinal parasite in stool specimens submitted to public health
laboratories in the United States. Studies have demonstrated the occurrence of
diarrhea and malabsorption when *G. lamblia* are present and the improvement or
disappearance of symptoms following treatment. Several waterborne epidemics
of giardiasis have been reported.

Etiology

Giardia lamblia is a flagellate with trophozoite and cyst stages. The trophozoite
is pear-shaped and measures 12-15 by 5-15 by 2-4 μm with two nuclei, a ventral
sucking disc and four flagella. Encystation occurs during transit through the intestine. Cysts measuring 8-12 by 7-10 μm have two to four nuclei depending on
maturity. Trophozoites inhabit the duodenum and upper jejunum and attach to the
mucosa by the suction disc.

Epidemiology

Giardiasis occurs throughout the world. It is both endemic and epidemic. The
prevalence in the United States has been calculated to be 7.4%. The mode of
transmission is most likely by fecal-oral contamination or by ingestion of cysts
present in water. Cysts remain viable in water for longer than 3 months and are

not destroyed by ordinary chlorination procedures. Between 1972 and 1977, 23 waterborne outbreaks of giardiasis affecting 7009 persons were reported in the United States. These occurred primarily in mountainous areas: the Rocky Mountains (particularly in Aspen, Colorado), New England, and the Pacific Northwest. Most outbreaks have occurred as the result of consuming untreated surface water or surface water with disinfection as the only treatment. Tap water has been implicated as the probable means of transmission in an outbreak among American travelers to Leningrad in which the attack rate was 23%.

After ingestion of cysts, excystation occurs in the duodenum; two trophozoites are formed which then mature in the duodenum and upper jejunum. Infection rates of 100% and 36.4% were reported following ingestion of 100-1 million cysts and 10-25 cysts, respectively, by human volunteers. The latent period in the experimental infections averaged 9 days. The usual incubation period in endemic cases is 15 days. Giardiasis has been reported in increased frequency among homosexual men.

Pathogenesis and Pathology

The reasons underlying the varied presentation from asymptomatic to severe symptoms are not clear. Possible explanations include differences in virulence, inoculum size, or immunity. Immunoglobulin A deficiency has been associated with an increased risk of giardiasis. Symptomatic giardiasis is common in grossly immunodeficient patients, whereas giardiasis in apparently healthy individuals is not related to unsuspected immunoglobulin deficiency.

Malabsorption of D-xylose and vitamin B_{12} occurs in 55-60% of patients with giardiasis. Several mechanisms have been postulated for the malabsorption: blockade of mucosa by the parasite, mechanical irritation, nutritional competition, villous atrophy, and bacterial overgrowth with bile salt deconjugation. Significant reductions in brush border enzymes have also been demonstrated in patients with giardiasis. Giardia usually do not invade beyond the bowel lumen. The mechanisms involved in the production of inflammation are not clear, although giardia might elaborate substances that are toxic to the tissues. Bacteria associated with giardia may also be responsible.

In symptomatic patients, a biopsy of the small intestine usually shows varying degrees and combinations of blunting of villi, acute and chronic inflammation of the lamina propria, and increased crypt epithelial mitoses thought to represent a response to epithelial injury. The inflammatory cells are usually polymorphonuclear, but occasionally eosinophils are seen. The mucosal lesions are usually patchy and much of the confusion in the literature regarding presence or absence of pathologic lesions may be explained by this feature. In asymptomatic patients the number and appearance of the villi are usually normal but the lamina propria is infiltrated with inflammatory cells. In patients with hypogammaglobulinemia, marked mucosal abnormalities and nodular lymphoid hyperplasia have been demonstrated.

Giardia may be seen in tissue sections but the familiar dorsal view is uncommon as a result of random orientation in the tissues. Giardia may appear elongated or have a sickle shape. Paired nuclei, if found, are a valuable diagnostic feature. Giardia are sometimes found attached to the epithelium. The easiest place to find organisms is in the mucus lying between the villi. Giardia can be demonstrated by hematoxylin-eosin or Giemsa stain.

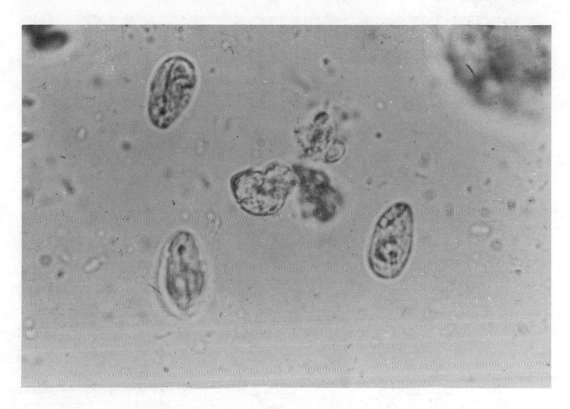

FIGURE 120.1   Cysts of *Giardia lamblia* in stool (iodine stain, 2050x).   Courtesy of J. E. Hall.

Diagnostic Features

Clinical

A wide spectrum of presentation is noted from asymptomatic or mild to very severe. Watery foul-smelling diarrhea is a common symptom. Patients may complain of epigastric or generalized crampy abdominal pain, flatulence, abdominal distension, nausea, anorexia, and weight loss. Steatorrhea occurs in 25–50% of patients. Less commonly, patients complain of belching, fatigue, and generalized weakness. Urticaria occasionally has been reported. Symptoms may last a short time or persist for months.

Laboratory

Careful examination of stools is important. A total of three specimens of stool obtained every other day should be examined. Use of concentration methods for stool examination improves the sensitivity. Cysts are usually seen in well-formed stool (Figure 120.1). In the presence of diarrhea with rapid transit time, trophozoites are usually seen (Figure 120.2). Barium, antimicrobials, and antacids can temporarily mask the presence of parasites. If the concentrated stool samples

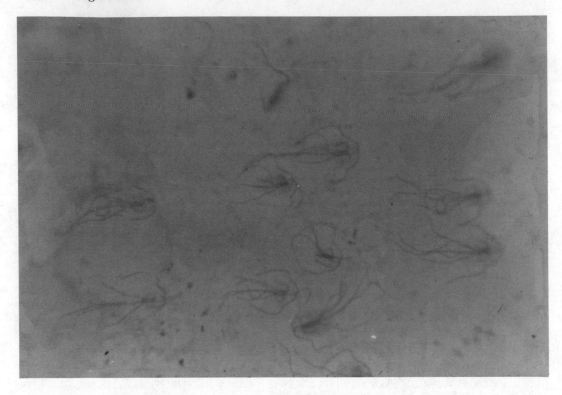

FIGURE 120.2   Trophozoites of *Giardia lamblia* in stool (silver impregnation technique for demonstrating flagella, 2050x). Courtesy of J. E. Hall.

are negative in a patient clinically suspected of having giardiasis, examination of a duodenal aspirate or jejunal biopsy for Giemsa-stained imprint smears and histopathology should be carried out.

Roentgenologic abnormalities in giardiasis are nonspecific. Abnormalities consisting of thickening of mucosal folds are most apparent in the duodenum and jejunum. At present no serologic test for the diagnosis of giardiasis is available. In one study, 29 of 30 patients with symptomatic giardiasis had increased indirect immunofluorescent antibody titers. The test was specific and reproducible.

Differential Diagnosis

In general, diarrhea caused by bacteria and viruses is not prolonged, whereas that caused by giardiasis may be. Also, fever and bloody diarrhea, which may occur with invasive bacterial disease, do not usually occur with giardiasis. Parasites other than ameba cause diarrhea infrequently. Stool examination and proctoscopy when necessary will help make the diagnosis. Noninfectious causes of diarrhea, e.g., drugs or laxatives, also need to be considered in the differential. Patients with Crohn's disease may present with watery diarrhea. With epigastric pain and flatulence, peptic ulcer or gallbladder disease should be considered.

Treatment

Quinacrine hydrochloride is considered the treatment of choice. The recommended dosage for adults is 100 mg three times a day for 7 days. For children, the usual dosage is 2 mg/kg three times a day. Side effects of quinacrine include psychosis, nausea, vomiting, skin rashes, fever, and yellow discoloration of skin and urine. Metronidazole is used as an alternate therapy, but is not approved for this use by the Food and Drug Administration. Metronidazole is better tolerated than quinacrine. The usual recommended dosage for adults is 250 mg three times a day for 7-10 days. Some studies have reported cure rates of more than 90% with the use of metronidazole. Some of the side effects include nausea, vomiting, diarrhea, headache, metallic taste in the mouth, and disulfiram-like reactions. Other drugs which are efficacious in the treatment of giardiasis include tinidazole and nimorazole, neither of which is licensed in the United States.

Stool examination should be repeated after completion of treatment. A small percentage of patients may require retreatment.

Prevention

Avoiding ingestion of potentially contaminated water or food is important. In endemic areas, water should be boiled for 10 min or purified with iodine compounds. Ordinary chlorination does not destroy cysts. Treatment of the asymptomatic cyst-passer is considered useful for preventing the spread of infection to others. There are no chemoprophylactic agents or vaccines available.

Complications and Prognosis

In general, the prognosis is very good. It may be difficult to eradicate *G. lamblia* in patients with immunodeficiency. Complications are rare. Long-standing infestation with malabsorption may produce nutritional deficiencies.

Selected Bibliography

Ament, M. E. and Rubin, C. E.: Relation of giardiasis to abnormal intestinal structure and function in gastrointestinal immunodeficiency syndromes. *Gastroenterology* 62:216-226, 1972.

Craun, G. F.: Waterborne giardiasis in the United States: A review. *Am J Public Health* 69:817-819, 1979.

Hartong, W. A., Gourley, W. K., and Arvanitakis, C.: Giardiasis: Clinical spectrum and functional-structural abnormalities of the small intestinal mucosa. *Gastroenterology* 77:61-69, 1979.

Jones, E. G. and Brown, W. R.: Serum and intestinal fluid immunoglobulins in patients with giardiasis. *Dig Dis* 19:791-796, 1974.

Kavousi, S.: Giardiasis in infancy and childhood: A prospective study of 160 cases with comparison of quinacrine and metronidazole (Flagyl). *Am J Trop Med Hyg* 28:19-23, 1979.

Levi, G. C., Armando de Avila, C., and Amato Neto, V.: Efficacy of various drugs for treatment of giardiasis. A comparative study. *Am J Trop Med Hyg* 26: 564–565, 1977.

Mahmoud, A. A. F. and Warren, K. S.: Algorithms in the diagnosis and management of exotic disease. II. Giardiasis. *J Infect Dis* 131:621–623, 1975.

Mildvan, D., Gelb, A. M., and William, D.: Venereal transmission of enteric pathogens in male homosexuals, two case reports. *JAMA* 238:532–534, 1977.

Naik, S. R., Rau, N. R., and Vinayak, V. K.: A comparative evaluation of examinations of three stool samples, jejunal aspirate and jejunal mucosal impression smears in the diagnosis of giardiasis. *Ann Trop Med Parasitol* 72:491–492, 1978.

Rendtorff, R. C.: The experimental transmission of human intestinal protozoan parasites. II. *Giardia lamblia* cysts given in capsules. *Am J Hyg* 59:209–226, 1954.

Smith, J. W. and Wolfe, M. S.: Giardiasis. *Ann Rev Med* 31:373–383, 1980.

Tandon, B. N., Tandon, R. K., Satpathy, B. K., and Shriniwas: Mechanism of malabsorption in giardiasis: A study of bacterial flora and bile salt deconjugation in upper jejunum. *Gut* 18:176–181, 1977.

Visvesvara, G. S., Smith, P. D., Mealy, G. D., and Brown, W. R.: An immunofluorescence test to detect serum antibodies to *Giardia lamblia*. *Ann Int Med* 93: 802–805, 1980.

Yardley, J. H., Takano, J., and Hendrix, T. R.: Epithelial and other mucosal lesions of the jejunum in giardiasis. Jejunal biopsy studies. *Bull Johns Hopkins Hosp* 115:389–406, 1964.

Zinneman, H. H. and Kaplan, A. P.: The association of giardiasis with reduced intestinal secretory immunoglobulin A. *Dig Dis* 17:793–796, 1972.

121

TOXOPLASMOSIS
David L. Hoover, M.D.

Toxoplasma gondii, a coccidian protozoan, is an obligate intracellular parasite. Although the parasite is widely distributed among animal species, members of the cat family are the definitive host.

Microbiology

Sexual reproduction in the cat alimentary tract results in the formation of an oocyst which is shed in the feces and becomes infectious after a short maturation period in the soil. The oocyst may remain viable under moist conditions for several months. Humans acquire the parasite rarely from organ transplantation or leukocyte transfusion. Ingestion of cysts in undercooked meat and contamination of food by cat feces are the most common means of infection. Cockroaches and flies may transport oocysts from infected feces to food.

After ingestion and digestion of cysts or oocysts the parasite is liberated, replicates at the site of entry, and spreads to cells in various organs. Continued replication results in the death of parasitized cells. When replication ceases the cyst form may develop. The cyst may remain dormant for years only to convert back to the multiplying trophozoite under conditions of suppressed host immunity. Tissue cysts are susceptible to drying and are killed by heating to 60°C for 10-15 min.

Clinical Manifestations

Despite the fact that about one-half of the population are infected with toxoplasmosis by the age of 50, most cases go undiagnosed. The most commonly recognized acute form of the disease is localized lymphadenopathy, especially of the head and neck regions. The nodes are usually firm and nontender. Fever, rash, pharyngitis, hepatosplenomegaly, and atypical lymphocytosis may occur, causing confusion with infectious mononucleosis. Occasionally, more severe forms of the disease such as encephalitis, polymyositis, peri- or myocarditis, pneumonitis, or hepatitis may develop. Patients with retroperitoneal lymphadenopathy may present as a fever of unknown origin and have lymphangiograms suggestive of lymphoma. Diagnosis is best made serologically. Lymph node biopsy may show a characteristic infiltration by macrophages. Trophozoites may be seen rarely by Giemsa stain. The presence of cysts or isolation of the parasite from tissues is not sufficient to diagnose acute disease, since cysts may remain dormant but viable for many years. Acute toxoplasmosis usually resolves without specific therapy in several weeks.

Patients who are immunosuppressed by cytotoxic agents or steroids are at increased risk of developing disseminated disease. In 90% of the fatal cases, central nervous system involvement, including encephalitis, meningitis, or focal lesions, has been found. Myocarditis and pneumonitis also may occur. Clinical disease in such patients usually represents reactivation of latent infection, but primary infection may be acquired from leukocyte transfusion or organ transplant. Since antibody rises may be blunted, demonstration of characteristic histopathologic changes in tissues may be necessary for diagnosis. Inoculation of blood or other body fluids into mice or tissue culture can be used to isolate the organism. Untreated, the case-fatality rate of disseminated disease has been reported as high as 80%.

Congenital infection is the most important cause of morbidity and mortality from toxoplasma. Approximately 1:200 mothers will acquire primary infection during pregnancy. The fetus will be infected in 30-45% of these cases. Chronic maternal infection acquired before conception represents no threat to the fetus. First trimester infection is especially likely to result in abortion or stillbirth. A neonatal syndrome of retinochoroiditis, rash, jaundice, hepatosplenomegaly, intracranial calcifications, hydro- or microcephaly, and fever occurs in a few infected infants. Even those who are asymptomatically infected, however, may later suffer blindness, hearing impairment, mental retardation, or other neurologic sequelae.

Toxoplasmic retinochoroiditis usually occurs in patients with long-standing asymptomatic infection, including congenital infection. Retinal scars due to old, burned out disease often coexist with active lesions. The inflammatory reaction may be intense with accompanying iridocyclitis. Delayed hypersensitivity to parasite antigens is thought to be a critical aspect of the pathogenesis of symptomatic ocular disease. Certain diagnosis is rarely achieved. Antibody is present in low titer, and no rise or fall is consistently detectable except in the unusual case in which ocular disease accompanies acute, primary infection.

Diagnosis and Management

Antibody to *T. gondii* may be detected by several techniques. Differences in timing of antibody rises and falls (Table 121.1) are useful clinically. The dye test (DT) is the benchmark by which other tests are measured. The method requires a source of viable organisms, however, and is thus too cumbersome for routine use. The indirect fluorescent antibody test (IFAT), with accuracy and patterns of antibody rise and decline similar to the dye test, is the most widely available method. The IgM-specific IFAT (IgM IFAT) is useful in defining acute disease and neonatal infection. Antibody titers in the complement-fixation test are lower than in the IFAT, but the delay in appearance of this antibody may allow detection

TABLE 121.1   Onset of Duration of Antibodies to Toxoplasma Following Acute Infection

Test	Abbreviation	Onset/Rise	Duration
Dye test	DT	0-2 mo	Years
Indirect fluorescent antibody test	IFAT	0-2 mo	Years
IgM indirect fluorescent antibody test	IgM-IFAT	0-1 mo	3 wk to 5 mo
Complement fixation	CF	1-5 mo	Years
Indirect hemagglutination	IHA	2-5 mo	Years

of a rising titer which by other methods has already reached a high plateau. An indirect hemagglutination (IHA) test is both sensitive and specific, and detects antibody which rises later than those measured by the DT and IFAT.

Other diagnostic approaches are summarized in Table 121.2. Newly pregnant women should have a determination of toxoplasmal antibody titer performed. A positive titer should be checked with an IgM-IFAT to determine whether it represents a response to latent or to primary infection. Documentation of primary infection in the mother during pregnancy should suggest consideration of treatment for the mother and infant. Options concerning therapeutic abortion should also be discussed. Treatment during the first trimester should consist of triple-sulfonamides or sulfadiazine without pyrimethamine because the latter drug is teratogenic. Congenitally infected infants and immunocompromised patients should be treated with a combination of both drugs. Pyrimethamine should be given in a loading dose of 100-200 mg in adults, followed by a maintenance dosage of 1 mg/kg/day. Sulfadiazine or triple-sulfonamides also should be administered in a dosage of 20-25 mg/kg/day every 6 hr. Pyrimethamine interferes with folate metabolism; therefore folinic acid is required twice weekly during treatment. Treatment with folinic acid is necessary if the platelet count declines below 100,000/mm^3. Previously healthy individuals without immune deficiency will usually not require specific treatment unless multiple organs, especially heart or central nervous system, are involved. Patients with ocular toxoplasmosis which significantly threatens central vision should receive sulfa and pyrimethamine in addition to steroids.

Immunity and Prevention

Immunity to *Toxoplasma* can be transferred by lymphoid cells but not by serum alone. Antibody, however, enhances intracellular destruction of the parasite by macrophages. Activation of macrophages by lymphokines also results in enhanced antiparasitic capability. Similarly, suppression of cellular immunity by steroids

TABLE 121.2   Diagnostic Approaches to Toxoplasmosis

Presenting Syndrome	Test	Confirmatory Results
Acute disease	IFAT, CF, IHA IgM–IFAT	Rising titer Titer present
Acute disease, pregnancy	IgM–IFAT	Titer present
Ocular disease	IFAT, CF	Titer present
Compromised host, acute disease	IFAT, CF IgM–IFAT	Rising titer Titer present
Congenital disease, neonate	IFAT, IHA, CF	Stable or rising titer
	IgM–IFAT	Titer present

or cytotoxic drugs may permit reactivation of latent infection and the development of overwhelming disease.

Toxoplasmosis may be prevented by avoidance of undercooked meat and ingestion of oocysts. Pregnant women should not empty cat litter boxes and should practice scrupulous personal hygiene if cat contact is unavoidable. Serologic screening to detect primary gestational toxoplasmosis may lead to a decline in the occurrence of congenital infection.

Selected Bibliography

Alford, C. A., Jr., Stagno, S., and Reynolds, D. W.: Congenital toxoplasmosis: Clinical laboratory and therapeutic considerations, with special reference to subclinical disease. *Bull NY Acad Med* 50:160–181, 1968.

Anderson, S. E., Jr., and Remington, J. S.: Effect of normal and activated human macrophages on *Toxoplasma gondii*. *J Exp Med* 139:1154–1174, 1974.

Beach, P. G.: Prevalence of antibodies to *Toxoplasma gondii* in pregnant women in Oregon. *J Infect Dis* 140:780–783, 1979.

Desmonts, G. and Couvreur, J.: Congenital toxoplasmosis. A prospective study of 378 pregnancies. *N Engl J Med* 290:1110–1116, 1974.

Feldman, H. A.: Toxoplasmosis: An overview. *Bull N Y Acad Med* 50:110–127, 1974.

Frenkel, J. K.: Adoptive immunity to intracellular infection. *J Immunol* 98: 1309–1319, 1967.

Ganley, J. P. and Comstock, G. W.: Association of cats and toxoplasmosis. *Am J Epidemiol* 111:238-246, 1980.

Gump, D. W. and Holden, R. A.: Acquired chorioretinitis due to toxoplasmosis. *Ann Intern Med* 90:58-60, 1979.

Jones, T. C.: Macrophages and intracellular parasitism. *J Reticuloendothel Soc* 15:439-450, 1974.

Krick, J. A. and Remington, J. S.: Toxoplasmosis in the adult – an overview. *N Engl J Med* 298:550-553, 1978.

O'Connor, G. R.: Manifestations and management of ocular toxoplasmosis. *Bull N Y Acad Med* 50:192-210, 1974.

Remington, J. S.: Toxoplasmosis: Recent developments. *Ann Rev Med* 21:201-218, 1970.

Remington, J. S., Jacobs, L., and Kaufman, H. E.: Toxoplasmosis in the adult. *N Engl J Med* 262:180-186; 237-241, 1960.

Roth, J. A., Swigel, S. E., Levine, A. S., and Berard, C. W.: Fatal recurrent toxoplasmosis in a patient initially infected via a leukocyte transfusion. *Am J Clin Pathol* 56:601-605, 1971.

Ruskin, J. and Remington, J. S.: Toxoplasmosis in the compromised host. *Ann Intern Med* 84:193-199, 1976.

Ryning, F. W., McLeod, R., Maddox, J. C., Hunt, S., and Remington, J. S.: Probable transmission of *Toxoplasma gondii* by organ transplantation. *Ann Intern Med* 90:47-49, 1979.

Scott, R. J.: Toxoplasmosis. *Trop Dis Bull* 75:809-827, 1978.

Sheagren, J. N., Lunde, M. N., and Simon, H. B.: Chronic lymphadenopathic toxoplasmosis. A case with marked hyperglobulinemia and impaired delayed hypersensitivity responses during active infection. *Am J Med* 60:300-305, 1976.

Stray-Pederson, B.: Infants potentially at risk of congenital toxoplasmosis. *Am J Dis Child* 134:638-642, 1980.

Teutsch, S. M., Juranek, D. D., Sulzer, A., Dubey, J. P., and Sikes, R. K.: Epidemic toxoplasmosis associated with infected cats. *N Engl J Med* 300:695-699, 1979.

Vietzke, W. M., Gelderman, A. H., Grimley, P. M., and Valsamis, M. P.: Toxoplasmosis complicating malignancy. *Cancer* 21:816-827, 1968.

Wallace, G. W.: Intermediate and transport hosts in the natural history of *Toxoplasma gondii*. *Am J Trop Med Hyg* 22:456-464, 1973.

Weitberg, A. L., Alper, J. C., Diamont, I., and Fligiel, Z.: Acute granulomatous hepatitis in the course of acquired toxoplasmosis. *N Engl J Med* 300:1093-1096, 1979.

Welch, P. C., Masur, H., Jones, T. C., and Remington, J. S.: Serologic diagnosis of acute lymphadenopathic toxoplasmosis. *J Infect Dis* 142:256–264, 1980.

Wilson, C. B., Remington, J. S., Stagno, S., and Reynolds, D. W.: Development of adverse sequelae in children born with subclinical congenital *Toxoplasma* infection. *Pediatrics* 66:767–774, 1980.

122

PNEUMOCYSTIS CARINII
Robert H. Waldman, M.D.

Pneumocystis carinii is probably either a protozoan or fungus although its taxonomic position has not been delineated. The organism causes a serious, often fatal pneumonia in immunosuppressed patients. The disease caused by *P. carinii* is difficult to diagnose mainly because the organism cannot be cultured in the clinical laboratory. However, it can be treated successfully in a significant number of cases. The relationship between this organism and the immunosuppressed host is emphasized by the fact that 25 years ago the disease was not seen in this country; its occurrence has paralleled the prolongation of lives of patients with a variety of disorders, leaving them susceptible hosts to organisms which are avirulent or nonpathogenic in normal individuals.

Microbiology

As mentioned, the organism is either a protozoan or fungus. In its life cycle, it has trophozoite and cyst stages. Sporozoites develop within the cyst. The cyst stains best with Gomori's methenamine silver nitrate, but does not stain with hematoxylin-eosin, nor with Giemsa, Wright's, or Gram stains (Figures 122.1 and 122.2). As many as eight sporozoites may be found within one cyst.

The organism can be grown in certain tissue culture systems available mainly in research laboratories.

Epidemiology

The organism commonly infects immunosuppressed patients, accounting for approximately 40% of interstitial pneumonias in cancer patients. It is the most frequent cause of death of patients with acute lymphocytic leukemia in remission.

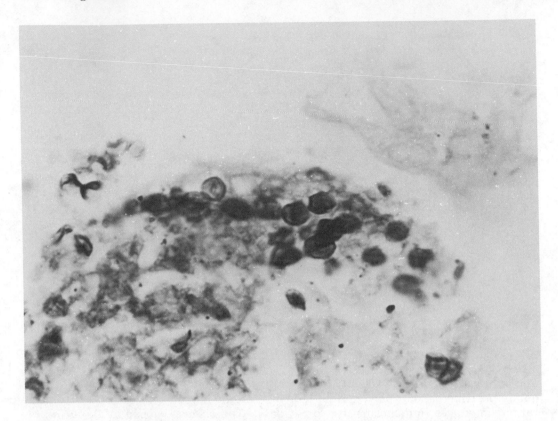

FIGURE 122.1 *Pneumocystis carinii* in the alveolar exudate of a 5-month-old boy with severe combined immunodeficiency disease, Swiss type. Grocott methenamine silver stain (500 x). (Courtesy of Dr. Jesse Jenkins, Dept. Pathology, West Virginia University.)

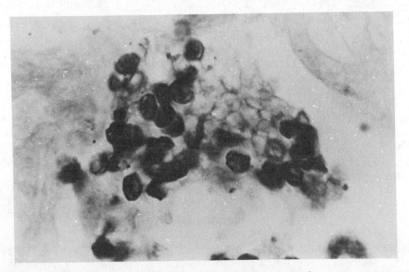

FIGURE 122.2 *Pneumocystis carinii* in alveolar exudate from 5-month-old child with combined immunodeficiency. Grocott methenamine silver stain (625 x).

The frequency increases in proportion to the extent and intensity of treatment with chemotherapy or irradiation. For example, in patients treated with one drug, approximately 5% become infected, while with four drugs, 28% are infected, and when mediastinal irradiation is added, the figure goes to 43%. Other factors which are related to an increased risk of the disease include having had *P. carinii* pneumonia previously (from this, one can conclude that there is little or no infection-induced immunity, and that some people seem to be more susceptible regardless of immunosuppressive therapy) and being malnourished (as indicated by a below-normal weight and a low serum albumin).

The disease was fairly common in postwar Europe, especially in children. With reconstruction in the late 1940s and early 1950s, the frequency of the disease declined in Europe. Recently, the disease has been seen in apparently healthy Vietnamese refugee children. There is one report of the disease in an apparently normal "American-born" child. The child was 7 months old, with no evidence of immune deficiency, and responded well to therapy. Unfortunately, the report does not indicate the racial, ethnic, or socioeconomic background of the child. In Africans with kwashiorkor, 8% had the organism in the lungs at autopsy, while none of the autopsied controls did. Serologic surveys suggest that *P. carinii* is a frequent cause of subclinical infection in normal people in the United States. In patients with the recently described acquired immune deficiency syndrome (AIDS), *P. carinii* pneumonia is a common infection.

The organism has been found in the lungs of a number of lower animals, including rats, dogs, sheep, goats, guinea pigs, rabbits, mice, monkeys, and horses. No relationship has been established between the animal reservoir and human disease. Present evidence suggests that infection is transmitted by the respiratory route and there are reports which indicate the possibility of person-to-person transmission. Until this question of person-to-person transmission has been settled, it is prudent to exercise care to prevent such spread when one is caring for a patient with *P. carinii* pneumonia in the hospital.

Pathology and Pathogenesis

The organism is limited almost exclusively to the lung, even in the most fulminant cases. It is found only rarely in the lungs of healthy people. As mentioned earlier, the disease is seen almost exclusively in children or adults with diseases which impair host defenses, or in whom immunosuppressive therapy is used.

The organisms multiply in the alveoli, eliciting an inflammatory response which includes transudation of a foamy proteinaceous material in which the cysts and alveolar cells with large and numerous vacuoles are trapped. In children afflicted with the disease, the cellular response is predominantly plasma cells, which led to the original terminology of the disease, i.e., interstitial plasma cell pneumonia. However, in the cases usually seen today, the inflammatory response consists primarily of lymphocytes, macrophages, and an occasional eosinophil. Polymorphonuclear leukocytes are rarely seen. Organisms are found in the cytoplasm of alveolar macrophages.

Diagnosis

Clinical

The European infantile form occurs in children from 2 to 6 months of age. Respiratory symptoms are usually preceded, by several days to weeks, by diarrhea. Pulmonary symptoms begin insidiously, with cough and tachypnea. Symptoms progress over 1-4 weeks to severe respiratory distress. The infants have little or no fever and the chest is usually normal on physical examination. A chest roentgenogram, however, shows hyperexpanded lungs with marked, diffuse bilateral granular infiltrates.

The disease which occurs in immunosuppressed patients often becomes manifest when the patient's steroid dosage is being decreased or discontinued. The onset is usually abrupt with the acute onset of fever and tachypnea, progressing rapidly to cyanosis and other signs of severe respiratory distress. Examination of the chest may show rales and rhonchi, or there may be no abnormalities. The chest roentgenogram may show one of several different patterns, but generally reveals diffuse alveolar disease.

Laboratory

Routine laboratory tests are of little diagnostic value. A definitive diagnosis can be made only by identification of the organism. Many different methods have been recommended for obtaining material for examination, including open lung biopsy, percutaneous transthoracic needle aspiration, lung lavage, or bronchial brushings. The method of choice depends upon the institution and the experience of the persons performing the procedure. As with other procedures in medicine, the yield of the procedure must be weighed against the associated morbidity and mortality.

Gallium scanning has been recently suggested as an accurate, noninvasive way of making the diagnosis. It has been suggested that a diffuse, generalized, abnormal accumulation of gallium, in marked contrast to the roentgenographic or clinical findings, is diagnostic of *P. carinii* pneumonia. Further experience with the technique must be accumulated before the gallium scan can be accepted as diagnostic without identifying the organism in pulmonary material.

The chest roentgenogram may be normal, but classically shows bilateral perihilar interstitial infiltrates, which later progress to involve the periphery. More unusual, but certainly occurring, are nodular, lobar, diffuse, or unilateral lesions, and even cavitation.

Active research is being carried out to develop a reliable serologic test. Complement-fixation, latex-agglutination, and immunofluorescent tests have been used, but none have been reliable enough to be useful clinically.

In the clinical setting in which pneumocystis infection is seen in the United States, the differential diagnosis is a difficult one and includes drug-induced interstitial fibrosis, infection with cytomegalovirus, *Aspergillus* or other fungi, unusual forms of bacterial bronchopneumonia, toxoplasmosis, or leukemic or other malignant infiltration.

Treatment

Until recently the treatment of choice was pentamidine isethionate, 4 mg/kg intramuscularly as a single daily dose. The problem with this drug has been toxicity, with up to 50% of patients developing nephrotoxicity, hepatotoxicity, hypotension, and hypoglycemia. The drug is available only through the Centers for Disease Control.

Trimethoprim-sulfamethoxazole (TMP-SMX) has several advantages over pentamidine isethionate. Trimethoprim-sulfamethoxazole is easier to administer, since it can be given either orally or parenterally at the same dosage level, is less toxic, and blood levels can be measured fairly easily. The recommended dose is 20/100 mg/kg given in four divided doses, for 14 days. Side effects are infrequent and mild, including rash and nausea. In critically ill patients, it is probably of value to measure the sulfamethoxazole blood levels. The therapeutic range is 100-150 µg/ml.

General supportive measures include oxygen and assisted ventilation, and some investigators have used a membrane oxygenator.

Since both pentamidine and the combination of TMP-SMX are effective, the question has been raised about the use of both forms of therapy. There is no evidence that the combination gives better results, and there is experimental evidence in an animal model that the results are less effective.

Prognosis

The European infantile form has an untreated fatality rate of about 50%. The form seen most commonly today has a 90-100% fatality rate if untreated or treated inappropriately. The use of pentamidine has lowered the mortality to approximately 60%. It appears as if the combination of TMP-SMX has an even better record, with the mortality probably approaching 20-30%. Most of the patients who die do so early in the course of treatment, and if patients survive 9 or more days of therapy, the survival is probably around 85%. In studies in which serologic testing has been done, the absence of serum antibody is a poor prognostic sign.

Prevention and Immunology

There is a great deal of interest recently in the use of trimethoprim-sulfamethoxazole as chemoprophylaxis in high-risk patients with malignancy. There has been a significant reduction in the frequency of *P. carinii* pneumonia by using approximately one-fourth the therapeutic dose. The only adverse effect which has been noted with this prophylactic regimen has been the development of oral candidiasis. A very serious potential problem, but one which has as yet not been encountered, is the development of resistant organisms. Which patients should be treated prophylactically? The current recommendation is that if the attack rate of *P. carinii* pneumonia in the susceptible population is less than 15%, then it is probably not worthwhile to give that patient population TMP-SMX. If the attack rate of *P. carinii* pneumonia in the susceptible population is higher than 15%, then chemoprophylaxis is recommended. Therefore, at each medical center, a review of the susceptible population must be updated frequently.

The protective mechanism in *P. carinii* pneumonia is not known, but from the types of patients who develop the disease, the fact that it is an intracellular parasite, and by analogy to other similar infectious diseases, it is probable that cell-mediated immunity is of primary importance.

The prospect for immunization against this disease is not good. This is based on the fact that reinfection is common, and it is a basic assumption that if active infection cannot induce immunity, then artificial stimulation of the immune system is not likely to be very potent. In addition, animal studies do not lead one to be very optimistic.

Selected Bibliography

Burke, B. A. and Good, R. A.: *Pneumocystis carinii* pneumonia. *Medicine* 52:23-50, 1973.

Byrd, R. B. and Horn, B. R.: Infection due to *Pneumocystis carinii* simulating lobar bacterial pneumonia. *Chest* 70:91-92, 1976.

Greenman, R. L., Goodall, P. T., and King, D.: Lung biopsy in immunocompromised hosts. *Am J Med* 59:488-496, 1975.

Hughes, W. T.: Current status of laboratory diagnosis of *Pneumocystis carinii* pneumonitis. *Crit Rev Clin Lab Sci* 6:145-170, 1975.

Hughes, W. T., Feldman, S., Chaudhary, S. C., Ossi, M. J., Cox, F., and Sanyal, S. K.: Comparison of pentamidine isethionate and trimethoprim-sulfamethoxazole in the treatment of *Pneumocystis carinii* pneumonia. *J Pediatr* 92:285-291, 1978.

Hughes, W. T., Feldman, S., and Sanyal, S. K.; Treatment of *Pneumocystis carinii* pneumonitis with trimethoprim-sulfamethoxazole. *Can Med Assoc J* 112:47S-50S, 1975.

Hughes, W. T., Kuhn, S., Chaudhary, S., Feldman, S., Verzosa, M., Aur, R. J. A., Pratt, C., and George, S. L.: Successful chemoprophylaxis for *Pneumocystis carinii* pneumonitis. *N Engl J Med* 297:1419-1426, 1977.

Kluge, R. M., Spaulding, D. M., and Spain, A. J.: Combination of pentamidine and trimethoprim-sulfamethoxazole in therapy of *Pneumocystis carinii* in rats. *Antimicrob Agents Chemother* 13:975-978, 1978.

Larter, W. E., John, T. J., Sieber, O. F., Jr., Johnson, H., Corrigan, J. J., Jr., and Fulginiti, V. A.: Trimethoprim-sulfamethoxazole treatment of *Pneumocystis carinii* pneumonitis. *J Pediatr* 92:826-978, 1978.

Lau, W. K. and Young, L. S.: Trimethoprim-sulfamethoxazole treatment of *Pneumocystis carinii* pneumonia in adults. *N Engl J Med* 295:716-718, 1976.

Pifer, L. L., Hughes, W. T., Stagno, S., and Woods, D.: *Pneumocystis carinii* infection: Evidence for high prevalence in normal and immunosuppressed children. *Pediatrics* 61:35-41, 1978.

Pifer, L. L., Woods, D., and Hughes, W. T.: Propagation of *Pneumocystis carinii* in Vero cell culture. *Infect Immun* 20:66-68, 1978.

Rao, M., Steiner, P., Victoria, M. S., James, P., Fikrig, S., Goldenberg, L., and Kassner, E. G.: *Pneumocystis carinii* pneumonia occurrence in a healthy American infant. *JAMA* 238:2301, 1977.

Rosen, P. P., Martini, N., and Armstrong, D.: *Pneumocystis carinii* pneumonia: Diagnosis by lung biopsy. *Am J Med* 58:794-802, 1975.

Singer, C., Armstrong, D., Rosen, P. P., and Schottenfeld, D.: *Pneumocystis carinii* pneumonia: A cluster of eleven cases. *Ann Intern Med* 82:772-777, 1975.

Walzer, P. D., Perl, D. P., Krogstad, D. J., Rawson, P. G., and Schultz, M. G.: *Pneumocystis carinii* pneumonia in the United States. *Ann Intern Med* 80:83-93, 1974.

123

MALARIA AND BABESIOSIS
Rashida A. Khakoo, M.D.

Malaria

Definition

Malaria is a disease with worldwide distribution; it is estimated that there are at least 150 million persons with this disease. One million children in Africa die annually of malaria. In developing countries, the impact of malaria in terms of morbidity and mortality is very significant. With increased international travel and immigration to nonendemic areas, malaria is no longer a "disease of the tropics." Physicians in nonendemic areas are also faced with chemoprophylaxis, diagnosis, and treatment of malaria. Increasing drug resistance of *Plasmodium falciparum* and insecticide resistance of the anopheles mosquito (the vector) have continued to pose problems in terms of malaria control.

Etiology

Malaria is caused by the protozoa plasmodia. Four species, *P. falciparum, P. vivax, P. malariae* and *P. ovale,* cause human infections. Malaria is transmitted by the bite of the female anopheles mosquito. Asexual stages of the plasmodia develop in man, and the sexual stages in the mosquito. Following the bite of the mosquito, sporozoites are injected into the bloodstream. They disappear from the bloodstream in about 30 min and appear in the hepatocytes. Here they develop into schizonts which liberate merozoites. The duration of the developmental cycle in the liver varies from 6 to 15 days, depending upon the species of plasmodium, being shortest for *P. falciparum* and longest for *P. malariae.* The stage of development in the liver is termed the exoerythrocytic stage. Persistence of the exoerythrocytic stages of *P. falciparum* and *P. malariae* does not occur. In contrast, *P. vivax* and *P. ovale* persist in the liver, resulting in future relapses.

The liberated merozoites invade erythrocytes. Erythrocytes negative for Duffy blood group antigens are resistant to invasion by *P. vivax*. A receptor associated with the Duffy factor may be involved in susceptibility. *Plasmodium falciparum* is capable of invading any erythrocytes irrespective of age. This accounts for the high parasite densities that may occur. *Plasmodium vivax* only attacks reticulocytes, whereas *P. malariae* only invades mature erythrocytes. The type of hemoglobin and enzyme content of erythrocytes also has bearing on resistance to malaria. Individuals heterozygous for HbS are relatively resistant to malaria. Impairment of parasite growth has been observed in erythrocytes containing fetal hemoglobin. It is controversial whether persons with thalassemia and glucose-6-phosphate dehydrogenase (G6PD) deficiency are less susceptible to malaria.

Once merozoites enter erythrocytes, they appear as blue, ring forms with a red chromatin dot in stained smears. An increase in the parasite cytoplasm results in the formation of the trophozoite. Ingested hemoglobin is processed in numerous cytoplasmic phagosomes to produce pigment. Later, the division of chromatin occurs, resulting in schizonts. Completion of division of both chromatin and cytoplasm results in the formation of mature schizonts containing merozoites. The rupture of schizonts leads to liberation of merozoites, which rapidly attach to and invade other erythrocytes. The developmental stages leading to the formation of the schizont and its rupture are called schizogony, usually requiring 48 hr for all species of plasmodia except *P. malariae* (72 hr).

The sexual stages in the erythrocyte begin with the development of the male and female gametocytes.

In *P. vivax, P. ovale,* and *P. malariae,* all forms of parasite development, from ring forms to schizonts and gametocytes, are found in the peripheral blood, whereas in *P. falciparum,* usually only ring forms and, later, gametocytes are seen. The development of intermediate stages of *P. falciparum* usually occurs in the capillaries of the viscera.

Male and female gametocytes are ingested by the female anopheline mosquito during a blood meal. Male gametes fertilize female gametes in the gut of the mosquito. The zygote develops into oocysts, each containing many sporozoites, the latter reaching the salivary glands from where they are injected into the bloodstream of humans via a bite.

Epidemiology

Malaria occurs worldwide, but particularly in countries in Africa, Asia, and Central and South America. The distribution of species varies in different parts of the world.

A global malaria eradication program was undertaken by the World Health Organization between 1951 and 1962, resulting in eradication in many areas. In the United States, return of military personnel during the Vietnam war resulted in approximately 3000 reported cases of malaria per year. The number of reported cases decreased after the Vietnam war era to approximately 200-300/year. Recently, there is again a resurgence of malaria. For 1980 and 1981, 3000 cases were reported to the Centers for Disease Control. The increase is secondary to cases occurring in immigrants from endemic areas and in travelers returning from endemic areas (improper or no chemoprophylaxis).

The usual incubation periods for malaria caused by *P. falciparum, P. vivax, P. malariae,* and *P. ovale* are 11-14 days, 11-15 days, 21-28 days, and 14-26 days, respectively.

Malaria may occur in the following settings in the United States: (a) travelers and military personnel returning from endemic areas, (b) immigrants or

visitors from endemic areas, (c) following transfusion of infected blood, (d) parenteral drug abuse and (e) transmission from mother to fetus (congenital).

Pathogenesis, Pathology, and Immunology

The pathogenesis of clinical manifestations of malaria is not clear. Fever coincides with the rupture of schizonts, with the liberation of pyrogen being postulated
but not demonstrated. Hemolysis of parasitized erythrocytes by rupture of schizonts leads to anemia. Recent studies indicate that immunologic factors also play
a role. Circulating immune complexes have been demonstrated during an attack of
malaria. Additionally, ^{59}Fe incorporation studies have indicated a mild degree of
bone marrow depression.

Splenomegaly is frequently seen in patients with an acute episode of malaria
and in those residing in endemic areas. The intensity of malaria in a given area is
defined by the percent of the population with enlarged spleens. Initially, the splenomegaly is thought to be due to congestion. Later, lymphoid and reticuloendothelial hyperplasia occur. The spleen is thought to play an important role in the
immune response to malaria. Immune humans and animals are rendered susceptible to malaria following splenectomy, and the recrudescence of asymptomatic infections may occur following splenectomy in humans.

Renal involvement in malaria consists of a transient nephritis which has usually been seen with *P. falciparum* infection. The renal biopsy demonstrates deposition of IgM, sometimes associated with complement and malarial antigen. Acute
tubular necrosis may also occur. Another major type of renal disease seen is the
nephrotic syndrome, which is associated with *P. malariae*. Deposition of IgG, IgM,
and complement occurs in a coarse, granular pattern. Antigen of *P. malariae* has
been demonstrated by immunofluorescence.

Complications resulting from plugging of the microvascular circulation are
seen in *P. falciparum*. Infected erythrocytes adhere to vascular endothelium, resulting in sluggish blood flow, tissue hypoxia, increased capillary permeability, and
edema.

Extensive studies in animal models and humans have been carried out to determine the immunologic mechanisms in malaria. Both humoral and cell-mediated
immune mechanisms are involved in retardation of intracellular proliferation of
plasmodia. Acquired immunity depends on the frequency of exposure to malaria.
Reduction of parasitemia in children has been demonstrated following the administration of immunoglobulins obtained from immune individuals. It is postulated
that the antibodies may interfere with binding of merozoites to the erythrocyte
receptor and their release from infected erythrocytes, blocking of entry of nutrients, increase in the rigidity of the erythrocyte membrane resulting in impaired
flow in capillaries, and premature lysis. Antibodies may also be important in opsonization prior to phagocytosis by macrophages.

In endemic areas, it has been observed that immunity to malaria develops
slowly. It is postulated that this might, in part, be related to immunosuppression
induced during malaria. Poor responses to other vaccines have been noted during
acute episodes of malaria. Pregnant patients in endemic areas are more likely to
develop acute malaria. The placenta usually shows heavy sequestration of parasites, most likely providing a barrier to invasion. The lower incidence of malaria
in children 3 months of age or younger may be explained by passive transfer of antibody from the mother, and the failure of fetal hemoglobin to support the growth
of the plasmodia.

Diagnostic Features

Clinical

In the United States, most patients with *P. falciparum* malaria present within the first 2 months of returning to the country. A few cases may occur up to a year later. In contrast, patients with *P. vivax, P. malariae,* and *P. ovale* infections may present up to a year or later if they have received chemoprophylaxis. Since the clinical picture is fairly nonspecific, malaria is often not considered initially. Occasionally, it is diagnosed by laboratory technicians reviewing a peripheral blood smear. Travel history in any febrile patient is important. Lack of expertise in examination of smears may lead to missing the diagnosis, or the species identification may not be accurate.

Patients usually present with the sudden onset of myalgias, arthralgias, chills, and fever, followed by drenching sweats. They also have accompanying headache and prostration. Although classically the temperature pattern for the different parasites is thought to be characteristic, the periodicity is not established early in the illness when the diagnosis ideally should be made. The temperature pattern in falciparum malaria may remain irregular. In *P. vivax* and *P. malariae* infections, once the periodicity of the parasite is established, the paroxysms may occur every 48 hr (benign tertian malaria) or every 72 hr (quartan malaria), respectively. In between paroxysms, the patient may feel very well or occasionally may continue to feel tired. During the paroxysm, the patient may complain of nausea, vomiting, and abdominal pain and diarrhea. If untreated, nonimmune patients or children may become severely ill with complications, particularly with *P. falciparum* or occasionally with *P. vivax* infections. Physical examination during a paroxysm of malaria demonstrates an ill-appearing patient. Splenomegaly is demonstrated in about half the patients, and hepatomegaly in a third. The patient may be mildly icteric, and occasionally moderately to severely jaundiced.

Some patients from endemic areas may be entirely asymptomatic in the face of demonstrable parasitemia (usually low grade).

Malaria following transfusion can be caused by any species but is more commonly caused by *P. malariae*. Prolonged persistence of asymptomatic parasitemia caused by *P. malariae* in the donor is the most likely reason.

When malaria occurs during pregnancy, development of severe anemia is a common problem. Premature labor or abortion may result. Low birth weight of babies born to infected mothers is seen, and is postulated to be secondary to parasitization of the placenta and interference in the transport of oxygen and nutrients. Congenital malaria is fairly uncommon in endemic areas.

Laboratory

The usual laboratory tests are nonspecific. The leukocyte count is often decreased, or occasionally may remain normal. The platelet count may be slightly or moderately decreased. Indirect bilirubinemia and a mild increase in serum glutamic oxaloacetic transaminase and lactic dehydrogenase may be seen. Urinalysis during a paroxysm may demonstrate mild proteinuria. Significant proteinuria will be demonstrated in patients with the nephrotic syndrome. Only mild elevations of blood urea nitrogen and creatinine may be seen secondary to dehydration, unless acute renal failure has supervened. Decreased hemoglobin and hematocrit will be present in patients with severe infections and in pregnant patients.

The most reliable way of making a diagnosis of malaria is by examination of the peripheral blood smear. Selected peripheral smears are demonstrated in Figures 123.1-123.3. With a lower degree of parasitemia, the thick smear is most

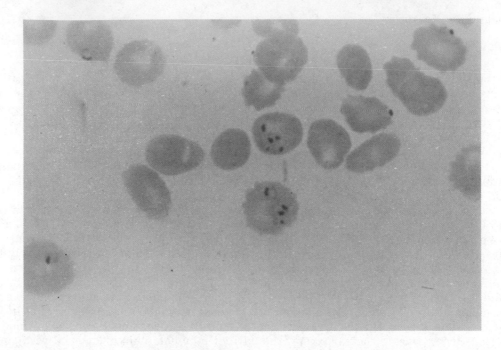

FIGURE 123.1   Peripheral blood smear demonstrating multiple ring forms of *P. falciparum.* (Courtesy of Koneman, E. W., Basham, L. R., and Buzbee, S. C.: *Laboratory Parasitology, Part IV: Malarial Parasites of Man,* 2nd ed., Famous Teachings in Modern Medicine, Medcom, Inc., New York, 1980.)

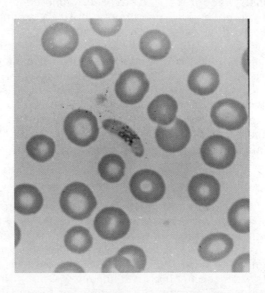

FIGURE 123.2   Typical crescent-shaped gametocyte of *P. falciparum* in the peripheral blood smear. (Courtesy of Koneman, E. W., Basham, L. R., and Buzbee, S. C.: *Laboratory Parasitology, Part IV: Malarial Parasites of Man,* 2nd ed., Famous Teachings in Modern Medicine, Medcom, Inc., New York, 1980.)

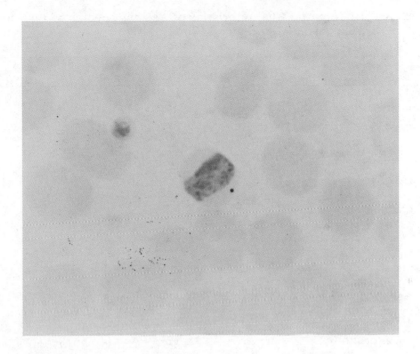

FIGURE 123.3   Typical band form seen with *P. malariae.* (Courtesy of Koneman, E. W., Basham, L. R., and Buzbee, S. C.: *Laboratory Parasitology, Part IV: Malarial Parasites of Man,* 2nd ed., Famous Teachings in Modern Medicine, Medcom, Inc., New York, 1980.)

helpful. Erythrocytes are lysed so the parasites are found lying free. Species identification is usually made from the Wright-Giemsa stained thin smear. Several slides should be examined by an experienced person. In trying to determine the species of plasmodium, particular attention should be paid to the size of the infected erythrocytes, forms of parasite within the erythrocytes, multiplicity of the ring form, type of chromatin dots (single vs. double), presence of dots in erythrocytes, number of merozoites, and morphology of gametocytes. Various differences are present in Table 123.1. Recently, the use of the dark-field technique has been reported in the diagnosis of malaria parasites in the peripheral blood.

A number of serologic tests are available for measuring antibodies against plasmodia. These are mostly helpful in epidemiologic studies and not for making a diagnosis of an acute episode in a patient. In cases of transfusion-associated malaria, determination of antibody titer in the donor is useful, since the degree of parasitemia, in general, is extremely low.

The differential diagnostic possibilities to be considered are many, since the clinical picture may be nonspecific (Table 123.2).

Treatment

Generally, drugs used in the treatment of malaria are either active against the erythrocytic forms, offering clinical cure, or those also having effect against the exoerythrocytic form, resulting in complete elimination. For *P. falciparum* and *P. malariae,* there are no persisting exoerythrocytic forms, so therapy is only

TABLE 123.1   Differential Characteristics of Various Species of Plasmodia in Thin Smear of Peripheral Blood

	P. falciparum	P. vivax	P. malariae	P. ovale
Multiple rings in erythrocytes	+	Rare	-	-
All forms of parasites in the peripheral blood	Not usually[1]	+	+	+
Double chromatin dots, accole[2] forms	+	-	-	-
Band forms	-	-	+	-
Crescent-shaped gametocytes	+	-	-	-
Number of merozoites	8-24	12-24	8-12	8-12
Enlarged erythrocytes	-	+	-	+
Schuffner's dots	-	+	-	+
Fimbriated and oval erythrocytes	-	-	-	+

[1] Usually stages beyond the ring forms with the exception of gametocytes are not seen. The rest of the stages are thought to develop in visceral capillaries

[2] Forms that appear on the smear to be plastered against the margin of the erythrocytes

directed against the erythrocytic form. In cases of *P. vivax* and *P. ovale,* after completion of therapy against the erythrocytic form, the treatment of exoerythrocytic forms is necessary to prevent relapses.

Chloroquine and other 4-aminoquinolines have been the mainstay of treatment of erythrocytic forms. Reports of chloroquine-resistant strains of *P. falciparum* appeared initially approximately 20 years ago. Resistant strains were mostly reported from Southeast Asia, Central, and South America. The number of countries from which resistant strains have been reported has been increasing. More recently, chloroquine-resistant *P. falciparum* strains have been reported from East Africa (Tanzania, Kenya, Uganda), Madagascar, Mozambique, and the Comoro Islands. The reports of resistance from increasing numbers of countries pose problems in the prophylaxis and treatment of malaria. The prevalence of strains with differing degrees of resistance varies in different parts of the world. In general, strains from South America are less resistant than those from Southeast Asia.

In the United States, recently, a fixed combination of sulfadoxine (500 mg) and pyrimethamine (50 mg), marketed as Fansidar, has become available. This

TABLE 123.2   Differential Diagnosis of Malaria and Associated Problems

Presenting Feature	Diagnostic Considerations
Fever, chills	Acute viral or bacterial infection
Jaundice, anemia, splenomegaly	Other causes of hemolytic anemia
Leukopenia, thrombocytopenia	Hematologic malignancy, other severe infections
Proteinuria, edema	Other causes of nephrotic syndrome
Acute renal failure	Other causes of acute renal failure
Hepatosplenomegaly, lymphocytic infiltration of hepatic sinusoids	Lymphoma
Altered mental status, seizures, coma	Viral or bacterial meningitis Encephalitis Reye's syndrome
Bilateral pulmonary infiltrates	Acute respiratory distress syndrome, related to shock from various causes

drug has been recommended for prophylaxis of malaria where chloroquine-resist-ant *P. falciparum* strains are suspected. It has also been used for the treatment of malaria suspected to be caused by chloroquine-resistant strains of *P. falciparum*. Lack of effectiveness of Fansidar in the treatment of chloroquine-resistant *P. falciparum* malaria has already been reported from Thailand, Papua New Guinea, Irian Jaya, and Brazil.

The currently recommended treatment of malaria is presented in Table 123.3. With rapid changes in this field, it is important to refer to the most updated in-formation.

Tetracycline has been used as part of combination therapy with quinine for the treatment of chloroquine-resistant *P. falciparum* malaria. Doxycycline alone, in a dose of 4 mg/kg for 7 days, has been used for the treatment of chloroquine-resistant *P. falciparum* in Malaya. With increasing drug resistance of *P. falciparum* (chloroquine, pyrimethamine-sulfadoxine and occasional cases of resistance to quinine), the search for new classes of agents continues. Mefloquine is a long-act-ing drug (half-life, 6-22 days) belonging to the class of quinolinementhols. The drug has minimal side effects and is effective against all strains of plasmodia, in-cluding those resistant to chloroquine and quinine. In China, a crude extract of a medicinal herb has been used for the treatment of malaria for centuries. The an-timalarial activity was rediscovered in 1971, and a purer crystalline extract, quinghaousu, has been studied. Its unique structure suggests that cross resistance with other antimalarial agents may not occur. In one study, quinghaousu cleared parasitemia more rapidly than mefloquine or intramuscular quinine. This property of rapid clearance of parasites may be useful in patients with high parasite counts.

TABLE 123.3   Treatment of Malaria

Type of Infection	Preparation	Salt (mg)/Base (mg)	Route	Adult Dose mg base	Pediatric Dose mg base	Side Effects	Comments
P. falciparum (chloroquine-sensitive) P. vivax P. malariae P. ovale	Chloroquine phosphate	500/300	p.o.	600 mg initially, then 300 mg at 6, 24 and 48 hr	10 mg/kg initially, then 5 mg/kg at 6, 24 and 48 hr	Gastrointestinal discomfort is common. Can be minimized by administering the drug with meals. Itching is sometimes seen even without urticaria. Ocular side effects seen with prolonged administration are not seen with short course	
	Chloroquine hydrochloride	50/40	IV, IM	3 mg/kg initially, then 3 mg/kg every 6 hr	2–3 mg/kg initially, no more than 5 mg/kg/24 hr	Hypotension and cardiac depression	Used when nausea, vomiting and altered mental status preclude oral therapy. IV preparation should be administered very slowly over 60 min. Monitor with vital signs and EKG. Change to p.o. as soon as possible
P. falciparum (chloroquine-resistant)	Quinine sulfate	650/540	p.o.	540 mg every 8 hr	10 mg/kg every 8 hr for 7 days	Tinnitus, ocular symptoms	
	or Quinine hydrochloride	600/490	IV, IM	490 mg every 8 hr	6 mg/kg every 8 hr		Used when nausea, vomiting and altered mental status preclude oral therapy. IV preparation should be administered very slowly over 60 min. Monitor with vital signs and EKG. Change to p.o. as soon as possible

			Adult dose	Pediatric dose	Toxicity	Remarks
+ Pyrimethamine	25	p.o.	25 mg twice a day x 3 days	< 10 kg- 5.25 mg/ day; 10-20 kg-12.5 mg/day; 20-40 kg- 25 mg/day		With recent demonstration of ineffectiveness of this regimen in different areas, it should be used judiciously. It should not be employed alone for the treatment of very ill or non-immune persons. Combination with quinine has been used. Avoid use in pregnancy, nursing mothers, and infants less than 2 months of age
+ Sulfadiazine	500	p.o.	500 mg every 6 hr for 5 days	100-200 mg/kg/ day in 4 divided doses every 6 hr (maximum 2 g/day)		
Pyrimethamine sulfadoxine (Fansidar)	50 500	p.o.	150 1500 (3 tablets)	2-4 months - 1/2 tablet; 4-8 years - 1 tablet; 9-14 years - 2 tablets		
P. vivax P. ovale Primaquine	26.3/15	p.o.	15 mg daily for 14 days	0.3 mg/kg daily for 14 days	Hemolytic anemia in patients with G6PD deficiency	Primaquine should be used after completion of treatment of the acute attack. In general, use of primaquine should be avoided in persons who have G6PD deficiency. Risk vs. benefit should be weighed in each case. In patients of African ancestry who are G6PD-deficient, 45 mg once a week for 8 weeks may be administered

Primaquine should be avoided during pregnancy |

Chloroquine can be safely used during pregnancy. Primaquine, pyrimethamine-sulfadoxine, and tetracycline should be avoided. Treatment of chloroquine-resistant *P. falciparum* is a real problem. However, the risk vs. benefit ratio usually dictates treatment of the patient. No specific recommendations have been made. Quinine can be an abortifacient, but should be tried alone first. In general, it is best for nonimmune pregnant patients to avoid travel to areas where chloroquine-resistant *P. falciparum* malaria has been reported. To avoid relapses of *P. vivax* or *P. ovale,* primaquine should be administered postpartum. During pregnancy, each episode should be treated with chloroquine.

Supportive or other treatment may be necessary, such as administration of intravenous fluids, and hemodialysis or peritoneal dialysis for those with acute renal failure not responding to conservative management. Ventilatory support may be needed in patients with acute respiratory distress syndrome. Exchange transfusion has been used concomitantly, with antimalarial therapy in a case of transfusion malaria when the diagnosis was delayed. Patients with cerebral malaria, depending on their mental status, may need other supportive measures. Dexamethasone has been demonstrated to have deleterious effects in a double-blind placebo-controlled trial.

Complications and Prognosis

The presence of complications is related to the degree of parasitemia, the species of plasmodia, and the immune status of the host. Cerebral malaria is usually caused by *P. falciparum* but has been reported with *P. vivax*. It is characterized by altered mental status, seizures, and coma. Meningeal and focal neurologic findings are rare. Acute renal failure is seen particularly with *P. falciparum*. Hemolysis, dehydration, hypotension, and disseminated intravascular coagulation are responsible. Peritoneal or hemodialysis may be required during the acute stage. Nephrotic syndrome secondary to malaria is associated with *P. malariae* infections. The degree of parasitemia is usually very low. Rarely, glomerulonephritis associated with *P. falciparum* infections has been reported. Intravascular hemolysis ("blackwater fever") has been reported to be both related and unrelated to the use of antimalarials. One of the other dreaded complications of *P. falciparum* malaria is the occurrence of adult respiratory distress syndrome.

Mortality in malaria is greater in nonimmune persons, particularly when the diagnosis is delayed, missed, or complications are present. Mortality is also related to parasite density. Higher densities and complications usually occur with *P. falciparum* infections, although they have been reported with *P. vivax* infections in nonimmune persons.

Prevention

Prevention consists of general measures and use of prophylactic agents. General preventive measures consist of avoiding as much contact with the vector as possible by remaining in well-screened areas during evening and night, use of mosquito net for sleeping, wearing clothing that reduces exposure, and use of mosquito repellents. Spraying of insecticide for the elimination of the vector has posed problems because of the development of resistance to the insecticide.

Although a number of cases of malaria can be prevented by appropriate chemoprophylaxis, there are many problems in this regard. In one study, half of the travelers to endemic areas did not receive chemoprophylaxis, and the remainder received inadequate chemoprophylaxis. Travelers either do not consult physicians or many physicians are not well-informed, themselves.

Currently recommended chemoprophylactic regimens are shown in Table 123.4. With these agents, the risks can be diminished, but may not be completely eliminated. Malaria should still be considered in a person who has traveled to an endemic area and presents with a febrile illness despite use of chemoprophylaxis.

Tremendous research is currently underway for studying various antigens of plasmodia and their suitability for production of vaccines. The use of hybridoma technology and cultivation of the *P. falciparum* in its sexual and asexual stages have facilitated the study of various antigens. A sporozoite vaccine has been the most studied in animal models and humans. Resistance to rechallenge has been demonstrated following repeated administration of the vaccine. It is felt that the antibody to sporozoites prevents attachment to host cells.

Babesiosis

Infections caused by a member of the genus *Babesia* have been recognized in animals for a long time. The first human case of babesiosis was reported in 1957, although intraerythrocytic organisms reported in 1904 by Wilson and Chowning during investigations of Rocky Mountain spotted fever most likely represented human cases. Severe cases were reported in Europe in asplenic patients. Cases in the United States have been reported mainly in otherwise healthy persons. Serologic studies have demonstrated the presence of asymptomatic infection. The clinical picture and results of the blood smear may be confused with malaria.

Babesia are small, intraerythrocytic protozoa. Although a number of species infect animals, *B. microti* is the major one reported to cause human infections in the United States, *B. divergens* and *B. bovis* in Europe. Babesia are transmitted by tick bites.

Babesia are well-known causes of disease in wild and domestic animals. In the United States, human cases have been reported from Nantucket Island, Martha's Vineyard, Shelter Island, the eastern tip of Long Island, Georgia, and California. *Babesia microti* infections in rodents are widespread in the United States, and the vector tick *Ixodes dammini* is also found in areas other than where cases have been reported, so the clustering of human cases in a limited number of areas is difficult to explain. It is postulated that frequent and close association of humans with infected ticks may be necessary. The reservoir for *B. microti* appears to be the white-footed or deer mouse. Babesia are present in 5% of nymphal ticks on Nantucket Island. The incubation period of babesiosis in humans is not well documented, but is probably 7–10 days following a tick bite. Babesiosis has been reported following transfusion of blood and platelets with an incubation period of 6–8 weeks. The donors were asymptomatic.

Illness usually starts gradually with malaise, anorexia, and fatigue. This is followed within several days to a week by fever, myalgias, sweats, and arthralgias. Depression and emotional lability have been noted occasionally. A history of tick bite is given by some patients. History of travel or residence in areas from where cases of babesia have been reported is important to obtain. Physical examination demonstrates increased temperature, splenomegaly in about half of the patients, and occasional hepatomegaly.

Evidence of hemolytic anemia is often present. The leukocyte count is either low or normal, but an increase in band forms may occur. Platelet counts may be decreased. Mild increases in serum glutamic oxaloacetic transaminase, alkaline phosphatase, and lactic dehydrogenase may occur.

The best way of making a diagnosis of babesiosis is to demonstrate intraerythrocytic trophozoites using the Giemsa stain of a peripheral blood smear. Extensive pseudopodial filaments, binucleate, or the classic quadrinucleate "tetrad" forms may be seen. Gametocytes and other stages seen with malaria are not found.

TABLE 123.4 Chemoprophylaxis for Malaria

Problems Against Which Prophylaxis is Being Recommended	Drugs and Dosages mg/Base – Adult	Pediatrics mg/Base	Comments
To prevent clinical attack			
P. falciparum (chloroquine-sensitive) *P. vivax* *P. ovale* *P. malariae*	Chloroquine phosphate p.o. 300 mg once a week 1–2 weeks before travel, for the duration of exposure and for 6 weeks following exposure	5 mg/kg once a week up to a maximum adult dose of 300 mg base administered in the same fashion as for adult	Other aminoquinoline preparations available in other countries but not in the United States. If the use of one or the other preparations is desired, a prescription should be given to the person
P. falciparum (chloroquine-resistant)	Pyrimethamine (25 mg) – sulfadoxine (500 mg) (Fansidar) 1–2 tablet once a week during and 6 weeks after exposure in a malarious area	0.5 mg/kg pyrimethamine plus 10 mg/kg sulfadoxine (up to maximum adult dose) administered in the same fashion as for adults	For detailed list of countries with chloroquine-resistant *P. falciparum*, refer to *MMWR* Vol. 31, April 16, 1982
	Chloroquine phosphate (same dose as above)		Concurrent use of chloroquine with Fansidar is recommended because (1) Fansidar alone may not be efficacious against chloroquine-sensitive strains, (2) the combination may retard the development of Fansidar resistance, and (3) the efficacy of Fansidar against non-falciparum species is not established
To prevent delayed attacks with			
P. vivax *P. ovale*	Primaquine 15 mg once a day for 14 days or 45 mg once a week for 8 weeks, generally on completion of a course of suppressive therapy or during the last weeks of therapy	0.3 mg/kg up to maximum adult dose once a day for 14 days or 0.9 mg once a week for 8 weeks administered in same fashion as for adults	Avoid use of primaquine in persons with G6PD deficiency and pregnant patients

The indirect immunofluorescent antibody test has been found to be sensitive, specific, and reproducible. It is useful for epidemiologic studies and the diagnosis of both symptomatic patients and asymptomatic-infected donors in cases of transfusion-associated babesiosis. Cross-reactions are seen in sera from patients with malaria and among the various species of babesia.

Inoculation of hamsters with blood from patients in whom the smear is negative is useful in some cases. Screening of drugs against babesia is also carried out in this experimental model.

The major differential diagnosis is malaria, since the clinical picture may be very similar, blood smear findings may be misinterpreted, and serologic cross-reactions occur. Epidemiologic history is important. Other differential diagnoses include causes of hemolytic anemia and hemoglobinuria, prolonged febrile illness secondary to other infections, inflammatory conditions, or malignancy. With a history of tick bite, other illnesses transmitted by ticks may be considered, such as tularemia. Rocky Mountain spotted fever, because of its characteristic clinical appearance, should not be a problem to differentiate.

Treatment is not required for every patient, since the disease can be mild and self-limited. Treatment is usually only necessary for very ill patients. Patients who have undergone splenectomy or who are immunosuppressed would generally be more ill and require treatment. The combination of quinine with pyrimethamine in a patient with presumed malaria, but who really had babesiosis, was effective. Recently, the combination of clindamycin and quinine has been demonstrated to result in the rapid eradication of parasites. Although the experience is very limited, this combination is currently the treatment of choice.

The mortality rate is high in splenectomized patients; however, in general, babesiosis is a benign, self-limited disease. Hemolysis and disseminated intravascular coagulation may occur.

Persons living in areas where babesiosis occurs should avoid exposure to ticks and quickly remove those which become attached. The risk of transmission increases with the duration of tick attachment. For reducing the risk of transfusion-related babesia, the current policy of the American Red Cross is not to accept blood from (1) anyone with a history of babesiosis, or (2) permanent residents of the Shelter or Nantucket Islands. Donor blood is known to remain infective after 2 weeks of storage in a refrigerator.

Selected Bibliography

Malaria

Aronsson, B., Bengtsson, E., Bjorkman, A., Pehrson, P. O., Rombo, L., and Wahlgren, M.: Chloroquine-resistant falciparum malaria in Madagascar and Kenya. *Ann Trop Med Parasitol* 75:367-373, 1981.

Bray, R. S. and Anderson, M. J.: Falciparum malaria and pregnancy. *Trans Royal Soc Trop Med Hyg* 73:427-431, 1979.

Bruce-Chwatt, L. J.: Transfusion malaria. *Bull WHO* 50:337-346, 1974.

Centers for Disease Control: Prevention of malaria in travelers, 1982. *MMWR* 31:3S-28S, 1981.

Centers for Disease Control: Revised recommendations for malaria chemoprophylaxis for travelers to East Africa. *MMWR* 31:328-330, 1982.

Gardner, A. L., Weinstein, R. A., and Lincoln, L. J.: Failure of chloroquine prophylaxis in *Plasmodium falciparum* from East Africa. *JAMA* 246:979-980, 1981.

Hall, A. P.: The treatment of malaria. *Brit Med J* 1:323-328, 1976.

Heineman, H. S.: The clinical syndrome of malaria in the United States. *Arch Intern Med* 129:607-616, 1972.

Hurwitz, E. S., Johnson, D., and Campbell, C. C.: Resistance of *Plasmodium falciparum* malaria to sulfadoxine-pyrimethamine (Fansidar) in a refugee camp in Thailand. *Lancet* 1:1068-1070, 1981.

Jiang, J-B., Guo, X-B., Li, G-Q., Kong, Y-C., and Arnold, K.: Antimalarial activity of mefloquine and quinghaosu. *Lancet* 2:285-288, 1982.

Jilly, P.: Anemia in parturient women, with special reference to malaria infection of the placenta. *Ann Trop Med Parasitol* 63:109-116, 1969.

Khusmith, S., Druilhe, P., and Gentilini, M.: Enhanced *Plasmodium falciparum* merozoite phagocytosis by monocytes from immune individuals. *Inf Immun* 35:874-879, 1982.

McQuay, R. M., Silberman, S., Mudrik, P., and Keither, L.E.: Congenital malaria in Chicago. A case report and a review of published reports (USA). *Am J Trop Med Hyg* 16:258-266, 1967.

Miller, L. H., Mason, S. J., Clyde, D. F., and McGinniss, M. H.: The resistance factor to *Plasmodium vivax* in blacks. The Duffy blood-group genotype, Fy Fy. *N Engl J Med* 295:302-304, 1976.

Ojo-Amaize, E. M., Salimonu, L. S., Williams, A. I. O., Akinwolere, O. A. O., Shabo, R., Alm, G. V., and Wigzell, H.: Positive correlation between degree of parasitemia, interferon titers, and natural killer cell activity in *Plasmodium falciparum*-infected children. *J Immunol* 127:2296-2300, 1981.

Pazzaglia, G. and Woodward, W. E.: An analysis of the relationship of host factors to clinical falciparum malaria by multiple regression techniques. *Am J Trop Med Hyg* 31:202-210, 1982.

Perrein, L. H., Mackey, L. J., and Miescher, P. A.: The hematology of malaria in man. *Sem Hematol* 19:70-82, 1982.

Ponnampalam, J. T.: Doxycycline in the treatment of falciparum malaria among aborigine children in West Malaysia. *Trans Royal Soc Trop Med Hyg* 75:372-377, 1981.

Quinn, T. C., Jacobs, R. F., Mertz, G. J., Hook, E. W., and Locklsey, R. M.: Congenital malaria: A report of four cases and a review. *J Pediatr* 101:229-232, 1982.

Reacher, M., Freeman, J., Campbell, C. C., Doberstyn, E. B., and Brandling-Bennett, A. D.: Drug therapy for *Plasmodium falciparum* malaria resistant to pyrimethamine-sulfadoxine (Fansidar). A study of alternate regimens in Eastern Thailand. *Lancet* 2:1066-1068, 1981.

Stone, W. J., Hanchett, J. E., and Knepshield, J. H.: Acute renal insufficiency due to falciparum malaria. *Arch Intern Med* 129:620-628, 1972.

Taylor, D. W. and Siddiqui, W. A.: Recent advances in malarial immunity. *Ann Rev Med* 33:69-96, 1982.

Trenholme, G. M. and Carson, P. E.: Therapy and prophylaxis of malaria. *JAMA* 240:2293-2295, 1978.

Voller, A.: Immunopathology of malaria. *Bull WHO* 50:177-186, 1974.

Warrell, D. A., Looareesuwan, S., Warrell, M. J., Kasemsarn, P., Intaraprasert, R., Bunnag, D., and Harinasuta, T.: Dexamethasone proves deleterious in cerebral malaria. A double-blind trial in 100 comatose patients. *N Engl J Med* 306:313-319, 1982.

Weniger, B. G., Blumberg, R. S., Campbell, C. C., Jones, T. C., Mount, D. L., and Friedman, S. M.: High-level chloroquine resistance of *Plasmodium falciparum* malaria acquired in Kenya. *N Engl J Med* 307:1560-1562, 1982.

Wernsdorder, W. H.: Prospects for the development of malaria vaccines. *Bull WHO* 59:335-341, 1981.

Wilson, R. J.: How the malarial parasite enters the red blood cell. *Nature* 295:368-360, 1982.

Woodruff, A. W., Ansdell, V. E., and Pettitt, L. D.: Cause of anemia in malaria. *Lancet* 1:1055-1057, 1979.

Wyler, D. J.: Malaria - Resurgence, resistance and research (Part 1). *N Engl J Med* 308:875-878, 1983.

Wyler, D. J.: Malaria - Resurgence, resistance and research (Part 2). *N Engl J Med* 308:934-940, 1983.

Yarrish, R. L., Janas, J. S., Nosanchuk, J. S., Steigbigel, R. T., and Nusbacher, J.: Transfusion malaria: Treatment with exchange transfusion after delayed diagnosis. *Arch Intern Med* 142:187-188, 1982.

Babesiosis

Benach, J. L., Habicht, G. S., and Hamburger, M. I.: Immunoresponsiveness in acute babesiosis in humans. *J Infect Dis* 146:369-380, 1982.

Bredt, A. B., Weinstein, W. M., and Cohen, S.: Treatment of babesiosis in asplenic patients. *JAMA* 245:1938-1939, 1981.

Cahill, K. M., Benach, J. L., Reich, L. M., Bilmes, E., Zins, J. H., Siegel, F. P., and Hochweis, S.: Red cell exchange: Treatment of babesiosis in a splenectomized patient. *Transfusion* 21:193-198, 1981.

Centers for Disease Control: Clindamycin and quinine treatment for *Babesia microti* infections. *MMWR* 32:65-72, 1983.

Chisholm, E. S., Ruebush, T. K., Sulzer, A. J., and Healy, G. R.: *Babesia microti* infection in man: Evaluation of an indirect immunofluorescent antibody test. *Am J Trop Med Hyg* 27:14-19, 1978.

Filstein, M. R., Benach, J. L., White, D. J., Brody, B. A., Goldman, W. D., Bakal, C. W., and Schwartz, R. S.: Serosurvey for human babesiosis in New York. *J Infect Dis* 141:518-521, 1980.

Healy, G. R.: Babesia infections in man. *Hosp Pract* 14:107-116, 1979.

Jacoby, G. A., Hunt, J. V., Kosinski, K. S., Demirjian, Z. N., Huggins, C., Etkind, P., Marcus, L. C., and Spielman, A.: Treatment of transfusion - transmitted babesiosis by exchange transfusion. *N Engl J Med* 303:1098-1100, 1980.

Marcus, L. C., Valigorsky, J. M., Fanning, W. L., Joseph, T., and Glick, B.: A case report of transfusion-induced babesiosis. *JAMA* 248:465-467, 1982.

Miller, L. H., Neva, F. A., and Gill, F.: Failure of chloroquine in human babesiosis (*Babesia microti*). Case report and chemotherapeutic trials in hamsters. *Ann Intern Med* 88:200-202, 1978.

Piesman, J. and Spielman, A.: Human babesiosis on Nantucket Island: Prevalence of *Babesia microti* in ticks. *Am J Trop Med Hyg* 29:742-746, 1980.

Ruebush, T. K.: Human babesiosis in North America. *Tran Royal Soc Trop Med Hyg* 74:149-152, 1980.

Ruebush, T. K., Cassaday, P. B., Marsh, H. J., Lisker, S. A., Voorhees, D. B., Mahoney, E. B., and Healy, G. R.: Human babesiosis on Nantucket Island. Clinical features. *Ann Intern Med* 86:6-9, 1977.

Ruebush, T. K., Juranek, D. D., Chisholm, E. S., Snow, P. C., Healy, G. R., and Sulzer, A. J.: Human babesiosis on Nantucket Island. Evidence for self-limited and subclinical infections. *N Engl J Med* 297:825-827, 1977.

Teutsch, S. M., Etkind, P., Burwell, E. L., Sato, K., Dana, M. M., Fleishman, P. R., and Juranek, D. D.: Babesiosis in postsplenectomy hosts. *Am J Trop Med Hyg* 29:738-741, 1980.

Ward, P. A. and Jack, R. M.: The entry process of babesia merozoites into red cells. *Am J Path* 109-113, 1981.

Wittner, M., Rowin, K. S., Tanowitz, H. B., Hobbs, J. F., Saltzman, S., Wenz, B., Hirsch, R., Chisholm, E., and Healy, G. R.: Successful chemotherapy of transfusion babesiosis. *Ann Intern Med* 96:601-604, 1982.

124

TRICHOMONAS
Robert H. Waldman, M.D.

Trichomonads are flagellated protozoans, three species of which are found in humans, but only one of these is pathogenic. *Trichomonas vaginalis* is found in the urogenital tract and causes vaginitis in women and less frequently, urethritis in men. Two other species found in humans are nonpathogenic, *T. hominis* and *T. lenax.*

Trichomonas vaginalis is pear-shaped with four flagella and moves in a jerky, rotating motion. It does not survive at a pII lower than 4.5. The organism can be cultured on egg yolk medium.

Trichomonas vaginalis causes about one-third of the cases of vaginitis and is about as common as gonorrhea. It is transmitted primarily by sexual intercourse but also by fomites. The organism has been recovered from sites outside the genitourinary tract in immunocompromised patients.

The frequency of asymptomatic carriage of the organism varies between 20 and 70%. Symptomatic women note an increase in vaginal discharge, often described as copious, yellow-green, foul-smelling, and frothy. Patients complain of itching and/or burning of the labia, and have dyspareunia and/or dysuria. The onset of symptoms is commonly during or immediately following a menstrual period. On examination the vagina and cervix usually appear granular and erythematous, with petechiae. Males are usually asymptomatic, but may develop acute or chronic urethritis or prostatitis.

A wet mount of cervicovaginal secretions in saline is adequate for making the diagnosis. Motile, oval, flagellated organisms are seen under low-power microscopy. Adding a drop of methylene blue helps identify the organisms. If the slide is allowed to dry, organisms become rounded and immotile. Douching within 24 hr before obtaining the specimen reduces the chance of obtaining a positive result. Although it is almost never necessary, vaginal secretions may be cultured for the organism and are almost always positive. The Papanicolaou smear is also

usually positive for the organism. A swab also should be sent for culture for gonococcus, since the two infections may coexist.

Only documented cases should be treated. Metronidazole is the drug of choice
and may be given in several different regimens, all of which are effective. It may
be given 250 mg p.o., t.i.d. for 10 days, with or without 500 mg vaginal suppository
daily, also for 10 days. Another regimen is a single 2 g oral dose. Oral metronidazole should not be used during pregnancy because the drug may be teratogenic, although this has never been documented in humans. If the symptoms are troublesome, treatment may be started after the first trimester, or vaginal suppositories
may be used alone. Because metronidazole has Antabuse-like activity, patients
should be advised not to consume alcohol during treatment. An alternative drug is
tinidazole, which may be given as a single dose, 1.4-1.8 g orally. Whichever therapeutic regimen is chosen, there is an approximately 80% cure rate with one
course, and most of the other 20% respond with a second course. It is advised that
the sexual partner of the patient be treated to avoid possible reinfection. An important but unresolved question is whether or not an asymptomatic patient should
be treated. Since the disease is, at its worst, benign and self-limited, with no
known sequelae, I recommend treating only symptomatic patients and their partners.

Selected Bibliography

Catterall, R. D.: Trichomonal infections of the genital tract. *Med Clin N Am* 56:
    1203, 1972.

Dykers, J. R.: Single-dose metronidazole for trichomonal vaginitis. A follow up.
    N Engl J Med 295:395, 1976.

Fleury, F. J., Van Bergen, W. S., Prentice, R. L., Russell, J. G., Singleton, J. A.,
    and Standard, J. V.: Single dose of two grams of metronidazole for *Tricho-
    monas vaginalis* infection. *Am J Obstet Gynecol* 128:320, 1977.

Masur, H., Hook, E., III, and Armstrong, D.: A *Trichomonas* species in a mixed
    microbial meningitis. *JAMA* 236:1978, 1976.

125

TRYPANOSOMIASIS
Robert H. Waldman, M.D.

Trypanosomes are flagellated protozoans which cause two very distinct diseases, American trypanosomiasis (Chagas' disease) and African trypanosomiasis (sleeping sickness) (Table 125.1). These two diseases have nothing in common except that the organisms which cause them are trypanosomes; therefore they will be discussed separately.

Chagas' Disease

Chagas' disease is caused by *Trypanosoma cruzi*. The disease has two forms, acute and chronic (Table 125.2). The disease is found in rural areas of Central and South America. Infected animals have been detected in the United States, but there have been no human cases. There is, however, serologic evidence of subclinical infections occurring in the United States.

The parasites are excreted in the feces of reduviid bugs during biting, and inoculation occurs through the bite, an abrasion, or mucous membranes. The reduviid bug is also known as the kissing bug, because it has a tendency to bite around the face. It feeds at night.

Reservoirs are domestic animals, such as cats and dogs, and wild animals, such as rats and raccoons. Wild animals are only of importance to human infection if they live near places of residence. The disease has also been reported to be transmitted by blood transfusions, transplacentally, and by contaminated food.

The acute form of the disease is seen mainly in children in endemic areas. Within several days of being bitten, an indurated, erythematous lesion appears at the site. This lesion has been named the chagoma. It is commonly found around the eye, and causes unilateral conjunctivitis, periocular edema, and preauricular lymphadenopathy. Together these findings are called Romaña's sign. A few weeks

TABLE 125.1   Trypanosomiasis

Disease	Geography	Vector	Parasite	Diagnosis
Sleeping sickness	Africa	*Glossina*		
(Subacute to chronic)	(Guinea, Ghana, Nigeria, Gambia, Sierra Leone, Zaire)	(*G. palpalis*)	*T. gambiense*	Giemsa stain for or-ganisms: tissue or lymph node "juice," CSF, blood
(Acute)	(Tanzania, Uganda, Zambia, Rhodesia)	(*G. morsitans*)	*T. rhodesiense*	
Chagas' disease	Central and South America	Reduviid bug	*T. cruzi*	Organisms in blood or lymph node "juice," blood culture in NNN medium

TABLE 125.2   Clinical Characteristics of Chagas' Disease

Acute disease

Incubation period: 1-3 wk

Age: children 1-5 yr old

Skin: chagoma (erythematous, warm mass at site of and within hours of bite), persists for 2-3 mo, most commonly on cheek or around eye, with unilateral edema of eye, regional lymphadenopathy

Cardiac: arrhythmias, congestive heart failure

Autonomic neuropathy: megaesophagus, megacolon

Moderate hepato- and/or splenomegaly

Epistaxis

Convulsions

Chronic disease

Cardiac: arrhythmias, CHF

Autonomic neuropathy

---

after the appearance of the chagoma, parasitemia occurs. The organisms infect and divide mainly in cells of mesenchymal origin. Patients develop fever, rash, hepatosplenomegaly, and lymphadenopathy. They develop nonpitting edema of the skin, and tender subcutaneous nodules. In the more severe cases, they develop myocarditis and meningoencephalitis, either of which may lead to death.

Laboratory diagnosis is made by observing the motile trypanosomes in wet mounts of blood. The organisms may also be demonstrated using the Giemsa stain, the sensitivity of which may be increased using the concentrating method of lysing the erythrocytes and centrifugation. The organism may be cultured on Nicolle, Novy, MacNeal (NNN) medium. Serologic diagnosis may be made using the complement-fixation test, a rise in titer being diagnostic in the acute form of the disease.

The prognosis is good, with the acute form usually being self-limited.

The chronic form is seen in patients who usually have no history of having had clinically apparent preceding acute disease. It occurs in older children and young adults. The most frequent manifestation of the chronic form is cardiac disease, pathologically a mononuclear-cell myocarditis. This is manifested by biventricular hypertrophy and conduction disturbances. The other main manifestation of the disease is gastrointestinal denervation leading to impaired motility and dilatation.

The diagnosis of the chronic form of the disease usually cannot be made by observing the organism on wet mount or stain of peripheral blood, nor by culturing the organism. Furthermore, the complement-fixation test is not helpful, since a positive titer only indicates that the patient had acute infection at some time in the past. Xenodiagnosis is successful in about 20% of the patients. Reduviid bugs, known to be free of infection, are allowed to feed on suspected cases. After 1 month, the feces of the insect are inspected for the organism. After 2 months, the insects are sacrificed and the intestinal contents are examined. Other methods of diagnosing the chronic form are intraperitoneal injection of blood from a suspected case into mice, with examination of the heart after 1 month; and the intradermal injection of a soluble protein extract of the organism.

Fatalities in the chronic form of the disease are a result of arrhythmias or congestive heart failure.

Treatment of Chagas' disease is not very effective. The drug of choice is nifurtimox, which has significant side effects, including psychosis and peripheral neuropathy, and hemolysis in patients with glucose-6-phosphate dehydrogenase (G6PD) deficiency. Patients should be treated medically for congestive heart failure and cardiac arrhythmias, and surgery may be necessary for relief of megacolon.

African Trypanosomiasis

Sleeping sickness is caused by *T. gambiense* and *T. rhodesiense* (Table 125.3). The latter causes a more acute and rapidly fatal disease. These organisms are transmitted to humans by the tsetse fly.

There are two phases of the disease, the acute and the central nervous system phases. After an incubation period of 1-3 weeks, patients develop fever and ulcer at the site of the bite of the tsetse fly. This is followed shortly by a morbilliform rash, lymphadenopathy, splenomegaly, headache, and early encephalitic symptoms (Table 125.4). Patients have prominent posterior cervical lymphadenopathy, known as Winterbottom's sign. They may also demonstrate delayed pain over the distribution of a nerve following a light tap on the nerve. This is particularly noticeable with the ulnar nerve, and is known as Kerandel's sign.

With *T. rhodesiense* infection patients develop myocarditis and rapid central nervous system involvement. With *T. gambiense* meningoencephalitis develops more slowly, over a period of months to years. Patients show lassitude, tremors, and progress to apathy and somnolence. Thereafter they become emaciated and lapse into coma.

In about 40% of the patients, the diagnosis can be made by visualizing the moving parasite in a wet mount of blood. A thin smear stained with Wright's or Giemsa is used to definitely identify the organism. A concentration method can be used to improve the sensitivity. Organisms may be seen in spinal fluid or bone marrow aspirate. The most sensitive method, however, is examination of material

TABLE 125.3   Comparison of *T. rhodesiense* and *T. gambiense* Infection

Feature	*T. rhodesiense*	*T. gambiense*
Severity of encephalitis	Less	More
Visceral involvement, including heart	More	Less
Lymphadenopathy	Less	More

TABLE 125.4   Clinical Features of Sleeping Sickness

Skin nodule	At site of bite Firm, tender, may ulcerate; persists 2-3 wk; precedes other manifestation of illness by weeks to years
Fever	2-3-wk duration, accompanied by erythematous skin eruption
Headache	Weeks to months
Lymphadenopathy	Symmetric; predominantly cervical; persists for several months
Hepatosplenomegaly	
Parasitemia	Frequently visible on blood smear
Sleeping stage	Early: lassitude, apathy, fatigue; later: asleep most of time; terminal coma
Hyperesthesia	Kerandel's sign: severe pain over area of nerve distribution following light tap on nerve

aspirated from an enlarged lymph node. In CNS disease the spinal fluid may or may not contain the organisms, but there is almost always spinal fluid pleocytosis and/or an elevated protein content. A helpful, though not diagnostic finding is markedly elevated IgM levels in spinal fluid and blood in patients with African trypanosomiasis.

The treatment of the acute phase of disease is suramin, and for the central nervous system phase, melarsoprol. The most important method of prevention of the disease is to protect against insect bites by using mosquito netting, by wearing long sleeves, and by avoiding bright-colored clothing. Pentamidine is effective as chemoprophylaxis, but should only be used for travelers who will have intense and prolonged exposure in an endemic area.

Selected Bibliography

Earlam, R. J.: Gastrointestinal aspects of Chagas' disease. *Am J Dig Dis* 17: 559, 1972.

Spencer, H. C., Jr., Gibson, J. J., Jr., Brodsky, R. E., and Schultz, M. G.: Imported African trypanosomiasis in the United States. *Ann Intern Med* 82: 633, 1975.

126

LEISHMANIA
Robert H. Waldman, M.D.

Leishmaniasis is a significant cause of morbidity and mortality in several under-developed countries (Table 126.1). The host is infected with the flagellated extracellular form of the parasite, the promastigote, via the bite of the sand fly. Promastigotes are rapidly phagocytized by macrophages, and the parasite transforms into the nonflagellated intracellular form, the amastigote. Disease is caused by multiplication of amastigotes within macrophages.

Three forms of the disease occur, cutaneous, mucocutaneous, and visceral. These three forms of disease are caused by four species of *Leishmania: L. donovani,* which causes the visceral disease; *L. tropica,* which causes the cutaneous form; and *L. braziliensis* and *L. mexicana* which cause the mucocutaneous form.

The female *Phlebotomas* sand fly acquires the parasite while feeding from infected skin or blood and transmits to another host, also while feeding. Sand flies are weak fliers, live near the ground commonly in cracks in walls of houses and in rubble. Leishmaniasis has also been transmitted congenitally and by blood transfusions.

Kala-Azar

Visceral leishmaniasis (kala-azar), also known as tropical splenomegaly and Dumdum fever, is a chronic disease caused by *L. donovani* infecting the reticuloendothelial system throughout the body. Most cases are found in India and China. Infected humans are probably the most important reservoir of the disease. It is an endemic disease, usually of children and young adults.

The flagellate forms of the parasite are injected by the insect and enter tissue macrophages where they transform into nonflagellated forms and divide. They disseminate and enter the cells of the reticuloendothelial system, where the

TABLE 126.1 Human Leishmaniasis

Disease	Type	Geography	Etiology	Reservoir
Kala-azar	Visceral	India Mediterranean East Africa Middle East South America	*L. donovani*	Human Dog, fox Human, rodent Jackal Dog, fox, human
Oriental sore	Old World cutaneous	Middle East, India, Mediterranean and North Africa	*L. tropica*	Gerbil, dog, and human
Chiclero ulcer	New World cutaneous	Mexico, British Honduras, and Amazon River basin	*L. mexicana*	Forest rodent
Espundia		Central and South America	*L. braziliensis*	Forest rodent
Uta		Peru		Dog

infected macrophages proliferate, and lead to hypertrophy. The results of this macrophage proliferation are splenomegaly, bone marrow replacement, and infiltration of the villi of the small intestines, along with other changes. The skin usually is not affected in kala-azar.

The incubation period is about 3-6 months. The diagnosis is clinical: in an endemic area the combination of prolonged fever, weight loss, weakness, splenomegaly, hepatomegaly, leukopenia, anemia, hyperglobulinemia, and hypoalbuminemia, is indicative of visceral leishmaniasis. Patients commonly have a chronic cough, bleeding diathesis, immune-complex glomerulonephritis, progressive emaciation, and abdominal distention. The hyperglobulinemia is marked, with total globulins in the range of 7-9 g/dl. The white blood cell count is usually less than $4000/mm^3$. The differential diagnosis includes malaria, salmonella infection, tuberculosis, pneumonia, and lymphoma.

Definitive diagnosis is made by demonstrating the organism. The Leishman-Donovan body is a small, 2- to 4-μm, ovoid organism, which is seen on using Giemsa stain. Bone marrow is the best source of material for demonstrating the organism (Table 126.2). It can be cultured on NNN medium, but this is not terribly helpful because it takes 1-4 weeks to grow.

The treatment is pentavalent antimonials and the response is variable, depending upon the region. Kala-azar in India responds well, but in Sudan the organism is resistant. The drug of choice is antimony sodium stibogluconate. It is given intramuscularly or intravenously, 600 mg daily. The duration of therapy depends upon the susceptibility of the organism and may be as short as 6 days, or as long as a month. Pentamidine is more effective, but also more toxic, and should be used in resistant cases. The dosage is 4 mg/kg intramuscularly q.o.d. Amphotericin B is also effective but toxic, and should be given in a total dosage of 1-1.5 g over several weeks.

General supportive measures are important, and include a high-protein, high-calorie diet, vitamin supplementation, and transfusions as needed. Splenectomy is usually contraindicated.

If untreated, 90% of patients die of kala-azar. With treatment, the mortality is only about 5%. Deaths are due to secondary bacterial infection, usually pneumonia, or bleeding and severe anemia. Although treatment has markedly reduced mortality, relapses are fairly common.

Recovery from the disease leads to complete and long-lasting immunity. There is good evidence that this is a result of the development of cell-mediated immunity.

TABLE 126.2   Demonstration of *L. donovani* in Various Tissue Specimens in Patients with Kala-Azar

Specimen	Approximate % Positive
Bone marrow aspirate	90
Splenic puncture	90
Liver biopsy	70
Buffy coat of blood	60

The disease is prevented by control of insect vectors. DDT is very effective when breeding places, both inside and outside the home, are sprayed. Insect repellents give only temporary protection. It is also important to eliminate the reservoirs of the disease, by eliminating the animal reservoirs and treating infected humans.

Cutaneous Leishmaniasis

Old World cutaneous leishmaniasis, also known as oriental sore or Delhi boil, is caused by *L. tropica*. It is transmitted by the bite of the sand fly and possibly also by direct contact. It is endemic but occasional epidemics also occur.

The organism infects monocytes, polymorphonuclear leukocytes, and endothelial cells of the capillaries of the skin, leading to a granulomatous reaction which causes ischemia and the formation of a necrotic ulcer. Secondary bacterial infection is important in the pathogenesis of the disease. There is great variability in the extent of the disease. Some patients have self-healing sores in which there is marked lymphocyte infiltration and few organisms. On the other hand, some patients have diffuse, progressive involvement, and these lesions have few lymphocytes and many organisms. These latter lesions tend to be nodular and similar to lepromatous leprosy. The pathogenesis also is similar and this form probably represents an inadequate cell-mediated immune response.

The incubation period is 2-6 months. A pruritic erythematous papule develops at the site of inoculation, usually on an exposed part of the body. This papule slowly grows and ulcerates, reaching a size of 2 cm or larger. The ulcer has well-defined and raised borders, is usually single, and heals spontaneously after several months, leaving a depigmented scar. The ulcer is accompanied by regional tender lymphadenopathy.

The diagnosis is confirmed by identifying the organism, either by staining a smear from scraping or aspiration of the edge of the ulcer, or by culturing the material on NNN medium at 22°C. It should be emphasized that material must be obtained from the edge of the ulcer because the base is usually negative. The leishmanin skin test is positive except in patients with diffuse cutaneous disease. The diagnosis can also be made serologically using an agglutination test.

The differential diagnosis includes blastomycosis, yaws, systemic lupus erythematosus, and syphilis.

The treatment is antimony sodium stibogluconate, neostibosan, or pentamidine. Cryotherapy is also effective. Permanent immunity follows the infection.

Mucocutaneous Leishmaniasis

New World cutaneous leishmaniasis, also called espundia, is seen in Central and South America, with very rare cases in Texas. It is a disfiguring disease because, in addition to skin lesions, it involves the mucous membranes of the nose, mouth, and pharynx. It is caused by either *L. braziliensis* or *L. mexicana*. With regard to the skin involvement, the disease is very similar to that caused by *L. tropica*.

Transmission is by sand flies and also possibly by direct contact and/or auto-inoculation. There are several animal reservoirs of the organism. The greatest concentration of the disease is in Brazil and Peru and the greatest prevalence is in forest workers, especially those involved in construction work. The time of greatest risk of acquiring the disease is during the hot season just after heavy rains.

The incubation period is 10 days to 3 months and as mentioned earlier, the skin ulcer is very much like that of the oriental sore except that satellite lesions are more common, and the ulcers are much slower to heal.

The mucosal lesions may accompany the skin ulcer or appear months to years later. Frequently patients give no history of having had a cutaneous lesion. The mucosal lesion is progressive, destructive of cartilage, but usually does not involve bone.

One can identify or isolate organisms in early lesions, but later this becomes difficult or impossible. The diagnosis then can be made by skin test or serologic testing. The disease may be confused with leprosy.

The lesions heal after years of progression and partial healing. Death may result from secondary bacterial infection and/or malnutrition, the latter from scarring and destruction which may make it difficult for the patient to eat.

The treatment is pentavalent antimonials or amphotericin B. After the mucosal lesions have been present for a few months, chemotherapy is ineffective.

The disease may be prevented by using insect repellents, screening of housing, and insecticide spraying. This has been extremely difficult to accomplish, however, because of the rural and sylvatic nature of the exposure.

Selected Bibliography

DeBrito, T., Hoshino-Shimizu, S., Amato Neto, V., Duarte, I. S., and Penna, D. O.: Glomerular involvement in human kala-azar. *Am J Trop Med Hyg* 24:9, 1975.

Geraci, J. E., Wilson, W. R., and Thompson, J. H.: Visceral leishmaniasis (kala-azar) as a cause of fever of unknown origin. *Mayo Clin Proc* 55:455, 1980.

Pampiglione, S., Manson-Bahr, P. E. C., LaPlaca, M., Borgatti, M. A., and Musumeci, S.: Studies in Mediterranean leishmaniasis. 3. The leishmanin skin test in kala-azar. *Trans Roy Soc Trop Med Hyg* 69:60, 1975.

Radwanski, Z. K., Bryceson, A. D. M., Preston, P. M., and Dumonde, D. C.: Immunofluorescence studies of *Leishmania enriettii* infection in the guinea pig. *Trans Roy Soc Trop Med Hyg* 68:124, 1974.

Shaw, P.K., Quigg, L. T., Allain, D. S., Juranek, D. D., and Healy, G. R.: Autochthonous dermal leishmaniasis in Texas. *Am J Trop Med Hyg* 25:788, 1976.

Singer, C., Armstrong, D., Jones, T. C., and Spiro, R. N.: Imported mucocutaneous leishmaniasis in New York City: Report of a patient treated with amphotericin B. *Am J Med* 59:444, 1975.

G. Helminths

127

NEMATODES
Robert H. Waldman, M.D.

The helminths, or worms, are divided into the Nematoda, or roundworms; the
Trematoda, or flukes; and the Cestoda, or tapeworms (Tables 127.1-127.3). The
helminths differ from other organisms which cause human disease in that they do
not multiply as adults in the human.

Intestinal Forms (Tables 127.4 and 127.5)

Enterobiasis

Enterobius, or pinworm, is a common infestation, especially of children, which is
very mild but can be extremely irritating.

Pinworm has a very simple life cycle compared with most of the other nematodes. The adults live in the cecum and ascending colon. The gravid female migrates to the perianal area, usually at night, and on contact with air, releases her
eggs over the perianal skin. The female continues to migrate for a time, causing
the itching which leads to scratching and picking up of the eggs on the hands and
under the fingernails. The eggs are usually viable for 2-3 days, but under ideal
conditions of low humidity and temperature, may remain viable for 1-2 months.
By direct hand-to-mouth transmission, the eggs are ingested and passed to the
upper small intestine where they hatch. Transmission may also occur indirectly,
by eggs becoming airborne from contaminated clothing, towels, etc., and rarely
there is retroinfection, where eggs may hatch in the perianal area and larvae migrate up the colon. After hatching in the small intestine, the organisms migrate
and mature to their place of residence as adults, the large intestine. The entire
time of this life cycle is about 15 days under optimum conditions.

TABLE 127.1   Classification of Helminths

Nematodes:	roundworms
Trematodes:	flukes
Cestodes:	tapeworms

TABLE 127.2   Estimated Worldwide Prevalence of Some Human Parasitic Diseases

Parasite	Number of People
Hookworm	700 million
Whipworm	350 million
Filariasis	300 million
Schistosomiasis	200 million
Malaria	150 million
Chagas' disease	12 million

TABLE 127.3   Characteristics of Helminthic Diseases Which Account for Tropical Distribution

Warm temperature and high humidity favor survival and multiplication

Vertebrate or invertebrate hosts, such as insects, snails, crustacea

Vectors (e.g., mosquitoes, biting flies) have access to people because of lack of preventive measures

Poor sanitation enables eggs or larvae passed in feces or urine to be transmitted to another host

Use of human excreta for fertilizer (night soil)

Food habits: eating raw or partially cooked fish, shellfish, meat, etc.

TABLE 127.4   Life Cycle of Intestinal Nematodes

Species	Route of Infection	Migration	Site of Larval Development	Infective Form
E. vermicularis	Mouth	Intestinal	Perianal	Egg
T. trichiura	Mouth	Intestinal	Soil	Egg
A. lumbricoides	Mouth	Pulmonary	Soil	Egg
N. americanus and A. duodenale	Skin	Pulmonary	Soil	Filariform larva
S. stercoralis	Skin	Pulmonary	Soil and intestine	Filariform larva

TABLE 127.5   Diagnosis and Indications for Treatment of Intestinal Nematodes

Species	Symptoms	Diagnosis	Indications for Treatment
E. vermicularis	Perianal pruritus	Eggs on perianal skin by "Scotch-tape" test	Symptoms and diagnosis in one member of a family
T. trichiura	None, or non-specific GI and/or anemia if infection is heavy	Eggs in feces	Symptoms
A. lumbricoides	None usually, or nonspecific GI	Eggs in feces	Finding eggs (worms may cause obstruction)
N. americanus and A. duodenale	None usually, anemia if heavy infection	Eggs in fresh stool sample, larvae in older sample	Symptoms or anemia
S. stercoralis	Mild to severe GI	Eggs in feces	Finding eggs (may disseminate at some later time)

Humans are the only host and it is estimated that 20-30% of all children world-wide are infected at any one time. Infections usually occur in groups living in close proximity, and very commonly, all members of a family are infected.

Pathologically there is no lesion, since the pinworm does not penetrate the intestinal mucosa. It has been postulated that the worm plays a role in appendicitis, but there is no good evidence for this. Rarely, the worm may migrate up the female genital tract and into the peritoneal cavity setting up a mild inflammatory response. There is some evidence that girls with pinworm infection may have a higher frequency of urinary tract infection as a result of scratching, with attendant inflammation, edema, and contamination of the external meatus.

Clinically, the disease may be asymptomatic or cause perianal pruritus, which may be intense. Girls may also develop vaginitis. Secondary symptoms of sleeplessness, irritability, etc., are not uncommon. There is no eosinophilia in pinworm infestation.

The diagnosis is made by using the "Scotch-tape" test. The test is done by putting a piece of Scotch tape, made into a circle, sticky side out, onto a microscope slide. This is touched to the perianal area in several locations. The Scotch tape is then placed, sticky side down, onto another microscope slide and examined for ova. The test is less likely to be positive if conducted in the doctor's office because children are commonly given a bath before being brought to the doctor. Therefore, the test should be done at home in the morning, before the patient bathes or defecates.

Treatment of the whole family should be carried out whenever the diagnosis is made. There are several treatment regimens which are effective and the choice depends upon side effects, drug availability, and convenience of the dosage regimen. Mebendazole is given in a single 100 mg dose and its use has been associated with side effects on only very rare occasions. The drug may be repeated in 2 weeks if necessary. Pyrvinium pamoate is given as a single dose of 5 mg/kg (maximum 350 mg), and has moderately frequent gastrointestinal side effects. Pyrantel pamoate is given as a single dose of 11 mg/kg (maxim 1 g), and may be repeated in 2 weeks if necessary. It also has gastrointestinal side effects, plus occasional rises in liver enzymes, headache, and dizziness. Piperazine citrate has been used most extensively in the treatment of pinworm. The recommended dosage is 65 mg/kg (maximum of 2.5 g/day) as a single daily dose for 7 days. Treatment may be repeated in 2 weeks if necessary. The side effects include cerebellar ataxia, nausea, vomiting, and urticaria. Piperazine should not be used in patients taking phenothiazines. Thiabendazole can be given in a dosage of 25 mg/kg twice, for 1 day only, and may be repeated 1-2 weeks later. The side effects of thiabendazole are minor but frequent: nausea, vomiting, diarrhea, headache, vertigo, and drowsiness.

Pinworm can be prevented with good hygiene, i.e., careful hand-washing. If it is established in a family the affected children should shower daily with thorough washing of the perianal region, their fingernails should be cut short, and possibly their clothing, towels, etc., soaked in ammonia (1 cup in 5 gal of water) for 1 hr, or boiled, and their toys soaked in ammonia or sterilized in the oven.

Trichuriasis

Trichuris, or whipworm, is found worldwide, but most commonly in warm, moist areas, where the sanitation is poor. After ingestion of eggs which hatch in the upper duodenum the larvae attach to small intestinal villi. When they have matured the parasites leave their first resting spot and pass distally to the proximal large intestine where they live for up to 20 years. The eggs are passed to the feces where they embryonate in 10 days to several months.

The worm gets its name from its whip-like shape. The eggs are barrel-shaped, with the characteristic "mucoid plug" at both ends. The egg is also double-shelled, and the outer shell is usually bile-stained. The eggs are sensitive to direct sunlight and drying.

The adult worms partially imbed in the colonic mucosa, usually to approximately 60% of their total length. A small worm burden produces no pathology, but a large number leads to mechanical irritation and hemorrhagic colitis. Thus most patients are asymptomatic, but heavy infestation leads to diarrhea which may be mucoid or bloody, and patients may occasionally develop rectal prolapse. Symptomatic patients usually have abdominal pain, tenderness, weight loss, and may develop weakness and lethargy.

Laboratory findings are a moderate eosinophilia, especially in severe infections; the diarrheal stool may contain eosinophilia and Charcot-Leyden crystals. Patients are commonly anemic. If there is a heavy infestation, one may see the worms when using sigmoidoscopy. The diagnosis is usually made by identifying characteristic eggs in the feces, and it is important to do a quantitative egg count to determine the significance of the infection. If there are few eggs, trichuriasis is probably not the cause of the symptoms in the patient.

The treatment of choice is mebendazole, one 100 mg tablet twice a day for 3 days in both adults and children. Treatment may be repeated in 3 weeks. This drug is also effective against ascariasis, hookworm, and enterobiasis. An alternative drug is difetarsone. The adult dosage is 1 g b.i.d. for 10 days, and in children the dosage should be reduced proportionally to their surface area. Side effects are vomiting and diarrhea.

Whipworm can be prevented by good sanitation, particularly by avoiding the eating of raw vegetables in areas where night soil is used, and by preventing children from defecating on the ground near living quarters.

Ascariasis

Ascariasis, the infection caused by the largest of the worms infecting humans, *Ascaris lumbricoides,* is common worldwide especially in areas with poor sanitation. It has a prevalence of 90% in some areas. In the United States it is also common but has its highest prevalence in Appalachia and the southern and Gulf states.

Adult worms are found in the lumen of the middle portion of the small intestines, where they live for about 6 months. Eggs pass in the feces and if deposited in the soil become infective in about 3 weeks. The best soil for survival and development of infectivity in the eggs is shaded clay. After ingestion, the eggs hatch in the small intestine and the larvae penetrate the mucosa traveling via the lymphatics and venous system to the lungs. In the lungs they penetrate the alveoli, migrate up the trachea, and are swallowed. They then mature to adults and come to rest in the small intestine. The whole cycle takes an average of 2 months.

The adult is white, cream, or pink, measuring 15 35 cm in length, with the female being slightly larger than the male. The eggs are highly resistant to extremes of temperature and to drying.

Pathologically there are three stages in the life cycle where damage may be done. The first is very minor, and consists of minute hemorrhages at the points where larvae penetrate the small intestinal mucosa. The second is the pneumonitis that may occur, especially with heavy infection. The third is with respect to the adult worms, which normally cause no pathology; however, with very heavy infestation, partial or complete obstruction of the intestines may occur. Very rarely, perforation, appendicitis, or bile duct obstruction by the adult worms may occur. Also, the adult worm may, to a minor extent, interfere with digestion and absorption of protein.

The clinical manifestations also correspond to the three phases of the life cycle. Fever may be present during the migration of the larvae, but symptoms are usually absent or minimal. During the pulmonary phase, cough, hemoptysis, and evidence on physical examination of pneumonitis are fairly common. Patients are usually diagnosed as having viral or mycoplasmal pneumonia.

The adult intestinal phase is usually asymptomatic but a few patients may have colicky epigastric or periumbilical pain. A rare manifestation of the disease during the intestinal phase is asthma, which is the result of a hypersensitivity reaction to antigen liberated from the worms.

Moderate eosinophilia is seen, especially during the pulmonary phase. Although rarely observed, because they are rarely looked for, larvae can be seen if sputum is examined during the pulmonary phase. The diagnosis is usually made by a history of the patient having passed worms in the stool, or demonstrating eggs in the feces. The diagnosis may also be made by roentgenographic examination following a barium meal since the worms will create filling defects, and barium may be seen in the alimentary canals of the worms.

Treatment should be carried out in all cases in which the diagnosis has been made to prevent the complications, particularly intestinal obstruction. The drugs of choice are pyrantel pamoate, mebendazole, or piperazine. Both pyrantel and mebendazole have few side effects. The advantage of pyrantel is that it is given as a single dose of 11 mg/kg. The advantage of mebendazole is that it is also effective against trichuriasis, which commonly coinfects the same patients. Mebendazole is given in 100 mg dose twice a day for 3 days, the same dosage being used for both adults and children.

Hookworm

Hookworm is a common nematode infestation found worldwide, but particularly concentrated in tropical and subtropical areas. There are two species, *Ancylostoma duodenale* and *Necator americanus.* The former is found mainly in southern Europe, northern Africa, northern India, China, and Japan. The latter is found mainly in southern Asia, central and southern Africa, and the Americas. It is found in all age groups and is especially common where human feces is used for fertilizer, in which case infection results from working the fields.

Hookworms are pink or creamy, 8-13-mm long, the female being larger than the male. Eggs are passed in the feces and hatch in a few days, forming rhabditiform larvae. Both the eggs and larvae are quite susceptible to freezing temperatures and drying of the soil. The rhabditiform larvae mature into filariform larvae, which is the form which penetrates the skin of humans. Penetration is not easy, but is aided by the common occurrence of contaminated mud being caked onto the feet.

Following penetration, the filariform larvae go via the circulation to the lung, where they penetrate the alveoli, pass up the respiratory tract and are swallowed. They mature into the adults which attach to the small intestinal mucosa. The complete cycle takes 5 weeks or longer. Adults live in the small intestines for up to 15 years, but most of them are eliminated in 1-2 years.

Disease is almost entirely a result of blood loss, which is proportional to the number of worms. An infested person loses about 0.5 ml of blood per worm per day. The development of symptoms is thus a result of the size of the worm burden, along with the nutritional status of the patient, since adequate iron and other nutrient intake will negate the effects of all but the heaviest of infestations. Very heavy infestation will also lead to some interference with absorption, contributing to malnutrition and avitaminosis. Larval penetration of the skin may cause a pruritic maculopapular rash, lasting up to 2 weeks, known as ground itch. The pulmonary stage is asymptomatic or causes very mild pulmonary symptoms. Children with a heavy infestation and a poor diet may develop a pot-bellied appearance, and demonstrate geophagy.

Eosinophilia is common. The anemia is usually hypochromic and microcytic, but also a mixed pattern with macrocytosis is seen. The diagnosis is made by identifying eggs in the stool, but rhabditiform larvae may be seen as well if the stool has not been examined promptly. This may cause some confusion in differentiating hookworm from strongyloidiasis, since the larvae appear similar, and the diagnosis of strongyloidiasis is usually made by identification of larvae in the stool. Another complicating factor is that the two infections may coexist.

The prognosis of hookworm infection is variable, from excellent in mild cases, to being a significant socioeconomic factor where productivity is decreased due to weakness and lethargy, to causing mental and physical retardation in children.

There is no convincing evidence that immunity develops in this disease. There is evidence for racial differences in susceptibility, since heavy infestations are less common in blacks.

Preventive measures are very effective and include the obvious, good public health and hygiene. These measures are easy to state, but difficult to attain in underdeveloped parts of the world, e.g., wearing shoes and eating a balanced diet. In areas with heavy infestation, mass treatment programs have been somewhat sucessful in reducing the reservoir. The drug tetrachloroethylene has been used.

Treatment should be undertaken only in patients who are symptomatic. Patients should be given iron, a good diet, and transfusions, as necessary. The drugs of choice are mebendazole and pyrantel pamoate.

Mebendazole has the advantages of having the lowest frequency of side effects and being effective against both ascariasis and whipworm infection. The disadvantage of mebendazole is the frequency of dosage, requiring a 100 mg b.i.d. for 3 days.

Strongyloides

Strongyloides stercoralis is unique among the nematode infestations in that it causes a mild to moderately severe illness in normals, but may also cause an extremely severe, disseminated, and life-threatening disease in patients with altered host defenses.

The helminth is prevalent in warm, humid climates, and is a common infestation particularly in persons living under unhygienic conditions (Table 127.6).

The life cycle of strongyloides is the most complicated of any nematode that parasitizes humans (Figure 127.1). Humans are infected by the filariform larva which penetrates the skin, usually in people who walk barefoot in contaminated soil. The larva travels to the lungs, then up the trachea, to be swallowed. During the passage the filariform larva matures. The female burrows submucosally in the duodenum and upper jejunum where she lays eggs. The eggs hatch and become rhabditiform larvae which usually pass in the feces. Hyperinfection may occur when the rhabditiform larva mature to filariform larvae in the lower intestines, penetrate the colonic mucosa, and begin the life cycle again. A variant of hyperinfection is autoinfection, which occurs under poor sanitary conditions when filariform larva penetrate the perianal skin. Thus, the host may maintain the infestation indefinitely. Predisposing factors for hyperinfection are decreased bowel motility and an impaired immune response.

In the normal host, the clinical picture of strongyloidiasis is extremely variable from completely asymptomatic to fairly severe gastrointestinal symptoms.

TABLE 127.6   Strongyloidiasis in World War II Ex-prisoners of War

Persistence of infestation	20% of all prisoners in Burma-Thailand camps
Recurrent pruritic rash	25% of all prisoners in Burma-Thailand
Other symptoms:	Abdominal crampy pain Diarrhea Heartburn
Persistence in those with symptoms	50%

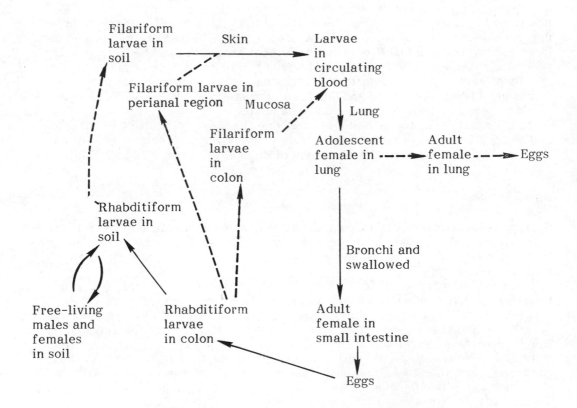

FIGURE 127.1   Life cycle of *Strongyloides*.

Most commonly patients have intermittent, dull, aching pain or a burning sensation to the right of the midline. The symptoms are exacerbated by food or alcohol. Patients often have nonspecific symptoms of nausea, anorexia, and weight loss. Less commonly, patients develop generalized urticaria.

From the life cycle, it is not unexpected that patients frequently have pulmonary symptoms. These may be more intense because occasionally the larvae mature in the respiratory tract and the adult female may lay eggs in the lung. The manifestations are most commonly cough, wheezing, and infiltrates on chest roentgenographic examination. Strongyloidiasis is one of the causes of the syndrome of pulmonary infiltrates and eosinophilia (PIE syndrome).

In immunosuppressed patients, in addition to intestinal involvement, one may see hyperinfection, a much heavier worm burden limited to the organs usually involved, i.e., the respiratory and gastrointestinal tracts; or disseminated infection, in which case larvae are found in other organs of the body. In the latter situation, strongyloides can disseminate to virtually any organ. Usually, gastrointestinal and pulmonary symptoms are severe, including vomiting, abdominal pain, gastrointestinal hemorrhage, diffuse pneumonia, and respiratory insufficiency. Filariform larvae have been reported in the brain and spinal cord, liver, spleen, heart, pancreas, various muscles, lymph nodes, and skin.

In the normal host, eosinophilia is prominent. However, in the immunosuppressed individual, one finds eosinopenia. It is not known in the latter situation which is cause and which effect, i.e., if the eosinopenia predisposes to hyperinfection and dissemination, or if these events cause the eosinopenia.

Diagnosis is made by finding larvae in stool or duodenal aspirate. Recovery of organisms is improved by using the culture method of Harada and Mori.

In the normal individual, mild but nagging symptoms may persist for many years. There is circumstantial evidence that the infestation may persist for over 40 years. This is an important point, and explains how patients who have not been exposed to the worm in recent years, may develop severe infection when they become immunosuppressed. In a sense, this is analogous to reactivation of tuberculosis or the various herpes viruses.

In immunosuppressed individuals, disseminated infection has a 90% fatality. Adding to the problem of widespread organ involvement is that severe infestation leads to recurrent, often polymicrobial, bacteremias. This is caused by breaks in the mucosal barrier of the colon and carriage of bacteria in and on the larvae as they penetrate the colon.

Treatment of the normal and immunosuppressed host is with thiabendazole, at a dosage of 25 mg/kg b.i.d. (maximum 3 g/day). In the normal host treatment should be for 2 days, and in the immunosuppressed patient, for at least 5 days (Table 127.7). In the immunosuppressed patient, in addition to administering thiabendazole, corticosteroid dosage should be decreased, if possible, and care should be taken to maintain optimal nutrition.

To prevent the severe infection, it has been suggested that all susceptible individuals, i.e., patients who have compromised host defenses, should be checked for the infestation by routine examination of stool.

There is evidence that we are normally protected against dissemination by intact cell-mediated immune responses, and probably also by the eosinophil (Table 127.8), but the exact mechanisms of protection are unknown.

Cutaneous Larva Migrans

Cutaneous larva migrans, also known as creeping eruption, is a dermatitis caused by the burrowing of certain nematode larvae. The dermatitis marks the course of

TABLE 127.7   Effect of Treatment on Mortality – *Strongyloides* Hyperinfection

Group	% Mortality
No treatment	100
Treatment ≥ 72 hr	32

TABLE 127.8   Eosinophilia and Mortality in Patients with *Strongyloides* Hyperinfection

% Eosinophils	% Mortality
< 8	84
≥ 8	27

the migrating larvae, and is seen as a linear, or curvilinear, papulovesicular pruritic lesion. It results from skin contact with soil containing filariform larvae, usually of the dog and cat hookworm, *Ancylostoma braziliense*. It characteristically follows contact with warm, moist, and sandy soil which has been contaminated with animal excreta. It is most common along the Atlantic and Gulf coasts, from Maryland to Texas.

The disease is mild and self-limited, but may be complicated by secondary bacterial infection, from scratching, or an occasional patient may develop a generalized hypersensitivity reaction to antigens released by dead and dying larvae. This reaction may persist for many weeks, and is characterized by generalized urticaria and pharyngeal edema.

Treatment of creeping eruption is thiabendazole, which may be given either orally or used topically.

Other

Some other minor helminthic infestations should be mentioned. The first of these is trichostrongyliasis, which is found in Asia and the USSR. This nematode imbeds in the mucosa of the upper small intestine.

Capillariasis, caused by *Capillaria philippinensis,* is a chronic wasting disease seen in the Philippines and Thailand. The life cycle is similar to strongyloides and the worm is acquired by eating raw fresh water fish. Patients develop diarrhea, abdominal pain, and edema, and they gradually deteriorate until they die in 2-4 months. The treatment is mebendazole or thiabendazole at high doses for an extended length of time. Patients are also helped by parenteral feeding.

Angiostrongylus cantonensis causes eosinophilic meningitis. This is a disease of rats with the larvae developing in mollusks and certain fish, fresh water shrimp and crabs being the carrier. Humans develop the disease by ingesting inadequately cooked snails or the carrier. The disease occurs in Hawaii, other Pacific islands, Southeast Asia, Australia, and Cuba. After being ingested, the larvae migrate to

the central nervous system where they die, setting up the eosinophilic inflammatory reaction. Patients have severe headache, stiff neck, and paresthesias. The
typical case has 150-1500 cells/mm^3 in the spinal fluid with 20% or more being eosinophils. Peripheral eosinophilia may be minimal or completely absent. The prognosis is usually good, with only occasional deaths. Patients improve over a few
weeks, although paresthesias may persist for several months. There is no treatment which has been effective, but some authorities recommend thiabendazole
25 mg/kg b.i.d. for 3 days.

Anisakiasis is contracted from eating raw, undercooked, or pickled infected
fish, usually herring. The disease is found in Japan and parts of Europe, although
there have been a few cases seen in the United States. The ingested worms remain in the intestinal lumen and patients are usually asymptomatic and only dis-
cover they have the infestation upon vomiting up a worm or passing one in the feces. On occasion, the worm may become invasive leading to abdominal pain which
leads to the diagnosis of an acute abdomen. Thus the diagnosis is usually made at
surgery, and pathologically one sees an eosinophilic granulomatous tissue reaction.
There is no medical therapy available. The disease can be prevented by cooking
the fish at 60°C or higher for 5 min or longer, or by freezing the fish below -20°C
for 60 hr or more.

Tissue Forms

Trichinosis

Trichinosis is the most important tissue round worm. It is caused by *Trichinella
spiralis,* and results from ingestion of inadequately cooked infected meat. Almost
all persons with trichinosis have no or only very mild symptoms, and illness is seen
only in those who are very heavily infected (Table 127.9).

Following ingestion of infected meat, i.e., muscle with encysted larvae in it,
adult worms develop in the intestines, a process taking 1-7 days. The adults reproduce, and newborn larvae penetrate the intestinal mucosa, and enter the venous circulation and lymphatics. They migrate mainly to striated muscle where
they encyst (Figure 127.2).

The distribution of trichinosis is worldwide, except for Australia and some
Pacific islands. Humans are usually infected following the eating of pork or bear
meat. Pork is a common source of the infection because of the practice of using
garbage as a source of food for swine. This garbage often contains contaminated
meat. The prevalence of the disease has gone down dramatically in the United
States with outlawing the feeding of raw garbage to swine. Beef is a very rare
source of the infection, and most cases have probably been due to adulteration of
beef by pork.

**TABLE 127.9   Approximate % of Humans with Evidence* of
Trichinosis at Autopsy**

1930	16
1960	4

*By examination of diaphragmatic muscle

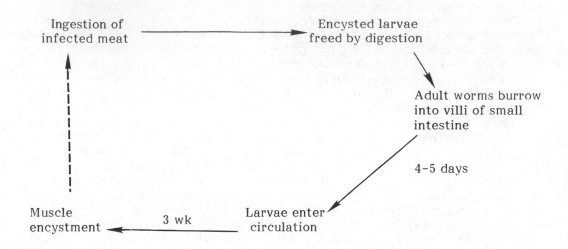

FIGURE 127.2   Life cycle of trichinosis.

The diagnosis of trichinosis is probable in the presence of the triad of myalgia, periorbital edema and eosinophilia, especially in the presence of a history of eating poorly cooked pork or bear meat. During the intestinal phase of the infestation patients almost always are asymptomatic although there are occasional nonspecific gastrointestinal symptoms reported. During the muscle phase early on, there is edema and weakness, as well as fever. Eosinophilia is quite marked and may reach more than 90%. Less common findings are headache, cough, dyspnea, dysphagia, and a macular or urticarial rash (Table 127.10).

TABLE 127.10   Clinical Findings in Trichinosis

Finding	Approximate % of Patients
Fever	90
Myalgias	90
Malaise	80
Periorbital edema	75
Headache	50
Rash	20
Peripheral edema	20
Diarrhea	15
Nausea	15
Subconjunctival hemorrhages	10
Splinter hemorrhages	10

Muscle enzymes are usually elevated. A reliable diagnosis may be made serologically using the bentonite flocculation test available from the Centers for Disease Control. Serum must be submitted to CDC through the State Health Department, and the test does not become positive until about 3 weeks following infection.

A positive muscle biopsy is the most accurate way to make the diagnosis. The highest yield is obtained from a biopsy specimen taken from the clinically involved muscle near its tendinous insertion, the location of the highest density of cysts. The biopsy should be done after the third week of infection when larvae are maximum in number and size.

The illness persists for about 3 weeks after which complete recovery without significant sequelae is the rule. There are occasional fatalities usually due to myocardial involvement.

Most patients should not be treated; however, in the very seriously ill patient, prednisone, 40-60 mg/day, is recommended. Some authorities recommend thiabendazole also; however, the efficacy of this drug has not been proved, and it has significant side effects.

Trichinosis is a very good example of successful host defenses against a multicellular parasite. Eosinophils and neutrophils attach to newborn larvae and cause their destruction. The activity of these phagocytic cells appears to be IgG antibody-dependent, but complement-independent. The eosinophil appears to be more potent in this cytotoxic activity than does the neutrophil. Expulsion of the adult worms from the intestines occurs within 1-3 weeks of infection, thus removing the source of larvae, and appears to be immunologically mediated, dependent upon both B and T lymphocytes.

Visceral Larva Migrans (Table 127.11)

This process is caused by larval migration of animal nematodes. It is found most commonly in young children who ingest the larvae of the dog or cat roundworm. *Toxocara canis* is very common in dogs in the United States, who are infected in utero and begin passing eggs at about 3 weeks of age, with the number of eggs in the feces declining at about 6 months of age. *Toxocara cati* is less of a problem.

Eggs passed in the stools become infective in about 3 weeks and remain viable for several months. Thus humans do not have to be in direct contact with an infected dog or cat. Humans become infected by ingesting soil with infective eggs. A common source is soil from public playgrounds, and a study of such soil from parks in Britain revealed that about one-fourth had viable ova.

After ingestion, the eggs hatch, and the larvae penetrate the small intestine entering the portal and systemic circulation. Because of their small size, they may pass through the pulmonary circulation and disseminate. Most are trapped in the liver. The larvae exit the small vessels where they lodge and are unable to complete their life cycle.

Patients develop fever, cough, wheezing, rales, hepatomegaly, and intense eosinophilia. There are undoubtedly many patients with light infections who are asymptomatic. Less common symptoms are nausea, vomiting, weight loss, ataxia, convulsions, and findings of myocarditis. Eosinophilia is intense, with a cell count up to $80,000/mm^3$. The diagnosis is usually made on the basis of the clinical findings, particularly hepatomegaly, in a child with a history of pica, and intense eosinophilia. Immunologic tests have been developed, with the precipitin test being quite specific but not very sensitive. More recently, work has been done on development of an ELISA test. A liver biopsy is occasionally indicated, but the infecting larvae are difficult to demonstrate because they continue to move beyond the area of eosinophilic granulomatous inflammation.

TABLE 127.11   Visceral Larva Migrans

	Visceral Form	Ocular Form
Age	1–5 yr	5–20
History of pica	+	Unusual
Symptoms	Malaise, weight loss, wheezing, cough, fever, seizures	Failing vision
Signs	Hepatomegaly, pruritic rash, abnormal behavior	Strabismus, whitish retinal granuloma, endophthalmitis, uveitis
Laboratory	Leukocytosis, eosinophilia (usually > 30%), hypergammaglobulinemia (including ↑ IgE), ↑ isohemagglutinin titers, pulmonary infiltrates	Usually normal
Prognosis	Usually benign, but rare deaths due to severe neurologic or myocardial involvement	Unnecessary enucleation because of misdiagnosis of retinoblastoma
Treatment	Corticosteroids in severe cases	Corticosteroids, thiabendazole, and diethylcarbamazine unproven efficacy

A complication of the disease is the development of ocular lesions, months to years later. These are characterized by granulomas or endophthalmitis.

The prognosis is good, although a few deaths have been reported. There is no evidence that drug treatment is effective, although some authorities recommend the use of thiabendazole, 25 mg/kg b.i.d. for 5 days, or diethylcarbamazine, 12 mg/kg/day, in four divided doses, for 3 weeks, in severe cases, with the addition of corticosteroids in patients with eye involvement.

Dracunculiasis

Guinea worm is a common infestation in some parts of the world, specifically areas of Africa, India, and the Middle East. It is a very sensitive indicator of the level of sanitation since its transmission involves contamination of the water supply. In some villages it affects up to 40% of the farmers. It is transmitted by water contamination by the cyclops, a small crustacean which serves as the intermediate host for *Dracunculus medinensis.* Although guinea worm infestation has a very low mortality, it causes significant morbidity when the worm emerges through the skin, usually on the lower part of the legs. This occurs approximately 1 year after an individual becomes infected. The disease is rapidly controlled by the very simple maneuver of filtering drinking water through double-thickness cotton cloth.

Filariasis (Tables 127.12-127.15)

The various types of filariasis are different from the other worm infestations in that they require insects as an intermediate host with the vector ingesting microfilariae when feeding on people. No human filarial parasites are found in the continental United States, except in immigrants.

TABLE 127.12   Filariae Causing Human Disease

W. bancrofti
B. malayi
O. volvulus
L. loa

TABLE 127.13   Filarial Infections

Parasite	Vector	Microfilaria
W. bancrofti	Mosquitoes	Sheathed, nocturnal, peripheral blood
O. volvulus	Black flies	Skin, subcutaneous tissues, unsheathed
L. loa	Tabanid flies	Sheathed, diurnal, peripheral blood

TABLE 127.14   Characteristics of Life Cycles of Filariae

Adults inhabit tissues or body cavities, where females produce eggs

Microfilariae are produced when eggs embryonate and the embryos uncoil

Microfilariae may or may not retain the eggshell, resulting in "sheathed" or "unsheathed" characteristic

Microfilariae develop in a bloodsucking insect vector

TABLE 127.15   Conditions Necessary for Maintaining Endemicity of Filariasis

---

Adequate human reservoir: cases with microfilariae in blood

Adequate vector: suitable mosquitoes in the area of infected humans, feeding at correct time

---

Onchocerciasis

Onchocerciasis caused by *Onchocerca volvulus* is known as river blindness, and is transmitted by buffalo gnats (black flies). The disease is characterized by subcutaneous nodules, dermatitis, and blindness. It is found in Central America and tropical Africa. The microfilariae are rarely found in peripheral blood but are mainly in the subcutaneous nodules, in the skin near the parent organisms, or in the eye. Adults live up to 15 years and the microfilariae for up to 30 months. The fly is capable of spreading the infection in about 6 days after ingesting microfilariae. After injecting infective larvae into a new host, the life cycle in the human requires about 15-18 months until the patient has microfilariae which can be ingested by another fly.

The characteristic clinical finding, the subcutaneous nodule, follows a pruritic rash, and slowly grows to reach full size, 2-3 cm, in 3-4 years. These nodules show a low-grade inflammatory reaction with many eosinophils and abundant microfilariae. The patient may have a few to over 100 nodules. A nodule itself usually causes few symptoms unless present near a joint in which case it may limit motion and/or be painful.

The most devastating problem is caused by the migration of microfilariae to the eye, resulting in chronic iritis and iridocyclitis with eventual development of blindness. In some communities in Africa, half of the adult males are blind. Another complication of onchocerciasis is "hanging groin" and hernia: this is a skin sac containing a mass of sclerosed inguinal or femoral lymph nodes.

Laboratory examinations reveal a moderate eosinophilia in about one-third of the patients. The diagnosis is made by identifying microfilariae in skin or in nodules. Material may be obtained by skin biopsy or by scarification, i.e., serosanguinous transudate obtained from superficial skin incisions. The microfilariae are identified by Giemsa stain. The Mazzotti test is carried out by giving 50 mg of diethylcarbamazine orally, this drug causes intense pruritus in about 24 hr in patients with onchocerciasis. Occasionally, microfilariae may be seen in the urine.

With experience the diagnosis can be made by observing the pathognomonic superficial punctate keratitis.

A very effective mode of treatment is excision of the tumors, but this is impractical when there are a very large number. Drug treatment is somewhat dangerous in patients who have ocular involvement, because they may develop an inflammatory reaction which may lead to further eye damage. Suramin is effective but reactions are common, including fever, headache, myalgias, arthralgias, abdominal pain, hyperesthesias of the soles of the feet, and pruritus. Most of the reactions can be handled symptomatically. Treatment should be stopped if the symptoms are severe or if the patients develop peripheral edema or evidence for nephrotoxicity. The first dose should be 100-200 mg (test), then 1 g should be given each week for five more doses. The drug is administered intravenously. Suramin kills the adult parasite.

Diethylcarbamazine, on the other hand, kills the microfilariae, but not the adults. It is particularly likely to lead to worsening of ocular disease. Mebendazole is also effective.

The only preventive measure of definite value is the use of DDT to control the vector. Insect repellants are of doubtful value.

Loa loa

Loa loa, often known as calabar swelling, is characterized by transient subcutaneous swellings. The disease is transmitted by tabanid flies, also known as deer flies, in the western and central African rain forest. Only the female tabanid flies bite, and their preferred habitat is darker areas, i.e., in heavily forested regions.

The female fly injects mature larvae which reside in subcutaneous tissue and slowly develop into adults. The adult female worm liberates sheathed microfilariae into the blood stream in a diurnal pattern, with the highest concentration being found in the middle of the day. Adults live for 15 years or longer. The disease is caused by the constant migration of adults, which produces the main characteristic of the disease, transient swelling. The swellings are more common over the back, axilla, groin, breast, penis, scalp, and around the eye.

There is a suggestion that nonhuman primates serve as a reservoir for this disease.

Lymphatic-Dwelling Filaria

These are the most common filarial infections, and are caused by three parasites, with very similar life cycles and clinical manifestations, and with overlapping geographic distributions. The most common is *Wuchereria bancrofti,* which is found in most tropical areas, including the West Indies, South America, Central and North Africa, the Middle East, India, and Southeast Asia. At one time it was common in the southeast United States, as far north as Charleston, South Carolina. *Brugia malayi* is found in Southeast Asia, and *Brugia timori* in Indonesia. The intermediate hosts, various mosquito species, introduce the infective larvae while biting. The larvae take about 1 year to mature into adults which reside in the lymphatic system. Adults are thread-like and creamy white, measuring 40-100 mm in length, the female longer than the male. The female produces microfilariae which circulate in the bloodstream. There are differences between the various species, and within species depending upon the geographic location, with respect to when the microfilariae are found most abundantly in the bloodstream. The *W. bancrofti* microfilariae circulate mainly at night; however in the South Pacific it has been observed that there is no diurnal variation; *B. malayi* is also mainly nocturnal. The time from mosquito injection of larvae to production of microfilariae is 3-12 months.

The pathology and clinical findings are caused by inflammation induced by the adult worm and depend upon where the worms are located and the degree of secondary bacterial infection. The microfilariae are mainly innocuous, although they may produce tropical eosinophilia as a result of entrapment in the lung. The disease caused by these filariae has been divided into an early or inflammatory phase and a late or obstructive phase.

The early, inflammatory phase begins 3 months or more after infection, and is characterized by lymphadenitis, lymphangitis, orchitis, epididymitis, fever, rigors, and urticaria. Patients develop pain, swelling, redness, and stiffness of the affected part of the body. The painful swelling usually persists for only 7-10 days, then disappears leaving only a persistently swollen lymph node. Pathologically, there is eosinophilic granulomatous inflammation. In contrast to bacterial lymphangitis, in filariasis the inflammation is descending, rather than ascending.

The late, obstructive phase results from chronic, recurrent infection, obstruction of the lymphatics, and secondary bacterial infection. Patients develop elephantiasis of extremities, the breast, or external genitalia. Lymph varices are common, and present as soft, painless, lobulated swellings. Other common findings are hydrocele, chylous ascites, and chyluria, the latter from lymphatic obstruction of the retroperitoneal area.

The diagnosis is made by identifying microfilaria in the blood, which may be accomplished by examining a thick blood smear. The yield may be increased by concentration procedures, i.e., centrifugation or filtration, or by administering 100 mg diethylcarbamazine, and drawing blood 1 hr later. There are usually no microfilaria in the blood during the obstructive phase of the disease. Biopsy of lesions should be avoided, since this exacerbates lymphatic obstruction.

Prevention is difficult, since mosquito control is so hard to attain. There has been some success with mass treatment of infected populations, and various regimens of diethylcarbamazine citrate have been attempted. One approach is 5 mg/kg given once weekly.

The treatment of choice is also diethylcarbamazine, which decreases or eliminates the microfilariae very quickly and may also kill the adults. Reactions are common, mainly due to toxic substances released by the dying parasites, and include fever, malaise, vertigo, urticaria, headache, and a bullous skin rash. Reactions can be controlled with corticosteroids, but these should be used only in the most severe reactions because so many patients have secondary bacterial infections, and the steroids will adversely affect the outcome of these. For milder reactions, antihistamines have been somewhat effective. The dosage of diethylcarbamazine citrate is 5 mg/kg as a single dose or in three divided doses daily for 3 weeks. *Brugia malayi* is more sensitive and therefore can be treated with half this dosage. Other treatment modalities are the use of corticosteroids in elephantiasis, the steroids causing transient improvement. Hydroceles are improved by the injection of sclerosing agents. The treatment of chyluria is bed rest, if possible.

Tropical pulmonary eosinophilia is thought to be filarial, but definite association with a particular species has not been made. This disease is characterized by paroxysmal asthma, often nocturnal. Patients have blood and pulmonary eosinophilia. The evidence that it is filarial is the finding of increased filarial antibody titers and improvement with treatment with diethylcarbamazine.

Animal filarial parasites may rarely infect humans. The filarial heartworm of the dog may cause asymptomatic pulmonary nodules in humans, but no treatment is necessary.

Selected Bibliography

Anderson, D. C., Greenwood, R., Fishman, M., and Kagan, I. G.: Acute infantile hemiplegia with cerebrospinal fluid eosinophilic pleocytosis: An unusual case of visceral larva migrans. *J Pediatr* 86:247, 1975.

Bass, D. A. and Szejda, P.: Mechanisms of killing of newborn larva of *Trichinella spiralis* by neutrophils and eosinophils: Killing by generators of hydrogen peroxide in vitro. *J Clin Invest* 64:1558, 1979.

Blumenthal, D. S.: Current concepts. Intestinal nematodes in the United States. *N Engl J Med* 297:1437, 1977.

Botero, D. and Castaño, A.: Comparative study of pyrantel pamoate, bephenium hydroxynaphthoate, and tetrachlorethylene in the treatment of *Necator americanus* infections. *Am J Trop Med Hyg* 22:45, 1973.

Bradley, S. L., Dines, D. E., and Brewer, N. S.: Disseminated *Strongyloides stercoralis* in an immunosuppressed host. *Mayo Clin Proc* 53:332, 1978.

Bryceson, A. D. M., Warrell, D. A., and Pope, H. M.: Dangerous reactions to treatment of onchocerciasis with diethylcarbamazine. *Br Med J* 1:742, 1977.

Cahill, K. M.: Thiabendazole in massive strongyloidiasis. *Am J Trop Med Hyg* 16:451, 1967.

Clark, P. S., Brownsberger, K. M., Saslow, A. R., Kagan, I. G. Noble, G. R., and Maynard, J. E.: Bear meat trichinosis. Epidemiologic, serologic and clinical observations from two Alaskan outbreaks. *Ann Intern Med* 76:951, 1972.

Connor, D. H.: Current concepts in parasitology. Onchocerciasis. *N Engl J Med* 298:379, 1978.

Coolidge, C., Weller, P. F., Ramsey, P. G., Ottesen, E. A., Beaver, P. C., and von Lichtenberg, F. C.: Zoonotic *Brugia* filariasis in New England. *Ann Intern Med* 90:341, 1979.

de la Riva, H., Escamilla, D. G., and Frati, A. C.: Acute massive intestinal bleeding caused by hookworm. *JAMA* 246:68, 1981.

Garcia, E. G.: Treatment of trichuriasis with oxantel. *Am J Trop Med Hyg* 25:914, 1976.

Higgenbottam, T. W. and Heard, B. E.: Opportunistic pulmonary strongyloidiasis complicating asthma treated with steroids. *Thorax* 31:266, 1976.

Hopkins, D. and Foege, W.: Guinea worm disease. *Science* 212:495, 1981.

Jones, W. E., Schantz, P. M., Foreman, K., Smith, L. K., Witte, E. J., Schooley, D. E., and Juranek, D.: Human toxocariasis in a rural community. *Am J Dis Child* 134:967, 1980.

Kazura, J. W.: Host defense mechanisms against nematode parasites: Destruction of newborn *Trichinella spiralis* larvae by human antibodies and granulocytes. *J Infect Dis* 143:712, 1981.

Kazura, J. W. and Aikawa, M.: Host defense mechanisms against *Trichinella spiralis* infection in the mouse: Eosinophil-mediated destruction of newborn larvae in vitro. *J Immunol* 124:355, 1980.

Keystone, J. S. and Murdoch, J. K.: Diagnosis and treatment. Drugs 5 years later: Mebendazole. *Ann Intern Med* 91:582, 1979.

Krupp, I. M.: Hemagglutination test for the detection of antibodies specific for ascaris and toxocara antigens in patients with suspected visceral larva migrans. *Am J Trop Med Hyg* 23:378, 1974.

Kuberski, T.: Eosinophils in the cerebrospinal fluid. *Ann Intern Med* 91:70, 1979.

Kuberski, T. and Wallace, G. D.: Clinical manifestations of eosinophilic meningitis due to *Angiostrongylus cantonensis*. *Neurology* 29:1566, 1979.

Margolis, H. S., Middaugh, J. P., and Burgess, R. D.: Arctic trichinosis: Two Alaskan outbreaks from walrus meat. *J Infect Dis* 139:102, 1979.

Miller, M. J., Krupp, I. M., Little, M. D., and Santos, C.: Mebendazole. An effective antihelminthic for trichuriasis and enterobiasis. *JAMA* 230:1412, 1974.

Moens, M., Dom, J., Burke, W. E., Schlossberg, S., and Schuermans, V.: Levamisole in ascariasis: A multicenter controlled evaluation. *Am J Trop Med Hyg* 27: 897, 1978.

Most, H.: Current concepts in parasitology. Trichinosis - preventable yet still with us. *N Engl J Med* 298:1178, 1978.

Most, H.: Treatment of common parasitic infections of man encountered in the United States. *N Engl J Med* 287:495, 698, 1972.

Muller, R.: Guinea worm disease: Epidemiology, control and treatment. *Bull WHO* 57:683, 1979.

Nawalinski, T. A. and Schad, G. A.: Arrested development in *Ancylostoma duodenale:* Course of self-induced infection in man. *Am J Trop Med Hyg* 23:855, 1974.

Neva, F. A.: Parasitic diseases of the GI tract in the United States. *Disease-a-Month,* pp. 2-44, (June) 1972.

Neva, F. A. and Ottesen, E.A.: Tropical (filarial) eosinophilia. *N Engl J Med* 298: 1129, 1978.

Pearson, R. D., Irons, R. P., Sr., and Irons, R. P., Jr.: Chronic pelvic peritonitis due to the pinworm *Enterobius vermicularis*. *JAMA* 245:1340, 1981.

Phillip, M., Parkhouse, R. M. E., and Ogilvie, B. M.: Changing proteins on the surface of a parasite nematode. *Nature* 287:538, 1980.

Pinkus, G. S., Coolidge, C., and Little, M. D.: Intestinal anisakiasis: First case report from North America. *Am J Med* 59:145, 1975.

Powell, R. W., Moss, J. P., Nagar, D., Melo, J. C., Boram, L. H., Anderson, W. H., and Cheng, S. H.: Strongyloidiasis in immunosuppressed hosts. Presentation as massive lower gastrointestinal bleeding. *Arch Intern Med* 140:1061, 1980.

Punyagupta, S., Juttijudata, P., and Bunnag, T.: Eosinophilic meningitis in Thailand: Clinical studies of 484 typical cases probably caused by *Angiostrongylus cantonensis*. *Am J Trop Med Hyg* 24:921, 1975.

Purtilo, D. T., Meyers, W. M., and Conner, D. H.: Fatal strongyloidiasis in immunosuppressed patients. *Am J Med* 56:488, 1974.

Rivas-Alcalá, A. R., Taylor, H. R., Ruvalcaba-Macias, A. M., Mackenzie, C. D., Greene, B. M., Domíguez-Vásquez, A., Luge-Pfeiffer, C., and Beltran, H. F.: Chemotherapy of onchocerciasis: A controlled comparison of mebendazole, levamisole, and diethylcarbamazine. *Lancet* 2:485, 1981.

Sargent, R. G., Savory, A. M., Mina, A., and Lee, P. R.: A clinical evaluation of mebendazole in the treatment of trichuriasis. *Am J Trop Med Hyg* 23:375, 1974.

Schantz, P. M. and Glickman, L. T.: Current concepts in parasitology. Toxocaral visceral larva migrans. *N Engl J Med* 298:436, 1978.

Scoggin, C. H. and Call, N. B.: Acute respiratory failure due to *Strongyloides stercoralis* infection – association with ectopic ACTH syndrome and depressed cell-mediated immunity. *Arch Intern Med* 138:1005, 1978.

Scowden, E. B., Schaffner, W., and Stone, W. J.: Overwhelming strongyloidiasis. *Medicine* 57:85, 1978.

Scragg, J. N. and Proctor, E. M.: Mebendazole in the treatment of severe symptomatic trichuriasis in children. *Am J Trop Med Hyg* 26:198, 1977.

Seah, S. K., Hucal, G., and Law, C.: Dogs and intestinal parasites: A public health problem. *Can Med Assoc J* 112:1191, 1975.

Simon, R. D.: Pinworm infestation and urinary tract infection in young girls. *Am J Dis Child* 128:21, 1974.

Spillman, R. K.: Pulmonary ascariasis in tropical communities. *Am J Trop Med Hyg* 24:791, 1975.

Warren, K. S.: Helminthic diseases endemic in the United States. *Am J Trop Med Hyg* 23:723, 1974.

Wolfe, M. S. and Wershing, J. M.: Mebendazole. Treatment of trichuriasis in Bahamian children. *JAMA* 230:1408, 1974.

Zinkham, W. H.: Visceral larva migrans: A review and reassessment indicating two forms of clinical expression: Visceral and ocular. *Am J Dis Child* 132: 627, 1978.

128

CESTODES
Robert H. Waldman, M.D.

The cestodes, or tapeworms (Table 128.1), are mainly benign, although a few patients develop complications; in addition, their treatment is safe and effective (Table 128.2).

Diphyllobothrium latum

The fish tapeworm, *D. latum,* is the largest of the tapeworms affecting humans, reaching a length of 10 m. Humans are infected following ingestion of inadequately cooked fish containing the plerocercoid stage. The fish most commonly infected are pike, yellow perch, salmon, trout, and whitefish (smoked salmon should not cause infection). The plerocercoid stage develops into the adult tapeworm in 3-5 weeks.

In North America the disease is found around the Great Lakes and in Alaska, and Canada. Other areas where the disease is commonly found are Finland, northern USSR, Switzerland, Japan, Manchuria, Chile, Argentina, and Australia. The incidence of the disease seems to be falling.

Disease is usually asymptomatic, although patients may have some nonspecific gastrointestinal symptoms. Vitamin B_{12} deficiency may develop, because the tapeworm competes for this vitamin. However, only about 0.1% of infected patients develop macrocytic anemia.

The diagnosis is made by identifying the eggs in the feces, or alternatively one can find proglottids, i.e., segments of the tapeworm, after purging the patient.

The treatment, which is highly effective, is niclosamide, 2 g as a single dose. The disease can be prevented by adequate cooking of fish (all parts of the fish at 56°C or higher for 5 min or longer), freezing (minus 18°C for 24 hr or longer) or by soaking in a brine solution. Sanitary disposal of human feces will also prevent spread of the disease.

1104

TABLE 128.1   Human Tapeworms

Of major importance

T. *saginata* (beef tapeworm)
T. *solium* (pork tapeworm)
D. *latum* (fish tapeworm)
H. *nana* (dwarf tapeworm)

Minor

H. *diminuta*
D. *caninum*

TABLE 128.2   Human Cestode Infections

Organism	Disease	Usual Organ Involvement
T. *solium*	Cysticercosis	Muscle, CNS, eyes
E. *granulosus*	Cystic hydatid disease	Liver, lungs
E. *multilocularis*	Alveolar hydatid disease	Liver
E. *oligarthrus*	Polycystic hydatid disease	Liver
Taenia spp	Coenurosis	CNS, eyes, subcutaneous
Spirometra spp	Sparganosis	Subcutaneous, eyes

Taenia solium

The most dangerous tapeworm is *T. solium,* or the pork tapeworm (Table 128.3). Two different types of disease are caused by the pork tapeworm: intestinal, which is benign; and cysticercosis (which is tissue invasion), which is dangerous.

The intestinal disease almost never causes symptoms. The proglottids have very little motility and therefore do not migrate to areas where they may cause obstruction. The disease should be differentiated from the beef tapeworm, because of the danger of cysticercosis. Despite the fact that the intestinal disease is benign, patients should be treated, again to prevent cysticercosis. The treatment is niclosamide, 2 g on an empty stomach. The question of the use of a purgative is controversial, those who recommend it arguing that it will reduce the likelihood of regurgitation of eggs. Cysticercosis can develop in patients with intestinal pork tapeworm by either endo- or exoinfection. The former is by regurgitation of eggs, the latter by the transfer of eggs from the anus to the mouth via the hands.

TABLE 128.3   Diseases Caused by *T. solium*

	Intestinal	Cysticercosis
Stage ingested	Cysticerci from inadequately cooked pork	Eggs (food contaminated by infected person, or autoinfection)
Cysticerci	Ingested	Subcutaneous tissues, skeletal muscles, brain, eye, heart, lungs, liver
Adult worm	Intestines	–
Eggs	Feces	Ingested
Symptoms	Abdominal pain, weight loss	Depends on organ involved
Treatment	Niclosamide 2 g in single dose, purgative 3-4 hr later	Surgery, as necessary; no chemotherapy effective

In cysticercosis, the eggs hatch in the stomach and duodenum, and oncospheres migrate to various tissues. Cysticerci develop in about 10 weeks, and induce an inflammatory reaction resulting in a fibrous capsule which eventually usually calcifies. The cysts are 0.5-2 cm in diameter. There is usually no inflammatory response until the cysts die and degeneration begins. Therefore there is usually a long interval between infection and development of signs and symptoms. Diagnosis is made from the excised cysts. The signs and symptoms depend upon the tissue in which the cysts are located, but one of the most dangerous manifestations is central nervous system involvement in which a picture of chronic meningitis is seen.

Pork tapeworm and cysticercosis develop in areas where pork is eaten uncooked and in which pigs are exposed to human feces. This occurs most commonly in Latin America, southern Africa, and Southeast Asia. In Mexico, 2% of the swine are infected. There are no indigenous cases in the United States. Worldwide, the prevalence appears to be falling. The disease is prevented by swine inspection, adequate cooking of pork, prompt treatment of human carriers, and proper disposal of human feces. The risk of cysticercosis in medical personnel is minimal, but care should be taken in handling feces from patients with pork tapeworm.

Taenia saginata

Taenia saginata, which develops to a length of 4-10 m, results from the ingestion of undercooked beef containing cysticerci. The proglottids of the beef tapeworm are motile, and are passed in the stool. They contain eggs which have a long survival. They are ingested by an intermediate host, usually cattle, which develop the cysticerci in muscle.

Disease is found in all parts of the world where raw beef is eaten (Table 128.4). Since this practice is increasing, especially among more affluent populations, the prevalence is increasing. It is usually seen in young adults, who eat more raw beef.

Most patients are asymptomatic, but a few may have abdominal pain, nausea, weight loss, and weakness. Patients may also notice an increased appetite and notice the passing of proglottids or note a crawling perianal sensation. Some patients may have a mild eosinophilia.

The diagnosis is impossible in the first 3 months of infestation, since proglottids will not be found in the stool, unless the tapeworm is seen when the patient has gastrointestinal roentgenographic studies. The best specimen for making the diagnosis is a perianal swab. Species identification is important, as mentioned earlier in the discussion of pork tapeworm, but it can only be made by examination of a proglottid or scolex (the head of the tapeworm by which it is attached to the intestinal mucosa) because the eggs of the pork and beef tapeworm are identical.

The treatment of choice is niclosamide, 2 g on an empty stomach. This drug is safe and gives a > 90% cure. Alternative drugs are paromomycin, quinacrine, and inorganic tin compounds.

Untreated, the tapeworm lives for many years and reinfection is common. Complications are unusual but proglottids, being motile, may obstruct the appendix or the pancreatic or biliary ducts. Human cysticercosis caused by the beef tapeworm only rarely occurs, there having been a handful of cases reported. Beef tapeworm can be prevented by routine beef inspection and by freezing or adequately cooking beef. Human carriers should be treated promptly.

Hymenolepis nana

Hymenolepis nana is the most common human tapeworm, and humans are the only host. Infection results from self-inoculation or person-to-person transmission. The eggs do not survive well, so close contact is necessary. It is seen most commonly in children in warm climates, or in institutionalized individuals. In India, the prevalence has been noted to be as high as 20% in some areas.

Hymenolepis nana is small averaging 20 mm in length. Mature proglottids disintegrate in the ileum, liberating eggs which either pass out in the feces, or

TABLE 128.4   Prevalence of T. saginata

Area	Prevalence (%)		
	Human	Cattle	
U.S.	0.02	0.06	About one-third of patients have never been abroad; most infected cattle in the Southwest states
Europe	0.2	4	
East Africa	As high as 30 in some areas	10	

develop into oncospheres which live in the intestinal villi. The oncospheres develop into cysticercoids which invade the mucosa and after maturation, pass back out into the lumen and mature further into the adult form. This cycle takes approximately 16 days, causing autoinfection and persistent infection.

Most patients are asymptomatic; however the cysticercoids destroy villi leading to an enteritis, which may cause gastrointestinal symptoms, weight loss, loss of energy, and apathy. The diagnosis is made by identifying the eggs in the feces.

The treatment is niclosamide, 2 g/day for 7 days, leading to a > 90% cure. The dosage for children is 60-80 mg/kg. In institutions where the infestation is established, everyone should be treated with two courses of niclosamide. An alternative drug is paromomycin, 45 mg/kg for 7 days.

There is evidence of some sort of host defense mechanism against the parasite. It is less prevalent in adults and self-cure eventually occurs in nearly all cases.

Other Tapeworms

Hymenolepis diminuta is usually found in rodents which swallow insects containing cysticercoids. Humans are infected in the same way. This tapeworm is found primarily in Papua New Guinea and Iran, where up to 2% of children have been found to harbor the parasite.

Dipylidium caninum is usually seen in canines and felines and is contracted from fleas and lice.

Hydatid Disease

Hydatid disease (Table 128.5) is caused by one of two echinococcal organisms, the more common *Echinococcus granulosus* and *E. multilocularis*.

TABLE 128.5   Organ Involvement in Hydatid Disease

Organ	Approximate % of Cases
Liver	40
Lung	30
Subcutaneous	10
Female genital	3
Spleen	2
Bones	2
Orbit	2
Parotid glands and neck	2
Breast	1
Kidney	1

In infection with *E. granulosus,* eggs are passed in dog feces, where they contaminate pastures and water supplies. The eggs are ingested by the intermediate host, usually sheep, but occasionally humans. Oncospheres migrate to the liver and lungs where cysts develop. The disease is most common in sheep-raising areas, such as the western states, Alaska, and Canada. There is some evidence that the disease is increasing in incidence.

Patients may be asymptomatic, or may have symptoms resulting from the development of cysts. In the lung they cause chest pain, cough, and hemoptysis. Chest x-ray may show solitary or multiple nodules. Next to liver and lung the most common symptomatic site is bone, where pathologic fractures may develop. Cysts may also develop in the central nervous system. Cysts may become secondarily infected and may rupture, leading to sepsis or anaphylaxis in reaction to antigens from the parasite present in the cyst fluid. If the cysts rupture into a bronchus, patients may drown from the fluid. In less severe cases, one may see air-fluid levels on chest x-ray.

Eosinophilia is present in less than one-fourth of the patients. A serologic test is available, which is positive in about 85%. If surgical material is available, a touch preparation of the specimen may demonstrate proglottids. Needle aspiration should not be done because leakage of cyst fluid may cause anaphylaxis.

Treatment is surgical; there is no effective medical therapy.

Echinococcus multilocularis is also a canine infestation, with the intermediate host being small mammals such as mice. It is found in cooler northern climates, such as the upper Midwest of the United States, Alaska, Canada, and Northern Europe. In *E. multilocularis* infestation the cysts do not become encapsulated, and therefore they progressively invade, resulting in a "honeycomb" cyst. The liver is the most commonly affected organ, leading to jaundice and portal hypertension. The treatment is surgical, although mebendazole has been reported to be somewhat effective.

Selected Bibliography

Danziger, J. and Bloch, S.: Tapeworm cyst infestations of the brain. *Clin Radiol* 26:141, 1975.

Latovitzki, N., Abrams, G., Clark, C., Mayeux, R., Ascherl, G., and Sciarra, D.: Cerebral cysticercosis. *Neurology* 28:838, 1978.

Most, H.: Treatment of common parasitic infections of man encountered in the United States. *N Engl J Med* 287:495, 698, 1972.

Most, H., Yoeli, M., Hammond, J., and Scheinessan, G. P.: Yomesan (niclosamide) therapy of *Hymenolepis nana* infections. *Am J Trop Med Hyg* 20:206, 1971.

Pawlowski, Z. and Schultz, M. G.: Taeniasis and cysticercosis *(Taenia saginata).* *Adv Parasitol* 10:269, 1972.

Stanley, J. D. and Jordan, M. C.: Clinical aspects of CNS cysticercosis. *Arch Intern Med* 140:1309, 1980.

Varela-Diaz, V. M., Coltorti, E. A., Prezioso, U., Lopez-Lemes, M. H., Guisantes, J. A., and Yarzabal, L. A.: Evaluation of three immunodiagnostic tests for human hydatid disease. *Am J Trop Med Hyg* 24:312, 1975.

Yarzabal, L. A., Schantz, P. M., and Lopez-Lemes, M. H.: Comparative sensitivity and specificity of the Casoni intradermal and the immunoelectrophoresis tests for the diagnosis of hydatid disease. *Am J Trop Med Hyg* 24:843, 1975.

129

TREMATODES
Robert H. Waldman, M.D.

Schistosomiasis

There are several medically important trematode or fluke infections, the most important of which is schistosomiasis, a disease not found in the United States, but one of the greatest causes of significant morbidity in many parts of the world. In fresh water, schistosome eggs hatch and become miracidia (Figure 129.1). This form penetrates snails and develops into cercariae, which penetrate human skin and develop into schistosomes. These circulate, maturing in the portal system before migrating to their final resting place, venules around the intestines or urinary bladder, depending upon the species (Table 129.1). The eggs laid by the adult female may then pass into the lumen of the intestines or urinary bladder, or into the circulatory system of the host.

The clinical forms of the disease are shown in Table 129.2. The chronic form is the most important and results from heavy deposition of eggs. In infection with *Schistosoma mansoni* and *S. japonicum,* the eggs lead to a granulomatous reaction in the liver which may result in portal hypertension. With the development of this complication, there is shunting of eggs to the lung, where the reaction may lead to pulmonary hypertension. The disease caused by schistosomes is prehepatic, and therefore liver function is normal.

The diagnosis is made in a patient who has had appropriate exposure, compatible symptoms, hepatosplenomegaly, eosinophilia, and identifiable eggs. In addition to demonstrating schistosome eggs, it is important to do a quantitative egg count with respect to deciding whether or not treatment should be undertaken, as outlined later. The optimum time to identify eggs in the urine is between 10 a.m. and 2 p.m. If the disease is suspected and eggs are not found in feces, a biopsy of rectal mucosa may be indicated. A serologic test has been developed, but is not helpful because of the high incidence of false-positive results.

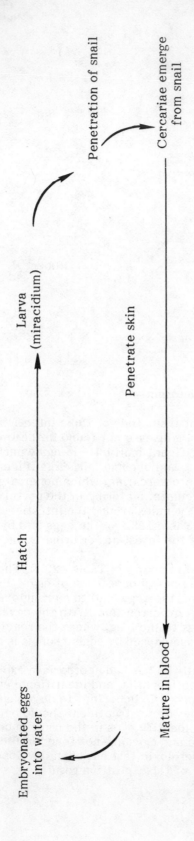

FIGURE 129.1 Life cycle of schistosomiasis.

TABLE 129.1   *Schistosoma* spp

Species	Geographical Distribution	Mature Adults	Eggs	Treatment
S. *mansoni*	Africa, Middle East, S. America, Caribbean	Mesenteric venules	Liver or feces	Niridazole or oxamniquine
S. *japonicum*	Japan, China, Philippines	Mesenteric venules	Liver or feces	Niridazole
S. *haematobium*	Africa, Middle East	Venules in bladder or mesentery	Urine or liver	Metrifonate

TABLE 129.2   **Clinical Stages of Schistosomiasis**

Dermatitis	Within 1-2 days of cercarial penetration
Katayama fever	4-8 wk after primary infection Fever, cough, hepatosplenomegaly, myalgias, urticaria, eosinophilia
Chronic	S. *haematobium:* hematuria, dysuria, frequency, hydronephrosis S. *mansoni* and S. *japonicum:* fever, abdominal pain, diarrhea, hepatosplenomegaly, portal hypertension, pulmonary hypertension Less common: intestinal polyps, bladder carcinoma, focal neurologic abnormalities

Treatment of schistosomiasis is far from ideal. The available drugs are toxic and of limited effectiveness. Therefore, some authorities recommend treating only heavily infected individuals, e.g., those with ten or more eggs per gram of stool, or patients who are symptomatic. On the other hand, the argument has been made that there is not a perfect correlation between number of eggs in feces and the intensity of infection, and moreover, a single pair of organisms could lead to eggs being deposited in a vital area. Proponents of the latter approach recommend treating all patients with schistosomiasis. Whichever approach is taken, it is recommended that treatment be undertaken only when there is definite proof of infection, except in the rare individual with suspected central nervous system disease, in whom treatment cannot await definite proof. Those who propose treating only heavily infected and symptomatic individuals have as their aim of treatment to diminish, but not eradicate all of the organisms. The rationale is that, since reinfection is common, a few organisms remaining maintain immunity.

The three species vary in their susceptibility to treatment, and there is also variation within a single species. *Schistosoma japonicum* is generally the most resistant, occasionally necessitating the use of the most toxic of the antischistosome drugs, antimony potassium tartrate, which is given intravenously. Preferred alternatives as first line drugs, because of less toxicity, are niridazole and stibocaptate. The former may be used as treatment for all three species of schistosomes and is given orally in a dosage of 25 mg/kg/day, in two divided doses, for 7 days. Its side effects are gastrointestinal and dizziness. Stibocaptate is given intramuscularly at a dosage of 8 mg/kg once a week for 5 weeks. Its side effects are gastrointestinal, headache, pain at the site of injection, and cardiotoxicity. All are about 50% effective in treating *S. japonicum,* and none has been established to be safe in pregnancy.

Infection with *S. mansoni* has been effectively treated with a relatively new compound oxamniquine, but this drug has not been fully evaluated. Infection with *S. haematobium* should not be treated with antimonials, and the drug of choice is niridazole, or alternatively, metrifonate.

There is no specific therapy for Katayama fever (reaction probably due to antigen release), but steroids have been used to suppress symptoms. Surgical treatment of the complications of schistosomiasis should be approached cautiously because with medical therapy lesions often resolve more than would have been predicted. Portocaval shunts are usually unnecessary.

Since the treatment of schistosomiasis is less than ideal, it is obvious that the answer to the problems presented by this disease is prevention. Molluscicides and other environmental approaches theoretically would be the most reasonable approach, but results have been disappointing. Low-dose hycanthone for mass use has been reported to be beneficial, if only temporarily. Travelers should be advised to be cautious about swimming in fresh waters in endemic areas.

Swimmers Itch

Swimmers itch is caused by exposure to the cercariae from those species which infect humans, or those which do not cause human schistosomiasis. The disease is caused by penetration of the cercariae, which then die without causing systemic infection. The dead cercariae cause a dermatitis. In the United States the disease is caused by nonhuman-infecting schistosomes only, and this explains the fact that in some areas 25% of people have antischistosomal antibody in their serum.

Paragonimiasis

Lung fluke infection results from eating uncooked, infected crabs or crayfish in which the metacercariae of *Paragonimus westermani* or less commonly, another species, are present. The disease is most common in the Orient, where *P. westermani* is found. Other species are found in West Africa and Central and South America.

After the metacercariae are ingested, they encyst in the duodenum. Thereafter they pass through the intestinal wall, migrate through the peritoneal cavity, through the diaphragm, and penetrate the lung. Less commonly, the organism may migrate to other organs, such as the central nervous system or skin. Five to six weeks later, the organisms are mature, and eggs are laid.

The host mounts an inflammatory reaction to the organisms and eggs, first neutrophilic and eosinophilic, later monocytic. Finally, a fibrous capsule is laid down.

Patients usually do not appear ill, and complain only of cough, pleuritic pain, night sweats, and brownish or blood-tinged sputum. Laboratory examination reveals a high eosinophil count, and chest roentgenograms shows infiltrates which later may cavitate, a pleural reaction with or without an effusion, and occasionally a pneumothorax. Examination of the gelatinous sputum reveals eggs. Eggs may also be in the stool as a result of being swallowed and surviving transit through the gastrointestinal tract. The main differential diagnosis is tuberculosis, but it must be remembered that the two diseases may coexist. Although the major diagnostic test is identification of the eggs, a complement-fixation test is available.

The treatment is bithionol, 30–50 mg/kg q.o.d. for 10-15 doses, or praziquantel, which is not yet available in the United States.

Clonorchiasis

The Chinese liver fluke, or *Clonorchis sinensis,* results in human disease after ingestion of encysted metacercariae in inadequately cooked fresh water fish. Larvae migrate to the common bile duct where maturation occurs. Adults persist for an average of 8 years. Rarely adults are found in the gallbladder or the pancreatic duct. Within 2-3 weeks of ingestion of metacercaria the adult female is laying eggs.

The disease is endemic in the Orient and Southeast Asia. The prevalence is very high in some areas, for example, 65-80% in Hong Kong.

Damage is done by the inflammatory reaction to the parasites and leads to fibrosis of bile ducts. Patients are usually asymptomatic. There may be, however, an acute illness which develops soon after infestation, with the patient having fever, chills, right upper-quadrant abdominal tenderness and hepatomegaly. The chronic stage is also usually asymptomatic, although patients may develop bacterial cholangitis, pancreatitis, cholelithiasis, portal hypertension, or cholangiocarcinoma.

During the acute stage of illness patients may demonstrate leukocytosis, eosinophilia, and an elevated alkaline phosphatase. The diagnosis is made by demonstration of eggs in the feces or by duodenal aspiration. The diagnosis should be strongly suspected in patients with appropriate geographic and dietary exposure, and a compatible clinical picture.

Asymptomatic patients should not be treated. Symptomatic ones should be given chloroquine phosphate, 250 mg t.i.d. for 6 weeks. Treatment is only moderately successful, and this dosage causes frequent side effects. Surgery may be necessary for drainage of the biliary system.

The disease can be prevented by adequate cooking of fish. The disease is also related to the common practice of fertilizing fish ponds with human feces. This can be overcome by storing the feces for a few days before fertilization, or by adding ammonium sulfate to the feces.

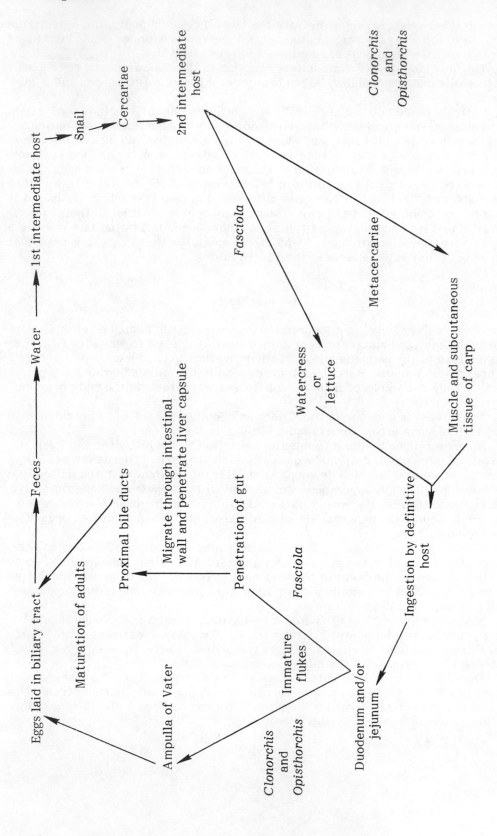

FIGURE 129.2   Life cycle of liver flukes.

Opisthorchiasis

Opisthorchiasis is very similar to clonorchiasis, and is caused by *Opisthorchis felineus* and *O. viverrini*. Opisthorchiasis is endemic in Russia, Eastern Europe, Thailand, and Laos.

Fascioliasis

Fascioliasis is caused by the liver fluke of sheep and cattle, *Fasciola hepatica*. Humans are infected by ingesting cysts attached to wild watercress or other aquatic plants. Following ingestion, the parasite burrows through the intestinal wall, then migrates through the peritoneal cavity, and penetrates the liver. It then eats its way through the liver parenchyma into a bile duct, where it matures in 3-4 months (Figure 129.2).

Fascioliasis is endemic in Europe, China, Africa, and Central and South America, related to areas and periods of high rainfall. The organism is rare in the United States.

Pathologically there is dilatation of the bile ducts, but obstruction is uncommon.

During the enterohepatic stage the patient may have fever, right upper-quadrant abdominal pain and hepatomegaly. Less common are pruritus, urticaria, and jaundice. The disease is difficult to diagnose in this acute stage because there is no egg production. Laboratory examination reveals a marked eosinophilia of up to 60%. The diagnosis is usually made on the basis of geography, diet, and the presence of fever, eosinophilia, and hepatomegaly.

The treatment of choice is bithionol, 30-50 mg/kg q.d. or q.o.d., for 10-15 doses. An alternative to bithionol is dehydroemetine, 65 mg intramuscularly, daily for 12 days. Both bithionol and dehydroemetine are only moderately effective. The disease can be prevented by discontinuing the practice of eating wild watercress and excluding livestock from areas where watercress is cultivated.

Halzoun is a disease in the Middle East caused by ingestion of raw sheep or goat liver containing flukes. Patients complain of dysphagia and dyspnea from the pharyngeal mass secondary to the lodged flukes.

Selected Bibliography

Bassily, S., Farid, Z., Higashi, G. I., and Watten, R. H.: Treatment of complicated schistosomiasis mansoni with oxamniquine. *Am J Trop Med Hyg* 27:1284, 1978.

Caulfield, J. P., Korman, G., Butterworth, A. E., Hogan, M., and David, J. R.: Partial and complete detachment of neutrophils and eosinophils from schistosomula: Evidence for the establishment of continuity between a fused and normal parasite membrane. *J Cell Biol* 86:64, 1980.

Ellner, J. J . and Mahmoud, A. A. F.: Killing of schistosomula of *Schistosoma mansoni* by normal human monocytes. *J Immunol* 123:949, 1979.

Kazura, J. W., Fanning, M. M., Blumer, J. T., and Mahmoud, A. A. F.: Role of cell-generated hydrogen peroxide in granulocyte-mediated killing of schistosomula of *Schistosoma mansoni* in vitro. *J Clin Invest* 67:93, 1981.

Nwokob, A. and Volkmer, K. J.: Single dose therapy of paragonomiasis with me-
    nichlopholan. *Am J Trop Med Hyg* 26:688, 1977.

Omer, A. H. S.: Oxamniquine for treating *Schistosoma mansoni* infection in Sudan.
    Br Med J 2:163, 1978.

Polderman, A. M. and Manshande, J. P.: Failure of targeted mass treatment to
    control schistosomiasis. *Lancet* 1:27, 1981.

Weller, T. H.: Manson's schistosomiasis: Frontiers in vivo, in vitro, and in the
    body politic. *Am J Trop Med Hyg* 25:208, 1976.

130

ACQUIRED IMMUNE DEFICIENCY SYNDROME (AIDS)
Robert M. D'Alessandri, M.D.

Since 1981, over 1500 cases of an acquired immune deficiency syndrome (AIDS) have been reported to the CDC. Included in these reports are cases of Kaposi's sarcoma in persons under 60 years of age, and cases with life-threatening opportunistic infections with no underlying cause or history of immune deficiency. Since the etiology at present is not clear, and new information is accumulating rapidly, a separate section describing current knowledge regarding this syndrome was planned for this edition. It is probable that by the time of publication, the etiology of this syndrome will be more completely understood.

Etiology

Although the etiology of AIDS is not known, there are several likely possibilities. At present, the most likely candidate is a retrovirus similar to the human T-cell leukemia virus (HTLV). HTLV plays a causal role in epidemic T-cell leukemia in Japan. This virus is similar to the feline retrovirus which causes leukemia, aplastic anemia, and other disorders of impaired immune function in cats.

Other possible agents include cytomegalovirus and Epstein-Barr virus. The hypothesis that CMV may be the etiologic agent was based on the fact that CMV has been shown to cause at least transient immunosuppression in infected hosts. In addition, it was believed that frequent reexposures and reinfections associated with sexual promiscuity may lead to a more profound immune suppression with the subsequent development of malignancy and/or opportunistic infections. However, most now feel that the frequent association of CMV infections in AIDS patients is probably a result of the immunosuppression rather than the cause. The frequent finding of E-B virus infection is explained in the same manner.

Another view holds that exposure to multiple antigens with agents that suppress immunity, such as hepatitis B, CMV, E-B virus, etc., may be responsible for this syndrome. Certainly more research is needed to identify the cause of the immune suppression in patients with AIDS.

Epidemiology

In 1981, the CDC became aware of a clustering of cases of *Pneumocystis carinii* pneumonia and Kaposi's sarcoma in homosexuals. Shortly thereafter, CDC formed a task force to undertake surveillance and conduct epidemiologic studies for these disorders. To date, over 1500 cases of AIDS have been reported to CDC and the number of reported cases appears to be doubling every 6 months. Initially it was thought that the disease affected only homosexuals or bisexuals. Subsequent reports have indicated that intravenous drug abusers, hemophiliacs, newborns of affected mothers, and Haitians also appear to be at particular risk.

Over 80% of all cases have been reported from metropolitan areas on the east and west coasts. New York City, San Francisco, and Los Angeles account for the greatest majority of these cases. The geographic clustering suggests that causal factors related to lifestyle and/or environment are important.

In general, the population most at risk appears to be homosexuals (72% of cases) with frequent sexual experiences (often more than 100 different sexual partners per year). The ages most affected are between 15 and 60 years, with the greatest preponderance in the fourth decade. Although most cases occur in men, approximately 5-10% of cases occur in women. Recent reports indicate that AIDS may be transmitted between heterosexual men and women. In addition, Haitians (4% of cases) appear to be at higher risk, although the reasons for this are not known.

Intravenous drug abusers (17% of cases) and patients with hemophilia (1% of cases) are also at increased risk of developing AIDS. Another group at particular risk are prisoners. The increased incidence of homosexuality and drug abuse in this population may account for the increased risk of developing AIDS. This has led to the belief that AIDS may be spread by contaminated needles and blood products. All of this suggests that AIDS is caused by a transmissable agent.

The distribution of AIDS cases parallels that of hepatitis B infection. However, there have been no documented cases among health care or laboratory personnel caring for AIDS patients or handling laboratory specimens. To date, no cases of person-to-person transmission have been identified other than through intimate contact or blood transmission.

Clinical Manifestations

Although the presentation of this syndrome is extremely varied, the major elements of AIDS include the development of an illness associated with a defect in cell-mediated immunity, occurring in a person with no known cause of diminished resistance to that disease. Such diseases include *Pneumocystis carinii* pneumonia; Kaposi's sarcoma; opportunistic infections due to one or more of the following: *Aspergillus,* atypical mycobacteria, *Candida, Cryptococcus,* CMV, herpes simplex virus, *Nocardia, Strongyloides,* toxoplasma, etc.; progressive multifocal leukoencephalopathy; cryptosporidiosis; or extensive mucocutaneous herpes simplex infection of more than 5 weeks' duration.

Excluded from consideration are patients receiving (or having received) immunosuppressive therapy or patients with Hodgkin's disease or other lymphomas.

Other conditions which may predispose individuals to certain diseases seen in patients with AIDS should be excluded on a case-by-case basis.

Individuals with AIDS and Kaposi's sarcoma are younger and tend to have a more progressive form of the disease. In patients with classical Kaposi's sarcoma, plaques or nodules most commonly occur on the extremities, but may occur anywhere on the skin or mucous membranes. The disease generally follows an indolent and protracted course, and dissemination occurs uncommonly. In addition, the disease is rare in individuals under 50 years of age. The current outbreak of Kaposi's sarcoma in patients with AIDS is highly unusual. Not only is the age group much younger (fourth decade), but also the clinical course is much more aggressive, with a mortality of close to 50%. Extracutaneous lesions involving the lymph nodes, gastrointestinal tract, and lungs are much more common and follow the pattern of the disease seen in younger African patients.

In addition to these diseases, there has been described a condition of persistent, generalized lymphadenopathy among homosexuals. The characteristics of this are: (1) lymphadenopathy of at least 3 months' duration, involving two or more extra-inguinal sites, and confirmed on physical exam by the physician; (2) absence of any current illness or drug use known to cause lymphadenopathy; and (3) presence of reactive hyperplasia in a lymph node biopsy if performed. Approximately 70% of these patients have associated constitutional symptoms of fatigue (70%), fever (50%), night sweats (44%), and weight loss of 5 or more pounds (28%). In addition, hepatomegaly and/or splenomegaly is noted in over one-fourth of patients. Of interest is the fact that many of these patients have eventually developed Kaposi's sarcoma or a major opportunistic infection. The finding of persistent lymphadenopathy may be merely a manifestation of the underlying immunologic disorder. These patients require careful observation for the development of more clearly defined and commonly recognized diseases associated with AIDS.

Ocular findings may occur early and should alert physicians to the possibility of AIDS. These findings include cotton-wool spots and optic nerve-head swelling, and may be associated with the infectious complications rather than directly related to either the etiologic agent or the underlying immune deficiency.

Diagnosis

At the present time, the diagnosis of AIDS is predominantly a clinical one. The presence of a disease associated with a defect in cell-mediated immunity (CMI) in a person with no known cause of impaired CMI defines the presence of AIDS. As noted previously, excluded from this definition are those individuals receiving immunosuppressive therapy, patients with lymphoma, and individuals with conditions which may predispose them to diseases associated with a defect in CMI.

Although there are no specific tests available to diagnose AIDS, there have been certain consistently abnormal laboratory results in patients with AIDS. There is a significant elevation of the frequency of the HLA-DR5 haplotype in homosexual as well as nonhomosexual men with Kaposi's sarcoma. Homosexuals with Kaposi's sarcoma and other AIDS patients tend to have lower white blood cell counts and reduced circulating lymphocytes. Of greatest importance is the finding of a reduced helper to suppressor T-cell ratio. This has been a consistent finding in patients with AIDS and is considered necessary to make the diagnosis. Although studies have demonstrated these immunologic abnormalities in homosexuals without AIDS, the magnitude is significantly greater in affected homosexuals.

The major defect appears to be a selective impairment of the ability to induce a CMI response. There is sparing of the inductive function for humoral responses. There may also be a defect in the normal expression of suppressor cell activity, creating an autoimmune-like state as a result of defective immunoregulation. Defects in cellular cytotoxicity and the finding of a polyclonal gammopathy are unexplained components of AIDS.

Treatment

Since the etiology of AIDS is unknown, treatment must be directed at the infectious complications of the disease. Thus, AIDS patients present a major therapeutic challenge because of the frequent presence of multiple opportunistic infections and because of the limited availability of treatment modalities. For many of the infections in AIDS patients, available treatment is inadequate, especially in the immune-suppressed host.

The best treatment would appear to be prevention. Although optimum control awaits identification of the etiologic agent, several public health measures have been recommended: (1) Sexual contact should be avoided with persons known or suspected to have AIDS. Members of high-risk groups should be aware that multiple sexual partners increase the risk of developing AIDS. (2) As a temporary measure, members of groups at increased risk for AIDS should refrain from donating blood or plasma. (3) Studies should be conducted to develop effective screening tests and procedures in identifying and excluding blood and plasma with a high probability of transmitting AIDS. (4) Physicians should adhere strictly to indications for transfusions. Autologous blood transfusions are recommended. (5) Safer blood products for hemophiliacs should be developed.

Prognosis

The prognosis for patients with AIDS is poor. Approximately half of all reported cases had *Pneumocystis carinii* pneumonia without Kaposi's sarcoma and 45% of these patients died. Nearly one-third of all AIDS patients were reported to have Kaposi's sarcoma alone, and mortality in this group was 20%. Approximately 7% of patients had both *Pneumocystis* pneumonia and Kaposi's sarcoma with mortality at 60%. Other opportunistic infections accounted for about 10-12% of patients with a mortality rate of about 50%. The high case fatality rate in patients with this disease indicates the seriousness of this public health problem.

It must be remembered that the magnitude of the present problem is greatly understated by the data. Many individuals presenting with interstitial pneumonia may go undiagnosed because a biopsy is not performed, or because empiric therapy is given. The benign appearance of early Kaposi's sarcoma lesions may lead to delay or failure to diagnose this condition. There are data that a lesser degree of immune suppression is widely present in the homosexual community which may, in time, lead to the development of other neoplastic or infectious complications. Therefore, physicians treating high-risk groups must be aware of the possibility of opportunistic infections and malignancies in these patients.

Future Developments

It would appear that the identification of the causative agent of AIDS is at hand. This would represent the first major breakthrough in the control of this condition. Following this, attempts at identifying, by a simple laboratory procedure, those at high risk of transmitting the disease would go far to prevent transmission by blood products.

If indeed the causative agent proves to be a virus, the likelihood of developing effective chemotherapy in the near future is probably small. It would appear that prevention, either by public health measures, or by the development of a vaccine, would offer the most hope for the future.

Selected Bibliography

Follansbee, S. E., Busch, D. F., Wofsy, C. B., Coleman, L., Gullet, J., Aurigemma, G. P., Ross, T., Hadley, W. K., and Drew, W. L.: An outbreak of *Pneumocystis carinii* pneumonia in homosexual men. *Ann Int Med* 96:705-713, 1982.

Harris, C., Small, C. B., Klein, R. S., Friedland, G. H., Moll, B., Emeson, E. E., Spigland, I., and Steigbigel, N. H.: Immunodeficiency in female sexual partners of men with the acquired immunodeficiency syndrome. *N Engl J Med* 308:1181-1184, 1983.

Haverkos, H. W. and Curran, J. W.: The current outbreak of Kaposi's sarcoma and opportunistic infections. *Ca-A Canc J Clin* 32:330-339, 1982.

Persistent, generalized lymphadenopathy among homosexual males. *MMWR* 31 (19), May, 1982.

A cluster of Kaposi's sarcoma and *Pneumocystis carinii* pneumonia among homosexual male residents of Los Angeles and Orange Counties, California. *MMWR* 31(23), June, 1982.

Prevention of acquired immune deficiency syndrome (AIDS). *MMWR* 32(8), March, 1983.

Stahl, R. E., Friedman-Kein, A., Dubin, R., Marmor, M., and Zolla-Pazner, S.: Immunologic abnormalities in homosexual men. *Am J Med* 73:171-178, 1982.

APPENDIX

Epidemiologic Features of More Common and/or Important Infectious Diseases

Disease	Agent	Transmission	Incubation Period	Prevention and Control
Viral				
Adenovirus	(More than 30 serotypes)	Droplets, contact: respiratory tract, eye	2-10 days	Live, attenuated oral vaccine, experimental
Chickenpox	Varicella-zoster virus	Respiratory droplets: crusts from lesions	2-3 wk	Human hyperimmune globulin after exposure in high-risk individuals; isolation of cases
Common cold	Nearly 200 different viruses and strains	Airborne droplets and by touching contaminated objects	1-4 days	Experimental vaccines and antiviral drugs
Cytomegalic inclusion	Cytomegalovirus	Respiratory, blood transfusions, in utero	1-3 mo	None
Dengue	Aedes aegypti mosquito bite	Aedes aegypti mosquito bite	3-15 days	Mosquito control
Encephalitis	St. Louis, Venezuelan, Eastern and Western equine	Mosquito bite, and other arthropods	4-21 days	Mosquito and other appropriate insect control; experimental vaccines

(Cont'd)

Disease	Agent	Transmission	Incubation Period	Prevention and Control
Hepatitis	A	Fecal-oral	15–35 days	Care in handling feces, blood, other secretions, and possibly contaminated objects; gamma globulin after exposure; experimental vaccine being tested
	B	Blood and blood products; secretions (e.g., saliva, semen)	3–20 wk	Care in handling contaminated blood and secretions; hyperimmune globulin after exposure; vaccine
	C, D, etc.	Unknown – Probably similar to hepatitis B in most respects		
Herpes simplex		Droplets, saliva		Probably none except possibly antiviral drugs
Infectious mononucleosis	E-B virus	Contact with external secretions	7–14 days	None
Influenza	Types A, B, and C	Respiratory	1–4 days	Inactivated vaccine administered parenterally; experimental live, attenuated vaccines administered via the respiratory tract; chemoprophylaxis: amantadine and isoprinosine may be of some benefit

Disease	Agent	Transmission	Incubation	Prevention/Control
Meningitis	Enteroviruses, herpes simplex	Fecal and respiratory	1 to several days	Immunization against poliovirus; experimental antiviral drugs
Mumps	–	Respiratory	2-3 wk	Live vaccine
Poliomyelitis	Types I, II, III	Fecal and respiratory	1-3 wk	Immunization
Rabies	–	Saliva of infected animal	10 days to 6 mo	Active and passive immunization; animal immunization and other control practices aimed at stray and wild animals
Rubella		Respiratory	2-3 wk	Immunization
Smallpox	Varicla	Respiratory, contact with lesions	7-16 days	Unnecessary: disease has been eradicated
Yellow fever		Bite of infected mosquito	3-6 days	Immunization, mosquito control
Bacterial				
Actinomycosis	*A. israelii* (anaerobe), and *Nocardia asteroides* (aerobe)	Endogenous (oral) / Exogenous		Good dental hygiene
Anthrax	*B. anthracis*	Contact, inhalation, or ingestion of contaminated animal tissue	1-4 days	Sterilization of infected tissue, hides, etc.

(Cont'd)

Disease	Agent	Transmission	Incubation Period	Prevention and Control
Brucellosis	*Brucella abortus, B. suis, B. melitensis, B. canis*	Contact with infected animals, ingestion of milk products	1 wk to several months	Immunization of animals, pasteurization of milk products
Chancroid	*H. ducreyi*	Sexual contact	1–10 days	Exposure prevention
Cholera	*V. cholerae*	Contaminated water and food	Hours to few days	Improved sanitation; vaccine of marginal benefit
Diphtheria	*C. diphtheriae*	Respiratory: from patients or carriers	2–5 days	Isolation of cases; active and passive immunization
Dysentery	Shigellae	Contaminated water and food	1–7 days	Identification and enteric isolation of cases; good hygiene
Gas gangrene	Clostridia	Contamination of wounds	Hours	Complete wound debridement; penicillin, antitoxin of questionable benefit
Gonorrhea	*N. gonorrhoeae*	Mucous membrane contact	1–8 days	Exposure prevention; identification and treatment of cases, symptomatic and asymptomatic, and contacts
Granuloma inguinale	*Calymmatobacterium granulomatis*	Sexual contact	Days to months	Exposure prevention

Disease	Organism	Transmission	Incubation	Prevention/Control
Impetigo	Staphylococci and streptococci	Contact with lesions, inoculation with person's own indigenous flora	1-5 days	Hygiene
Leprosy	M. leprae	Personal contact	Years	Treatment of active cases
Lymphogranuloma venereum	C. trachomatis	Venereal contact	1-5 wk	Exposure prevention, treatment of cases
Meningococcal meningitis	N. meningitidis	Respiratory	2-10 days	Avoid overcrowded conditions, rifampin or minocycline (sulfonamides for sensitive strains), vaccines for types A and C
Nongonococcal urethritis	C. trachomatis	Venereal contact		Exposure prevention, treatment of cases
Pertussis	B. pertussis	Respiratory	5-10 days	Immunization
Plague	Y. pestis	Infected rodents, fleas; pus from lesions; sputum	2-10 days	Rodent and flea control; treatment of cases and contacts
Pneumonia	Pneumococci, staphylococci, Haemophilus spp, klebsiellae, streptococci	Indigenous flora		Pneumococcal polysaccharide vaccine
Psittacosis	C. psittaci	Excreta of infected birds	5-15 days	Eliminate contact with infected birds

(Cont'd)

Disease	Agent	Transmission	Incubation Period	Prevention and Control
Relapsing fever	*Borrelia recurrentis, B. duttoni*	Bite of ticks, lice; infected insect feces; infected rodents	3-12 days	Lice and tick control
Syphilis	*T. pallidum*	Contact with infectious lesion; transplacental	2-4 wk	Exposure prevention; identification and treatment of cases
Tetanus	*C. tetani*	Contamination of wounds	Few days to several weeks	Immunization: active and passive; wound debridement
Trachoma	*C. trachomatis*	Contact with infectious discharges		Hygiene; treatment of cases
Tuberculosis	*M. tuberculosis*	Respiratory	Weeks to years	Isolation (for 7-10 days) and treatment of cases; BCG; antituberculous chemoprophylaxis
Tularemia	*P. tularensis*	Contact with infected animals (e.g., rabbit), or ticks, deerfly	1-10 days	Avoid contact
Typhoid fever	*S. typhi*	Contaminated water or food	10-14 days	Good sanitation, vaccine of marginal value

Disease	Organism	Transmission	Incubation	Prevention/Control
Weil's disease	*Leptospira interrogans*	Food or water contaminated with animal (e.g., rat) urine	4-19 days	Good sanitation
Fungal				
Blastomycosis	*B. dermatitidis*	Inhalation		None
Coccidioidomycosis	*C. immitis*	Inhalation	1-3 wk	Dust control in endemic areas
Ringworm	*Microsporum, Trichophyton,* and other fungi	Lesions: human and animal; contaminated objects		Hygiene
Protozoan				
Amebic dysentery	*E. histolytica*	Infected food or water	Days to months	Sanitation, control of carriers
Leishmaniasis	*L. donovani*	Insect bite	Weeks to months	Insect control
Malaria	*P. vivax, P. malariae, P. falciparum, P. ovale*	Female *Anopheles* mosquito bite	Variable	Mosquito control, treatment of cases, chemoprophylaxis

(Cont'd)

Disease	Agent	Transmission	Incubation Period	Prevention and Control
Helminths				
Ascariasis	*A. lumbricoides*	Fecal	2 mo	Sanitation
Filariasis	*Wuchereria*	Infected arthropods	Weeks to years	Control of vectors, treatment of cases
Hookworm	*Ancylostomiasis duodenale, Necator americanus*	Skin contact with contaminated soil	2–10 wk	Sanitation, wearing of shoes
Trichinosis	*T. spiralis*	Insufficiently cooked infected meat	5–8 days	Adequate cooking or freezing

INDEX